HEAD AND NECK CANCERS

HEAD AND NECK CANCERS

Evidence-Based Treatment

Editors

Athanassios Argiris, MD, PhD, FACP
Professor, Department of Medical Oncology
Thomas Jefferson University
Philadelphia, Pennsylvania;
Adjunct Professor of Medicine
University of Texas Health Science Center at San Antonio
San Antonio, Texas;
Consultant Medical Oncologist
Hygeia Hospital
Athens, Greece

Robert L. Ferris, MD, PhD, FACS
Director, UPMC Hillman Cancer Center
Hillman Professor of Oncology
Associate Vice-Chancellor for Cancer Research
Co-Director, Tumor Microenvironment Center
Professor of Otolaryngology, of Immunology, and of Radiation Oncology
University of Pittsburgh
Pittsburgh, Pennsylvania

David I. Rosenthal, MD, FACR, FASTRO
Professor
Section Chief, Head and Neck Radiation Oncology
Director, Head and Neck Translational Research Department of Radiation Oncology
The University of Texas MD Anderson Cancer Center
Houston, Texas

demosMEDICAL
An Imprint of Springer Publishing

Visit our website at www.springerpub.com

ISBN: 9780826137777
e-book ISBN: 9780826137784

Acquisitions Editor: David D'Addona
Compositor: Exeter Premedia Services Pvt Ltd.

Medicine is an ever-changing science. Research and clinical experience are continually expanding our knowledge, in particular our understanding of proper treatment and drug therapy. The authors, editors, and publisher have made every effort to ensure that all information in this book is in accordance with the state of knowledge at the time of production of the book. Nevertheless, the authors, editors, and publisher are not responsible for errors or omissions or for any consequences from application of the information in this book and make no warranty, expressed or implied, with respect to the contents of the publication. Every reader should examine carefully the package inserts accompanying each drug and should carefully check whether the dosage schedules mentioned therein or the contraindications stated by the manufacturer differ from the statements made in this book. Such examination is particularly important with drugs that are either rarely used or have been newly released on the market.

Library of Congress Cataloging-in-Publication Data

Names: Argiris, Athanassios, editor. | Ferris, Robert L., editor. | Rosenthal, David I., editor.
Title: Head and neck cancers: evidence-based treatment / editors, Athanassios Argiris, Robert L. Ferris, David I. Rosenthal.
Description: New York: Demos Medical Publishing/Springer Publishing Company, [2018] | Includes bibliographical references and index.
Identifiers: LCCN 2018005800| ISBN 9780826137777 (alk. paper) | ISBN 9780826137784 (e-book)
Subjects: | MESH: Head and Neck Neoplasms—therapy | Head and Neck Neoplasms—pathology
Classification: LCC RC280.H4 | NLM WE 707 | DDC 616.99/491—dc23
LC record available at https://lccn.loc.gov/2018005800

Printed in the United States of America.
18 19 20 21 22 / 5 4 3 2 1

Contents

Contributors

David J. Adelstein, MD, Professor of Medicine, Cleveland Clinic Lerner College of Medicine of Case Western Reserve University; Staff Physician, Department of Hematology and Medical Oncology, Cleveland Clinic Taussig Cancer Institute, Cleveland, Ohio

Moran Amit, MD PhD, Fellow, Department of Head and Neck Surgery, Division of Surgery, The University of MD Anderson Cancer Center, Houston, Texas

Athanassios Argiris, MD, PhD, FACP, Professor, Department of Medical Oncology, Thomas Jefferson University, Philadelphia, Pennsylvania; Adjunct Professor of Medicine, University of Texas Health Science Center at San Antonio, San Antonio, Texas; Consultant Medical Oncologist, Hygeia Hospital, Athens, Greece

Shirin Attarian, MD, Fellow, Division of Oncology, Department of Medicine, Albert Einstein College of Medicine/Montefiore Medical Center, Bronx, New York

Julie E. Bauman, MD, MPH, Professor of Medicine, Chief, Division of Hematology and Oncology, Associate Director, Translational Research, University of Arizona Cancer Center, Tuscon, Arizona

Jacques Bernier, MD, PhD, Department of Radiation Oncology, Oncology Institute of Southern Switzerland, San Giovanni Hospital, Bellinzona, Switzerland

Pierre Blanchard, MD, PhD, Department of Radiation Oncology, The University of Texas MD Anderson Cancer Center, Houston, Texas

Paolo Bossi, MD, Head and Neck Medical Oncology Unit, Fondazione IRCCS Istituto Nazionale Tumori, Milan, Italy

Karim Boudadi, MD, Clinical Associate and Assistant Professor-Hematology/Medical Oncology, Department of Oncology, Johns Hopkins University, Baltimore, Maryland

Ruud H. Brakenhoff, PhD, Professor of Head and Neck Cancer Genomics, Tumor Biology Section, Department of Otolaryngology-Head and Neck Surgery, Cancer Center Amsterdam, Amsterdam, the Netherlands

Barbara A. Burtness, MD, Professor of Medicine, Co-Director, Developmental Therapeutics Research Program, Yale University School of Medicine and Yale Cancer Center, New Haven, Connecticut

Oscar S. H. Chan, FRCR, Honorary Associate Consultant, Department of Clinical Oncology, Pamela Youde Nethersole Eastern Hospital, Hong Kong

Steven B. Chinn, MD, MPH, Assistant Professor Head and Neck Surgical Oncology, Department of Otolaryngology-Head and Neck Surgery, Head and Neck Surgical Oncology, Microvascular Reconstructive Surgery, University of Michigan, Ann Arbor, Michigan

Anthony J. Cmelak, MD, Professor of Radiation Oncology, Senior Medical Director, Radiation Oncology Satellites, Department of Radiation Oncology, Vanderbilt-Ingram Cancer Center, Nashville, Tennessee

Yanqun Dong, MD, PhD, Radiation Oncology Resident, Department of Radiation Oncology, Fox Chase Cancer Center, Philadelphia, Pennsylvania

Avraham Eisbruch, MD, Professor of Radiation Oncology, Department of Radiation Oncology, University of Michigan, Ann Arbor, Michigan

Adel K. El-Naggar, MD, PhD, Professor, Department of Pathology, Kenneth D. Muller Professorship, The University of Texas MD Anderson Cancer Center, Houston, Texas

Tomohiro Enokida, MD, PhD, Department of Head and Neck Medical Oncology, National Cancer Center Hospital East, Kashiwa, Chiba, Japan

Antoine Eskander, MD, ScM, FRCS(C), Assistant Professor, Department of Otolaryngology—Head and Neck Surgery, University of Toronto, Sunnybrook Health Sciences Centre and Odette Cancer Centre; Surgical Oncologist, Endocrine Surgery, Michael Garron Hospital, Toronto, Ontario, Canada

Carole Fakhry, MD, MPH, Associate Professor, Department of Otolaryngology-Head and Neck Surgery, Johns Hopkins University School of Medicine, Baltimore, Maryland

Farhoud Faraji, PhD, Medical Student, MD/PhD Program, Saint Louis University School of Medicine, St. Louis, Missouri

Robert L. Ferris, MD, PhD, FACS, Director, UPMC Hillman Cancer Center; Hillman Professor of Oncology; Associate Vice-Chancellor for Cancer Research; Co-Director, Tumor Microenvironment Center; Professor of Otolaryngology, of Immunology, and of Radiation Oncology, University of Pittsburgh, Pittsburgh, Pennsylvania

Arlene A. Forastiere, MD, Professor of Oncology, Department of Oncology, Johns Hopkins University, Baltimore, Maryland

Steven J. Frank, MD, Professor, Department of Radiation Oncology, The University of Texas MD Anderson Cancer Center, Houston, Texas

Thomas J. Galloway, MD, Associate Professor, Department of Radiation Oncology, Fox Chase Cancer Center, Philadelphia, Pennsylvania

Adam S. Garden, MD, Professor, Department of Radiation Oncology, The University of Texas MD Anderson Cancer Center, Houston, Texas

Jessica L. Geiger, MD, Assistant Professor of Medicine, Cleveland Clinic Lerner College of Medicine of Case Western Reserve University; Associate Staff, Department of Hematology and Medical Oncology, Cleveland Clinic Taussig Cancer Institute, Cleveland, Ohio

Neil D. Gross, MD, Professor, Department of Head and Neck Surgery, Division of Surgery, The University of Texas MD Anderson Cancer Center, Houston, Texas

G. Brandon Gunn, MD, Associate Professor, Department of Radiation Oncology, The University of Texas MD Anderson Cancer Center, Houston, Texas

Patrick K. Ha, Professor, Department of Otolaryngology, University of California San Francisco, San Francisco, California

Robert I. Haddad, MD, Associate Professor of Medicine at Harvard Medical School, Department of Medical Oncology, Dana-Farber Cancer Institute, Boston, Massachusetts

Missak Haigentz, Jr., MD, Section Chief of Oncology, Morristown Medical Center, Atlantic Health System, Morristown, New Jersey; Adjunct Clinical Professor of Medicine (Oncology) and Otorhinolaryngology-Head & Neck Surgery, Albert Einstein College of Medicine, Bronx, New York

Glenn J. Hanna, MD, Instructor of Medicine at Harvard Medical School, Department of Medical Oncology, Dana-Farber Cancer Institute, Boston, Massachusetts

Ryuichi Hayashi, MD, Department of Head and Neck Surgery, National Cancer Center Hospital East, Kashiwa, Chiba, Japan

F. Christopher Holsinger, MD, FACS, Professor and Chief, Division of Head and Neck Surgery, Department of Otolaryngology-Head and Neck Surgery, Stanford University Medical Center, Palo Alto, California

Katherine A. Hutcheson, PhD, Associate Professor, Department of Head and Neck Surgery, Section of Speech Pathology and Audiology, The University of Texas MD Anderson Cancer Center, Houston, Texas

Jennifer M. Johnson, MD, PhD, Assistant Professor, Department of Medical Oncology, Thomas Jefferson University, Philadelphia, Pennsylvania

Lisa Ann Kachnic, MD, FASTRO, Professor and Cornelius Vanderbilt Chair of Radiation Oncology, Department of Radiation Oncology, Vanderbilt University Medical Center, Nashville, Tennessee

Jens P. Klussmann, Dr. med., Professor and Chairman, Department of Otorhinolaryngology, Head and Neck Surgery, University of Cologne, Cologne, Germany

Christien A. Kluwe, MD, Radiation Oncology Resident, Department of Radiation Oncology, Vanderbilt-Ingram Cancer Center, Nashville, Tennessee

Shlomo A. Koyfman, MD, Radiation Oncologist, Department of Radiation Oncology, Taussig Cancer Institute, Cleveland Clinic, Cleveland, Ohio

Rajesh V. Lalla, DDS, PhD, Associate Professor, Section of Oral Medicine; Associate Dean for Research, University of Connecticut School of Dental Medicine, Farmington, Connecticut

Ka On Lam, FRCR, Clinical Assistant Professor, Department of Clinical Oncology, The University of Hong Kong, Hong Kong

Corey J. Langer, MD, FACP, Professor of Medicine at the Hospital of the University of Pennsylvania, Department of Medicine, Division of Hematology Oncology, Penn Medicine, Philadelphia, Pennsylvania

Anne W. M. Lee, MD, Professor, Department of Clinical Oncology, The University of Hong Kong and The University of Hong Kong-Shenzhen Hospital, Hong Kong

Jae Lee, MD, PhD, Clinical Resident, Department of Radiation Oncology, University of Michigan, Ann Arbor, Michigan

Nancy Y. Lee, MD, Vice Chair, Department of Radiation Oncology; Service Chief, Head and Neck Radiation Oncology; Director, Proton Therapy, Memorial Sloan Kettering Cancer Center, New York, New York

Jan S. Lewin, PhD, Professor, Department of Head and Neck Surgery, Chief, Section of Speech Pathology and Audiology, The University of Texas MD Anderson Cancer Center, Houston, Texas

Lisa Licitra, MD, Head and Neck Medical Oncology Unit, Fondazione IRCCS Istituto Nazionale Tumori, Milan, Italy

Derrick T. Lin, MD, FACS, Chief, Division of Head and Neck Oncology, Massachusetts Eye and Ear Infirmary, Clinical Surgical Director, Center for Head and Neck Cancers, Massachusetts General Hospital; Co-Director, Cranial Base Center, Massachusetts Eye and Ear Infirmary/Massachusetts General Hospital; Daniel Miller Associate Professor of Otolaryngology, Harvard Medical School, Boston, Massachusetts

Jean-Pascal Machiels, MD, PhD, Professor, Department of Medical Oncology and Head and Neck Surgery, Institut Roi Albert II, Cliniques Universitaires Saint-Luc and Institut de Recherche Clinique et Expérimentale, Université Catholique de Louvain, Brussels, Belgium

Jon Mallen-St. Clair, MD, PhD, Attending Surgeon, Head and Neck Oncologic and Microvascular Reconstructive Surgery, Cedars-Sinai Medical Group, Los Angeles, California

Takashi Maruo, MD, PhD, Department of Head and Neck Surgery, National Cancer Center Hospital East, Kashiwa, Chiba, Japan

Angela L. Mazul, PhD, MPH, Assistant Professor, Department of Otolaryngology/Head and Neck Surgery, Washington University School of Medicine, St. Louis, Missouri

Loren K. Mell, MD, Chief, Head and Neck Malignancy Service; Associate Professor, Department of Radiation Medicine and Applied Sciences, Moores Cancer Center, University of California San Diego, La Jolla, California

Jessica Moskovitz, MD, Fellow, Department of Otolaryngology, University of Pittsburgh, Pittsburgh, Pennsylvania

Jennifer Moy, MD, Physician, Department of Otolaryngology, University of Pittsburgh, Pittsburgh, Pennsylvania

Wai Tong Ng, MD, Consultant, Department of Clinical Oncology, Pamela Youde Nethersole Eastern Hospital, Hong Kong

Susumu Okano, MD, PhD, Department of Head and Neck Medical Oncology, National Cancer Center Hospital East, Kashiwa, Chiba, Japan

Andrew F. Olshan, PhD, Barbara Sorenson Hulka Distinguished Professor in Cancer Epidemiology, Department of Epidemiology, University of North Carolina at Chapel Hill, Chapel Hill, North Carolina

Heather A. Osborn, MD, FRCSC, Assistant Professor, Department of Otolaryngology—Head and Neck Surgery, Yale University, New Haven, Connecticut

Jong Chul Park, MD, Assistant in Medicine, Department of Hematology and Oncology, Massachusetts General Hospital Cancer Center, Boston, Massachusetts

Douglas E. Peterson, DMD, PhD, Professor and Chair, Section of Oral Medicine, University of Connecticut School of Dental Medicine, Farmington, Connecticut

James W. Rocco, MD, PhD, FACS, Professor and Chairman, Department of Otolaryngology-Head and Neck Surgery, Wexner Medical Center, James Cancer Hospital, Solove Research Institute, The Ohio State University, Columbus, Ohio

Cristina P. Rodriguez, MD, Associate Professor, Division of Medical Oncology, Department of Medicine, University of Washington, Seattle, Washington

Richard Blake Ross, BS, Medical Student, Department of Radiation Oncology, Taussig Cancer Institute, Cleveland Clinic, Cleveland, Ohio

Nabil F. Saba, MD, FACP, Professor, Hematology and Medical Oncology, Emory University School of Medicine; Director, Head and Neck Medical Oncology Program, Winship Cancer Institute of Emory University, Atlanta, Georgia

Anirudh Saraswathula, BA, Medical Student, Department of Otolaryngology-Head and Neck Surgery, Stanford University School of Medicine, Palo Alto, California

Sandra Schmitz, MD, PhD, Associate Professor, Department of Medical Oncology and Head and Neck Surgery, Institut Roi Albert II, Cliniques Universitaires Saint-Luc and Institut de Recherche Clinique et Expérimentale, Université Catholique de Louvain, Brussels, Belgium

Emmanuel Seront, MD, PhD, Medical Oncologist, Institut Roi Albert II, Service d'Oncologie Médicale, Cliniques Universitaires Saint-Luc and Institut de Recherche Clinique et Expérimentale (Pole MIRO), Université Catholique de Louvain, Brussels, Belgium; Service d'Oncologie Médicale, Centre Hospitalier de Jolimont, Haine Saint Paul, Belgium

Jussi Sillanpaa, PhD, Memorial Sloan Kettering Cancer Center, Middletown, New Jersey

Denis Soulières, MD, Hematologist and Medical Oncologist, Department of Hematology and Medical Oncology, CHUM, University of Montreal, Montreal, Quebec, Canada

Sharon A. Spencer, MD, Professor and Chief of Medical Services, Hazelrig Salter Radiation Oncology Center, Department of Radiation Oncology—University of Alabama at Birmingham School of Medicine, Birmingham, Alabama

Sophie Stock-Martineau, MD, Fellow, Department of Hematology and Medical Oncology, CHUM, University of Montreal, Montreal, Quebec, Canada

Erich M. Sturgis, MD, MPH, Professor, Department of Head and Neck Surgery, Division of Surgery, The University of Texas MD Anderson Cancer Center, Houston, Texas

Rathan M. Subramaniam, MD, PhD, MPH, FRANZCR, FACNM, Robert W. Parkey MD Distinguished Professor of Radiology, Professor and Chief, Division of Nuclear Medicine, Medical Director of the Cyclotron and Molecular Imaging Programs, Program Director of Nuclear Medicine Residency and PET/CT Fellowships, Departments of Radiology, Clinical Sciences and Advanced Imaging Research Center, The University of Texas Southwestern Medical Center, Dallas, Texas

Henry C. K. Sze, FRCR, Associate Consultant, Department of Clinical Oncology, Pamela Youde Nethersole Eastern Hospital, Hong Kong

Makoto Tahara, MD, PhD, Department of Head and Neck Medical Oncology, National Cancer Center Hospital East, Kashiwa, Chiba, Japan

Theodoros N. Teknos, MD, FACS, Clinical Professor, Otolaryngology, CWRU School of Medicine; President and Scientific Director, UH Seidman Cancer Center, Cleveland, Ohio

Minh Tam Truong, MD, Chief of Radiation Oncology, Department of Radiation Oncology, Boston Medical Center; Associate Professor and Chair of Radiation Oncology, Boston University School of Medicine, Boston, Massachusetts

C. Jillian Tsai, MD, PhD, Director, Head and Neck Radiation Oncology Research, Memorial Sloan Kettering Cancer Center, New York, New York

Meghan T. Turner, MD, Assistant Professor, Department of Otolaryngology-Head and Neck Surgery, West Virginia University School of Medicine, Morgantown, West Virginia

Steffen Wagner, Dr. rer. nat., Group Leader, Head and Neck Cancer Research, Department of Otorhinolaryngology, Head and Neck Surgery, University of Giessen, Giessen, Germany

Randal S. Weber, MD, Chief Patient Experience Officer; Professor of Head and Neck Surgery, Department of Head and Neck Surgery, The University of Texas MD Anderson Cancer Center, Houston, Texas

Michelle D. Williams, MD, Associate Professor, Department of Pathology, The University of Texas MD Anderson Cancer Center, Houston, Texas

Sue S. Yom, MD, PhD, Associate Professor of Clinical Radiation Oncology, Department of Radiation Oncology, University of California San Francisco, San Francisco, California

Sadamoto Zenda, MD, PhD, Department of Radiation Oncology, National Cancer Center Hospital East, Kashiwa, Chiba, Japan

Jose P. Zevallos, MD, MPH, Joseph B. Kimbrough Professor of Head and Neck Surgery, Department of Otolaryngology/Head and Neck Surgery, Washington University School of Medicine, St. Louis, Missouri

Preface

Head and neck cancers are challenging diseases that require complex management and exemplify the value of collaboration among multiple specialties. Very appropriately, we the Editors are representatives of each of the three major treatment modalities. The genesis of this work was driven by recognition that, despite evolution in various approaches and new emerging data, high quality clinical care is optimal when there is mutual respect of each other's discipline, and when each patient has a treatment recommendation made by multidisciplinary input.

When discussing the need for a new textbook we recognized and agreed that critical developments have been transforming the field of head and neck oncology. Indeed, in the past few years there have been significant advances in our understanding of the molecular biology, immune evasion, and genetic landscape of head and neck cancers, as well as the multidisciplinary management of these malignancies, including immunotherapy, targeted therapies, precision radiation therapy, robotic surgery, and supportive care capabilities. With the rising epidemic of human papillomavirus-associated oropharyngeal cancer, customizing treatment is of utmost importance, in particular taking into consideration long-term treatment effects. A major breakthrough worth reiterating has been the introduction of immunotherapy as a standard therapy that establishes the significance of host immune response in the initiation and progression of squamous cell carcinoma of the head and neck. Taken together, these developments provide the basis and justify the timely publication of "Head and Neck Cancers: Evidence-Based Treatment".

This textbook captures key advances and aims to become a quick and handy reference tool for head and neck cancer management issues, and features didactic patient cases in each site-specific management chapter. We anticipate that physicians involved in the care of these patients will find the material relevant to their clinical practice. Evidence-based approaches are emphasized throughout the textbook. The chapters have been authored by internationally recognized experts, with a focus on multi-modality representation. We are thankful and much obliged to their diligent and thoughtful contributions.

Finally, we owe a debt of gratitude to our patients. Their journeys and life stories are teaching us to become better doctors.

Athanassios Argiris, MD, PhD, FACP
Robert L. Ferris, MD, PhD, FACS
David I. Rosenthal, MD, FACR, FASTRO

SECTION I

Epidemiology, Biology, Diagnosis, and Staging

1

Head and Neck Cancer Epidemiology

Angela L. Mazul

Erich M. Sturgis

Andrew F. Olshan

Jose P. Zevallos

Head and neck cancers are a heterogeneous group of tumors arising from sites within the upper aerodigestive tract and from salivary glands and the nasopharynx, oropharynx, oral cavity, larynx, and hypopharynx. The vast majority of cancers arising from the upper aerodigestive tract are squamous cell carcinomas. While they share a general histology, these tumors often differ with respect to etiology and epidemiology. In this chapter, we review the epidemiology of nasopharyngeal, oropharyngeal, oral cavity, laryngeal, and salivary gland cancers.

The World Health Organization (WHO) estimated population rates for head and neck cancer in 2012 (1). Four head and neck cancer categories are available: lip, oral cavity (*International Classification of Diseases* [*ICD*]-10: C00-08), nasopharynx (ICD-10: C11), other pharynx (ICD-10: C09-10, C12-14), and larynx (ICD-10: C32). Worldwide age-standardized rates by site are displayed in Table 1.1 and mapped in Figure 1.1.

NASOPHARYNGEAL CARCINOMA

BURDEN OF DISEASE

Nasopharyngeal carcinomas (NPCs) are neoplasms that arise from the nasopharyngeal epithelium. Despite being in the same tissue type as other head and neck cancers, distinct differences exist between NPC and carcinoma of other regions. There are three different histological types of nasopharyngeal cancer: keratinizing squamous cell carcinoma and nonkeratinizing carcinoma, which is further characterized as differentiated or undifferentiated.

Overall, NPC is rare. In 2012, 86,000 incident cases of nasopharyngeal cancer were diagnosed worldwide and resulted in approximately 50,000 deaths (1). However, there are distinct patterns of incidence throughout different geographical regions in the world. NPC incidence is low in the United States and Europe (0.5 to 2 per 100,000) (2). In contrast, high-incidence regions such as southern China have an age-adjusted incidence that has been reported to be as high as 25 per 100,000 (3,4). Other high- or intermediate-incidence regions include Southeast Asia (5,6), North Africa (7,8), the Middle East (9), and the Arctic (10). The vast majority of NPCs in high-incidence areas are nonkeratinizing, with more undifferentiated than differentiated cases (11). Keratinizing squamous cell carcinoma is the most common histological type in low-incidence regions such as the United States (11).

Several previous studies have investigated the changes in NPC incidence in immigrants from high-incidence regions to low-incidence

TABLE 1.1

Age-Standardized Rates of Head and Neck Cancer Per 100,000 by Geographic Region

	Nasopharynx	Other Pharynx	Lip, Oral Cavity. I	Larynx
World	1.2	1.9	4	2.1
WHO Africa region	1	0.8	2.7	1.2
WHO Americas region	0.4	1.9	4.1	2.5
WHO East Mediterranean region	0.9	1.1	4.6	2.5
WHO Europe region	0.4	2.7	4.6	3.3
WHO Southeast Asia region	1.2	3.6	6.4	2.2
WHO Western Pacific region	2	0.8	2	1.2
IARC membership (24 countries)	0.4	2.8	5.4	2.5
Middle East and Northern Africa	1.3	0.6	2.2	2.9
Africa	1.1	0.8	2.6	1.4
Sub-Saharan Africa	0.9	0.9	2.7	1.1
Eastern Africa	1.5	0.8	3.6	1.2
Middle Africa	0.9	1.1	2.6	0.8
Northern Africa	1.6	0.7	2.3	2.2
Southern Africa	0.2	2.5	4	2.7
Western Africa	0.5	0.3	1.5	0.7
Latin America and Caribbean	0.3	1.5	3.3	2.7
Caribbean	0.3	2.2	3.2	4.2
Central America	0.1	0.6	2.1	2.1
South America	0.3	1.7	3.8	2.8
Northern America	0.5	2.5	5.1	2.4
Asia	1.6	1.8	3.8	1.8
Eastern Asia	1.8	0.7	1.7	1.2
Southeast Asia	4.3	1.6	3.2	1.5
South–Central Asia	0.4	3.8	7.3	2.6
Western Asia	0.9	0.6	2.1	3.6
Europe	0.4	2.9	4.8	3.2
European Union (EU-28)	0.4	3.2	4.9	3.1
Central and Eastern Europe	0.4	2.6	5	3.6

(continued)

TABLE 1.1 (*continued*)

Age-Standardized Rates of Head and Neck Cancer Per 100,000 by Geographic Region

	Nasopharynx	Other Pharynx	Lip, Oral Cavity. I	Larynx
Northern Europe	0.3	2.1	4.4	1.9
Southern Europe	0.5	1.9	3.9	3.7
Western Europe	0.3	4.5	5.5	2.7
Oceania	0.5	1.8	7.4	1.6
Australia/New Zealand	0.5	1.9	5.9	1.6
Melanesia	0.2	1.8	19	1.5
Micronesia/Polynesia	2	1	2.7	1
Micronesia	2.7	0	2.4	0
Polynesia	1.4	1.9	3	1.8

IARC, International Agency for Research on Cancer; WHO, World Health Organization.

regions. Incidence rates are stable among people who migrate from high-incidence countries to low-incidence countries and remain elevated compared to the native population (12–14). However, the NPC risk declines proportionally with duration of residence (15) and with each subsequent generation (13). Interestingly, non-Hispanic White males born in China or the Philippines have a higher risk of NPC compared with those born in the United States (16). However, these results should be interpreted with caution because migrants are self-selected and may represent a low-risk population from within the native source population.

Regardless of high-incidence or low-incidence populations, NPC incidence is about three to four times higher in males than in females (10). There are remarkable differences in incidence by age depending on geographic location. In southern China the incidence peaks between ages 40 and 59, after which there is a significant decline (3,17), suggesting an early life exposure. Another incidence peak is observed among adolescents and young adults in the Middle East and North Africa (18), as well as among African Americans in the United States (19). In low-incidence population, there appear to be two incidence peaks, one in early adolescence and another in the fourth or fifth decade of life (19,20).

RISK FACTORS

Epstein–Barr Virus

The Epstein Barr virus (EBV) is a DNA virus that is ubiquitous worldwide. Over 90% of the adult population has been infected with EBV, which persists latently. In Hong Kong, 100% of the children seroconvert by 10 years of age (21). Because EBV does not readily infect the epithelium, the current belief is that EBV establishes dormancy in the premalignant epithelium, which is then the initiating event for NPC (22). EBV is most commonly found in NPC with nonkeratinizing histological features, especially undifferentiated NPC (23,24). Although most people have been exposed, only a small proportion will develop NPC. Thus, host genetics and environmental exposures must also contribute to EBV-associated NPC, suggesting EBV is a necessary, but not sufficient cause.

EBV has been associated with NPC when patients with nasopharyngeal cancer were found to express antibodies against EBV (25,26). Subsequent studies have shown that IgG and IgA antibodies against EBV antigens are a feature of NPC and associated with clinical presentation of the disease (27–29). Additionally, IgA antibodies against EBV capsid antigen is a strong predictor of an NPC diagnosis (30). EBV is classified

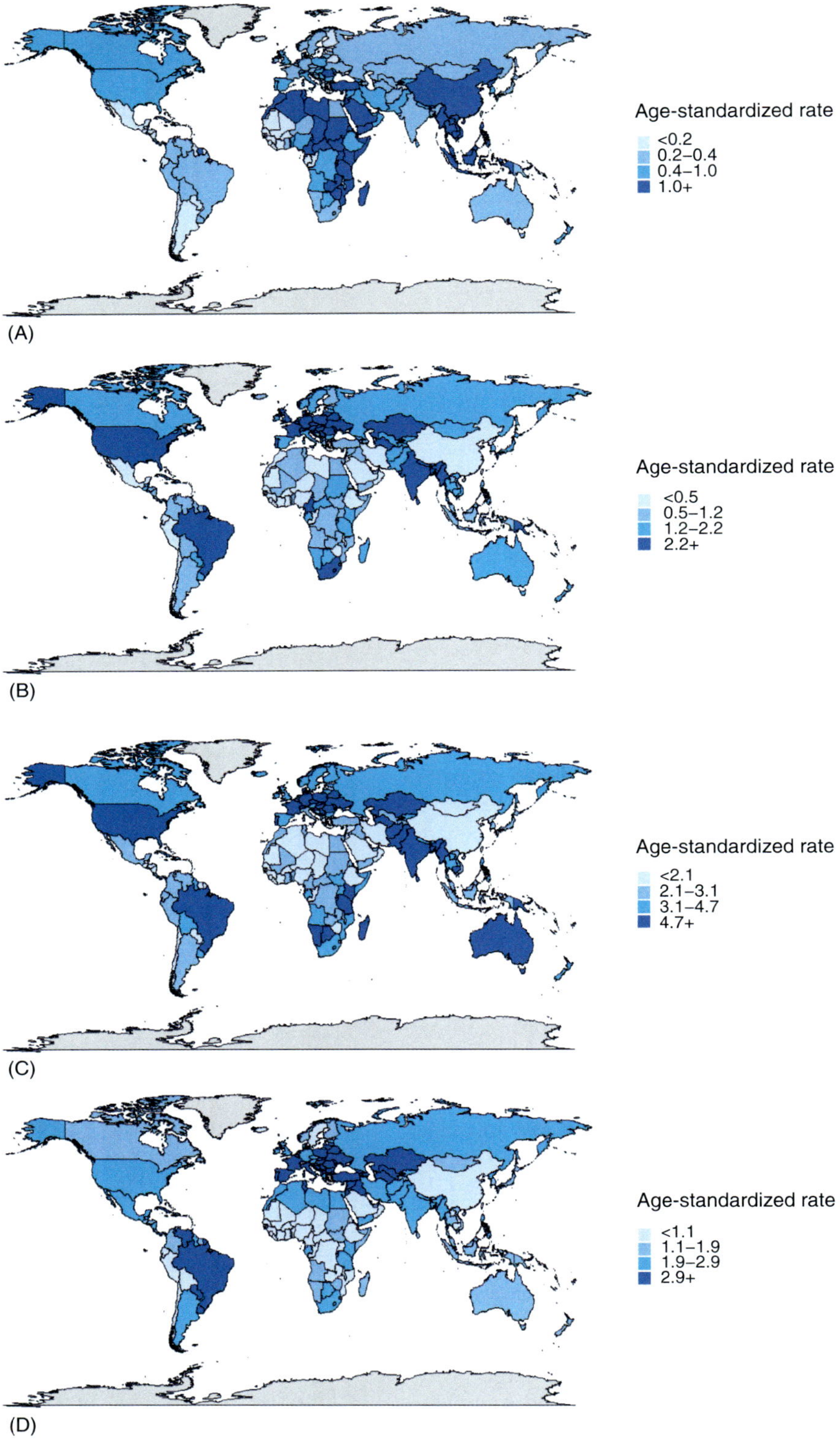

FIGURE 1.1 Maps of age-standardized rates per 100,000 for cancer of the (A) nasopharynx, (B) other pharynx, (C) lip, oral cavity, and (D) larynx.

into two categories based on genetic differences in the EBV nuclear antigen sequence, EBV type 1 (B95-8 strain) and EBV type 2 (AG876 strain) (31–33). Extensive research has been conducted to determine if genetic variability in EBV is at least partially responsible for the geographic distribution of NPC. EBV type 1 is more prevalent worldwide, but especially in Caucasian and Asian populations, while EBV type 2 is more common among African populations (34). Latent membrane protein 1 (LMP1), one of the most important EBV proteins, is able to induce phenotypic changes in epithelial cells (35) and is overexpressed in the majority of NPC cases (36). Two variants of *LMP1* have been previously described. The most frequent variant is a 30-bp deletion in the C-terminus of *LMP1* (del-*LMP1*), which has been associated with increased tumorigenesis in vitro and mouse studies (37–40). Additionally, in a meta-analysis, del-*LMP1* is more prevalent in NPC cases than in the population for Asian populations, but not for European and North African populations (41). However, few studies have been conducted in non-Asian populations and these results should be taken with caution. The second variation is the loss of a XhoI restriction site in *LMP1* and is most commonly found in nasopharyngeal tumors from Asian and U.S. non-Hispanic White populations (41,42), but is largely absent in North African populations (41). There is evidence that XhoI restriction site loss is more prevalent in China than Western populations (43) and may be associated with geographic variation rather than NPC.

Salt-Preserved Products

Salt-preserved fish, a staple food in many high-incidence areas, is the most common nonviral exposure associated with NPC (10). Many studies have reported a strong association between consuming Chinese-style salt-preserved fish and NPC, with odds ratios (ORs) ranging from 1.8 to 7.5 comparing high consumption (daily or ≥1/week) with no consumption (44–58). The difference in effect estimation is likely due to the duration of consumption and the age at first consumption as well as differences in population (i.e., low incidence versus high incidence) (59). Salted fish is frequently used as weaning food for infants in endemic areas and studies have shown that childhood exposure increases the risk of NPC (46,50,59). Additionally, NPC has been associated with other types of salt-preserved foods such as meats, eggs, fruits, and vegetables in Asian populations as well as in North African and North American populations (52,60–62). Thus, dietary differences may explain a portion of the geographic distribution associated with NPC.

A biologic basis exists for the association between salted foods and NPC, and the carcinogenicity of salt-preserved fish has been demonstrated in animal models. Rats fed salt-preserved fish were significantly more likely to develop malignant nasal and nasopharyngeal tumors (63,64). This may be due to the partial putrefaction and subsequent accumulation of nitrosamines commonly associated with salt-preservation (65–67). Despite this overwhelming evidence of an association, no prospective studies have been conducted on salt-preserved fish and risk of NPC.

Smoking

There are conflicting data on the association between tobacco use and risk of NPC. Several previous case–control studies suggest that smokers have a two- to sixfold increased risk of NPC compared to nonsmokers (56,58,68–72). However, other studies have shown a null association (48,52,73,74). This discrepancy could be due to differences in the study population and histological types because most studies reporting a stronger positive association were conducted in low-incidence populations where nonkeratinizing NPCs are more common (69–72). Although few studies have looked at histology specifically, two previous studies show a stronger association between smoking and keratinizing NPC compared to nonkeratinizing NPC (69,75).

Genetics

Currently, many studies are examining genetic factors associated with NPC, especially in genes involved in host immunity such as human leukocyte antigen (HLA). Studies have consistently linked NPC with the *HLA-A* genes (76–78). Since the distribution of the *HLA-A* alleles appears to be consistent with the distribution of NPC, these may be a marker for geographical distribution (79). However, in a meta-analysis, rs2517713 located near the *HLA-A* gene was strongly associated with a 40% decrease risk of NPC, suggesting there may be a true association with *HLA-A* (79).

PREVENTION

Given the strong risk factors for NPC, there is potential for effective primary and secondary prevention. Since EBV plays an important role in the development of NPC, as well as other cancers such as gastric carcinoma, Hodgkin lymphoma, and Burkitt lymphoma, an EBV vaccine would be a very effective method of primary prevention. Although a few nonprimate models have shown protection against EBV-induced lymphoma and EBV replication (80,81), the results of clinical trials with an EBV vaccine have not been promising (82–84).

Secondary prevention through screening of high-risk populations has been proposed in high-incidence regions such as southern China. Patients with stage I and stage II NPC have a 5-year survival rate of up to 90%, suggesting that early detection leads to better survival (85). Recently, a cluster randomized screening trial with combined EBV viral capsid antibody (VCA/IgA) and EBV nuclear antigen (EBNA 1/IgA) measured by ELISA and physical examination was started in southern China. Although the trial is still ongoing, preliminary results are encouraging. Among the 41 NPC cases detected, 38 were serologically determined to be high risk while 7 were positive through the physical examination (86). Additionally, the majority of the cases in the screening trial were diagnosed at early stages and before they manifested clinical symptoms. Additional studies are needed to determine the benefits and cost-effectiveness of widespread screening efforts (87).

OROPHARYNGEAL CARCINOMA

BURDEN OF DISEASE/INCIDENCE

Oropharyngeal squamous cell carcinoma (OPSCC) includes cancers arising from the tonsils, base of tongue, soft palate, and lateral and posterior pharyngeal walls. Over the past 30 years, there has been a significant change in the epidemiology of OPSCC. While the incidence of squamous cell carcinoma at all other head and neck cancer sites has declined over the past several decades, the incidence of OPSCC has increased precipitously. According to data from the Surveillance, Epidemiology, and End Results (SEER) registry (88), the overall incidence of cancers of the tonsil and oropharynx among people aged 50 to 74 has increased from to 4.9 per 100,000 in 1975 to 8.3 per 100,000 in 2013. While the rates remained relatively stable between 1975 and 1999, a pronounced increase occurred between 2000 and 2013 (annual percentage change = 2.9, $p < .05$). Among males, the incidence increased from 6.1/100,000 to 14.1/100,000 over the same time period, with the highest rate occurring among non-Hispanic Whites compared to African Americans or other racial/ethnic groups. Furthermore, this incidence trend has been most pronounced among non-Hispanic White males between ages 40 and 59 (88).

It is well established that the rapid increase in OPSCC incidence noted in the United States and other developed nations is attributable to human papillomavirus (HPV) infection. In fact, the majority of incident OPSCC cases in the United States (60% to 70%) are now HPV-associated (89,90). A similar pattern has been demonstrated across other developed nations, with higher rates of HPV-associated OPSCC occurring primarily in younger males (91). The rise in HPV-associated OPSCC incidence began in the 1990s (92) and has been attributed largely to changing sexual practices beginning in the 1960s (91). HPV-associated OPSCC has become a significant public health problem and is projected to overtake cervical cancer as the most common HPV-related malignancy in the United States by 2020 (90).

The demographics of head and neck cancer have changed significantly as a result of the increase in HPV-associated OPSCC. When compared to head and neck cancer caused by tobacco and alcohol use, patients with HPV-associated OPSCC are generally younger with a predominance of cases occurring in the fifth and sixth decades of life (91,93). Furthermore, a significant percentage of HPV-associated OPSCC occurs in never smokers (93). Previous research has suggested that HPV-associated OPSCC is significantly more common in non-Hispanic Whites compared to African Americans. However, more recent studies suggest that incidence rates among African Americans and females may have been understated (94). In a large retrospective cohort study on OPSCC, D'Souza et al. demonstrate similar trends in HPV-associated OPSCC incidence between males and females (94). They also demonstrate an increase in HPV-associated OPSCC in both Whites and non-Whites (94). It has also been suggested that HPV-associated OPSCC is associated with higher socioeconomic status when compared to HPV-negative head and neck cancer (95).

HPV-associated OPSCC is characterized by significantly better oncologic outcomes compared to stage- and site-matched HPV-negative head and neck cancer. HPV-associated tumors respond more effectively to treatment and demonstrate a 5-year overall survival between 70% and 90% in recent case series (96,97). While the majority of HPV-associated OPSCC have excellent oncologic outcomes, there is a subset of patients who fail to respond to therapy. A history of tobacco exposure attenuates the excellent prognosis typically associated with HPV-associated OPSCC (89,98).

RISK FACTORS

Tobacco and Alcohol Use

Like head and neck squamous cell carcinoma in other sites (oral cavity, larynx, and hypopharynx), OPSCC has traditionally been associated with tobacco and alcohol exposure. The combined use of heavy tobacco and alcohol use results in an exponentially increased risk of head and neck squamous cell carcinoma, including OPSCC. In the era of HPV-associated OPSCC, approximately 30% to 40% of incident OPSCC cases in the United States are associated with tobacco and alcohol use. These cancers generally have a poor outcome compared to HPV-associated OPSCC (89).

Oral HPV Infection

HPVs comprise approximately 150 DNA viruses that infect epithelial tissues of the skin and mucosa. Human papillomavirus infection is ubiquitous, with at least 13 well-established high-risk HPV types associated with malignancies of the cervix, anogenital region, and the oropharynx. Alpha HPV types, particularly HPV16, account for the vast majority of cancers in humans. Non-HPV16 types, including HPV18, HPV33, and HPV35 collectively account for less than 10% of OPSCC cases in the United States (99). Oral HPV infection has been demonstrated as a causal factor in the development of HPV-associated OPSCC. In a large prospective case–control study, Agalliu et al. established a temporal relationship between oral infection with high-risk HPV and the development of HPV-associated OPSCC (100,101). HPV-associated OPSCC has a latency period of 20 to 30 years; patients are typically exposed to HPV infection in their 20s and 30s but do not develop malignancy until the fifth or sixth decade of life (102,103).

The overall prevalence of oral HPV infection among adults in the United States is approximately 7%, and 1% for high-risk HPV infection (102). Oral HPV infection is sexually transmitted and the risk of both oral HPV infection and HPV-associated OPSCC is directly associated with the number of lifetime sexual partners and number of oral sexual partners (104,105). Additionally, there is a strong association between tobacco exposure and risk of oral HPV Infection (102). Oral HPV infection has a bimodal age distribution, with the highest rates of infection occurring in the early 30s and again in the sixth decade of life (102). Investigators have previously hypothesized that the early peak in HPV prevalence corresponds to infection associated with sexual debut while the second peak may be related to reactivation of dormant HPV infection as a result of immunosenescence (102,106).

While oral high-risk HPV infection is a necessary cause of HPV-associated OPSCC, a small fraction of exposed individuals develop cancer. This suggests additional host factors associated with susceptibility to HPV-associated OPSCC. In a recent genome-wide association study (GWAS) of oral and pharyngeal squamous cell carcinoma, Lesseur et al. demonstrate several novel susceptibility loci associated with head and neck cancer (107). Specifically, a variant at class II HLA region was significantly associated with risk of HPV-associated OPSCC, underscoring the potential importance of host immunity on the risk of HPV-associated OPSCC and the need for further exploration (107).

PREVENTION AND SCREENING

HPV vaccination has been a public health success, resulting in a dramatic decline in HPV-associated cervical cancer over the past several decades. The increasing rise of HPV-associated OPSCC underscores the importance in continued public health efforts at vaccination, and there is growing evidence that HPV vaccination is effective at reducing the risk of oral HPV infection (103,106,108). Three HPV vaccines are currently available in the United States: Cervarix is a bivalent vaccine against HPV16 and HPV 18, Gardasil is a quadrivalent vaccine against HPV16, HPV18, HPV6, and HPV 11, and Gardasil 9 is a nonavalent that provides protection against HPV16, 18, 33, 45, 52, 58, 6, and 11. These vaccines are approved for females aged 9 to 26 and males aged 9 to 15 (109). There are ongoing efforts increase awareness of the importance of HPV vaccination for both males and females.

Several recent studies have examined the possible role of tonsillectomy in secondary prevention for oropharyngeal cancer (110,111). In a study of the Danish Cancer Registry, Fahkry et al. noted a decrease in tonsil cancer in patients with a history of undergoing tonsillectomy (110). These results should be interpreted with caution for several different reasons. First, residual lymphoid tissue in the base of tongue remains susceptible to HPV infection and HPV-associated malignancy (111,112). Furthermore, it is generally considered that the morbidity and cost of surgery preclude the use of prophylactic tonsillectomy as an effective means of secondary prevention (112).

ORAL CAVITY CARCINOMA

INCIDENCE/BURDEN OF DISEASE

Anatomically the oral cavity consists of the mucosal lip, oral tongue, floor of the mouth, mandibular and maxillary gingivae, retromolar trigone, buccal mucosa, and hard palate subsites. Although oropharynx is occasionally included, it is important to separate them due to differing etiology, treatment, and management. Although other cancers such as salivary gland malignancies, sarcomas, mucosal melanomas, and lymphomas can also arise within the oral cavity, squamous cell carcinomas compose over 90% of oral cavity cancer and are the focus of this chapter.

Cancers of the oral cavity represent the most common cancers of the upper aerodigestive tract, accounting for approximately 30%. In the United States, the incidence of oral cavity squamous cell carcinoma (OCSCC) is much higher among Black males (9.65 per 100,000, age-standardized to the 1960 population) compared to White males (7.16 per 100,000). However, there is little racial difference among women (0.74 per 100,000 among White females and 0.79 per 100,000 for Black females) (113). Globally there are an estimated 300,000 cases of cancer of the lip and oral cavity in 2012 with the majority occurring in men. About 145,000 deaths were due to OCSCC in 2012. The highest incidence is seen in the South Pacific with Melanesia having 22.9 per 100,000 per year for men (114).

The overall 5-year survival for OCSSC is about 60% but can range from 10% to 80% depending on different factors. Five-year survival for early-stage tumors can be as high as 80%. In contrast, survival for late-stage tumors is about 10% (115).

Although OCSCC incidence has declined over the years (116), an increase in incidence has been observed among young females (117). These tumors are not HPV-associated, and the etiology remains unclear (118).

RISK FACTORS

Tobacco and Alcohol Use

A strong association has been consistently demonstrated between OCSCC and tobacco use (119). Over a quarter of oral cancers are attributable to smoking (120). In the largest pooled analysis to date from the International Head and Neck Cancer Epidemiology (INHANCE) Consortium, cigarette smokers have 2.83 times the risk of OCSCC compared with noncigarette smokers (121). Even low cigarette use (>0–3 cigarettes a day) is associated with a 50% increased risk of OCSCC (122). Using the 11 case–control studies from INHANCE based in the United States, Wyss et al. demonstrated a 3-fold and 1.8-fold increase in the risk of OCSCC associated with snuff and smokeless tobacco use, respectively, among never cigarette users (123). However, this association did not persist among ever cigarette users. Similar associations are seen in INHANCE with pipe and cigar smokers. An association is only seen for either pipe or cigar smokers (OR: 2.83 and 2.51, respectively) and OCSCC among noncigarette smokers (121).

High alcohol consumption is also a major risk factor for OCSCC. In an INHANCE study of different types of alcohol, OCSCC had the strongest association of all head and neck cancer sites, likely due to its proximity (124). They also found little difference between beer and liquor consumption (OR nondrinkers versus >30 drinks: 6.4 and 5.9, respectively) and a weaker association with wine (OR: 3.2), which is likely due to residual confounding due to socioeconomic status (125). However, among never smokers, the magnitude of the association is greatly diminished (120).

Although the literature is inconsistent about the magnitude of the interaction, there appears to be a synergistic association between alcohol and tobacco use (126–128). In INHANCE, among those who smoke more than 20 cigarettes a day and consume more than 3 drinks a day, there is a 14-fold increase in the risk of OCSCC (126). Additionally, in this population, 23.5% of OCSCC can be attributable to both alcohol and cigarette smoking (126).

Betel Quid

Betel quid is a mixture of substances wrapped in a betel leaf and placed in the mouth. It usually contains either tobacco and sliced fresh or dried areca nut or both. Betel quid is very common in Southeast Asia and the Pacific Islands and used by 600 million people worldwide (129). The betel quid has been strongly associated with risk of oral squamous cell carcinoma (130). According to a recent review of existing data on this association, Merchant and Pitiphat demonstrated a 7-fold increase in the risk of oral cancer associated with betel use without tobacco and a 15-fold increased risk when betel was combined with tobacco (131).

Betel quid has been classified as an oral carcinogen in humans by the International Agency for Research on Cancer, with evidence for a dose–response relationship (132). Although the exact mechanism has yet to be elucidated (133), endogenous nitrosation has been demonstrated in betel quid chewers, with consequent production of potentially carcinogenic nitrosamines, such as 3-methylnitrosopropionitrile. Reactive oxygen species generation in the oral cavity due to auto-oxidation of polyphenols contained in areca nut and enhanced by the alkaline pH from slaked lime has been reported (131).

Dietary Factors/Oral Hygiene

Diets rich in fruits and vegetables have been inversely associated with OCSCC. Similarly, diets high in red and processed meats are associated with increased risk of OCSCC (134). The increased association between diet and OCSCC may be mediated through damage to the DNA through exposure in foods such as free radicals or nitrosamines. However, the protective association may be due to antioxidants and phytonutrients that could also prevent DNA damage (135). Another analysis found that folate consumption is associated with decreased risk of OCSCC with little interaction with alcohol or tobacco (136).

Dental health has also been associated with OCSCC in many studies (137). In the largest study to date, poor dental health is associated with an almost three times increase in the risk of OCSCC (138). The mechanisms for this association could be due to inflammation and disruption of the oral microbiota or could be due to general well-being. Interestingly, mouthwash has been associated with a small increase in the risk of OCSCC (137,139). This could be due to the alcohol that is present in many mouthwash formulations.

Oral HPV Infection

Although HPV infection has been definitively linked with oropharyngeal cancer, its role in OCSCC is highly debated (140,141). Many studies find HPV in 10% to 25% of OCSCC, but unlike oropharyngeal cancer (141), the survival has been contradictory suggesting better survival (142,143), worse survival (144,145), or no difference in survival (145). To date, there is no clear molecular evidence that OCSCC is driven by HPV since the presence of HPV does not necessarily indicate biologically active HPV.

PREVENTION

There is no accepted and validated method for oral cancer screening. No population screening programs for OCSCC have been implemented and the U.S. Preventive Services Task Force does not currently recommend screening. In a 2008 survey of U.S. adults, 29.4% reported ever having an oral cancer examination. Visual examination for leukoplakia and erythroplakia lesions, the most commonly used method to detect lesions, can be augmented by toluidine blue, brush biopsy, and fluorescence staining.

LARYNX CANCER

BURDEN OF DISEASE

Cancer of the larynx includes tumors of the glottis, supraglottis, subglottis, and laryngeal cartilage. Most larynx tumors are squamous cell carcinomas. Because of similar clinical management, hypopharynx tumors, albeit rare, are sometimes included with larynx tumors in epidemiologic analyses. An estimated 13,150 new cases of laryngeal cancer cases will be diagnosed in 2018 (146). This constitutes about 22% of all head and neck cancers. Based on SEER data (2008–2012), the age-adjusted incidence rates are higher in men (5.8 per 100,000) than women (1.2 per 100,000). Black men had a higher rate (8.8 per 100,000). For both sexes combined, lower rates were found among Hispanics (2.3 per 100,000), American Indians/Alaskan Natives (2.3 per 100,000), and Asians/Pacific Islanders (1.2 per 100,000) (147). In the United States, based on SEER data, men have a much higher mortality rate (1.9 per 100,000) than women (0.4 per 100,000) (147). Black males had a higher mortality rate (3.6 per 100,000) than White males (1.8 per 100,000). In the United States incidence and death rates have been decreasing (2003–2012, average annual percent change for incidence −2.6% and −2.2% for mortality). This pattern, largely due to the parallel trend in decreased smoking, was seen for all race/ethnic groups. International patterns, based on the International Agency for Research on Cancer GLOBOCAN 2012 data, showed higher incidence rates among men and more economically developed countries (114). The highest incidence rates were found in the Caribbean (7.9 per 100,000), Central and Eastern Europe (7.8), Southern Europe (7.2), and Western Asia (6.5). Mortality rates also followed a similar geographic pattern. Globally, incidence rates have been declining since 1980.

RISK FACTORS

The major risk factor for larynx cancer is tobacco use, but other exposures have been associated with an increased or decreased risk in epidemiologic studies.

Tobacco

Tobacco smoking is a well-established risk factor for larynx cancer; only lung cancer has a stronger association (148). In relative terms, the association with tobacco smoking is stronger in women than men but represents a lower absolute risk. The decrease in laryngeal cancer incidence and mortality has been attributed to the decline in smoking, especially among men. Pipe and cigar smoking has been associated with an increased risk of larynx cancer (149,150). Passive smoke exposure has also been associated with an increased risk (151). Quitting smoking has been shown to significantly reduce risk up to 20 years after cessation (152). Variation in the association of tobacco use has been reported for larynx subsites with stronger effects seen for hypopharynx and supraglottic tumors (121,153).

Alcohol and Diet

Several studies have reported a modest independent effect of alcohol consumption after adjustment for tobacco use or among never smokers (153). Consumption of fruits and vegetables has consistently been associated with a decreased risk of larynx cancer, while consumption of meat and eggs has increased risk (134,154). Dietary patterns described as “prudent” or patterns with greater intake of fruits and vegetables and lean proteins have a reduced risk, and patterns described as the “Western” diet or those with higher consumption of fried foods, high fat, and processed meats have an elevated risk (155,156).

Other Exposures and Factors

A number of occupations, industries, and related exposures have been associated with an increased risk of larynx cancer including asbestos, solvents, formaldehyde, wood dust, metal-related occupations, paint and print workers, textile workers, plastic and rubber manufacturing, agriculture, and crop protection chemical and pesticide manufacturing (153). HPV has been associated with larynx cancer in some studies, but not with the consistency and strength of association found in studies of other head and neck cancer sites, most notably oropharynx cancer (157). Multiple studies have reported an association between lower body mass index (BMI) and an elevated risk of larynx cancer (158,159), and a recent study suggested an association with higher BMI. However, the effect of lower BMI has been attributed to residual confounding of tobacco smoking, the influence of the disease, and study design (160). Poor oral health has been linked with an elevated risk in one study (161). Earlier studies have suggested an association between gastrointestinal reflux (gastroesophageal reflux disease [GERD]) and hypopharynx or larynx cancer, but recent studies have not supported these findings (162,163).

Family history of head and neck and other cancers has been associated with an elevated risk of larynx cancer (164). A variety of candidate genes and associated single nucleotide polymorphisms (SNPs) have been found to increase or decrease the risk of larynx cancer (165–167). Candidate pathways examined have included DNA repair, carcinogen metabolism, alcohol metabolism, and immune response. A GWAS reported associations with SNPs in alcohol-metabolizing genes (168). A recent Chinese GWAS reported associations with three other variants (169).

PREVENTION

Primary prevention measures to reduce tobacco use remain a clear priority. Chemoprevention studies using alpha-tocopherol and beta-carotene supplements do not show a benefit for the reduction of second primary tumors upper aerodigestive tract cancers including laryngeal cancer (169).

SALIVARY GLAND CANCER

BURDEN OF DISEASE

Salivary gland cancers are a diverse group of neoplasms that can be found in any of the major salivary glands (parotid, submandibular, and sublingual) or minor salivary glands, which are widely distributed throughout the upper aerodigestive tract. The majority of salivary gland neoplasms are benign; only 20% are malignant. For both benign and malignant tumors considered together, the incidences of salivary gland tumors have been reported to range from 0.4 to 13.5 cases per 100,000 population per year (170). The incidences of salivary gland cancer in different regions of the world range from 0.1 to 3.2 cases per 100,000 population per year in men and 0.1 to 1.8 cases per 100,000 population per year in women (171). However, because many prior reports only account for cancers of the major salivary glands, the true incidence of salivary gland cancer may be higher (171). Moreover, because the disease is rare and its diagnosis is challenging, it is difficult to determine whether the considerable geographic variations in incidence are caused by different tumor registration policies or indicate real region-to-region differences. However, population studies have suggested that susceptibility to different histological subtypes of salivary gland cancer may differ by ethnicity (172,173).

Salivary gland cancers are relatively rare in the United States, accounting for 11% of cancers of the oral cavity and pharynx and 0.3% of cancers of all sites combined (174). Salivary gland cancers are more common in U.S. men (mean annual incidence, 1.7 cases per 100,000 population) than in U.S. women (mean annual incidence, 1.0 case per 100,000 population). Over the past 40 years, the annual percentage change in incidence of salivary gland cancer has steadily increased by 0.6% each year. For both men and women, the incidence of salivary gland cancer increases with age, and a majority of patients are diagnosed after 50 years of age (172,174). An estimated 700 deaths related to salivary gland cancer occur in the United States each year (0.4 deaths per 100,000 population for men and 0.1 deaths per 100,000 population for women), and the average annual mortality rate is 1.4 deaths per 100,000 population in patients more than 65 years old. The 5-year relative survival rate for salivary gland cancer varies from 93% in patients with localized disease to 65% in patients with regional spread to 38% in patients with distant metastases.

Salivary gland cancer comprises an extremely heterogeneous group of tumors, including approximately 40 histological types of epithelial tumors. In theSEER registry, mucoepidermoid carcinoma is the most common subtype, accounting for 18% of major salivary gland cancers, followed by adenoid cystic carcinoma, which accounts for 11%, and acinic cell carcinoma, which accounts for 10% (172). Regardless of histological subtype, 80% of major salivary gland cancers arise in the parotid glands, while most minor salivary gland cancers arise in the palate.

The proportion of histological subtypes of salivary gland cancer varies by anatomic site and population. For example, in the U.S. population, 62% of mucoepidermoid carcinomas, 57% of adenoid cystic carcinomas, and 92% of acinic cell carcinomas occur in the major salivary glands (175). Among children and adolescents (<20 years old) with salivary gland cancer in the SEER population, 49% had mucoepidermoid carcinoma, 35% had acinic cell carcinomas, and 5% had adenoid cystic carcinomas; in contrast, among adults with salivary gland cancer in the SEER population, 24% had mucoepidermoid carcinoma, 11% had acinic cell carcinoma, and 13% had adenoid cystic carcinoma (176). Acinic cell carcinoma is more common among women at younger ages, and mucoepidermoid carcinoma is more common among men than among women (172).

RISK FACTORS

Although the etiology of salivary gland cancer is not well understood, a number of factors have been implicated as potential causes.

Radiation Exposure

Exposure to ionizing radiation is one of the well-established risk factors for both benign and malignant salivary gland tumors. The most compelling evidence implicating ionizing radiation comes from the Life Span Study cohort of survivors of the atomic bombs in Hiroshima and Nagasaki (177–180). Compared to individuals not exposed to radiation from the bombs, atomic bomb survivors had 11 times the risk of malignant salivary gland tumors and 3.5 times the risk of benign salivary tumors; furthermore, a significant linear dose–response relationship was found (177,179). The dose–response relationship was strongest for mucoepidermoid carcinomas and for Warthin tumors (179).

Therapeutic radiation has been linked to an increased risk of salivary gland cancer. In childhood cancer survivors, a dose–response relationship has been established, and the risk of salivary gland cancer was seven times as high in survivors treated with high doses of radiotherapy as in survivors who received no radiotherapy (181). A 30% increased risk for secondary salivary gland cancer was found in adult cancer survivors treated with radiotherapy (182). Additional evidence linking salivary gland cancer with therapeutic irradiation comes from studies of children treated with scalp irradiation for tinea capitis (183,184), patients treated with iodine-131 for hyperthyroidism (185,186), patients who underwent repeated dental radiography (187–189), and bone marrow transplant recipients (190–192).

An observation of higher incidence of salivary gland cancer in the southern region than in the central and northern regions of the SEER registries led to the suggestion that exposure to ultraviolet radiation might be a risk factor for salivary gland cancer (193). However, this observation may have been due to misclassification of metastatic cutaneous squamous cell carcinoma as primary salivary gland cancer. Cutaneous squamous cell carcinoma that metastasizes to lymph nodes of the parotid gland is commonly misclassified as primary parotid cancer. In the SEER population, squamous cell carcinoma accounted for 14% of salivary gland cancers (19% among men) (193), while in other single-institution case series with more precise site classification, squamous cell carcinoma accounted for very few primary parotid cancers (194–196). Retrospective studies evaluating parotid gland tumors showed that in most cases in which metastases were initially misdiagnosed as primary salivary gland cancer, the primary tumor was a squamous cell carcinoma, and fewer than 25% of cases of squamous cell carcinoma of the parotid gland were consistent with a possible true primary squamous cell carcinoma of the salivary gland (197–200).

Occupational Exposures

The evidence linking salivary gland cancer to occupational exposures is sparse. Several studies showed an increased risk of salivary gland cancer (particularly minor salivary gland cancer of the paranasal sinuses) in workers in rubber manufacturing, plumbing, and some types of woodworking and in workers with occupational exposure to nickel compounds/alloys, silica dust, and asbestos (201–205). The elevated risks were largely limited to workers exposed in the early years of the 20th century or in developing countries, where the exposure dose was substantially higher.

Viral Exposures

Several viruses have been implicated in the etiology of salivary gland cancer. A strong association has been found between EBV and lymphoepithelial carcinoma of the salivary glands, although this association has been demonstrated only among Asians and Greenlandic Inuits (206,207). While HPV and HIV type 1 have been found in salivary gland tumors, there is no convincing evidence to support a causal association between these viruses and development of salivary gland cancer (208–210).

PREVENTION

Prevention of salivary gland cancer will require a better understanding of the etiology of the disease. Minimizing exposure to ionizing radiation and avoiding the aforementioned occupational exposures might reduce the likelihood of developing salivary gland cancer, but the preventive effect is uncertain for this rare disease. There is no screening paradigm for salivary gland cancer, though further understanding of environmental and genetic risk factors might allow screening in a highly selected group.

REFERENCES

1. Ferlay J, Soerjomataram I, Ervik M. GLOBOCAN, Cancer Incidence and Mortality Worldwide: IARC Cancer Base No. 11 [Internet]. Lyon, France: International Agency for Research on Cancer; 2013.
2. Yu MC, Yuan J-M. Epidemiology of nasopharyngeal carcinoma. *Semin Cancer Biol.* 2002;12(6):421–429. doi:10.1016/S1044579X02000858
3. Jia WH, Huang QH, Liao J, et al. Trends in incidence and mortality of nasopharyngeal carcinoma over a 20-25 year period (1978/1983-2002) in Sihui and Cangwu counties in southern China. *BMC Cancer.* 2006;6:178. doi:10.1186/1471-2407-6-178
4. Parkin DM, Bray F, Ferlay J, et al. Global cancer statistics, 2002. *CA Cancer J Clin.* 2005;55(2):74–108.
5. Kataki AC, Simons MJ, das AK, et al. Nasopharyngeal carcinoma in the northeastern states of India. *Chin J Cancer.* 2011;30(2):106–113.

6. Chong VH, Telisinghe PU, Lim E, et al. Declining incidence of nasopharyngeal carcinoma in Brunei Darussalam: a three decade study (1986-2014). *Asian Pac J Cancer Prev*. 2015;16(16):7097–7101.
7. Zanetti R, Tazi MA, Rosso S. New data tells us more about cancer incidence in North Africa. *Eur J Cancer*. 2010;46(3):462–466. doi:10.1016/j.ejca.2009.11.012
8. Hamdi Cherif M, Serraino D, Mahnane A, et al. Time trends of cancer incidence in Setif, Algeria, 1986-2010: an observational study. *BMC Cancer*. 2014;14:637. doi:10.1186/1471-2407-14-637.
9. Abdulamir AS, Hafidh RR, Abdulmuhaimen N, et al. The distinctive profile of risk factors of nasopharyngeal carcinoma in comparison with other head and neck cancer types. *BMC Public Health*. 2008;8(1):400. doi:10.1186/1471-2458-8-400
10. Chang ET, Adami HO. The enigmatic epidemiology of nasopharyngeal carcinoma. *Cancer Epidemiol Biomarkers Prev*. 2006;15(10):1765–1777. doi:10.1158/1055-9965.EPI-06-0353
11. Tao Q, Chan AT. Nasopharyngeal carcinoma: molecular pathogenesis and therapeutic developments. *Expert Rev Mol Med*. 2007;9(12):1–24. doi:10.1017/S1462399407000312
12. Rottenberg Y, et al. Risk of nasopharyngeal carcinoma penetrates across immigrant generations: a migrant cohort study of 2.3 million Jewish Israeli adolescents. *Int J Cancer*. 2017;140(5):1060–1067. doi:10.1002/ijc.30525
13. Buell P. The effect of migration on the risk of nasopharyngeal cancer among Chinese. *Cancer Res*. 1974;34(5):1189–1191.
14. Mousavi SM, Sundquist J, Hemminki K. Nasopharyngeal and hypopharyngeal carcinoma risk among immigrants in Sweden. *Int J Cancer*. 2010;127(12):2888–2892. doi:10.1002/ijc.25287
15. McCredie M, Williams S, Coates M. Cancer mortality in East and Southeast Asian migrants to New South Wales, Australia, 1975-1995. *Br J Cancer*. 1999;79(7-8):1277–1282. doi:10.1038/sj.bjc.6690205
16. Buell P. Race and place in the etiology of nasopharyngeal cancer: a study based on California death certificates. *Int J Cancer*. 1973;11(2):268–272.
17. Lee AW, Foo W, Mang O, et al. Changing epidemiology of nasopharyngeal carcinoma in Hong Kong over a 20-year period (1980-99): an encouraging reduction in both incidence and mortality. *Int J Cancer*. 2003;103(5):680–685. doi:10.1002/ijc.10894
18. Obafunwa JO, Bhatia PL. Nasopharyngeal carcinoma in Plateau State, Nigeria: a pathological study. *Eur J Surg Oncol*. 1991;17(4):335–337.
19. Richey LM, Olshan AF, George J, et al. Incidence and survival rates for young blacks with nasopharyngeal carcinoma in the United States. *Arch Otolaryngol Head Neck Surg*. 2006;132(10):1035–1040. doi:10.1001/archotol.132.10.1035
20. Bray F, Haugen M, Moger TA, et al. Age-incidence curves of nasopharyngeal carcinoma worldwide: bimodality in low-risk populations and aetiologic implications. *Cancer Epidemiol Biomarkers Prev*. 2008;17(9):2356–2365. doi:10.1158/1055-9965.EPI-08-0461
21. Kangro HO, Osman HK, Lau YL, et al. Seroprevalence of antibodies to human herpesviruses in England and Hong Kong. *J Med Virol*. 1994;43(1):91–96.
22. Tsao SW, Tsang CM, To KF, et al. The role of Epstein-Barr virus in epithelial malignancies. *J Pathol*. 2015;235(2):323–333. doi:10.1002/path.4448
23. Raab-Traub N, Flynn K, Pearson G, et al. The differentiated form of nasopharyngeal carcinoma contains Epstein-Barr virus DNA. *Int J Cancer*. 1987;39(1):25–29.
24. Nicholls JM, Agathanggelou A, Fung K, et al. The association of squamous cell carcinomas of the nasopharynx with Epstein-Barr virus shows geographical variation reminiscent of Burkitt's lymphoma. *J Pathol*. 1997;183(2):164–168.
25. Old LJ, Boyse EA, Oettgen HF, et al. Precipitating antibody in human serum to an antigen present in cultured burkitt's lymphoma cells. *Proc Natl Acad Sci USA*. 1966;56(6):1699–1704.
26. Henle W, Henle G, Ho HC, et al. Antibodies to Epstein-Barr virus in nasopharyngeal carcinoma, other head and neck neoplasms, and control groups. *J Natl Cancer Inst*. 1970;44(1):225–231.
27. de-Thé G, Ho JH, Ablashi DV, et al. Nasopharyngeal carcinoma. IX. Antibodies to EBNA and correlation with response to other ebv antigens in chinese patients. *Int J Cancer*. 1975;16(5):713–721.
28. Henle G, Henle W. Epstein-Barr virus-specific IgA serum antibodies as an outstanding feature of nasopharyngeal carcinoma. *Int J Cancer*. 1976;17(1):1–7.
29. Wara WM, Wara DW, Phillips TL, et al. Elevated IGA in carcinoma of the nasopharynx. *Cancer*. 1975;35(5):1313–1315.
30. Chien YC, Chen JY, Liu MY, et al. Serologic markers of Epstein-Barr virus infection and nasopharyngeal carcinoma in Taiwanese men. *N Engl J Med*. 2001;345(26):1877–1882. doi:10.1056/NEJMoa011610
31. Palser AL, Grayson NE, White RE, et al. Genome diversity of Epstein-Barr virus from multiple tumor types and normal infection. *J Virol*. 2015;89(10):5222–5237. doi:10.1128/JVI.03614-14
32. Baumforth KR, Young LS, Flavell KJ, et al. The Epstein-Barr virus and its association with human cancers. *Mol Pathol*. 1999;52(6):307–322.
33. Zimber U, Adldinger HK, Lenoir GM, et al. Geographical prevalence of two types of Epstein-Barr virus. *Virology*. 1986;154(1):56–66.
34. Chang CM, Yu KJ, Mbulaiteye SM, et al. The extent of genetic diversity of Epstein-Barr virus and its geographic and disease patterns: a need for reappraisal. *Virus Res*. 2009;143(2):209–221. doi:10.1016/j.virusres.2009.07.005
35. Temple RM, Zhu J, Budgeon L, et al. Efficient replication of Epstein-Barr virus in stratified epithelium in vitro. *Proc Natl Acad Sci USA*. 2014;111(46):16544–16549. doi:10.1073/pnas.1400818111
36. vera-Sempere FJ, Burgos JS, Botella MS, et al. Immunohistochemical expression of Epstein-Barr virus-encoded latent membrane protein (LMP-1) in paraffin sections of EBV-associated nasopharyngeal carcinoma

in Spanish patients. *Eur J Cancer B Oral Oncol.* 1996;32B(3):163–168.

37. Tao Q, Ambinder RF, Swinnen LJ. Epstein-Barr virus (EBV) variant with a 30-bp deletion at the carboxyl terminus (amino acids 346-355) of latent membrane protein-1 (LMP1) gene is able to transform cells and evade immune surveillance. *Am J Pathol.* 1998;152(5):1398–1399.
38. Li SN, Chang YS, Liu ST. Effect of a 10-amino acid deletion on the oncogenic activity of latent membrane protein 1 of Epstein-Barr virus. *Oncogene.* 1996;12(10):2129–2135.
39. Miller WE, Edwards RH, Walling DM, et al. Sequence variation in the Epstein-Barr virus latent membrane protein 1. *J Gen Virol.* 1994;75 (Pt 10)(Pt 10):2729–2740. doi:10.1099/0022-1317-75-10-2729
40. Mainou BA, Raab-Traub N. LMP1 strain variants: biological and molecular properties. *J Virol.* 2006;80(13):6458–6468. doi:10.1128/JVI.00135-06
41. da Costa VG, Marques-Silva AC, Moreli ML. The Epstein-Barr virus latent membrane protein-1 (LMP1) 30-bp deletion and XhoI-polymorphism in nasopharyngeal carcinoma: a meta-analysis of observational studies. *Syst Rev.* 2015;4:46. doi:10.1186/s13643-015-0037-z
42. See HS, Yap YY, Yip WK, et al. Epstein-Barr virus latent membrane protein-1 (LMP-1) 30-bp deletion and Xho I-loss is associated with type III nasopharyngeal carcinoma in Malaysia. *World J Surg Oncol.* 2008;6:18. doi:10.1186/1477-7819-6-18
43. Neves M, Marinho-Dias J, Ribeiro J, et al. Epstein-Barr virus strains and variations: Geographic or disease-specific variants? *J Med Virol.* 2017;89(3). doi:10.1002/jmv.24633
44. Henderson BE, Louie E, Soohoo Jing J, et al. Risk factors associated with nasopharyngeal carcinoma. *N Engl J Med.* 1976;295(20):1101–1106. doi:10.1056/NEJM197611112952003
45. Henderson BE, Louie E. Discussion of risk factors for nasopharyngeal carcinoma. *IARC Sci Publ.* 1978;20(20):251–260.
46. Geser A, Charnay N, Day NE, et al. Environmental factors in the etiology of nasopharyngeal carcinoma: report on a case-control study in Hong Kong. *IARC Sci Publ.* 1978;20(20):213–229.
47. Armstrong RW, Eng AC. Salted fish and nasopharyngeal carcinoma in Malaysia. *Soc Sci Med.* 1983;17(20):1559–1567.
48. Yu MC, Ho JH, Lai S-H, Henderson BE. Cantonese-style salted fish as a cause of nasopharyngeal carcinoma: report of a case-control study in Hong Kong. *Cancer Res.* 1986;46(2):956–961.
49. Yu MC, Mo C-C, Chong W-X, et al. Preserved foods and nasopharyngeal carcinoma: a case-control study in Guangxi, China. *Cancer Res.* 1988;48(7):1954–1959.
50. Yu MC, Huang T-B, Henderson BE. Diet and nasopharyngeal carcinoma: a case-control study in Guangzhou, China. *Int J Cancer.* 1989;43(6):1077–1082.
51. Ning J-P, Yu MC, Wang Q-S, et al. Consumption of salted fish and other risk factors for nasopharyngeal carcinoma (NPC) in Tianjin, a low-risk region for NPC in the People's Republic of China. *JNCI J Natl Cancer Inst.* 1990;82(4):291–296.
52. Sriamporn S, Vatanasapt V, Pisani P, et al. Environmental risk factors for nasopharyngeal carcinoma: a case-control study in northeastern Thailand. *Cancer Epidemiol Biomarkers Prev.* 1992;1(5):345–348.
53. Zheng CX, Yan L, Nilsson B, et al. Epstein-Barr virus infection, salted fish and nasopharyngeal carcinoma: a case-control study in Southern. *Acta Oncol.* 1994;33(8):867–872.
54. Armstrong RW, Imrey PB, Lye MS, et al. Nasopharyngeal carcinoma in Malaysian Chinese: salted fish and other dietary exposures. *Int J Cancer.* 1998;77(2):228–235.
55. Zou J, Sun Q, Akiba S, et al. A case-control study of nasopharyngeal carcinoma in the high background radiation areas of Yangjiang, China. *J Radiat Res.* 2000;41(suppl):53–62.
56. Guo X, Johnson RC, Deng H, et al. Evaluation of non-viral risk factors for nasopharyngeal carcinoma in a high-risk population of Southern China. *Int J Cancer.* 2009;124(12):2942–2947. doi:10.1002/ijc.24293
57. Yuan JM, Wang XL, Xiang YB, et al. Preserved foods in relation to risk of nasopharyngeal carcinoma in Shanghai, China. *Int J Cancer.* 2000;85(3):358–363.
58. Yang XR, Diehl S, Pfeiffer R, et al. Chinese and American Genetic Epidemiology of NPC Study Team. Evaluation of risk factors for nasopharyngeal carcinoma in high-risk nasopharyngeal carcinoma families in Taiwan. *Cancer Epidemiol Biomarkers Prev.* 2005;14(4):900–905. doi:10.1158/1055-9965.EPI-04-0680
59. Ward MH, Pan WH, Cheng YJ, et al. Dietary exposure to nitrite and nitrosamines and risk of nasopharyngeal carcinoma in Taiwan. *Int J Cancer.* 2000;86(5):603–609.
60. Jeannel D, Hubert A, de Vathaire F, et al. Diet, living conditions and nasopharyngeal carcinoma in Tunisia—a case-control study. *Int J Cancer.* 1990;46(3):421–425.
61. Farrow DC, Vaughan TL, Berwick M, et al. Diet and nasopharyngeal cancer in a low-risk population. *Int J Cancer.* 1998;78(6):675–679.
62. Friborg JT, Melbye M. Cancer patterns in Inuit populations. *Lancet Oncol.* 2008;9(9):892–900. doi:10.1016/s1470-2045(08)70231-6
63. Yu MC, Nichols PW, Zou X-N, et al. Induction of malignant nasal cavity tumours in Wistar rats fed Chinese salted fish. *Br J Cancer.* 1989;60(2):198–201.
64. Huang DP, Ho JH, Saw D, et al. Carcinoma of the nasal and paranasal regions in rats fed Cantonese salted marine fish. *IARC Sci Publ.* 1978;20(20):315–328.
65. Huang DP, Ho JHC, Webb KS, et al. Volatile nitrosamines in salt-preserved fish before and after cooking. *Food Cosmet Toxicol.* 1981;19(2):167–171.
66. Al Bulushi I, Poole S, Deeth HC, et al. Biogenic amines in fish: roles in intoxication, spoilage, and nitrosamine formation—a review. *Crit Rev Food Sci Nutr.* 2009;49(4):369–377.

67. Anderson LM, Souliotis VL, Chhabra SK, et al. N-nitrosodimethylamine-derived O(6)-methylguanine in DNA of monkey gastrointestinal and urogenital organs and enhancement by ethanol. *Int J Cancer*. 1996;66(1):130–134.
68. Friborg JT, Yuan JM, Wang R, et al. A prospective study of tobacco and alcohol use as risk factors for pharyngeal carcinomas in Singapore Chinese. *Cancer*. 2007;109(6):1183–1191.
69. Vaughan TL, et al. Nasopharyngeal cancer in a low-risk population: defining risk factors by histological type. *Cancer Epidemiol Biomarkers Prevention*. 1996;5(8):587–593.
70. Chow WH, Mclaughlin JK, Hrubec Z, et al. Tobacco use and nasopharyngeal carcinoma in a cohort of US veterans. *Int J Cancer*. 1993;55(4):538–540.
71. Zhu K, Levine RS, Brann EA, et al. A population-based case-control study of the relationship between cigarette smoking and nasopharyngeal cancer (United States). *Cancer Causes Control*. 1995;6(6):507–512.
72. Nam JM, McLaughlin JK, Blot WJ. Cigarette smoking, alcohol, and nasopharyngeal carcinoma: a case-control study among U.S. whites. *J Natl Cancer Inst*. 1992;84(8):619–622.
73. Zheng X, Yan L, Nilsson B, et al. Epstein-Barr virus infection, salted fish and nasopharyngeal carcinoma. A case-control study in southern China. *Acta Oncol*. 1994;33(8):867–872.
74. Ning J-P, Yu MC, Wang Q-S, Henderson BE. Consumption of salted fish and other risk factors for nasopharyngeal carcinoma (NPC) in Tianjin, a low-risk region for NPC in the People's Republic of China. *J Natl Cancer Inst*. 1990;82(4):291–296.
75. Polesel J, Franceschi S, Talamini R, et al. Tobacco smoking, alcohol drinking, and the risk of different histological types of nasopharyngeal cancer in a low-risk population. *Oral Oncol*. 2011;47(6):541–545.
76. Hildesheim A, Wang CP. Genetic predisposition factors and nasopharyngeal carcinoma risk: a review of epidemiological association studies, 2000-2011: Rosetta Stone for NPC: genetics, viral infection, and other environmental factors. *Semin Cancer Biol*. 2012;22(2):107–116. doi:10.1016/j.semcancer.2012.01.007
77. Bei J-X, Jia W-H, Zeng Y-X. Familial and large-scale case-control studies identify genes associated with nasopharyngeal carcinoma. *Semin Cancer Biol*. 2012;22(2):96–106. doi:10.1016/j.semcancer.2012.01.012
78. Burt RD, Vaughan TL, McKnight B, et al. Associations between human leukocyte antigen type and nasopharyngeal carcinoma in Caucasians in the United States. *Cancer Epidemiol Biomarkers Prev*. 1996;5(11):879–887.
79. Su W-H, Chiu C-C, Yao Shugart Y. Heterogeneity revealed through meta-analysis might link geographical differences with nasopharyngeal carcinoma incidence in Han Chinese populations. *BMC Cancer*. 2015;15:598. doi:10.1186/s12885-015-1607-0
80. Cui X, Cao Z, Chen Q, et al. Rabbits immunized with Epstein-Barr virus gH/gL or gB recombinant proteins elicit higher serum virus neutralizing activity than gp350. *Vaccine*. 2016;34(34):4050–4055.
81. Cohen JI. Epstein–barr virus vaccines. *Clin Transl Immunology*. 2015;4(1):e32. doi:10.1038/cti.2014.27
82. Rees L, Tizard EJ, Morgan AJ, et al. A phase I trial of epstein-barr virus gp350 vaccine for children with chronic kidney disease awaiting transplantation. *Transplantation*. 2009;88(8):1025–1029. doi:10.1097/TP.0b013e3181b9d918
83. Moutschen M, Léonard P, Sokal EM, et al. Phase I/II studies to evaluate safety and immunogenicity of a recombinant gp350 Epstein-Barr virus vaccine in healthy adults. *Vaccine*. 2007;25(24):4697–4705. doi:10.1016/j.vaccine.2007.04.008
84. Sokal EM, Hoppenbrouwers K, Vandermeulen C, et al. Recombinant gp350 vaccine for infectious mononucleosis: a phase 2, randomized, double-blind, placebo-controlled trial to evaluate the safety, immunogenicity, and efficacy of an Epstein-Barr virus vaccine in healthy young adults. *J Infect Dis*. 2007;196(12):1749–1753.
85. Chua DTT, Sham JST, Kwong DLW, Au GKH. Treatment outcome after radiotherapy alone for patients with Stage I-II nasopharyngeal carcinoma. *Cancer*. 2003;98(1):74–80. doi:10.1002/cncr.11485
86. Liu Z, Ji M-F, Huang Q-H, et al. Two Epstein-Barr virus-related serologic antibody tests in nasopharyngeal carcinoma screening: results from the initial phase of a cluster randomized controlled trial in Southern China. *Am J Epidemiol*. 2013;177(3):242–250. doi:10.1093/aje/kws404
87. Yang S, Wu S, Zhou J, Chen XY. Screening for nasopharyngeal cancer. *Cochrane Database Syst Rev*. 2015;31(6). doi:10.1002/14651858.CD008423.pub2
88. Surveillance E. End Results (SEER) Program SEER*Stat Database: Incidence - SEER 9 Regs Research Data, Nov 2015 Sub (1973-2013) - Linked To County Attributes - Total U.S., 1969-2014 Counties, National Cancer Institute, DCCPS, Surveillance Research Program, Surveillance Systems Branch, released April 2016, based on the November 2015 submission.
89. Ang KK, Harris J, Wheeler R, et al. Human papillomavirus and survival of patients with oropharyngeal cancer. *N Engl J Med*. 2010;363(1):24–35. doi:10.1056/NEJMoa0912217
90. Chaturvedi AK, Engels EA, Pfeiffer RM, et al. Human papillomavirus and rising oropharyngeal cancer incidence in the United States. *J Clin Oncol*. 2011;29(32):4294–4301. doi:10.1200/JCO.2011.36.4596
91. Chaturvedi AK, Anderson WF, Lortet-Tieulent J, et al. Worldwide trends in incidence rates for oral cavity and oropharyngeal cancers. *J Clin Oncol*. 2013;31(36):4550–4559. doi:10.1200/JCO.2013.50.3870
92. Ernster JA, Sciotto CG, O'Brien MM, et al. Rising incidence of oropharyngeal cancer and the role of oncogenic human papilloma virus. *Laryngoscope*. 2007;117(12):2115–2128. doi:10.1097/MLG.0b013e31813e5fbb

93. Young D, Xiao CC, Murphy B, et al. Increase in head and neck cancer in younger patients due to human papillomavirus (HPV). *Oral Oncol*. 2015;51(8):727–730. doi:10.1016/j.oraloncology.2015.03.015
94. D'Souza G, Westra WH, Wang SJ, et al. Differences in the prevalence of human papillomavirus (HPV) in head and neck squamous cell cancers by sex, race, anatomic tumor site, and HPV detection method. *JAMA Oncol*. 2016;December 8 [epub ahead of print]. doi:10.1001/jamaoncol.2016.3067
95. Dahlstrom KR, Bell D, Hanby D, et al. Socioeconomic characteristics of patients with oropharyngeal carcinoma according to tumor HPV status, patient smoking status, and sexual behavior. *Oral Oncol*. 2015;51(9):832–838. doi:10.1016/j.oraloncology.2015.06.005
96. O'Sullivan B, Huang SH, Siu LL, et al. Deintensification candidate subgroups in human papillomavirus-related oropharyngeal cancer according to minimal risk of distant metastasis. *J Clin Oncol*. 2013;31(5):543–550. doi:10.1200/JCO.2012.44.0164
97. Quon H, Richmon JD. Treatment deintensification strategies for HPV-associated head and neck carcinomas. *Otolaryngol Clin North Am*. 2012;45(4):845–861. doi:10.1016/j.otc.2012.04.007
98. Sandulache VC, Hamblin J, Lai S, et al. Oropharyngeal squamous cell carcinoma in the veteran population: association with traditional carcinogen exposure and poor clinical outcomes. *Head Neck*. 2015;37(9):1246–1253. doi:10.1002/hed.23740
99. Mazul AL, Rodriguez-Ormaza N, Taylor JM, et al. Prognostic significance of non-HPV16 genotypes in oropharyngeal squamous cell carcinoma. *Oral Oncol*. 2016;61:98–103. doi:10.1016/j.oraloncology.2016.08.019
100. Agalliu I, Wang T, Burk RD. β- and γ-Human papillomavirus types and smoking in head and neck cancer—reply. *JAMA Oncol*. 2016;2(5):687–688. doi:10.1001/jamaoncol.2016.0973
101. Agalliu I, Gapstur S, Chen Z, et al. Associations of oral α-, β-, and γ-human papillomavirus types with risk of incident head and neck cancer. *JAMA Oncol*. 2016;599. doi:10.1001/jamaoncol.2015.5504
102. Gillison ML, Broutian T, Pickard RK, et al. Prevalence of oral HPV infection in the United States, 2009-2010. *JAMA*. 2012;307(7):693–703. doi:10.1001/jama.2012.101
103. D'Souza G, Dempsey A. The role of HPV in head and neck cancer and review of the HPV vaccine. *Prev Med*. 2011;53(Suppl 1):S5–S11. doi:10.1016/j.ypmed.2011.08.001
104. D'Souza G, Agrawal Y, Halpern J, et al. Oral sexual behaviors associated with prevalent oral human papillomavirus infection. *J Infect Dis*. 2009;199(9):1263–1269. doi:10.1086/597755
105. Heck JE, Berthiller J, Vaccarella S, et al. Sexual behaviours and the risk of head and neck cancers: a pooled analysis in the International Head and Neck Cancer Epidemiology (INHANCE) consortium. *Int J Epidemiol*. 2010;39(1):166–181. doi:10.1093/ije/dyp350
106. Guo T, Eisele DW, Fakhry C. The potential impact of prophylactic human papillomavirus vaccination on oropharyngeal cancer. *Cancer*. 2016;122(15):2313–2323. doi:10.1002/cncr.29992
107. Lesseur C, Diergaarde B, Olshan AF, et al. Genome-wide association analyses identify new susceptibility loci for oral cavity and pharyngeal cancer. *Nat Genet*. 2016;48(12):1544–1550. doi:10.1038/ng.3685
108. Beachler DC, Kreimer AR, Schiffman M, et al. Costa Rica HPV Vaccine Trial (CVT) Group. Multisite HPV16/18 Vaccine Efficacy Against Cervical, Anal, and Oral HPV Infection. *J Natl Cancer Inst*. 2016;108(1):djv302. doi:10.1093/jnci/djv302
109. Herrero R, González P, Markowitz LE. Present status of human papillomavirus vaccine development and implementation. *Lancet Oncol*. 2015;16(5):e206–e216. doi:10.1016/S1470-2045(14)70481-4
110. Fakhry C, Andersen KK, Christensen J, et al. The impact of tonsillectomy upon the risk of oropharyngeal carcinoma diagnosis and prognosis in the Danish Cancer Registry. *Cancer Prev Res*. 2015;8(7):583–589. doi:10.1158/1940-6207.CAPR-15-0101
111. Zevallos JP, Mazul AL, Rodriguez N, et al. Previous tonsillectomy modifies odds of tonsil and base of tongue cancer. *Br J Cancer*. 2016;114(7):832–838. doi:10.1038/bjc.2016.63
112. Misiukiewicz K, Posner M. Role of prophylactic bilateral tonsillectomy as a cancer preventive strategy. *Cancer Prev Res*. 2015;8(7):580–582. doi:10.1158/1940-6207.CAPR-15-0153
113. Simard EP, Torre LA, Jemal A. International trends in head and neck cancer incidence rates: differences by country, sex and anatomic site. *Oral Oncol*. 2014;50(5):387–403. doi:10.1016/j.oraloncology.2014.01.016
114. Ferlay J, Soerjomataram I, Dikshit R, et al. Cancer incidence and mortality worldwide: sources, methods and major patterns in GLOBOCAN 2012. *Int J Cancer*. 2015;136(5):E359–E386. doi:10.1002/ijc.29210
115. Amit M, Yen TC, Liao CT, et al. Improvement in survival of patients with oral cavity squamous cell carcinoma: an international collaborative study. *Cancer*. 2013;119(24):4242–4248. doi:10.1002/cncr.28357
116. Carvalho AL, Nishimoto IN, Califano JA, et al. Trends in incidence and prognosis for head and neck cancer in the United States: a site-specific analysis of the SEER database. *Int J Cancer*. 2005;114(5):806–816. doi:10.1002/ijc.20740
117. Muller K, Kazimiroff J, Fatahzadeh M, et al. Oral human papillomavirus infection and oral lesions in HIV-positive and HIV-negative dental patients. *J Infect Dis*. 2015;212(5):760–768. doi:10.1093/infdis/jiv080
118. Patel SC, Carpenter WR, Tyree S, et al. Increasing incidence of oral tongue squamous cell carcinoma in young white women, age 18 to 44 years. *J Clin Oncol*. 2011;29(11):1488–1494. doi:10.1200/JCO.2010.31.7883
119. World Health Organization and International Agency for Research on Cancer. Tobacco smoke and involuntary smoking. Vol. 83. 2004: IARC.

120. Hashibe M, Brennan P, Benhamou S, et al. Alcohol drinking in never users of tobacco, cigarette smoking in never drinkers, and the risk of head and neck cancer: pooled analysis in the International Head and Neck Cancer Epidemiology Consortium. *J Natl Cancer Inst.* 2007;99(10):777–789. doi:10.1093/jnci/djk179
121. Wyss A, Hashibe M, Chuang SC, et al. Cigarette, cigar, and pipe smoking and the risk of head and neck cancers: pooled analysis in the International Head and Neck Cancer Epidemiology Consortium. *Am J Epidemiol.* 2013;178(5):679–690. doi:10.1093/aje/kwt029
122. Berthiller J, Straif K, Agudo A, et al. Low frequency of cigarette smoking and the risk of head and neck cancer in the INHANCE consortium pooled analysis. *Int J Epidemiol.* 2016;45(3):835–845. doi:10.1093/ije/dyv146
123. Wyss AB, Hashibe M, Lee YA, et al. Smokeless Tobacco Use and the Risk of Head and Neck Cancer: Pooled Analysis of US Studies in the INHANCE Consortium. *Am J Epidemiol.* 2016;703–716. doi:10.1093/aje/kww075
124. Baan R, Straif K, Grosse Y, et al. WHO International Agency for Research on Cancer Monograph Working Group. Carcinogenicity of alcoholic beverages. *Lancet Oncol.* 2007;8(4):292–293.
125. Purdue MP, Hashibe M, Berthiller J, et al. Type of alcoholic beverage and risk of head and neck cancer—a pooled analysis within the INHANCE Consortium. *Am J Epidemiol.* 2009;169(2):132–142. doi:10.1093/aje/kwn306
126. Hashibe M, Brennan P, Chuang SC, et al. Interaction between tobacco and alcohol use and the risk of head and neck cancer: pooled analysis in the International Head and Neck Cancer Epidemiology Consortium. *Cancer Epidemiol Biomarkers Prev.* 2009;18(2):541–550. doi:10.1158/1055-9965.EPI-08-0347
127. Radoï L, Menvielle G, Cyr D, et al. ICARE Study Group. Population attributable risks of oral cavity cancer to behavioral and medical risk factors in France: results of a large population-based case-control study, the ICARE study. *BMC Cancer.* 2015;15:827. doi:10.1186/s12885-015-1841-5
128. Radoï L, Paget-Bailly S, Cyr D, et al. Tobacco smoking, alcohol drinking and risk of oral cavity cancer by subsite: results of a French population-based case-control study, the ICARE study. *Eur J Cancer Prev.* 2013;22(3):268–276. doi:10.1097/CEJ.0b013e3283592cce
129. IARC Working Group on the Evaluation of Carcinogenic Risks to Humans. Betel-quid and areca-nut chewing and some areca-nut derived nitrosamines. *IARC Monogr Eval Carcinog Risks Hum.* 2004;85:1–334.
130. Gupta B, Johnson NW. Systematic review and meta-analysis of association of smokeless tobacco and of betel quid without tobacco with incidence of oral cancer in South Asia and the Pacific. *PLOS ONE.* 2014;9(11):e113385. doi:10.1371/journal.pone.0113385
131. Merchant AT, Pitiphat W. Total, direct, and indirect effects of paan on oral cancer. *Cancer Causes Control.* 2015;26(3):487–491. doi:10.1007/s10552-014-0516-x
132. Kim L, King T, Agulnik M. Head and neck cancer: changing epidemiology and public health implications. *Oncology.* 2010;24(10):915–924.
133. Petti S. Lifestyle risk factors for oral cancer. *Oral Oncol.* 2009;45(4-5):340–350. doi:10.1016/j.oraloncology.2008.05.018
134. Chuang SC, Jenab M, Heck JE, et al. Diet and the risk of head and neck cancer: a pooled analysis in the INHANCE consortium. *Cancer Causes Control.* 2012;23(1):69–88. doi:10.1007/s10552-011-9857-x
135. Chainani-Wu N, Epstein J, Touger-Decker R. Diet and prevention of oral cancer: strategies for clinical practice. *J Am Dent Assoc.* 2011;142(2):166–169.
136. Galeone C, Edefonti V, Parpinel M, et al. Folate intake and the risk of oral cavity and pharyngeal cancer: a pooled analysis within the INHANCE Consortium. *Int J Cancer.* 2015;136(4):904–914. doi:10.1002/ijc.29044
137. Ahrens W, Pohlabeln H, Foraita R, et al. Oral health, dental care and mouthwash associated with upper aerodigestive tract cancer risk in Europe: the ARCAGE study. *Oral Oncol.* 2014;50(6):616–625. doi:10.1016/j.oraloncology.2014.03.001
138. Hashim D, Sartori S, Brennan P, et al. The role of oral hygiene in head and neck cancer: results from International Head and Neck Cancer Epidemiology (INHANCE) consortium. *Ann Oncol.* 2016;27(8):1619–1625. doi:10.1093/annonc/mdw224
139. Boffetta P, Hayes RB, Sartori S, et al. Mouthwash use and cancer of the head and neck: a pooled analysis from the International Head and Neck Cancer Epidemiology Consortium. *Eur J Cancer Prev.* 2016;25(4):344–348. doi:10.1097/CEJ.0000000000000179
140. Syrjänen S, Lodi G, von Bültzingslöwen I, et al. Human papillomaviruses in oral carcinoma and oral potentially malignant disorders: a systematic review. *Oral Dis.* 2011;17(Suppl 1):58–72. doi:10.1111/j.1601-0825.2011.01792.x
141. Isayeva T, Li Y, Maswahu D, et al. Human papillomavirus in non-oropharyngeal head and neck cancers: a systematic literature review. *Head Neck Pathol.* 2012;6(Suppl 1):104–120. doi:10.1007/s12105-012-0368-1
142. Schwartz SR, Yueh B, McDougall JK, et al. Human papillomavirus infection and survival in oral squamous cell cancer: a population-based study. *Otolaryngol Head Neck Surg.* 2001;125(1):1–9. doi:10.1067/mhn.2001.116979
143. Elango KJ, Suresh A, Erode EM, et al. Role of human papilloma virus in oral tongue squamous cell carcinoma. *Asian Pac J Cancer Prev.* 2011;12(4):889–896.
144. Kozomara R, Jović N, Magić Z, et al. p53 mutations and human papillomavirus infection in oral squamous cell carcinomas: correlation with overall survival. *J Craniomaxillofac Surg.* 2005;33(5):342–348. doi:10.1016/j.jcms.2005.05.004
145. Duray A, Descamps G, Decaestecker C, et al. Human papillomavirus DNA strongly correlates with a poorer prognosis in oral cavity carcinoma. *Laryngoscope.* 2012;122(7):1558–1565. doi:10.1002/lary.23298

146. Siegel RL, Miller KD, Jemal A. Cancer Statistics, 2018. *CA Cancer J Clin.* 2018;68:7–30.
147. Howlader N, et al. SEER *Cancer Statistics Review*, 1975–2012. Bethesda, MD: National Cancer Institute; 2015.
148. IARC Working Group on the Evaluation of Carcinogenic Risks to Humans. Tobacco smoke and involuntary smoking. *IARC Monogr Eval Carcinog Risks Hum.* 2004;83:1–1438.
149. Henley SJ, Thun MJ, Chao A, et al. Association between exclusive pipe smoking and mortality from cancer and other diseases. *J Natl Cancer Inst.* 2004;96(11):853–861.
150. Shapiro JA, Jacobs EJ, Thun MJ. Cigar smoking in men and risk of death from tobacco-related cancers. *J Natl Cancer Inst.* 2000;92(4):333–337.
151. Lee YC, Boffetta P, Sturgis EM, et al. Involuntary smoking and head and neck cancer risk: pooled analysis in the International Head and Neck Cancer Epidemiology Consortium. *Cancer Epidemiol Biomarkers Prev.* 2008;17(8):1974–1981. doi:10.1158/1055-9965.EPI-08-0047
152. Bosetti C, Gallus S, Peto R, et al. Tobacco smoking, smoking cessation, and cumulative risk of upper aerodigestive tract cancers. *Am J Epidemiol.* 2008;167(4):468–473. doi:10.1093/aje/kwm318
153. Olshan AF, Divaris K. Occupation and other risk factors for head and neck cancer. In AF Olshan, ed. *Epidemiology, Pathogenesis, and Prevention of Head and Neck Cancer.* New York, NY: Springer; 2010:137–154.
154. Lucenteforte E, Dietary factors. In AF Olshan, ed. *Epidemiology, Pathogenesis, and Prevention of Head and Neck Cancer.* New York, NY: Springer; 2010:117–136.
155. Bradshaw PT, Siega-Riz AM, Campbell M, et al. Associations between dietary patterns and head and neck cancer: the Carolina head and neck cancer epidemiology study. *Am J Epidemiol.* 2012;175(12):1225–1233. doi:10.1093/aje/kwr468
156. de Stefani E, Boffetta P, Correa P, et al. Dietary patterns and risk of cancers of the upper aerodigestive tract: a factor analysis in Uruguay. *Nutr Cancer.* 2013;65(3):384–389. doi:10.1080/01635581.2013.761254
157. Chaturvedi A, Gillison ML. Human papillomavirus and head and neck cancer. In AF Olshan, ed. *Epidemiology, Pathogenesis, and Prevention of Head and Neck Cancer.* New York, NY: Springer; 2010:87–116.
158. Gaudet MM, Olshan AF, Chuang SC, et al. Body mass index and risk of head and neck cancer in a pooled analysis of case-control studies in the International Head and Neck Cancer Epidemiology (INHANCE) Consortium. *Int J Epidemiol.* 2010;39(4):1091–1102. doi:10.1093/ije/dyp380
159. Etemadi A, O'Doherty MG, Freedman ND, et al. A prospective cohort study of body size and risk of head and neck cancers in the NIH-AARP diet and health study. *Cancer Epidemiol Biomarkers Prev.* 2014;23(11):2422–2429. doi:10.1158/1055-9965.EPI-14-0709-T
160. Gaudet MM, Kitahara CM, Newton CC, et al. Anthropometry and head and neck cancer:a pooled analysis of cohort data. *Int J Epidemiol.* 2015;44(2):673–681. doi:10.1093/ije/dyv059
161. Guha N, Boffetta P, Wünsch Filho V, et al. Oral health and risk of squamous cell carcinoma of the head and neck and esophagus: results of two multicentric case-control studies. *Am J Epidemiol.* 2007;166(10):1159–1173. doi:10.1093/aje/kwm193
162. Macfarlane TV, Macfarlane GJ, Thakker NS, et al. Role of medical history and medication use in the aetiology of upper aerodigestive tract cancers in Europe: the ARCAGE study. *Ann Oncol.* 2012;23(4):1053–1060. doi:10.1093/annonc/mdr335
163. Busch EL, Zevallos JP, Olshan AF. Gastroesophageal reflux disease and odds of head and neck squamous cell carcinoma in North Carolina. *Laryngoscope.* 2016;126(5):1091–1096. doi:10.1002/lary.25716
164. Negri E, Boffetta P, Berthiller J, et al. Family history of cancer: pooled analysis in the International Head and Neck Cancer Epidemiology Consortium. *Int J Cancer.* 2009;124(2):394–401. doi:10.1002/ijc.23848
165. Wang L-E, et al. Host susceptibility and molecular epidemiology. In AF Olshan, ed. *Epidemiology, Pathogenesis, and Prevention of Head and Neck Cancer* New York, NY: Springer; 2010;155–185.
166. Wang Y, Chu X, Meng X, et al. Association of X-ray repair cross complementing group 1 Arg399Gln polymorphisms with the risk of squamous cell carcinoma of the head and neck: evidence from an updated meta-analysis. *PLOS ONE.* 2013;8(10):e77898. doi:10.1371/journal.pone.0077898
167. Hakenewerth AM, Millikan RC, Rusyn I, et al. Joint effects of alcohol consumption and polymorphisms in alcohol and oxidative stress metabolism genes on risk of head and neck cancer. *Cancer Epidemiol Biomarkers Prev.* 2011;20(11):2438–2449. doi:10.1158/1055-9965.epi-11-0649
168. McKay JD, Truong T, Gaborieau V, et al. A genome-wide association study of upper aerodigestive tract cancers conducted within the INHANCE consortium. *PLOS Genet.* 2011;7(3):e1001333. doi:10.1371/journal.pgen.1001333
169. Wei Q, Yu D, Liu M, et al. Genome-wide association study identifies three susceptibility loci for laryngeal squamous cell carcinoma in the Chinese population. *Nat Genet.* 2014;46(10):1110–1114. doi:10.1038/ng.3090
170. Thompson L. World Health Organization classification of tumours: pathology and genetics of head and neck tumours. *Ear Nose Throat J.* 2006;85(2):74.
171. Bray F, Ferlay J, Laversanne M, et al. Cancer Incidence in Five Continents: Inclusion criteria, highlights from Volume X and the global status of cancer registration. *Int J Cancer.* 2015;137(9):2060–2071. doi:10.1002/ijc.29670
172. Boukheris H, Curtis RE, Land CE, et al. Incidence of carcinoma of the major salivary glands according to the WHO classification, 1992 to 2006: a population-

based study in the United States. *Cancer Epidemiol Biomarkers Prev*. 2009;18(11):2899–2906. doi:10.1158/1055-9965.EPI-09-0638
173. Bjørndal K, Krogdahl A, Therkildsen MH, et al. Salivary gland carcinoma in Denmark 1990-2005: a national study of incidence, site and histology. Results of the Danish Head and Neck Cancer Group (DAHANCA). *Oral Oncol*. 2011;47(7):677–682. doi:10.1016/j.oraloncology.2011.04.020
174. Howlader N, et al. *SEER Cancer Statistics Review, 1975-2013*. National Cancer Institute.
175. Li N, Xu L, Zhao H, et al. A comparison of the demographics, clinical features, and survival of patients with adenoid cystic carcinoma of major and minor salivary glands versus less common sites within the Surveillance, Epidemiology, and End Results registry. *Cancer*. 2012;118(16):3945–3953. doi:10.1002/cncr.26740
176. Sultan I, Rodriguez-Galindo C, Al-Sharabati S, et al. Salivary gland carcinomas in children and adolescents: a population-based study, with comparison to adult cases. *Head Neck*. 2011;33(10):1476–1481. doi:10.1002/hed.21629
177. Thompson DE, Mabuchi K, Ron E, et al. Cancer incidence in atomic bomb survivors. Part II: solid tumors, 1958-1987. *Radiat Res*. 1994;137(2, Suppl):S17–67.
178. Land CE, Saku T, Hayashi Y, et al. Incidence of salivary gland tumors among atomic bomb survivors, 1950-1987. Evaluation of radiation-related risk. *Radiat Res*. 1996;146(1):28–36.
179. Saku T, Hayashi Y, Takahara O, et al. Salivary gland tumors among atomic bomb survivors, 1950-1987. *Cancer*. 1997;79(8):1465–1475.
180. Belsky JL, Tachikawa K, Cihak RW, et al. Salivary gland tumors in atomic bomb survivors, Hiroshima-Nagasaki, 1957 to 1970. *JAMA*. 1972;219(7):864–868.
181. Boukheris H, Stovall M, Gilbert ES, et al. Risk of salivary gland cancer after childhood cancer: a report from the Childhood Cancer Survivor Study. *Int J Radiat Oncol Biol Phys*. 2013;85(3):776–783. doi:10.1016/j.ijrobp.2012.06.006
182. Berrington de Gonzalez A, Curtis RE, Kry SF, et al. Proportion of second cancers attributable to radiotherapy treatment in adults: a cohort study in the US SEER cancer registries. *Lancet Oncol*. 2011;12(4):353–360. doi:10.1016/S1470-2045(11)70061-4
183. Shore RE, Albert RE, Pasternack BS. Follow-up study of patients treated by X-ray epilation for Tinea capitis; resurvey of post-treatment illness and mortality experience. *Arch Environ Health*. 1976;31(1):21–28.
184. Modan B, Baidatz D, Mart H, et al. Radiation-induced head and neck tumours. *Lancet*. 1974;1(7852):277–279.
185. Hall P, Holm LE, Lundell G, et al. Tumors after radiotherapy for thyroid cancer. A case-control study within a cohort of thyroid cancer patients. *Acta Oncol*. 1992;31(4):403–407.
186. Hoffman DA, McConahey WM, Fraumeni JF, et al. Cancer incidence following treatment of hyperthyroidism. *Int J Epidemiol*. 1982;11(3):218–224.
187. Preston-Martin S, Henderson BE, Bernstein L. Medical and dental x rays as risk factors for recently diagnosed tumors of the head. *Natl Cancer Inst Monogr*. 1985;69:175–179.
188. Preston-Martin S, White SC. Brain and salivary gland tumors related to prior dental radiography: implications for current practice. *J Am Dent Assoc*. 1990;120(2):151–158.
189. Preston-Martin S, Thomas DC, White SC, et al. Prior exposure to medical and dental x-rays related to tumors of the parotid gland. *J Natl Cancer Inst*. 1988;80(12):943–949.
190. Boukheris H, Ron E, Dores GM, et al. Risk of radiation-related salivary gland carcinomas among survivors of Hodgkin lymphoma: a population-based analysis. *Cancer*. 2008;113(11):3153–3159. doi:10.1002/cncr.23918
191. Manzitti C, Mereu P, Haupt R, et al. Parotid carcinoma after autologous bone marrow transplantation for relapsed nephroblastoma. *J Pediatr Hematol Oncol*. 2003;25(8):672–673.
192. Perkins JL, Neglia JP, Ramsay NK, et al. Successful bone marrow transplantation for severe aplastic anemia following orthotopic liver transplantation: long-term follow-up and outcome. *Bone Marrow Transplant*. 2001;28(5):523–526. doi:10.1038/sj.bmt.1703177
193. Spitz MR, Sider JG, Newell GR, et al. Incidence of salivary gland cancer in the United States relative to ultraviolet radiation exposure. *Head Neck Surg*. 1988;10(5):305–308.
194. Wahlberg P, Anderson H, Biörklund A, et al. Carcinoma of the parotid and submandibular glands--a study of survival in 2465 patients. *Oral Oncol*. 2002;38(7):706–713.
195. Batsakis JG, McClatchey KD, Johns M, Regazi J. Primary squamous cell carcinoma of the parotid gland. *Arch Otolaryngol*. 1976;102(6):355–357.
196. Spitz MR, Batsakis JG. Major salivary gland carcinoma. Descriptive epidemiology and survival of 498 patients. *Arch Otolaryngol*. 1984;110(1):45–49.
197. Ying YL, Johnson JT, Myers EN. Squamous cell carcinoma of the parotid gland. *Head Neck*. 2006;28(7):626–632. doi:10.1002/hed.20360
198. Nuyens M, Schüpbach J, Stauffer E, et al. Metastatic disease to the parotid gland. *Otolaryngol Head Neck Surg*. 2006;135(6):844–848. doi:10.1016/j.otohns.2006.05.010
199. Flynn MB, Maguire S, Martinez S, et al. Primary squamous cell carcinoma of the parotid gland: the importance of correct histological diagnosis. *Ann Surg Oncol*. 1999;6(8):768–770.
200. Shemen LJ, Huvos AG, Spiro RH. Squamous cell carcinoma of salivary gland origin. *Head Neck Surg*. 1987;9(4):235–240.
201. Horn-Ross PL, Ljung BM, Morrow M. Environmental factors and the risk of salivary gland cancer. *Epidemiology*. 1997;8(4):414–419.

202. Straif K, Weiland SK, Bungers M, et al. Exposure to nitrosamines and mortality from salivary gland cancer among rubber workers. *Epidemiology.* 1999;10(6):786–787.
203. Swanson GM, Belle SH. Cancer morbidity among woodworkers in the U.S. automotive industry. *J Occup Med.* 1982;24(4):315–319.
204. Zheng W, Shu X-O, Ji B-T, Gao Y-T. Diet and other risk factors for cancer of the salivary glands:a population-based case-control study. *Int J Cancer.* 1996;67(2):194–198. doi:10.1002/(SICI)1097-0215(19960717)67:2<194::AID-IJC8>3.0.CO;2-O
205. Sturgis EM, Pytynia KB. After the smoke clears: environmental and occupational risks for carcinoma of the upper aerodigestive tract. *Cancer J.* 2005;11(2):96–103.
206. Tsai CC, Chen CL, Hsu HC. Expression of Epstein-Barr virus in carcinomas of major salivary glands: a strong association with lymphoepithelioma-like carcinoma. *Hum Pathol.* 1996;27(3):258–262.
207. Saemundsen AK, Albeck H, Hansen JP, et al. Epstein-Barr virus in nasopharyngeal and salivary gland carcinomas of Greenland Eskimoes. *Br J Cancer.* 1982;46(5):721–728.
208. Vageli D, Sourvinos G, Ioannou M, et al. High-risk human papillomavirus (HPV) in parotid lesions. *Int J Biol Markers.* 2007;22(4):239–244.
209. Boland JM, McPhail ED, García JJ, et al. Detection of human papilloma virus and p16 expression in high-grade adenoid cystic carcinoma of the head and neck. *Mod Pathol.* 2012;25(4):529–536. doi:10.1038/modpathol.2011.186
210. Shebl FM, Bhatia K, Engels EA. Salivary gland and nasopharyngeal cancers in individuals with acquired immunodeficiency syndrome in United States. *Int J Cancer.* 2010;126(10):2503–2508. doi:10.1002/ijc.24930

2

Pathology of HNSCC

Michelle D. Williams
Adel K. El-Naggar

Head and neck squamous cell carcinoma (HNSCC) accounts for over 90% of the tumors encountered and arises from the surface epithelium. The majority of the upper aerodigestive tract structures are lined by epithelialized squamous mucosa. The multilayered squamous epithelial lining is formed of sequential differentiation from basal cells with higher nuclear to cytoplasmic (N/C) ratios along the basement membrane to squamous cells with increased cytoplasm and a lower N/C ratio, finally terminating superiorly with a flatted anuclear cell layer. The remainder of the mucosa in nasal and sinonasal sites is lined by respiratory mucosa.

Clinical findings of leukoplakia and erythroplakia do not specifically correlate with any single pathologic diagnosis and require histologic evaluation to determine the associated pathology.

ORAL PREMALIGNANT LESIONS

Clinically oral premalignant lesions are recognized as leukoplakia (white) and erythroplakia (red). Histologically, dysplasia is defined by progressive cellular alteration in morphology and loss of polarity of the squamous epithelial lining. Dysplasia is graded based on the extent of cytologic and architectural alterations of the epithelial lining into three grades: mild dysplasia, alterations limited to the lower third; moderate alterations involving the lower two thirds of the epithelial thickness; and severe dysplasia/carcinoma in situ with alterations involving the entire thickness (Figure 2.1) (1). Squamous dysplasia and subsequent carcinoma arise from accumulative genetic alterations including loss of heterozygosity of chromosomal regions and gain in others. Although several genetic mutations have been linked to the development of oral dysplasias including *p53*, *p16*, *PI3K*, and *Notch1*, none of them are validated for clinical use, nor do they predict which lesions will progress to invasive carcinoma.

SQUAMOUS CELL CARCINOMA

Squamous cell carcinoma (SCC) is the most frequent epithelial malignancy of the upper aerodigestive tract. SCC displays remarkable phenotypic variations and can be classified into conventional and distinct phenotypes. Conventional SCC is also the most common form encountered and is graded into well, moderate, and severe based on the degree of cytologic and architectural recapitulation of the normal mucosa (Figure 2.2). This form commonly arises in the oral cavity, nasal cavity, and larynx.

VARIANTS OF SQUAMOUS CELL CARCINOMA

Verrucous Carcinoma

Presenting as broad-based warty growths, verrucous carcinoma histologically shows

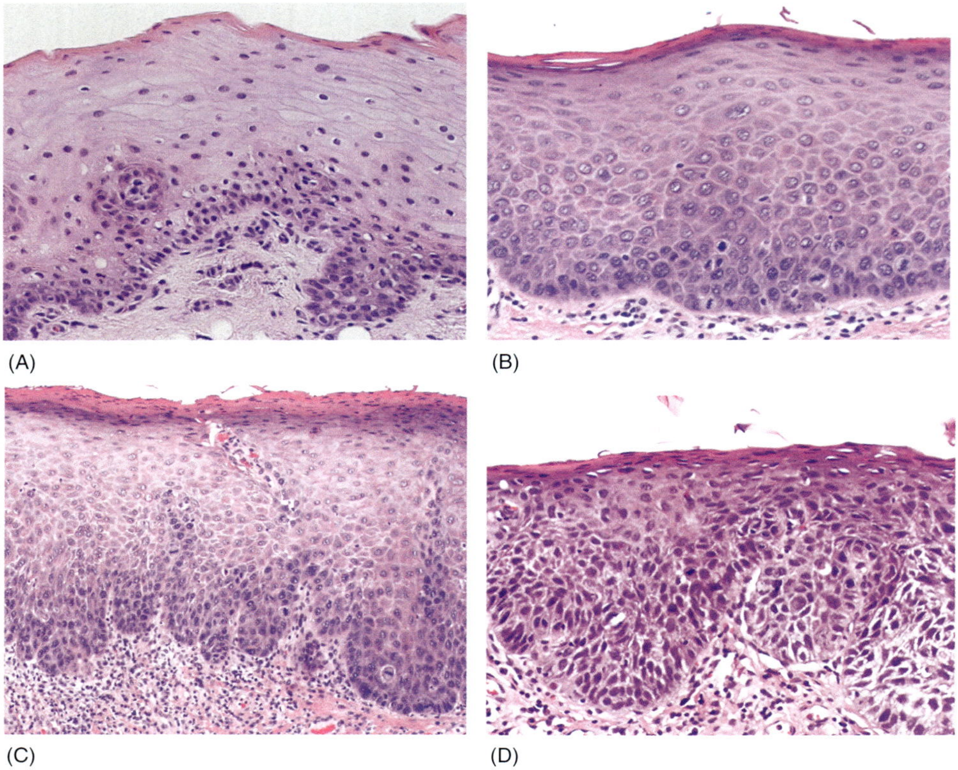

FIGURE 2.1 Increasing cytologic and architectural changes in the progression of squamous mucosa (upper left) through to carcinoma in situ (lower right). The squamous epithelium shows normal maturation (A), basalar atypic in mild dysplasia (B), increased architectural and cytologic enlargement in moderate dysplasia (C), and full thickness cytologic alterations in carcinoma in situ (D).

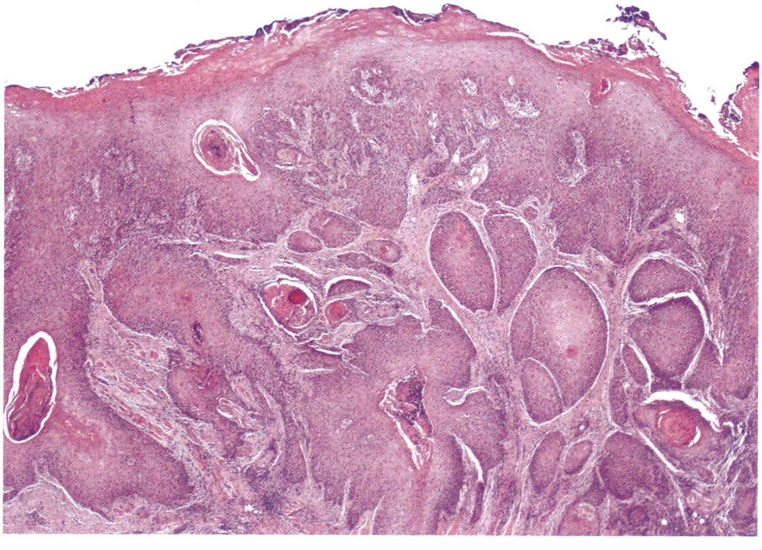

FIGURE 2.2 Conventional well-differentiated squamous carcinoma with invasive broad nests.

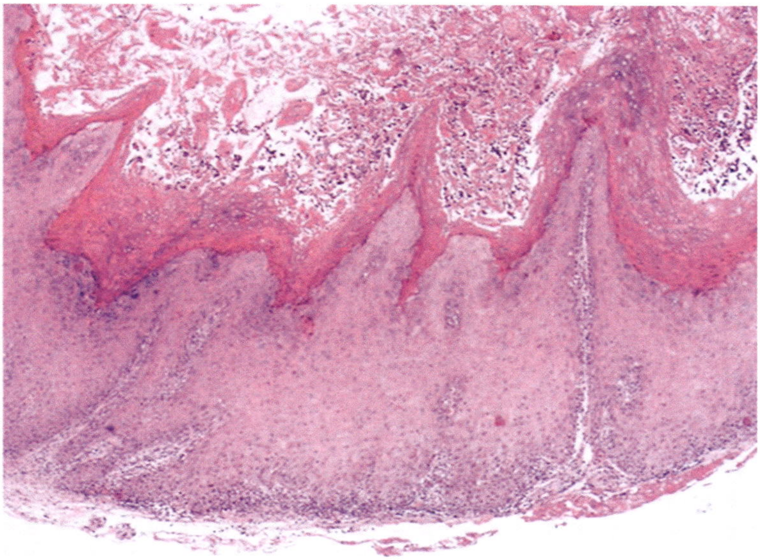

FIGURE 2.3 Verrucous carcinoma shows exophytic growth with spires and a broad pushing base with minimal cytologic alterations.

well-differentiated squamous mucosa with pushing broad nests into the underlying stroma with local destruction (Figure 2.3) (2,3). Although uncommon, verrucous carcinoma typically affects the gin-giva, larynx, or oral tongue. In its pure form verrucous carcinoma has a minimal metastatic potential; however, it is often coexistent with a conventional SCC, which is critical to diagnosis for treatment to prevent local and regional recurrence.

Papillary Squamous Carcinoma

Papillary SCC is defined as an exophytic SCC with finger-like projections lined by cancer cells with and without squamous differentiation around a fibrovascular core (Figure 2.4). Invasion can be difficult to evaluate unless complete excision is performed. This variant typically arises in the larynx or sinonasal sites and may be less aggressive than conventional SCC (4).

Basaloid Squamous Carcinoma

Basaloid SCC is a distinct high-grade subtype of SCC with monomorphic, hyperchromatic tumor cells with scant cytoplasm, often central tumor nest necrosis, and prominent collagen-like material deposition (Figure 2.5). This unique variant has a predilection for the oropharynx, larynx, and hypopharynx, and may be encountered in the sinonasal region. Only the subset of basasloid SCCs that arise within the oropharynx may be associated with human papillomavirus (HPV) (5). Morphologically these tumors must be differentiated from solid adenoid cystic and neuroendocrine carcinomas.

Sarcomatoid Squamous Carcinoma

This high-grade variant is characterized by transformation of epithelial to sarcoma-like malignancy. Coexisting conventional SCC component aids in the diagnosis of this variant from true mesenchymal tumors (sarcomas) (6). Morphologic evaluation combined with evidence for the expression of keratin intermediate filaments, even focal, supports this classification. Tumors may present as exophytic masses typically arising in the larynx or tongue, which may protend a better clinical course over the endophytic form (Figure 2.6). The differential diagnosis of this variant includes sarcoma and pseudosarcomatous reactive proliferative lesions. Clinical and ancillary markers are critical to excluding these entities. Other terminologies used for this entity include spindle cell SCC and historically carcinosarcoma.

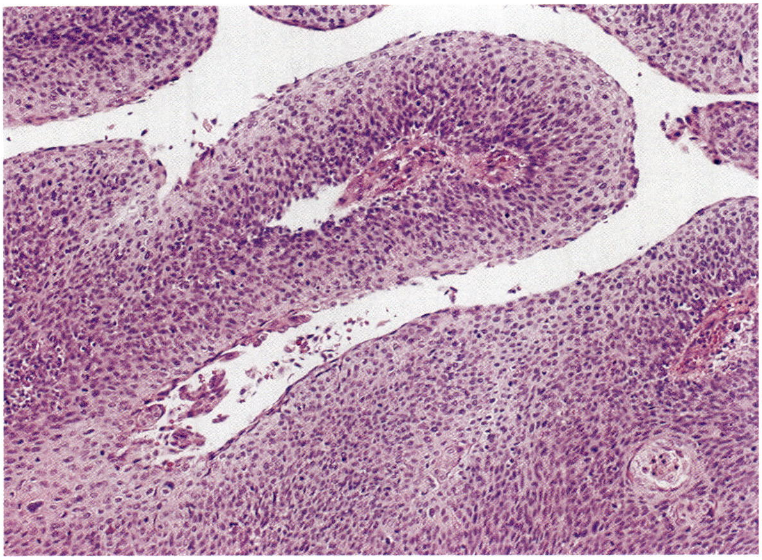

FIGURE 2.4 Papillary squamous cell carcinoma shows an exophytic growth pattern with fibrovascular cores lined by full-thickness atypical squamous cells.

VIRUS-ASSOCIATED SQUAMOUS CARCINOMAS

Oropharyngeal Squamous Carcinoma

SCCs of the oropharynx are increasingly associated with HPV (7). Clinical and pathologic features vary compared to conventional SCC; see Table 2.1. Morphologically HPV-associated SCC show more uniform basaloid cells often with minimal keratinization (8). This phenotype should not be confused with the basaloid SCC variant that is distinct and solid adenoid cystic carcinoma. Tumors often originate in the epithelium of the crypts of the palatine and lingual

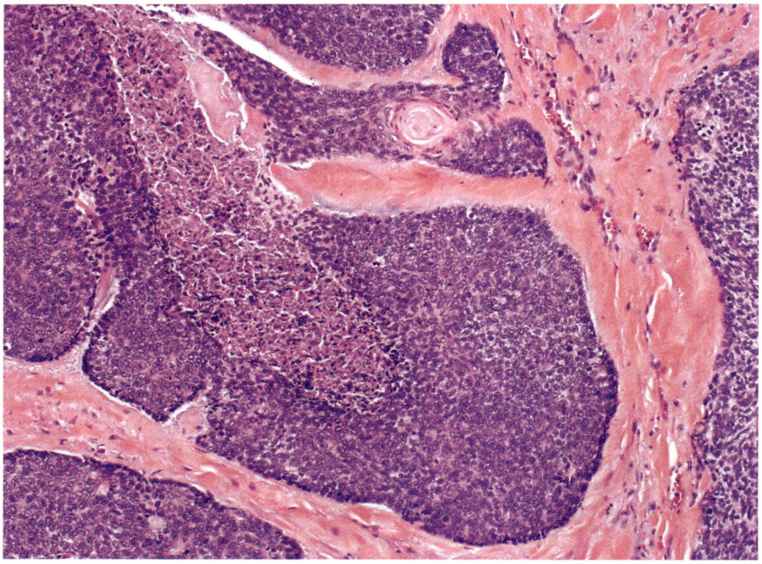

FIGURE 2.5 Basaloid squamous cell carcinoma grows in nests with intervening dense basement membrane. Focal abrupt keratinization and central necrosis also occur.

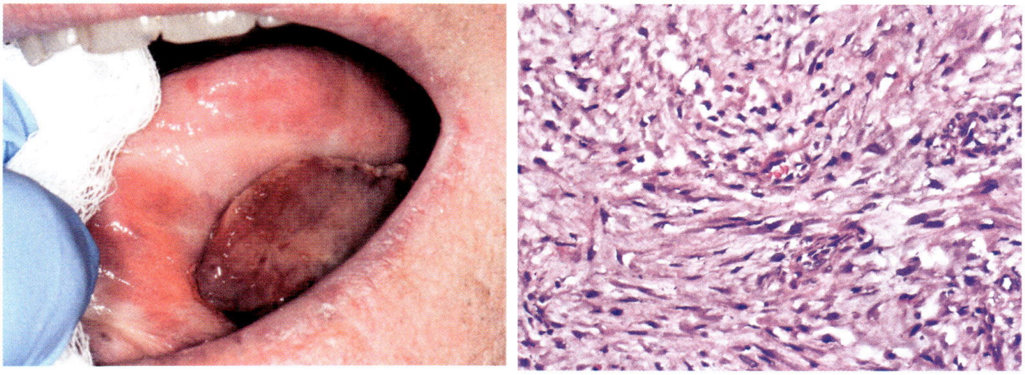

(A) (B)

FIGURE 2.6 Sarcomatoid carcinoma may occur as a gross polypoid mass (A); the tumor cells are spindled without nest formation mimicking sarcoma (B).

tonsils. A subset of tumors present as exophytic masses. Tumors not uncommonly present with cystic nodal metastases (9). p16 immunostaining with or without direct HPV viral testing is now part of standard clinical care (Figure 2.7). The eighth edition of the American Joint Committee on Cancer (AJCC) *Cancer Staging Manual* includes p16/HPV status in stratifying oropharyngeal SCC for staging (10).

Nasopharyngeal Carcinoma

Undifferentiated carcinomas with lymphoid stroma of the nasopharynx are associated with Epstein–Barr virus (EBV) in the majority of patients. They can be graded into differentiated and undifferentiated subtypes, World Health Organization (WHO) types I and II, respectively (1). Undifferentiated morphology is the most commonly encountered histology,

TABLE 2.1

Clinical and Pathologic Factors in Conventional and HPV-Associated Squamous Cell Carcinoma

Factors	HPV-Associated SCC	SCC (Conventional/ Tobacco Related)
Associated with	High-risk HPV types 16>>18> others*	Tobacco exposure
Age at onset (mean)	53 years	57 years
Sex	M:F (2.8:1)	M:F (1.5:1)
Location (subsites)	Tonsils, base of tongue	Oral cavity, larynx
Lymph nodes	30%–60% at presentation Often cystic metastases; maybe bilateral	Prognostic factor
Prognosis (3 years)	82%	57%
Pathologic	Often nonkeratinizing	Usually keratinizing
Morphology	High nuclear to cytoplasmic ratio, monotonous	Surface dysplasia often present

*Incidence and HPV types identified vary globally; risk factors for developing persistent HPV.
HPV, human papillomavirus; SCC, squamous cell carcinoma.

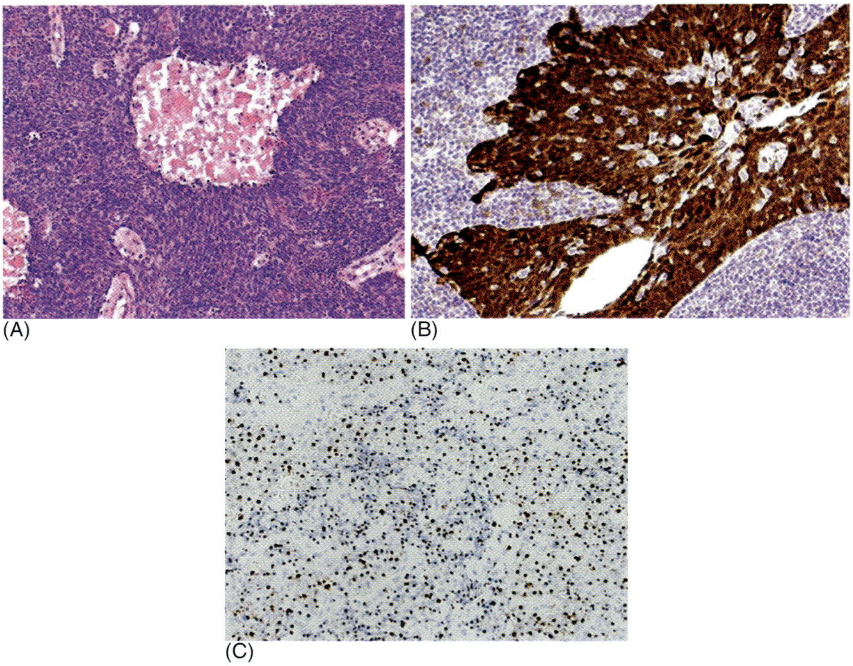

FIGURE 2.7 HPV-associated oropharyngeal squamous cell carcinoma often shows a nonkeratinizing pattern (A). p16 immunohistochemical study highlights the tumor cells diffusely (B). HPV direct assessment for high-risk type 16 may be performed by RNA or DNA probes by in situ hybridization (C).

HPV, human papillomavirus.

showing large open elongated nuclei with nucleoli in sheets and nests within an associated lymphocytic infiltrate and lymphocytic stroma (Figure 2.8). WHO type I is conventional SCC with varying degrees of keratinization and is graded into well, moderately, and poorly differentiated. A small subset of nasopharyngeal carcinomas may be HPV positive for which the significance remains to be fully studied (11).

UNKNOWN PRIMARY HISTOLOGIC EVALUATION

A common presentation for head and neck cancer is a palpable neck mass representing metastatic SCC in a lymph node (Figure 2.9). Pathologic evaluation of the neck mass by fine needle aspiration (FNA) biopsy allows for a diagnosis to be rendered. Clinical and radiographic evaluations are utilized to locate the primary tumor. Pathologic assessment for HPV and EBV can assist with identifying tumors likely to arise in the oropharynx and nasopharynx, respectively. Additionally the eighth edition of AJCC *Cancer Staging Manual* added an unknown primary chapter with staging recommendations, which vary based on these testing results (10).

PATHOLOGIC EVALUATION

Margin Assessment

Margin assessment is a critical component for determining the adequacy of an oncologic resection. Two methods are commonly utilized to assess margins including "cavity-based" tissue sampling or "resection-based" specimen sampling. The surgeon may submit margins from the cavity after the resection specimen has been removed. In this manner, the distance from the tumor to the margin cannot be directly measured and tissue margins are reported as positive or negative for tumor. Advocates of this method note better correlation of findings by anatomic area submitted. Some studies have noted higher rates of recurrences when the cavity-based approach was utilized over evaluation of the resection specimen, which may reflect the need for more thorough tissue submission by the surgeon utilizing the cavity-based approach

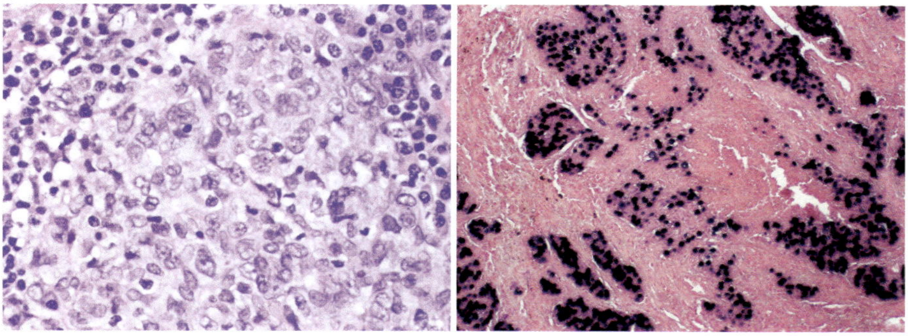

(A) (B)

FIGURE 2.8 Nasopharyngeal carcinoma, undifferentiated pattern, is composed of large cells with clear nuclei and nucleoli admixed with a lymphoid stroma (A). EBER in situ hybridization detects EBV RNA showing diffuse tumor positivity (B).

EBER, EBV-encoded small RNA; EBV, Epstein–Barr virus.

(12). Alternatively margins may be assessed from the resection specimen by the pathologist. Serially sectioning the tumor allows for distance from the tumor edge to the margins to be measured grossly and under the microscope in three dimensions. Review of the resection specimen by the pathologist with the surgeon can augment communication of areas of concern by both parties and further allow for anatomic correlation of such sites.

Histologic Risk Features and Staging

Beyond the diagnosis, relevant histopathologic risk factors include evaluation for the presence of perineural invasion (tumor within the perineurim) and lymphovascular involvement. Perineural invasion is a known risk factor for local recurrence (Figure 2.10) (13). Intraoperative assessment of nerve branches may aid in surgical resection to obtain negative

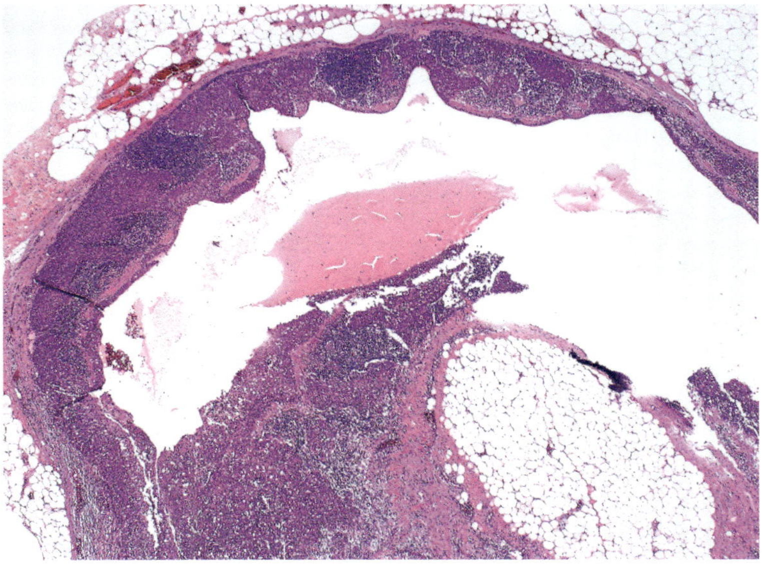

FIGURE 2.9 Unknown primary squamous carcinomas may present as cystic masses within a neck lymph node; this pattern is commonly encountered with HPV-associated oropharyngeal primary squamous carcinomas.

HPV, human papillomavirus.

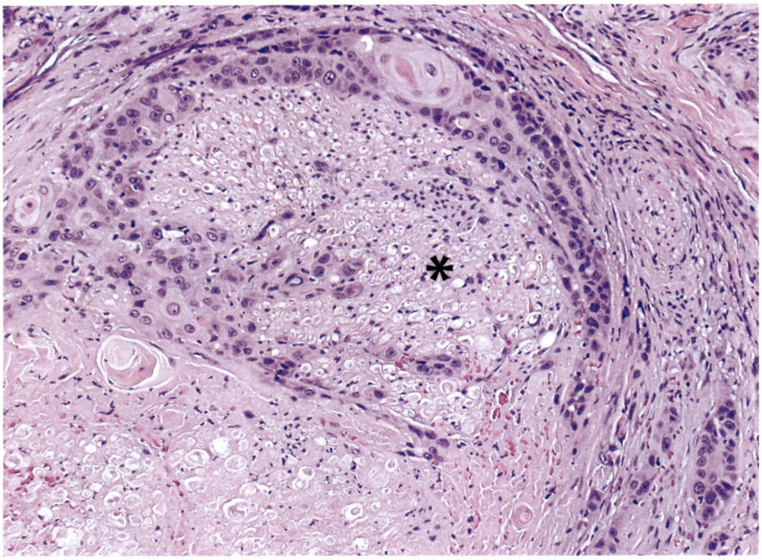

FIGURE 2.10 Perineural invasion is prominent with squamous carcinoma cells surrounding and invading the nerve(*).

margins when perineural invasion is identified or suspected by imaging, from clinical findings, or on biopsy. Lymphovascular invasion may signify risk for regional lymph node metastases or local spread typically submucosally around the primary site (Figure 2.11).

Tumor and Nodal Staging

The eighth edition of the AJCC manual for staging head and neck cancers incorporates changes recognizing the more favorable biology in HPV-associated tumors as well as the adverse

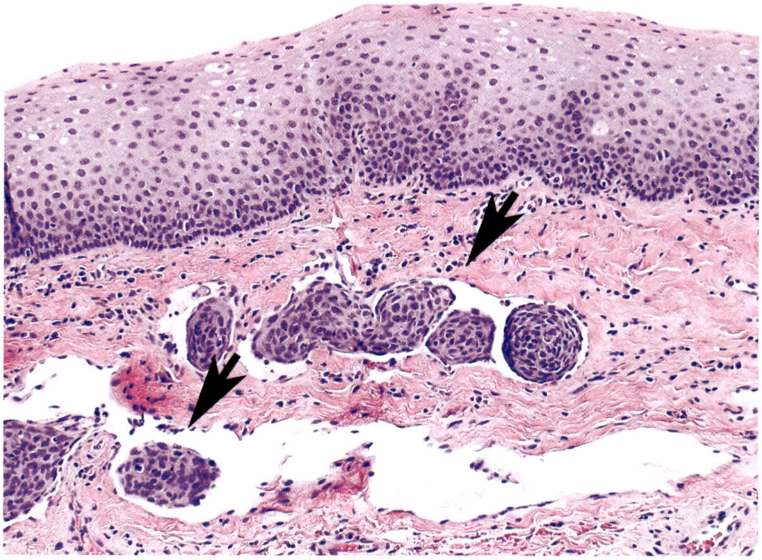

FIGURE 2.11 Lymphovascular invasion is present with tumor cells (arrows) percolating in the submucosal vascular space. The overlying squamous mucosa is normal.

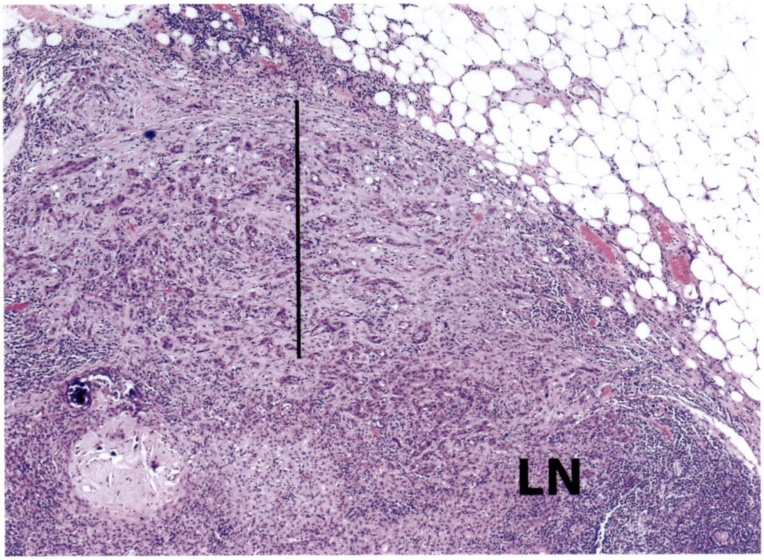

FIGURE 2.12 Extranodal extension: Following tumor metastasis to a lymph node (LN) the tumor may grow and invade into the surrounding fibroadipose tissue (as marked with line).

outcomes often associated with patients whose tumors have extranodal extension (ENE) (10,14,15). In brief, major updates include separate staging chapters for HPV-associated oropharynx tumors versus non-HPV-associated oropharyngeal tumors, and guidance for staging unknown primary tumors. In addition to tumor size and extent of tumor invasion into adjacent structures, the depth of invasion now is also considered in determining the T classification in oral cavity and lip SCC. This parameter coincides with the known risk for occult metastases with increasing tumor depth (16). Depth of invasion is measured from the basement membrane of the adjacent normal epithelium and should be distinguished from tumor thickness, which is from the top of the tumor including any exophytic component. Tumor thickness is utilized in skin cancer staging. Other parameters that are being collected for future analyses include the pattern of tumor invasion and significance of tumor-related inflammatory infiltrates.

A major shift in the eighth edition of the AJCC manual includes the presence of ENE in the determination of the nodal "N" classification for the majority of head and neck sites (10,17). Nodal staging does not incorporate ENE for HPV-associated oropharynx and nasopharynx tumors. The definition of ENE is the presence of tumor cells extending beyond the lymph node capsule into the surrounding soft tissues (Figure 2.12). Although ENE is generally considered a risk factor, the evaluation of this feature is inconsistent and remains subjective.

Posttreatment Histologic Evaluation

Histologic evaluation of head and neck sites after treatment leads to particular challenges. Mucosal biopsies often show ulceration and reactive "pseudoepitehliomatous hyperplasia" of the mucosa with downward growth into the stroma mimicking invasion. Similarly, the underlying stromal cells develop radiation atypia with enlargement and hyperchromasia of the nuclei, which should not be mistaken for sarcomatoid change and tumor. The salivary tissue, whether it be in the deep base of tongue, palate, or floor of mouth will show atrophy with loss of acini and secondary squamous metaplasia and hyperplasia of the residual duct structure, which may be overcalled as recurrent tumor. This particular pitfall must be avoided by looking for residual lobular structure in the tissue and awareness of this histologic change secondary to therapy. Moreover, the abnormal juxtaposition of mucosa lying on bone and within the bone marrow space is a frequent pathologic finding associated with osteoradionecrosis. Therefore, a bone biopsy of suspected osteonecrosis diagnosed as recurrent SCC should be carefully rereviewed and discussed to ensure reactive mucosa within the bone is truly differentiated from SCC, which should have increased pleomorphism and irregular growth patterns.

As neoadjuvant chemotherapy trials are undertaken, posttherapy changes of varying degrees will be encountered in the primary tumor. Partial and complete histologic response will show dense fibrosis, scattered giant cells, and possible keratin debris with or without residual SCC. Thorough histologic evaluation of the pretreatment surgical bed is warranted as correlation with complete versus partial response may have prognostic value.

Neck Dissections After Radiation

Lymph node dissection may occur after definitive radiation such as for oropharyngeal primary SCCs. Neck dissections of the radiation field may show decreased lymph nodes, partial or complete fibrosis of the lymph nodes representing successfully treated metastatic tumor, or necrosis, parakeratosis, and giant cell reaction with or without viable residual tumor cells (Figure 2.13). A distinction should be made if viable SCC cells are identified, which has prognostic significance. Immunohistochemical markers for cytokeratins and proliferative markers such as Ki-67 proliferation marker are problematic as nonviable debris may show reactivity to keratins and the background tissue is full of reparative cells (lymphocytes, blood vessels, giant cells), which are proliferative but not indicative of viable tumor.

Head and Neck Biopsies

The initial step in the diagnosis of head and neck cancers is a tissue biopsy for histopathologic evaluation. For many sites in the head and neck region, biopsies are performed as an examination under anesthesia, and adequacy of tissue sampled may be evaluated by intraoperative consultation (frozen section). Factors that may limit initial biopsy adequacy include tumor necrosis, inflammatory/reactive changes around tumors, and tumor deep to normal tissues (particularly in lymphoid tissue of base of tongue or tonsil). Additionally by initially examining the tissue for confirmation, concern for lymphoma, which on occasion mimics SCC particularly in Waldeyer's ring, may lead to additional directed biopsies for flow cytometric analysis (which requires fresh tissue).

Confounding Factors and Mimics of Carcinoma

Mucosal biopsies may be challenging to fully classify pathologically secondary to their superficial nature, lacking stroma for evaluation of invasion, when the orientation of the biopsy and surface ulceration precludes grading of

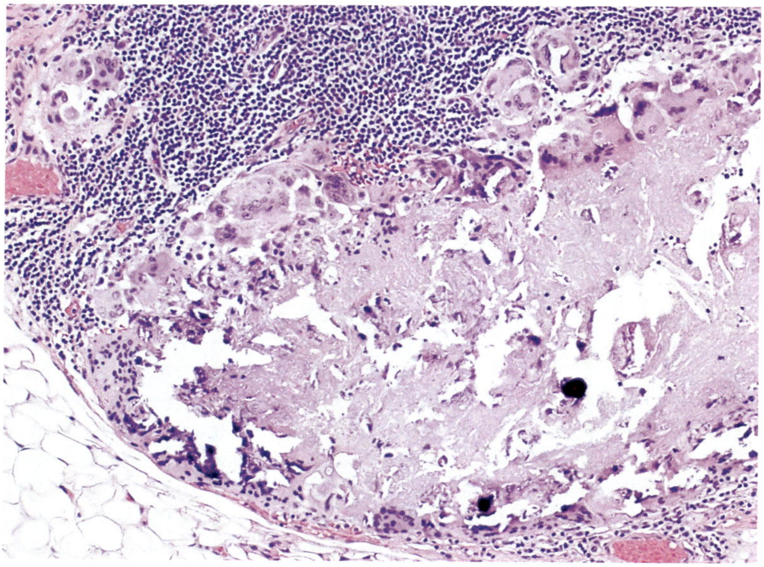

FIGURE 2.13 Therapy-related changes in a lymph node after radiation therapy with prominent giant cell reaction, necrosis, and fibrosis.

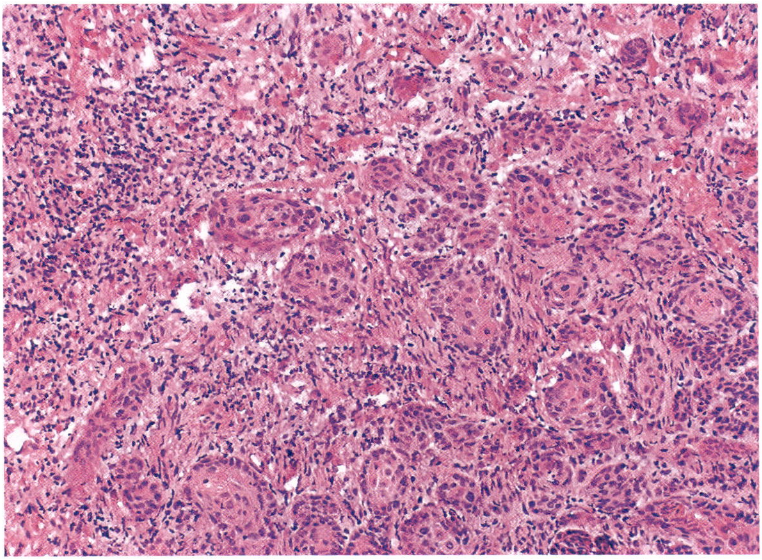

FIGURE 2.14 Metaplastic changes within the salivary units may mimic squamous carcinoma following trauma or therapy.

dysplasia and ulceration, which leads to inflammation and reactive epithelial changes.

Several histologic features may mimic SCC. Pseudoepitheliomatous hyperplasia with elongation of the rete ridges admixed with inflammation commonly occurs associated with gingivitis and is also associated with granular cell tumor. Squamous metaplasia of the salivary ducts occurs secondary to trauma, following radiation therapy leading to sialoadenitis (inflammation of the salivary units (Figure 2.14)). Frequent locations include within the submucosa of the palate, base of tongue, and floor of mouth. Clinical correlation is essential to aid in avoiding overcalling squamous biopsies as malignant in the aforementioned conditions.

CYTOLOGIC EVALUATION—FNA BIOPSY

FNA biopsy allows for rapid evaluation of neck nodes and can be used in conjunction with interventional radiology or ultrasound for deep lesions. FNA utilizes 23- to 27-gauge needles to aspirate cells for immediate microscopic evaluation, which allows for triaging material for ancillary studies such as for cultures or flow cytometric assessment when lymphoma is in the differential diagnosis. Microscopic evaluation of FNAs relies on the cellular characteristics to diagnose malignancy. Ancillary studies including immunohistochemical evaluation may be utilized in poorly differentiated neoplasms to aid in defining tumor lineage and establishing possible sites for the primary tumor.

FNA may also be utilized in the posttreatment setting with caution. In oropharyngeal SCC where the primary treatment modality is often radiation therapy, failure of the neck nodes to fully resolve may lead to evaluation for persistent disease. In this setting, the FNA may show necrosis and parakeratosis, consistent with treated tumor, or even rare atypical forms, which do not specifically denote definitive viable residual tumor. Similarly a negative FNA is only selective sampling and does not fully sample the residual nodule; thus, further follow-up and correlation are required.

ANCILLARY STUDIES IN HNSCC

Beyond the hematoxylin and eosin (H&E) –stained tissue section for morphologic assessment, immunohistochemical and in situ hybridization testing may be utilized for the following studies.

POORLY DIFFERENTIATED NEOPLASMS OF UNCERTAIN LINEAGE AND UNKNOWN PRIMARIES

If a tumor encountered in the neck as an unknown primary is so poorly differentiated that the lineage of the tumor is not clear, immunohistochemical studies allow for excluding other tumor types for which treatment and prognosis may be distinct from HNSCC. Immunohistochemical studies use directed antibodies to specific proteins that most commonly associate with a tumor's lineage. SCC is typically positive for cytokeratins, cytokeratins 5/6, p63/p40, and often expresses epidermal growth factor receptor (EGFR). These markers, however, are not specific for SCC, and caution should be used when utilizing them for tumor classification as overlap may occur in salivary gland tumors and tumors in other sites. Melanoma should be excluded utilizing lineage specific markers S100 tyrosinase, HMBE, and/or Mart1, which will be negative in SCC.

BIOMARKERS IN HNSCC

The most common biomarker in HNSCC is the presence or absence of HPV specifically in oropharyngeal SCC (10,18). p16 is considered a surrogate marker for high-risk HPV when utilized in the correct setting, specifically in primary oropharyngeal tumors and level II or III neck nodes (19,20). Immunohistochemical evaluation for p16 is more readily available in a variety of clinical settings. Interpretation of p16 for correlation with HPV should show strong, diffuse staining in both the cytoplasm and nuclear in at least 70% of the tumor cells Lower levels of p16 expression are considered negative for HPV association. Low-risk HPV testing plays no role in SCC. Additionally HPV/p16 testing should not be routinely performed in other subsites in the head and neck (i.e., outside oropharynx). Moreover, p16 expression is not specific for HPV association outside oropharyngeal SCC and caution should be used in testing of unknown primaries for p16 alone (21).

HPV specific testing is often performed on formalin-fixed paraffin tumor sections by in situ hybridization for either viral RNA or DNA techniques. This method allows for the pathologist to localize the signal within the tumor cells for confirmation of HPV high-risk subtypes either individually or as a screening panel cocktail, such as high-risk types 16, 18, 31, 33, 35, 41, and 48, which are known to be pathogenic in humans. Other methodologies utilizing cytology and extracted nucleic acids including polymerase chain reaction (PCR) are also available in some laboratories (22).

EBV may be tested for by either immunohistochemistry for the latent membrane protein (LMP) or for EBV-encoded small RNAs (EBERs), which are noncoding RNAs expressed in EBV-infected tumor cells. In nasopharyngeal carcinomas EBER testing is preferred as LMP is less sensitive in detecting the virus in these tumors.

EGFR is another pathway known to be altered in HNSCC and is targeted by therapeutic agents. Expression is typically elevated; however, EGFR testing is not routinely performed. Molecular alterations, specifically a splice variant or in-frame deletion of exons 2 to 7, may occur, known as EGFRvIII. This deletion causes truncation of the extracellular domain of EGFR leading to ligand-independent constitutive activity. Other mechanisms may also be contributing EGFR altered expression (23).

REFERENCES

1. El-Naggar AK, Chan JKC, Grandis JR, Takata T, Slootweg PJ. eds. *WHO Classification of Head and Neck Tumours*. 4th ed. IARC: Lyon. 2017.
2. Ferlito A, Recher G. Ackerman's tumor (verrucous carcinoma) of the larynx: a clinicopathologic study of 77 cases. *Cancer*. 1980;46(7):1617–1630. doi:10.1002/1097-0142(19801001)46:7<1617::AID-CNCR2820460722>3.0.CO;2-T
3. Echanique KA, Desai SV, Marchiano E, et al. Laryngeal verrucous carcinoma. *Otolaryngol Head Neck Surg*. 2017;156(1):38–45. doi:10.1177/0194599816662631
4. Thompson LD, Wenig BM, Heffner DK, Gnepp DR. Exophytic and papillary squamous cell carcinomas of the larynx: a clinicopathologic series of 104 cases. *Otolaryngol Head Neck Surg*. 1999;120:718–724. doi:10.1053/hn.1999.v120.a92773
5. Begum S, Westra WH. Basaloid squamous cell carcinoma of the head and neck is a mixed variant that can be further resolved by HPV status. *Am J Surg Pathol*. 2008;32:1044–1050. doi:10.1097/PAS.0b013e31816380ec
6. Gerry D, Fritsch VA, Lentsch EJ. Spindle cell carcinoma of the upper aerodigestive tract: an analysis of 341 cases with comparison to conventional squamous cell carcinoma. *Ann Otol Rhinol Laryngol*. 2014;123:576–583. doi:10.1177/0003489414525337
7. Kreimer AR, Clifford GM, Boyle P, et al. Human papillomavirus types in head and neck squamous cell carcinomas worldwide: a systematic review. *Cancer Epidemiol Biomarkers Prev*. 2005;14(2):467–475. doi:10.1158/1055-9965.EPI-04-0551

8. El-Mofty SK, Patil S. Human papillomavirus (HPV)-related oropharyngeal non-keratinizing squamous cell carcinoma: characterization of a distinct phenotype. *Oral Surg Oral Med Oral Pathol Oral Radiol Endod.* 2006;101:339–345. doi:10.1016/j.tripleo.2005.08.001
9. Goldenberg D, Sciubba J, Koch WM. Cystic metastasis from head and neck squamous cell cancer: a distinct disease variant? *Head Neck.* 2006;28:633–638. doi:10.1002/hed.20381
10. Amin MB (editor-in-chief). *AJCC Cancer Staging Manual.* 8th ed. New York, NY: Springer. 2017. doi:10.3322/caac.21388
11. Lo EJ, Bell D, Woo JS, et al. Human papillomavirus and WHO type I nasopharyngeal carcinoma. *Laryngoscope.* 2010;120(10):1990–1997. doi:10.1002/lary.21649
12. Maxwell JH, Thompson LD, Brandwein-Gensler MS, et al. Early oral tongue squamous cell carcinoma: sampling of margins from tumor bed and worse local control. *JAMA Otolaryngol Head Neck Surg.* 2015;141(12):1104–1110. doi:10.1001/jamaoto.2015.1351
13. Chinn SB, Spector ME, Bellile EL, et al. Impact of perineural invasion in the pathologically N0 neck in oral cavity squamous cell carcinoma. *Otolaryngol Head Neck Surg.* 2013;149(6):893–899. doi:10.1177/0194599813506867
14. Ang KK, Harris J, Wheeler R, et al. Human papillomavirus and survival of patients with oropharyngeal cancer. *N Engl J Med.* 2010;363(1):24–35. doi:10.1056/NEJMoa0912217
15. Sinha P, Kallogjeri D, Gay H, et al. High metastatic node number, no extracapsular spread or N-classification is a nod-related prognosticator in transorally resected, neck dissected p16 positive oropharynx cancer. *Oral Oncol.* 2015;51(5);514–520. doi:10.1016/j.oraloncology.2015.02.098
16. International Consortium for Outcome Research (ICOR) in Head and Neck Cancer, Ebrahimi A, Gil Z, et al. Primary tumor staging for oral cancer and a proposed modification incorporating depth of invasion: an international multicenter retrospective study. *JAMA Otolaryngol Head Neck Surg.* 2014;140(12):1138–1148. doi:10.1001/jamaoto.2014.1548
17. Dünne AA, Müller HH, Eisele DW, et al. Meta-analysis of the prognostic significance of perinodal spread in head and neck squamous cell carcinomas (HNSCC) patients. *Eur J Cancer.* 2006;42(12):1863–1868. doi:10.1016/j.ejca.2006.01.062
18. O'Sullivan B, Huang SH, Su J, et al. Development and validation of a staging system for HPV-related Oropharyngeal cancer by the ICON-S: a multicenter cohort study. *Lancet Oncol.* 2016;17(4);440–451. doi:10.1016/S1470-2045(15)00560-4
19. El-Naggar AK, Westra WH. p16 expression as a surrogate marker for HPV-related oropharyngeal carcinoma: a guide for interpretative relevance and consistency. *Head Neck.* 2012;34(4):459–461. doi:10.1002/hed.21974
20. Zafereo ME, Xu L, Dahlstrom KR, et al. Squamous cell carcinoma of the oral cavity often overexpresses p16 but is rarely driven by human papillomavirus. *Oral Oncol.* 2016;56:47–53. doi:10.1016/j.oraloncology.2016.03.003
21. Beadle BM, William WN Jr, McLemore MS, Sturgis EM, Williams MD. p16 expression in cutaneous squamous carcinomas with neck metastases: a potential pitfall in identifying unknown primaries of the head and neck. *Head Neck.* 2013;35(11):1527–1533. doi:10.1002/hed.23188
22. Schache AG, Liloglou T, Risk JM, et al. Evaluation of human papilloma virus diagnostic testing in oropharyngeal squamous cell carcinoma: sensitivity, specificity, and prognostic discrimination. *Clin Cancer Res.* 2011;17(19):6262–6271. doi:10.1158/1078-0432.CCR-11-0388
23. Bossi P, Resteghini C, Paielli N, et al. Prognostic and predictive value of EGFR in head and neck squamous cell carcinoma. *Oncotarget.* 2016;7(45):74362–74379. doi:10.18632/oncotarget.11413

3

The Genomic Landscape of HNSCC

Steffen Wagner
Jens P. Klussmann
Ruud H. Brakenhoff

CANCER AND SOMATIC GENETIC ALTERATIONS

Since the 1990s, it was broadly accepted that cancer arises by an accumulation of somatic genetic changes. These genetic alterations were deciphered by studying cancer and their recognizable precursor stages at the molecular level. The number of genetic changes roughly increases in parallel to the morphological severity of the lesions, and although there seems a certain order, the accumulation was considered more important than the order (1,2). Most of these concepts are still valid in 2018, although the complexity has been tremendously enhanced by the rapidly increasing knowledge during the past few years. The relatively simple linear genetic progression models became more complex and more variable (3).

Smoking and excessive alcohol consumption are important risk factors for head and neck squamous cell carcinoma (HNSCC), causing gene mutations, and these tumors still form the bulk of HNSCC. However, a subgroup of tumors is caused by infection with the human papillomavirus (HPV), and the incidence of these tumors has also increased. Hence, exogenous factors play an important role in HNSCC.

Notwithstanding these causative exogenous carcinogens, it is important to realize that by every cell division somatic mutations occur and accumulate (4). From the first cell division in the developing embryo, mutations start to accumulate. DNA replication is not foolproof, causing mutations to occur from the day of conception, and when the wrong genes are hit, cancer may result. However, when certain critical genes are hit, such as *TP53* and other genes in cell cycle regulation or DNA maintenance, replication stress may develop and the accumulation of genetic changes will dramatically increase in such cells (5). After a couple of mutations in critical control genes, the carcinogenic process may drive itself (6). To summarize, there is an intrinsic risk for cancer development by accumulating somatic mutations in every cell division, but exogenous factors that trigger or increase genetic alterations boost the cancer risk.

MUTATIONS, COPY NUMBER ALTERATIONS, AND EPIGENETIC CHANGES

Somatic genetic changes are broadly defined. The term "mutations" links to genes, and usually relates to genetic alterations at the base pair level, stretching from a single nucleotide to small deletions and insertions (indels).

However, many genetic changes encompass gains and losses of almost entire chromosomes. How critical these huge losses and gains are in the development of cancer remains somewhat elusive, but for sure they add to the inactivation of tumor suppressor genes and activation of oncogenes (3,7). The *CDKN2A* locus encoding p16^{INK4A} is frequently lost usually by a large chromosomal loss at 9p21 on one allele and a focal loss around the *CDKN2A* gene, or a mutation or epigenetic event in the gene itself, on the second allele. Hence, we can assume that these chromosomal losses clearly play a role.

The more frequent gene amplifications (up to 10–20 copies) are also relevant. There are frequent amplifications in HNSCC at chromosome locus 11q13 where the *CCND1* gene is residing encoding cyclinD1 or at the 7p12 locus of the epidermal growth factor receptor (EGFR) gene (7), both bona fide oncogenes in HNSCC. What is less clear is the precise role of the large chromosomal gains that increase gene copy numbers just twofold.

Besides mutations and chromosomal alterations, epigenetic alterations occur frequently. At the DNA level these encompass methylations at CpG sequences, most particularly in the promoter region of genes, thereby shutting them off. Also, the *CDKN2A* gene is frequently inactivated by methylation. However, many more epigenetic alterations are described that encompass, for example, histone code modifications. The DNA is wrapped around histone octamers, and these proteins play an active role in the expression of the genes in the vicinity of where they bind to the DNA strand. These histones can be acetylated and methylated at different amino acid residues, with major effects on gene expression (8).

Last but not least are the microRNAs (miRNAs). These small noncoding RNAs of approximately 22 nucleotides can bind to the 3′ untranslated region (3′UTR) in the mRNA of genes targeting them for degradation by the RISC complex. Hence, one miRNA may target a multitude of genes. Many changes in miRNA expression are reported in cancer, including HNSCC. In addition, major changes in general miRNA biogenesis have been described in cancer (9).

DRIVERS AND PASSENGERS

Since modern cancer genomics was initiated by large-scale Sanger sequencing of cancer genomes (10), and emerged rapidly by next-generation sequencing methods (7), a major problem became apparent. Many somatic mutations were identified, but mostly not in cancer driver genes but in so-called passenger genes. As indicated earlier, during every cell division cells accumulate mutations and this holds true for tumor cells as well. Hence, the number of mutations will increase, but not all are in genes that drive cancer progression. In 2013 this problem of drivers and passengers was comprehensively evaluated, and some solutions were suggested (11). It became apparent that there is a considerable mutational heterogeneity between tumors causing bias in the mutational profiles, and which is not corrected for to weigh whether a mutated gene is indeed a driver gene in a particular cancer. A most important factor of this mutational heterogeneity was a consequence of the tumor type and exposure to mutagens, as some tumors such as melanomas were shown to accumulate many mutations, while others show hardly any mutations. In addition, the type of mutations differs between tumors: in melanomas frequent TT-dimers occur causing a specific mutational profile. Summarized, some mutations are just more likely to occur in a particular tumor type.

Most remarkable was the observation that the number of mutations accumulates in genome regions that replicate late during S-phase encompassing the regions that are not actively transcribed. Hence, genes in these locations are found to become frequently mutated, but usually do not encompass cancer driver genes. The authors suggested that nucleotide shortage may play a role here.

When the authors developed a correction algorithm that takes all the biases into account, and used that on the sequencing data of 178 lung squamous cell carcinomas (SCCs), the number of candidate cancer driver genes reduced from 450 to 11 (11). Hence, mutation data should be interpreted with great caution to identify potential cancer genes. Obviously, the frequency with which mutations occur in genes underpins their relevance as cancer drivers, but in those cases that genes are mutated infrequently, additional functional studies should elucidate the role of these genes.

CLASSIFICATION OF HNSCC

The very large majority of head and neck cancers (>90%) are SCCs that arise in the mucosal linings of the upper aerodigestive tract, and in a single cell type, suggesting that it is a relatively homogeneous disease. However, HNSCC is a remarkably heterogeneous disease, and this led to several subclassifications of the disease in relation to anatomy, etiology, and clinical or molecular characteristics. Some of these are overlapping. In this section, we describe these classifications and take one as the main topic in the subsequent chapter.

ANATOMICAL CLASSIFICATION OF HEAD AND NECK CANCERS BY SUBSITE

In combination with histology (morphology) obtained from microscopic tumor examination, anatomical classification is used routinely in cancer registries to describe the kind (morphology, behavior, and grading) and origin of neoplasms, which can be used as tool for epidemiology, health management, and clinical purposes. Nine subsites of head and neck cancer are distinguished according to anatomical localization and molecular properties ($p16^{INK4A}$ expression and HPV status) of the disease (12). In Table 3.1 the major subsites of head and neck cancers are listed including corresponding *International Classification of Diseases for Oncology*, third edition (*ICD-O-3*) codes and the further molecular subclassification in the case of oropharyngeal and hypopharyngeal cancer.

In consideration of risk factors, each subsite has its particular set of usually more than one environmental factor that contributes to the genetic alterations associated with carcinogenesis. For example, sunlight exposure is more relevant for cancers of the lip than for laryngeal or oropharyngeal cancers, for which lifestyle factors

TABLE 3.1

The Major Sites of Head and Neck Cancer With Corresponding *ICD-O-3* Codes and Molecular Subclassification

	Anatomical Subsite	Molecular Classification	*ICD-O-3* Codes
1	Lip and oral cavity		C00.0-6, C00.8-9, C02.0-3, C02.8-9, C03.0-1, C03.9, C04.0-1, C05.0, C05.8-9, C06.0-2, C06.8-9
2	Major salivary glands		C07.9, C08.0-1, C08.8-9
3	Nasopharynx		C11.0-3, C11.8-9
4	Oropharynx	$p16^{INK4A}$-positive, HPV-mediated	C01.9, C02.4, C05.1-2, C09.0-1, C09.8-9, C10.0, C10.2-3, C10.8-9, C11.1
5	Oropharynx and hypopharynx	$p16^{INK4A}$-negative, HPV-unrelated	C01.9, C02.4, C05.1-2, C09.0-1, C09.8-9, C10.0, C10.2-3, C10.8-9, C11.1 and C12.9, C13.0-2, C13.8-9
6	Nasal cavity and paranasal sinuses		C30.0, C31.0-1
7	Larynx		C10.1, C32.0-2, C32.8-9
8	Mucosal melanoma of the head and neck		C00.0-6, C00.8-9, C01.9, C02.0-4, C02.8-9, C03.0-1, C03.9, C04.0-1, C04.8-9, C05.0-2, C05.8-9, C06.0-2, C06.8-9, C09.0-1, C09.8-9, C10.0-3, C10.8-9, C11.0-3, C11.8-9, C12.9, C13.0-2, C13.8-9, C14.0, C14.2, C14.8, C30.0, C31.0-1, C32.0-2, C32.8-9
9	Cutaneous squamous cell carcinoma of the head and neck		C00.0-2, C44.0, C44.2-4, C44.8

ICD-O-3, I*International Classification of Diseases for Oncology*, third edition.

such as tobacco and alcohol exposure or viral infection have the highest impact. HPV-related tumors are typically found in the oropharynx and even more particularly in the tonsils, which is discussed in more detail in the following.

In summary, head and neck cancers are diverse concerning anatomical localization and contributing risk factors. The current knowledge shows that HPV-related cancers in the head and neck region are primarily localized within the oropharynx, mainly within the tonsil (13). Up to a certain extent, HPV-negative cancers of the oropharynx might be very comparable to nonoropharyngeal head and neck cancers, but HPV-related cancers of the oropharynx are a true distinct disease entity, and classification on the basis of HPV status is the leading topic in this chapter.

SUBTYPES IN HNSCC BASED ON GENE EXPRESSION

Initially microarray hybridizations and later RNA sequencing studies allowed researchers to identify all genes in a tissue that are expressed. These gene expression profiles have been explored in different tumor types including HNSCC by several groups. In 2004, four expression subtypes were defined in HNSCC by cDNA microarray hybridization, resembling those in lung cancer found before (14,15). In a later study, four comparable profiles were identified using Agilent 44K microarrays, and these groups were classified and termed as basal, mesenchymal, atypical, and classical gene expression subtypes (16). While HPV status was not included in the earlier study, an enrichment of HPV-associated gene expression was observed in the atypical subtype with elevated expression of *CDKN2A*, *LIG1*, and the transcription factor *RPA2* (16,17). The basal gene expression profile showed signatures found in basal cells from airway epithelium (e.g., high *COL17A1* expression associated with the extracellular matrix production, and high *TGFA*, *EGFR*, and *TP63* expression) (16,18). Genes associated with epithelial-to-mesenchymal transition (EMT), mesenchymal markers, and transcription/growth factors were enriched in the mesenchymal subtype, while genes enriched in the classical subtype were associated with exposure to cigarette smoke, xenobiotic metabolism genes, and transcription factors (16). Also four subtypes were identified in a third study using Illumina Expression BeadChips (19). Although one cluster closely matched the classical gene expression profile, the other clusters correlated less well with the former studies. This could illustrate the heterogeneity of HNSCC regarding gene expression, but may also indicate differences in collecting and processing of samples and the used profiling platforms. However, an important finding of this study was that the samples containing transcriptionally inactive HPV16 DNA shared characteristics with HPV-negative samples regarding gene expression and frequency of *TP53* mutations, indicating that the presence of HPV16 DNA is not indicative for a role of the virus. Further, the so-called disruptive *TP53* mutations and an immune response–related gene expression cluster were associated with lymph node metastasis, independent of HPV status (19).

Five subtypes of HNSCC, including two biologically distinct HPV subtypes, were identified by Keck and coworkers in 2015 in a clinically homogeneous cohort of 134 locoregionally advanced HNSCCs with 44% HPV-positive tumors. All patients were treated with concurrent chemoradiotherapy. Gene expression profiling was done using Agilent 4x44Kv2 expression arrays and combined with previously published and publicly available data, generating a final dataset of more than 900 patients. One of the subtypes showed an immune and mesenchymal phenotype and contained both HPV-positive and HPV-negative tumors, while the other subgroup resembled the classical expression pattern according to prior nomenclature in other cancer types and molecular characteristics (20–22), but also contained both HPV-positive and HPV-negative tumors. A basal expression subgroup encompassed the remaining HPV-negative samples with significant enrichment of hypoxia-responsive genes (e.g. *HIF1A*, *CA9*, and *VEGF*), neuregulin signaling (including *EGFR*, *AREG NRG1*), and overexpression of epithelial marker genes like P-cadherin (*CDH3*) and cytokeratins (*KRT1*, *KRT9*). In contrast to the basal expression subgroup, both HPV-positive subtypes showed low expression and no copy number events for *EGFR/HER* ligands (23).

Several gene expression signatures have been established from microarray and RNA-Seq studies. However, none of these approaches could be implemented in the standard of care for HNSCC so far. A recent study demonstrates the use of formalin-fixed paraffin embedded (FFPE) oropharyngeal squamous cell carcinoma (OPSCC) tumor tissue for mutation and transcriptional profiling by using Ion Torrent

AmpliSeq cancer panel tNGS and NanoString gene expression assays (24). In this pilot study, 230 cancer-relevant genes were analyzed in four HPV-positive and four HPV-negative samples. The expression of several genes was highly likely to correlate with HPV status (e.g. *WNT1*, *PDGFA*, and *OGG1*). Further, by unsupervised hierarchical clustering six groups of differentially expressed genes were identified in this dataset. Technical replicates of this gene expression study proved a reproducible pattern of gene expression for each tumor with respect to the underlying biology (24) and it may be assumed that the ability to use FFPE samples will advance gene expression studies.

The expression profiling either by protein or RNA expression suggests differential benefit of target specific therapies for different patient groups with HNSCC. Tumors with high and amplified levels of EGFR may qualify for cetuximab treatment. Especially in sight of current antibody-based therapies, this might be of translational importance and further efforts are needed for biomarker development and improvement of personalized care for patients with HNSCC in the future.

In summary, there are several ways to classify head and neck tumors, based on anatomical subsite, based on gene expression profiles, but most prominent at present is the classification on the basis of HPV status, at least in the oropharynx. HPV-positive tumors are different at the molecular level and show a very different clinical behavior, which recently led to an adaptation in the staging (25) and clinical trials to de-intensify therapy. The role of HPV in nonoropharyngeal tumors is less clear, but all in all we separate HNSCC primarily in HPV-negative and HPV-positive tumors, and discuss the genomic landscape likewise.

HPV-NEGATIVE AND HPV-POSITIVE HNSCC: CARCINOGENESIS

HPV-NEGATIVE TUMORS

Most HNSCC patients present with tumors de novo. However, there are precancerous lesions in the mucosal linings of the upper aerodigestive tract that are either white (leukoplakia) or red (erythroplakia) areas of the mucosa. These lesions may progress and develop into SCCs (26). Leukoplakia is the most common precursor lesion of oral squamous carcinomas and its prevalence varies between 0.1 and 0.5% (27,28). The standard policy is to treat the lesion when possible and analyze the specimen or a biopsy by microscopic examination for dysplasia, graded as mild, moderate, or severe. Although consensus criteria have been defined by the World Health Organization (WHO), it remains problematic to make an objective categorization of dysplasia owing to a high inter- and intraobserver variation. Patients are subsequently monitored by active surveillance and biopsy on indication.

The percentage of oral leukoplakias that develop into cancer depends on various factors such as the study population, the definition of leukoplakia used, and the length of the observation time, but an annual transformation rate of 1% to 2% per year is a reasonable assumption (26). Risk factors for progression are female gender, size, and the presence and grade of dysplasia.

Besides these recognizable lesions in the mucosal linings, it has been well established that mucosal abnormalities may exist that are only visible under the microscope. When tumors are diagnosed and excised, the specimen is transferred to the pathology laboratory to perform definitive staging and investigate the surgical margins for tumor invasion. The pathologist also scores for changes in the mucosal epithelium, and grades these as mild, moderate, or severe dysplasia. Particularly severe dysplasia is considered as a preneoplastic change in the mucosal epithelium. Already in 1953, the term "field cancerization" was proposed to describe these dysplastic changes that might also explain the high propensity that local recurrences develop after HNSCC treatment and the high risk that multiple independent tumors develop in the mucosal linings of the upper aerodigestive tract (29).

In the nineties, these precancerous changes were comprehensively studied with genetic markers, and it was shown that the number of genetic changes runs more or less in parallel to the severity of the lesions. This led to the first genetic progression model of head and neck cancer (2). Loss of heterozygosity at chromosomes 3p, 9p, and 17p appeared to occur in dysplasia, apparently reflecting early carcinogenesis, while other alterations at 11q, 4q, and 8 were typically present in carcinomas, likely corresponding to a relatively late phase in carcinogenesis.

These genetic markers were employed to study the presence of genetically altered mucosal epithelial cells, also coined as "fields" in relation to the field cancerization concept of Slaughter et al. (29). Indeed many more premalignant changes characterized by tumor-associated genetic changes were observed, and shown to be clinically relevant as they formed an important source of local recurrences and second primary tumors at least in surgically treated patients (30–32). Most recent studies have identified these same genetic changes at chromosome arms 3p and 9p together with mutations in *TP53* as the best predictors of malignant transformation in leukoplakia (33) and in surgical margins (34).

The tumor suppressor gene on chromosome arm 9p is *CDKN2A* encoding the $p16^{INK4A}$ protein, which binds and disrupts the cyclinD/CDK4-6 complex that drives cells through the G1-S checkpoint. The $p16^{INK4A}$ cell cycle inhibiting protein is frequently inactivated in HNSCC by mutation or methylation in combination with chromosomal loss, or by homozygous deletion (7,68). On chromosome 17p13 the *TP53* gene is located that is also frequently inactivated in HNSCC, mostly by missense mutations combined with allelic loss. Somatic mutations are found in 60% to 80% of the tumors (7,35–37). Hence, there is quite some information on the precancerous fields and the molecular changes in these fields, although more detailed DNA sequencing data are still lacking.

Furthermore, there is only very limited data on what precedes the development of these fields. Van Houten et al. described small p53-positive focal patches in tumor-adjacent mucosal epithelium (35), and showed that these indeed contained mutations, but not related to the index tumor of these patients. These mutated p53-positive patches were considered equivalent to the "clones" or "clonal units" and defined as a family of daughter cells that originate from an adult stem cell that makes up that part of the squamous epithelium, and that has now become detectable by the mutation in p53. These p53 mutated clonal units were considered to represent the first oncogenic changes in the mucosa, and formed together with the genetically defined fields the basis of the hypothetical patch–field–tumor–metastasis progression model for HNSCC development (3). This model was deduced from the existing descriptive studies but recent data in engineered mouse models support such a model. By Axin2 lineage tracing experiments the stem cells and the patches they form have been shown recently, at least in mouse skin (38).

The initial genetic progression model, later adapted and simplified, are elementary linear models (3). However, the plethora of new candidate cancer genes that are mutated in HNSCC will make these simple linear models much more complex and diverse, and the research field has to deal with the fact that there are likely multiple ways that lead to mucosal epithelial cell transformation.

In most recent molecular profiling studies it was shown that another subgroup of tumors exists that is characterized by very few copy number alterations. This subgroup of HPV-negative and *TP53* wild type tumors typically displays *HRAS* and *CASP8* mutations and a more favorable prognosis (7). In previous studies, it was shown that this group is diploid, proficient in DNA mismatch repair and seems to occur more frequently in females without a history of smoking and alcohol consumption (39).

HPV-POSITIVE TUMORS

HPV infection causes a subgroup of tumors, most particularly those arising in the oropharynx. HPV-positive OPSCCs form a separate disease entity that led to an adapted staging system (25). In addition, several studies to de-escalate therapy have been initiated and the results are awaited. Most assays to test for HPV in tumor specimen are based on the detection of viral DNA. There are many HPV types that may cause cancer, but most prominent is HPV16, particularly in the head and neck region. As mentioned earlier, the virus encodes two oncogenes E6 and E7. The E7 protein binds the pocket proteins pRb, P130, and p107 thereby creating an S-phase environment in the cell. Usually an unscheduled S-phase with high E2F activity causes p53 activation by p14 inhibition of MDM2 and induction of apoptosis, and therefore the virus expresses the oncoprotein E6 that targets p53 for degradation. Hence, the virus hits precisely the same pathways as is noted in HPV-negative tumors: the p53–p21 pathway and the p16–cyclinD1–Rb pathway. Typically in HPV-positive tumors, $p16^{INK4A}$ is active and often overexpressed, while cyclinD1 at 11q13 is not amplified and p53 is wild type (7,40,41). Hence, at the genetic level, most prominent in HPV-positive tumors is the absence of *TP53* mutations as well as the absence of the loss of chromosome arms 3p and 9p and the amplification of 11q13, while these changes are very common in HPV-negative tumors.

Both E6 and E7 expression remains critical in HPV-positive HNSCC cell lines (42) and the cancer-associated phenotype caused by inactivation of the p53 and pRb pathways in oropharyngeal keratinocytes is at least cellular immortalization (43). This phenotype would also fit with the timing of the genetic events early in the progression of HPV-negative HNSCC as abrogation of the p53 and pRb pathways by loss of 9p21, the location of *CDKN2A* as well as *TP53* mutations are frequently found in the precursor fields (2,30,44), and are considered as the earliest genetic changes. In HPV-positive HNSCC these same pathways are likely also the first to be inactivated by the viral E6 and E7 oncoproteins, strongly suggesting that HPV infection is indeed the initial carcinogenic event as it is in cervical cancer (45).

The key precursor lesions in the mucosal linings are leukoplakias, and it was therefore logical to study HPV presence in these lesions, but the results are highly discordant. A major problem in the different studies is the false positive results by the applied ultrasensitive HPV DNA assays. Most reliable studies suggest a very low prevalence of less than 1%; this is reviewed by Ha and Califano (46). Given the second observation that 3p and 9p losses of heterozygosity are the key genetic changes predicting malignant transformation of leukoplakias (33), although these alterations are typically absent in HPV-positive tumors (40), we consider progressing leukoplakia lesions as being HPV-negative, and they should not be considered the precursor lesion of HPV-mediated carcinogenesis.

Are there any other indications for HPV-induced precancerous changes in the upper aerodigestive tract? They are very common in the cervix, and in fact the target lesion for screening (45). The highest attributable fraction of HPV in the head and neck is found in the tonsils, and therefore both precancerous changes and sites of infection are expected in the tonsils. Several studies have been carried out with the largest reporting on over 4,000 tonsils of which over 3,300 could be analyzed. No HPV was found (47). Hence, the precursor lesions of HPV-driven carcinogenesis in the upper aerodigestive tract are still an enigma. There have been indications that tonsillar cancers may be surrounded by $p16^{INK4A}$-positive mucosal fields, but these might have been superficially growing tumors and without proper genetic analysis of these lesions this remains unclear (48).

Finally, it was also studied using HPV assays whether HPV-positive tumors in the oropharynx are surrounded by large fields of infected cells, a surrogate for the fields of genetically altered cells that precede HPV-negative tumors. It was assumed that HPV infection is the first carcinogenic event in HPV-positive tumors, as it is in the cervix, and that HPV presence and E6 transcripts could be used to study the presence of these fields surrounding HPV-positive tumors. Remarkably, in none of the analyzed tumor-free surgical margins E6 transcripts could be detected. Again, strongly suggesting that HPV-induced field cancerization seems not to occur in the upper aerodigestive tract. Alternatively, HPV infection may also not be the first carcinogenic event (49). In contrast to HPV-mediated carcinogenesis in the cervix that can be followed by inspection and biopsies of the acetowhite lesions, there are at present no indications for HPV-related precancerous changes in the upper aerodigestive tract. Hence, the molecular pathogenesis of HPV-induced squamous cancers in the upper aerodigestive tract remains unsolved, and currently relies on the extrapolation of data collected in the invasive carcinomas.

HPV-NEGATIVE AND HPV-POSITIVE HNSCC: PROTEIN EXPRESSION, GENETICS, AND EPIGENETICS

A most interesting feature of head and neck cancers in comparison to other tumor entities is the existence of virus and chemical agent driven cancer within one anatomically well-defined sublocalization (the oropharynx) in a somewhat balanced numerical ratio. For example, in lung cancer, smoking is the dominant risk factor while viral infection is negligible. In contrast, almost 100% of cervical carcinomas are associated with HPV infection. During the past year it became evident that HPV-related OPSCCs are a distinct entity with characteristic molecular and clinical features such as superior survival of patients. Consequently, it was to be expected that HPV was introduced for classification of oropharyngeal cancer in the latest version of American Joint Committee on Cancer (AJCC) staging albeit HPV status is determined only by $p16^{INK4A}$ immunostaining as a surrogate and not in combination with HPV testing (12).

The choice to rely on $p16^{INK4A}$ immunostaining was that it is easier to standardize compared to viral oncogene (mainly E6 and E7) mRNA detection, and that it is a good although not perfect surrogate marker. Overexpression of p16^{INK4A} protein is indirectly linked to the oncogenetic activity of HPV encoded protein E7. In contrast, CDKN2A, the gene encoding p16^{INK4A}, it is one of the most frequently inactivated tumor suppressor genes in HPV-negative tumors (50,51).

DIFFERENTIAL PROTEIN EXPRESSION IN HPV-POSITIVE AND HPV-NEGATIVE HNSCC

The most prominent protein markers in HNSCC include p53, EGFR, and VEGF. The 53 kDa nuclear phosphoprotein p53 is coded by the tumor suppressor gene *TP53*. It is one of the most important tumor suppressors involved in DNA synthesis/repair and programmed cell death and, when activated, inhibits the cell cycle by induction of p21. Expression of p53 is usually not detected in healthy cells owing to its short half-life, but it is frequently observed in cancer cells. Accumulation of p53 occurs by enhanced expression upon cellular stress, for example, induction by carcinogenic processes. However, several mutational hot spots within *TP53* in cancer cells have been identified, which lead to mutated protein with abrogated tumor suppression function. Therefore, selection processes cause tumor cells to accumulate *TP53* mutations. Although not fully understood, the consequence of more *TP53* mutations/higher p53 expression level could be a worse prognosis. These findings are superimposed by effects of HPV-induced carcinogenesis, and right now, it is unclear whether *TP53* mutations have prognostic impact independently from HPV status. Some studies do report this (52), but the studied cohorts are somewhat small and based on heterogeneous patient populations. HPV-positive tumors rarely contain *TP53* mutations compared to HPV-negative tumors (40) and prognosis is usually better. Although pointing in the same direction, underlying mechanisms differ. In HPV-driven cancers, viral E6 oncoprotein expression impedes p53 function via binding and recruitment of ubiquitinating proteins and labeling p53 for proteasomal degradation. Therefore, no selection pressure to acquire *TP53* mutations exists in HPV-driven cancers. However, as already mentioned another protein marker (p16^{INK4A}) is overexpressed in HPV-related cancers. The p16^{INK4A} tumor suppressor protein is generally inactivated by mutation, methylation, and losses in HPV-negative tumors. In HPV-driven tumors, p16^{INK4A} expression is usually detectable in the majority (>70%) of tumor cells by immunohistochemistry, with a strong, diffuse expression pattern in both nucleus and cytoplasm (classical pattern of HPV-induced transformation) (48,50,53,54). Inactivation of retinoblastoma (Rb) by the HPV E7 oncoprotein overcomes cell cycle arrest and E7 enhances p16^{INK4A} expression by inducing epigenetic changes (55). However, it has to be mentioned that HPV-independent p16^{INK4A} overexpression is described for different cancers and about 5% of oropharyngeal cancers (50), probably by alternative alterations in the p16-signaling pathway (e.g., inactivation of retinoblastoma). Previous studies have shown that respective disadvantages of HPV detection by polymerase chain reaction (PCR; low specificity) or by p16^{INK4A} immunohistochemistry (HPV-independent overexpression) can be ruled out by the combination of both techniques.

MUTATIONS AND COPY-NUMBER ABERRATION (CNA) PROFILES

Complex karyotypes are frequent in HNSCC, including several numeric and structural alterations. A high variability and heterogeneity among cells indicates selection processes and clonal evolution in HNSCC. This led to one of the first genetic progression models for HNSCC, in which chromosomal changes (gains, losses, and translocations) accumulate in an ordered manner with resulting growth advantage of a favored cell population (2). In a 2014 review, cytogenetic aberrations in HNSCC have been summarized (56).

The current knowledge indicates that certain genetic alterations are shared by HNSCC irrespective of HPV status, while others are restricted to either HPV-negative or HPV-positive HNSCC (57). This has been largely confirmed by data from The Cancer Genome Atlas (TCGA) consortium. For example, amplification of the 3q26-28 region, containing *PIK3CA*, *TP63*, and *SOX2* are frequent to both (7). Deletion (14%) or mutation (8%) of *TRAF3* (tumor necrosis factor receptor–associated factor 3), which is involved in innate and acquired antiviral immune response, was found in high frequency in HPV-positive HNSCC (7). In this context, higher mutation rates in *CYLD* (cylindromatosis lysine 63 deubiquitinase) have also been identified in HPV-positive HNSCC and both aberrations correlated with *NFκB* (nuclear factor kappa-light-chain-enhancer of activated B cells) activation, episomal HPV status of tumors, and improved patient survival (58).

Amplifications of *EGFR* and *FGFR1* appear to be restricted to HPV-negative HNSCC, which is confirmed by other studies (7,59–61).

A comparison of HPV-positive and HPV-negative tumors was done for mutations and CNAs in 617 cancer-associated genes in 120 matched tumor/normal samples (42.5% HPV-positive tumors) (62). In contrast to the general expectation, mutational burden did not differ between HPV positive and HPV negative. The mutational spectrum of HPV-negative tumors resembles that of published lung SCC analyses with high mutation frequency in *TP53*, *CDKN2A*, *MLL2*, *CUL3*, *NSD1*, *PIK3CA*, and *NOTCH* genes. In HPV-positive tumors a unique profile with high mutation rates in *DDX3X*, *FGFR2/3* and aberrations in *PIK3CA*, *KRAS*, *MLL2/3*, and *NOTCH1* was found (62).

A most important progress in recent years was the publication of 279 head and neck cancer genomes characterized by next-generation sequencing and array analysis by TCGA consortium (7). In this dataset, 36 cases were identified to be HPV positive. The analysis confirmed differential genetic patterns described earlier. Further, frequent structural changes in TRAF3, a gene at chromosomal region 14q32 and frequently involved in antiviral immune responses were found in HPV-positive tumors. In contrast, amplifications of *EGFR* and *FGFR1* appear to be restricted to HPV-negative HNSCC (7,59–61). *TpC* mutations were found more frequent in HPV-positive tumors, although the total number of somatic mutations was not different between HPV-positive and HPV-negative tumors. Missense mutations in *PIK3CA* coding for the catalytic subunit of PI3-kinase were identified in HPV-positive tumors as well as amplifications of *E2F1*. PI3-kinase activity activates AKT signaling and *PIK3CA* mutations in HPV-positive tumors have been reported before [e.g., in 8/33 HPV-positive tumors analyzed (63)]. Data from TCGA and other studies have recently been summarized to describe the genetic landscape of HPV-associated HNSCC, including structural alterations, mutation signatures, viral integration, and their relation to cellular pathways (64).

Although latest sequencing results are a great progress for cancer research, one has to mention that total numbers of analyzed samples are still small. For example, the aforementioned mutation in *KRAS* was found in 5.8% of HPV-positive tumors (3/51 patients) (62), and this finding could not be validated in another study (65).

Among the best known and highly validated differences between HPV-negative and HPV-positive HNSCC are somatic mutations in the *TP53* gene, which are found in 60% to 80% of HPV-negative but are virtually absent in HPV-positive tumors (7,35–37). This reflects the low selection pressure to acquire *TP53* mutations in HPV-positive cancers due to p53 inactivation by the HPV E6 oncoprotein.

Although the majority of HNSCCs are either driven by HPV or harbor *TP53* mutations, a remaining 20% cases seem to have p53 wild type (39). It might be that other genes in the p53 pathway are altered in selected cases (66) or that p53-independent tracks of malignant progression are followed. For example, this subgroup of HPV-negative and *TP53* wild type tumors typically show *HRAS* and *CASP8* mutations, as was recently shown by molecular profiling studies (7).

HPV-driven tumors with E6 transcription were shown to have a different genetic pattern (e.g., absence of chromosome arms 3p, 9p loss, and 11q13 amplification) compared to HPV-negative HNSCC with respect to loss of heterozygosity analysis and microarray comparative genomic hybridization (40,41,67). The genes located at 9p and 11q13 are *CDKN2A* and *CCND1*, and both are established cancer genes in HPV-negative HNSCC and often affected by genetic alterations (7,41,68). In HPV-positive HNSCC, chromosomal instability seems to be associated with HPV DNA integration into the host´s genome and, albeit being linked to cancer progression in general, is associated with favorable prognosis in tonsillar cancer (69).

In the classical view of HPV-related carcinogenesis, integration of the viral DNA into the host genome disrupts control of E6 and E7 activity by inactivating E2 protein by linearizing the HPV genome within this E2 coding open reading frame. Although this model appears to be reasonable, in an analysis of 73 HPV-associated OPSCCs, episome-derived PCR products were only detected for more than 60% of samples (70). Also, HNSCC cell line analysis indicated that viral oncogene expression was independent of viral copy number and the presence of viral integration. One of the studied cell lines did not show HPV DNA integration at all, indicating that HPV DNA integration is not a necessary event in carcinogenesis (71). Very recently, RNA-Seq and whole genome sequence data from TCGA HNSCC samples were analyzed for the possible HPV genome states (episomal only, integrated state, and a state in which the viral genome exists as a hybrid episome with human DNA). All three states were split relatively evenly and more strikingly, about three quarters of HPV16-positive HNSCC contain episomal viral genomes (72).

EPIGENETICS AND miRNAS

Epigenetic alterations, either DNA methylation or histone modifications of viral and host genomes, are two important processes effecting gene expression. Especially the role of DNA methylation in HPV-positive OPSCC is well established, and affects not only pathogenesis of OPSCC but also clinical behavior of tumors. Gene promoter methylation often causes transcriptional silencing of tumor suppressor genes involved in DNA damage repair, detoxification, cell cycle regulation, and apoptosis, and may be as important as inactivation of genes by deletion or somatic mutation (73,74).

Viral E2 protein expression and binding to E2 binding sites (E2BSs) in the viral genome are important regulators of E6 and E7 expression during the normal HPV life cycle. Loss of E2 function during carcinogenesis is considered a prerequisite for consistent activation of viral oncogene expression and malignant transformation (75). Methylation marks at E2BS in the upstream regulatory region of E6 and E7 regulate transcription in the presence of intact E2 expression, which is particularly important in tumors with episomal (nonintegrated) HPV (76,77). Distinct patterns of DNA methylation in the host genome are described for viral driven cancers including HPV (78–80). Since DNA methylation profiles persist or even increase during disease progression, this is of particular clinical relevance. A trend toward a higher level of gene promoter methylation in HPV-related as compared to HPV-negative OPSCC was shown, which is most likely due to accelerated expression and enzymatic activity of DNA methyltransferases (DNMTs) (80–84). In patients with HPV-associated SCCs distinct subgroups were identified based on viral DNA integration and the E2BS methylation status, causally linked with viral oncogene expression (70,76,77). Recently, a methylation signature for HPV-related cancers was determined based on quantitative evaluation of differentially methylated regions in the proximal promoter of five host genes (*ALDH1A2*, *OSR2*, *IRX4*, *GRIA4*, and *GATA4*), predicting the clinical outcome of HNSCC patients, including HPV-related OPSCC (78,85).

MiRNAs are the best studied noncoding RNAs involved in gene regulation since their discovery in 1993 (86). After their processing from 60 to 70 nucleotide, long hairpin-like precursors, miRNAs are incorporated together with DICER1 and Argonaute (AGO) proteins in the miRNA-induced silencing complex (miRISC). This complex is guided by sequence complementary of the miRNA to its target mRNAs, and causing gene suppression by targeted mRNA degradation and translational repression. Although altered miRNA expression is known in various cancers and carcinogenic processes, invasion and metastasis, less is known in head and neck cancer. A definite conclusion from the large-scale profiling studies is hampered by the fact that miRNAs do not have "one" target and one function. Because of their small size of about 22 bases, miRNA may bind to more or less conserved target sequences and target genes themselves can have several binding sites for one or different miRNAs. This generates rather complex networks of molecular interactions regulated by miRNAs. Although only partially documented, most cellular pathways involved in carcinogenesis of head and neck cancers are influenced by miRNA regulation.

Several differentially expressed miRNAs have been described until now for HPV-negative and -positive HNSCC and with the technical progress, their number and reliability of data will certainly rise. Hsa-miR-363 is among the best known miRNAs found to be upregulated in HPV-positive compared to HPV-negative HNSCCs (87–89). Among others, its predicted target sequences are within *CDKN1A* (cyclin-dependent kinase inhibitor 1), *CASP3* (Caspase-3), and *CD274* (programmed cell death 1 ligand 1), indicating regulatory function in apoptosis, cell cycle, transcriptional regulation, and immunity. Downregulation in HPV-positive compared to HPV-negative HNSCC was reported for hsa-miR-125a, -143, -145, -199a, -126, -181b, and -31 in at least two studies each (87–91). The most prominent target genes are: *CD34* (hematopoietic progenitor cell antigen CD34), *CDKN1A*, *TP53* (p53), *ERBB2* (receptor tyrosine-protein kinase erbB-2), *KRAS* (GTPase KRas), *SOX2* (transcription factor SOX-2), *MET* (hepatocyte growth factor receptor), *MTOR* (serine/threonine-protein kinase mTOR), *HIF1A* (hypoxia-inducible factor 1-alpha), *VEGFA* (vascular endothelial growth factor A), *PIK3R2* (phosphatidylinositol 3-kinase regulatory subunit beta), *TERT* (telomerase reverse transcriptase), BCL2 (apoptosis regulator Bcl-2), and *FOXP3* (forkhead box protein P3). Other miRNAs reported in at least two studies are hsa-miR-26b, -29a, -155, and -222 (87–91). Predicted target sequences are within genes already mentioned or with similar important functions. However, expression data are conflicting for these miRNAs indicating the need for further investigations in this field of gene regulation. Although miRNA regulation is highly complex, miRNAs may serve as diagnostic and prognostic markers and miRNA-mediated gene regulation could be the target of future therapy concepts.

HPV-NEGATIVE AND HPV-POSITIVE HNSCC: ALTERED PATHWAYS

For development and progression of every malignant disease, a critical set of cellular pathways has to be dysregulated. Although involved factors may differ depending on the originating tissue and impact of environmental factors (chemicals, radiation, or carcinogenic viruses), a basic set of pathways seems comparable for most cancers. Generally, proliferation and cellular survival are increased, while cell cycle control is changed, and DNA-repair and linked apoptotic programs are suppressed (Figure 3.1). This is achieved by the action of the major HPV oncoproteins E6 and E7 in HPV-induced carcinogenesis, and is independent from inactivation of anticancer sentinels like p53 on the genetic level. Further steps involve dedifferentiation of tumor cells and activation of immune escape mechanisms. Downregulation of *HLA-A* and *–B* alleles has been reported for HPV-driven cancers in 1995 (92) and recent sequencing data point to enrichment of mutations in *HLA* and *beta-2-microglobulin* genes in HPV-positive HNSCC (7). This is particularly interesting, since attraction and activation of CD56[+] natural killer cells is expected by HLA I loss and higher numbers of CD56[+] natural killer cells were reported in HPV-associated OPSCC recently, and correlate with improved survival independently from HPV status (93).

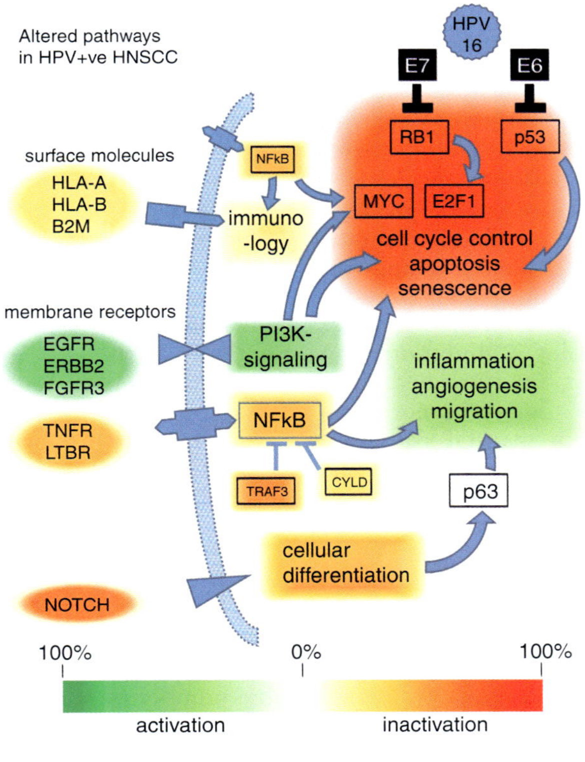

FIGURE 3.1 Molecular pathways frequently altered in HPV-positive HNSCC.
HNSCC, head and neck squamous cell carcinoma.

Further, an increased disturbance in NOTCH signaling was observed in both HPV-positive and HPV-negative HNSCC (7,59), indicating a certain need for dedifferentiation in carcinogenesis for both entities. For development of invasive properties, downregulation of cell surface adhesion molecules and activation of extracellular matrix degrading enzymes have to take place. Further, enhanced angiogenesis and adaptation of metabolic processes regarding changing environmental conditions during tumor growth or migration of tumor cells, is needed for tumor progression.

The driving forces, details of the molecular participants, and potentially the sequence of events differ between HPV-positive and HPV-negative HNSCC. Therefore, a detailed knowledge of molecular processes is needed for disease classification and development of more specific and effective treatment concepts for distinct tumor types.

IMPLICATIONS FOR THERAPEUTIC TARGETING

Molecular and genetic classification of patients´ tumors will help to guide treatment decisions in the future. Further, the increasing knowledge of altered pathways in HNSCC by investigating underlying genetic alterations will lead to the prediction of novel therapeutic targets and reevaluation of already known target/therapy combinations, which in clinical trials with genetically unselected patients, have not been as successful as expected (e.g., EGFR-directed therapies). As a prerequisite, genetic profiling of patients has to become possible by routine, which can be assumed regarding developments in high-throughput sequencing technologies.

Generally, oncogenic alterations are more susceptible to pharmacologic inhibition than changes in tumor suppressors or related pathways. HPV-positive HNSCC might be more eligible for therapeutic targeting than HPV-negative HNSCC, as they appear to be more homogeneous regarding altered pathways and activation of cancer-associated pathways seems to be more frequent. To date, the most obvious candidates are PIK3CA and CDK4/CDK6 pathways, due to high rates of *PIK3CA* mutations and *CCND1* amplifications. Furthermore, suitable therapeutics are already available for interfering with both pathways. *STAT3* might be another promising therapeutic target. Hyperactivation of the STAT3 transcription factor is a hallmark of HNSCC, although oncogenic mutations are not described. STAT3 activation is driven by upstream growth factor receptors like Janus kinase (JAK) and EGFR and associated with oncogenic behavior and resistance to standard therapeutics in HNSCC (94).

Options to interfere with dysregulated pathways in cancer are numerous and have been recently summarized for HNSCC (95,96). However, as HPV-negative HNSCC is mainly caused by tumor suppressor gene inactivation, synthetic lethal interactions with other genes need to be explored. Logical candidates might be the remaining genes regulating the head and neck cancer cell cycle. In tumors the G1/S checkpoint is inactivated by the abrogation of pRb and p53 pathways, and molecules such as Wee1 kinase that keep the cyclinB/CDK1 complex inactivated till cell division occurs, are now becoming regulation nodes (97). Increasing data of genetic alterations driving carcinogenesis, functional analysis of the cancer genes, and future development of methods for their therapeutic targeting will provide further options for the treatment of HNSCC. It remains to be seen whether novel targeted treatment options have the power to complement or replace conventional therapy, and the immunotherapies that are discussed in other chapters.

SUMMARY

The genomic landscape of head and neck cancer is known in greatest detail. The main classification in our view at present is between HPV-positive and HPV-negative tumors, certainly in the oropharynx as these tumors differ enormously with respect to etiology, molecular changes, patient characteristics, and most importantly, clinical outcome. HPV-positive tumors are staged differently in TNM8 (12), and likely may be treated differently in time. Within the oral cancers, there is also a subgroup of tumors that are devoid of copy-number changes, and this group needs to be characterized in more detail.

The most important driver pathways in head and neck cancer are p53-p21, p16-cyclinD1-Rb, EGFR-PI3K-AKT, TGF-beta, and NOTCH1. Many other genes have been found mutated in much lower frequencies and are likely to play a role, but precisely how and in which pathways remains to be investigated. Disappointingly, the number of oncogenes involved in HNSCC is very limited. *EGFR* and *PIK3CA* seem the main oncogenes involved but only in subsets of tumors. Oncogenes are interesting targets for therapy, but HNSCC seems more a disease of inactivated tumor suppressor genes, which are no direct targets, enforcing the exploration of other strategies. But new opportunities have emerged. Head and neck cancers belong to the group of tumors with a relatively high mutational load, which may make them susceptible to immunotherapies. Thus far, treatment is still mainly based on stage and site, and not on genetic or other molecular classifications. This may change on short notice for the oropharyngeal tumors that are caused by HPV.

REFERENCES

1. Fearon ER, Vogelstein B. A genetic model for colorectal tumorigenesis. *Cell*. 1990;61:759–767. doi:10.1016/0092-8674(90)90186-I
2. Califano J, van der Riet P, Westra W, et al. Genetic progression model for head and neck cancer: implications for field cancerization. *Cancer Res*. 1996;56:2488–2492.
3. Leemans CR, Braakhuis BJ, Brakenhoff RH. The molecular biology of head and neck cancer. *Nat Rev Cancer*. 2011;11:9–22.
4. Tomasetti C, Vogelstein B. Cancer etiology. Variation in cancer risk among tissues can be explained by the number of stem cell divisions. *Science*. 2015;347:78–81.
5. Bartkova J, Hořejší Z, Koed K, et al. DNA damage response as a candidate anti-cancer barrier in early human tumorigenesis. *Nature*. 2005;434:864–870.
6. van Harn T, Foijer F, van Vugt M, et al. Loss of Rb proteins causes genomic instability in the absence of mitogenic signaling. *Genes Dev*. 2010;24:1377–1388.
7. Cancer Genome Atlas Network. Comprehensive genomic characterization of head and neck squamous cell carcinomas. *Nature*. 2015;517:576–582.
8. Allis CD, Jenuwein T. The molecular hallmarks of epigenetic control. *Nat Rev Genet*. 2016;17:487–500.
9. Lin S, Gregory RI. MicroRNA biogenesis pathways in cancer. *Nat Rev Cancer*. 2015;15:321–333.
10. Wood LD, Parsons DW, Jones S, et al. The genomic landscapes of human breast and colorectal cancers. *Science*. 2007;318:1108–13.
11. Lawrence MS, Stojanov P, Polak P, et al. Mutational heterogeneity in cancer and the search for new cancer-associated genes. *Nature*. 2013;499:214–218.
12. Amin MB, Edge S, Greene F, et al. eds. *AJCC Cancer Staging Manual* (8th ed). New York, NY: Springer; 2017.
13. Klussmann JP, Weissenborn SJ, Wieland U, et al. Prevalence, distribution, and viral load of human papillomavirus 16 DNA in tonsillar carcinomas. *Cancer*. 2001;92:2875–2884.
14. Garber ME, Troyanskaya OG, Schluens K, et al. Diversity of gene expression in adenocarcinoma of the lung. *Proc Natl Acad Sci USA*. 2001;98:13784–13789.
15. Chung CH, Parker JS, Karaca G, et al. Molecular classification of head and neck squamous cell carcinomas using patterns of gene expression. *Cancer Cell*. 2004;5:489–500.
16. Walter V, Yin X, Wilkerson MD, et al. Molecular subtypes in head and neck cancer exhibit distinct patterns of chromosomal gain and loss of canonical cancer genes. *PLOS ONE*. 2013;8:e56823.
17. Slebos RJ, Yi Y, Ely K, et al. Gene expression differences associated with human papillomavirus status in head and neck squamous cell carcinoma. *Clin Cancer Res*. 2006;12:701–709.
18. Hackett NR, Shaykhiev R, Walters MS, et al. The human airway epithelial basal cell transcriptome. *PLOS ONE*. 2011;6:e18378.
19. Wichmann G, Rosolowski M, Krohn K, et al. The role of HPV RNA transcription, immune response-related gene expression and disruptive TP53 mutations in diagnostic and prognostic profiling of head and neck cancer. *Int J Cancer*. 2015;137:2846–2857.
20. Verhaak RG, Hoadley KA, Purdom E, et al. An integrated genomic analysis identifies clinically relevant subtypes of glioblastoma characterized by abnormalities in PDGFRA, IDH1, EGFR, and NF1. *Cancer Cell*. 2010;17:98–110.
21. Wilkerson MD, Yin X, Hoadley KA, et al. Lung squamous cell carcinoma mRNA expression subtypes are reproducible, clinically important, and correspond to normal cell types. *Clin Cancer Res*. 2010;16:4864–4875.
22. Sørlie T, Tibshirani R, Parker J, et al. Repeated observation of breast tumor subtypes in independent gene expression data sets. *Proc Natl Acad Sci USA*. 2003;100:8418–8423.
23. Keck MK, Zuo Z, Khattri A, et al. Integrative analysis of head and neck cancer identifies two biologically distinct HPV and three non-HPV subtypes. *Clin Cancer Res*. 2015;21:870–881.
24. Saba NF, Wilson M, Doho G, et al. Mutation and transcriptional profiling of formalin-fixed paraffin embedded specimens as companion methods to immunohistochemistry for determining therapeutic targets in oropharyngeal squamous cell carcinoma (OPSCC): a pilot of proof of principle. *Head Neck Pathol*. 2015;9:223–235.
25. O'Sullivan B, Huang SH, Su J, et al. Development and validation of a staging system for HPV-related oropharyngeal cancer by the International Collaboration on Oropharyngeal cancer Network for Staging (ICON-S): a multicentre cohort study. *Lancet Oncol*. 2016;17:440–451.
26. Brouns E, Baart J, Karagozoglu K, et al. Malignant transformation of oral leukoplakia in a well-defined cohort of 144 patients. *Oral Dis*. 2014;20:e19–e24.
27. Napier SS, Speight PM. Natural history of potentially malignant oral lesions and conditions: an overview of the literature. *J Oral Pathol Med*. 2008;37:1–10.
28. van der Waal I. Potentially malignant disorders of the oral and oropharyngeal mucosa; terminology, classification and present concepts of management. *Oral Oncol*. 2009;45:317–323.
29. Slaughter DP, Southwick HW, Smejkal W. Field cancerization in oral stratified squamous epithelium; clinical implications of multicentric origin. *Cancer*. 1953;6:963–968.

30. Tabor MP, Brakenhoff RH, van Houten VM, et al. Persistence of genetically altered fields in head and neck cancer patients: biological and clinical implications. *Clin Cancer Res.* 2001;7:1523–1532.
31. Tabor MP, Brakenhoff RH, Ruijter-Schippers HJ, et al. Genetically altered fields as origin of locally recurrent head and neck cancer: a retrospective study. *Clin Cancer Res.* 2004;10:3607–3613.
32. Tabor MP, Brakenhoff RH, Ruijter-Schippers HJ, et al. Multiple head and neck tumors frequently originate from a single preneoplastic lesion. *Am J Pathol.* 2002;161:1051–1060.
33. Zhang L, Poh CF, Williams M, et al. Loss of heterozygosity (LOH) profiles—validated risk predictors for progression to oral cancer. *Cancer Prev Res (Phila).* 2012;5:1081–1089.
34. Graveland AP, Golusinski PJ, Buijze M, et al. Loss of heterozygosity at 9p and p53 immunopositivity in surgical margins predict local relapse in head and neck squamous cell carcinoma. *Int J Cancer.* 2011;128:1852–1859.
35. van Houten VM, Tabor MP, van den Brekel MW, et al. Mutated p53 as a molecular marker for the diagnosis of head and neck cancer. *J Pathol.* 2002;198:476–486.
36. Balz V, Scheckenbach K, Götte K, et al. Is the p53 inactivation frequency in squamous cell carcinomas of the head and neck underestimated? Analysis of p53 exons 2-11 and human papillomavirus 16/18 E6 transcripts in 123 unselected tumor specimens. *Cancer Res.* 2003;63:1188–1191.
37. Poeta ML, Manola J, Goldwasser MA, et al. TP53 mutations and survival in squamous-cell carcinoma of the head and neck. *N Engl J Med.* 2007;357:2552–2561.
38. Lim X, Tan SH, Koh WLC, et al. Interfollicular epidermal stem cells self-renew via autocrine Wnt signaling. *Science.* 2013;342:1226–1230.
39. Smeets SJ, Brakenhoff RH, Ylstra B, et al. Genetic classification of oral and oropharyngeal carcinomas identifies subgroups with a different prognosis. *Cell Oncol.* 2009;31:291–300.
40. Braakhuis BJM, Snijders PJF, Keune W-JH, et al. Genetic patterns in head and neck cancers that contain or lack transcriptionally active human papillomavirus. *J Natl Cancer Inst.* 2004;96:998–1006.
41. Smeets SJ, Braakhuis BJ, Abbas S, et al. Genome-wide DNA copy number alterations in head and neck squamous cell carcinomas with or without oncogene-expressing human papillomavirus. *Oncogene.* 2006;25:2558–2564.
42. Rampias T, Sasaki C, Weinberger P, Psyrri A. E6 and e7 gene silencing and transformed phenotype of human papillomavirus 16-positive oropharyngeal cancer cells. *J Natl Cancer Inst.* 2009;101:412–423.
43. Smeets SJ, van der Plas M, Schaaij-Visser TB, et al. Immortalization of oral keratinocytes by functional inactivation of the p53 and pRb pathways. *Int J Cancer.* 2011;128:1596–1605.
44. Braakhuis BJ, Tabor MP, Kummer JA, et al. A genetic explanation of Slaughter's concept of field cancerization: evidence and clinical implications. *Cancer Res.* 2003;63:1727–1730.
45. Steenbergen RD, Snijders PJ, Heideman DA, Meijer CJ. Clinical implications of (epi)genetic changes in HPV-induced cervical precancerous lesions. *Nat Rev Cancer.* 2014;14:395–405.
46. Ha PK, Califano JA. The role of human papillomavirus in oral carcinogenesis. *Crit Rev Oral Biol Med.* 2004;15:188–196.
47. Palmer E, Newcombe RG, Green AC, et al. Human papillomavirus infection is rare in nonmalignant tonsil tissue in the UK: implications for tonsil cancer precursor lesions. *Int J Cancer.* 2014;135:2437–2443.
48. Mooren JJ, Gultekin SE, Straetmans JM, et al. P16(INK4A) immunostaining is a strong indicator for high-risk-HPV-associated oropharyngeal carcinomas and dysplasias, but is unreliable to predict low-risk-HPV-infection in head and neck papillomas and laryngeal dysplasias. *Int J Cancer.* 2014;134:2108–2117.
49. Rietbergen MM, Braakhuis BJ, Moukhtari N, et al. No evidence for active human papillomavirus (HPV) in fields surrounding HPV-positive oropharyngeal tumors. *J Oral Pathol Med.* 2014;43:137–142.
50. Prigge ES, Toth C, Dyckhoff G, et al. $p16^{INK4a}$/Ki-67 co-expression specifically identifies transformed cells in the head and neck region. *Int J Cancer.* 2015;136:1589–1599.
51. Gültekin SE, Sengüven B, Klussmann JP, Dienes HP. $P16^{INK\ 4a}$ and Ki-67 expression in human papilloma virus-related head and neck mucosal lesions. *Invest Clin.* 2015;56:47–59.
52. Lindenbergh-van der Plas M, Brakenhoff RH, Kuik DJ, et al. Prognostic significance of truncating TP53 mutations in head and neck squamous cell carcinoma. *Clin Cancer Res.* 2011;17:3733–3741.
53. Reuschenbach M, Roos J, Panayotopoulos D, et al. Characterization of squamous cell cancers of the vulvar anterior fourchette by human papillomavirus, p16INK4a, and p53. *J Low Genit Tract Dis.* 2013;17:289–297.
54. Klussmann JP, Gültekin E, Weissenborn SJ, et al. Expression of p16 protein identifies a distinct entity of tonsillar carcinomas associated with human papillomavirus. *Am J Pathol.* 2003;162:747–753.
55. McLaughlin-Drubin ME, Park D, Munger K. Tumor suppressor $p16^{INK4A}$ is necessary for survival of cervical carcinoma cell lines. *Proc Natl Acad Sci USA.* 2013;110:16175–16180.
56. Gollin SM. Cytogenetic alterations and their molecular genetic correlates in head and neck squamous cell carcinoma: a next generation window to the biology of disease. *Genes Chromosomes Cancer.* 2014;53:972–990.
57. Wagner S, Würdemann N, Hübbers C, et al. HPV-assoziierte kopf-hals-carzinome: mutationssignaturen und genomische abberrationen [HPV-associated head and neck cancer: mutational signature and genomic aberrations]. *HNO.* 2015;63:758–767.
58. Hajek M, Sewell A, Kaech S, et al. *TRAF3/CYLD* mutations identify a distinct subset of human papillomavirus-associated head and neck squamous cell carcinoma. *Cancer.* 2017;123:1778–1790.
59. Agrawal N, Frederick MJ, Pickering CR, et al. Exome sequencing of head and neck squamous cell carcinoma

reveals inactivating mutations in *NOTCH1*. *Science.* 2011;333:1154–1157.
60. Stransky N, Egloff AM, Tward AD, et al. The mutational landscape of head and neck squamous cell carcinoma. *Science.* 2011;333:1157–1160.
61. Lechner M, Frampton GM, Fenton T, et al. Targeted next-generation sequencing of head and neck squamous cell carcinoma identifies novel genetic alterations in HPV+ and HPV- tumors. *Genome Med.* 2013;5:49.
62. Seiwert TY, Zuo Z, Keck MK, et al. Integrative and comparative genomic analysis of HPV-positive and HPV-negative head and neck squamous cell carcinomas. *Clin Cancer Res.* 2015;21:632–641.
63. Sewell A, Brown B, Biktasova A, et al. Reverse-phase protein array profiling of oropharyngeal cancer and significance of PIK3CA mutations in HPV-associated head and neck cancer. *Clin Cancer Res.* 2014;20:2300–2311.
64. Hayes DN, Van Waes C, Seiwert TY. Genetic landscape of human papillomavirus-associated head and neck cancer and comparison to tobacco-related tumors. *J Clin Oncol.* 2015;33:3227–3234.
65. Prigge E-S, Urban K, Stiegler S, et al. No evidence of oncogenic *KRAS* mutations in squamous cell carcinomas of the anogenital tract and head and neck region independent of human papillomavirus and p16^{INK4a} status. *Hum Pathol.* 2014;45:2347–2354.
66. Berns K, Hijmans EM, Mullenders J, et al. A large-scale RNAi screen in human cells identifies new components of the p53 pathway. *Nature.* 2004;428:431–437.
67. Klussmann JP, Mooren JJ, Lehnen M, et al. Genetic signatures of HPV-related and unrelated oropharyngeal carcinoma and their prognostic implications. *Clin Cancer Res.* 2009;15:1779–1786.
68. Reed AL, Califano J, Cairns P, et al. High frequency of *p16 (CDKN2/MTS-1/INK4A)* inactivation in head and neck squamous cell carcinoma. *Cancer Res.* 1996;56:3630–3633.
69. Mooren JJ, Kremer B, Claessen SM, et al. Chromosome stability in tonsillar squamous cell carcinoma is associated with HPV16 integration and indicates a favorable prognosis. *Int J Cancer.* 2013;132:1781–1789.
70. Olthof NC, Speel EJ, Kolligs J, et al. Comprehensive analysis of HPV16 integration in OSCC reveals no significant impact of physical status on viral oncogene and virally disrupted human gene expression. *PLOS ONE.* 2014;9:e88718.
71. Olthof NC, Huebbers CU, Kolligs J, et al. Viral load, gene expression and mapping of viral integration sites in HPV16-associated HNSCC cell lines. *Int J Cancer.* 2015;136:E207–E218.
72. Nulton TJ, Olex AL, Dozmorov M, et al. Analysis of the cancer genome atlas sequencing data reveals novel properties of the human papillomavirus 16 genome in head and neck squamous cell carcinoma. *Oncotarget.* 2017;8(11):17684–17699.
73. Rodriguez-Paredes M, Esteller M. Cancer epigenetics reaches mainstream oncology. *Nat Med.* 2011;17:330–339.
74. Azad N, Zahnow CA, Rudin CM, Baylin SB. The future of epigenetic therapy in solid tumours—lessons from the past. *Nat Rev Clin Oncol.* 2013;10:256–266.
75. Thierry F. Transcriptional regulation of the papillomavirus oncogenes by cellular and viral transcription factors in cervical carcinoma. *Virology.* 2009;384:375–379.
76. Chaiwongkot A, Vinokurova S, Pientong C, et al. Differential methylation of E2 binding sites in episomal and integrated HPV 16 genomes in preinvasive and invasive cervical lesions. *Int J Cancer.* 2013;132:2087–2094.
77. Reuschenbach M, Huebbers CU, Prigge ES, et al. Methylation status of HPV16 E2-binding sites classifies subtypes of HPV-associated oropharyngeal cancers. *Cancer.* 2015;121:1966–1976.
78. Kostareli E, Holzinger D, Bogatyrova O, Hielscher T, et al. HPV-related methylation signature predicts survival in oropharyngeal squamous cell carcinomas. *J Clin Invest.* 2013;123:2488–2501.
79. Minarovits J, Demcsak A, Banati F, Niller HH. Epigenetic dysregulation in virus-associated neoplasms. *Adv Exp Med Biol.* 2016;879:71–90.
80. Lechner M, Fenton T, West J, et al. Identification and functional validation of HPV-mediated hypermethylation in head and neck squamous cell carcinoma. *Genome Med.* 2013;5:15.
81. Sartor MA, Dolinoy DC, Jones TR, et al. Genome-wide methylation and expression differences in HPV(+) and HPV(-) squamous cell carcinoma cell lines are consistent with divergent mechanisms of carcinogenesis. *Epigenetics.* 2011;6:777–7787.
82. Lleras RA, Smith RV, Adrien LR, et al. Unique DNA methylation loci distinguish anatomic site and HPV status in head and neck squamous cell carcinoma. *Clin Cancer Res.* 2013;19:5444–5455.
83. Schlecht NF, Ben-Dayan M, Anayannis N, et al. Epigenetic changes in the *CDKN2A* locus are associated with differential expression of P16INK4A and P14ARF in HPV-positive oropharyngeal squamous cell carcinoma. *Cancer Med.* 2015;4:342–353.
84. Chalertpet K, Pakdeechaidan W, Patel V, et al. Human papillomavirus type 16 E7 oncoprotein mediates CCNA1 promoter methylation. *Cancer Sci.* 2015;106:1333–1340.
85. Kostareli E, Hielscher T, Zucknick M, et al. Gene promoter methylation signature predicts survival of head and neck squamous cell carcinoma patients. *Epigenetics.* 2016;11:61–73.
86. Lee RC, Feinbaum RL, Ambros V. The C. elegans heterochronic gene *lin-4* encodes small RNAs with antisense complementarity to *lin-14*. *Cell.* 1993;75:843–854.
87. Lajer CB, Nielsen FC, Friis-Hansen L, et al. Different miRNA signatures of oral and pharyngeal squamous cell carcinomas: a prospective translational study. *Br J Cancer.* 2011;104:830–840.
88. Lajer CB, Garnaes E, Friis-Hansen L, et al. The role of miRNAs in human papilloma virus (HPV)-associated cancers: bridging between HPV-related head and neck cancer and cervical cancer. *Br J Cancer.* 2012;106:1526–1534.
89. Wald AI, Hoskins EE, Wells SI, et al. Alteration of microRNA profiles in squamous cell carcinoma of the head and neck cell lines by human papillomavirus. *Head Neck.* 2011;33:504–512.

90. Miller DL, Davis JW, Taylor KH, et al. Identification of a human papillomavirus-associated oncogenic miRNA panel in human oropharyngeal squamous cell carcinoma validated by bioinformatics analysis of the Cancer Genome Atlas. *Am J Pathol.* 2015;185: 679–692.
91. Gao G, Gay HA, Chernock RD, et al. A microRNA expression signature for the prognosis of oropharyngeal squamous cell carcinoma. *Cancer.* 2013;119:72–80.
92. Keating PJ, Cromme FV, Duggan-Keen M, et al. Frequency of down-regulation of individual HLA-A and -B alleles in cervical carcinomas in relation to TAP-1 expression. *Br J Cancer.* 1995;72:405–411.
93. Wagner S, Wittekindt C, Reuschenbach M, et al. CD56-positive lymphocyte infiltration in relation to human papillomavirus association and prognostic significance in oropharyngeal squamous cell carcinoma. *Int J Cancer.* 2016;138:2263–2273.
94. Geiger JL, Grandis JR, Bauman JE. The STAT3 pathway as a therapeutic target in head and neck cancer: Barriers and innovations. *Oral Oncol.* 2016;56:84–92.
95. Parsel SM, Grandis JR, Thomas SM. Nucleic acid targeting: towards personalized therapy for head and neck cancer. *Oncogene.* 2016;35:3217–3226.
96. Ausoni S, Boscolo-Rizzo P, Singh B, et al. Targeting cellular and molecular drivers of head and neck squamous cell carcinoma: current options and emerging perspectives. *Cancer Metastasis Rev.* 2016;35:413–426.
97. Moser R, Xu C, Kao M, et al. Functional kinomics identifies candidate therapeutic targets in head and neck cancer. *Clin Cancer Res.* 2014;20:4274–4288.

4

HPV-Related Head and Neck Cancer Biology

Farhoud Faraji
Carole Fakhry

Human papillomavirus (HPV) was first detected in human malignancies of the head and neck over 30 years ago (1,2). Yet less than a decade has passed since its formal recognition as an etiologic agent in head and neck squamous cell carcinoma (HNSCC) (3). More recently, a subset of HPV-related HNSCC, HPV-related oropharyngeal squamous cell carcinoma (HPV-positive OPC), has been recognized as a distinct neoplastic entity and one of only a few malignancies that continues to increase in incidence (4–6).

HNSCC comprises a heterogeneous group of tumors arising from the squamous epithelium of the upper aerodigestive tract (7). HNSCC is clinically divided by anatomic subsite into tumors arising from the oral cavity, nasopharynx, oropharynx, hypopharynx, and larynx. While HPV has been detected in HNSCC of all subsites (8), it exhibits a tendency to transform the squamous epithelium overlying the palatine and lingual tonsils, constituents of oropharyngeal lymphoid tissue known collectively as Waldeyer's ring (7,9,10).

The emergence of HPV-positive OPC as a distinct neoplastic entity has led to paradigm shifts in the staging and treatment of this subset of HNSCC. HPV-positive OPC is markedly more responsive to treatment than HPV-negative HNSCC and HPV-positive tumor status confers a significant survival advantage (11,12). However, current staging recommendations were developed in the context of HPV-negative HNSCC (13). Indeed, the 7th edition of the American Joint Committee on Cancer *Cancer Staging Manual* (AJCC-7th) (14), are inadequate to stratify prognosis in HPV-positive OPC (13,15–17). This observation has resulted in efforts to define an independent clinical staging strategy specific for HPV-positive OPC (16,18–21).

The current therapeutic standard of care was established prior to the widespread recognition that HPV-positive OPC exhibited improved prognosis relative to HPV-negative OPC (22–25). These therapeutic regimens may be more intense than necessary for HPV-positive disease (26). Clinical trials have thus been implemented to test therapeutic de-intensification protocols striving to mitigate long-term toxicities associated with the current standard of care for HNSCC while maintaining high response rates (27). The success of de-intensification protocols hinges on the accurate selection of patients at low risk of disease progression.

Key questions remain regarding the clinical impact of HPV-related HNSCC. The influence of HPV status remains unclear in nonoropharyngeal HNSCC (28,29). Recent studies are beginning to clarify whether HPV acts as an oncogenic driver in nonoropharyngeal HNSCC, and if HPV-positive nonoropharyngeal HNSCC also confers improved survival (30). Second, despite its favorable prognosis, greater than one-third of patients with HPV-positive OPC who respond to current therapeutic modalities experience recurrence in 8 years (31). The successful implementation of therapeutic de-intensification will rely on correctly identifying patients at high risk for recurrence. Whether the current paradigm of staging patients based on tumor status, lymph node involvement, and distant metastatic status (TNM) will be adequate to predict recurrence in HPV-positive OPC remains unanswered.

This chapter reviews evidence supporting the conclusion that HPV-positive HNSCC is a distinct neoplastic process from HPV-negative HNSCC and discusses ongoing efforts toward novel strategies to predict prognosis in HPV-positive OPC.

A DISTINCT ENTITY

This section reviews epidemiologic and molecular evidence establishing HPV-positive HNSCC as a distinct neoplastic entity.

EPIDEMIOLOGY

Divergent Risk Factor Profiles in HPV-Positive and HPV-Negative HNSCC

Most HNSCCs result from exposure to one of two independent but complementary classes of risk factors: chemical and infectious. Alcohol and tobacco are classical risk factors of HNSCC and sources of chemical carcinogens that give rise to HPV-negative HNSCC (32–34). HPV constitutes the primary infectious cause of HPV-positive HNSCC (35).

Chemical mutagens contained in tobacco inactivate key HNSCC tumor suppressors, rendering tobacco use a strong, independent risk factor in HPV-negative HNSCC (36–39). Alcohol is another source of carcinogens (32) and an independent risk factor for HPV-negative HNSCC (33,34). Although rare in the West, the cultural practice of chewing "paan" (areca nut with lime folded in betel leaf) is another important independent HNSCC risk factor in parts of Asia and East Africa (40–42).

Alcohol and tobacco were established as independent risk factors of HNSCC in a pooled analysis of 15 case-control studies. This study examined HNSCC risk in tobacco smokers among never-users of alcohol (1587 cases, 4051 controls), and alcohol use among never-users of tobacco (1072 cases, 5775 controls) (34). In never-users of alcohol, those who had ever smoked were two times more likely to develop HNSCC. A dose–response relationship was also observed, with subjects who smoked 31–40 cigarettes per day significantly more likely to develop HNSCC than those who smoked 1–10 cigarettes per day (odds ratio [OR]: 4.5 vs. 1.8). Dose–response relationships were also observed for duration in years and cumulative tobacco consumed in pack-years. Among never-users of tobacco, participants who had ever used alcohol exhibited a modest but statistically significant increase in risk (OR: 1.18). Heavy alcohol consumption of greater than four drinks per day was associated with 2.8-fold increase in risk (34).

HPV is the most common sexually transmitted infection in the United States and the primary infectious cause of HNSCC (43,44). Nearly 200 types of HPV have been described based on the sequence diversity of the viral gene encoding the L1 capsid protein (45). Of these, oncogenic (serotypes 16, 18, 31, 33, 45, 51, 52, 56, 58, 59, and 68) and nononcogenic types (11, 32, 44, 53, 57, and 81) have been detected in HNSCC tumor samples (46–50). Yet, a single type, HPV16, is found in 87%–96% of HPV-positive OPC and 68%–74% of HPV-positive non-OPC (8,50,51).

Compared to HPV-negative disease, HPV-positive HNSCC is more common in younger patients and those with a history of high-risk sexual behaviors (6,52). Number of lifetime oral sexual partners is the strongest and most specific risk factor in HPV-positive HNSCC (52,53). A pooled analysis of four case-control studies with participants from 12 countries over five continents (5,642 cases, 6,069 controls) found a history of four or more oral–genital sex partners most strongly increased the risk of squamous cell carcinoma of the tonsil and base of tongue, anatomic subsites of the oropharynx (54). Younger age at sexual debut, increasing number of vaginal sexual partners, history of oral–anal sex, and a history of same-sex sexual contact among men also increased risk for HPV-positive OPC (54).

High-risk sexual behavior is an independent risk factor for oral HPV infection. Lifetime history of greater than 10 oral sex or 25 vaginal sex partners resulted in a respective increase in oral HPV infection of 5.2-fold or 3.9-fold (53). A large cross-sectional study (n = 5579) conducted as part of the National Health and Nutrition Examination Survey (NHANES) extended these findings, demonstrating that individuals who ever performed oral or vaginal sex were at 2.2-fold or 5.4-fold greater risk of oral HPV infection, respectively (55). The NHANES study also found that HPV16 represented the most prevalent oral HPV infection of the 37 tested HPV types, accounting for 27% of high-risk HPV types and 15% of all detected oral HPV type-specific infections (55). Considered together with data indicating oral HPV infection is associated with a 53-fold greater risk of HPV-positive HNSCC (52), these findings support the sexual transmission of oral HPV infection.

Although not central to HPV-related oncogenesis, tobacco and alcohol exposure can modify risk in HPV-positive HNSCC. Compared to HPV-negative HNSCC, patients with HPV-positive HNSCC are less likely to report a history of heavy tobacco use (52). Current tobacco users, however, are three times more likely to have oral HPV16 infection compared to never or former tobacco users (56). Moreover, serum and urinary levels of tobacco-related metabolites display dose–response relationships with increasing odds of HPV16 infection (56). Similarly, heavy alcohol consumption increases risk of oral HPV infection, with greater than 21 drinks per week resulting in a 19-fold greater risk of oral HPV infection (57). The increased prevalence of oral HPV infection in current tobacco and heavy alcohol users suggests an indirect means by which tobacco and alcohol use increases risk for HPV-positive HNSCC.

In summary, the risk factor profiles contributing to carcinogenesis in HPV-positive and HPV-negative HNSCC are largely distinct. Sexual behavior is the most important risk factor in HPV-positive HNSCC, while heavy tobacco and alcohol use are the strongest risk factors in HPV-negative HNSCC. Diverging trends in the incidences of HPV-positive and HPV-negative HNSCC are generally attributed to societal shifts that have driven changes in exposures to these risk factors.

Incidence Trends in HPV-Positive and HPV-Negative HNSCC

Direct assessment of long-term trends of HPV-positive HNSCC has been impeded by the absence of HPV status in historical epidemiologic datasets. Investigations into incidence trends of HPV-related HNSCC have thus relied on observations that HPV was most consistently associated with HNSCC arising from Waldeyer's ring (58,59). These studies considered HNSCC arising from oropharyngeal subsites (base of tongue, palatine tonsils, and lingual tonsils) as HPV-related and HNSCC arising from nonoropharyngeal subsites (oral cavity, larynx, and hypopharynx) as HPV-unrelated (60). Supporting this approach, a recent worldwide meta-analysis found HPV to be a likely cause of HNSCC in 40% of oropharyngeal tumors but only 19% of laryngeal and hypopharyngeal tumors and 7% of oral cavity tumors (8).

Over the past four decades, shifts have been observed in the distribution of anatomic subsites of HNSCC. Incidence rates of HNSCC arising from HPV-related subsites have increased while HNSCC arising from HPV-unrelated subsites have declined (60). Consistently, direct testing of tumor HPV status of 271 OPC tumors in the United States from 1984 to 2004 revealed that the incidence of HPV-positive OPC increased by 225%, while the incidence of HPV-negative OPC declined by 50% (61). These changes in incidence have been attributed to a successful public health campaign resulting in diminishing tobacco use, and a shift in sexual practices that increase risk of exposure to HPV.

Epidemiologic data linking the rise in incidence rates of HPV-positive HNSCC to cohorts born in the latter half of the 20th century offer another line of evidence implicating sexual behavior in HPV-related carcinogenesis (60,62). Analyses of the Surveillance, Epidemiology, and End Results (SEER) data from 1975 to 2011 found that men aged 40 to 70 years showed significant increases in the incidence of OPC in successive birth cohorts after 1940 (60,62). This birth cohort effect coincided with trends in sexual behavior likely to increase sexual transmission of HPV. Sexual behavior over the 20th century has trended toward younger age at sexual debut and an increase in the average number of sexual partners (63–65). A cross-sectional analysis of sexual practices and oral HPV infection showed that age cohort no longer associated with oral HPV infection after accounting for oral sexual behavior (66). This observation supported the notion that trends in the incidence of HPV-positive OPC in more recent birth cohorts are a result of trends of increased exposure to oral HPV infection.

Meanwhile, the declining incidence of HPV-negative HNSCC has been largely attributed to worldwide declines in tobacco and alcohol consumption. In the United States, smoking and alcohol consumption have declined by 42% and 20%, respectively (15,67). An international survey examining incidence trends of HPV-unrelated and HPV-related HNSCC subsites found that countries exhibiting decreasing trends in HPV-unrelated HNSCC also displayed significant declines in squamous cell carcinoma of the lung, a strongly tobacco-related tumor (68).

MOLECULAR PATHOPHYSIOLOGY

Distinctions between HPV-positive and HPV-negative HNSCC extend beyond risk factor profiles to key differences in the molecular pathophysiology of these HNSCC subtypes. *TP53*, the most mutated tumor suppressor gene in malignancy (69), whose gene product is the p53 protein, is also commonly mutated in HNSCC (38,70). Early molecular investigations showed that *TP53* mutation in HNSCC was strongly correlated with smoking (71,72). This is consistent with smoking as a major risk factor for HPV-negative tumors, as tobacco smoke contains numerous chemicals extensively shown to cause oncogenic mutations, including specific mutations in *TP53* (73–75). These early investigations also revealed that *TP53* mutations occurred at markedly lower rates in HPV-positive tumors (71,72). Comprehensive genome profiling of HNSCC has confirmed these findings and demonstrated that HPV-positive HNSCC displays a significantly lower overall mutation rate and far fewer mutations in canonical oncogenic driver genes (76–78).

The reduced mutational burden of HPV-positive HNSCC is likely related to a lower incidence of heavy alcohol and tobacco use in this patient population (52), and HPV-driven tumorigenesis may not require mutation of key tumor suppressor genes. The HPV genome encodes viral oncogenes that inactivate host cellular tumor suppressive pathways. HPV oncoprotein E6 binds the p53 and marks it for proteolytic degradation (79). The oncogenic activity of HPV oncoprotein E7 involves the targeting of the retinoblastoma tumor suppressor protein, Rb, for degradation (80). Rb serves to sequester the mitogenic transcription factor E2F in the cytoplasm; its degradation results in the translocation of E2F into the nucleus and expression of proliferative genes (81,82). The degradation of Rb also initiates a regulatory cascade that induces compensatory upregulation of another tumor suppressor, $p16^{INK4A}$ (p16) (83). This paradigm forms the basis of p16 immunohistochemistry as one method for attributing HPV as the etiologic driver of OPC (84). Interestingly, while p16 is diffusely expressed in HPV-positive HNSCC, homozygous deletion of the gene locus encoding p16, *CDKN2A*, is frequently observed in HPV-negative tumors and is strongly associated with tobacco and alcohol use (78,85,86). Distinctions between HPV-positive and HPV-negative HNSCC exist in the molecular pathophysiology of these diseases as well as their risk factor profile and epidemiology. Further elucidation of these distinctions and integrating molecular findings with clinical presentations may facilitate clinicians' ability to determine prognosis and optimally manage patients with HPV-positive HNSCC.

PROGNOSIS OF HPV-RELATED HNSCC

PROGNOSIS OF HPV-POSITIVE OPC

The effect of HPV on survival represents its most significant impact on clinical practice. HPV-positive tumor status at diagnosis is well established as a favorable prognostic indicator in OPC. However, the effect of HPV on survival in nonoropharyngeal HNSCC subsites remains incompletely understood. Early studies establishing the causal relationship of HPV in HNSCC noted improved disease-specific survival associated with HPV-positive HNSCC (6,87).

The survival benefit of HPV-positive OPC was directly demonstrated in a prospective study of 96 patients with stage III or IV HNSCC treated with induction chemotherapy followed by definitive chemoradiotherapy (CRT) as part of an Eastern Cooperative Oncology Group (ECOG) 2399 phase II trial (12). In this study, all HPV-positive HNSCC were confined to the oropharynx; HPV-negative tumors were derived from the oropharynx (41%) or larynx (59%). After median follow-up of 39 months, patients with HPV-positive disease were found to exhibit better progression-free survival (PFS) and overall survival (OS). Two-year PFS in HPV-positive versus HPV-negative HNSCC was 86% versus 51%; 2-year OS was 95% versus 62%. Multivariate analysis found that HPV status reduced risk of death 64% and was prognostic independent of age, tumor stage, or ECOG performance status (12).

Since this report, other prospective studies have consistently observed survival benefits for HPV-positive OPC relative to HPV-negative OPC (11,88). Meta-analysis of 42 studies found that, compared to HPV-negative HNSCC, patients with HPV-positive disease displayed

54% better OS (89). Multivariate analysis of pooled data showed HPV-positive disease was associated with a 72% reduction in disease-specific death, independent of age and tumor stage (89). Thus, over the past several years, multiple lines of evidence have demonstrated the favorable effect of HPV-positive status on OPC.

PROGNOSIS OF HPV-POSITIVE NON-OPC

Clinical Cohort Studies

Recent studies are beginning to elucidate the impact of HPV status on survival in nonoropharyngeal HNSCC. Using p16 as a surrogate marker for tumor HPV status (90) in a large Danish cohort, Lassen and colleagues compared the effect of p16-status on survival in stage III/IV OPC and non-OPC (28). Consistent with previous findings, p16-positive OPC (n = 425) was associated with dramatically improved locoregional control (80% vs. 52%), event-free survival (67% vs. 31%), and OS (80% vs. 37%) at 5 years compared to p16-negative OPC (n = 390). Conversely, p16-status showed no effect on survival in hypopharyngeal and laryngeal HNSCC (p16-positive n = 65, p16-negative n = 414). These findings do, however, require the consideration of important caveats. Reliance on p16 as a sole surrogate for HPV status presents a major limitation in discerning the role of HPV in non-OPC survival. Although p16- and HPV status show high concordance (~90%) in OPC (11), p16-status exhibited an unacceptably low positive predictive value for HNSCC subsites with low fractions of HPV-driven tumors (91). In the study by Lassen et al., only 13% of non-OPC were positive for p16. Considering other reports on the relationship of p16 and HPV status (29), even fewer non-OPC tumors in this study would likely be HPV-positive, complicating conclusions of HPV status on survival in non-OPC. Indeed, the small number of p16-positive non-OPC tumors may have lacked the statistical power to observe survival effects of p16 status. Data have since arisen, suggesting that p16 status may be a prognostic indicator in both OPC (92) and non-OPC (29,93).

Secondary analysis of three Radiation Therapy Oncology Group (RTOG) trials, which comprise prospectively collected data from randomized controlled trials representing higher quality data than a retrospective cohort, provided the first evidence that positive p16 status may be prognostic in non-OPC (29). In this study, HPV and p16 status were ascertainable in 297 and 322 patients, respectively, of 683 eligible patients with oral cavity, hypopharyngeal, and laryngeal HNSCC enrolled in RTOG trials 0129, 0234, and 0522. In combined analysis of non-OPC subsites, p16-positive tumors exhibited better PFS and OS than p16-negative tumors after adjustment for known prognostic factors, including age, sex, T stage, and N stage (hazard ratio [HR] (adj PFS) = 0.63, HR (adj OS) = 0.56). Comparison of p16-status in non-OPC to OPC demonstrated a survival hierarchy dependent on both anatomic subsite and p16-status. The class of HNSCC showing the most favorable prognosis was p16-positive OPC (5-year PFS = 69%, OS = 80%) followed by p16-positive non-OPC (5-year PFS = 55%, OS = 64%). The poorest survival was observed in p16-negative HNSCC, with p16-negative OPC and non-OPC demonstrating no significant differences (5-year PFS = 37% and 34%, OS = 46% and 44%, respectively) (29). Although shedding insight into the role of p16 status on the outcome of non-OPC, this analysis was limited in its ability to resolve the role of HPV status in non-OPC survival. The implementation of more effective markers of HPV status in these tumors are thus key to firmly establishing the effect of HPV status on survival in non-OPC.

A recent multi-institutional retrospective study (n = 860) implemented combined testing for p16 and HPV16 status to investigate the role of HPV status on survival in HNSCC in a population intentionally oversampled for women and non-Whites (94,95). While patients with HPV-positive OPC demonstrated significantly improved survival compared to HPV-negative OPC (5-year OS = 79% vs. 42%, 10-year OS = 58% vs. 29%), patients with HPV-positive and HPV-negative non-OPC had similar survival (5-year OS = 56% vs. 52%, 10-year OS = 42% vs. 36%) (95). Similarly, p16 status was predictive of survival in OPC but not in non-OPC. HPV-positive OPC also demonstrated a nonsignificant trend toward improved recurrence-free survival (RFS) compared to HPV-negative OPC (5-year RFS: 86% vs. 77%, p = .14). Interestingly, this study also found differences in survival with respect to sex and race. After adjustment for HPV status, age, tobacco use, and disease stage, women with OPC but not non-OPC exhibited a significant reduction (45%) in risk of death. Indeed, HPV status and female sex were independent favorable prognostic factors on multivariate analysis (95).

Integrative Analysis of Molecular and Clinical Data

Understanding the intricacies of HPV-positive HNSCC at multiple scales, from epidemiologic to molecular, will facilitate the development of novel risk assessment and therapeutic strategies. Recent efforts have been directed toward developing molecular tools capable of identifying HPV etiology in HNSCC with high confidence. Analysis of The Cancer Genome Atlas (TCGA) multicenter cohort provided the most direct and mechanistic view into the survival impact of HPV at oropharyngeal and nonoropharyngeal subsites (30). In this study, Chakravarthy and colleagues interrogated ribonucleic acid (RNA)-sequencing data from 520 TCGA HNSCC tumors for HPV transcripts. HNSCC tumor RNA found to contain HPV transcripts were defined as HPV-positive samples. This method of identifying HPV-etiologic tumors is equivalent in principle to the current "gold standard": amplification of HPV-specific RNA in tumor samples by quantitative reverse transcriptase polymerase chain reaction (96,97).

Chakravarthy et al. then employed differential gene expression analysis and machine learning algorithms to identify a 159-gene expression signature (GES) common to HPV-driven tumors across diverse tissue types, including squamous cell carcinoma of the uterine cervix, HNSCC, and vulvar intraepithelial neoplasia. Both infection of cultured keratinocytes with HPV and forced expression of HPV E6 and E7 oncogenes in mesenchymal stem cells induced expression of this 159-GES (30). Pathway analysis demonstrated that upstream regulators of the 159-GES included p53 inhibition, a canonical effect of E6 activity, and E2F activation, a canonical effect of E7-mediated Rb degradation (30). Collectively, this constellation of in vivo and in vitro findings strongly suggested that this 159-GES was directly regulated by viral oncogenes and represented a reliable method to attribute HPV as the etiologic factor in tumors that expressed this signature. Indeed, implementing the 159-GES to segregate HPV-positive and -negative HNSCC samples in TCGA resulted in high-fidelity clustering of HPV-positive samples independent of anatomic subsite (30).

In addition to similar patterns of virus-mediated gene expression, HPV-positive OPC and non-OPC exhibited (a) similar genome-wide methylation patterns, which distinguished HPV-positive and HPV-negative HNSCC (30), and (b) a characteristic mutational pattern attributable to dysregulated activity of the cytidine deaminase APOBEC (98). Finally, HPV-positive non-OPC were also found to display a basaloid morphology (30), a histologic feature long associated with HPV-positive OPC (99). These findings collectively provided the most direct evidence to date supporting the notion that HPV-positive tumors are indeed caused by HPV, independent of anatomic subsite.

The identification of HPV-driven HNSCC in the molecularly and clinically well-defined TCGA dataset allowed for direct evaluation and integrative mechanistic analysis of the influence of HPV on OPC and non-OPC. Comparison of HPV transcript-positive HNSCC by subsite showed that only HPV-positive OPC was associated with improved OS while HPV-positive non-OPC showed similar survival to HPV-negative HNSCC. The difference in prognosis of HPV-positive OPC and non-OPC despite high molecular and cellular similarity was found be associated with differences in lymphocyte infiltration and activation. Indeed, previous studies have reported associations between tumor-infiltrating lymphocytes (TILs) and survival in HPV-positive OPC (100). Chakravarthy et al. demonstrated that compared to HPV-positive non-OPC, HPV-positive OPC tumors contained increased TILs on microscopic examination and increased expression of T-cell specific transcripts, such as CD4, CD8A, and CD8B on RNA analysis. Further examination of tumor RNA demonstrated that HPV-positive OPC tumors were enriched for immune checkpoint transcripts while HPV-positive non-OPC tumors showed depletion of these transcripts. Based on these findings, it can be reasonably concluded that although viral etiology plays a role in both HPV-positive OPC and non-OPC, it is not sufficient to confer a favorable prognosis. The unique prognosis of HPV-positive OPC may reflect physiologic differences in the nonoropharyngeal squamous epithelium of the upper aerodigestive tract and that of the specialized epithelium lining Waldeyer's ring (101–103).

Impact of HPV Status on Survival After First Event of Tumor Progression

Improved survival in patients with HPV-positive OPC also extends to patients who develop recurrent or metastatic (R/M) disease. In secondary analysis of RTOG 0129 and 0522, patients with p16-positive OPC who experienced disease progression exhibited significantly better prognosis than those with p16-negative OPC (104). HPV status has been reported to be independently associated with improved OS in R/M OPC who underwent salvage therapy (105,106). Although more data are necessary to elucidate the role of HPV status on survival in R/M OPC, current results suggest that select patients with HPV-positive R/M OPC are suitable candidates for curative-intent salvage therapy.

TRENDS IN THE MANAGEMENT OF HPV-RELATED OPC

Current multimodality treatment of OPC includes combinations of surgery, radiation therapy (RT), and chemotherapy. These therapeutic strategies were developed prior to the establishment of HPV-positive OPC as a distinct HNSCC subtype. The evolution of treatment paradigms in HNSCC has revolved around a balance of therapeutic response and treatment-related morbidity. This evolution in treatment has continued upon recognition of HPV-positive OPC as a distinctly treatment-sensitive HNSCC subtype. Ongoing clinical trials are focused on de-intensifying components of multimodality therapy, with the goal of mitigating acute and long-term therapeutic toxicity yet maintaining high response rates (107).

NONSURGICAL MANAGEMENT

The traditional mainstay of HNSCC therapy regardless of anatomic subsite involved primary surgical resection, often followed by RT (108). The oropharyngeal anatomy, however, is uniquely challenging to access surgically. Operative approaches for advanced-stage OPC require large incisions often accompanied by mandibulotomy or mandibular swing. These procedures have historically carried high rates of morbidity and require tracheostomy and gastrostomy (109). The treatment paradigm for HNSCC, however, began to evolve when large prospective trials (not specifically evaluating OPC) demonstrated definitive RT resulted in similar outcomes with considerably less morbidity than primary surgery (110,111).

A pooled analysis of 51 series compared outcomes of OPC treated with definitive RT versus primary surgery (112). Consistent with results reported for laryngeal HNSCC, definitive RT of OPC resulted in similar 5-year locoregional control, cause-specific survival, and OS with dramatically lower rates of severe and fatal complications (112). Definitive RT regimens have since been investigated intensively in OPC, demonstrating that hyperfractionation regimens—in which the total dose of radiation is divided into more frequent treatments of smaller doses—and accelerated fractionation regimens—in which the total dose of radiation is delivered in a shorter period (113)—both resulted in improved local control and survival (114). Unfortunately, compared with conventional fractionation, altered fractionation also increases risk of acute toxicity and requirement for gastrostomy tube placement (115).

The adoption of definitive RT as the mainstay of organ-preserving therapy in HNSCC has been accompanied by the concurrent administration of chemotherapy to radiation, known as CRT. Platinum- and taxane-based chemotherapeutics are effective radiosensitizers (116,117). In HNSCC of the larynx, CRT resulted in similar or improved locoregional control and survival compared to RT alone (118). CRT has also been found to improve locoregional control and survival compared to RT of advanced-stage OPC, although this study did not account for HPV status (25). Like advances in RT, increased control rates in CRT were accompanied by increases in toxicity (119). The Head and Neck Intergroup Phase III trial of standard RT versus two CRT regimens in unresectable HNSCC found that grade 3 or worse toxicity occurred in 52% RT-only patients but in 89% and 77% of patients receiving the two CRT regimens (24).

HPV status, however, had not yet been recognized as a prognostic factor in landmark trials leading to current therapeutic standards of care, precluding interpretation of these trials with respect to HPV status. Observations that HPV-positive OPC exhibited high response rates and significantly improved survival independently of treatment modality suggested that current therapeutic regimens were overly intense in a subset of HPV-positive OPC (120). The rising HPV-attributable fraction of OPC and its favorable effect on survival have thus led efforts to reevaluate therapeutic strategies for HPV-positive OPC (107).

RESURGENCE OF PRIMARY SURGICAL MANAGEMENT: A ROLE FOR MINIMALLY INVASIVE SURGERY

Advances in minimally invasive surgical techniques have reignited investigation into surgery as a possible means to mitigate high rates of severe acute and late toxicity associated with CRT (111). Both transoral laser microsurgery (TLM) and transoral robotic surgery (TORS) offer access to previously transorally inaccessible oropharyngeal tumors and show promising oncologic results with diminished morbidity profiles.

TLM and TORS are distinct modes of transoral endoscopic-assisted surgery. TLM employs endoscopic or microscopic visualization and carbon dioxide laser to transect and segmentally excise tumor (121). TORS with the da Vinci™ Surgical System carries several advantages, including three-dimensional visualization, miniaturized jointed instrumentation, and tremor filtering (122). Multiple groups have reported promising oncologic results with TORS as primary therapeutic modality in OPC (123–125).

Retrospective analyses of multicenter TLM cohorts showed comparable oncologic results to nonsurgical therapy but with better functional outcomes (121,126,127). Haughey and colleagues analyzed prospectively collected data from 204 patients who underwent TLM for OPC at three tertiary care centers in the United States (126). The analysis included tumor stages T1 to T4; 124 and 167 evaluable tumors were HPV and p16-positive, respectively. In addition to TLM, 97% of patients also underwent neck dissection, and 74% received adjuvant RT (58%) or CRT (16%). Investigators demonstrated a 2-year OS of 89% and a disease-specific survival of 91% for all tumor stages combined. Survival outcomes for TLM followed by adjuvant therapy were comparable to those observed in organ-preserving CRT (128). As might be expected, the intensity of adjuvant therapy revealed an inverse relationship between oncologic and functional outcomes. Patients receiving no adjuvant therapy showed the poorest survival rates but the most favorable swallowing outcomes; those receiving RT had intermediate survival rates and swallowing outcomes; and patients who received adjuvant CRT showed the most favorable survival but the poorest swallowing outcomes (126). Notably, local, regional, and distant recurrences were observed in node-positive disease of all tumor stages. Although HPV- or p16-positive OPC exhibited significantly better OS than HPV- or p16-negative OPC, disease-specific survival was not reported, and analysis of recurrent disease was not stratified by HPV or p16 status (126). A following retrospective analysis of 153 OPC patients who underwent TLM confirmed findings by Haughey et al. and demonstrated that HPV-positivity reduced 3-year risk of death and recurrence by 71% and 77%, respectively (127).

Weinstein and colleagues at the University of Pennsylvania reported the first prospective trial implementing TORS in OPC. Forty-seven patients with stage III/IV OPC were treated with primary TORS and staged neck dissection. Adjuvant therapy strategy was based on pathologic features, including stage, margin status, and extranodal extension. Disease-specific survival and disease-free survival at 2 years were 90% and 79%, respectively. These results were comparable to control rates reported for primary CRT of OPC (123,129–131). Importantly, tailoring adjuvant treatment to pathologic results allowed 38% of patients in the Weinstein et al. cohort to avoid adjuvant chemotherapy and 11% to avoid adjuvant therapy altogether. TORS has been touted to have superior functional outcomes to CRT. Only 1 of 47 (2.4%) patients treated with TORS was gastrostomy tube dependent at 1 year, while long-term gastrostomy tube dependency rates for CRT ranged from 9%–38% (119,129–131).

A systematic review compared oncologic and functional outcomes reported in TORS over 12 studies (n = 772) to intensity-modulated radiotherapy (IMRT) with or without concurrent chemotherapy in eight studies (n = 1287) as the primary treatment for OPC (132). Consistent with findings reported by Weinstein and colleagues (123), 2-year OS ranges were similar among patients treated with TORS (82%–94%) and IMRT (84%–96%). Disease-free survival at 2 years for IMRT across three studies ranged from 82% to 90% and was reported in a single TORS study at 79% (132). In addition, accumulating evidence supports improved swallowing and overall quality of life for patients treated with TORS compared to those treated with CRT (124,133,134).

More recently, the University of Pennsylvania group investigated the impact of HPV-positive OPC status on the oncologic outcomes of TORS (135). In this study, a significantly greater portion of HPV-positive patients (n = 37) were more likely to present with stage IV disease (51% vs. 31%) but better performance status and fewer comorbidities than HPV-negative patients (n = 13). Although these differences complicate interpretation of the impact of HPV status on oncologic outcomes of TORS, patients with HPV-positive OPC exhibited 2-year OS of 80%, identical to that observed in HPV-negative OPC. The HPV-positive group experienced two (5.4%) distant metastases but no local or regional recurrences.

TORS is emerging as a therapeutic modality with excellent oncologic and functional outcomes in OPC. Yet despite promising outcomes observed with novel therapeutic strategies, a portion of HPV-positive patients remains at risk for recurrence, distant metastasis, and poor prognosis, regardless of treatment modality. Further progress in the treatment of HPV-positive OPC thus necessitates novel strategies to classify risk of recurrence and overall prognosis.

TRENDS IN HPV-RELATED OPC STAGING

Groome and colleagues delineated four criteria for developing an effective TNM staging system (136). These criteria provide a framework through which performance of the currently accepted staging system for HNSCC—the AJCC-7th—and recently proposed staging systems may be evaluated. To be clinically useful, TNM stage groups must demonstrate: (a) hazard consistency—patients in the same stage group should exhibit similar survival rates; (b) hazard discrimination—patients in different groups should show significantly different survival rates; (c) outcome prediction—the staging system should predict prognosis with some consistency; and (d) balance—the distribution of patients into staging groups should be balanced (136).

Several teams have independently shown that AJCC-7th fails to meet the Groome criteria for HPV-positive OPC (16,20,21,137). First, staging HPV-positive OPC patients with AJCC-7th does not segregate patients into groups with significantly different prognoses. Compared to HPV-negative HNSCC, patients with HPV-positive OPC are more likely to present with smaller primary tumors and more advanced nodal disease (137,138). This unique aspect of HPV-positive OPC leads to an unbalanced distribution of patients into staging groups, with 93%–95% of patients classified as stage III/IV by AJCC-7th (16,21,137). Finally, AJCC-7th staging groups have repeatedly been shown incapable of predicting survival in HPV-positive OPC. This dissociation of staging and prognosis has led to recent attempts to devise a novel clinical staging system for HPV-positive OPC (17).

TOWARD A NEW STAGING SYSTEM FOR HPV-POSITIVE OPC

Early suggestions that a redesigned staging system might better predict prognosis in HPV-positive OPC derived from a reanalysis of RTOG 0129 to evaluate the impact of HPV status on survival in stage III/IV OPC (11). In this study, Ang and colleagues' multivariate analysis found age, race, performance status, tumor stage, nodal stage, and tobacco use to be significant determinants of OS and PFS. Ang et al. then implemented recursive partitioning analysis (RPA), a statistical algorithm that identifies variables that best partition risk groups and generates a tree-structured hierarchical staging model, to segregate patients into survival groups based on clinical variables significantly associated with survival (139). RPA resulted in three risk groups based on tumor (T) stage, nodal (N) stage, HPV status, and cumulative lifetime pack-years of tobacco smoked (py). Patients classified as low risk were either HPV-positive, any T and N stage, and <10 py (Group 1) or HPV-positive, any T stage, N0-N2a, and >10 py (Group 2). Intermediate-risk patients were classified as either HPV-positive, any T stage, N2b-N3, and >10 py (Group 3) or HPV-negative T2-3, any N stage, and <10 py (Group 4). High-risk patients were classified as either HPV-negative, T4, any N stage, and <10 py (Group 5) or HPV-negative, any T stage, any N stage, and >10 py (Group 6) (Table 4.1, Row A). This classification system divided patients into three well-balanced and well separated risk strata. Low-, intermediate-, and high-risk patients comprised 43%, 30%, and 27% of patients, respectively (Table 4.2, Row A). OS at 3 years for low-, intermediate-, and high-risk was 93%, 71%, and 46%, respectively (Figure 4.1). In summary, Ang and colleagues found HPV-positive patients to be low risk unless presenting with both advanced nodal disease and >10 py history of smoking, in which case they were classified with low risk HPV-negative tumors. In this early example, HPV status was considered a prognostic factor rather than a distinguishing disease feature. Subsequent staging proposals strived to classify risk specifically for HPV-positive OPC.

TABLE 4.1

Characteristics of Proposed HPV-Positive OPC Staging Systems and Study Features

Study	*n*	Method	Validation	Design	Primary Treatment *n* (%)
A. Ang et al. (2010) (11)	266	RPA	None	Secondary analysis of RTOG 0129: Prospective multicenter randomized controlled trial	Radiation + chemo: 266 (100%)
B. Huang et al. (2015) (16)	573	RPA RPA + age + pack-years	1) Internal: Bootstrap 2) Imputation of HPV-unknown samples Failed external validation by Dahlstrom et al.	Retrospective single institution	Radiation +/− chemo: 573 (100%)
C. MDACC Dahlstrom et al. (2016) (20)	661	RPA	Imputation of HPV-unknown samples	Retrospective single institution	Radiation +/− chemo: 649 (98%) Surgery: 12 (2%)
D. ICON-S O'Sullivan et al. (2016) (21)	t: 661 v: 1246	AHR	External: Multicenter, multinational cohort	Retrospective multicenter multinational	Radiation+/− chemo: 1873 (98%) Surgery: 34 (2%)
E. Hussain et al. (2017) (144)	5,626	RPA	Internal: Bootstrap	Retrospective National Cancer Database	Radiation +/− chemo: 3175 (56%) Surgery: 2350 (42%)

Note: Each study proposing a staging system for HPV-positive OPC is listed by row (A–E). Characteristics of each study are listed including number of patients in each study cohort (*n*), statistical method for partitioning risk groups (method), approach for validating staging system (validation), overall study design, and differences in primary treatment.

AHR, adjusted hazard ratio; chemo, chemotherapy; ICON-S, International Collaboration on Oropharyngeal cancer Staging; MDACC, MD Anderson Cancer Center; OPC, oropharyngeal cancer; RPA, recursive partitioning analysis; t, ICON-S training cohort; v, ICON-S validation cohort.

The initial efforts by Ang and colleagues to account for HPV status in survival raise important lessons for devising a novel staging system. First, limitations of the risk stratification method by Ang et al. included its relatively small sample size (n = 266), resulting in very small populations in Group 2 (n = 26), Group 4 (n = 15), and Group 5 (n = 8). Stratification of 266 patients into six groups, some of which are relatively small, has the inherent risk of being overly reliant on outliers, or "overfitting" (140). Second, Ang et al. did not validate their risk stratification system in an external dataset (141). Careful consideration of overfitting and validation of any proposed staging system on independent data will be central to implementing a novel system that faithfully stratifies risk in HPV-positive OPC.

The attempt by Huang and colleagues at the Princess Margaret Cancer Centre (PMCC) to refine the AJCC-7th TNM staging groups for HPV-positive OPC highlighted the importance of external validation in devising a reproducible staging system (16). Employing

TABLE 4.2

Proposed HPV-Positive OPC Staging Systems: Staging Criteria and Patient Distributions

	Risk Group 1		Risk Group 2		Risk Group 3		Risk Group 4		Risk Group 5	
Study	**Criteria**	**n (%)**	**Criteria**	**n (%)**	**Criteria**	**n (%)**	**Criteria**	**n (%)**	**Criteria**	**n (%)**
A. Ang et al. 2010 (11)	HPV-pos ≤10 PY - or - HPV-pos N0 – N2a >10 PY	178 (43%)	HPV-pos N2b – N3 >10 PY - or - HPV-neg T2 – T3 <10 PY	79 (30%)	HPV-neg, T4 - or - HPV-neg >10 PY	73 (27%)	–	–	–	–
B. Huang et al. 2015 (16)	T1 – T3 N0 – N2b	335 (58%)	T1 – T3 N2c	91 (16%)	T4 - or - N3	147 (26%)	M1	0	–	–
	T1 – T3 N0 – N2c ≤20 PY	283 (49%)	T1 – T3 N0 – N2c >20 PY	143 (25%)	T4 - or - N3 ≤70 YO	120 (21%)	T4 - or - N3 >70 YO	27 (5%)	M1	0
C. <u>MDACC</u> Dahlstrohm et al. 2016 (20)	T1 N0 – N2*	195 (30%)	T2 N0 – N2*	219 (33%)	T1 – T2, N3* - or - T3	171 (26%)	T4	76 (11%)	M1	0

(continued)

TABLE 4.2 (*continued*)

Proposed HPV-Positive OPC Staging Systems: Staging Criteria and Patient Distributions

	Risk Group 1		Risk Group 2		Risk Group 3		Risk Group 4		Risk Group 5	
Study	**Criteria**	**n (%)**	**Criteria**	**n (%)**	**Criteria**	**n (%)**	**Criteria**	**n (%)**	**Criteria**	**n (%)**
D. ICON-S O'Sullivan et al. 2016 (21)	T1 – T2 N0 – N2b	t: 277 (42%) v: 685 (55%)	T1 – T2 N2c - or - T3 N0 – N2b	t: 221 (33%) v: 343 (28%)	T4 - or - N3	t: 163 (25%) v: 218 (17%)	M1	0	–	–
E. Hussain et al. 2016 (144)	T1 – T2 N0 – N2a	2,001 (36%)	T1 – T2 N2b – N3	2,183 (39%)	T3, N0 – N3	872 (15%)	T4a – T4b N0 – N3	570 (10%)	M1	0

Each study is listed by row (A – E). TNM stage groupings are collectively labeled as "risk groups" to collate study-specific differences in TNM stage assignments. Increasing risk group reflects worsening prognosis: risk group 1 (most favorable) to 5 (worst prognosis). Each risk group is divided into one column summarizing its inclusion criteria and a second column reporting the number and percentage of patients meeting inclusion criteria. All T stages correspond to AJCC-7th edition T stage definitions for HNSCC. All N stages correspond to AJCC-7th edition definitions for HNSCC except for N stages labeled with asterisk (*), which correspond to AJCC-7th edition N stage definitions for NPC.

PY, pack years smoked; YO, years old in age; t, ICON-S training cohort; v, ICON-S validation cohort.

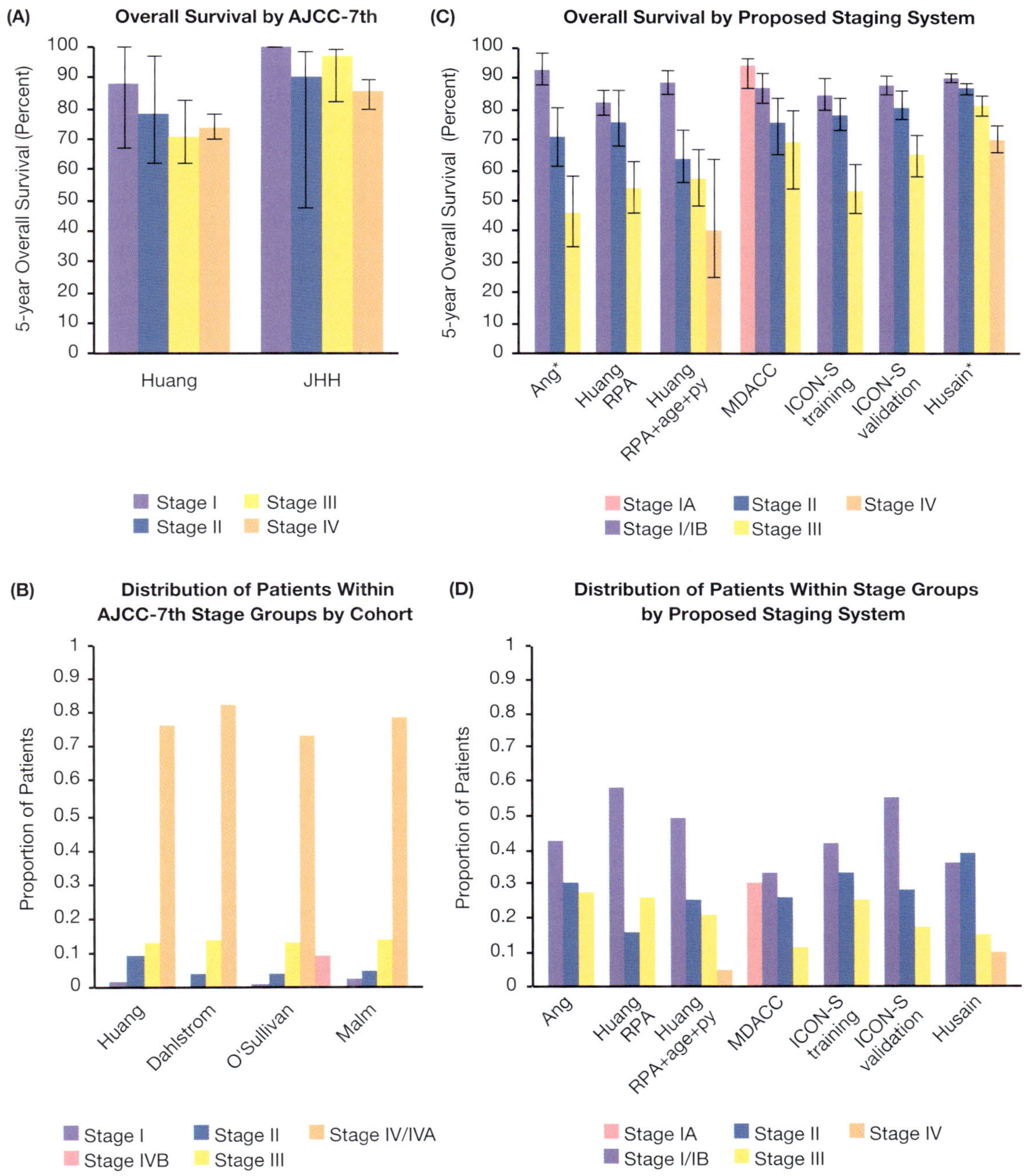

FIGURE 4.1 Survival stratification and patient distribution by existing and proposed staging systems. (A) AJCC-7th staging system is incapable of discriminating prognosis for HPV-positive OPC in neither Princess Margaret Cancer Centre (Huang) nor Johns Hopkins Hospital (Malm) cohorts. (B) AJCC-7th staging system classifies the vast majority of patients as stage III and IV. (C) Comparison of prognosis discrimination in proposed staging systems. (D) All proposed staging systems show better distribution of patients across stage groups. MDACC staging system divides stage I into IA and IB. All other staging systems propose single stage I group.

Note: See text for further discussion and use of abbreviations.

*Ang and Husain studies report 3-year overall survival.

AJCC-7th, 7th edition of the American Joint Committee on Cancer; MDACC, MD Anderson Cancer Center.

two separate methods, RPA and Cox regression-based adjusted hazards ratios (AHR), Huang et al. reorganized AJCC-7th T and N stages into two new TNM staging schema that appeared to improve prognostication of HPV-positive OPC. For example, AJCC-7th currently defines TNM stage I disease to only include patients who present with T1N0M0 disease. The Huang RPA stage I group, however, encompassed all patients presenting with T1 to T3, N0 to N2b, M0 disease. Validation of the Huang staging schema was performed with internal validation by the bootstrap method (Tables 4.1 and 4.2, Row B). In other words, these data were validated on the same dataset used to generate the staging schema. Bootstrap validation entails testing the performance of a model, the TNM staging schema proposed by Huang in the present case, on a random subset of the original cohort used to generate the model (142). Random sampling is performed iteratively, 1,000 iterations in the present case, after which bootstrap scores are aggregated to assess the overall performance of the model. Huang et al. also validated their data on another dataset with formally unknown HPV status that was imputed based on the "clinical behavior" of individual samples. Given that the true HPV status of imputed samples is ultimately unascertainable, validation through imputation remains a questionable strategy. Indeed, the staging schema proposed by Huang et al. failed external validation (20).

Dahlstrom and colleagues at the MD Anderson Cancer Center (MDACC) also proposed a staging system (20). Noting parallels in early nodal involvement in HPV-positive OPC and nasopharyngeal carcinoma (NPC), another virally mediated tumor of the head and neck, the MDACC staging system incorporated N categories from NPC. N staging categories in NPC are simplified compared to HNSCC and reflect the propensity of NPC patients to present with advanced nodal disease (143). NPC lymph node categories are defined as: N1, any number of positive unilateral lymph nodes smaller than 6 cm; N2, positive bilateral lymph nodes smaller than 6 cm; and N3, any lymph node greater than 6 cm in greatest dimension or presence of positive supraclavicular lymph nodes (Tables 4.1 and 4.2, Row C). Incorporating the NPC N categories, Dahlstrom et al. implemented RPA to develop a staging system found to predict PFS and OS (Figure 4.1). Like Huang et al., this staging system was validated on OPC patients with imputed HPV status (20).

The International Collaboration on Oropharyngeal cancer Staging (ICON-S) represents the largest-scale effort in the development and validation of a new staging system for HPV-positive OPC (21). This multicenter, multinational effort was designed to develop a staging system in one cohort, the "training cohort," that would be validated in an independent cohort, the "validation cohort." The training cohort comprised 661 patients from PMCC in Canada. The validation cohort included a combined 1246 patients from four American cancer centers (MDACC, Memorial Sloan Kettering Cancer Center, Cleveland Clinic Taussig Cancer Institute, and University of Colorado Cancer Center) and two European hospitals (Rigshospitalet Copenhagen University Hospital and Maastricht University Medical Centre). Implementation of RPA and AHR methods resulted in the same RPA- and AHR-based staging schema previously described by Huang et al. (16). The AHR method also identified a second, novel model initially termed AHR_{new} and subsequently named ICON-S after outperforming the original RPA and AHR schema in training and validation cohorts (Tables 4.1 and 4.2, Row D).

In ICON-S, stage I was defined as T1–T2N0–N2b, stage II as T1–T2N2c or T3N0–N2c, stage III as patient presenting with T4 or N3 disease, and stage IV as any disease presenting with distant metastasis. Similar to the MDACC staging system (20), ICON-S simplified and relabeled nodal categorization to resemble that of NPC. As such, ICON-S N1, N2, and N3 respectively correspond to AJCC-7th N0–N2b, N2c, and N3 disease. OS at 5 years in the training and validation cohorts were 85% (95% confidence intervals: 81–90) and 88% (85–91) in ICON-S stage I, 78% (73–84) vs. 81% (77–86) in ICON-S stage II, and 53% (46–62) vs. 65% (58–72) in ICON-S stage III (Figure 4.1).

In addition to representing the first externally reproducible proposed staging system, ICON-S also satisfied the Groome criteria (136). Demonstrating both hazard discrimination and outcome prediction, each successive step up in ICON-S stage resulted in a significant drop in survival. The relatively narrow, minimally overlapping 95% confidence intervals confirmed that ICON-S was hazard consistent. Finally, ICON-S exhibited reasonable balance in the distribution of patients across stages, with a respective 42% and 55% of patients training and validation cohorts classified as ICON-S stage I, 33% and 28% classified as stage II, and 25% and 17% classified as stage III. Taken together, these data indicate that ICON-S represents the most rigorously validated and most robust clinical staging system proposed yet proposed.

ICON-S was, however, limited by the relatively small proportion (~2%) of patients in training and validation cohorts who underwent primary surgical treatment. Acknowledging recent trends toward primary surgical treatment of HPV-positive OPC, Husain and colleagues analyzed data from the National Cancer Database (NCDB) to develop a staging system for HPV-positive OPC that included approximately equal portions of patients who underwent primary surgical and nonsurgical intervention (144). Of the 5,626 patients, 42 underwent primary surgery while 56% were treated nonsurgically. RPA on this group identified distinct staging system with stage IA defined as T1-2N0-2a, stage IB as T1-2N2b-3; stage II as T4a-bN0-3, stage III as T4a-bN0-3, and stage IV reserved for patients presenting with distant metastatic disease (Tables 4.1 and 4.2, Row E). In addition, Husain et al. applied ICON-S to the NCBD cohort and found that it discriminated 3-year OS (Figure 4.1). The Husain RPA staging system was subjected to internal cross-validation but was not validated on an external cohort. Given that internal validation methods cannot truly overcome overfitting bias, it is not surprising that Husain et al. concluded that their staging system outperformed ICON-S. Nonetheless, this report provided further validation of ICON-S in a diversely treated cohort.

The ICON-S and MDACC schema were also applied to a heterogeneously treated HPV-positive OPC cohort of 435 patients at Johns Hopkins Hospital (JHH) (137). This study evaluated the performance of the two staging systems in discriminating OS and PFS (Figure 4.2). On the JHH cohort, ICON-S showed significant stratification across four stage groups with respect to OS at 5 years (stage I: 92%; II: 87%; III: 74%; IV: 40%). However, direct comparison of stage I and stage II disease showed no difference in OS. ICON-S also demonstrated significant stratification across stage groups with respect to PFS at 5 years (stage I: 85%; II: 70%; III: 56%; IV: 0%). Importantly, after adjusting for age, smoking history, and primary treatment modality, patients with ICON-S stage II disease were twice as likely to experience disease progression than ICON-S stage I disease. The MDACC staging system also significantly stratified JHH patients with respect to OS (stage IA: 95%; IB: 91%; II:

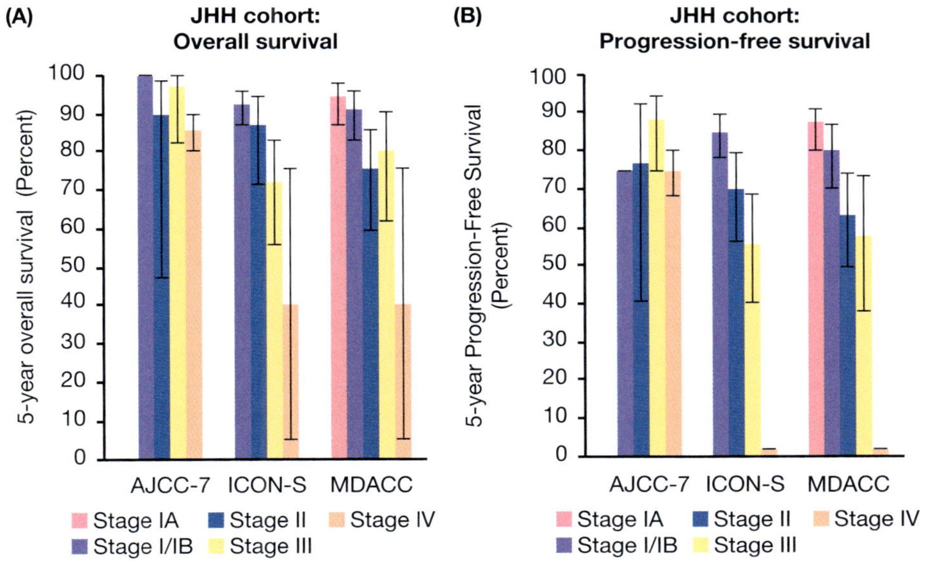

FIGURE 4.2 Comparison of AJCC-7th, ICON-S, and MDACC in the Johns Hopkins Cohort. In the Johns Hopkins Hospital (JHH) cohort, ICON-S shows superior risk stratification to the MDACC staging system with respect to both (A) overall survival and (B) progression-free survival. AJCC-7th edition exhibits no prognostic value in the JHH cohort.

Note: See text for further discussion and use of abbreviations.

AJCC-7th, 7th edition of the American Joint Committee on Cancer; ICON-S, International Collaboration on Oropharyngeal cancer Staging; MDACC, MD Anderson Cancer Center.

76%; III: 80%; IV: 40%) and PFS (IA: 88%; IB: 80%; II: 63%; III: 58%; IV: 0%). However, after adjustment for other prognostic covariates, neither stages IA and IB nor stages II and III were statistically distinguishable with respect to risk of death or progression. The JHH report provided the third independent validation of ICON-S and evidence supporting the superiority of ICON-S to the MDACC staging system.

Beyond confirming the validity of ICON-S, this study provided the first evidence showing ICON-S also fulfilled the Groome criteria with respect to PFS, bringing to light the limits of risk-prediction based purely on clinical parameters. ICON-S classified 65% of patients in JHH cohort as stage I. Although the overwhelming majority of these patients demonstrated excellent OS, 15% of stage I experienced disease progression within 5 years. This subset of patients, who appear to have excellent prognosis but go on to recur even with the current-intensity therapeutic approaches, presents the greatest challenge to patient selection for treatment de-intensification and underscores the need for higher resolution markers for recurrent disease.

Efforts toward the development of a clinically useful staging system for HPV-positive OPC have culminated in the revision of staging criteria in the 8th edition of the *AJCC Cancer Staging Manual* (AJCC-8th) (145). AJCC-8th now formally recognizes HPV-positive OPC as a unique malignancy and has defined a novel staging system for it. Given that p16-positive status is an independent prognostic marker in OPC and strongly correlates with HPV-positive status in OPC, the AJCC-8th staging system for HPV-positive OPC applies to all p16-positive OPC (52,61,146). The AJCC-8th staging system for HPV-positive OPC closely resembles ICON-S (21). The N stage categories and TNM stage groupings set forth by AJCC-8th are identical to those proposed by ICON-S. With respect to tumor stage, AJCC-8th disposes of Tis, defines T0 as tumors of unknown primary (a designation only restricted to HPV-positive OPC and Epstein–Barr virus–positive NPC), and merges T4a and T4b into T4, as these categories demonstrate no difference in survival. Since HPV-positive OPC is often treated nonsurgically, the AJCC-8th staging system may be reliably implemented by clinical TNM assessment.

In addition, AJCC-8th defines a separate, more detailed surgical pathology-based (pTNM) system to classify risk in patients undergoing surgical treatment. The pTNM system defines three (pN0-pN2) instead of four (cN0-cN3) nodal groups. Patients with one to four pathologically confirmed positive lymph nodes (pN1) were found to have better prognosis compared to those with five or more positive lymph nodes (pN2). This addition to the staging system lays the groundwork for identifying patients most likely to benefit from postoperative adjuvant treatment. However, the authors acknowledged that prospective study will be necessary to understand the implications and utility of the pTNM system (145).

EMERGING BIOMARKERS

A variety of prognostic biomarkers have established roles in clinical oncology. Though a nascent field, emerging markers in circulating blood and primary tumors of HPV-positive OPC patients are showing early promise in predicting risk of recurrence and death. Interestingly, both biomarkers implicate aspects of immune function.

Two independent groups have identified increased titers of circulating antibodies to HPV16 proteins to be correlated with risk of recurrence (147,148). In a retrospective study of HPV16-positive OPC patients, pretreatment as well as early (0–6 months) and late (>6 months) posttreatment serum samples were taken from 43, 34, and 52 patients, respectively (147). Mean serum anti-E6, and E7 titers were observed to fall steadily from pretreatment to late posttreatment time points. In addition, higher levels of anti-E6 levels were associated with an increased risk of recurrence in univariate analysis as well as after adjustment for alcohol consumption, smoking, and TNM stage (147).

A second retrospective study compared circulating anti-E6/E7 levels in 52 HPV-positive OPC patients uniformly treated with CRT (148). Of these patients, 22 developed recurrent disease while 30 patients did not recur after minimum 30 months of follow-up. No differences in T stage, N stage, or smoking status were found between patients who developed recurrence and those who did not. Serum was collected from all patients prior to treatment and at 3-month intervals after completion of therapy. Although both recurrent and nonrecurrent patients showed reductions in anti-E6 and anti-E7 over time, patients who developed recurrent disease had significantly higher levels of both antibodies than nonrecurrent patients. Next, the authors defined clearance as the ratio of anti-E6/E7 at nearest time point preceding recurrence to baseline in order to evaluate if differences in anti-E6/E7 clearance were associated with recurrence. This ratio was found to be significantly elevated for anti-E7 in patients who experienced recurrence, suggesting that patients susceptible to recurrence showed diminished clearance of anti-E7 (148). These observations suggest that longitudinal evaluation of anti-E6/E7 trends warrant further investigation as biomarkers in prospective trials.

The abundance of lymphocytes detected in tumor samples upon microscopic examination (TILs) represents another potential marker of prognosis in HPV-positive OPC. In a multicenter retrospective analysis of 270 patients, high abundance of TILs was associated with favorable OS (100). Investigators found that 96% of patients with TIL_{high} tumors were alive at 3 years, compared to 59% of patients with TIL_{low} tumors. Although the role of TILs has not been directly investigated with respect to recurrence, the prognostic effect of TIL abundance on OS has since been replicated in an independent dataset (30).

In a follow-up study, the same group of investigators implemented a systems biology approach on publicly available gene expression data to identify molecular correlates of TIL abundance (149). By defining putatively coregulated gene expression networks, the authors found that the expression of genes that were members of networks associated with lymphocyte activation and favorable prognosis were inversely correlated with genes in networks related to aerobic glycolysis and regulated by established cancer-associated genes epidermal growth factor receptor (EGFR) and hypoxia-inducible factor 1-alpha (HIF1A) (149). Although not considered a prevalent feature of disease, tumor hypoxia and HIF activation are observed in a subset of HPV-positive OPC associated with poor prognosis (150,151). These findings not only suggest a potential of HIF1 inhibition (152) as novel targeted treatment strategy in HPV-positive OPC but also highlight the immense potential of more deeply understanding the underlying biology of HPV-positive OPC in the context of recurrence and survival.

CONCLUSIONS

Significant strides have been made in the understanding of HPV-positive HNSCC over the past decade. HPV-positive OPC is established as a disease entity unique from HPV-negative HNSCC with distinct pathophysiology, epidemiology, and disease natural history. Recognition of HPV-positive OPC is leading to the development of novel therapeutic strategies and clinical staging criteria specific to this disease entity. However, clinical factors may yet prove inadequate in patient selection for therapeutic de-intensification. Emerging evidence suggests that insights into the molecular and cellular pathobiology of recurrent and metastatic HPV-positive OPC hold the key for developing higher resolution, higher confidence modalities to predict recurrence, and poor prognosis.

REFERENCES

1. de Villiers E-M, Weidauer H, Otto H, Zur Hausen H. Papillomavirus DNA in human tongue carcinomas. *Int J Cancer*. 1985;36(5):575–578. doi:10.1002/ijc.2910360510
2. Syrjänen K, Syrjänen S, Pyrhönen S. Human papilloma virus (HPV) antigens in lesions of laryngeal squamous cell carcinomas. *ORL J Otorhinolaryngol Relat Spec*. 1982;44(6):323–334. doi:10.1159/000275612
3. IARC Working Group on the Evaluation of Carcinogenic Risks to Humans. Human papillomaviruses. *IARC Monogr Eval Carcinog Risks Hum*. 2007;90:1–636. https://monographs.iarc.fr/ENG/Monographs/vol90/mono90.pdf
4. Jemal A, Simard EP, Dorell C, et al. Annual Report to the Nation on the Status of Cancer, 1975-2009, featuring the burden and trends in human papillomavirus(HPV)-associated cancers and HPV vaccination coverage levels. *J Natl Cancer Inst*. 2013;105(3):175–201. doi:10.1093/jnci/djs491
5. Patel MA, Blackford AL, Rettig EM, et al. Rising population of survivors of oral squamous cell cancer in the United States. *Cancer*. 2016;122(9):1380–1387. doi:10.1002/cncr.29921
6. Gillison ML, Koch WM, Capone RB, et al. Evidence for a causal association between human papillomavirus and a subset of head and neck cancers. *J Natl Cancer Inst*. 2000;92(9):709–720. doi:10.1093/jnci/92.9.709
7. Pai SI, Westra WH. Molecular pathology of head and neck cancer: implications for diagnosis, prognosis, and treatment. *Annu Rev Pathol*. 2009;4:49–70. doi:10.1146/annurev.pathol.4.110807.092158
8. Ndiaye C, Mena M, Alemany L, et al. HPV DNA, E6/E7 mRNA, and $p16^{INK4a}$ detection in head and neck cancers: a systematic review and meta-analysis. *Lancet Oncol*. 2014;15(12):1319–1331. doi:10.1016/S1470-2045(14)70471-1
9. Paz IB, Cook N, Odom-Maryon T, et al. Human papillomavirus (HPV) in head and neck cancer. An association of HPV 16 with squamous cell carcinoma of Waldeyer's tonsillar ring. *Cancer*. 1997;79(3):595–604. doi:10.1002/(SICI)1097-0142(19970201)79:3<595::AID-CNCR24>3.0.CO;2-Y

10. Syrjänen S. HPV infections and tonsillar carcinoma. *J Clin Pathol.* 2004;57(5):449–455. doi:10.1136/jcp.2003.008656
11. Ang KK, Harris J, Wheeler R, et al. Human papillomavirus and survival of patients with oropharyngeal cancer. *N Engl J Med.* 2010;363(1):24–35. doi:10.1056/NEJMoa0912217
12. Fakhry C, Westra WH, Li S, et al. Improved survival of patients with human papillomavirus-positive head and neck squamous cell carcinoma in a prospective clinical trial. *J Natl Cancer Inst.* 2008;100(4):261–269. doi:10.1093/jnci/djn011
13. Ward MJ, Mellows T, Harris S, et al. Staging and treatment of oropharyngeal cancer in the human papillomavirus era. *Head Neck.* 2015;37(7):1002–1013. doi:10.1002/hed.23697
14. Edge SB, Byrd D, Compton C, et al., eds. *AJCC Cancer Staging Manual.* 7th ed. New York, NY: Springer Publishing; 2010. http://www.springer.com/us/book/9780387884424
15. Dahlstrom KR, Calzada G, Hanby JD, et al. An evolution in demographics, treatment, and outcomes of oropharyngeal cancer at a major cancer center: a staging system in need of repair. *Cancer.* 2013;119(1):81–89. doi:10.1002/cncr.27727
16. Huang SH, Xu W, Waldron J, et al. Refining American Joint Committee on Cancer/Union for International Cancer Control TNM stage and prognostic groups for human papillomavirus-related oropharyngeal carcinomas. *J Clin Oncol.* 2015;33(8):836–845. doi:10.1200/JCO.2014.58.6412
17. Keane FK, Chen YH, Neville BA, et al. Changing prognostic significance of tumor stage and nodal stage in patients with squamous cell carcinoma of the oropharynx in the human papillomavirus era. *Cancer.* 2015;121(15):2594–2602. doi:10.1002/cncr.29402
18. Gillison ML. Human papillomavirus and prognosis of oropharyngeal squamous cell carcinoma: implications for clinical research in head and neck cancers. *J Clin Oncol.* 2006;24(36):5623–5625. doi:10.1200/JCO.2006.07.1829
19. Rios Velazquez E, Hoebers F, Aerts HJ, et al. Externally validated HPV-based prognostic nomogram for oropharyngeal carcinoma patients yields more accurate predictions than TNM staging. *Radiother Oncol.* 2014;113(3):324–330. doi:10.1016/j.radonc.2014.09.005
20. Dahlstrom KR, Garden AS, William WN Jr, et al. Proposed staging system for patients with HPV-related oropharyngeal cancer based on nasopharyngeal cancer N categories. *J Clin Oncol.* 2016;34(16):1848–1854. doi:10.1200/JCO.2015.64.6448
21. O'Sullivan B, Huang SH, Su J, et al. Development and validation of a staging system for HPV-related oropharyngeal cancer by the International Collaboration on Oropharyngeal cancer Network for Staging (ICON-S): a multicentre cohort study. *Lancet Oncol.* 2016;17(4):440–451. doi:10.1016/S1470-2045(15)00560-4
22. Bernier J, Domenge C, Ozsahin M, et al. European Organization for Research and Treatment of Cancer Trial 22931. Postoperative irradiation with or without concomitant chemotherapy for locally advanced head and neck cancer. *N Engl J Med.* 2004;350(19):1945–1952. doi:10.1056/NEJMoa032641
23. Cooper JS, Pajak TF, Forastiere AA, et al. Radiation Therapy Oncology Group 9501/Intergroup. Postoperative concurrent radiotherapy and chemotherapy for high-risk squamous-cell carcinoma of the head and neck. *N Engl J Med.* 2004;350(19):1937–1944. doi:10.1056/NEJMoa032646
24. Adelstein DJ, Li Y, Adams GL, et al. An intergroup phase III comparison of standard radiation therapy and two schedules of concurrent chemoradiotherapy in patients with unresectable squamous cell head and neck cancer. *J Clin Oncol.* 2003;21(1):92–98. doi:10.1200/JCO.2003.01.008
25. Calais G, Alfonsi M, Bardet E, et al. Randomized trial of radiation therapy versus concomitant chemotherapy and radiation therapy for advanced-stage oropharynx carcinoma. *J Natl Cancer Inst.* 1999;91(24):2081–2086. doi:10.1200/JCO.2003.01.008
26. O'Sullivan B, Huang SH, Siu LL, et al. Deintensification candidate subgroups in human papillomavirus-related oropharyngeal cancer according to minimal risk of distant metastasis. *J Clin Oncol.* 2013;31(5):543–550. doi:10.1200/jco.2012.44.0164
27. Bhatia A, Burtness B. Human papillomavirus-associated oropharyngeal cancer: defining risk groups and clinical trials. *J Clin Oncol.* 2015;33(29):3243–3250. doi:10.1200/JCO.2015.61.2358
28. Lassen P, Primdahl H, Johansen J, et al. Impact of HPV-associated p16-expression on radiotherapy outcome in advanced oropharynx and non-oropharynx cancer. *Radiother Oncol.* 2014;113(3):310–316. doi:10.1016/j.radonc.2014.11.032
29. Chung CH, Zhang Q, Kong CS, et al. p16 protein expression and human papillomavirus status as prognostic biomarkers of nonoropharyngeal head and neck squamous cell carcinoma. *J Clin Oncol.* 2014;32(35):3930–3938. doi:10.1200/JCO.2013.54.5228
30. Chakravarthy A, Henderson S, Thirdborough SM, et al. Human papillomavirus drives tumor development throughout the head and neck: improved prognosis is associated with an immune response largely restricted to the oropharynx. *J Clin Oncol.* 2016;34(34):4132–4141. doi:10.1200/JCO.2016.68.2955
31. Nguyen-Tan PF, Zhang Q, Ang KK, et al. Randomized phase III trial to test accelerated versus standard fractionation in combination with concurrent cisplatin for head and neck carcinomas in the Radiation Therapy Oncology Group 0129 trial: long-term report of efficacy and toxicity. *J Clin Oncol.* 2014;32(34):3858–3867. doi:10.1200/JCO.2014.55.3925
32. Seitz HK, Stickel F. Molecular mechanisms of alcohol-mediated carcinogenesis. *Nat Rev Cancer.* 2007;7(8):599–612. doi:10.1038/nrc2191
33. Blot WJ, Mclaughlin JK, Winn DM, et al. Smoking and drinking in relation to oral and pharyngeal cancer. *Cancer Res.* 1988;48(11):3282–3287. http://cancerres.aacrjournals.org/content/48/11/3282.long
34. Hashibe M, Brennan P, Benhamou S, et al. Alcohol drinking in never users of tobacco, cigarette smoking

in never drinkers, and the risk of head and neck cancer: pooled analysis in the International Head and Neck Cancer Epidemiology Consortium. *J Natl Cancer Inst.* 2007;99(10):777–789. doi:10.1093/jnci/djk179
35. Marur S, D'Souza G, Westra WH, Forastiere AA. HPV-associated head and neck cancer: a virus-related cancer epidemic. *Lancet Oncol.* 2010;11(8):781–789. doi:10.1016/S1470-2045(10)70017-6
36. Hecht SS. Tobacco carcinogens, their biomarkers and tobacco-induced cancer. *Nat Rev Cancer.* 2003;3(10):733–744. doi:10.1038/nrc1190
37. Applebaum KM, Furniss CS, Zeka A, et al. Lack of association of alcohol and tobacco with HPV16-associated head and neck cancer. *J Natl Cancer Inst.* 2007;99(23):1801–1810. doi:10.1093/jnci/djm233
38. Boyle JO, Hakim J, Koch W, et al. The incidence of p53 mutations increases with progression of head and neck cancer. *Cancer Res.* 1993;53(19):4477–4480. http://cancerres.aacrjournals.org/content/53/19/4477
39. Brennan JA, Boyle JO, Koch WM, et al. Association between cigarette smoking and mutation of the p53 gene in squamous-cell carcinoma of the head and neck. *N Engl J Med.* 1995;332(11):712–717. doi:10.1056/NEJM199503163321104
40. Balaram P, Sridhar H, Rajkumar T, et al. Oral cancer in southern India: the influence of smoking, drinking, paan-chewing and oral hygiene. *Int J Cancer.* 2002;98(3):440–445. doi:10.1002/ijc.10200
41. Mack TM. The new pan-Asian paan problem. *Lancet.* 2001;357(9269):1638–1639. doi:10.1016/S0140-6736(00)04860-1
42. Merchant A, Husain SS, Hosain M, et al. Paan without tobacco: an independent risk factor for oral cancer. *Int J Cancer.* 2000;86(1):128–131. doi:10.1002/(SICI)1097-0215(20000401)86:1<128::AID-IJC20>3.0.CO;2-M
43. Satterwhite CL, Torrone E, Meites E, et al. Sexually transmitted infections among US women and men: prevalence and incidence estimates, 2008. *Sex Transm Dis.* 2013;40(3):187–193. doi:10.1097/OLQ.0b013e318286bb53
44. Plummer M, de Martel C, Vignat J, et al. Global burden of cancers attributable to infections in 2012: a synthetic analysis. *Lancet Glob Health.* 2016;4(9):e609–e616. doi:10.1016/S2214-109X(16)30143-7
45. de Villiers EM. Cross-roads in the classification of papillomaviruses. *Virology.* 2013;445(1-2):2–10. doi:10.1016/j.virol.2013.04.023
46. Anantharaman D, Gheit T, Waterboer T, et al. Human papillomavirus infections and upper aero-digestive tract cancers: the ARCAGE study. *J Natl Cancer Inst.* 2013;105(8):536–545. doi:10.1093/jnci/djt053
47. Michaud DS, Langevin SM, Eliot M, et al. High-risk HPV types and head and neck cancer. *Int J Cancer.* 2014;135(7):1653–1661. doi:10.1002/ijc.28811
48. Viens LJ, Henley SJ, Watson M, et al. Human Papillomavirus-Associated Cancers—United States, 2008–2012. *Morb Mortal Wkly Rep.* 2016;65(26):661–666. doi:10.15585/mmwr.mm6526a1
49. Steinau M, Saraiya M, Goodman MT, et al. Human papillomavirus prevalence in oropharyngeal cancer before vaccine introduction, United States. *Emerg Infect Dis.* 2014;20(5):822–828. doi:10.3201/eid2005.131311
50. Kreimer AR, Clifford GM, Boyle P, Franceschi S. Human papillomavirus types in head and neck squamous cell carcinomas worldwide: a systematic review. *Cancer Epidemiol Biomarkers Prev.* 2005;14(2):467–475. doi:10.1158/1055-9965.EPI-04-0551
51. Mehanna H, Beech T, Nicholson T, et al. Prevalence of human papillomavirus in oropharyngeal and nonoropharyngeal head and neck cancer—systematic review and meta-analysis of trends by time and region. *Head Neck.* 2013;35(5):747–755. doi:10.1002/hed.22015
52. Gillison ML, D'Souza G, Westra W, et al. Distinct risk factor profiles for human papillomavirus type 16-positive and human papillomavirus type 16-negative head and neck cancers. *J Natl Cancer Inst.* 2008;100(6):407–420. doi:10.1093/jnci/djn025
53. D'Souza G, Agrawal Y, Halpern J, et al. Oral sexual behaviors associated with prevalent oral human papillomavirus infection. *J Infect Dis.* 2009;199(9):1263–1269. doi:10.1086/597755
54. Heck JE, Berthiller J, Vaccarella S, et al. Sexual behaviours and the risk of head and neck cancers: a pooled analysis in the International Head and Neck Cancer Epidemiology (INHANCE) consortium. *Int J Epidemiol.* 2010;39(1):166–181. doi:10.1093/ije/dyp350
55. Gillison ML, Broutian T, Pickard RK, et al. Prevalence of oral HPV infection in the United States, 2009-2010. *JAMA.* 2012;307(7):693–703. doi:10.1001/jama.2012.101
56. Fakhry C, Gillison ML, D'Souza G. Tobacco use and oral HPV-16 infection. *JAMA.* 2014;312(14):1465–1467. doi:10.1001/jama.2014.13183
57. Smith EM, Ritchie JM, Summersgill KF, et al. Human papillomavirus in oral exfoliated cells and risk of head and neck cancer. *J Natl Cancer Inst.* 2004;96(6):449–455. doi:10.1093/jnci/djh074
58. Gillison ML. Human papillomavirus-associated head and neck cancer is a distinct epidemiologic, clinical, and molecular entity. *Semin Oncol.* 2004;31(6):744–754. doi:10.1053/j.seminoncol.2004.09.011
59. Begum S, Cao D, Gillison M, et al. Tissue distribution of human papillomavirus 16 DNA integration in patients with tonsillar carcinoma. *Clin Cancer Res.* 2005;11(16):5694–5699. doi:10.1158/1078-0432.CCR-05-0587
60. Chaturvedi AK, Engels EA, Anderson WF, Gillison ML. Incidence trends for human papillomavirus-related and -unrelated oral squamous cell carcinomas in the United States. *J Clin Oncol.* 2008;26(4):612–619. doi:10.1200/JCO.2007.14.1713
61. Chaturvedi AK, Engels EA, Pfeiffer RM, et al. Human papillomavirus and rising oropharyngeal cancer incidence in the United States. *J Clin Oncol.* 2011;29(32):4294–4301. doi:10.1200/JCO.2011.36.4596
62. Gillison ML, Chaturvedi AK, Anderson WF, Fakhry C. Epidemiology of human papillomavirus-positive head and neck squamous cell carcinoma. *J Clin Oncol.* 2015;33(29):3235–3242. doi:10.1200/JCO.2015.61.6995

63. Turner CF, Danella RD, Rogers SM. Sexual behavior in the United States 1930–1990: trends and methodological problems. *Sex Transm Dis.* 1995;22(3):173–190. https://journals.lww.com/stdjournal/Abstract/1995/05000/Sexual_Behavior_in_the_United_States,_1930_1990_.9.aspx
64. Bajos N, Bozon M, Beltzer N, et al. Changes in sexual behaviours: from secular trends to public health policies. *AIDS.* 2010;24(8):1185–1191. doi:10.1097/QAD.0b013e328336ad52
65. Finer LB. Trends in premarital sex in the United States, 1954–2003. *Public Health Rep.* 2007;122(1):73–78. doi:10.1177/003335490712200110
66. D'Souza G, Cullen K, Bowie J, et al. Differences in oral sexual behaviors by gender, age, and race explain observed differences in prevalence of oral human papillomavirus infection. *PLOS ONE.* 2014;9(1):e86023. doi:10.1371/journal.pone.0086023
67. Greenfield TK, Midanik LT, Rogers JD. A 10-year national trend study of alcohol consumption, 1984-1995: is the period of declining drinking over? *Am J Public Health.* 2000;90(1):47–52. https://www.ncbi.nlm.nih.gov/pmc/articles/PMC1446127/
68. Chaturvedi AK, Anderson WF, Lortet-Tieulent J, et al. Worldwide trends in incidence rates for oral cavity and oropharyngeal cancers. *J Clin Oncol.* 2013;31(36):4550–4559. doi:10.1200/JCO.2013.50.3870
69. Hollstein M, Sidransky D, Vogelstein B, Harris CC. p53 mutations in human cancers. *Science.* 1991;253(5015):49–53. doi:10.1126/science.1905840
70. Somers KD, Merrick MA, Lopez ME, et al. Frequent p53 mutations in head and neck cancer. *Cancer Res.* 1992;52(21):5997–6000. http://cancerres.aacrjournals.org/content/52/21/5997.long
71. Brachman DG, Graves D, Vokes E, et al. Occurrence of p53 gene deletions and human papilloma virus infection in human head and neck cancer. *Cancer Res.* 1992;52(17):4832–4836. http://cancerres.aacrjournals.org/content/52/17/4832.long
72. Koch WM, Lango M, Sewell D, et al. Head and neck cancer in nonsmokers: a distinct clinical and molecular entity. *Laryngoscope.* 1999;109(10):1544–1551. doi:10.1097/00005537-199910000-00002
73. Kier LD, Yamasaki E, Ames BN. Detection of mutagenic activity in cigarette smoke condensates. *Proc Natl Acad Sci USA.* 1974;71(10):4159–4163. http://www.pnas.org/content/71/10/4159
74. Pfeifer GP, Denissenko MF, Olivier M, et al. Tobacco smoke carcinogens, DNA damage and p53 mutations in smoking-associated cancers. *Oncogene.* 2002;21(48):7435–7451. doi:10.1038/sj.onc.1205803
75. Alexandrov LB, Ju YS, Haase K, et al. Mutational signatures associated with tobacco smoking in human cancer. *Science.* 2016;354(6312):618–622. doi:10.1126/science.aag0299
76. Stransky N, Egloff AM, Tward AD, et al. The mutational landscape of head and neck squamous cell carcinoma. *Science.* 2011;333(6046):1157–1160. doi:10.1126/science.1208130
77. Agrawal N, Frederick MJ, Pickering CR, et al. Exome sequencing of head and neck squamous cell carcinoma reveals inactivating mutations in NOTCH1. *Science.* 2011;333(6046):1154–1157. doi:10.1126/science.1206923
78. Cancer Genome Atlas Network. Comprehensive genomic characterization of head and neck squamous cell carcinomas. *Nature.* 2015;517(7536):576–582. doi:10.1038/nature14129
79. Scheffner M, Werness BA, Huibregtse JM, et al. The E6 oncoprotein encoded by human papillomavirus types 16 and 18 promotes the degradation of p53. *Cell.* 1990;63(6):1129–1136. doi:10.1016/0092-8674(90)90409-8
80. Boyer SN, Wazer DE, Band V. E7 protein of human papilloma virus-16 induces degradation of retinoblastoma protein through the ubiquitin-proteasome pathway. *Cancer Res.* 1996;56(20):4620–4624. http://cancerres.aacrjournals.org/content/56/20/4620.long
81. Ikeda MA, Jakoi L, Nevins JR. A unique role for the Rb protein in controlling E2F accumulation during cell growth and differentiation. *Proc Natl Acad Sci USA.* 1996;93(8):3215–3220. http://www.pnas.org/content/93/8/3215.long
82. Nevins JR. E2F: a link between the Rb tumor suppressor protein and viral oncoproteins. *Science.* 1992;258(5081):424–429. doi:10.1126/science.1411535
83. Serrano M, Hannon GJ, Beach D. A new regulatory motif in cell-cycle control causing specific inhibition of cyclin D/CDK4. *Nature.* 1993;366(6456):704–707. doi:10.1038/366704a0
84. Singhi AD, Westra WH. Comparison of human papillomavirus in situ hybridization and p16 immunohistochemistry in the detection of human papillomavirus-associated head and neck cancer based on a prospective clinical experience. *Cancer.* 2010;116(9):2173. doi:10.1002/cncr.25033
85. Reed AL, Califano J, Cairns P, et al. High frequency of *p16 (CDKN2/MTS-1/INK4A)* inactivation in head and neck squamous cell carcinoma. *Cancer Res.* 1996;56(16):3630–3633. http://cancerres.aacrjournals.org/content/56/16/3630.long
86. Kraunz KS, Mcclean MD, Nelson HH, et al. Duration but not intensity of alcohol and tobacco exposure predicts $p16^{INK4A}$ homozygous deletion in head and neck squamous cell carcinoma. *Cancer Res.* 2006;66(8):4512–4515. doi:10.1158/0008-5472.CAN-05-3748
87. Mellin H, Friesland S, Lewensohn R, et al. Human papillomavirus (HPV) DNA in tonsillar cancer: clinical correlates, risk of relapse, and survival. *Int J Cancer.* 2000;89(3):300–304. doi:10.1002/1097-0215(20000520)89:3<300::AID-IJC14>3.0.CO;2-G
88. Rischin D, Young RJ, Fisher R, et al. Prognostic significance of $p16^{INK4A}$ and human papillomavirus in patients with oropharyngeal cancer treated on TROG 02.02 phase III trial. *J Clin Oncol.* 2010;28(27):4142–4148. doi:10.1200/JCO.2010.29.2904
89. O'Rorke MA, Ellison MV, Murray LJ, et al. Human papillomavirus related head and neck cancer survival: a systematic review and meta-analysis. *Oral Oncol.* 2012;48(12):1191–1201. doi:10.1016/j.oraloncology.2012.06.019

90. El-Naggar AK, Westra WH. p16 expression as a surrogate marker for HPV-related oropharyngeal carcinoma: a guide for interpretative relevance and consistency. *Head Neck*. 2012;34(4):459–461. doi:10.1002/hed.21974
91. Lingen MW, Xiao W, Schmitt A, et al. Low etiologic fraction for high-risk human papillomavirus in oral cavity squamous cell carcinomas. *Oral Oncol*. 2013;49(1):1–8. doi:10.1016/j.oraloncology.2012.07.002
92. Lewis JS, Thorstad WL, Chernock RD, et al. p16 positive oropharyngeal squamous cell carcinoma: an entity with a favorable prognosis regardless of tumor HPV status. *Am J Surg Pathol*. 2010;34(8):1088–1096. doi:10.1097/PAS.0b013e3181e84652
93. Coordes A, Lenz K, Qian X, et al. Meta-analysis of survival in patients with HNSCC discriminates risk depending on combined HPV and p16 status. *Eur Arch Otorhinolaryngol*. 2016;273(8):2157–2169. doi:10.1007/s00405-015-3728-0
94. D'Souza G, Westra WH, Wang SJ, et al. Differences in the prevalence of human papillomavirus (HPV) in head and neck squamous cell cancers by sex, race, anatomic tumor site, and HPV detection method *JAMA Oncol*. 2016 Dec 8. doi:10.1001/jamaoncol.2016.3067
95. Fakhry C, Westra WH, Wang SJ, et al. The prognostic role of sex, race, and human papillomavirus in oropharyngeal and nonoropharyngeal head and neck squamous cell cancer. *Cancer*. 2017;123(9):1566–1575. doi:10.1002/cncr.30353
96. Adelstein DJ, Ridge JA, Gillison ML, et al. Head and neck squamous cell cancer and the human papillomavirus: summary of a National Cancer Institute State of the Science Meeting, November 9-10, 2008, Washington, D.C. *Head Neck*. 2009;31(11):1393–1422. doi:10.1002/hed.21269
97. Chung CH, Gillison ML. Human papillomavirus in head and neck cancer: its role in pathogenesis and clinical implications. *Clin Cancer Res*. 2009;15(22):6758–6762. doi:10.1158/1078-0432.CCR-09-0784
98. Henderson S, Chakravarthy A, Su X, et al. APOBEC-mediated cytosine deamination links *PIK3CA* helical domain mutations to human papillomavirus-driven tumor development. *Cell Rep*. 2014;7(6):1833–1841. doi:10.1016/j.celrep.2014.05.012
99. Begum S, Westra WH. Basaloid squamous cell carcinoma of the head and neck is a mixed variant that can be further resolved by HPV status. *Am J Surg Pathol*. 2008;32(7):1044–1050. doi:10.1097/PAS.0b013e31816380ec
100. Ward MJ, Thirdborough SM, Mellows T, et al. Tumour-infiltrating lymphocytes predict for outcome in HPV-positive oropharyngeal cancer. *Br J Cancer*. 2014;110(2):489–500. doi:10.1038/bjc.2013.639
101. Howie AJ. Scanning and transmission electron microscopy on the epithelium of human palatine tonsils. *J Pathol*. 1980;130(2):91–98. doi:10.1002/path.1711300205
102. Perry M, Whyte A. Immunology of the tonsils. *Immunol Today*. 1998;19(9):414–421. doi:10.1016/S0167-5699(98)01307-3
103. Kang SYC, Kannan N, Zhang L, et al. Characterization of epithelial progenitors in normal human palatine tonsils and their HPV16 E6/E7-induced perturbation. *Stem Cell Reports*. 2015;5(6):1210–1225. doi:10.1016/j.stemcr.2015.09.020
104. Fakhry C, Zhang Q, Nguyen-Tan PF, et al. Human papillomavirus and overall survival after progression of oropharyngeal squamous cell carcinoma. *J Clin Oncol*. 2014;32(30):3365–3373. doi:10.1200/JCO.2014.55.1937
105. Joseph AW, Guo T, Hur K, et al. Disease-free survival after salvage therapy for recurrent oropharyngeal squamous cell carcinoma. *Head Neck*. 2016;38(suppl 1):E1501–E1509. doi:10.1002/hed.24268
106. Guo T, Qualliotine JR, Ha PK, et al. Surgical salvage improves overall survival for patients with HPV-positive and HPV-negative recurrent locoregional and distant metastatic oropharyngeal cancer. *Cancer*. 2015;121(12):1977–1984. doi:10.1002/cncr.29323
107. Kelly JR, Husain ZA, Burtness B. Treatment de-intensification strategies for head and neck cancer. *Eur J Cancer*. 2016;68:125–133. doi:10.1016/j.ejca.2016.09.006
108. Marks SC. Surgical management of head and neck cancer. *Hematol Oncol Clin North Am*. 1999;13(4):655–678. doi:10.1016/S0889-8588(05)70084-8
109. Spiro RH, Gerold FP, Strong EW. Mandibular "swing" approach for oral and oropharyngeal tumors. *Head Neck Surg*. 1981;3(5):371–378. doi:10.1002/hed.2890030505
110. The Department of Veterans Affairs Laryngeal Cancer Study Group. Induction chemotherapy plus radiation compared with surgery plus radiation in patients with advanced laryngeal cancer. *N Engl J Med*. 1991;324:1685–1690. doi:10.1056/NEJM199106133242402
111. Forastiere AA, Goepfert H, Maor M, et al. Concurrent chemotherapy and radiotherapy for organ preservation in advanced laryngeal cancer. *N Engl J Med*. 2003;349(22):2091–2098. doi:10.1056/NEJMoa031317
112. Parsons JT, Mendenhall WM, Stringer SP, et al. Squamous cell carcinoma of the oropharynx: surgery, radiation therapy, or both. *Cancer*. 2002;94(11):2967–2980. doi:10.1002/cncr.10567
113. Bernier J. Alteration of radiotherapy fractionation and concurrent chemotherapy: a new frontier in head and neck oncology? *Nat Clin Pract Oncol*. 2005;2(6):305–314. doi:10.1038/ncponc0201
114. Bourhis J, Overgaard J, Audry H, et al. Hyperfractionated or accelerated radiotherapy in head and neck cancer: a meta-analysis. *Lancet*. 2006;368(9538):843–854. doi:10.1016/S0140-6736(06)69121-6
115. Trotti A, Bellm LA, Epstein JB, et al. Mucositis incidence, severity and associated outcomes in patients with head and neck cancer receiving radiotherapy with or without chemotherapy: a systematic literature review. *Radiother Oncol*. 2003;66(3):253–262. doi:10.1016/S0167-8140(02)00404-8

116. Al-Sarraf M, Pajak TF, Byhardt RW, et al. Postoperative radiotherapy with concurrent cisplatin appears to improve locoregional control of advanced, resectable head and neck cancers: RTOG 88-24. *Int J Radiat Oncol Biol Phys*. 1997;37(4):777–782. doi:10.1016/S0360-3016(96)00614-1
117. Nabell L, Spencer S. Docetaxel with concurrent radiotherapy in head and neck cancer. *Semin Oncol*. 2003;30(6, suppl 18):89–93. doi:10.1053/j.seminoncol.2003.11.017
118. Forastiere AA, Zhang Q, Weber RS, et al. Long-term results of RTOG 91-11: a comparison of three nonsurgical treatment strategies to preserve the larynx in patients with locally advanced larynx cancer. *J Clin Oncol*. 2013;31(7):845–852. doi:10.1200/JCO.2012.43.6097
119. Machtay M, Moughan J, Trotti A, et al. Factors associated with severe late toxicity after concurrent chemoradiation for locally advanced head and neck cancer: an RTOG analysis. *J Clin Oncol*. 2008;26(21):3582–3589. doi:10.1200/JCO.2007.14.8841
120. Fischer CA, Zlobec I, Green E, et al. Is the improved prognosis of p16 positive oropharyngeal squamous cell carcinoma dependent of the treatment modality? *Int J Cancer*. 2010;126(5):1256–1262. doi:10.1002/ijc.24842
121. Steiner W, Fierek O, Ambrosch P, Hommerich CP, Kron M. Transoral laser microsurgery for squamous cell carcinoma of the base of the tongue. *Arch Otolaryngol Head Neck Surg*. 2003;129(1):36–43. doi:10.1001/archotol.129.1.36
122. Weinstein GS, O'Malley BW, Hockstein NG. Transoral robotic surgery: supraglottic laryngectomy in a canine model. *Laryngoscope*. 2005;115(7):1315–1319. doi:10.1097/01.MLG.0000170848.76045.47
123. Weinstein GS, O'Malley BW, Cohen MA, Quon H. Transoral robotic surgery for advanced oropharyngeal carcinoma. *Arch Otolaryngol Head Neck Surg*. 2010;136(11):1079–1085. doi:10.1001/archoto.2010.191
124. Genden EM, Desai S, Sung CK. Transoral robotic surgery for the management of head and neck cancer: a preliminary experience. *Head Neck*. 2009;31(3):283–289. doi:10.1002/hed.20972
125. Hurtuk A, Agrawal A, Old M, et al. Outcomes of transoral robotic surgery: a preliminary clinical experience. *Otolaryngol Head Neck Surg*. 2011;145(2):248–253. doi:10.1177/0194599811402172
126. Haughey BH, Hinni ML, Salassa JR, et al. Transoral laser microsurgery as primary treatment for advanced-stage oropharyngeal cancer: a United States multicenter study. *Head Neck*. 2011;33(12):1683–1694. doi:10.1002/hed.21669
127. Wilkie MD, Upile NS, Lau AS, et al. Transoral laser microsurgery for oropharyngeal squamous cell carcinoma: a paradigm shift in therapeutic approach. *Head Neck*. 2016;38(8):1263–1270. doi:10.1002/hed.24432
128. Cmelak AJ, Li S, Goldwasser MA, et al. Phase II trial of chemoradiation for organ preservation in resectable stage III or IV squamous cell carcinomas of the larynx or oropharynx: results of Eastern Cooperative Oncology Group Study E2399. *J Clin Oncol*. 2007;25(25):3971–3977. doi:10.1200/JCO.2007.10.8951
129. Rusthoven KE, Raben D, Ballonoff A, et al. Effect of radiation techniques in treatment of oropharynx cancer. *Laryngoscope*. 2008;118(4):635–639. doi:10.1097/MLG.0b013e31815fdf0e
130. de Arruda FF, Puri DR, Zhung J, et al. Intensity-modulated radiation therapy for the treatment of oropharyngeal carcinoma: the Memorial Sloan-Kettering Cancer Center experience. *Int J Radiat Oncol Biol Phys*. 2006;64(2):363–373. doi:10.1016/j.ijrobp.2005.03.006
131. Lawson JD, Otto K, Chen A, et al. Concurrent platinum-based chemotherapy and simultaneous modulated accelerated radiation therapy for locally advanced squamous cell carcinoma of the tongue base. *Head Neck*. 2008;30(3):327–335. doi:10.1002/hed.20694
132. de Almeida JR, Byrd JK, Wu R, et al. A systematic review of transoral robotic surgery and radiotherapy for early oropharynx cancer: a systematic review. *Laryngoscope*. 2014;124(9):2096–2102. doi:10.1002/lary.24712
133. Maxwell JH, Mehta V, Wang H, et al. Quality of life in head and neck cancer patients: impact of HPV and primary treatment modality. *Laryngoscope*. 2014;124(7):1592–1597. doi:10.1002/lary.24508
134. More YI, Tsue TT, Girod DA, et al. Functional swallowing outcomes following transoral robotic surgery vs primary chemoradiotherapy in patients with advanced-stage oropharynx and supraglottis cancers. *JAMA Otolaryngol Head Neck Surg*. 2013;139(1):43–48. doi:10.1001/jamaoto.2013.1074
135. Cohen MA, Weinstein GS, O'Malley BW, et al. Transoral robotic surgery and human papillomavirus status: oncologic results. *Head Neck*. 2011;33(4):573–580. doi:10.1002/hed.21500
136. Groome PA, Schulze KM, Mackillop WJ, et al. A comparison of published head and neck stage groupings in carcinomas of the tonsillar region. *Cancer*. 2001;92(6):1484–1494. doi:10.1002/1097-0142(20010915)92:6<1484::AID-CNCR1473>3.0.CO;2-W
137. Malm IJ, Fan CJ, Yin LX, et al. Evaluation of proposed staging systems for human papillomavirus-related oropharyngeal squamous cell carcinoma. *Cancer*. 2017;123(10):1768–1777. doi:10.0.3.234/cncr.30512
138. Straetmans JM, Olthof N, Mooren JJ, et al. Human papillomavirus reduces the prognostic value of nodal involvement in tonsillar squamous cell carcinomas. *Laryngoscope*. 2009;119(10):1951–1957. doi:10.1002/lary.20593
139. Strobl C, Malley J, Tutz G. An introduction to recursive partitioning: rationale, application, and characteristics of classification and regression trees, bagging, and random forests. *Psychol Methods*. 2009;14(4):323–348. doi:10.1037/a0016973

140. Hawkins DM. The problem of overfitting. *J Chem Inf Comput Sci*. 2004;44(1):1–12. doi:10.1021/ci0342472
141. Gillison ML. Human papillomavirus and oropharyngeal cancer stage. *J Clin Oncol*. 2016;34(16):1833–1835. doi:10.1200/JCO.2016.66.6081
142. Efron B, Tibshirani R. Statistical data analysis in the computer age. *Science*. 1991;253(5018):390–395. doi:10.1126/science.253.5018.390
143. Sham JS, Choy D, Wei WI. Nasopharyngeal carcinoma: orderly neck node spread. *Int J Radiat Oncol Biol Phys*. 1990;19(4):929–933. doi:10.1016/0360-3016(90)90014-B
144. Husain ZA, Chen T, Corso CD, et al. A comparison of prognostic ability of staging systems for human papillomavirus-related oropharyngeal squamous cell carcinoma. *JAMA Oncol*. 2017;3(3):358–365. doi:10.1001/jamaoncol.2016.4581
145. Lydiatt WM, Patel SG, O'Sullivan B, et al. Head and Neck cancers—major changes in the American Joint Committee on Cancer eighth edition cancer staging manual. *CA Cancer J Clin*. 2017;67(2):122–137. doi:10.3322/caac.21389
146. Mehanna H, Jones TM, Gregoire V, Ang KK. Oropharyngeal carcinoma related to human papillomavirus. *BMJ*. 2010;340:c1439. doi:10.1136/bmj.c1439
147. Fakhry C, Qualliotine JR, Zhang Z, et al. Serum Antibodies to HPV16 early proteins warrant investigation as potential biomarkers for risk stratification and recurrence of HPV-associated oropharyngeal cancer. *Cancer Prev Res*. 2016;9(2):135–141. doi:10.1158/1940-6207.CAPR-15-0299
148. Spector ME, Sacco AG, Bellile E, et al. E6 and E7 antibody levels are potential biomarkers of recurrence in patients with advanced-stage human papillomavirus-positive oropharyngeal squamous cell carcinoma. *Clin Cancer Res*. 2017;23(11). doi:10.1158/1078-0432.CCR-16-1617
149. Ottensmeier CH, Perry KL, Harden EL, et al. Upregulated glucose metabolism correlates inversely with CD8+ T-cell infiltration and survival in squamous cell carcinoma. *Cancer Res*. 2016;76(14):4136–4148. doi:10.1158/0008-5472.CAN-15-3121
150. Hanns E, Job S, Coliat P, et al. Human papillomavirus-related tumours of the oropharynx display a lower tumour hypoxia signature. *Oral Oncol*. 2015;51(9):848–856. doi:10.1016/j.oraloncology.2015.06.003
151. Samuels SE, Eisbruch A, Beitler JJ, et al. Management of locally advanced HPV-related oropharyngeal squamous cell carcinoma: where are we? *Eur Arch Otorhinolaryngol*. 2016;273(10):2877–2894. doi:10.1007/s00405-015-3771-x
152. Semenza GL. Targeting HIF-1 for cancer therapy. *Nat Rev Cancer*. 2003;3(10):721–732. doi:10.1038/nrc1187

5

Imaging of Head and Neck Cancers

Rathan M. Subramaniam

EPIDEMIOLOGY

Head and neck cancer is the sixth most frequent cancer worldwide with a current estimation of incidence being about 600,000 per year and deaths resulting in about 300,000 per year (1). Most head and neck cancers (90%–95%) are squamous cell carcinomas arising from mucosal linings of the upper aerodigestive tract. Other rare cancers that may involve the head and neck region include salivary tumors, thyroid cancers, lymphoma, and melanoma. Tobacco use and alcohol use are the most important risk factors for most head and neck cancers. However, the human papillomavirus (HPV) has been recognized as a major etiologic factor for a subset of head and neck squamous cell cancers (HNSCCs) arising from the oropharynx (2,3).

Early diagnosis and accurate staging are essential for treatment planning and can strongly influence prognosis. In addition, with early identification tumor recurrence can often be treated with additional surgery or reirradiation. The use of advanced imaging with CT, MRI, and PET/CT has greatly improved staging, therapy assessment, and monitoring for disease recurrence.

ANATOMY

The anatomy of the head and neck is very complex. It is imperative for physicians to have knowledge of head and neck anatomy to accurately localize the disease process and assess its relationship to adjacent structures. The extracranial head and neck can be divided into various anatomical spaces by fascial planes, with different contents giving rise to various types of head and neck cancers.

The suprahyoid neck is divided into the pharyngeal mucosal space, the masticator space, the parapharyngeal space, the parotid space, the carotid space, the retropharyngeal space, and the perivertebral space including the vertebrae (4). The infrahyoid neck spaces consist of the visceral space (including the trachea, esophagus, thyroid, and parathyroid glands), the carotid space, the retropharyngeal space, and the perivertebral space, which extend downward from the suprahyoid neck. The carotid, perivertebral, and retropharyngeal spaces are long vertical spaces extending from the skull base into the chest. The retropharyngeal space is a potential space bounded anteriorly by the visceral fascia and posteriorly by the prevertebral fascia and extends from the base of the skull to the posterior mediastinum to the level of the carina. The perivertebral space includes the longus colli muscles, the paraspinal muscles, vertebrae, vertebral artery and vein, and the spinal cord. Knowledge of these spaces and their displacement patterns helps in localization of the tumors to the various spaces and aids in diagnosis. These spaces also act as potential pathways for spread of disease. Malignant tumors can grow across spaces and are transpatial or tumors can be multispatial in different spaces simultaneously, such as lymphoma.

For clinical purposes, the head and neck is divided into anatomical and functional areas. These include the (a) nasal cavity and nasopharynx; (b) oral cavity; (c) oropharynx (tongue base, soft palate, and palatine tonsils); (d) larynx; (e) hypopharynx; and (f) thyroid gland and salivary glands.

HEAD AND NECK TUMORS

The vast majority (>90%) of the head and neck tumors arise from the epithelial surface of the upper aerodigestive tract and are HNSCC. The second common group of tumors consists of glandular tumors arising in the major and minor salivary glands and in the thyroid gland. Melanoma and nonmelanoma skin cancer of the head and neck are considered a separate group. Other rare tumors of head and neck include lymphoma, sarcoma, and paragangliomas.

IMAGING MODALITIES

COMPUTED TOMOGRAPHY

CT is the most commonly used first-line imaging modality for head and neck cancer. It has many advantages—widely available, easily performed, cheap, reproducible, short imaging time so motion artifacts are minimal, thin slices and the ability for multiplanar reconstruction, superior evaluation of bony structures than other modalities, and it can be used to evaluate the whole body, if needed (5). The disadvantages include limited soft tissue resolution (compared to MRI), need for iodinated contrast, radiation dose, and amalgam streak artifacts, which can obscure pathology. *For imaging the primary tumor, CT is the modality of choice, except for imaging small mucosal lesion or perineural spread or bone marrow involvement (where MRI has an advantage).*

MAGNETIC RESONANCE IMAGING

MRI is a relatively commonly available modality and provides many advantages including no radiation, excellent soft tissue resolution and multiplanar imaging, visualization of blood vessels without contrast injection, and sensitivity for detecting marrow involvement and perineural spread of tumor (6). In addition, functional information using diffusion-weighted imaging (DWI) sequence and contrast enhanced dynamic imaging can be obtained. Disadvantages include—cost, long imaging time, multitude of artifacts (motion, field distortion, flow, susceptibility) degrading images and obscuring pathology, and the need for gadolinium-based contrast agents.

POSITRON EMISSION TOMOGRAPHY/ COMPUTED TOMOGRAPHY

PET/CT is increasingly commonly available. Advantages include whole body staging in a single sitting as the scan field of view covers from skull base to midthigh, extremely sensitive for tumor detection (7) and various biological mechanisms are probed in detecting tumors such as glucose metabolism (with ^{18}F fluorodeoxyglucose [^{18}F-FDG]) or somatostatin receptor expression (with ^{68}Ga DOTATATE) for detecting neuroendocrine tumors, medullary thyroid cancers, and paragangliomas or amino acid transport with ^{18}F fluciclovine and relatively short imaging time (20–30 min). The disadvantageous include its spatial resolution limit (about 5 mm), patient preparation time depending on the PET radiopharmaceutical used, cost, and radiation dose. *It is the modality of choice for detecting neck lymph nodal and distant metastases for staging and posttherapy assessment after concurrent chemoradiation.*

POSITRON EMISSION TOMOGRAPHY/ MAGNETIC RESONANCE IMAGING

The newest hybrid imaging modality—PET/MRI—combines those two functional imaging modalities (8). Though it is only available in leading academic centers now, its advantages include primary tumor delineation, especially small lesions; neck nodal and distant metastasis detection; and excellent soft tissue resolution; it is extremely sensitive for bone marrow involvement, perineural spread, and multiparametric information (such as standardized uptake value [SUV], total tumor burden from PET, and apparent diffusion coefficient from MRI, which improves the accuracy and predictive capabilities of imaging markers). However, its value in the clinical setting over PET/CT is yet to be validated, systematically. Its disadvantages include longer scan time (60 min or more) and cost.

ULTRASOUND

This is a valuable imaging modality for assessment of neck lymph nodes, especially to obtain tissue when the node is well visualized (9) and to assess the tumor vascularity and vessels. It is widely available and cheap, the resolution is high, and no radiation is involved. The disadvantages include operator dependency, difficulty to visualize lesions behind bone and air interfaces, and incomplete mapping of large lesions in a single plane.

NUCLEAR MEDICINE

In addition to PET/CT and PET/MRI, general nuclear medicine imaging is valuable for staging differentiated thyroid cancers before and after ^{131}I ablation (10) and for mapping the sentinel lymph nodes in head and neck skin malignancies such as melanoma (11). Single photon emission computed tomography (SPECT)/CT is valuable in detecting and accurately identifying the sentinel lymph nodes in head and neck (12).

VALUE OF IMAGING

Surgeons can visualize the tumors arising from the mucosal surfaces of the upper aerodigestive tract. The most important value of imaging is to map out the submucosal extent and tumor spread, which is invisible by endoscopic examination. Key roles of imaging for patient management in head and neck cancer are (a) to detect the primary site of tumor (unknown primary); (b) to define the extent of the primary tumor and invasion of adjacent structures—neurovascular or bone or muscle involvement; (c) to detect neck nodal metastases; (d) to detect distant metastases; (e) to facilitate radiation therapy planning; (f) to assess therapy response; and (g) to detect recurrences for salvage therapy.

PRETREATMENT STRATEGY

IMAGING FEATURES OF TUMOR

CT or MRI is commonly used as the first-line imaging modality. Tumors appear as soft tissue thickening of the mucosa or soft tissue mass on CT and usually enhance with intravenous contrast and may exhibit low-density areas suggestive of tumor necrosis. On MRI, tumors are either hypo- or isointense to muscle on T1 weighted sequence and hyperintense to muscle on T2 weighted sequence. Fat is hyperintese on T1 weighted images and is helpful to differentiate tumors from normal anatomy, especially detecting marrow involvement as well as neurovascular encasement. Tumors usually enhance with gadolinium intravenous contrast agent. DWI is very valuable in detecting tumor, especially in the posttherapy settings, when postsurgical changes and inflammation make it very difficult to assess. Bony erosion is best seen in thin slice CT with disruption of the cortex. Bone sclerosis can be seen with tumor infiltration or reactive osteitis and medullary involvement is best seen in T2 weighted sequence with increased signal, though nonspecific as this can be seen in edema, inflammation, and coexisting periodontal disease.

^{18}F-FDG PET/CT is increasingly used at baseline, especially for neck nodal and distant metastatic staging, and routinely used for posttherapy assessment, as the modality of choice, after concurrent chemoradiation, when available. HNSCC usually demonstrates intense, focal FDG uptake, which allows tumor staging as well as accurate posttherapy assessment. The FDG uptake can be variable based on tumor type with intense uptake seen in HNSCC to minimal uptake seen in well-differentiated mucoepidermoid carcinoma. Necrotic areas of tumor usually demonstrate mild or no FDG uptake. Intense ^{68}Ga DOTATATE uptake is usually seen in somatostatin receptor–expressing tumors such as medullary carcinoma of thyroid and paragangliomas.

Perineural spread of tumor can be recognized with both MRI (sensitive) and PET/CT (specific). On MRI, the nerve is thickened as well as demonstrates gadolinium enhancement. Atrophy of the muscles or enhancement of the muscles supplied by the nerve can also be seen as a secondary effect. On PET/CT, intense FDG uptake can be seen along the nerve, though this is a late sign as the resolution of PET is currently limited to about 5 mm. Hence, this is specific when identified in PET/CT, but not sensitive. In addition, compensatory increased FDG uptake may be seen in the synergistic or antagnostic muscles. CT may demonstrate enlargement of the foramina.

FDG PET/CT has the best accuracy among all imaging modalities for detection of neck nodal metastases (13). Focal increased FDG uptake, above blood pool, in an anatomically normal appearing lymph node with normal size and fatty hilum, would be suspicious for metastases, until proved otherwise. When the focal FDG uptake is above the FDG uptake of liver, it is highly accurate (14) for nodal metastases. Inflammatory uptake, especially after concurrent chemoradiation therapy, tends to be diffuse. On CT, nodal enlargement (>1.5 cm in short axis diameter for level II lymph nodes and >1 cm for all other levels), loss of fatty hilum, a round configuration (rather than oval shape), and enhancement are suggestive of nodal involvement. Ultrasound is also useful in identifying nodal metastases. Peripheral nodal vascularity and microcalcifications are two valuable features to identify nodal involvement, in addition to shape, irregular borders, and loss of fatty hilum. Pericapsular tumor spread, an adverse feature of patient outcomes in head and neck cancer, can be recognized by strandings extending outward from the lymph nodes into the adjacent perinodal fat, especially recognized in contrast-enhanced CT or MRI or ultrasound. However, the concordance between the imaging finding of extracapsular spread and pathological finding needs further investigation.

STAGING—TUMOR, NODE, AND METASTASIS (TNM)

The anatomically based TNM staging system, which was first reported in the 1940s, was first adapted by the Union for International Cancer Control (UICC) in 1968. It is universally accepted in clinical practice for staging head and neck cancers and facilitating appropriate therapy planning and predicting prognosis. Head and neck region comprises a variety of anatomical sites and the T staging varies based on anatomical sites (15).

The nodal staging is based on site, number, and laterality of involved nodes relative to the primary tumor. Important prognostic features such as necrosis, extracapsular spread, and FDG avidity of metastatic nodes are not considered in the N classification. In addition, retropharyngeal nodal involvement, which affects management, is not included in the classification. N staging for most of the head and neck tumors, except for nasopharynx and thyroid cancers, is similar. N0—no node involvement, N1—single ipsilateral lymph node <3 cm in greatest diameter, N2a—single ipsilateral lymph node 3 to 6 cm, N2b—multiple ipsilateral lymph nodes <6 cm, N2c—contralateral or bilateral lymph nodes <6 cm, and N3—any lymph node >6 cm.

For nasopharyngeal cancers, N0—no lymph node involvement; N1—ipsilateral single lymph node above the supraclavicular fossa or uni- or bilateral retropharyngeal lymph node(s) <3 cm; N2a—ipsilateral single lymph node 3 to 6 cm; N2b—multiple ipsilateral lymph nodes <6 cm; N2c—ipsi- or contralateral multiple lymph nodes <6 cm above supraclavicular fossa; N3a—ipsi- or bilateral lymph node(s) >6 cm; N3b—extension to the supraclavicular fossa. For thyroid cancers, N1a—level VI and N1b—uni- or bilateral (levels I–V) or retropharyngeal or level VII lymph nodes.

Distant metastatic staging will determine therapy decisions. M0—no evidence for distant metastatic staging and M1—spread of tumor to lymph nodes or other organs beyond regional neck lymph nodes.

Unknown primary tumors account for 1% to 4% of all head and neck tumors. The main course of treatment for patients with an unknown primary site with neck nodal metastases is neck dissection and adjuvant radiation therapy for entire mucosal surface from skull base to clavicle. Detecting a primary site is important for selecting appropriate therapy in patients presenting with unknown primary tumor to avoid unnecessary comorbidities. Unknown primary is evaluated with a CT or MRI neck in the first instance. According to the National Comprehensive Cancer Network (NCCN) 2017 guidelines for head and neck cancer (16), ^{18}F-FDG PET/CT should be considered for diagnostic workup of unknown primary tumors and metastatic neck lymph nodes, if CT or MRI neck fails to identify a primary site (Figure 5.1). In a meta-analysis of 7 studies comprising 246 patients, Zhu et al. (17) evaluated the diagnostic accuracy of ^{18}F-FDG PET/CT and the authors demonstrated that the primary tumor detection rate varied from 28% to 79% with 97% sensitivity and 68% specificity. Patients with HNSCC have a higher risk for second primary cancers.

Metastasis to the cervical lymph nodes is an important prognostic factor in HNSCC. ^{18}F-FDG PET/CT provides the highest accuracy in identifying cervical nodal metastases (Figure 5.2). A meta-analysis of 32 studies suggested that the sensitivity and specificity of PET for the detection of cervical lymph node spread from squamous cell carcinoma of the head and neck were 79% and 86%, respectively, and was superior to CT or MRI (13). However, the sensitivity of FDG PET/CT for cN0 neck was thought to be suboptimal. The recently accrual completed, National Cancer Institute (NCI) sponsored ACRIN 6685 study shows the utility of FDG PET/CT in the setting of cN0 neck (18). This prospective, nonrandomized study evaluates the negative predictive value (NPV) for node negativity in newly diagnosed 287 patients with T2-T4 HNSCC. In all patients,

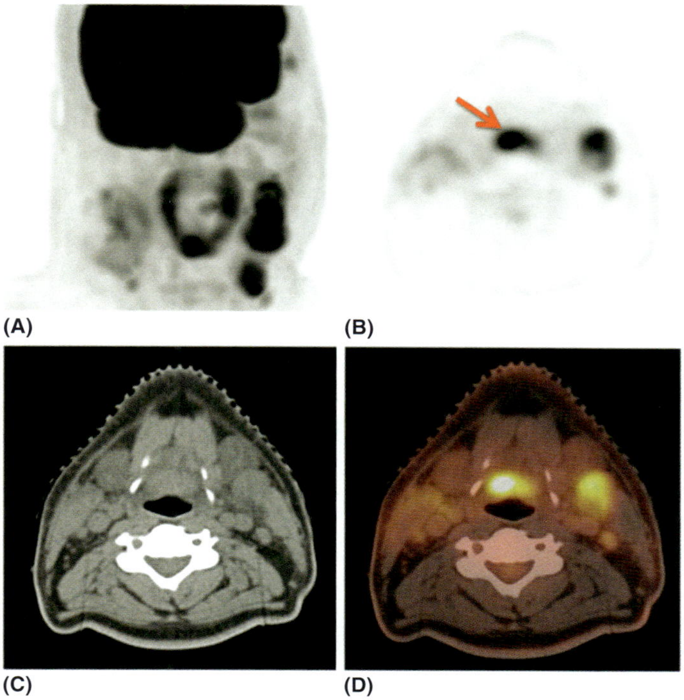

FIGURE 5.1 Detection of unknown primary. FDG PET/CT performed for identification of unknown primary in a 57-year-old presenting with metastatic cervical lymphadenopathy demonstrated FDG avid focus in the base of tongue (right side, arrow), confirmed on histology as moderately differentiated SCC. MIP image (A), transaxial PET image (B), CT image (C), fused PET/CT image (D) demonstrate focal FDG uptake in base of tongue (arrow) with bilateral level II enlarged and FDG avid lymph nodes (36).

FDG, fluorodeoxyglucose, MIP, maximum intensity projection; SCC, squamous cell cancer.

one side was cN0 verified with neck CT or MRI who were willing to undergo an elective neck dissection. In this report, high NPV has been demonstrated with FDG PET/CT for node negativity for bilateral necks with 0.90 (95% confidence interval [CI]: 0.83–0.95) and specific to the N0 sides 0.92 (95% CI: 0.86–0.97). This may obviate the need for elective neck dissection in cN0 neck, if the FDG PET/CT is negative in HNSCC patients.

The presence of distant metastases is an important prognostic factor in patients with head and neck cancer. The validity of the following as high-risk factors for the development of distant metastases has been confirmed: three or more lymph node metastases, bilateral lymph node metastases, lymph nodes larger than 6 cm, low jugular lymph node metastases, and regional recurrence (19). Lung metastasis is the most frequent metastatic site and CT chest (sensitivity and specificity 73% and 80%, respectively) is valuable in detecting lung metastases. However, ^{18}F-FDG PET/CT is recommended as first-line imaging for detecting distant metastases, as it covers the entire body from skull base to midthigh (Figure 5.3). A meta-analysis by Xu et al. (20) suggested that 209 of 1,445 (14.4%) patients had a distant metastasis or a second primary tumor, with PET showing a sensitivity of 87.5% and an overall specificity of 95% in the initial M staging of HNSCC.

PREDICTING PATIENT OUTCOMES

High FDG avidity on pretherapy FDG PET/CT has been shown in meta-analyses to be significantly associated with worse survival outcomes in patients with HNSCC (21,22). Zhang et al. (21) concluded that increased SUVmax of the primary tumor is a poor prognostic factor and has a potential value in predicting local control, disease-free survival, and overall survival (OS). Other PET-derived parameters for the primary tumor such as metabolic tumor volume (MTV) and total lesion glycolysis (TLG) have also been studied in a meta-analysis by Pak et al.

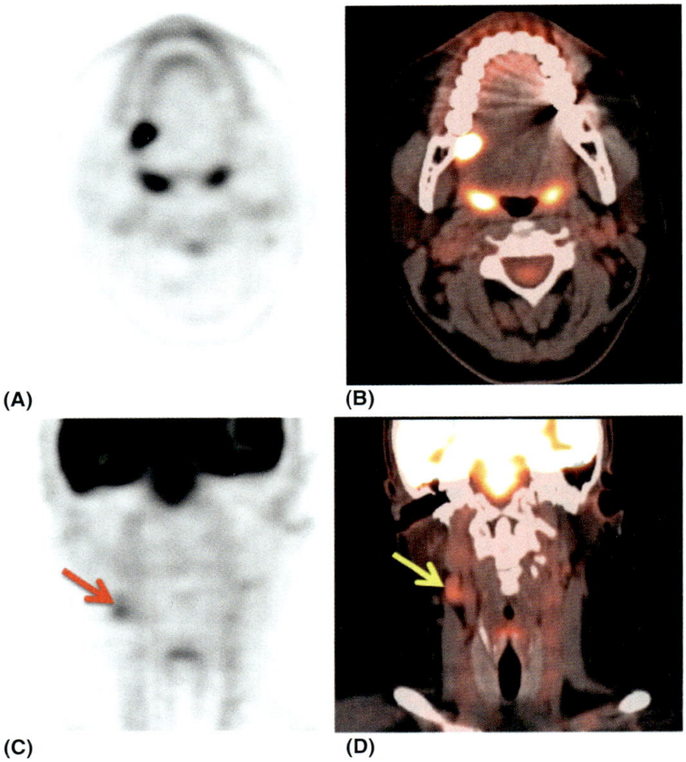

FIGURE 5.2 Initial staging. FDG PET/CT for initial staging in a 38-year-old female with newly diagnosed moderately differentiated SCC of the tongue and a clinically N0 neck. There is an intensely FDG avid right lateral tongue mass on transaxial PET image (A) and fused transaxial PET–CT image (B). FDG avid, morphologically normal and nonenlarged right level II cervical lymph node (measuring 7 mm in short axis with SUVmax 4.2) seen on coronal PET (C, arrow) as well as on fused coronal PET/CT image (D, arrow), found positive for metastatic carcinoma on histopathology (pT1pN1) (36).

FDG, fluorodeoxyglucose; SCC, squamous cell carcinoma; SUV, standardized uptake value.

(22). They reviewed 13 studies including 1,180 patients and found these volumetric measurements to be valuable prognostic markers for predicting future recurrence, progression, or both. However, it is important to note that SUV and consequently all other PET-derived quantitative parameters suffer from lack of standardization of the acquisition and processing protocols. Significant efforts are under way in standardizing PET/CT to utilize these imaging markers in clinical practice and in clinical trials (23).

POSTTREATMENT STRATEGY

THERAPY RESPONSE ASSESSMENT

In a landmark prospective, randomized, controlled trial of 564 patients with advanced head and neck cancer (no metastatic disease) published in 2016, Mehanna et al. (24) showed ^{18}F-FDG PET/CT performed at 12 weeks following completion of chemoradiotherapy could direct neck dissection (Figures 5.4 and 5.5). Specifically, neck dissection performed only if ^{18}F-FDG PET/CT posttherapy showed incomplete or equivocal response resulted in similar patient quality of life and survival at lower cost than when neck dissection was planned because of stage N2 or N3 disease. Authors recommended that the patients with an equivocal FDG uptake with HPV-negative disease should proceed to neck dissection. Authors pointed out patients with HPV-positive cancers having enlarged nodes with no FDG uptake after chemoradiotherapy may be closely followed up with serial CT or PET/CT. This strategy of avoiding surgical complications may be more cost-effective than neck dissection.

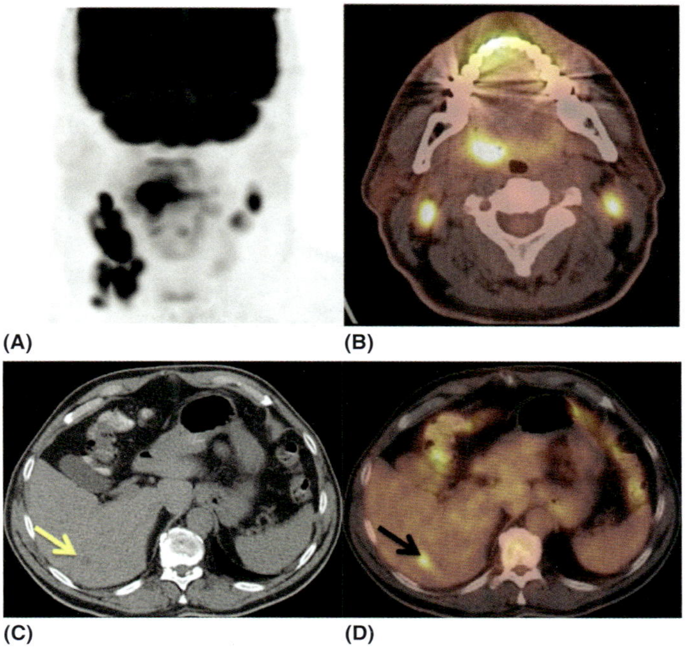

FIGURE 5.3 Initial staging. FDG PET/CT for initial staging demonstrates FDG avid right palatine tonsillar mass, FDG avid bilateral level II and right level III cervical lymph nodes on MIP image (A) and fused transaxial PET/CT image (B) as well as 11 mm FDG avid right hepatic lesion in segment 6 on fused transaxial PET/CT image (D, arrow) with subtle hypodensity on noncontrast transaxial CT (C, arrow) upstaging the disease to clinical stage T2N2cM1 (histology—moderately differentiated p16 positive SCC) (36).

FDG, fluorodeoxyglucose; MIP, maximum intensity projection; SCC, squamous cell carcinoma.

One of the limitations in evaluating ^{18}F-FDG PET/CT effectiveness posttherapy for patients with HNSCC is the lack of a universal scoring system for result classification. A five-point qualitative posttherapy assessment scoring system (Hopkins criteria) (14) has been proposed for head and neck ^{18}F-FDG PET/CT (Table 5.1). The Hopkins criteria have strong inter-reader agreement, has excellent NPV, and is predictive of PFS and OS in this patient population. Specifically, the overall agreement between readers was 86%, the NPV was 91%, and using a Kaplan–Meier survival analysis, the PFS and OS between patients classified as negative for residual tumor by the five-point scale compared with those classified as positive were statistically significant. The hazard ratio (HR) was 0.05 (95% CI: 0.02–0.11) for PFS and 0.046 (95% CI: 0.018–0.120) for OS.

In a meta-analysis of 51 studies comprising 2,335 patients, Gupta and colleagues (25) evaluated the diagnostic performance of posttreatment FDG PET/CT scan. The impact of timing of posttreatment FDG PET/CT was also assessed before and after 12 weeks. The pooled sensitivity (79.9% and 72.7%), specificity (87.5% and 87.6%), NPV (95.1% and 94.5%), and positive predictive value (PPV; 58.6% and 52.1%) of FDG PET/CT were reported for the primary site and the neck nodes, respectively. Sensitivity was higher in both primary tumor (91.9% vs. 73.6%, p = .12) and neck nodes (90.4% vs. 62.5%, p < .001) in scans performed greater than or equal to 12 weeks compared to those less than 12 weeks. Similarly, Isles and colleagues (26) performed a meta-analysis of 27 studies to evaluate the effectiveness of PET in detection of recurrence or residual HNSCC after cisplatin-based chemoradiation (CRT). They reported pooled sensitivity, specificity, PPV, and NPV of 94%, 82%, 75%, and 95%, respectively. Considering the effect of the timing of scans, they indicated that the sensitivity is significantly higher for scans performed greater than 10 weeks after CRT compared with those performed less than 10 weeks (p = .002).

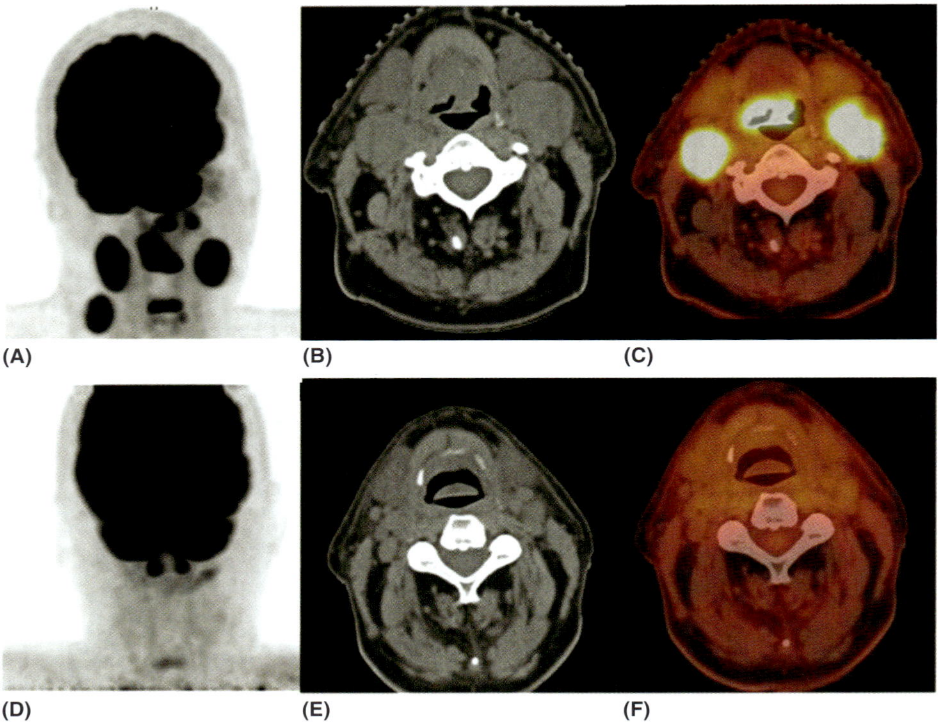

FIGURE 5.4 Posttherapy assessment. FDG PET/CT for initial staging in a 72-year-old man demonstrates FDG avid oropharyngeal mass with FDG avid bilateral level II, right level III cervical lymph nodes seen on MIP image (A), transaxial CT (B), and fused transaxial PET/CT image (C) (stage IVb disease). FDG PET/CT 3 months after completion of definitive CRT demonstrates resolution of FDG avid oropharyngeal mass seen on MIP image (D), resolution of the FDG avid bilateral cervical lymphadenopathy with a remaining left level II 1.2 cm residual node (E) with mild FDG uptake (F), below liver FDG uptake. The neck was negative on clinical examination and the patient had no recurrence on a 12-month follow-up (36).

CRT, isplatin-based chemoradiation; FDG, fluorodeoxyglucose; MIP, maximum intensity projection.

FDG PET/CT findings in posttherapy assessment are time and therapy dependent. An increase in FDG uptake occurs in recently radiated tissues, which may last 12 to 16 weeks. To ensure a balance between the disadvantages of early and late imaging, the first posttreatment FDG PET/CT scan to assess therapy response is recommended at least 10 to 12 weeks after radiation therapy to minimize radiation-related inflammatory uptake and at least after 3 weeks (before the next cycle) completion of chemotherapy. In order to minimize the effects of therapy-related inflammation, it is preferable to allow a minimum of 10 to 12 weeks to elapse between the time of chemoradiotherapy and imaging. Performing the ^{18}F-FDG PET/CT sooner than 10 to 12 weeks after completion of treatment may be associated with lower sensitivity and specificity. When imaging is performed 12 months after therapy, the sensitivity of ^{18}F-FDG PET/CT for the detection of recurrent disease has been reported to be as high as 100%. Also, use of contrast-enhanced ^{18}F-FDG PET/CT with an additional head and neck acquisition may improve the specificity of locoregional recurrence.

DETECTING RECURRENCES AND FOLLOW-UP

The NCCN guidelines suggest clinical surveillance every 1 to 3 months for the first year following therapy, every 2 to 4 months for the second year following therapy, and every 4 to 6 months for the subsequent 3 years (16). Imaging of the primary site of disease is recommended within 6 months of therapy. CT and MRI are commonly the imaging modalities chosen. However, interpretation may be limited by changes from therapy. There have been

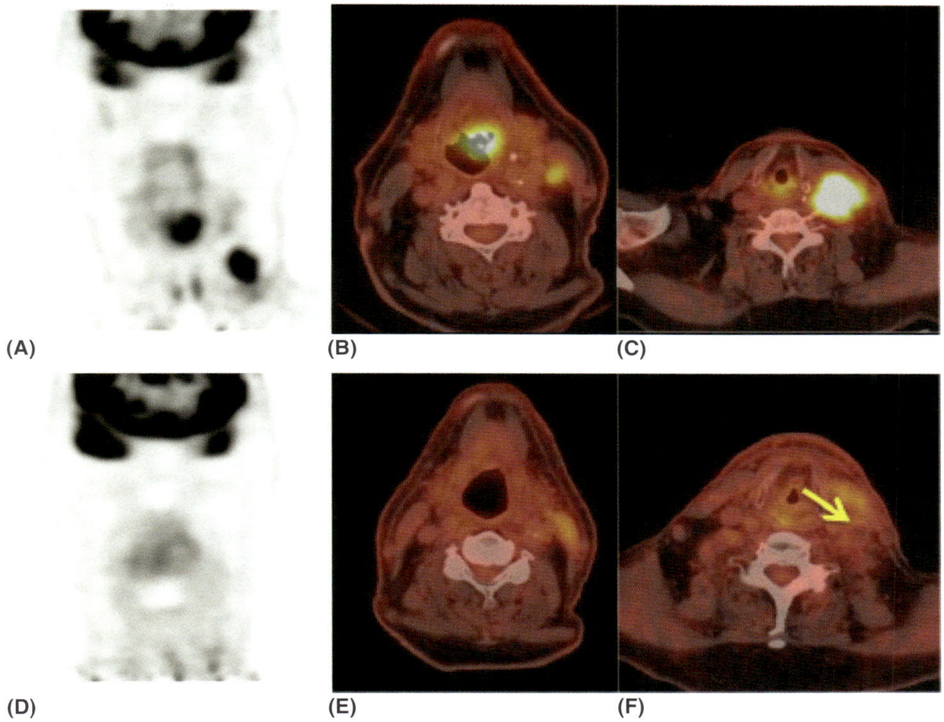

FIGURE 5.5 Posttherapy assessment. Pretreatment FDG PET/CT in a 76-year-old man demonstrates FDG avid left palatine tonsillar mass with extension to the left base of tongue and across midline on MIP image (A) as well as fused transaxial PET/CT image (B) with FDG avid left cervical lymph nodes most prominent being left level III nodal mass on fused transaxial PET/CT images (B and C) (stage T3N2cM0). FDG PET/CT 3 months after CRT with carboplatin/Taxol demonstrates resolution of FDG avid left base of tongue mass as seen on MIP image (D) and fused transaxial PET/CT image (E) as well as resolution of the FDG avid left cervical lymphadenopathy with a remaining left level III 1.2-cm residual necrotic node with no FDG uptake (36).

CRT, cisplatin-based chemoradiation; FDG, fluorodeoxyglucose; MIP, maximum intensity projection.

several studies suggesting ^{18}F-FDG PET/CT is valuable for assessing patients with HNSCC after therapy. Meta-analyses have suggested a high sensitivity and specificity of ^{18}F-FDG PET/CT for detecting residual or recurrent head and neck cancer after therapy (80%–94% and 80%–95%, respectively).

No recommendation is available for an imaging strategy in follow-up. The best clinical strategy is to perform imaging when clinical signs or symptoms are suggestive of recurrence. Routine surveillance imaging without clinical suspicion should be strongly avoided. Most of the recurrences or distant metastases occur during the first 2 years after completion of therapy (Figure 5.6). Patients with HPV-positive oropharyngeal SCC have a better clinical outcome and prognosis (27). Though the disease recurrence is less common in HPV-positive orpharyngeal squamous cell cancer (SCC), up to 36% of patients experience treatment failure within 8 years. There is controversy over the pattern and timing of recurrence in HPV-positive versus HPV-negative cohorts. The pattern and timing of recurrences and distant metastases may be different in patients with HPV-positive disease with late metastases (after 2 years of completion of therapy) and "disseminated type" seen in many solid organs and skeleton (28,29) (Figure 5.7). However, the secondary analysis of RTOG 0129 and RTOG 0522 found that 41% of HPV-positive and 38% of HPV-negative oropharyngeal carcinoma (OPC) displayed isolated distant metastatic disease at first progression (30). Median time to distant metastasis did not differ based on p16 status (11.9 vs. 12.4 months). p16-positive and p16-negative OPCs were found to

TABLE 5.1

Hopkins Criteria—Head and Neck PET/CT Therapy Assessment Standardized Method

Score	FDG Uptake Pattern	Response Category
1	FDG uptake at the primary site and nodes, less than IJV	Complete metabolic response
2	Focal FDG uptake at the primary site and nodes greater than IJV, but less than liver	Likely complete metabolic response
3	Diffuse FDG uptake at the primary site or nodes is greater than IJV or liver	Likely postradiation inflammation
4	Focal FDG uptake at the primary site or nodes, greater than liver	Likely residual tumor
5	Focal and intense FDG uptake at the primary site or nodes	Residual tumor FDG, fluorodeoxyglucose; IJV, internal jugular vein.

Scores 1, 2, and 3, which represent complete metabolic response, likely complete metabolic response, and likely postradiation inflammation, respectively, were considered negative for tumor. Scores 4 and 5, which represent likely residual tumor and residual tumor, respectively, were considered positive for tumor. A new lesion would be considered as progressive disease.

have similar anatomical distribution of distant metastasis (lung: 73% vs. 70%; bone: 14.6% vs. 15.2%; liver: 8.3% vs. 15.2%; other 16.7% vs. 12.1%). Despite these similarities, patients with HPV-positive disease showed significantly improved OS relative to those with HPV-negative disease (2.6 vs. 0.8 years, respectively). There is also evidence that HPV-positive patients with a negative PET/CT within 6 to 12 months of completion of therapy

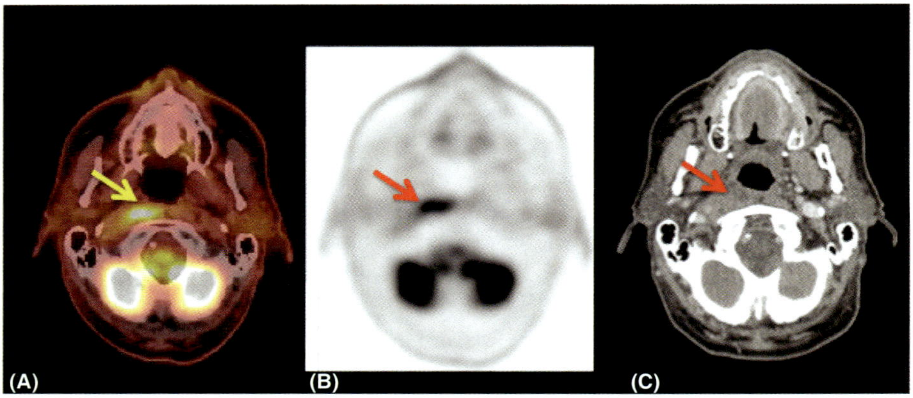

FIGURE 5.6 Recurrence detection. Pretreatment FDG PET/CT in a 68-year-old man showed intensely FDG avid mass in the right base of the tongue with associated hypermetabolic right lateral retropharyngeal and right cervical level II to V lymphadenopathy with resolution on 3-month post-CRT FDG PET study. However, a new asymmetric focus of FDG avidity in the right side of nasopharynx on the 9-month follow-up PET scan—(A) transaxial fused PET/CT image, (B) transaxial PET image—correlating with low attenuation lesion on contrast CT neck (C) was proved to be recurrent SCC (36).

CRT, cisplatin-based chemoradiation; FDG, fluorodeoxyglucose; SCC, squamous cell carcinoma.

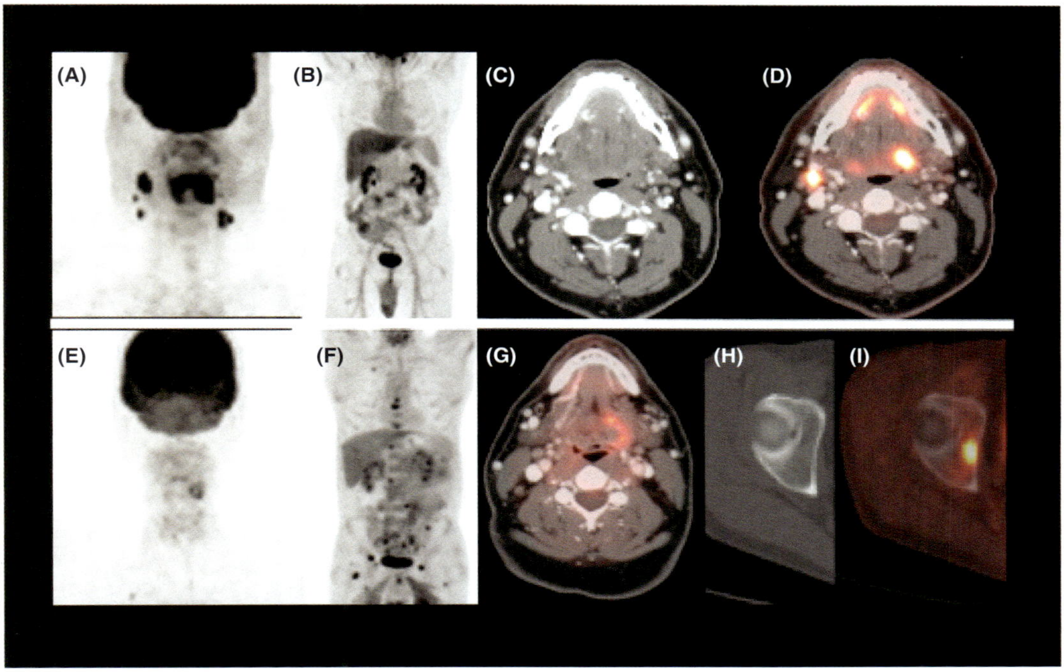

FIGURE 5.7 Disease recurrence with distant metastases. 46-year-old man with a history of HPV-positive squamous cell carcinoma of the left base of tongue, stage T1N2cM0. Staging scan with MIP of head and neck (A) and whole body (B), axial IV contrast CT (C) and fused contrast-enhanced PET/CT (D). Primary site had SUVmax 10.52, SUV peak 7.74, MTV 5.91 mL, and TLG 32.11 g with locoregional nodal metastasis in bilateral neck nodes. The patient was treated with definitive chemoradiation with cisplatin, fractional dose 200 cGy with 35 fractions for a total dose of 70 Gy. Contrast-enhanced PET/CT scan 4 months after the end of treatment showed recurrent disease. Restaging scan with MIP of the head and neck (E), whole body (F) demonstrated significant progression with recurrent disease in the left base of tongue (G), and multiple intense foci of FDG uptake scattered throughout the axial skeleton, including right acetabulum (I) with no obvious corresponding CT (H) abnormalities. This case is an example of distant metastasis occurring in unusual sites (multiple skeletal sites) and with a "disseminating phenotype." HPV status may have more of an influence on the pattern rather than incidence of delayed distant spread, surfacing at distant sites rarely targeted by HPV-negative cancers, may be related to repression of viral oncogene expression, which induce massive apoptosis and restoration of p53 and pRb tumor suppressor pathways (2).

FDG, fluorodeoxyglucose; HPV, human papillomavirus; MIP, maximum intensity projection; MTV, metabolic tumor volume; SUV, standardized uptake value; TLG, total lesion glycolysis.

have a median 28 months of progression-free survival (PFS) (31). These observations suggest that the frequency of follow-up PET/CT (or any imaging) can be reduced in patients with HPV-positive oropharyngeal SCC.

RECENT ADVANCES

In recent years, integrated PET/MRI systems have become possible in clinical settings. Schaarschmidt et al. (32) evaluated the accuracy of integrated ^{18}F-FDG PET/MR, ^{18}F-FDG PET/CT, and MR imaging in initial tumor diagnosis and recurrence in 25 patients with histopathologically confirmed HNSCC. They found no significant differences in T and N staging and cancer recurrence among the three modalities ($p > .017$). Although ^{18}F-FDG PET/MR had higher sensitivity than MR imaging in tumor recurrence, accuracy was found to be equivalent to the FDG PET/CT. However, it should be noted that PET/MRI provides unique opportunities for multiparametric imaging such as interrogating a lesion with FDG metabolism (SUVmax) and apparent diffusion coefficient (ADC) (33).

Recent studies demonstrate FDG PET has the potential to predict the tumor heterogeneity. Kwon et al. indicated that the intratumoral heterogeneity of ^{18}F-FDG uptake is an important prognostic factor for OS as well as demonstrating that SUVmax, MTV, TLG, and heterogeneity factor of the primary tumor were significant prognostic factors in oral cavity cancer (34). Mena et al. (35) investigated 105 HPV-positive oropharyngeal squamous cell carcinoma (OPSCC) patients, retrospectively. They demonstrated that, intratumoral metabolic heterogeneity using ^{18}F-FDG PET/CT was a prognostic factor for event-free survival with primary HPV-positive OPSCC. Similarly Oh et al. investigated that in a small group of patients with hypopharyngeal squamous cell cancer (HPSCC) who underwent cisplatin-based induction chemotherapy followed by definitive chemoradiation therapy (CRT). The authors showed that textural features derived baseline ^{18}F-FDG PET images may be predictive of response to CRT and survival in HPSCC and intratumoral heterogeneity may identify patients at risk for low response rates and poor DFS and OS outcomes. Accordingly, the abnormal textural feature of tumor coarseness may be useful for predicting response and survival after CRT in HPSCC patients.

CONCLUSIONS

Imaging plays a central role in detecting head and neck cancers and staging, facilitating therapy decisions, assessing therapy response, detecting recurrences, and following up patients. CT, MRI and PET/CT are the common imaging modalities deployed appropriately, based on the clinical context. NCCN guidelines recommend CT or MRI neck for primary tumor and local disease, PET/CT for stage III and IV disease staging, detecting unknown primary, and therapy response assessment 10 to 12 weeks after concurrent chemoradiation therapy. If posttherapy FDG PET/CT is negative, planned neck dissection is avoided. Imaging is best performed in the context of clinical suspicion of recurrence or metastases in follow-up, than for routine surveillance.

REFERENCES

1. Jemal A, Bray F, Center MM, et al. Global cancer statistics. *CA Cancer J Clin*. 2011;61(2):69–90. doi:10.3322/caac.20107
2. Subramaniam RM, Alluri KC, Tahari AK, Aygun N, Quon H. PET/CT Imaging and human papilloma virus-positive oropharyngeal squamous cell cancer: evolving clinical imaging paradigm. *J Nucl Med*. 2014.
3. Ang KK, Harris J, Wheeler R, et al. Human papillomavirus and survival of patients with oropharyngeal cancer. *N Engl J Med*. 2010;363(1):24–35.
4. Chong VF, Mukherji SK, Goh CH. The suprahyoid neck: normal and pathological anatomy. *J Laryngol Otol*. 1999;113(6):501–508.
5. Mukherji SK, Pillsbury HR, Castillo M. Imaging squamous cell carcinomas of the upper aerodigestive tract: what clinicians need to know. *Radiology*. 1997;205(3):629–646.
6. Badger D, Aygun N. Imaging of perineural spread in head and neck cancer. *Radiol Clin North Am*. 2017;55(1):139–149.
7. Subramaniam R, Truong M, Peller P, Sakai O, Mercier G. Fluorodeoxyglucose–positron-emission tomography imaging of head and neck squamous cell cancer. *Am J Neuroradiol*. 2010;31(4):598–604.
8. Platzek I. (18)F-Fluorodeoxyglucose PET/MR imaging in head and neck cancer. *PET Clin*. 2016;11(4):375–386.
9. Khokhar MT, Day KM, Sangal RB, et al. Preoperative high-resolution ultrasound for the assessment of malignant central compartment lymph nodes in papillary thyroid cancer. *Thyroid*. 2015;25(12):1351–1354.
10. Padma S, Sundaram PS. Radioiodine as an adjuvant therapy and its role in follow-up of differentiated thyroid cancer. *J Cancer Res Ther*. 2016;12(3):1109–1113.
11. Tardelli E, Mazzarri S, Rubello D, et al. Sentinel lymph node biopsy in cutaneous melanoma: standard and new technical procedures and clinical advances. A systematic review of the literature. *Clin Nucl Med*. 2016;41(12):e498–e507.
12. Jimenez-Heffernan A, Ellmann A, Sado H, et al. Results of a prospective multicenter international atomic energy agency sentinel node trial on the value of SPECT/CT over planar imaging in various malignancies. *J Nucl Med*. 2015;56(9):1338–1344.
13. Kyzas PA, Evangelou E, Denaxa-Kyza D, Ioannidis JP. 18F-fluorodeoxyglucose positron emission tomography to evaluate cervical node metastases in patients with head and neck squamous cell carcinoma: a meta-analysis. *J Natl Cancer Inst*. 2008;100(10):712–720.
14. Marcus C, Ciarallo A, Tahari AK, et al. Head and neck PET/CT: therapy response interpretation criteria (Hopkins Criteria)-interreader reliability, accuracy, and survival outcomes. *J Nucl Med*. 2014;55(9):1411–1416.
15. Edge SB, Byrd DR, Compton CC, et al. eds. *AJCC Cancer Staging Manual*. 7th ed. France: Springer; 2010 [cited 2014 Jun 12]. Retrieved from http://www.springer.com/medicine/surgery/
16. NCCN Clinical Practice Guidelines in Oncology - Head and Neck Cancers. version 2.2017- May 8, 2017.
17. Zhu L, Wang N. ^{18}F-fluorodeoxyglucose positron emission tomography-computed tomography as a diagnostic tool in patients with cervical nodal metastases of unknown primary site: a meta-analysis. *Surg Oncol*. 2013;22(3):190–194.

18. Stack BC, Duan F, Sicks J, et al. The negative predictive value (NPV) of FDG-PET/CT in the head and neck squamous cell carcinoma (HNSCC) N0 patient, the first report of the ACRIN 6685 trial. *J Clin Oncol* 2017;35 (suppl; abstr 6041).
19. Peters TT, Senft A, Hoekstra OS, et al. Pretreatment screening on distant metastases and head and neck cancer patients: validation of risk factors and influence on survival. *Oral Oncol.* 2015;51(3):267–271.
20. Xu G-Z, Guan D-J, He Z-Y. ^{18}FDG-PET/CT for detecting distant metastases and second primary cancers in patients with head and neck cancer. A meta-analysis. *Oral Oncol.* 2011;47(7):560–565.
21. Zhang B, Li X, Lu X. Standardized uptake value is of prognostic value for outcome in head and neck squamous cell carcinoma. *Acta Oto-laryngol.* 2010;130(7):756–762.
22. Pak K, Cheon GJ, Nam HY, et al. Prognostic value of metabolic tumor volume and total lesion glycolysis in head and neck cancer: a systematic review and meta-analysis. *J Nucl Med.* 2014;55(6):884–890.
23. Radiological Society of North America. Quantitative imaging biomarkers alliance. Retrieved from www.rsna.org/QIBA.
24. Mehanna H, Wong WL, McConkey CC, et al. PET-CT Surveillance versus neck dissection in advanced head and neck cancer. *N Engl J Med.* 2016;374(15):1444–1454.
25. Gupta T, Master Z, Kannan S, et al. Diagnostic performance of post-treatment FDG PET or FDG PET/CT imaging in head and neck cancer: a systematic review and meta-analysis. *Eur J Nucl Med Mol Imaging.* 2011;38(11):2083–2095.
26. Isles MG, McConkey C, Mehanna HM. A systematic review and meta-analysis of the role of positron emission tomography in the follow up of head and neck squamous cell carcinoma following radiotherapy or chemoradiotherapy. *Clin Otolaryngol.* 2008;33(3):210–222.
27. Sedghizadeh PP, Billington WD, Paxton D, et al. Is p16-positive oropharyngeal squamous cell carcinoma associated with favorable prognosis? A systematic review and meta-analysis. *Oral Oncol.* 2016;54:15–27.
28. Huang SH, Perez-Ordonez B, Liu FF, et al. Atypical clinical behavior of p16-confirmed HPV-related oropharyngeal squamous cell carcinoma treated with radical radiotherapy. *Int J Radiat Oncol Biol Phys.* 2012;82(1):276–283.
29. Sinha P, Thorstad WT, Nussenbaum B, et al. Distant metastasis in p16-positive oropharyngeal squamous cell carcinoma: a critical analysis of patterns and outcomes. *Oral Oncol.* 2014;50(1):45–51.
30. Faraji F, Eisele DW, Fakhry C. Emerging insights into recurrent and metastatic human papillomavirus-related oropharyngeal squamous cell carcinoma. *Laryngoscope Investig Otolaryngol.* 2017;2(1):10–18.
31. Taghipour M, Marcus C, Califano J, Fakhry C, Subramaniam RM. The value of follow-up FDG-PET/CT in the management and prognosis of patients with HPV-positive oropharyngeal squamous cell carcinoma. *J Med Imaging Radiat Oncol.* 2015;59(6):681–686.
32. Schaarschmidt BM, Heusch P, Buchbender C, et al. Locoregional tumour evaluation of squamous cell carcinoma in the head and neck area: a comparison between MRI, PET/CT and integrated PET/MRI. *Eur J Nucl Med Mol Imaging.* 2016;43(1):92–102.
33. Rasmussen JH, Norgaard M, Hansen AE, et al. Feasibility of multiparametric imaging with PET/MR in head and neck squamous cell carcinoma. *J Nucl Med.* 2017;58(1):69–74.
34. Kwon SH, Yoon J-K, An Y-S, et al. Prognostic significance of the intratumoral heterogeneity of ^{18}F-FDG uptake in oral cavity cancer. *J Surg Oncol.* 2014;110(6):702–706.
35. Mena E, Taghipour M, Sheikhbahaei S, et al. Value of intratumoral metabolic heterogeneity and quantitative 18F-FDG PET/CT parameters to predict prognosis in patients with HPV-positive primary oropharyngeal squamous cell carcinoma. *Clin Nucl Med.* 2017;42(5):e227–e234.
36. Goel R, Moore W, Sumer B, et al. Clinical practice in PET/CT for the management of head and neck squamous cell cancer. *AJR Am J Roentgenol.* 2017;209(2):289–303.

SECTION II

Established and Emerging Treatment Modalities

6

Advances in Radiation Therapy Techniques for HNSCC: Image-Guided RT Stereotactic, IMRT-VMAT, MRI-Linac and Simulation

Jussi Sillanpaa

C. Jillian Tsai

Nancy Y. Lee

Photon-based (x-ray and gamma ray) radiation therapy techniques for head and neck cancer have undergone rapid development in the past decades. Improvements in pretreatment imaging, image guidance, and treatment delivery have changed clinical practices considerably. This chapter outlines recent developments in x-ray based treatment techniques. Another major change in radiation therapy technology is the growing use of proton therapy; that is described in a dedicated Chapter 7.

RADIATION THERAPY SIMULATION

Radiation therapy simulation is the process in which a patient is positioned and immobilized, and diagnostic quality imaging is obtained from which a radiation therapy treatment plan is derived. This is performed in a dedicated simulation suite, and is now typically computed tomography based.

COMPUTED TOMOGRAPHY

Contrast-enhanced CT, with a typical slice thickness of 1–3 mm and no CT gantry tilt, is the primary imaging modality for simulating most patients. CT images have excellent spatial resolution, have good visualization of the bony anatomy and airways, and provide the electron density information needed for megavoltage dose calculations. CT is a low-cost modality with fast scanning time and is universally available. However, metal objects, such as dental fillings, could cause artifacts in CT images. In addition, some patients may not be able to tolerate iodinated contrast agents.

CT scanners especially designed for radiation treatment planning, with a big (approx. 85 cm) bore and a large reconstruction field of view, are available from all major manufacturers. Patients are simulated in a supine position, on a flat table top similar to that in the treatment machine. A multislice CT scanner makes the acquisition of scans with thin slice thicknesses much easier and reduces patient motion artifacts; however, a single slice CT is usually sufficient for many scanning techniques. Immobilization is usually achieved by using thermoplastic masks indexed to the treatment machine couch. If optical tracking is used, such as AlignRT (1), the masks are left partially open to leave most of the patient's face uncovered.

If the oral cavity is in the radiation field and the patient has a large number of metal dental fillings, a mouth guard is sometimes utilized. The rubber mouth guard, made prior to the simulation, fits over the teeth and can absorb some of the scattered radiation from the fillings, thus potentially sparing the oral mucosa. The effects of the mouth guard are hard to quantify and they do not enjoy universal popularity. There has not been enough evidence suggesting its significance in reducing oral toxicities from radiation therapy. However, the mouth guards do reduce metal artifacts in the simulation CT scan, making it easier to define treatment volumes. Software is also used to reduce metal artifacts; see following text.

A custom-made positioning stent is sometimes used to displace the tongue from radiation target areas to reduce toxicity or to immobilize it to properly expose the target tumor (Figure 6.1). For example, a mouth opening tongue depressing stent may be used for postoperative oral tongue cancer cases to secure the target volume, and a tongue lateralizing stent may be used during unilateral postoperative radiation therapy for parotid salivary cancer. A recent trial randomizing 30 oral tongue cancer patients to conventional radiation therapy with or without using a positioning stent demonstrated significantly improved stimulated and unstimulated salivary flow as well as quality of life in the group of patients treated with the use of stents (2). Of note, stents and mouth guards affect patient positioning and should be worn throughout the treatment course.

Unless the patient has a history of severe reactions to iodinated contrast media, a contrast injection is commonly used to enhance the soft tissue differentiation. Typically 100–150 mL of contrast agent is utilized. A delay of approximately 1 minute between the contrast injection and the beginning of the scan is used to allow the tissues to take up the contrast agent. The tumor usually takes up more contrast agent than surrounding soft tissue, allowing improved target delineation. In most cases, contrast uptake is not large enough to have an adverse effect on the accuracy of dose calculations; if this is a concern, a noncontrast CT may also be acquired.

Dual-energy CT scanners are a very promising recent development. Dual energy means that two scans at widely separated energies (e.g., 80 kVp and 140 kVp) are acquired simultaneously. The low-energy scan has a high noise level, but bones and contrast media can be clearly distinguished from other materials, because of increased probability of photoelectric interaction. The high-energy scan has less noise but a lower enhancement level. The high- and low-energy scans may be combined in linear or nonlinear ways; reconstructions at

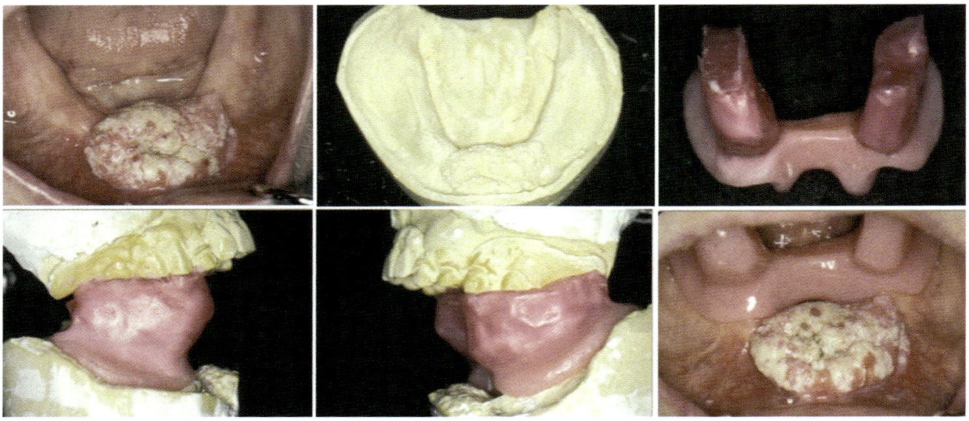

FIGURE 6.1 An 88-year-old patient with recurrent floor of mouth squamous cell carcinoma undergoing re-irradiation. A custom mouth-opening stent was fabricated to properly immoblize the tongue and jaws as well as to expose the gross tumor.

Source: Photos courtesy of Dr. Joesph M Huryn, DDS, FAAMP, Chief of the Dental Service, Memorial Sloan Kettering Cancer Center.

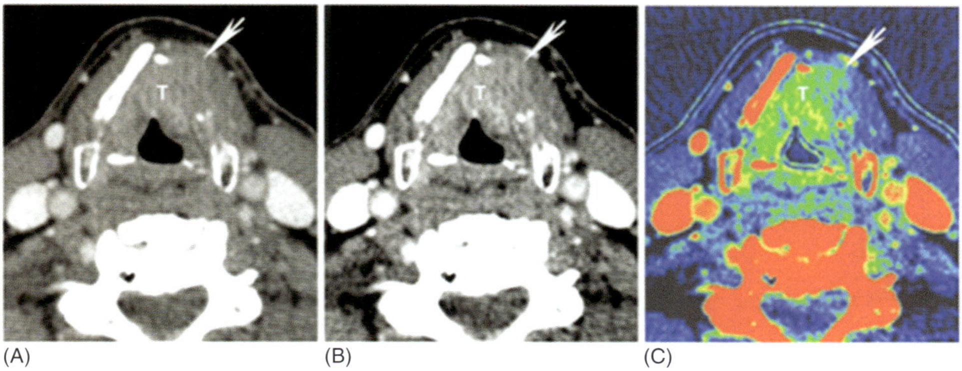

FIGURE 6.2 Virtual monochromatic images ([A] 65 keV, [B] 40 keV) and an iodine-water decomposition (C) constructed from a dual-energy CT scan (4). The laryngeal tumor (T) is more conspicuous in (B); the edge of the extralaryngeal tumor component, indicated by the arrow, is also more clearly seen in (B) and (C), while (A) has lower image noise.

virtual tube potentials between the two extremes can also be created; as demonstrated in Figure 6.2, these can be very helpful in tissue delineation (3,4). A virtual noncontrast image can also be reconstructed without additional scanning (5), thus reducing the scanning time and imaging dose and minimizing movement between the contrast and noncontrast images. The determination of tissue electron densities for dose calculation can also be made more accurate when a dual-energy scanner is utilized (6). Dual-energy CT scanning is a rapidly developing field that holds great promise for head and neck imaging.

The use of dynamic contrast-enhanced (DCE) CT techniques, such as CT perfusion, has also been proposed to better help define radiation target volumes. In these techniques, several images sets are acquired at different time points after the contrast injection, and a model describing the time-dependent contrast uptake is fitted to each region. Variation in the model parameters allows for tumor/normal tissue delineation. In DCE techniques for head and neck tumors reported in the literature (7,8) the patient is injected with iodinated contrast agent and CT scans are then acquired in cine mode (i.e., without moving the scanner table), using a low, 80 kVp tube potential to maximize the photoelectric interactions in the contrast material and the highest temporal resolution available. The scans are started 10 seconds after the contrast injection and are performed until 50 seconds after the injection. A time-contrast enhancement curve is then constructed for each voxel, which is used to create blood flow, blood volume, mean transit time, and permeability–surface area product maps. These maps can then be used to identify abnormal structures, such as pathologic lymph nodes, see Figure 6.3. DCE techniques have not yet attained wide popularity.

Artifacts from high-Z objects, such as dental fillings, may diminish the CT image quality significantly. Recently, many scanner manufacturers have brought to market metal artifact reduction algorithms, including O-MAR by Philips Healthcare, iMAR by Siemens Medical Systems, and MARS by GE Healthcare. These software packages utilize sophisticated image reconstruction techniques, typically based on iterative reconstruction, to reduce the metal artifacts. Dual-energy CT systems, such as Gemstone Spectral Imaging (GSI) by GE Healthcare, can also improve CT reconstruction accuracy.

Huang et al. (9,10) studied the performance of O-MAR, GSI, and MARS in the presence of metal objects. They scanned simple and anthropomorphic phantoms and created radiotherapy treatment plans on them; measurements taken with ion chambers and radiochromic film were compared with the dose calculations. The dose calculation effects could be divided into two causes—streak artifacts from the fillings and inaccurate metal object size representation in the CT images (the size of metal objects is overestimated), with the latter effect being the more important one for the head and neck phantom, see Figure 6.4. As shown in Figure 6.5, both MARS and O-MAR improved dose calculation accuracy. It was concluded that MARS reconstructions of the head and neck phantom were easier to contour, but its performance may be dependent on the size of the metallic implants.

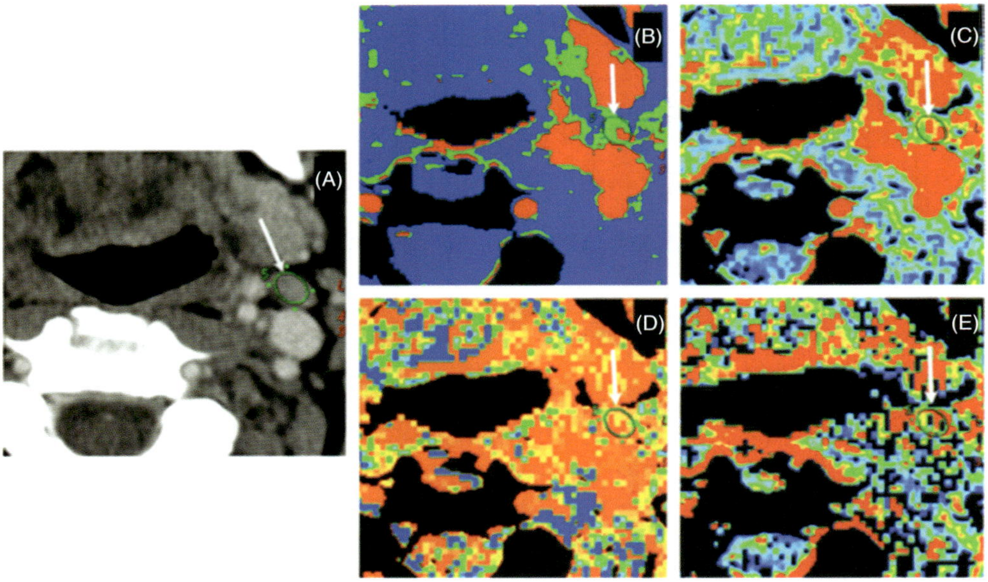

FIGURE 6.3 A laryngeal cancer patient with a suspicious lymph node ([A] regular CT, [B] blood flow, [C] blood volume, [D] mean transit time, [E] permeability surface map) (8). High values of blood flow and volume are strongly suggestive of malignancy; this was later confirmed on histologic examination.

Source: From Trojanowska A, Trojanowski P, Bisdas S, et al. Squamous cell cancer of hypopharynx and larynx—evaluation of metastatic nodal disease based on computed tomography perfusion studies. *Eur J Radiol.* 2012;81(5):1034–1039.

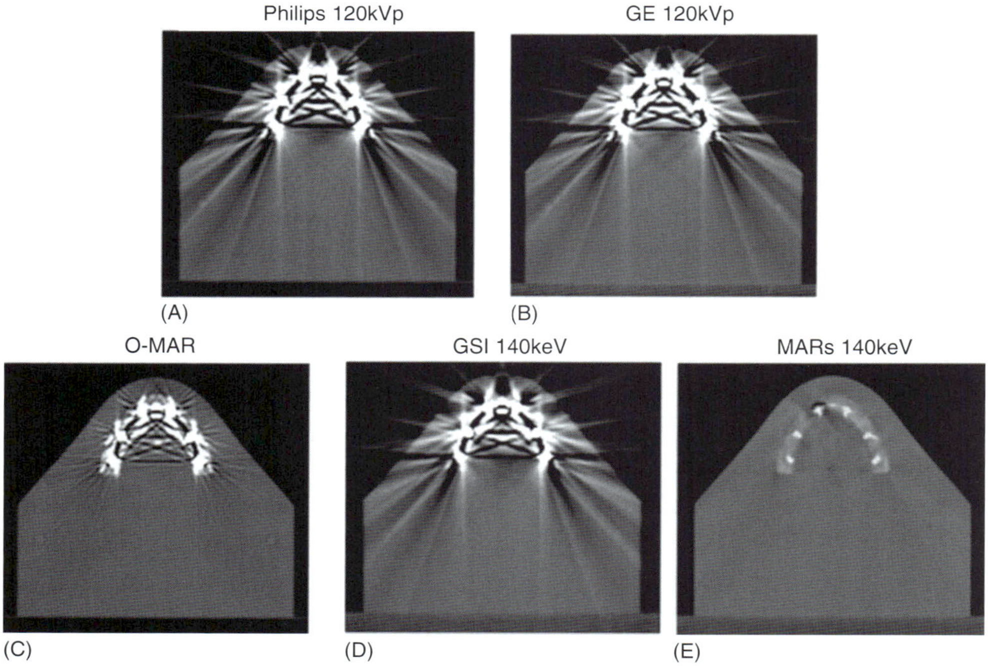

FIGURE 6.4 An anthropomorphic phantom with dental fillings set in cortical bone substitute, reconstructed using different metal artifact reduction strategies.

Source: From Huang JY, Followill DS, Howell RM, et al. Approaches to reducing photon dose calculation errors near metal implants. *Med Phys.* 2016;43(9):5117–5130.

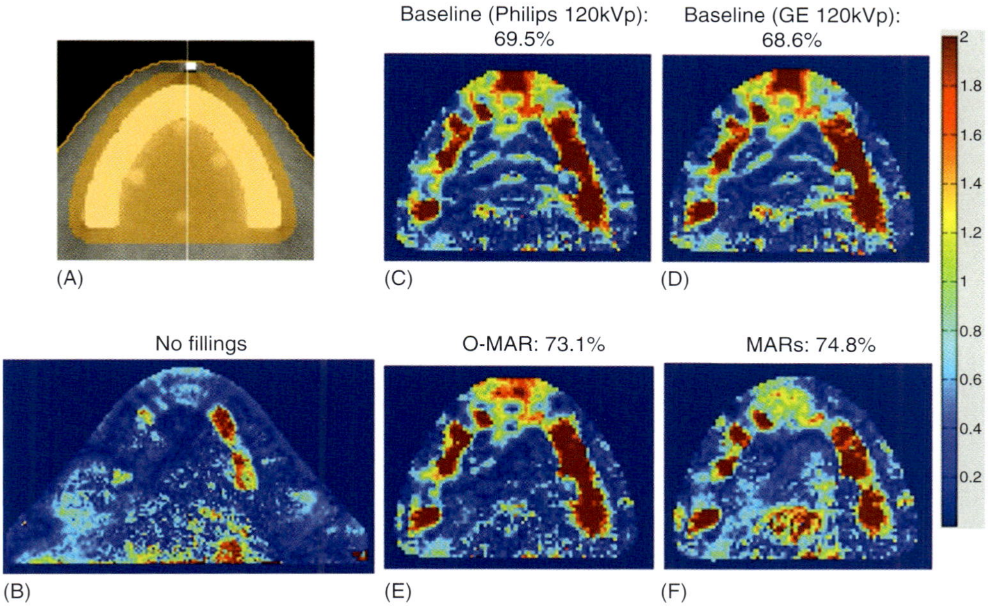

FIGURE 6.5 Radiochromic film dosimetry results for the phantom with dental fillings (A) (9). The percentages are the scores for gamma analysis with 3%, 3 mm passing criteria. When the fillings are removed (B), the score is 91.7%; the scores for with the dental fillings inserted and different CT reconstruction options (C-F) are noted in the figure.

Source: From Huang JY, Followill DS, Howell RM, et al. Approaches to reducing photon dose calculation errors near metal implants. *Med Phys*. 2016;43(9):5117–5130.

POSITRON EMISSION TOMOGRAPHY

PET scans with ^{18}F-fluorodeoxyglucose (FDG) co-registered to the conventional contrast CT simulation may improve the delineation of the primary lesion as well as the nodal metastases involved (11–13). There are two challenges for the use of PET-CT. One is that if the window-level is not accurate, the imaged volume will vary in size, and the other is the challenge of co-registration. A diagnostic imaging FDG PET is acquired with a curved scanner table top and a different patient position than the simulation CT, so registering them with the treatment planning CT scan may not be accurate. An image fusion program with a sophisticated deformable registration algorithm, such as MiM Vista (MiM Software, Cleveland, OH) or Velocity (Velocity Medical Solutions, Atlanta, GA), may help to improve co-registration. Another option is to acquire a PET scan specifically for treatment planning purposes, using a flat tabletop and the same patient immobilization as for the treatment planning CT. This kind of scan can be registered much more accurately with the primary CT data set, increasing the tissue contouring accuracy.

FDG PET highlights areas on increased glucose metabolism. It has higher sensitivity and specificity for detecting lymph node metastasis than CT or MRI. Although this is very helpful in identifying tumor spread, FDG is not a specific marker for cancer. Normal tissues, such as salivary glands, skeletal muscle, or brain, can also show uptake. Tissues with inflammation can exhibit high uptake as well and can lead to false positive findings. The PET resolution is much lower than in CT, making small lesions and bone destruction hard to characterize.

In addition to FDG, other kinds of radiotracers may be useful. Tracers for hypoxia are potentially useful, since hypoxic areas of the tumor are much more radioresistant and require higher doses to control them—identifying such regions and prescribing a higher dose for them may increase tumor control. A large number of hypoxia tracers are under investigation, including ^{62}Cu-diacetyl-bis(*N*-4-methyl-thiosemicarbazone) (Cu-ATSM) and ^{18}F-misonidazole (F-MISO). F-MISO is the most popular tracer in clinical practice. Several investigators have studied the feasibility of incorporating hypoxia PET imaging into radiotherapy treatment planning (14–19); for example, Hendrickson et al. studied the use of F-MISO scans to identify hypoxic regions for dose boosting. Intensity-modulated radiation therapy (IMRT) plans were created with simultaneous integrated boosts for hypoxic regions, resulting in a significant increase in predicted tumor control probability (19). When using hypoxia information for dose painting, the limitations of poor PET spatial resolution and possible time-dependent changes in hypoxia should be kept in mind; Lee et al. (14) studied hypoxia in patients with oropharyngeal cancer and found that while hypoxia is present in human papillomavirus positive patients, it resolves within 1 week of treatment in 48% of the cases either at the primary site or the lymph nodes. Figure 6.6 illustrates such a case; the hypoxic lymph node on the left side is resolved after one week of combined chemotherapy and radiation therapy. The 100% 2-year locoregional control rate achieved in their study suggests that intratreatment functional imaging could be used to de-escalate radiation dose in a clinical trial.

MAGNETIC RESONANCE IMAGING

MRI produces excellent soft tissue contrast and can be very valuable for target delineation. Modern MRI scanners with high magnetic field strength can produce image sets with good spatial resolution and signal-to-noise ratio in a reasonable imaging time. The imaging parameters can be adjusted according to the clinical need, making MRI a very versatile technique. The relatively long acquisition times mean that motion artifacts may be an issue. MRI also suffers from geometric distortion problems, which generally increase with increasing field strength. These artifacts may not be an issue for diagnostic purposes, but have the potential to cause significant contouring errors. A rigorous quality assurance program for image geometric integrity is thus strongly recommended (20). Some patients also have contraindications for MRI, including aneurysm clips and implanted medical devices.

Traditionally treatment planning MRI scans have been acquired on diagnostic units. Recently, dedicated MRI simulators have also become available (20,21). These systems incorporate a flat tabletop and lasers, as in a CT simulator, and can be used in addition to or instead of a CT simulator. The latter approach, which requires generation of electron densities from the MRI image, is not commonly used for head and neck patients. Using an MRI simulator makes the image registration task much easier. The bore of these units are still often smaller than those of the CT scanners, limiting the use of some immobilization devices.

The choice of receiver coil depends on the location of the tumor. A large number of pulse sequences, each with their own advantages and drawbacks, have been used (22–24). T1-weighted images have good contrast between fat or bone and soft tissue; the contrast between tumor, muscle, and lymphoid tissue, however, is usually poor. Gadolinium-based contrast can be used to shorten the T1 relaxation time

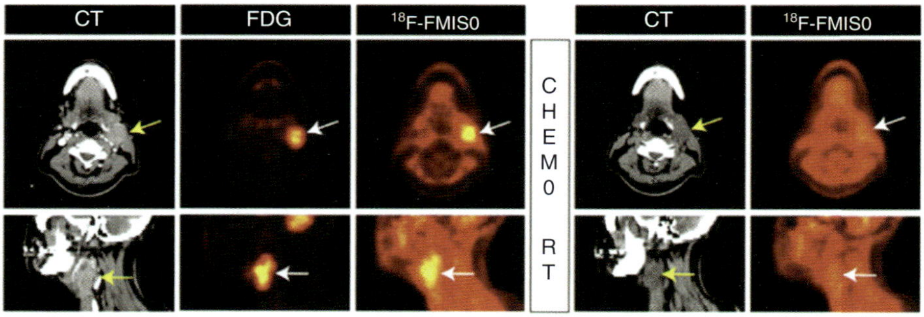

FIGURE 6.6 An F-MISO PET image of a patient with oropharyngeal cancer, registered with a CT scan and an FDG PET image (14). After 1 week of chemotherapy and radiation therapy (RT), the hypoxic volume is resolved.

FDG, ^{18}F-fluorodeoxyglucose; F-MISO, ^{18}F-misonidazole.

Source: From Lee N, Schoder H, Beattie B, et al. Strategy of using intratreatment hypoxia imaging to selectively and safely guide radiation dose de-escalation concurrent with chemotherapy for locoregionally advanced human papillomavirus-related oropharyngeal carcinoma. *Int J Radiat Oncol Biol Phys.* 2016;96(1):9–17.

of tumor, increasing the contrast to soft tissue. Postcontrast T1-weighted images with fat suppression are commonly used to determine the extent of the tumor. T1-weighted spin echo (SE) or turbo spin echo (TSE) sequences are commonly acquired. T2-weighted images are also useful, a TSE T2 scan with fat saturation is often acquired. T1-weighted gradient echo is another commonly used sequence.

MRI is most helpful in target delineation. The tumor volumes contoured on MRI are often quite different from those drawn on CT; typically the MRI identifies more suspect areas, resulting in larger contours (23,25,26). The accuracy of MRI image registration should always be considered when deciding on target volume margins.

Similar to CT, dynamic contrast-enhanced (DCE) MRI scans have also been used for head and neck cancer imaging. DCE MRI allows noninvasive assessment of permeability and blood flow, both of which are features of tumor hypoxia (27). It is also useful for detecting the lymph nodes involved (28) and differentiating tumor types (29).

TREATMENT PLANNING

INTENSITY-MODULATED RADIATION THERAPY (IMRT) VARIATIONS

With few exceptions, most head and neck cancers are treated with IMRT using 6 MV photons (some units use ^{60}Co). IMRT involves use of inverse treatment planning and a multileaf collimator (MLC). The radiation source is shaped by a collimator, which is mounted on a rotating gantry. Conventional radiation therapy utilized rectangular radiation fields shaped by the collimator jaws., The MLC uses multiple narrow rectangular leaves to shape the radiation field, and improves our ability to confine the shape of the radiation isodoses to the target volumes. There are many different ways to deliver IMRT, including step-and-shoot fields (MLC does not move when the radiation beam is on), sliding window fields (MLC moves when the beam is on), volumetric arc therapy (VMAT) (gantry and MLC move), and tomotherapy (gantry, couch, and MLC move). MLC leaf sizes vary, 2.5- to 5-mm leaves are typically available, at least in the center of the field. This results in a sufficiently fine resolution for head and neck patients. Compensator-based IMRT, which does not require an MLC, is also possible, but today is rarely used. Regardless of which delivery technique is used, a thorough quality assurance (QA) program is necessary (30,31).

DOSE CALCULATION

The head and neck region contains tissues of very different atomic compositions and electron densities, such as bones and airways. A dose calculation algorithm with an accurate inhomogeneity correction is therefore needed. A calculation grid voxel size of 1 to 2.5 mm is typically used; a fine calculation is important for head and neck plans, since many of the organs contoured have very small volumes (32).

Commonly used algorithms include collapsed cone convolution (CCC), the adaptive anisotropic algorithm (AAA), and Acuros and various Monte Carlo (MC) based algorithms. The Acuros and MC algorithms are considered to have the most accurate inhomogeneity calculations (33,34) but are usually also the slowest of the group. AAA and CCC calculate dose to water; MC and Acuros can be configured to calculate either dose to water or dose to medium. Although there is no universal agreement, most users of these algorithms appear to prefer reporting dose to tissue. Han et al. (35) studied the accuracy of the Acuros algorithm in the Radiological Physics Center's anthropomorphic head and neck phantom, while Kan et al. (36) studied AAA and Acuros in different phantoms, including a Rando anthropomorphic head and neck phantom. Both IMRT and VMAT plans were studied; the conclusion was that while both algorithms performed well, the Acuros results agreed better with radiochromic film and thermoluminescent dosimetry (TLD) measurements close to and inside inhomogeneities. Figure 6.7 shows the Radiological Physics Center phantom and the gamma scores that were achieved with different dose calculation algorithms and gamma criteria.

Small radiation fields, such as those used in radiosurgery, place even higher requirements on the dose calculation algorithm. Kan et al. (37) studied the accuracy of Acuros XB (AXB) and AAA dose calculation for nasopharyngeal carcinoma. They concluded that for small treatment fields, AAA and Acuros overestimated the dose at air/tissue interfaces by 41% and 6%, respectively, but the Acuros depth dose caught up well with the measured data 2 mm from the interface, see Figure 6.8. Testing using anthropomorphic phantoms showed that AAA

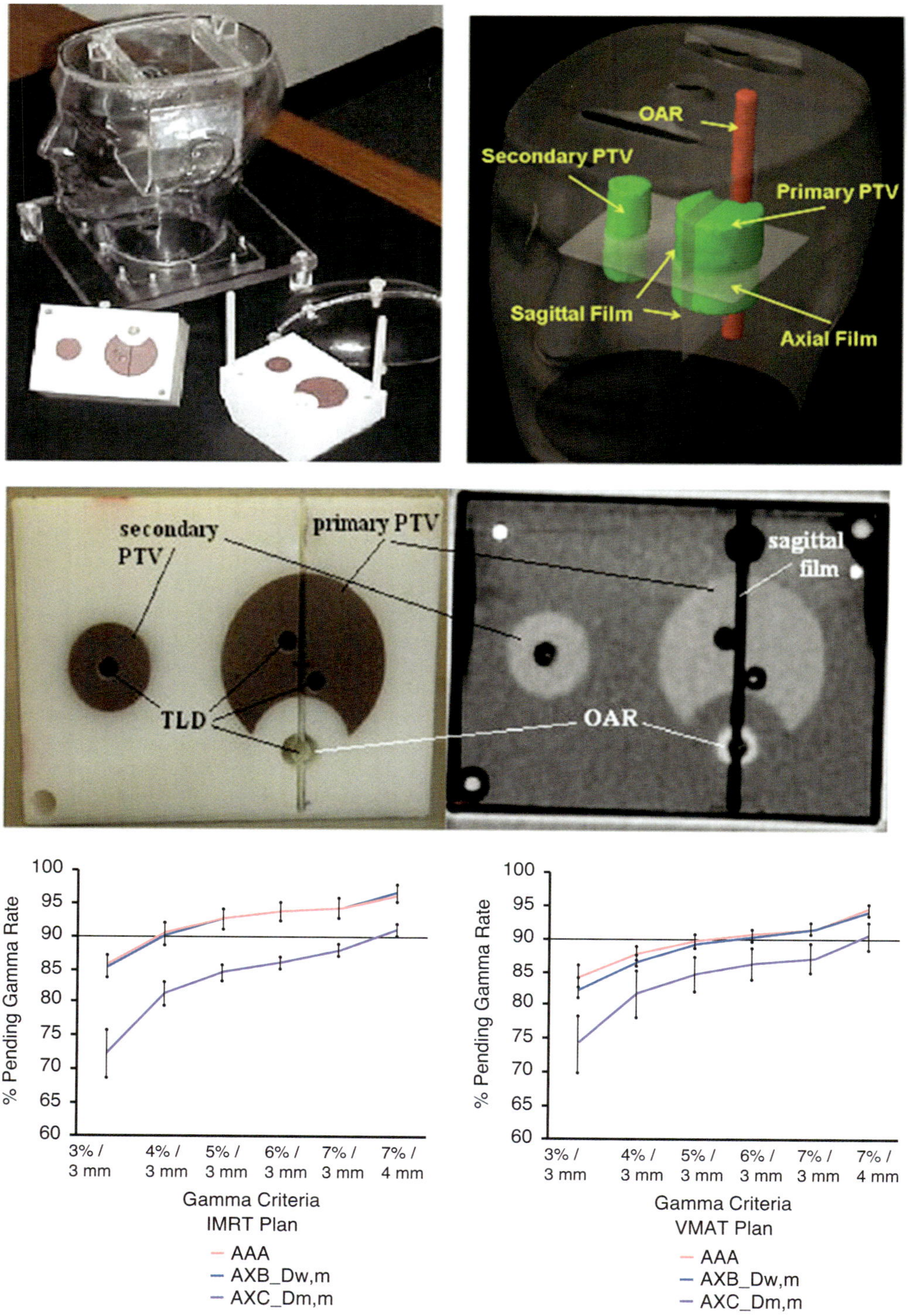

FIGURE 6.7 Top row: photograph and 3D rendering of the Radiological Physics Center phantom; middle row: close-up photograph and a CT image of the phantom; bottom row: the passing gamma score for VMAT and IMRT plans for different algorithms and choices of gamma parameters.

IMRT, intensity-modulated radiation therapy; OAR, organs at risk; PTV, planning treatment volume; VMAT, volumetric arc therapy.

Source: Adapted from Han T, Mourtada F, Kisling K, et al. Experimental validation of deterministic Acuros XB algorithm for IMRT and VMAT dose calculations with the Radiological Physics Center's head and neck phantom. *Med Phys.* 2012;39(4):2193–2202.

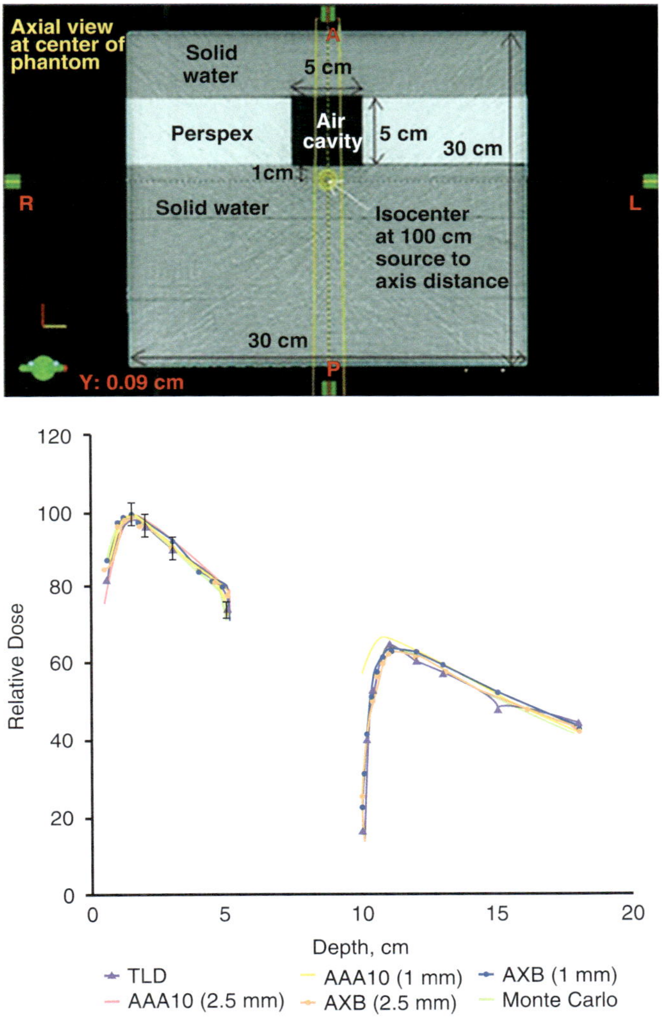

FIGURE 6.8 AAA and Acuros depth (AXB) doses calculated in an inhomogeneous phantom for a 2 x 2 field (37). Both algorithms have difficulties predicting the dose at the air–solid water interface, but the Acuros results agree significantly better with the measurements and Monte Carlo calculations.

Source: Adapted from Kan MW, Leung LH, Yu PK. Verification and dosimetric impact of Acuros XB algorithm on intensity modulated stereotactic radiotherapy for locally persistent nasopharyngeal carcinoma. *Med Phys.* 2012;39(8):4705–4714. With permission from John Wiley and Sons.

overestimated the doses by up to 10%, while the measured doses matched those of the AXB to within 3%.

INVERSE PLANNING AND OPTIMIZATION

IMRT plans are generated by inverse planning—the physician contours the targets (gross tumor volume (GTV), sets clinical treatment volumes (CTVs), notes organs at risk (OARs), specifies the dose limits to the target, and determines the critical structures and the field geometry. Dosimetrists or physicists assign fields (beams) and use the treatment planning software (TPS) to calculate the fluence distribution to be delivered from each field. Typically, the optimal fluence distribution is generated by the optimizer and converted into a deliverable MLC leaf sequence by the sequencer. The optimizer consists of the objective function, which is used to rank fluence distributions, and an algorithm used to minimize the objective function. The objective function is usually based on dose, but objectives based on tumor control probability, normal tissue complication probability, and equivalent uniform dose have also been used (38,39). These approaches will become more common once the dose response models become more sophisticated. The shape of the objective function is usually quadratic. It can be minimized using many different approaches, including gradient methods (40) and simulated annealing (41). The leaf sequencer converts the fluence distribution into a deliverable MLC sequence.

TREATMENT DELIVERY

CONVENTIONAL ACCELERATORS

Both the step-and-shoot and sliding window approaches have been used extensively in the treatment of head and neck cancer. The step-and-shoot method is the most robust delivery method and has the least demanding QA requirements—only the MLC leaf positioning needs to be checked, whereas for the sliding window technique the leaf speed is also important (42). The monitor unit (MU) of step-and-shoot plans is also low. The main drawbacks of the step-and-shoot method are that the desired dose distribution has to be approximated by discrete steps and the plan delivery time is often long (43). In order to be able to deliver sliding window fields, the MLC must allow interdigitation of the leaves. Almost all modern MLCs are capable of this. The size of the treatment fields often exceeds the limits of the MLC, in which case the field can be split into several subfields.

VMAT is a relatively recent technique, in which the treatment is delivered by 1–4 intensity-modulated arcs. Couch kicks are utilized more frequently than with conventional IMRT techniques. The QA requirements are also higher, since the gantry speed also affects the dose distribution. VMAT often produces treatment plans with quality comparable to conventional IMRT, but significantly lower MU (44). This results in shorter treatment time and hence less concern about patient motion, and a smaller risk of radiation-induced secondary malignancies. In certain situations, in which strong dose modulation is required around small OARs, a clinically acceptable plan may only be achievable with IMRT (45,46). Figure 6.9 illustrates the effect of the beam arrangement on the isodose distributions. A hybrid technique, consisting of VMAT arcs interspersed with IMRT fields, has been introduced recently (47); it may further extend the range of cases amenable to VMAT. Figure 6.10 shows an example of the hybrid technique.

The proximity of targets and critical organs and the potential for tumor regression or patient weight loss during treatment mandate accurate image guidance for treating head and neck patients. More accurate image guidance can also enable the use of smaller planning treatment volume (PTV) margins, reducing normal tissue complications and enabling dose escalation (48). A large number of guidance systems, based on x-rays, ultrasound, and infrared and visible light, are commercially available (49); some can be used both for patient setup and intrafraction motion management. Typically, image guidance is achieved by an orthogonal planar kV x-rays and kV conebeam CT (CBCT). Diagnostic CT units in the treatment vault ("CT on rails") provide excellent image quality (50), but are expensive and, sometimes, slow and cumbersome to use.

Major LINAC manufacturers market accelerators with integrated kV CBCT systems. The image quality of the CBCT system does not equal that of diagnostic CT units—the conebeam geometry produces significantly more scatter than a fan beam, resulting in reduced low contrast resolution and increased cupping artifacts, among other effects. These effects make treatment planning and dose calculations on CBCT images difficult, although CBCT is still very useful for patient positioning. The low contrast resolution is often sufficient to allow setup on the basis of soft tissue, and rotations can also be accounted for. CBCT also allows for tracking patient weight loss, tumor regression, and other changes that may necessitate replanning for the patient (51). A CBCT can be acquired either at every fraction or once or twice a week—the imaging dose to radiosensitive organs from daily CBCT scans can total over 300 cGy over the course of treatment (52). The CBCT imaging parameters and the frequency of imaging should, therefore, be carefully considered.

The accuracy of CBCT-based setup has been studied by several authors. Den et al. (53) studied the effect of daily CBCT guidance on head and neck PTV margins, and concluded that PTV margins could be reduced to 2–3 mm, except for mobile targets, such as oral tongue. Oh et al. (54) analyzed 2,200 treatments of different tumor sites and found that the PTV margins required for head and neck patients were reduced to less than 4 mm when daily CBCT is used.

Another advantage of volumetric imaging by CBCT is that the image set may be co-registered

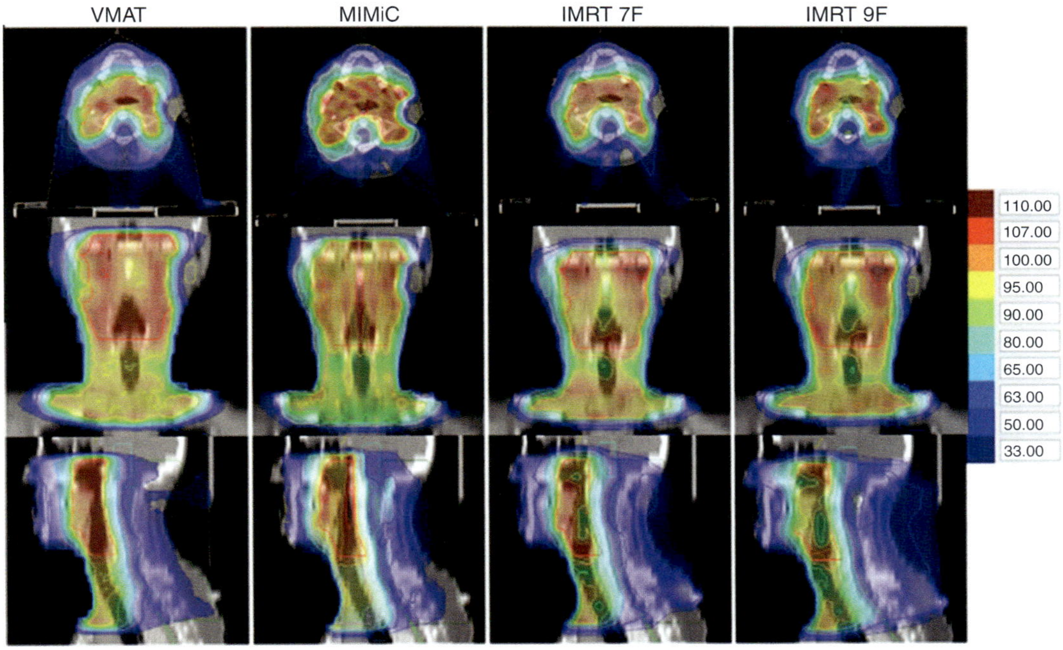

FIGURE 6.9 A comparison of different IMRT treatment planning approaches in a head and neck patient (46). The authors concluded that IMRT provided the best OAR sparing while VMAT was the most efficient treatment technique.

IMRT, intensity-modulated radiation therapy; OAR, organs at risk; VMAT, volumetric arc therapy

Source: From Stieler F, Wolff D, Schmid H, et al. A comparison of several modulated radiotherapy techniques for head and neck cancer and dosimetric validation of VMAT. *Radiother Oncol.* 2011;101(3):388–393.

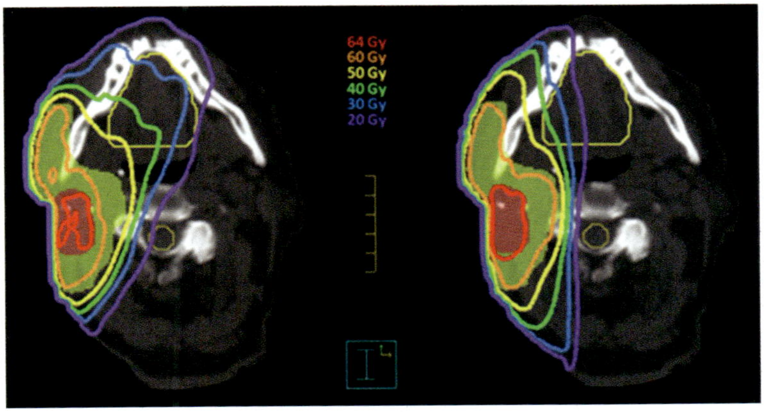

FIGURE 6.10 A comparison between VMAT (left) and a hybrid technique, incorporating VMAT arcs interspersed IMRT fields (right).

IMRT, intensity-modulated radiation therapy; VMAT, volumetric arc therapy.

Source: From Macfarlane M, Hoover DA, Wong E, et al. Evaluation of unified intensity-modulated arc therapy for the radiotherapy of head-and-neck cancer. *Radiother Oncol.* 2016;119(2):331–336.

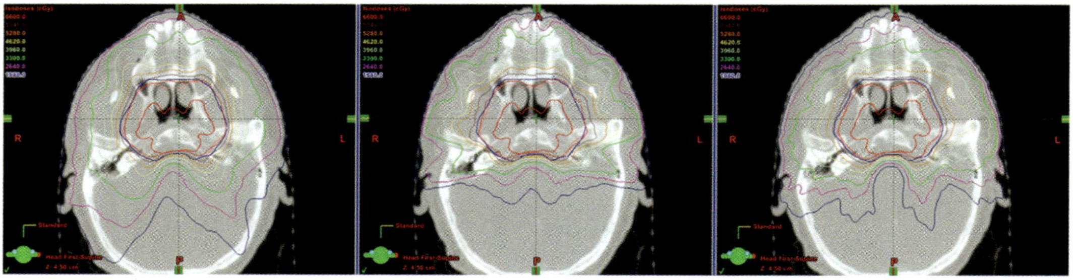

FIGURE 6.11 A patient with nasopharynx cancer, planned with RapidArc (left), IMRT (center), and TomoTherapy (right).

IMRT, intensity-modulated radiation therapy

Source: From Lee FK, Yip CW, Cheung FC, et al. Dosimetric difference amongst 3 techniques: TomoTherapy, sliding-window intensity-modulated radiotherapy (IMRT), and RapidArc radiotherapy in the treatment of late-stage nasopharyngeal carcinoma (NPC). *Med Dosim*. 2014;39(1):44–49.

to the original CT-based treatment plan to determine if changes in tumor size or location and patient factors such as weight loss or swelling may alter the intended radiation treatment plan, and, therefore, require adaptive treatment planning.

TOMOTHERAPY

A tomotherapy unit (Accuray Inc., Sunnyvale, CA) incorporates a 6 MV LINAC and a binary MLC (a leaf can be either fully open or fully closed). Similar to a spiral CT scan, helical tomotherapy is delivered while the treatment couch, gantry, and MLC move. Image guidance is achieved by acquiring a fan-beam MV CT scan, with the energy of the MV beam degraded to improve the contrast resolution. The treatment plans are generated on HiArt, a software package from Accuray. Tomotherapy has the potential to greatly limit dose critical structures. Lee et al. (55) compared RapidArc, IMRT, and tomotherapy plans for late-stage nasopharyngeal carcinoma. All the techniques achieved similar target coverage; the lens and mandible doses were significantly lower for tomotherapy, and RapidArc plans had the lowest MU, treatment time, and eye dose. Figure 6.11 shows a nasopharynx patient planned with the three techniques. Wiezorek et al. (56) compared tomotherapy, VMAT, and conventional IMRT for planning ten complex head and neck

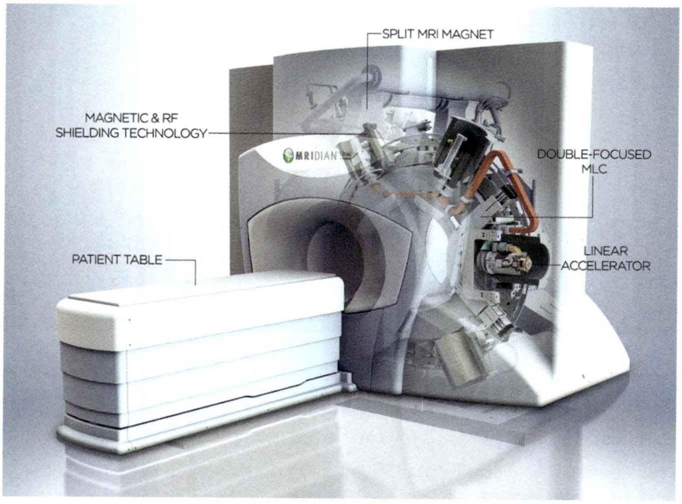

FIGURE 6.12 TheMRIdian MRI-guided treatment unit.

Source: Image courtesy of Viewray, Inc., Oakwood Village, OH.

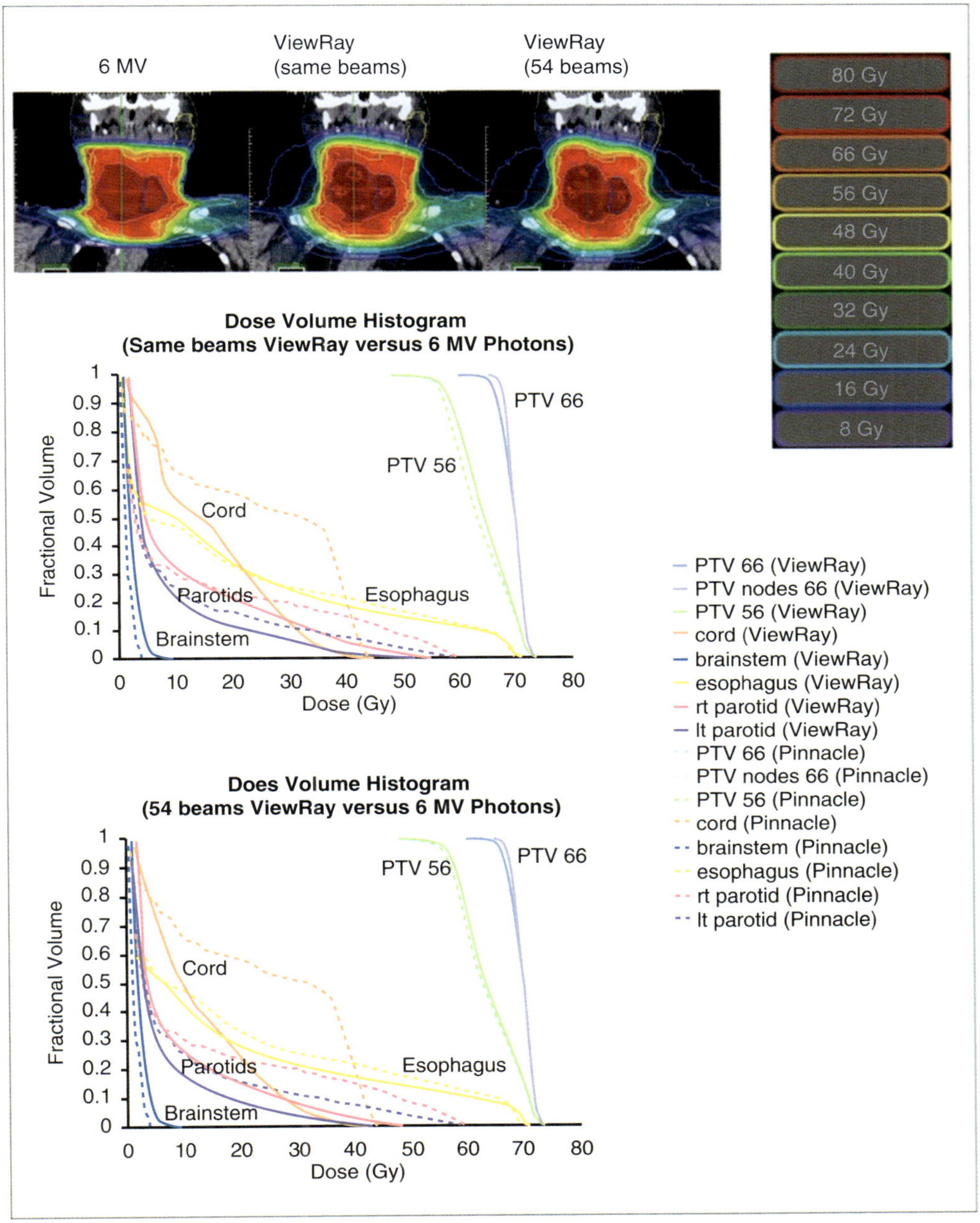

FIGURE 6.13 A comparison between 6 MV IMRT and MRIdian head and neck plans (65). Two MRIdian plans were constructed, one with the same beams as in the 6X plan, and a reoptimized plan with more beams.

IMRT, intensity-modulated radiation therapy.

Source: From Saenz DL, Paliwal BR, Bayouth JE. A dose homogeneity and conformity evaluation between ViewRay and pinnacle-based linear accelerator IMRT treatment plans. *J Med Phys*. 2014;39(2):64–70. With permission from Wolters Kluwer Medknow Publications.

patients. They found that tomotherapy appeared to be advantageous with respect to OAR sparing and treatment delivery efficiency, at the cost of a higher dose delivered to normal tissues. In addition, tomotherapy has also been used for reirradiation of recurrent head and neck cancer. Jeong et al. reported promising results for re-treatment of unresectable recurrences (57).

CYBERKNIFE

The Cyberknife (Accuray Inc., Sunnyvale, CA) is a smaller 6 MV X-band accelerator mounted on a robotic arm allowing greater degrees of movement freedom. It incorporates two orthogonal kV imagers for image guidance (58)—the same imaging system is used for intrafraction motion management. It can track either spine/skull or implanted fiducial markers. The robot provides the accelerator with six degrees of freedom. Changes in patient position are compensated by a combination of robot and couch movement. The treatment fields are shaped either by fixed cones, a variable aperture collimator (Iris), or an MLC, depending on the version of the accelerator.

Treatment planning is performed using the manufacturer's software (Multiplan), which has an optional Monte Carlo algorithm. The Cyberknife is mostly used for radiosurgery, but it can also be used for more conventional hypofractionated IMRT. This approach has become popular in the treatment of prostate cancer. In head and neck cancers, the Cyberknife is a relatively new technology and has been mostly used for reirradiation (59). It is also possible to incorporate a Cyberknife radiosurgical boost into a conventionally fractionated head and neck treatment (60).

MRI-GUIDED TREATMENT UNITS

An MRI-guided cobalt teletherapy unit (61) (MRIdian, by Viewray, Oakwood Village, OH) has received Food and Drug Administration (FDA) approval; several manufacturers are currently developing MRI-guided linear accelerators. The MRIdian incorporates three rotating Co-60 sources, each with a doubly focused MLC; this unit is depicted in Figure 6.12. The unit is capable of a dose rate of 550 cGy/min at the isocenter. The MRI is a 0.35 T split-bore whole body imaging system and can be used while the treatment beam is on. The unit comes with a Monte Carlo based treatment planning system that is capable of adapting the treatment plan to new MRI scans acquired on the treatment unit (62). This is a very promising feature for adapting treatment plans to patient weight loss or tumor regression (63,64). As seen in Figure 6.13, the quality of the head and neck plans is comparable to regular 6 MV IMRT plans, but the MRIdian plans show slightly increased inhomogeneity and volume receiving 20% of prescription dose (65), as shown in Figure 6.13. Because of their relative novelty, the literature on MRI-guided treatment units is not yet well developed and there are no outcome data available yet.

CONCLUSION

Recent advances in radiation therapy have the potential to improve survival and reduce the risk and severity of treatment complications. Advances in imaging will allow us to better identify specific areas requiring increased radiation doses due to, for example, hypoxia. They will also allow us to identify patients for whom dose de-escalation is a safe option. Improved imaging and patient positioning on the treatment machines will facilitate the use of smaller treatment margins, thereby reducing the probability of complications, and allow for on-the-fly adaptive planning based on tumor response and anatomic changes. Another major change in radiation therapy technology is the growing use of proton therapy that is described in a dedicated chapter. There are a large number of competing systems to achieve these goals; time will tell which of them will overcome the technological and economic barriers to succeed.

REFERENCES

1. Peng JL, Kahler D, Li JG, et al. Characterization of a real-time surface image-guided stereotactic positioning system. *Med Phys*. 2010;37(10):5421–5433. doi:10.1118/1.3483783
2. Mall P, Chand P, Singh BP, et al. Effectiveness of positioning stents in radiation-induced xerostomia in patients with tongue carcinoma: a randomized controlled trial. *Int J Prosthodont*. 2016;29(5):455–460.
3. Vogl TJ, Schulz B, Bauer RW, et al. Dual-energy CT applications in head and neck imaging. *AJR Am J Roentgenol*. 2012;199(5, suppl):S34–S39.
4. Lam S, Gupta R, Kelly H, et al. Multiparametric evaluation of head and neck squamous cell carcinoma using a single-source dual-energy CT with fast kVp switching: state of the art. *Cancers*. 2015;7(4):2201–2216.
5. Ginat DT, Mayich M, Daftari-Besheli L, et al. Clinical applications of dual-energy CT in head and neck imaging. *Eur Arch Otorhinolaryngol*. 2016;273(3):547–553.
6. Garcia LI, Azorin JF, Almansa JF. A new method to measure electron density and effective atomic number using dual-energy CT images. *Phys Med Biol*. 2016;61(1):265–279.
7. Faggioni L, Neri E, Bartolozzi C. CT perfusion of head and neck tumors: how we do it. *AJR Am J Roentgenol*. 2010;194(1):62–69.

8. Trojanowska A, Trojanowski P, Bisdas S, et al. Squamous cell cancer of hypopharynx and larynx—evaluation of metastatic nodal disease based on computed tomography perfusion studies. *Eur J Radiol.* 2012;81(5):1034–1039.
9. Huang JY, Followill DS, Howell RM, et al. Approaches to reducing photon dose calculation errors near metal implants. *Med Phys.* 2016;43(9):5117–5130.
10. Huang JY, Kerns JR, Nute JL, et al. An evaluation of three commercially available metal artifact reduction methods for CT imaging. *Phys Med Biol.* 2015;60(3):1047–1067.
11. Rumboldt Z, Gordon L, Gordon L, et al. Imaging in head and neck cancer. *Curr Treat Options Oncol.* 2006;7(1):23–34.
12. Vellayappan BA, Soon YY, Earnest A, et al. Accuracy of ^{18}F-flurodeoxyglucose-positron emission tomography/computed tomography in the staging of newly diagnosed nasopharyngeal carcinoma: a systematic review and meta-analysis. *Radiol Oncol.* 2014;48(4): 331–338.
13. Matsuura T, Nishimura Y, Nakamatsu K, et al. Clinical outcomes of IMRT planned with or without PET/CT simulation for patients with pharyngeal cancers. *Int J Clin Oncol.* 2017;22(1).
14. Lee N, Schoder H, Beattie B, et al. Strategy of using intratreatment hypoxia imaging to selectively and safely guide radiation dose de-escalation concurrent with chemotherapy for locoregionally advanced human papillomavirus-related oropharyngeal carcinoma. *Int J Radiat Oncol Biol Phys.* 2016;96(1): 9–17.
15. Chao KS, Bosch WR, Mutic S, et al. A novel approach to overcome hypoxic tumor resistance: Cu-ATSM-guided intensity-modulated radiation therapy. *Int J Radiat Oncol Biol Phys.* 2001;49(4):1171–1182.
16. Dirix P, Vandecaveye V, de Keyzer F, et al. Dose painting in radiotherapy for head and neck squamous cell carcinoma: value of repeated functional imaging with ^{18}F-FDG PET, ^{18}F-fluoromisonidazole PET, diffusion-weighted MRI, and dynamic contrast-enhanced MRI. *J Nucl Med.* 2009;50(7):1020–1027.
17. Thorwarth D, Eschmann SM, Paulsen F, et al. Hypoxia dose painting by numbers: a planning study. *Int J Radiat Oncol Biol Phys.* 2007;68(1):291–300.
18. Lee N, Nehmeh S, Schöder H, et al. Prospective trial incorporating pre-/mid-treatment [^{18}F]-misonidazole positron emission tomography for head-and-neck cancer patients undergoing concurrent chemoradiotherapy. *Int J Radiat Oncol Biol Phys.* 2009;75(1):101–108.
19. Hendrickson K, Phillips M, Smith W, et al. Hypoxia imaging with [F-18] FMISO-PET in head and neck cancer: potential for guiding intensity modulated radiation therapy in overcoming hypoxia-induced treatment resistance. *Radiother Oncol.* 2011;101(3):369–375.
20. Paulson ES, Erickson B, Schultz C, et al. Comprehensive MRI simulation methodology using a dedicated MRI scanner in radiation oncology for external beam radiation treatment planning. *Med Phys.* 2015;42(1):28–39.
21. Devic S. MRI simulation for radiotherapy treatment planning. *Med Phys.* 2012;39(11):6701–6711.
22. Hermans R. Medical radiology: diagnostic imaging. In: R Hermans, ed. *Head and Neck Cancer Imaging.* 2nd ed. Berlin, NY: Springer Publishing; 2012: xiv, 413.
23. Emami B, Sethi A, Petruzzelli GJ. Influence of MRI on target volume delineation and IMRT planning in nasopharyngeal carcinoma. *Int J Radiat Oncol Biol Phys.* 2003;57(2):481–488.
24. Poon I, Fischbein N, Lee N, et al. A population-based atlas and clinical target volume for the head-and-neck lymph nodes. *Int J Radiat Oncol Biol Phys.* 2004;59(5):1301–1311.
25. Rasch C, Keus R, Pameijer FA, et al. The potential impact of CT-MRI matching on tumor volume delineation in advanced head and neck cancer. *Int J Radiat Oncol Biol Phys.* 1997;39(4):841–848.
26. Chung NN, Ting LL, Hsu WC, et al. Impact of magnetic resonance imaging versus CT on nasopharyngeal carcinoma: primary tumor target delineation for radiotherapy. *Head Neck.* 2004;26(3):241–246.
27. Gaddikeri S, Gaddikeri RS, Tailor T, et al. Dynamic contrast-enhanced MR imaging in head and neck cancer: techniques and clinical applications. *AJNR Am J Neuroradiol.* 2016;37(4):588–595.
28. Fischbein NJ, Noworolski SM, Henry RG, et al. Assessment of metastatic cervical adenopathy using dynamic contrast-enhanced MR imaging. *AJNR Am J Neuroradiol.* 2003;24(3):301–311.
29. Lee FK, King AD, Ma BB, et al. Dynamic contrast enhancement magnetic resonance imaging (DCE-MRI) for differential diagnosis in head and neck cancers. *Eur J Radiol.* 2012;81(4):784–788.
30. Burman C, Chui CS, Kutcher G, et al. Planning, delivery, and quality assurance of intensity-modulated radiotherapy using dynamic multileaf collimator: a strategy for large-scale implementation for the treatment of carcinoma of the prostate. *Int J Radiat Oncol Biol Phys.* 1997;39(4):863–873.
31. Ling CC, Zhang P, Archambault Y, et al. Commissioning and quality assurance of RapidArc radiotherapy delivery system. *Int J Radiat Oncol Biol Phys.* 2008;72(2):575–581.
32. Srivastava SP, Cheng CW, das IJ. The dosimetric and radiobiological impact of calculation grid size on head and neck IMRT. *Pract Radiat Oncol.* 2017;7(3).
33. Wang L, Yorke E, Chui CS. Monte Carlo evaluation of 6 MV intensity modulated radiotherapy plans for head and neck and lung treatments. *Med Phys.* 2002;29(11):2705–2717.
34. Kan MW, Yu PK, Leung LH. A review on the use of grid-based Boltzmann equation solvers for dose calculation in external photon beam treatment planning. *Biomed Res Int.* 2013;2013:1–10.
35. Han T, Mourtada F, Kisling K, et al. Experimental validation of deterministic Acuros XB algorithm for IMRT and VMAT dose calculations with the Radiological Physics Center's head and neck phantom. *Med Phys.* 2012;39(4):2193–2202.
36. Kan MW, Leung LH, So RW, et al. Experimental verification of the Acuros XB and AAA dose calculation adjacent to heterogeneous media for IMRT and RapidArc of nasopharygeal carcinoma. *Med Phys.* 2013;40(3):031714.

37. Kan MW, Leung LH, Yu PK. Verification and dosimetric impact of Acuros XB algorithm on intensity modulated stereotactic radiotherapy for locally persistent nasopharyngeal carcinoma. *Med Phys.* 2012;39(8):4705–4714.
38. de Neve W, de Gersem W, Derycke S, et al. Clinical delivery of intensity modulated conformal radiotherapy for relapsed or second-primary head and neck cancer using a multileaf collimator with dynamic control. *Radiother Oncol.* 1999;50(3):301–314.
39. Choi B, Deasy JO. The generalized equivalent uniform dose function as a basis for intensity-modulated treatment planning. *Phys Med Biol.* 2002;47(20):3579–3589.
40. Spirou SV, Chui CS. A gradient inverse planning algorithm with dose-volume constraints. *Med Phys.* 1998;25(3):321–333.
41. Webb S. Optimization by simulated annealing of three-dimensional, conformal treatment planning for radiation fields defined by a multileaf collimator: II. Inclusion of two-dimensional modulation of the x-ray intensity. *Phys Med Biol.* 1992;37(8):1689–1704.
42. Fuks Z LS, Ling CC. *A Practical Guide to Intensity-Modulated Radiation Therapy*. Madison, WI: Medical Physics Publishing; 2003.
43. Chui CS, Chan MF, Yorke E, et al. Delivery of intensity-modulated radiation therapy with a conventional multileaf collimator: comparison of dynamic and segmental methods. *Med Phys.* 2001;28(12):2441–2449.
44. Pursley J, Damato AL, Czerminska MA, et al. A comparative study of standard intensity-modulated radiotherapy and RapidArc planning techniques for ipsilateral and bilateral head and neck irradiation. *Med Dosim.* 2017;42(1).
45. Studenski MT, Bar-Ad V, Siglin J, et al. Clinical experience transitioning from IMRT to VMAT for head and neck cancer. *Med Dosim.* 2013;38(2):171–175.
46. Stieler F, Wolff D, Schmid H, et al. A comparison of several modulated radiotherapy techniques for head and neck cancer and dosimetric validation of VMAT. *Radiother Oncol.* 2011;101(3):388–393.
47. Macfarlane M, Hoover DA, Wong E, et al. Evaluation of unified intensity-modulated arc therapy for the radiotherapy of head-and-neck cancer. *Radiother Oncol.* 2016;119(2):331–336.
48. Chen AM, Farwell DG, Luu Q, et al. Evaluation of the planning target volume in the treatment of head and neck cancer with intensity-modulated radiotherapy: what is the appropriate expansion margin in the setting of daily image guidance? *Int J Radiat Oncol Biol Phys.* 2011;81(4):943–949.
49. de Los Santos J, Popple R, Agazaryan N, et al. Image guided radiation therapy (IGRT) technologies for radiation therapy localization and delivery. *Int J Radiat Oncol Biol Phys.* 2013;87(1):33–45.
50. Zhang L, Garden AS, Lo J, et al. Multiple regions-of-interest analysis of setup uncertainties for head-and-neck cancer radiotherapy. *Int J Radiat Oncol Biol Phys.* 2006;64(5):1559–1569.
51. Boda-Heggemann J, Lohr F, Wenz F, et al. kV cone-beam CT-based IGRT: a clinical review. *Strahlenther Onkol.* 2011;187(5):284–291.
52. Ding GX, Coffey CW. Radiation dose from kilovoltage cone beam computed tomography in an image-guided radiotherapy procedure. *Int J Radiat Oncol Biol Phys.* 2009;73(2):610–617.
53. Den RB, Doemer A, Kubicek G, et al. Daily image guidance with cone-beam computed tomography for head-and-neck cancer intensity-modulated radiotherapy: a prospective study. *Int J Radiat Oncol Biol Phys.* 2010;76(5):1353–1359.
54. Oh YK, Baek JG, Kim OB, et al. Assessment of setup uncertainties for various tumor sites when using daily CBCT for more than 2200 VMAT treatments. *J Appl Clin Med Phys.* 2014;15(2):85–99.
55. Lee FK, Yip CW, Cheung FC, et al. Dosimetric difference amongst 3 techniques: TomoTherapy, sliding-window intensity-modulated radiotherapy (IMRT), and RapidArc radiotherapy in the treatment of late-stage nasopharyngeal carcinoma (NPC). *Med Dosim.* 2014;39(1):44–49.
56. Wiezorek T, Brachwitz T, Georg D, et al. Rotational IMRT techniques compared to fixed gantry IMRT and tomotherapy: multi-institutional planning study for head-and-neck cases. *Radiat Oncol.* 2011;6:20.
57. Jeong S, Yoo EJ, Kim JY, et al. Re-irradiation of unresectable recurrent head and neck cancer: using Helical Tomotherapy as image-guided intensity-modulated radiotherapy. *Radiat Oncol J.* 2013;31(4):206–215.
58. Hara W, Soltys SG, Gibbs IC. CyberKnife robotic radiosurgery system for tumor treatment. *Expert Rev Anticancer Ther.* 2007;7(11):1507–1515.
59. Yamazaki H, Ogita M, Himei K, et al. Reirradiation using robotic image-guided stereotactic radiotherapy of recurrent head and neck cancer. *J Radiat Res.* 2016;57(3):288–293.
60. Yamazaki H, Ogita M, Himei K, et al. Hypofractionated stereotactic radiotherapy using CyberKnife as a boost treatment for head and neck cancer, a multi-institutional survey: impact of planning target volume. *Anticancer Res.* 2014;34(10):5755–5759.
61. Wooten HO, Rodriguez V, Green O, et al. Benchmark IMRT evaluation of a Co-60 MRI-guided radiation therapy system. *Radiother Oncol.* 2015;114(3):402–405.
62. Acharya S, Fischer-Valuck BW, Kashani R, et al. Online magnetic resonance image guided adaptive radiation therapy: first clinical applications. *Int J Radiat Oncol Biol Phys.* 2016;94(2):394–403.
63. Raghavan G, Kishan AU, Cao M, et al. Anatomic and dosimetric changes in patients with head and neck cancer treated with an integrated MRI-tri-60Co teletherapy device. *Br J Radiol.* 2016;89(1067):20160624.
64. Olsen J, Green O, Kashani R. World's First Application of MR-Guidance for Radiotherapy. *Mo Med.* 2015;112(5):358–360.
65. Saenz DL, Paliwal BR, Bayouth JE. A dose homogeneity and conformity evaluation between ViewRay and pinnacle-based linear accelerator IMRT treatment plans. *J Med Phys.* 2014;39(2):64–70.

7

Proton Therapy

Pierre Blanchard

G. Brandon Gunn

Steven J. Frank

Radiation therapy is an essential component of the treatment strategy for head and neck cancer. Most such treatments are delivered via external beam photon therapy (EBRT). Despite technological improvements in the planning and delivery of EBRT such as intensity modulated radiotherapy (IMRT), significant debilitating acute and late toxic side effects are still common because most head and neck tumors are close to critical organ structures. Among the potential side effects, dry mouth, the need for a feeding tube during and after treatment, swallowing dysfunction resulting in chronic dysphagia or aspiration pneumonia, secondary malignancies, hormonal dysfunction, or osteoradionecrosis of the mandible in particular can significantly impair quality of life both during treatment and long afterward.

Reducing the integral radiation dose delivered to the body, that is, reducing the incidental dose to nontarget structures, can improve outcomes because most of these toxic effects follow a dose–response relationship. The use of proton beam therapy, given the unique physical properties of protons, is one way to reduce unnecessary incidental irradiation (1–3). Proton therapy is not experimental, and is Food and Drug Administration (FDA) cleared. The number of proton therapy facilities in the United States is rapidly growing. The aims of this chapter are to present (a) the physical aspects of proton therapy and dosimetric differences between intensity modulated proton therapy (IMPT) and photon IMRT using x-rays; (b) outcomes of proton therapy according to tumor site and treatment setting; (c) the comparative toxicity profiles for proton and photon EBRT; and (d) issues of patient selection and the cost-effectiveness of proton therapy in resource-constrained environments.

PHYSICS AND TREATMENT PLANNING

In proton beam therapy, a particle accelerator is used to create and accelerate a focused beam of protons that can be used for therapeutic purposes. Photons have no mass or charge and travel through the patient depositing higher energy upon entry into the body as a result of interactions with electrons resulting in a "dose-accumulation" effect. Protons travel fast through the body with minimal interactions and then increase interactions as the velocity of the protons is reduced with maximal energy deposited resulting in the "Bragg peak" and no exit dose. Integral dose delivered to the body is strongly reduced on proton plans relative to photon treatment plans, and numerous dosimetric comparisons have confirmed the reduction in dose to nontarget structures associated with proton therapy (4,5). Examples are given in Figure 7.1. In one dosimetric study, in which treatment plans for 25 patients with oropharyngeal carcinoma (OPC) treated with IMPT were compared with IMRT plans for the same patients or for other patients treated with IMRT using x-rays, the doses to the anterior oral cavity, the posterior oral cavity, the middle and inferior pharyngeal constrictors, the esophagus, swallowing structures, the brainstem, cerebellum, and central nervous system (CNS) structures involved in the nausea and vomiting response were significantly lower in the IMPT plans (4). In this chapter, the unit of measure for doses delivered by protons is the gray (Gy), which represents cobalt gray equivalent (CGE) dosing using a relative biological effectiveness (RBE) of 1.1. RBE refers to the biological effectiveness of protons compared with photons; it is the factor used to quantify the difference in the effective dose from protons compared with an equivalent biological dose of photons. Although some evidence exists to suggest that RBE is variable (6), the current practice is to use a uniform RBE value of 1.1. Therefore, in order to deliver the same dose in grays, the proton prescribed dose is reduced by 10% in order to give the same biologically effective dose as with x-rays in IMRT. This is called CGE dosing.

Proton treatments can be delivered by using passive scatter or active scanning techniques. In the passive scatter technique, the

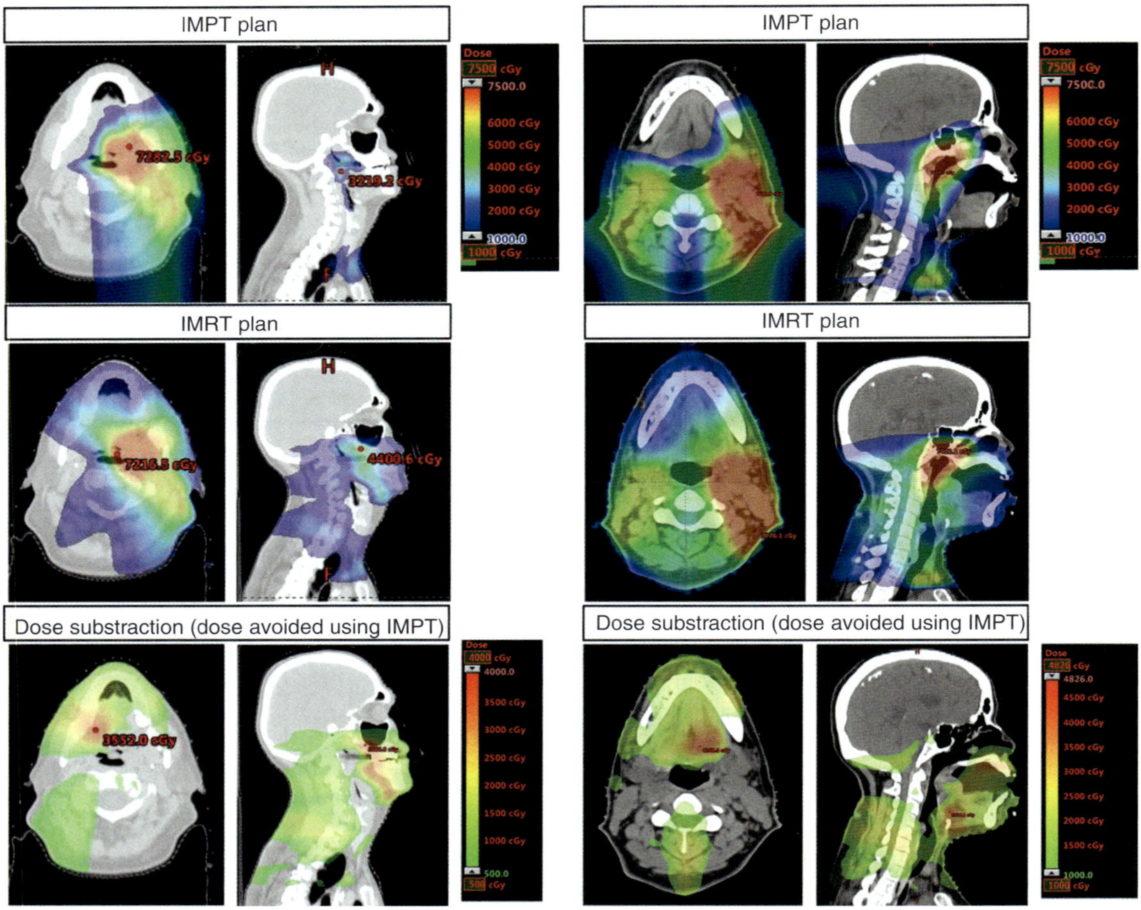

(A) 46 y/o male with T1N2b left sided tonsillar fossa p16+ squamous cell carcinoma

(B) 56 y/o female with T1N1 left sided nasopharyngeal carcinoma (four nodes in levels IIa, IIb, III and Va)

FIGURE 7.1 Examples of treatment plans with IMPT and IMRT for a tonsillar fossa cancer, nasopharyngeal cancer, and maxillary adenoid cystic carcinoma. The dose subtraction section shows the amount of radiation that can be avoided when treating with proton compared to photon.

IMPT, intensity modulated proton therapy; IMRT, intensity modulated radiotherapy.

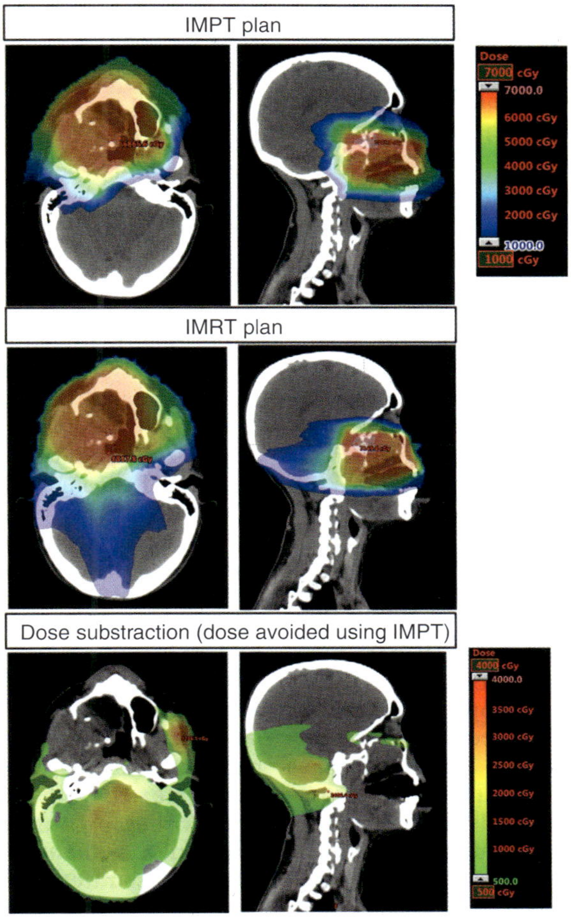

(C) 47 y/o female with T4N0 adenoid cystic carcinoma of the hard palate (surgery followed by adjuvant radiotherapy)

FIGURE 7.1 *(continued)*

proton beam is spread out by using scattering foils, and the beam is conformed laterally by using brass apertures and in terms of depth by using range compensators. This technique is less flexible than active scanning, requires patient-specific devices that are labor-intensive to create, generates secondary neutrons, and limits the capacity for adaptive replanning in the case of tumor or anatomic changes during treatment. In active scanning, also known as IMPT, magnets are used to deflect the proton beam to conform to the target volumes, and different layers are treated with different beam energies. This latter technique is currently the most widely used for proton therapy.

Treatment planning is done by using a multifield optimization algorithm that allows optimization of all spots from all fields simultaneously (7). Given the sensitivity of proton plans to physical and geometrical uncertainties, the robustness of the optimization with regard to changes in patient setup, anatomy, or beam range should be assessed before the plan is approved (8). The treatment delivery process at MD Anderson Proton Therapy Center includes verification of the accuracy of the dosimetry at least twice: on a second planning CT scan obtained the day before the treatment is begun and on a third scan obtained during the fourth week of treatment; this practice is considered optimal for off-line adaptive planning (9,10). For high-risk areas, weekly CT plan evaluation is done. If there are aberrations from the original plan, adaptive replanning is performed.

34. Bhattasali O, Holliday E, Kies MS, et al. Definitive proton radiation therapy and concurrent cisplatin for unresectable head and neck adenoid cystic carcinoma: a series of 9 cases and a critical review of the literature. *Head Neck*. 2016;38:E1472–E1480. doi:10.1002/hed.24262
35. Holliday EB, Esmaeli B, Pinckard J, et al. A multidisciplinary orbit-sparing treatment approach that includes proton therapy for epithelial tumors of the orbit and ocular adnexa. *Int J Radiat Oncol*. 2016;95:344–352.
36. Strojan P, Corry J, Eisbruch A, et al. Recurrent and second primary squamous cell carcinoma of the head and neck: when and how to reirradiate. *Head Neck*. 2015;37:134–150. doi:10.1002/hed.23542
37. Janot F, de Raucourt D, Benhamou E, et al. Randomized trial of postoperative reirradiation combined with chemotherapy after salvage surgery compared with salvage surgery alone in head and neck carcinoma. *J Clin Oncol*. 2008;26:5518–5523. doi:10.1200/JCO.2007.15.0102
38. Langendijk JA. Re-irradiation in head and neck cancer. In Nieder C, Langendijk J, eds. *Re-Irradiation: New Frontiers*. 2nd ed. Berlin: Springer International Publishing; 2017:151–168. doi:10.1007/174_2016_76
39. Stuschke M, Kaiser A, Abu-Jawad J, et al. Re-irradiation of recurrent head and neck carcinomas: comparison of robust intensity modulated proton therapy treatment plans with helical tomotherapy. *Radiat Oncol*. 2013;8:93. doi:10.1186/1748-717X-8-93
40. Phan J, Sio TT, Nguyen TP, et al. Reirradiation of head and neck cancers with proton therapy: outcomes and analyses. *Int J Radiat Oncol*. 2016;96:30–41. doi:10.1016/j.ijrobp.2016.03.053
41. Romesser PB, Cahlon O, Scher ED, et al. Proton beam reirradiation for recurrent head and neck cancer: multi-institutional report on feasibility and early outcomes. *Int J Radiat Oncol*. 2016;95:386–395. doi:10.1016/j.ijrobp.2016.02.036
42. Romesser PB, Cahlon O, Scher E, et al. Proton beam radiation therapy results in significantly reduced toxicity compared with intensity-modulated radiation therapy for head and neck tumors that require ipsilateral radiation. *Radiother Oncol*. 2016;118:286–292. doi:10.1016/j.radonc.2015.12.008
43. Ringash J. Survivorship and quality of life in head and neck cancer. *J Clin Oncol Off J Am Soc Clin Oncol*. 2015;33:3322–3327. doi:10.1200/JCO.2015.61.4115
44. Blanchard P, Volk RJ, Ringash J, et al. Assessing head and neck cancer patient preferences and expectations: a systematic review. *Oral Oncol*. 2016;62:44–53. doi:10.1016/j.oraloncology.2016.09.008
45. Van Der Laan HP, Van De Water TA, Van Herpt HE, et al. The potential of intensity-modulated proton radiotherapy to reduce swallowing dysfunction in the treatment of head and neck cancer: a planning comparative study. *Acta Oncol*. 2013;52:561–569. doi:10.3109/0284186X.2012.692885
46. Widder J, van der Schaaf A, Lambin P, et al. The quest for evidence for proton therapy: model-based approach and precision medicine. *Int J Radiat Oncol*. 2016;95:30–36. doi:10.1016/j.ijrobp.2015.10.004
47. Blanchard P, Wong AJ, Gunn GB, et al. Toward a model-based patient selection strategy for proton therapy: external validation of photon-derived normal tissue complication probability models in a head and neck proton therapy cohort. *Radiother Oncol*. 2016;121(3):381–386. doi:10.1016/j.radonc.2016.08.022
48. Thaker NG, Frank SJ, Feeley TW. Comparative costs of advanced proton and photon radiation therapies: lessons from time-driven activity-based costing in head and neck cancer. *J Comp Eff Res*. 2015;4:297–301. doi:10.2217/cer.15.32
49. Lievens Y, Pijls-Johannesma M. Health economic controversy and cost-effectiveness of proton therapy. *Semin Radiat Oncol*. 2013;23:134–141. doi:10.1016/j.semradonc.2012.11.005
50. Verma V, Mishra MV, Mehta MP. A systematic review of the cost and cost-effectiveness studies of proton radiotherapy. *Cancer*. 2016;122:1483–1501. doi:10.1002/cncr.29882
51. Peeters A, Grutters JPC, Pijls-Johannesma M, et al. How costly is particle therapy? Cost analysis of external beam radiotherapy with carbon-ions, protons and photons. *Radiother Oncol*. 2010;95:45–53. doi:10.1016/j.radonc.2009.12.002
52. Goitein M, Jermann M. The relative costs of proton and X-ray radiation therapy. *Clin Oncol*. 2003;15:S37–S50. doi:10.1053/clon.2002.0174
53. Ramaekers BLT, Grutters JPC, Pijls-Johannesma M, et al. Protons in head-and-neck cancer: bridging the gap of evidence. *Int J Radiat Oncol*. 2013;85:1282–1288. doi:10.1016/j.ijrobp.2012.11.006

8

Transoral Robotic Surgery: Advances and Applications

Meghan T. Turner
F. Christopher Holsinger
Robert L. Ferris

In the 1990s, several landmark, randomized clinical trials established "organ-sparing" chemoradiotherapy protocols as the primary treatment modality for many head and neck cancers. Following the VA Laryngeal Cancer Study and RTOG 91-11, chemoradiotherapy replaced total laryngectomy as the primary treatment of advanced laryngeal cancer (1,2). Later, results from the Groupe d'Oncologie Radiothérapie Tête et Cou (GORTEC) trial and others made definitive chemoradiotherapy the standard-of-care treatment for advanced stage oropharyngeal cancers (3–5). Finally, the Intergroup 0099 study on nasopharyngeal cancers established chemoradiotherapy as the standard-of-care for advanced nasopharyngeal carcinoma (6).

However, pooled data on organ preservation therapy (OPT) outcomes in the RTOG 91-11, RTOG 97-03, and RTOG 99-14 trials shows that 35% of head and neck cancer survivors have severe late toxicity (chronic grade 3/4 pharyngeal toxicity, gastrostomy dependence beyond 2 years, and/or treatment-related death within 3 years) (7). Additionally, it was noted that 60% of survivors treated with concurrent chemoradiotherapy suffer severe late-onset dysphagia, which was significantly higher than the incidence in those treated by surgery, radiation, or both (8). The true incidence of severe late-onset dysphagia is unknown. What is known is that it devastates survivors' quality of life and is refractory to treatment. Furthermore, the fibrosis following concurrent chemoradiotherapy makes salvage surgery technically and oncologically more difficult.

TRANSORAL ROBOTIC SURGERY

BACKGROUND

The advent of transoral endoscopic techniques renewed interest in surgery as a potential treatment for many aerodigestive squamous cell carcinomas (9). Steiner first began using endoscopic transoral laser microsurgery (TLM) to treat selected laryngeal and hypopharyngeal carcinomas in the 1980s. Since then, TLM has been used to treat advanced oropharyngeal squamous cell carcinoma (OPSCC) with control rates comparable to those for nonsurgical treatments (10–13). A multicenter trial with 204 OPSCC patients reported 3-year overall survival, disease-specific survival, and disease-free survival rates of 86%, 88%, and 82%, respectively, rivaling results of concurrent chemoradiotherapy trials (12). Despite successful outcomes in high-volume centers, TLM has not been widely adopted, for the following reasons: (a) line of sight surgery is technically challenging with respect to exposure and resection,

(b) it often requires division of the specimen, as opposed to en bloc resection, and (c) the aforementioned both increase the possibility of positive margins on pathologic examination.

In 2000, the Food and Drug Administration (FDA) approved use of the da Vinci robot (Intuitive Surgical, Sunnyvale, California) in general surgery. Applications in head and neck surgery were first explored in a porcine model of neck dissection in 2003 (14). However, Weinstein and colleagues at the University of Pennsylvania then pioneered the use of the da Vinci robot for transoral robotic surgery (TORS), and first reported on a canine model of supraglottic laryngectomy in 2005 (see Figure 8.1) (15). This was followed by a combined human cadaveric and canine study of oropharyngeal surgery feasibility in 2006 (16). This same group then performed the first human trials with two separate prospective case series: the first, 27 patients treated by radical tonsillectomy; and the second, 3 patients treated with TORS supraglottic laryngectomy. FDA approval for TORS was granted in 2009, and, subsequently, multi-institutional clinical trials have been performed or are under way.

TORS has gained popularity not only because of pioneers, but because of the surgical facility provided by the technology and the steep learning curve (17). The da Vinci system employs angled endoscopes for improved visualization and exposure over traditional techniques, as well as wristed, robotic instruments for easier and more precise dissection of the otherwise difficult to reach parapharyngeal and submandibular spaces. TORS is most superior compared to other surgical approaches in the base of tongue, where it provides binocular, three-dimensional, high-definition exposure and access from the circumvallate papillae to the vallecula (16). Critics of TORS cite the costliness of the da Vinci system and increased operative times as disadvantages. However, studies looking at learning curves and cost effectiveness have since been performed and find robotic approaches superior (17,18).

PROCEDURE

The patient is intubated and the tumor exposed as well as possible with the use of mouth gag retractors (i.e., Crowe-Davis, McGivor,

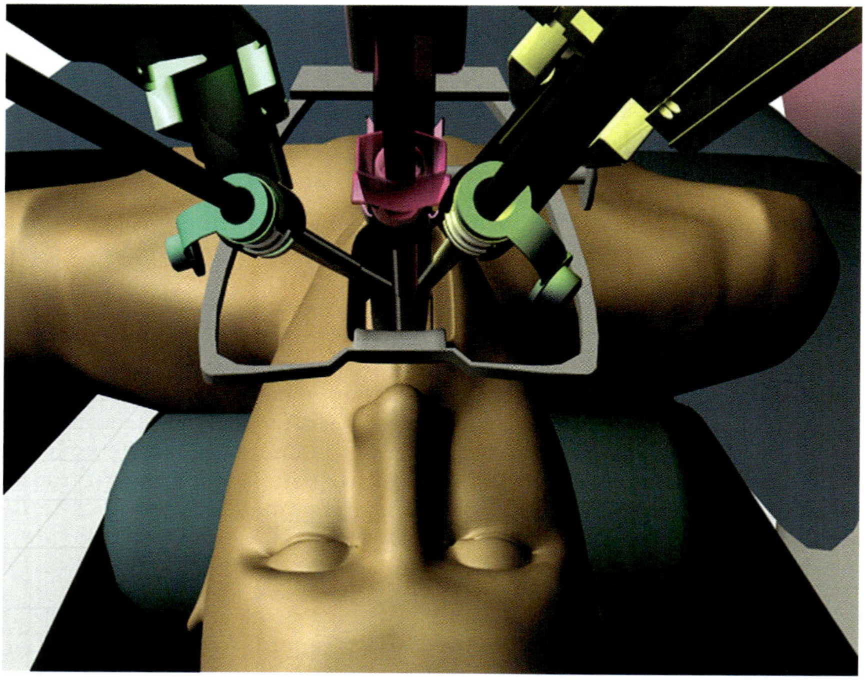

FIGURE 8.1 Positioning of the Feyh-Katzenbach mouth gag, cannulae, and camera (diagrammatic). The patient is in slight extension. The chosen mouth gag retractor is in position. The camera is positioned centrally (red cannula). The working arms are positioned laterally at approximately 30 degrees (green cannulae).

Source: ©[2017] Intuitive Surgical, Inc. Used with permission.

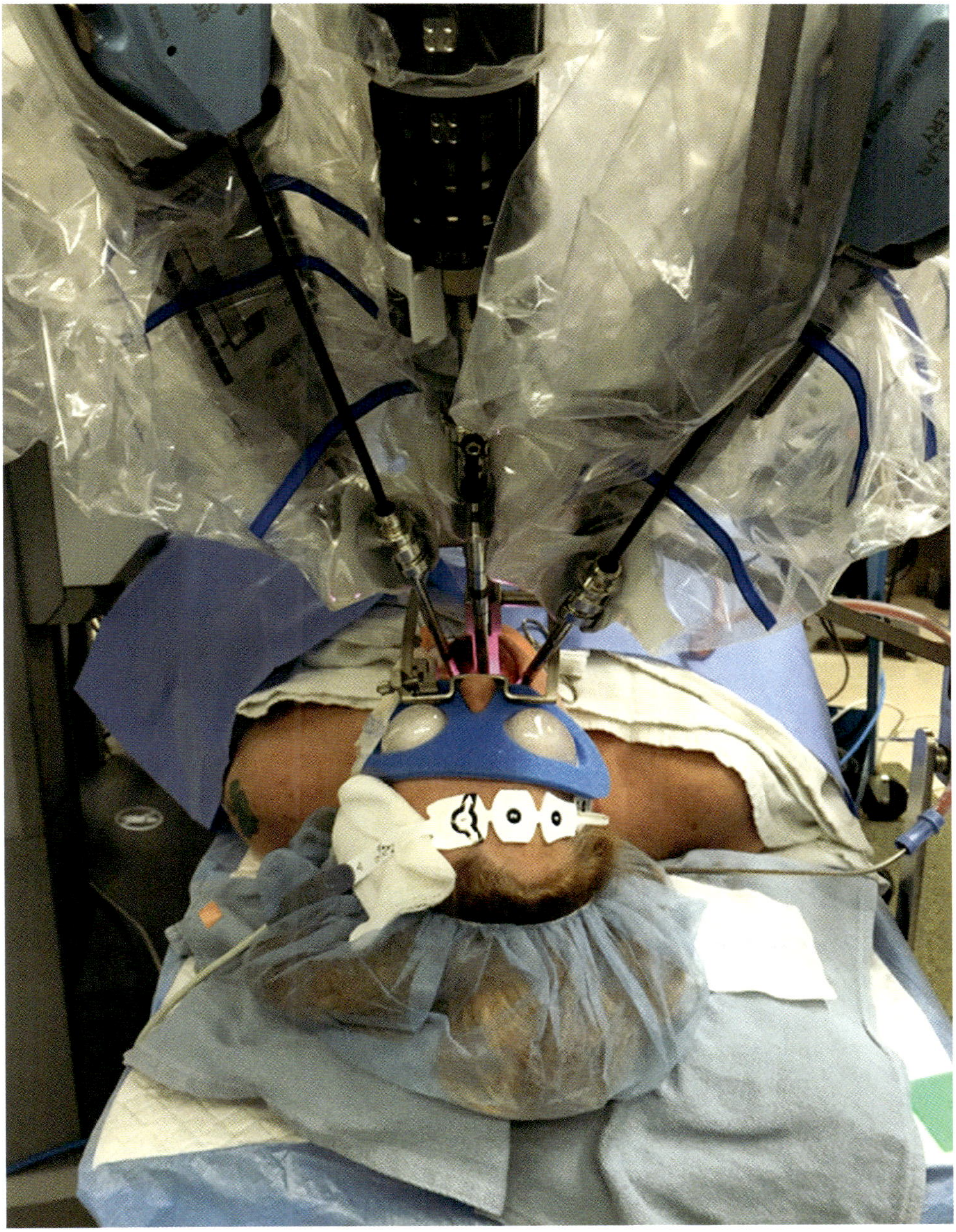

FIGURE 8.2 Transoral robotic surgery positioning (live example). Note the goggles placed to protect the patient's eyes from instruments. The BIS monitor is in place to monitor the level of conscious sedation in the setting of paralysis. The Feyh-Katzenbach mouth gag is in place and connected to the microsuspension system. The camera is in the center and the working arms positioned approximately 30 degrees from 12'clock.

BIS, bispectral index.

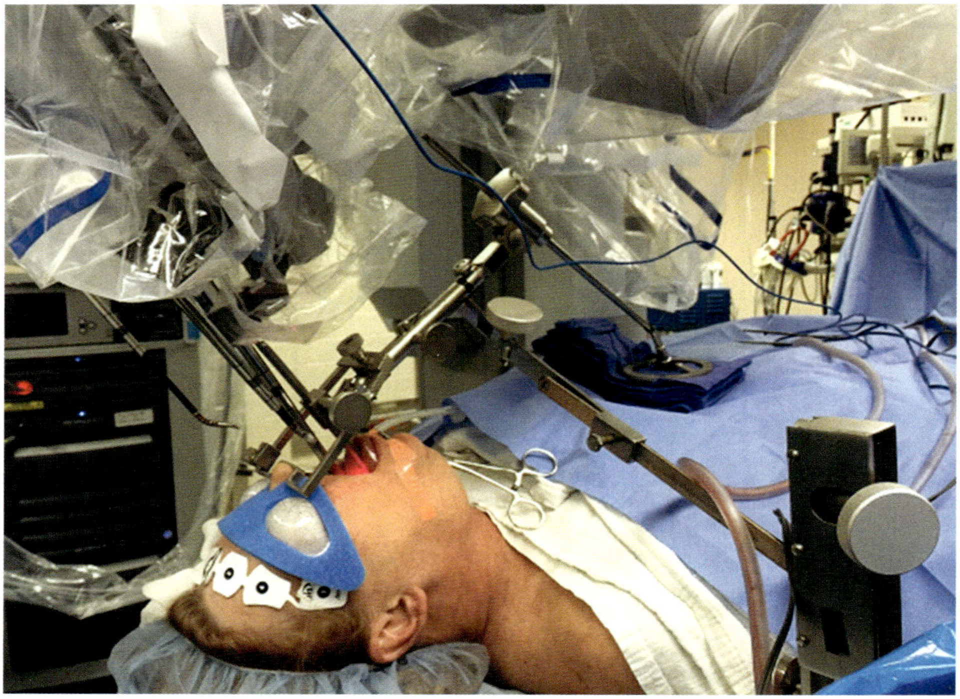

FIGURE 8.3 Note the position of the Feyh-Katzenbach mouth gag and microsuspension. Further stability is supplied by securing the microsuspension to the bedside with the Biomed arm.

Feyh-Katzenbach retractors). Next, the robot is "docked" near the patient's head at a 30-degree angle. The working arms (monopolar spatula cautery vs. laser, and forceps) and endoscope are then inserted transorally (see Figures 8.2 and 8.3). The operating surgeon sits at the remote console with binocular, high-definition, three-dimensional microscopy and tremor-free controls. The assistant provides countertraction, suction, and hemostasis at the patient's head (see Figure 8.4). Elective or therapeutic neck dissections may be performed concurrently, prior to, or after TORS, depending on indications for TORS and surgeon preference (19). For example, base of tongue (BOT) resection performed for cancer of the unknown primary may require a staged neck dissection, because the primary tumor may not be identified until final pathologic analysis. When possible, concurrent neck dissection allows for ligation of the external carotid artery branches (lingual, facial, and ascending pharyngeal), which significantly decreases the severity of postoperative bleeding (20).

TORS FOR OROPHARYNGEAL CANCER

BACKGROUND

Historically, surgical treatment of OPSCC often required large, morbid, open approaches to achieve oncologic en bloc extirpation. Open approaches included mandibular lingual release (21), transpharyngeal approaches (lateral or suprahyoid pharyngotomies) (22,23), and transmandibular approaches (midline labiomandibuloglossotomy or composite resection with segmental mandibulectomy) (24), all of which were associated with significant cosmetic and functional deficits. Because of the morbidity and complications associated with open approaches, organ-sparing concurrent chemoradiotherapy protocols became the standard of care for OPSCC.

The decreasing smoking incidence in the United States has brought about a parallel decreased incidence of aerodigestive squamous cell carcinoma, with two important exceptions,

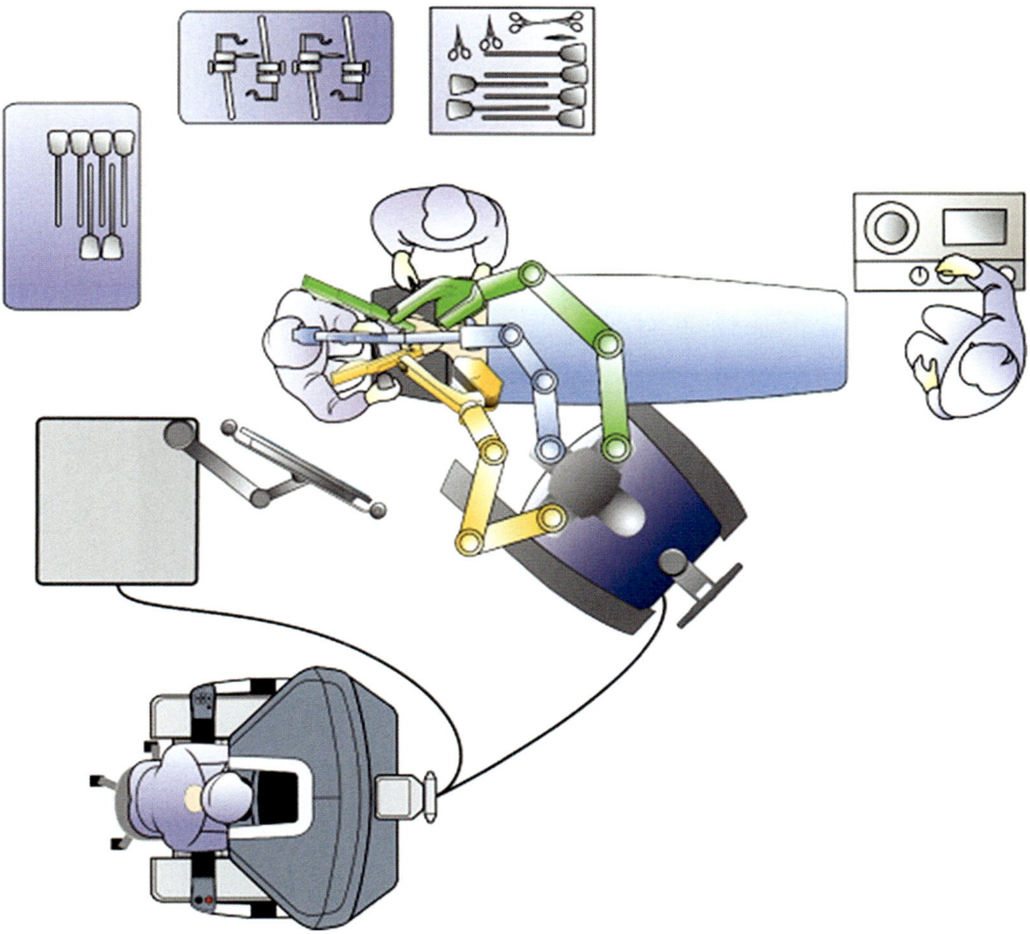

FIGURE 8.4 Diagrammatic representation of the standard TORS operating room setup.

TORS, transoral robotic surgery.

Source: ©[2014] Intuitive Surgical, Inc. Used with permission.

OPSCC and nasopharyngeal carcinoma (25). According to the Centers for Disease Control and Prevention (CDC), there are 11,726 new cases of OPSCC diagnosed annually in the United States. In 2003, human papillomavirus (HPV) was determined to be the causal agent in both a retrospective and prospective study (26,27). Between 1988 and 2004, there has been a 225% population-level increase in HPV-positive OPSCC and a 50% decline in HPV-negative OPSCC (26). Today, it is estimated that 70% of OPSCC cases are HPV-positive and this form appears epidemic around the world (Canada, the United Kingdom, Australia, Denmark, and Slovakia) (28).

Oropharyngeal cancer is no longer one disease, but two with two distinct patient populations. The first is the younger, HPV-positive patient, who is a nonsmoker and nondrinker (29) and who has a small, sometimes undetectable primary tumor, bulky lymph node metastases, and dramatically improved survival (see Figures 8.5 and 8.6) (4). The second, the HPV-negative patient, is older and has a large primary tumor, a history of tobacco and/or alcohol abuse, and a high risk of second primary cancers from field cancerization associated with substance use (30). HPV-positive OPSCC patients and their dramatically improved survival compared to their counterparts have challenged current treatment paradigms, because HPV-positive OPSCC represents a completely new disease. This group of patients is surviving to suffer the long-term toxicities from organ-sparing therapy and is calling its benefits into question. Viral-induced cancers such as HPV-positive OPSCC and Epstein–Barr

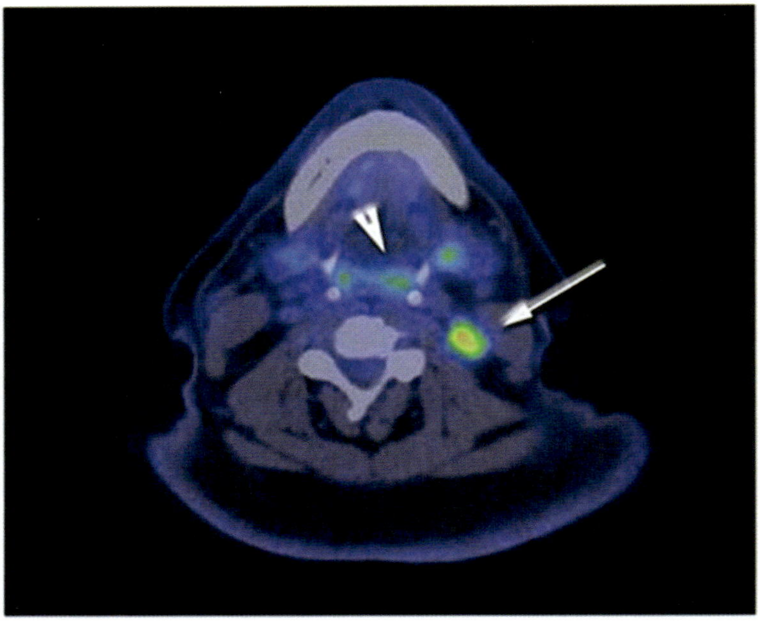

FIGURE 8.5 Oropharyngeal cancer patient. Arrowhead: primary. Long arrow: neck masses.

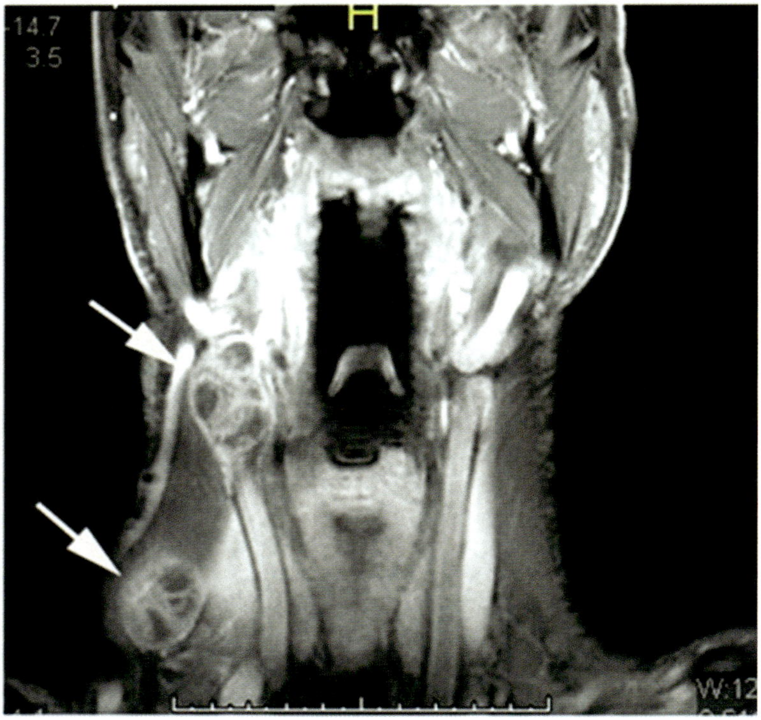

FIGURE 8.6 The "new" oropharyngeal cancer patient. Note the small primary tumor with asymmetric enhancement of the base of tongue. Also note the large, bulky cystic nodal conglomerates in the ipsilateral neck. Arrows: neck masses.

virus (EBV)-positive nasopharyngeal cancer have improved survival after initial response, regardless of progression of disease (31). TORS may improve care, prevent treatment-related toxicities, and improve quality of life in these typically younger patient groups.

PRIMARY TREATMENT FOR OROPHARYNGEAL CANCER

Oncologic outcomes following TORS for OPSCC have been reported in small series. The University of Pennsylvania group first reported series on TORS base of tongue resection in 2006, followed by TORS radical tonsillectomy in 2007 (16,32). After initial successes, they went on to perform the first prospective study on outcomes following TORS as the sole treatment without the use of adjuvant radiotherapy for OPSCC in 30 patients and reported 100% overall survival (OS) and 97% locoregional control at 2 years (33).

Several large, multicenter studies on TORS for OPSCC treatment have been performed. The largest, with 410 subjects, demonstrated 91.8% 2-year locoregional control and 94.5% disease-specific survival with only half of patients requiring adjuvant radiotherapy (31.3%) or chemoradiotherapy (21.3%) (34). A systematic review comparing 12 studies using TORS versus 8 studies using intensity modulated radiotherapy (IMRT) for early OPSCC was published reporting similar outcomes at 2 years (35). More recently in 2016, Morisod and Simon performed a systematic review with meta-analysis and found that 5-year OS and disease-specific survival were equivalent to nonsurgical treatments (36). Finally, Zevallos et al. reported effectiveness of TORS in practice by early adopters via data from the National Cancer Database and found that the positive margin rate was higher than reported in the multicenter study (20% versus 4.3%); the 30-day mortality rate remained low at 0.8%. The study highlighted the importance of surgeon experience, patient selection, and multidisciplinary care (37). Overall, TORS outcomes at high-volume centers compare favorably with those for IMRT as treatment for early-stage OPSCC in the literature (38).

Functional outcomes following TORS for OPSCC are also being studied. A recent systematic review by Hutcheson et al., including 12 papers with a total of 441 patients, found that gastrostomy-dependence rates following TORS were lower than those following IMRT (39). The same group looked at a subset of 89 patients who had MD Anderson Dysphagia Index scores, and found that patients undergoing TORS had better scores compared to those treated nonsurgically, 65.2–78.0 compared to 73.6–74.1, respectively.

SALVAGE TORS FOR OROPHARYNGEAL CANCER

Despite the improved prognosis of HPV-positive OPSCC, 25% of patients will experience recurrence after primary therapy (4,31). Interestingly, even in the salvage setting, HPV-positive patients still have improved OS compared to HPV-negative patients (31,40). Patients undergoing surgical salvage for recurrent OPSCC have improved survival compared to those undergoing nonsurgical salvage (40). Guo et al. recently performed a retrospective study including 86 patients with recurrent OPSCC and found that HPV-positive status and surgical salvage treatment (including TORS and open approaches) were positively associated with OS, but negative margin status at the time of salvage was associated with disease-free survival (see Figure 8.7) (41).

TORS in the salvage setting has been specifically studied for safety and efficacy and authors have found acceptable complication rate, even when routine microvascular free flap reconstruction to cover the carotid is omitted (31,42). For these reasons, salvage TORS may represent a better option for surgical salvage in select patients with recurrent OPSCC, who would otherwise require the traditional higher risk, open salvage open approaches and free tissue transfer reconstruction.

TORS FOR CANCER OF THE UNKNOWN PRIMARY

The incidence of cancer of unknown primary origin is rising; the majority eventually are discovered as small, clinically undetected, HPV-related oropharyngeal cancers (43). The major benefit of TORS in this setting is identification of the primary, which prevents wide field irradiation of the entire aerodigestive tract, pharyngeal constrictors, and necks required when the primary cannot be pathologically determined. Byrd et al. were able to localize 19 of 22 patients (86.4%) with nonlocalizing physical examinations and imaging using robotic surgery (18), similar to other groups (44,45). This

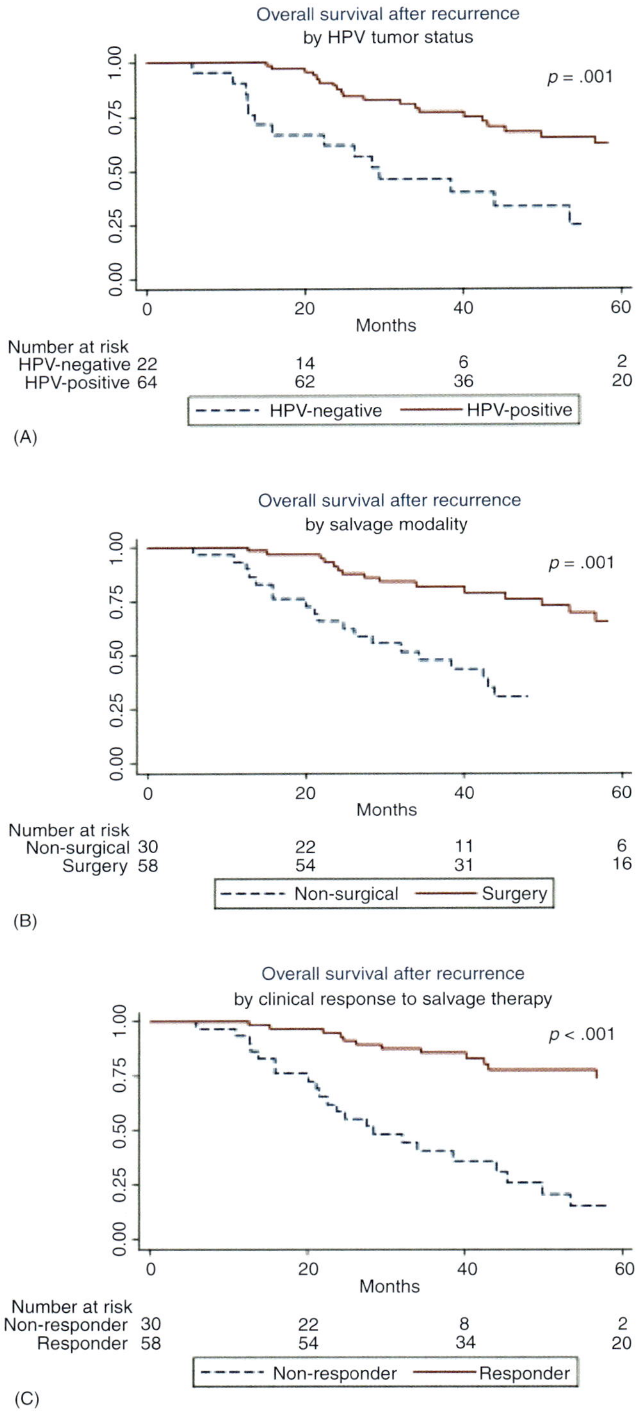

FIGURE 8.7 Kaplan–Meier estimates of overall survival after salvage therapy for patients with recurrent oropharyngeal squamous cell carcinoma by (A) HPV tumor status, (B) salvage modality, and (C) clinical response to salvage therapy.

Improved outcomes were observed for HPV-positive patients ($p = .001$), patients who underwent surgical salvage ($p = .001$), and patients who responded clinically to salvage therapy ($p < .001$).

HPV, human papillomavirus.

Source: Joseph AW, Guo T, Hur K, et al. Disease-free survival after salvage therapy for recurrent oropharyngeal squamous cell carcinoma. *Head Neck*. 2016;38(suppl 1):E1501–E1509. With permission from John Wiley and Sons.

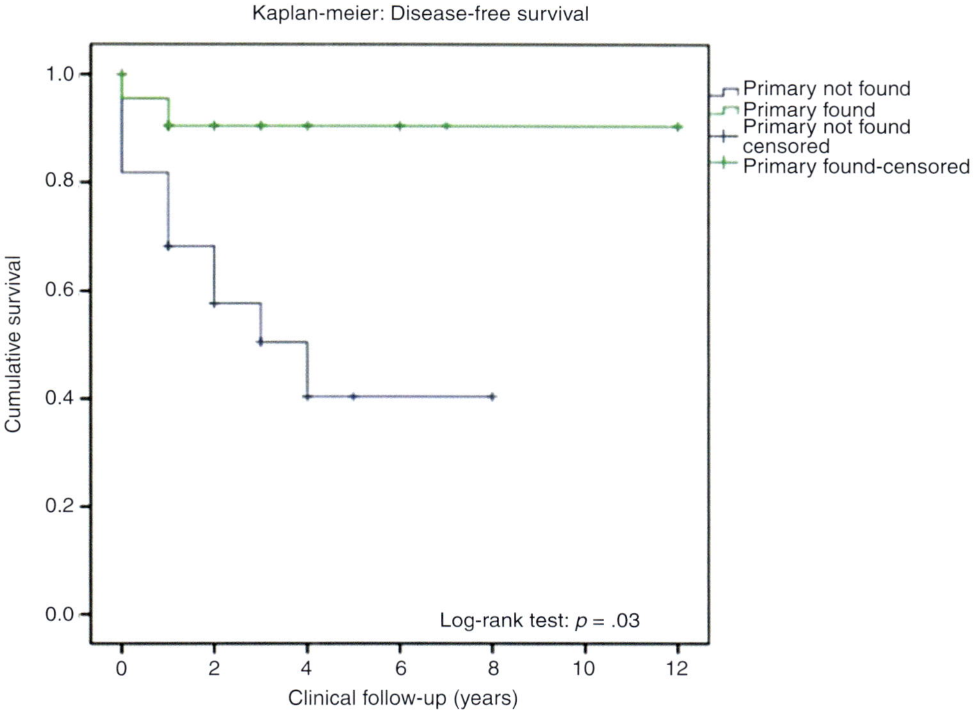

FIGURE 8.8 Kaplan–Meier curves for disease-free survival. Discovery of the primary was also associated with improved disease-free survival (HR: 0.25, 95% CI: 0.069–0.91, $p = .03$).

CI, confidence interval; HR, hazard ratio.

drops to 67% when physical examinations, imaging, and directed biopsies are negative. TORS lingual tonsillectomy, which is more conservative than base of tongue resections performed as treatment for a known primary, identifies the primary in 72% (18/25) of cases. More importantly, a retrospective case–control study by Davis et al. found that identification of the primary tumor is associated with significantly improved overall, cause-specific, and disease-free survival (see Figure 8.8) (46).

TORS FOR LARYNGEAL CANCER

BACKGROUND

Treatment of laryngeal cancer has evolved considerably in the past 20 years. Following the VA laryngeal cancer study and RTOG 91-11, organ-sparing definitive radiation and concurrent chemoradiotherapy protocols with salvage surgery for failure provided survival equivalent outcomes for advanced laryngeal cancer compared to primary total laryngectomy, and subsequently supplanted surgery as the standard of care (1,2). Therefore, surgery for laryngeal cancer was mostly limited to salvage total laryngectomy. However, salvage laryngectomy is fraught with postoperative complications and requires the addition of pectoralis muscle rotational flaps or microvascular free tissue transfer reconstruction to prevent complications with healing. The most vexing and common complication is postoperative salivary fistula, which occurs up to 65% of the time without some sort of additional reconstruction (47).

In response to organ-sparing protocols, surgeons started to explore open conservation, or partial, laryngeal surgery. Procedures include supraglottic, supracricoid laryngectomy with cricohyoidoepiglottopexy or cricohyoidopexy, and variations of vertical partial laryngectomy in attempts to preserve function and avoid radiation therapy. These approaches came with perioperative morbidity, dysphonia, dysphagia, and need for tracheostomy. The development of TLM for primary treatment of laryngeal cancer made open techniques less popular (48), since outcomes of TLM were improved and similar to definitive radiotherapy and chemoradiotherapy for early and advanced disease, respectively (49). In the United States where adoption of TLM was limited owing to the technical difficulty and concerns about achieving negative margins, primary nonsurgical therapy remains dominant and patients who recur are treated with salvage laryngectomy.

TORS FOR SUPGRAGLOTTIC CANCER

The advent of TORS for the treatment of early laryngeal cancer brought on renewed interest in transoral supraglottic laryngectomy for select laryngeal cancers in the United States. As previously stated, TORS was first reported feasible for supraglottic partial laryngectomy (SGPL) in 2005 (15). Since then, several groups have adopted the technique and reported successful outcomes (50–54). En bloc resection for primary tumors can be achieved with appropriate patient selection (see Figure 8.9). What is more, this procedure comes with a very low risk of fistula when performed without neck dissection.

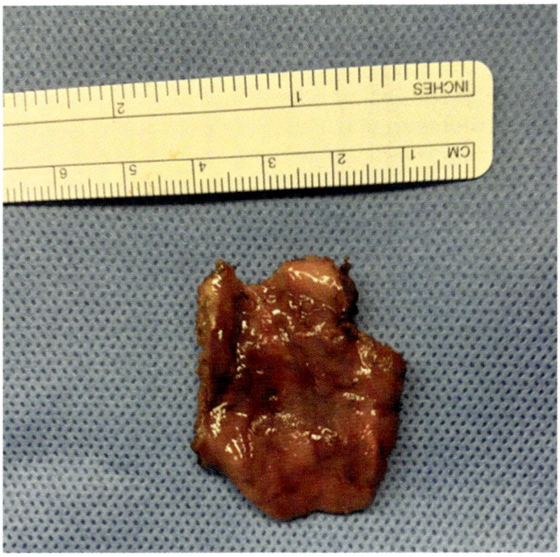

FIGURE 8.9 TORS supraglottic laryngectomy specimen. Note the typical shape of the epiglottis and aryepiglottic folds.

TORS, transoral robotic surgery.

Outcomes for TORS supraglottic laryngectomy have to be studied. Park et al. found that TORS supraglottic laryngectomy patients had shorter operating times, length of hospital stay, time to decannulation, and time to resumption of oral diet compared to open SGPL with an equal oncologic outcome (55). Tracheotomy and nasogastric/gastrostomy feeding practices vary in the literature according to surgeon preference, patient selection, and swallowing therapy protocols. According to a multicenter, European study on 84 patients undergoing TORS supraglottic laryngectomy, those patients with tracheotomy were likely decannulated within 2 weeks, and only 9.5% of patients required gastrostomy (56). These results were similar in other series (50–52,54). As in open partial laryngeal surgery, patient selection and early speech therapy are paramount in the treatment of early laryngeal cancer for TORS partial laryngeal surgery (55).

TORS FOR GLOTTIC CANCER

Traditionally, total laryngectomy is indicated as salvage therapy for recurrent or persistent laryngeal cancer following other treatments because of nests of persistent carcinoma in paralaryngeal soft tissues and the presence of submucosal spread that makes negative margin resection difficult with salvage partial laryngeal surgery (57). For this reason, Smith et al. first developed and described the TORS total laryngectomy procedure in a cadaver and went on to study its use in a small case series of five patients (see Figures 8.10 and 8.11) (58). In that original series, three patients with neck dissections developed fistula, but no patient had recurrence of disease and all patients were swallowing orally without gastrostomy. Since that time other authors have reported successful case series (59). Currently, pioneers recommend TORS total laryngectomy for salvage in patients needing narrow field laryngectomy for persistent or recurrent disease. Those patients needing concurrent neck dissection should have a total laryngectomy (58,60).

TORS FOR NASOPHARYNGEAL CANCER

BACKGROUND

In the past, surgical treatment of nasopharyngeal cancer required large open approaches to achieve

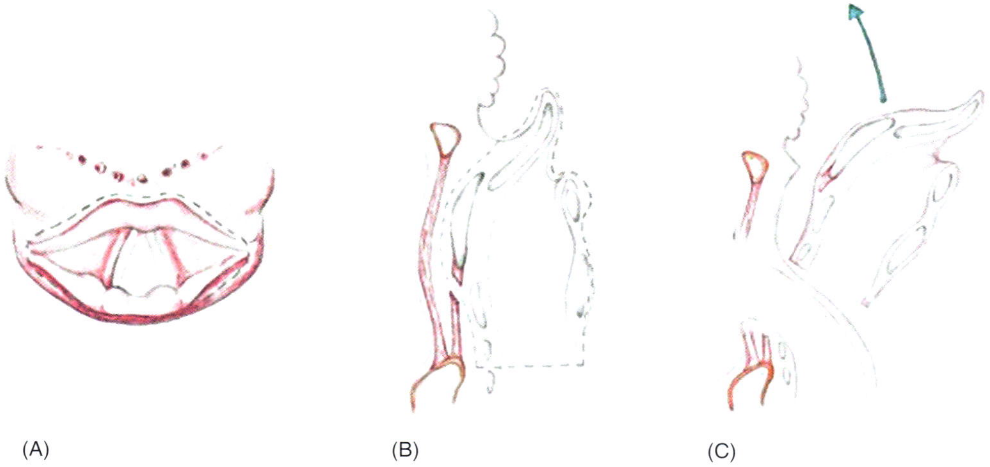

FIGURE 8.10 Transoral total laryngectomy anatomy.

Source: Dowthwaite S, Nichols AC, Yoo J, et al. Transoral robotic total laryngectomy: report of 3 cases. *Head Neck*. 2013;35(11):E338–E342. With permission from John Wiley and Sons.

en bloc resection with negative margins. Open approaches include the transpalatal approach (61,62), the infratemporal fossa approach (63), the maxillary swing approach (64), the midfacial degloving approach (65), and facial translocation. All of these approaches come with significant perioperative morbidity, and facial incisions and scarring. The Intergroup 0099 in the United States and subsequent studies in endemic populations changed the standard of care (6). Since then, the use of primary organ-sparing protocols for primary nasopharyngeal carcinoma treatment has been uncontested (66).

Nasopharyngeal carcinoma was recognized to have significant subtypes by the World Health Organization in 1978. Subsequently, the cancers have been classified differently based on the presence of keratinization and the EBV (67). Today, nasopharyngeal carcinoma is routinely diagnosed as EBV-positive and EBV-negative disease for purposes of management, prognostication, and surveillance. Screening for nasopharyngeal carcinoma is performed using the EBV-DNA (68). The gold-standard for confirmation of EBV-positive tumors the presence of EBER-1 using in-situ hybridization in analysis of

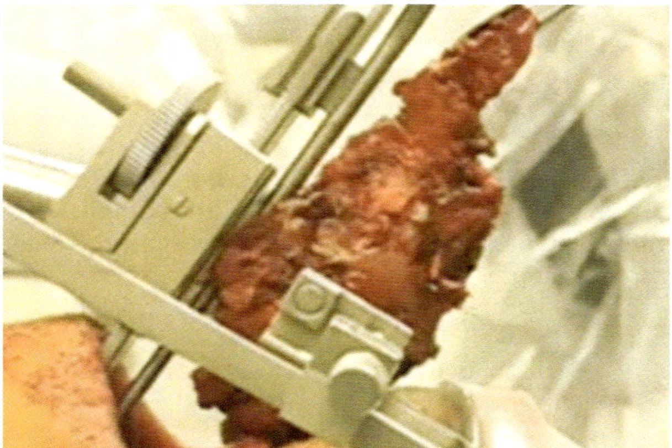

FIGURE 8.11 Transoral removal of the larynx with the robot moved out of position and the mouth retractor in place.

Source: Smith RV, Schiff BA, Sarta C, et al. Transoral robotic total laryngectomy. *Laryngoscope*. 2013;123(3):678–682. With permission from John Wiley and Sons.

pathologic specimens (67). Circulation plasma EBV-DNA levels are used to detect recurrence during surveillance and have a sensitivity and specificity of 96% and 93%, respectively (68–70).

Nasopharyngeal carcinoma, like OPSCC, has two distinct diseases and two distinct populations. The first is the younger, Southeast Asian, EBV-positive patient, who is a nonsmoker, nondrinker, with the nonkeratinizing subtype, bilateral bulky lymph node metastases, and improved survival. The second, is an older, Caucasian EBV-negative patient, who has a history of tobacco and/or alcohol abuse, keratinizing subtype, and poor response to chemoradiotherapy. Like the HPV-negative patient, the EBV-negative patient likely has a high risk of second primary cancers due to field cancerization caused by substance abuse (30,71). Again, viral-induced cancers such as HPV-positive OPSCC and EBV-positive nasopharyngeal cancer have improved survival with treatment (71). Concurrent chemoradiotherapy protocols should still be the standard of care for newly diagnosed nasopharyngeal cancer given the inoperability of nasopharyngeal primaries on presentation, nodes of Rouviere, and bulky bilateral neck nodes. Circulating EBV-DNA has been shown to correlate with tumor, node, and metastasis (TNM) staging, tumor control, and OS (66). However, salvage TORS may be indicated for recurrences, may improve care, may prevent treatment-related toxicities associated with nonsurgical salvage, and may improve quality of life in these typically younger patient groups.

TORS NASOPHARYNGECTOMY

TORS approaches to the skull base were first examined in cadaveric models by O'Malley and Weinstein (72). Transoral robotic nasopharyngectomy was first described in a cadaveric model by Ozer in 2008 and later modified by Tsang with the addition of lateral palatal flap approach to provide better access to the lateral parapharyngeal space in 2013 (73,74). The first human case report was later described by Wei and Ho in 2010 (see Figure 8.12) (75). The patient had no complications. Nasal packing to prevent epistaxis was removed without complication on the second postoperative day. The patient was eating on the fourth postoperative day. Tsang et al. have since done a prospective case series of patients undergoing robotic nasopharyngectomy as salvage surgery (76). The group operated on 12 patients and reported operative and postoperative outcomes: 9 of 12 patients had clear margins. Two-year local control, overall, and disease-free survival rates were 86%, 83%, and 61%, respectively. So far, the literature to date supports the use of TORS nasopharyngectomy in appropriately selected nasopharyngeal cancers requiring salvage following nonsurgical therapy.

TORS FOR PARAPHARYNGEAL SPACE TUMORS

BACKGROUND

Approximately 80% of tumors originating in the parapharyngeal space benign (77). Malignancies of parotid origin, lymphoma, and sarcoma do occur. Oropharyngeal and nasopharyngeal malignancies may also invade the parapharyngeal space secondarily. Still, benign tumors are far more common. Typically the treatment from primary parapharyngeal space tumors is surgery, which requires open transcervical, transparotid, orbitozygomatic, and transmandibular approaches if enough for adequate exposure (78). The traditional, transoral approach was originally described in the 1950s, but its use is controversial as it may put key neurovascular structures in the parapharyngeal space at risk because the exposure is limited compared to open approaches (79). TORS, however may improve access, shorten surgical times, avoid facial nerve injury, eliminate the need for an external incision, and require less manipulation of the tumor.

O'Malley et al. were the first to describe TORS for the treatment of parapharyngeal space tumors in 2010 in a prospective case series of 10 patients, and were successful in 9 of 10 cases (78). The authors reported no significant complications with regard to intraoperative tumor spillage or postoperative hemorrhage, infection, or trismus. Local control was 100%. Shortly after, Lee et al. reported on two successful cases of prestyloid neurogenic tumor removal without capsule rupture (80). Park et al. later described a series of TORS approach to the parpharyngeal space including 9 parapharyngeal tumors and 2 styloidectomies for Eagle's syndrome (81). Patients were swallowing immediately postoperatively, had minimal blood loss, and stayed in the hospital an average of 2.6 days prior to discharge. Later

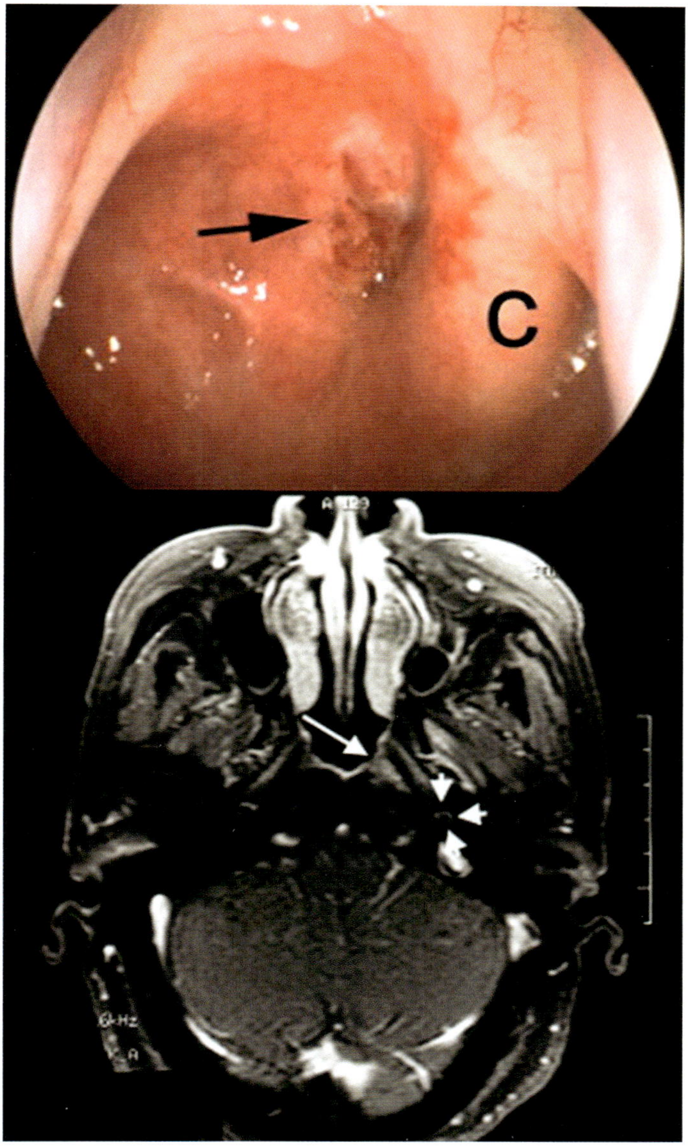

FIGURE 8.12 (Top) Endoscopic view of a small tumor situated in the left fossa of Rosenmüller (arrow) close to the medial crus (C) of the eustachian tube. (Bottom). MRI showing a small tumor (arrow) in the left lateral wall, not touching the carotid artery (arrowheads).

Source: Wei WI, Ho W-K. Transoral robotic resection of recurrent nasopharyngeal carcinoma. *Laryngoscope*. 2010;120(10):2011–2014. With permission from John Wiley and Sons.

Boyce et al. performed the largest single institution series of 17 patients and looked at technical limitations of TORS (82). They found that 11.7% of cases requires cervical incision to assist with dissection in the lateral and superior parapharyngeal space. Average total operative times were 140.5 minutes and average length of hospital stay was 1.8 days (range 1–7 days). All patients were on an oral diet. A systematic review of TORS for parapharyngeal space tumors was performed in 2014, with 44 patients undergoing TORS parapharyngeal space resection for TORS neoplasms. Mean length of stay was 3.0 days and mean time to resumption of normal diet was 1.0 days. TORS for the parapharyngeal space is safe in appropriate hands.

CONTROVERSIES IN TORS

OROPHARYNGEAL CANCER

The major argument favoring the use of TORS for OPSCC is to spare the HPV-positive patient with stage III or IV disease the debilitating side effects of concurrent chemoradiotherapy. Zevallos et al. recently reported effectiveness of TORS in practice by early adopters via data from the National Cancer Database and found a positive margin rate of 20%, which was more likely to be seen in T2 tumors and low-volume centers. This study also highlighted the importance of surgeon experience, patient selection, and multidisciplinary care in the treatment of oropharyngeal carcinoma (37). Reports of swallowing function (>2 years) after transoral laser surgery and robotic surgery are not well studied. However, several studies report low rates of immediate dysphagia and gastrostomy dependence (0%–7%) beyond the first year postsurgery (34,39,83). We will not know about the incidence of severe late dysphagia following TORS with or without adjuvant therapy for several more years.

Outside of a clinical trial, many OPSCC patients routinely receive chemoradiotherapy following TORS, which is one of the major arguments against primary surgical management (35). High rates of adjuvant chemoradiotherapy are attributable to the elevated incidence of nodal metastases and extracapsular spread (ECS) in HPV-positive neck dissection specimens. ECS was originally identified as a poor prognostic indicator in two randomized, controlled trials that have made it an indication for adjuvant chemoradiotherapy under the current standard of care (84). However, these studies were inherently flawed, because the majority of patients had OPSCC and the study results were not stratified by HPV status.

The incidence of ECS in surgically treated OPSCC has been studied using the National Cancer and Surveillance, Epidemiology, and End Results (SEER) databases and is estimated at 23% to 25% and increases with higher N stages (85,86). Recently, however, retrospective studies by Sinha et al. and Maxwell et al. demonstrate that this feature has no negative impact on survival in HPV-positive OPSCC, and may not require adjuvant chemoradiotherapy for curative treatment (85,87). In a study examining surgically treated early oropharyngeal cancer with both open and transoral techniques, Kass et al. reported that recurrence-free survival was 82%, and that HPV status and adjuvant radiotherapy were protective against recurrence, while nodal status and the addition of chemotherapy had no impact (88). More recently, Amini et al. looked at the National Cancer Database and found that ECS did not affect survival in surgically treated HPV-positive OPSCC patients (89). In the future, ECS may not be an indication for adjuvant chemoradiotherapy; however, level one evidence will be required to change the standard of care.

LARYNGEAL CANCER

Although TLM has widely been accepted as a technique for endoscopic partial laryngeal surgery, some proponents of TORS argue that the robotic approach is equally effective, and is faster owing to freedom of motion and the use of monopolar cautery. It is also more easily adopted (18). However, cases are frequently challenging due to anatomy and the decreased working space required for TORS (58). The Feyh-Katzenbach retractor's laryngeal blade is effective in many, but not all, patients for exposure of the supraglottis, and the freedom of motion for the da Vinci arms is restricted more inferiorly in the airway, which may hinder tumor resection (50). Ansarin et al. compared 10 early TLM cases to 10 early TORS cases, finding a higher rate of positive margins in the TORS group (90).

Salvage partial laryngeal surgery must be undertaken with caution due to the presence of invisible nest of cancer cells persistent in soft tissue and submucosal spread of visible recurrent lesion (57). This was a major criticism of partial laryngeal surgery and a reason for subsequent failures following salvage partial laryngeal surgery (91,92). This pitfall is true for TORS supraglottic laryngectomy, and likely applies to TORS total laryngectomy. However, in these cases salvage TORS total laryngectomy may overcome this risk and so far, seems to provide adequate control in the salvage setting. Opponents to this technique, also might argue that patients requiring salvage laryngectomy for a supraglottic primary should never have TORS total laryngectomy, because their risk of occult neck disease is too high and eliminates their candidacy for the procedure. Furthermore, TORS total laryngectomy is only very recently described and few surgeons have experience with the very advanced robotic approach. The outcomes of TORS total laryngectomy are limited to very small case series with limited follow-up. Future studies will be needed.

NASOPHARYNGEAL CANCER

Although some groups have reported success with salvage TORS nasopharyngectomy, there are several groups that would advocate for endonasal endoscopic resection of recurrent disease versus combined approaches. Opponents of TORS in the treatment of recurrent nasopharyngeal cancer might claim that most recurrence continues up into the skull base through foramen lacerum, and that this is only accessible with endoscopic techniques (93). Furthermore, identification and preservation of the carotid are easily accomplished transnasally. Transoral approaches require splitting the palate to achieve appropriate exposure, which could be associated with more morbidity, especially in the postirradiated patient (61). The choice of approach ultimately depends on surgeon experience and patient selection.

PARAPHARYNGEAL SPACE TUMORS

TORS for parapharyngeal space tumors is safe and successful as reported in the literature, but some surgeons might advocate for traditional open approaches. Opponents may say that the limited exposure in TORS puts critical neurovascular structures at greater risk, that the rate of tumor capsule rupture is too high (24%) (94), and that control of the carotid artery is better in transcervical approaches. However, champions would say that exposure using open approaches is equally poor when it comes to the superior medial extent of dissection, that complication rates are similar, and that TORS eliminates a cervical scar. While capsular disruption is undesirable, the literature is conflicting on the association between rupture/extracapsular dissection and recurrence (82,95). Follow-up of current series is too short to determine oncologic success of TORS for parapharyngeal space malignancy. Furthermore, there are very few reported cases of use in the treatment of malignancy.

Complication rates in the literature are similar between TORS and open approaches, and are related to dissection of the parapharyngeal space (94). However, given that TORS for the parapharyngeal space is a new procedure, surgeon experience and proper selection are paramount if TORS is to be employed.

TORS IN CLINICAL TRIALS

Medical and radiation oncologists are well aware of the toxicities of concurrent chemoradiotherapy protocols, and are exploring de-intensification of treatments via altered fractionation, decreased radiation doses, alternate chemotherapeutic agents with better side effect profiles, and immunotherapy regimens for HPV-positive OPSCC and nasopharyngeal carcinoma (96,97,98). Similarly, trials are under way in order to improve surgical treatment of OPSCC and de-escalation of adjuvant treatment (9,99).

The RTOG 1221 trial was designed to test the efficacy of TORS for early T stage, HPV-negative OPSCC. Though well conceived and supported by multiple centers across the nation, the study was forced to close in February 2015 owing to failure to enroll any patients after 15 months. Participating surgeons noted that HPV-negative OPSCC patients presented with advanced disease, which was not amenable to TORS. The efficacy of TORS for the treatment of HPV-negative disease, remains an important question, but the rarity of surgical candidates may mean that a large, retrospective, multi-institutional collaborative effort may be the only way to examine outcomes in this population.

The ADEPT (Adjuvant De-escalation, Extracapsular Spread, p16-positive, Transoral) trial was launched in 2013 with the goal of determining the role of chemotherapy in patients with HPV-positive OPSCC with ECS, using 2-year locoregional control and disease-free survival as end points. Unfortunately, this study recently closed because of low accrual rates (only 41 patients after 5 years). The presence of ECS on final pathologic examination in neck dissection specimens, therefore, still requires adjuvant chemoradiotherapy (100).

The PATHOS (Post-operative Adjuvant Treatment for HPV-positive Tumors) trial was initiated in 2014 to assess swallowing function following transoral resection (including TLM and TORS) of HPV-positive OPSCC, with varying intensity of adjuvant treatment protocols.

The aim is to personalize treatment, based on HPV status and pathology findings, and to optimize patient outcomes. The primary end point is 1-year swallowing determined by the MD Anderson Dysphagia Index. Other secondary end points are overall and disease-free survival. The study's estimated completion date is 2019.

The Eastern Cooperative Oncology Group (ECOG) 3311 trial is a national, phase II randomized, prospective trial studying the efficacy of TORS in the treatment of resectable, lateralized stage III or IV, HPV-positive OPSCC (cT1-T2, N1-2b) without matted nodes, followed by adjuvant therapy as guided by risk assessment (see Figure 8.13). Over 65 centers and 84 surgeons were credentialed to participate in the trial (15); 519 patients were enrolled in this large, randomized, National Cancer Institute (NCI) supported phase II trial, in order to determine safety and efficacy of de-intensification in the intermediate-risk pathologic group, using 2-year progression-free-survival as an end point. Approximately 66% of patients were eligible for reduced dose radiation, elimination of chemotherapy, or no adjuvant treatment. Of note, the trial passed all data and safety monitoring committee reviews without cessation for excess toxicity or futility. Data on oncologic

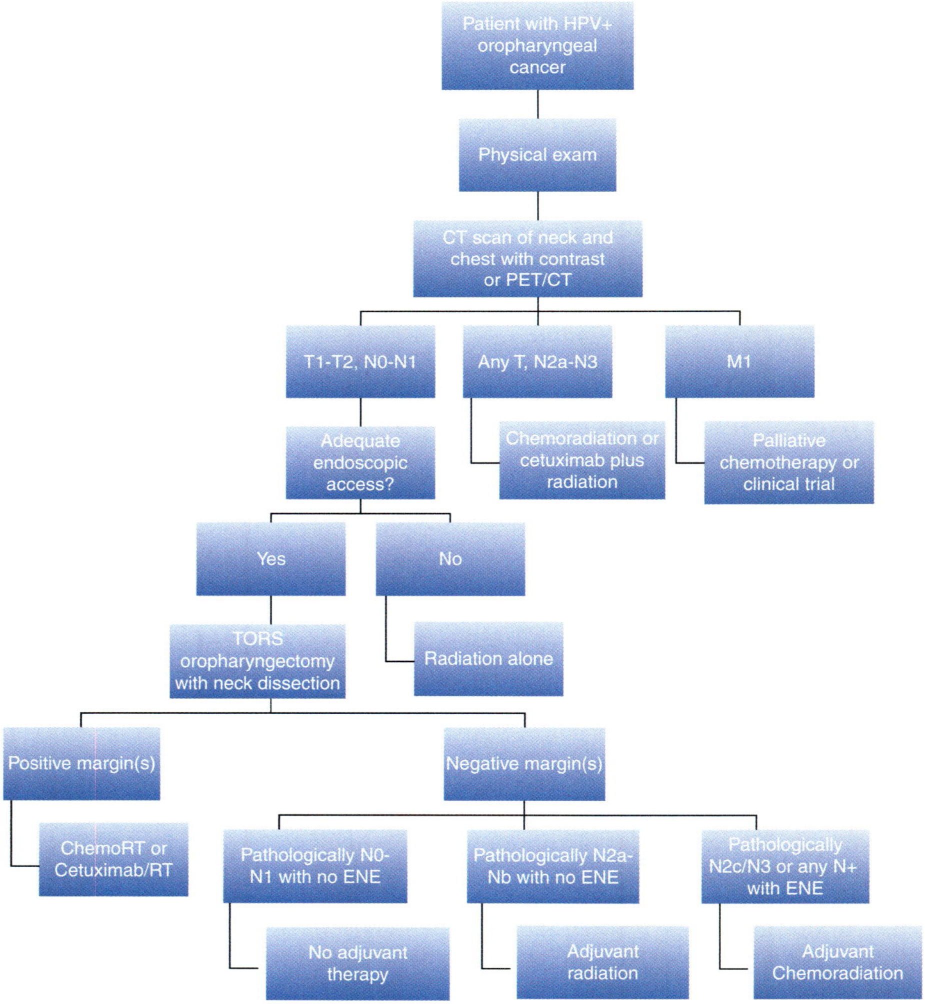

FIGURE 8.13 Flowchart delineating current diagnostic workup and treatment paradigm for oropharyngeal cancer.

ENE, extranodal extension; HPV, human papillomavirus; RT, radiation therapy; TORS, transoral robotic surgery.

and patient reported outcomes regarding quality of life and swallowing will be collected until 2020. The estimated clinical reporting date is 2020.

The ORATOR trial, a phase II trial of patients with HPV-positive and negative OPSCC, is under way, comparing TORS-based treatment to definitive radiotherapy with or without chemotherapy for early-stage oropharyngeal cancer. This is a single-institution, prospective trial in London, Ontario that just completed its needed enrollment of 68 patients. Primary end points are 1-year quality of life outcomes at 1 year posttreatment, while secondary end points include 1-year OS, progression-free survival, toxicity, as well as quality of life and swallow outcomes at 5 years posttreatment (99). While well designed, this study may require more patients to make more meaningful conclusions and may not be able to differentiate outcomes between HPV-positive and HPV-negative patients. The estimated completion date is June 2021.

CONCLUSIONS

Successful application and expansion of TORS procedures in head and neck surgery demands careful patient selection, the most important of which are technical feasibility, patient preferences, and overall health. Choice of robot type and tools is surgeon dependent. Careful workup including physical examination (particularly dentition, interincisoral opening, Mallampati score, assessment of the airway and exposure on flexible endoscopy, neck extension, as well as the presence and character of cervical metastases), imaging, and swallowing evaluation may influence candidacy for TORS. Patients need evidence-based counseling regarding risks and benefits of the different treatment modalities after discussion in a multidisciplinary tumor board. Contraindications to TORS are fixation of the mass on palpation, *obvious* ECS or need for trimodality therapy based on workup, and tumor surround more than 270 degrees of the internal carotid artery. Salvage TORS procedures should be undertaken by surgeons with extensive experience in primary TORS resections and with even more circumspection.

Specific contraindications for oropharyngeal cancers are retropharyngeal carotid arteries, significant palatal involvement, vallecula involvement requiring supraglottic resection, T4 tumors, and preoperative aspiration (32). Relative contraindications for oropharyngeal cancers are significant preoperative dysphagia or tumors that cross midline that may put the patient at risk for poor functional outcome (16).

For laryngeal cancers, exposure based on anatomy and fibrosis is the primary limiting factor; and, inadequate intraoperative exposure is an absolute contraindication for these cases. Preoperative pulmonary and swallowing function assessment is paramount, since patients will need to temporarily tolerate some degree of penetration/aspiration in the postoperative period; or, undergo total laryngectomy (open or robotic). With regard to the primary tumor, specific contraindications are involvement of the lateral piriform sinus, extralaryngeal invasion, or vessel invasion (101). Nodal disease is a relative contraindication, as it dramatically increases fistula rate. In such instances, the patient would be better served with total laryngectomy and free flap reconstruction.

For nasopharyngeal carcinoma, serum markers/radiography suspicion, and biopsy-proven recurrence are indications for salvage surgery. Surgery for recurrent tumors should be restricted to those less than 2 cm, and those involving only one eustachian tube (76). Bony invasion of the skull base and abutment to the carotid artery are other contraindications. Following strict criteria for patient selection, successful resection can be achieved.

For parapharyngeal space tumors, lateral and superior involvement with 10 mm of the skull base has been identified as high risk for capsule rupture and need for combined transcervical approach (see Figure 8.14) (82). It has also been noted that the classically described dumbbell tumor that traverses the stylomandibular tunnel is also not ideally suited for TORS resection and that such tumors likely require a transcervical approach. Preoperative trismus is a relative contraindication portends poor transoral exposure even under anesthesia.

In patients who require salvage TORS after chemotherapy/radiation, additional considerations include airway edema, postoperative hemorrhage (102), the potential for fistula, velopharyngeal insufficiency, and carotid exposure. In salvage TORS SGPL, airway edema and dysphagia are a major concern. Tracheotomy and gastrostomy are more often needed than in primary TORS. Salvage TORS has been reported successfully with an acceptable complication rate without routine reconstruction (42). Local flap or free tissue transfer is employed to minimize the chance for carotid blowout, restore

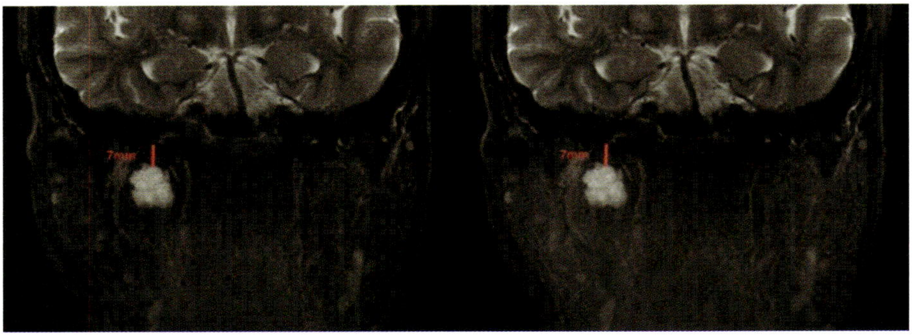

FIGURE 8.14 Inadequate distance from skull base.

Coronal T2-weighted MRI showing the parapharyngeal space neoplasm that had capsular fragmentation and was <10 mm from the skull base. The distance from the skull base is marked and measured at 7 mm.

Source: Boyce BJ, Curry JM, Luginbuhl A, Cognetti DM. Transoral robotic approach to parapharyngeal space tumors: case series and technical limitations. *Laryngoscope*. 2016;126(8):1776–1782. With permission from John Wiley and Sons.

tongue base bulk, and improve velopharyngeal closure in salvage oropharyngectomy, as radiation changes decrease the amount of parapharyngeal fat and hinder mobility via fibrosis (103).

In summary, TORS for head and neck cancer can achieve outcomes similar to “organ-sparing” techniques in appropriately selected patients. Surgery for treatment of cancer of the unknown primary may lead to identification of the primary, improved survival, and better quality of life. Surgery for oropharyngeal cancer may allow for de-intensification of adjuvant therapy and better long-term functional outcomes. Salvage TORS oropharyngectomy may provide superior functional and oncologic outcomes than other salvage treatments in select patients. TORS supraglottic laryngectomy provides similar functional and oncologic outcomes to radiotherapy in select patients. TORS total laryngectomy and TORS nasopharyngectomy are treatment options for selected patients with persistent disease following organ-sparing protocols, but represent very advanced robotic techniques. Prospective, randomized trials are under way to define the role of TORS in the future. The future will be interesting.

REFERENCES

1. Wolf GT, Fisher SG, Hong WK, et al. Induction chemotherapy plus radiation compared with surgery plus radiation in patients with advanced laryngeal cancer. *N Engl J Med*. 1991;324(24):1685–1690. doi:10.1056/NEJM199106133242402
2. Forastiere AA, Goepfert H, Maor M, et al. Concurrent chemotherapy and radiotherapy for organ preservation in advanced laryngeal cancer. *N Engl J Med*. 2003;349(22):2091–2098.
3. Calais G, Alfonsi M, Bardet E, et al. Randomized trial of radiation therapy versus concomitant chemotherapy and radiation therapy for advanced-stage oropharynx carcinoma. *J Natl Cancer Inst*. 1999;91(24):2081–2086.
4. Ang KK, Harris J, Wheeler R, et al. Human papillomavirus and survival of patients with oropharyngeal cancer. *N Engl J Med*. 2010;363(1):24–35.
5. Pignon JP, Le Maître A, Maillard E, Bourhis J. MACH-NC Collaborative Group. Meta-analysis of chemotherapy in head and neck cancer (MACH-NC): an update on 93 randomised trials and 17,346 patients. *Radiother Oncol*. 2009;92(1):4–14.
6. Al-Sarraf M, Leblanc M, Giri PG, et al. Chemoradiotherapy versus radiotherapy in patients with advanced nasopharyngeal cancer: phase III randomized Intergroup study 0099. *J Clin Oncol*. 1998;16(4):1310–1317.
7. Machtay M, Moughan J, Trotti A, et al. Factors associated with severe late toxicity after concurrent chemoradiation for locally advanced head and neck cancer: an RTOG analysis. *J Clin Oncol*. 2008;26(21):3582–3589.
8. Francis DO, Weymuller EA, Parvathaneni U, et al. Dysphagia, stricture, and pneumonia in head and neck cancer patients: does treatment modality matter? *Ann Otol Rhinol Laryngol*. 2010;119(6):391–397.
9. Holsinger FC, Ferris RL. Transoral endoscopic head and neck surgery and its role within the multidisciplinary treatment paradigm of oropharynx cancer: robotics, lasers, and clinical trials. *J Clin Oncol*. 2015;33(29):3285–3292.
10. Canis M, Martin A, Kron M, et al. Results of transoral laser microsurgery in 102 patients with squamous cell carcinoma of the tonsil. *Eur Arch Otorhinolaryngol*. 2013;270(8):2299–2306.

11. Canis M, Ihler F, Wolff HA, et al. Oncologic and functional results after transoral laser microsurgery of tongue base carcinoma. *Eur Arch Otorhinolaryngol.* 2013;270(3):1075–1083.
12. Haughey BH, Hinni ML, Salassa JR, et al. Transoral laser microsurgery as primary treatment for advanced-stage oropharyngeal cancer: a United States multicenter study. *Head Neck.* 2011;33(12):1683–1694.
13. Rich JT, Milov S, Lewis JS, et al. Transoral laser microsurgery (TLM) +/- adjuvant therapy for advanced stage oropharyngeal cancer: outcomes and prognostic factors. *Laryngoscope.* 2009;119(9):1709–1719.
14. Haus BM, Kambham N, Le D, et al. Surgical robotic applications in otolaryngology. *Laryngoscope.* 2003;113(7):1139–1144.
15. Weinstein GS, O'Malley BW, Hockstein NG. Transoral robotic surgery: supraglottic laryngectomy in a canine model. *Laryngoscope.* 2005;115(7):1315–1319.
16. O'Malley BW, Weinstein GS, Snyder W, Hockstein NG. Transoral robotic surgery (TORS) for base of tongue neoplasms. *Laryngoscope.* 2006;116(8):1465–1472.
17. Albergotti WG, Gooding WE, Kubik MW, et al. Assessment of surgical learning curves in transoral robotic surgery for squamous cell carcinoma of the oropharynx. *JAMA Otolaryngol Head Neck Surg.* 2017;143(6):542–548.
18. Byrd JK, Smith KJ, de Almeida JR, et al. Transoral robotic surgery and the unknown primary: a cost-effectiveness analysis. *Otolaryngol Head Neck Surg.* 2014;150(6):976–982.
19. Möckelmann N, Busch CJ, Münscher A, Knecht R, Lörincz BB. Timing of neck dissection in patients undergoing transoral robotic surgery for head and neck cancer. *Eur J Surg Oncol.* 2015;41(6):773–778.
20. Mandal R, Duvvuri U, Ferris RL, et al. Analysis of post-transoral robotic-assisted surgery hemorrhage: frequency, outcomes, and prevention. *Head Neck.* 2016;38(S1):E776–E782.
21. Stanley RB. Mandibular lingual releasing approach to oral and oropharyngeal carcinomas. *Laryngoscope.* 1984;94(94(5, Pt 1):596–600.
22. Pilcher LS. I. On lateral pharyngotomy for the extirpation of malignant tumors of the tonsillar region. *Ann Surg.* 1886;4(2):139–144.
23. Zeitels SM, Vaughan CW, Ruh S. Suprahyoid pharyngotomy for oropharynx cancer including the tongue base. *Arch Otolaryngol Head Neck Surg.* 1991;117(7):757–760.
24. Christopoulos E, Carrau R, Segas J, et al. Transmandibular approaches to the oral cavity and oropharynx. A functional assessment. *Arch Otolaryngol Head Neck Surg.* 1992;118(11):1164–1167.
25. Carvalho AL, Nishimoto IN, Califano JA, Kowalski LP. Trends in incidence and prognosis for head and neck cancer in the United States: a site-specific analysis of the SEER database. *Int J Cancer.* 2005;114(5):806–816.
26. Chaturvedi AK, Engels EA, Pfeiffer RM, et al. Human papillomavirus and rising oropharyngeal cancer incidence in the United States. *J Clin Oncol.* 2011;29(32):4294–4301.
27. Fakhry C, Westra WH, Li S, et al. Improved survival of patients with human papillomavirus-positive head and neck squamous cell carcinoma in a prospective clinical trial. *J Natl Cancer Inst.* 2008;100(4):261–269.
28. Chaturvedi AK, Anderson WF, Lortet-Tieulent J, et al. Worldwide trends in incidence rates for oral cavity and oropharyngeal cancers. *J Clin Oncol.* 2013;31(36):4550–4559.
29. Deschler DG, Richmon JD, Khariwala SS, et al. The "new" head and neck cancer patient-young, nonsmoker, nondrinker, and HPV positive: evaluation. *Otolaryngol Head Neck Surg.* 2014;151(3):375–380.
30. Slaughter DP, Southwick HW, Smejkal W. Field cancerization in oral stratified squamous epithelium; clinical implications of multicentric origin. *Cancer.* 1953;6(5):963–968.
31. Fakhry C, Zhang Q, Nguyen-Tan PF, et al. Human papillomavirus and overall survival after progression of oropharyngeal squamous cell carcinoma. *J Clin Oncol.* 2014;32(30):3365–3373.
32. Weinstein GS, O'Malley BW, Snyder W, et al. Transoral robotic surgery: radical tonsillectomy. *Arch Otolaryngol Head Neck Surg.* 2007;133(12):1220–1226.
33. Weinstein GS, Quon H, Newman HJ, et al. Transoral robotic surgery alone for oropharyngeal cancer: an analysis of local control. *Arch Otolaryngol Head Neck Surg.* 2012;138(7):628–634.
34. de Almeida JR, Li R, Magnuson JS, et al. Oncologic outcomes after transoral robotic surgery: A multi-institutional study. *JAMA Otolaryngol Head Neck Surg.* 2015;141(12):1043–1051.
35. de Almeida JR, Byrd JK, Wu R, et al. A systematic review of transoral robotic surgery and radiotherapy for early oropharynx cancer: a systematic review. *Laryngoscope.* 2014;124(9):2096–2102.
36. Morisod B, Simon C. Meta-analysis on survival of patients treated with transoral surgery versus radiotherapy for early-stage squamous cell carcinoma of the oropharynx. *Head Neck.* 2016;38(suppl 1):E2143–E2150.
37. Zevallos JP, Mitra N, Swisher-Mcclure S. Patterns of care and perioperative outcomes in transoral endoscopic surgery for oropharyngeal squamous cell carcinoma. *Head Neck.* 2016;38(3):402–409.
38. Eisbruch A, Harris J, Garden AS, et al. Multi-institutional trial of accelerated hypofractionated intensity-modulated radiation therapy for early-stage oropharyngeal cancer (RTOG 00-22). *Int J Radiat Oncol Biol Phys.* 2010;76(5):1333–1338.
39. Hutcheson KA, Holsinger FC, Kupferman ME, Lewin JS. Functional outcomes after TORS for oropharyngeal cancer: a systematic review. *Eur Arch Otorhinolaryngol.* 2015;272(2):463–471.
40. Guo T, Rettig E, Fakhry C. Understanding the impact of survival and human papillomavirus tumor status on timing of recurrence in oropharyngeal squamous cell carcinoma. *Oral Oncol.* 2016;52:97–103.
41. Joseph AW, Guo T, Hur K, et al. Disease-free survival after salvage therapy for recurrent oropharyngeal squamous cell carcinoma. *Head Neck.* 2016;38(suppl 1):E1501–E1509.

42. White H, Ford S, Bush B, et al. Salvage surgery for recurrent cancers of the oropharynx: comparing TORS with standard open surgical approaches. *JAMA Otolaryngol Head Neck Surg*. 2013;139(8):773–778.
43. Motz K, Qualliotine JR, Rettig E, et al. Changes in unknown primary squamous cell carcinoma of the head and neck at initial presentation in the era of human papillomavirus. *JAMA Otolaryngol Head Neck Surg*. 2016;142(3):223–228.
44. Durmus K, Rangarajan SV, Old MO, et al. Transoral robotic approach to carcinoma of unknown primary. *Head Neck*. 2014;36(6):848–852.
45. Fu TS, Foreman A, Goldstein DP, de Almeida JR. The role of transoral robotic surgery, transoral laser microsurgery, and lingual tonsillectomy in the identification of head and neck squamous cell carcinoma of unknown primary origin: a systematic review. *J Otolaryngol Head Neck Surg*. 2016;45(1):28.
46. Davis KS, Byrd JK, Mehta V, et al. Occult primary head and neck squamous cell carcinoma: Utility of discovering primary lesions. *Otolaryngol Head Neck Surg*. 2014;151(2):272–278.
47. Paydarfar JA, Birkmeyer NJ. Complications in head and neck surgery: a meta-analysis of postlaryngectomy pharyngocutaneous fistula. *Arch Otolaryngol Head Neck Surg*. 2006;132(1):67–72.
48. Steiner W. [Surgery of laryngeal cancer]. *MMW Munch Med Wochenschr*. 1982;124(9):198–203.
49. Hinni ML, Salassa JR, Grant DG, et al. Transoral laser microsurgery for advanced laryngeal cancer. *Arch Otolaryngol Head Neck Surg*. 2007;133(12):1198–1204.
50. Olsen SM, Moore EJ, Koch CA, et al. Transoral robotic surgery for supraglottic squamous cell carcinoma. *Am J Otolaryngol*. 2012;33(4):379–384.
51. Ozer E, Alvarez B, Kakarala K, et al. Clinical outcomes of transoral robotic supraglottic laryngectomy. *Head Neck*. 2013;35(8):1158–1161.
52. Lallemant B, Chambon G, Garrel R, et al. Transoral robotic surgery for the treatment of T1-T2 carcinoma of the larynx: preliminary study. *Laryngoscope*. 2013;123(10):2490.
53. Park YM, Kim WS, Byeon HK, et al. Surgical techniques and treatment outcomes of transoral robotic supraglottic partial laryngectomy. *Laryngoscope*. 2013;123(3):670–677.
54. Mendelsohn AH, Remacle M, van der Vorst S, et al. Outcomes following transoral robotic surgery: supraglottic laryngectomy. *Laryngoscope*. 2013;123(1):208–214.
55. Park YM, Byeon HK, Chung HP, et al. Comparison of treatment outcomes after transoral robotic surgery and supraglottic partial laryngectomy: Our experience with seventeen and seventeen patients respectively. *Clinical Otolaryngology*. 2013; 38(3):270–274.
56. Razafindranaly V, Lallemant B, Aubry K, et al. Clinical outcomes with transoral robotic surgery for supraglottic squamous cell carcinoma: Experience of a French evaluation cooperative subgroup of GETTEC. *Head Neck*. 2016;38(Suppl 1):E1097–E1101.
57. Kirchner JA. Growth and spread of laryngeal cancer as related to partial laryngectomy. *Laryngoscope*. 1975;85(9):1516–1521.
58. Smith RV, Schiff BA, Sarta C, et al. Transoral robotic total laryngectomy. *Laryngoscope*. 2013;123(3):678–682.
59. Krishnan G, Krishnan S. Transoral robotic surgery total laryngectomy: evaluation of functional and survival outcomes in a retrospective case series at a single institution. *ORL J Otorhinolaryngol Relat Spec*. 2017;79(4):191–201.
60. Dowthwaite S, Nichols AC, Yoo J, et al. Transoral robotic total laryngectomy: report of 3 cases. *Head Neck*. 2013;35(11):E338–E342.
61. Gy T, Yh H, Gz X, Ye M. Salvage surgery for nasopharyngeal carcinoma. *Arch Otolaryngol Head Neck Surg*. 1988;114(3):328–329.
62. Alonso WA, Black P, Connor GH, Uematsu S. Transoral transpalatal approach for resection of clival chordoma. *Laryngoscope*. 1971;81(10):1626–1631.
63. Fisch U. The infratemporal fossa approach for nasopharyngeal tumors. *The Laryngoscope*. 1983;93(1):36–44.
64. Wei WL, Lam KH, Sham JST. New approach to the nasopharynx: the maxillary swing approach. *Head Neck*. 1991;13(3):200–207.
65. Shah SR, Keshri A, Patadia S, et al. Stage III nasopharyngeal angiofibroma: improving results with endoscopic-assisted midfacial degloving and modification to the Fisch staging system. *J Cranio-Maxillofacial Surgery*. 2015;43(8):1678–1683.
66. Spratt DE, Lee N. Current and emerging treatment options for nasopharyngeal carcinoma. *Onco Targets Ther*. 2012;5:297–308.
67. Tsai S-T, Jin Y-T, Mann RB, Ambinder RF. Epstein-Barr virus detection in nasopharyngeal tissues of patients with suspected nasopharyngeal carcinoma. *Cancer*. 1998;82(8):1449–1453.
68. Chan KCA, Hung ECW, Woo JKS, et al. Early detection of nasopharyngeal carcinoma by plasma Epstein-Barr virus DNA analysis in a surveillance program. *Cancer*. 2013;119(10):1838–1844.
69. Allen Chan KC, Dennis Lo YM. Circulating EBV DNA as a tumor marker for nasopharyngeal carcinoma. *Semin Cancer Biol*. 2002;12(6):489–496.
70. Ym L, Chan LY, Kw L, et al. Quantitative analysis of cell-free Epstein-Barr virus DNA in plasma of patients with nasopharyngeal carcinoma. *Cancer Res*. 1999;59(6):1188–1191.
71. Cheung F, Chan O, Ng WT, et al. The prognostic value of histological typing in nasopharyngeal carcinoma. *Oral Oncol*. 2012;48(5):429–433.
72. O'Malley BW, Weinstein GS. Robotic anterior and midline skull base surgery: preclinical investigations. *Int J Rad Oncol Bio Phy*. 2007;69(2):S125–S128.
73. Ozer E, Waltonen J. Transoral robotic nasopharyngectomy: a novel approach for nasopharyngeal lesions. *Laryngoscope*. 2008;118(9):1613–1616.
74. Tsang RK, Mohr C. Lateral palatal flap approach to the nasopharynx and parapharyngeal space for transoral robotic surgery: a cadaveric study. *J Robot Surg*. 2013;7(2):119–123.

75. Wei WI, Ho W-K. Transoral robotic resection of recurrent nasopharyngeal carcinoma. *Laryngoscope*. 2010;120(10):2011–2014.
76. Tsang RK, To VS, Ho AC, et al. Early results of robotic assisted nasopharyngectomy for recurrent nasopharyngeal carcinoma. *Head Neck*. 2015;37(6): 788–793.
77. Fluur E. Parapharyngeal tumors. *Arch Otol Head Neck Surg*. 1964;80(5):557–565.
78. O'Malley Jr. BW, Quon H, Leonhardt FD, et al. Transoral robotic surgery for parapharyngeal space tumors. *ORL*. 2010;72(6):332–336.
79. Goodwin WJ, Chandler JR. Transoral excision of lateral parapharyngeal space tumors presenting intraorally. *Laryngoscope*. 1988;98(3):266–269.
80. Lee HS, Kim J, Lee HJ, et al. Transoral robotic surgery for neurogenic tumors of the prestyloid parapharyngeal space. *Auris Nasus Larynx*. 2012;39(4):434–437.
81. Park YM, de Virgilio A, Kim WS, et al. Parapharyngeal space surgery via a transoral approach using a robotic surgical system: transoral robotic surgery. *J Lap Advan Surg Tech*. 2013;23(3):231–236.
82. Boyce BJ, Curry JM, Luginbuhl A, Cognetti DM. Transoral robotic approach to parapharyngeal space tumors: case series and technical limitations. *Laryngoscope*. 2016;126(8):1776–1782.
83. Choby GW, Kim J, Ling DC, et al. Transoral robotic surgery alone for oropharyngeal cancer: quality-of-life outcomes. *JAMA Otolaryngol Head Neck Surg*. 2015;141(6):499–504.
84. Bernier J, Cooper JS, Pajak TF, et al. Defining risk levels in locally advanced head and neck cancers: a comparative analysis of concurrent postoperative radiation plus chemotherapy trials of the EORTC (#22931) and RTOG (# 9501). *Head Neck*. 2005;27(10):843–850.
85. Maxwell JH, Ferris RL, Gooding W, et al. Extracapsular spread in head and neck carcinoma: impact of site and human papillomavirus status. *Cancer*. 2013;119(18):3302–3308.
86. Cracchiolo JR, Baxi SS, Morris LG, et al. Increase in primary surgical treatment of T1 and T2 oropharyngeal squamous cell carcinoma and rates of adverse pathologic features: National Cancer Data Base. *Cancer*. 2016;122(10):1523–1532.
87. Sinha P, Lewis JS, Piccirillo JF, et al. Extracapsular spread and adjuvant therapy in human papillomavirus-related, p16-positive oropharyngeal carcinoma. *Cancer*. 2012;118(14):3519–3530.
88. Kass JI, Giraldez L, Gooding W, et al. Oncologic outcomes of surgically treated early-stage oropharyngeal squamous cell carcinoma. *Head Neck*. 2016;38(10): 1467–1471.
89. Amini A, Jasem J, Jones BL, et al. Predictors of overall survival in human papillomavirus-associated oropharyngeal cancer using the National Cancer Data Base. *Oral Oncol*. 2016;56:1–7.
90. Ansarin M, Zorzi S, Massaro MA, et al. Transoral robotic surgery vs transoral laser microsurgery for resection of supraglottic cancer: a pilot surgery. *Int J Robotics Comput Assis Surg*. 2014;10(1):107–112.
91. Kirchner JA. A historical and histological view of partial laryngectomy. *Bull NY Acad Med*. 1986;62(8):808–817.
92. Kirchner JA. Pathways and pitfalls in partial laryngectomy. *Annals of Otology, Rhinology & Laryngology*. 1984;93(4):301–305.
93. Yin Tsang RK, Ho WK, Wei WI. Combined transnasal endoscopic and transoral robotic resection of recurrent nasopharyngeal carcinoma. *Head Neck*. 2012;34(8):1190–1193.
94. Chan JYK, Tsang RK, Eisele DW, Richmon JD. Transoral robotic surgery of the parapharyngeal space: a case series and systematic review. *Head Neck*. 2015;37(2):293–298.
95. Hughes KV. 3rd, Olsen KD, McCaffrey TV. Parapharyngeal space neoplasms. *Head Neck*. 1995;17(2):124–130.
96. Ferris RL, Blumenschein G, Fayette J, et al. Nivolumab for recurrent squamous-cell carcinoma of the head and neck. *N Engl J Med Overseas Ed*. 2016;375(19):1856–1867.
97. Rosenthal DI, Harari PM, Giralt J, et al. Association of human papillomavirus and p16 status with outcomes in the IMCL-9815 phase iii registration trial for patients with locoregionally advanced oropharyngeal squamous cell carcinoma of the head and neck treated with radiotherapy with or without cetuximab. *J Clin Oncol*. 2016;34(12):1300–1308.
98. O'Sullivan B, Huang SH, Perez-Ordonez B, et al. Outcomes of HPV-related oropharyngeal cancer patients treated by radiotherapy alone using altered fractionation. *Radiotherapy Oncology*. 2012;103(1):49–56.
99. Nichols AC, Yoo J, Hammond JA, et al. Early-stage squamous cell carcinoma of the oropharynx: Radiotherapy vs. Trans-Oral Robotic Surgery (ORATOR)—study protocol for a randomized phase II trial. *BMC Cancer*. 2013;13(1):133.
100. Maxwell JH, Rath TJ, Byrd JK, et al. Accuracy of computed tomography to predict extracapsular spread in p16-positive squamous cell carcinoma. *Laryngoscope*. 2015;125(7):1613–1618.
101. Weinstein GS, O'Malley BW, Magnuson JS, et al. Transoral robotic surgery: a multicenter study to assess feasibility, safety, and surgical margins. *Laryngoscope*. 2012;122(8):1701–1707.
102. Mandal R, Duvvuri U, Ferris RL, et al. Analysis of post-transoral robotic-assisted surgery hemorrhage: frequency, outcomes, and prevention. *Head Neck*. 2016;38(suppl 1):776–782.
103. de Almeida JR, Park RC, Genden EM. Reconstruction of transoral robotic surgery defects: principles and techniques. *J Reconstr Microsurg*. 2012;28(7):465–472.

9

Induction Chemotherapy: Current and Emerging Role in HNSCC

Glenn J. Hanna

Robert I. Haddad

The treatment of locoregionally advanced head and neck squamous cell carcinoma (HNSCC) generally encompasses a multimodality approach, as single modality strategies fail to provide optimal disease control. One strategy that has fueled significant investigation has been an induction chemotherapy (IC) approach prior to either definitive radiation or surgery or prior to additional concurrent chemoradiotherapy (CRT); the latter is referred to as sequential therapy (ST) throughout this chapter. The rationale for applying an IC approach relates to an interest in maximizing tumor shrinkage and providing an early assessment of chemotherapy responsiveness, reducing the risk of distant metastatic spread, and capitalizing on principles of organ preservation in laryngeal and hypopharyngeal tumors (1). This chapter aims to review the historical approach to early induction strategies, which stemmed from attempts to improve laryngeal organ preservation, define the optimal IC regimen, present the available literature utilizing ST versus concurrent CRT approaches to treat locoregionally advanced HNSCC, and review alternative regimens and novel approaches incorporating IC.

In 2000, Pignon and colleagues published a meta-analysis of 63 trials including more than 10,000 patients with locoregionally advanced HNSCC demonstrating a trend toward improved overall survival (OS; absolute benefit of 4% at 5 years) in favor of incorporating chemotherapy into definitive treatment (2). These results were later updated in 2009 with the addition of 24 new trials (totaling over 16,000 patients) showing a continued absolute survival benefit of chemotherapy of 4.5% at 5 years (hazard ratio [HR]: 0.88, 95% confidence interval [CI]: 0.85–0.92, $p < .0001$), favoring a concurrent CRT approach (3). While the risk of death was lower in the concurrent CRT subgroup, the effect on the rate of distant metastatic spread was notable in the IC subgroup (HR: 0.73, 95% CI: 0.61–0.88, $p = .001$). The fact remains that chemotherapy is an important part of managing locoregionally advanced HNSCC, but defining the role of IC as part of multimodality therapy requires careful review of a complex literature.

Following the introduction of cisplatin in the 1970s, a series of single institution studies in newly diagnosed, advanced HNSCC patients emerged, which combined platinum with other agents in an IC approach prior to surgery or radiation, showing an important signal in tumor response rates (4–6). Later in the 1970s and early 1980s, a series of pilot studies were conducted at Wayne State University in Detroit, Michigan, which were designed to evaluate the use of multimodality therapy with various IC regimens to treat inoperable, locoregionally advanced HNSCC (7). A superior complete response (CR) rate of 54% (overall response rate [ORR] was 93%) was noted in the group receiving 120-hour infusional 5-fluorouracil (5-FU; 1,000 mg/m² on days 1–5) combined with cisplatin (100 mg/m² on day 1) chemotherapy, which translated into a significant OS benefit. These early studies proved the feasibility of a multimodality approach incorporating IC and highlighted the importance of clarifying the correct chemotherapy combination and number of cycles to optimize outcomes. Despite the benefits observed with the so-called Wayne State regimen of platinum and infusional 5-FU, a Southwest Oncology Group (SWOG) multicenter trial randomized patients with locoregionally advanced, operable HNSCC to a combination IC regimen (including cisplatin, methotrexate, bleomycin, and vincristine) followed by surgery and adjuvant radiation versus surgery followed by postoperative radiation alone (8). While the ORR to chemotherapy was 70% in the IC arm, median survival was longer in the group that had not received IC (30 vs. 18 months, *p* value not significant [NS]). Perioperative complications were similar in both arms. A similar multicenter National Cancer Institute (NCI) sponsored trial was conducted in operable, stage III and IV patients with locoregionally advanced HNSCC comparing IC with cisplatin plus bleomycin followed by surgery and radiation versus the same therapy followed by six cycles of maintenance cisplatin in the adjuvant setting versus standard surgery and radiation alone (9). Toxicity from chemotherapy was felt to be tolerable and IC resulted in an ORR of 37%. Disease-free survival (DFS) and OS were similar among all three groups but rates of distant failure were decreased in the maintenance cisplatin arm and time to first distant relapse was prolonged. Similarly, an Italian group began a multicenter, phase III study in 1986 of patients with stage III and IV HNSCC at all sites randomizing them to IC (cisplatin and infusional 5-FU) followed by radiation versus conventional laryngectomy and radiation (10). Results again demonstrated similar findings to the studies mentioned earlier: comparable survival rates and a decrease in distant failures favoring the IC arm. Interestingly, unresectable patients in the IC arm had improved DFS (49% vs. 28%, $p = .06$) and OS (30% vs. 19%, $p = .04$) in this study. At around the same time in 1986, the French were beginning to investigate the efficacy of neoadjuvant chemotherapy in patients with oropharyngeal HNSCC, randomized to either three cycles of IC followed by surgery and radiation versus surgery, radiation or a sequential approach (11). Chemotherapy consisted of cisplatin and infusional 5-FU using the preferred Wayne State regimen dosing. They reported a difference in OS favoring the IC arm when adjusted on initial therapy (radiation alone or surgery plus radiation), with a median OS of 5.1 years in the IC arm versus 3.3 years in the conventional arm ($p = .03$). While this trial was closed early due to other investigator interests, the benefit from IC they observed was similar to that demonstrated in the MACH-NC meta-analysis later published in 2000 (2).

These earlier trials confirmed the responsiveness of HNSCC to multiagent IC, but failed to show a survival benefit in operable patients. Some could argue that the optimal IC regimen was not utilized in all of these studies given outcomes with the Wayne State regimen. In addition, the first suggestions of improvement in distant failure rates were beginning to emerge with the use of IC. Whether the advantages of IC could offset the potential harm in delaying definitive surgery or radiation in this patient population was an important question, but toxicity from chemotherapy appeared manageable and failed to significantly impact surgical or radiation planning in these early trials.

INDUCTION CHEMOTHERAPY IN THE SETTING OF LARYNX AND HYPOPHARYNX PRESERVATION

An important rationale for the utilization of IC was the potential advantage of organ preservation in locoregionally advanced larynx and hypopharynx tumors, thus avoiding radical surgery. Following the historical results mentioned earlier, two initial larynx preservation trials were initiated: one in laryngeal cancer and the other in hypopharyngeal cancer. In 1991, the landmark Department of Veterans Affairs (VA) Laryngeal Cancer Study Group reported the results of a randomized, phase III trial in 332 patients with untreated stage III and IV laryngeal HNSCC comparing IC followed by radiation with conventional laryngectomy followed by postoperative radiation (12). Patients in the IC arm received two cycles of IC comprising cisplatin (100 mg/m² on day 1) and 5-FU (1,000 mg/m² per day on days 1–5). Patients with a response received a third cycle of IC followed by definitive radiation (66 to 76 Gy). Salvage laryngectomy was offered to those who failed to respond. A tumor CR rate of 31% was noted in the IC arm, and 54% had a partial response (PR). While the estimated 2-year OS was the same for both treatments (68%, p = .984), fewer distant failures were noted in the IC arm (p = .016). Perhaps most important, the larynx preservation rate (LPR) was 64% overall in the IC arm. These data suggested a new role for IC in locoregionally advanced laryngeal cancer, showing organ preservation was feasible without compromising survival.

The European Organization for Research and Treatment of Cancer (EORTC) published the results of a large, randomized phase III study a few years later comparing a larynx preservation approach using IC followed by definitive surgery or radiation to conventional surgery followed by postoperative radiation—but in a hypopharyngeal or piriform sinus cancer population (13). IC consisted of the same dosing of cisplatin and infusional 5-FU as in the VA larynx study and after two cycles, responders received a third cycle followed by 70 Gy of radiation (it should be noted that a CR at the primary site was required to proceed with nonsurgical management). Nonresponders underwent salvage laryngectomy and postoperative radiation. A CR rate of 43% was observed (54% had a clinical CR at the primary tumor site, 51% had a clinical CR in the neck) and the 3-year OS rate was 57% in the IC arm versus 43% in the conventional arm (HR: 0.86, 95% CI: 0.50–1.86, p = NS). Rates of distant failure in the IC arm were lower (25% vs. 36%, p = .041) and larynx preservation once again proved feasible without jeopardizing survival. This established IC followed by definitive therapy as a new reference arm in further cooperative group trials and fueled interest in comparing IC regimens with concurrent CRT approaches. Additionally, the 10-year results of this EORTC trial comparing larynx preservation with IC to conventional surgery and postoperative radiation were reported in 2012 (14). At a median follow-up of 10.5 years on the 194 eligible patients, 10-year OS was 13.1% in the IC arm compared with 13.8% in the conventional arm (p = NS)—suggesting similar OS, albeit poor, between arms and affording more than half of survivors larynx preservation. These two trials together further clarified that IC with a platinum-based doublet among favorable responders appeared to yield LPRs in the 40% to 60% range with comparable survival. However, information about larynx function and the use of single modality radiation was not available from these studies. This led to two additional larynx preservation trials aimed at further answering these questions.

In order to understand the contributions of chemotherapy and radiation to an organ preservation strategy in laryngeal cancer, the Radiation Therapy Oncology Group (RTOG) and the Head and Neck Intergroup initiated a large, randomized trial (RTOG 91-11) in patients with locoregionally advanced larynx cancer, which included cisplatin and 5-FU based IC followed by radiation for responders versus concurrent CRT with three cycles of bolus cisplatin (100 mg/m^2 on day 1) versus radiation alone with a primary end point of larynx preservation (15). At 2 years, the LPR was higher in the concurrent CRT arm (88%) compared with both the IC (75%, p = .005) and radiation alone arms (70%, p < .001). The rate of locoregional control (LRC) was also significantly improved in the concurrent CRT arm (78% vs. 61%, p = .004 and 56%, p < .001, respectively). Consistent with prior observations, both of the chemotherapy-containing arms decreased the rate of distant disease. However, OS was similar between all treatment groups. The toxicity profile of the chemotherapy arms was notable (81%–82%) compared with radiation alone. These findings taken together illustrate that concurrent CRT with cisplatin demonstrated improved LRC and LPRs compared with IC, despite no difference in survival. The long-term results of this study were published in 2013 (median follow-up of 10.8 years) and continued to show a significantly improved LPR favoring the concurrent CRT arm over the IC arm (HR: 0.58, 95% CI: 0.37–0.89, p = .005) (16,17). OS did not differ significantly between treatment groups in long-term follow-up; however, when OS was compared between the concurrent CRT and IC arms, there was some suggestion of long-term harm (more deaths unrelated to larynx cancer) associated with concurrent CRT (HR: 1.25, 95% CI: 0.98–1.161, p = .08). There was also evidence of a late emerging, nonstatistically significant but perhaps clinically meaningful, survival benefit in the IC arm whereby at 4.5 years the survival curves began to separate. Again, concurrent CRT and IC continued to show similar benefit in achieving distant control compared with radiation alone. In evaluating the composite end point of laryngectomy-free survival (LFS) there appeared to be no difference between the concurrent CRT and IC arms (23.5% vs. 28.9%; HR: 1.05,

95% CI: 0.83–1.34, p = .68), but LFS was significantly worse in the radiation-only arm. These long-term results continue to support the conclusion that while survival rates with an intact larynx appear similar in both concurrent CRT and IC subgroups, mere organ preservation and LRC outcomes appear to favor concomitant CRT. No differences in late toxicity with regard to speech or swallowing function were noted. These findings led to an update in national guidelines where both IC and concurrent CRT are considered appropriate as an initial approach for these patients.

Around the same time as RTOG 91-11, the EORTC 24954 trial was initiated as a randomized, phase III trial to investigate IC with platinum and 5-FU followed by radiation (control arm) versus an alternating IC and radiotherapy regimen in resectable, locoregionally advanced laryngeal and hypopharyngeal cancer (18). In the standard IC arm, two cycles of IC with cisplatin and infusional 5-FU at standard dosing were given and those with a 50% reduction in primary tumor size received an additional two cycles (total of four cycles) followed by 70 Gy of radiation. In the alternating arm, a total of four cycles of cisplatin and 5-FU (200 mg/m^2 per day instead of 1,000 mg/m^2 per day) were given alternating with 20 Gy of radiation during three 2-week intervals between chemotherapy dosing. Nonresponders underwent salvage surgery and postoperative radiation. At a median follow-up of 6.5 years, LFS was similar in both arms (HR: 0.85, 95% CI: 0.68–1.06, p = NS) as was median OS (4.4 years in the sequential arm vs. 5.1 years in the alternating arm). Grade 3 and 4 mucositis events were more frequent in the ST arm (32%).

As demonstrated by the trials summarized in Table 9.1, larynx preservation was an important milestone achieved with the introduction of IC in head and neck oncology. These trials clarified that a significant proportion of patients could be spared total laryngectomy without compromising survival and cure. From the MACH-NC meta-analysis we subsequently

TABLE 9.1

Organ Preservation Trials Incorporating an Induction Chemotherapy Approach in HNSCC

Trial	Enrollment	Regimens	LPR	OS	DFR
VA Larynx study (1991) (12)	n = 332 stage III, IV larynx	PF → RT, NR → TL + RT vs. TL → RT	64%	68% 68% (2 y)	11% 17%
EORTC (1996) (13)	n = 194 stage III, IV hypopharynx	PF → RT, NR → TL + RT vs. TL → RT	66%	57% 43% (3 y)	25% 36%
RTOG 91-11 (2003) (15)	n = 547 stage III, IV larynx	PF → RT, NR → TL + RT vs. CRT (P) vs. RT	75% 88% 70%	76% (2 y) 74% 75%	9% 8% 16%
EORTC 24954 (2009) (18)	n = 450 stage III, IV larynx, hypopharynx	PF → RT, NR → TL vs. PF + RT alternating	71% 77%	62.2% (3 y) 64.8%	15% 21%

CRT, concurrent chemoradiation; DFR, distant failure rate; LPR, larynx preservation rate; NR, nonresponders; OS, overall survival; P, cisplatin; PF, cisplatin + 5-fluorouracil; RT, radiation therapy; HNSCC, head and neck squamous cell carcinoma; TL, total laryngectomy.

established concomitant CRT with cisplatin as the standard of care for locoregionally advanced HNSCC—based on improvements in both LPR and LRC. We are reminded, however, of the late toxicity observed with concurrent CRT as presented in the long-term results of RTOG 91-11 and must continue to follow the late trend toward improved survival noted in the IC arm. It is also important to recognize the limitations of LPR as compared with LFS, OS, and other composite end points that capture survival in patients with a functional larynx. Another important limitation of some of the aforementioned early studies was the limited recruitment of resectable patients with advanced cervical nodal disease (N2 and N3). A new surge in interest to optimize IC for organ preservation was triggered by the addition of taxanes to IC regimens.

THE OPTIMAL INDUCTION CHEMOTHERAPY REGIMEN

As early as the late 1990s, taxane chemotherapy was shown to have activity in recurrent, metastatic HNSCC. Forastiere and colleagues reported a phase II study in which 30 patients with advanced, incurable HNSCC were treated with an infusional schedule of 250 mg/m^2 of paclitaxel at 3-week intervals until disease progression (19). Although an alternative infusion schedule was eventually proposed based on significant hematologic toxicity observed in the trial, the ORR was 40% (4 CRs and 8 PRs) with a median duration of response of 4.5 months. Docetaxel (T) was also shown to be an effective agent (ORRs 21%–42%) in incurable, advanced HNSCC but with febrile neutropenia observed as a dose-limiting toxicity (20,21). These initial observations with taxanes in head and neck cancer led to several trials combining these agents with a cisplatin plus 5-FU (PF) backbone in order to improve clinical and pathologic response rates to IC. Additionally, the nonoverlapping mechanism of action and acceptable toxicity profile of a PF-based combination facilitated experimental combinations with taxanes (particularly docetaxel).

Colevas and colleagues performed four consecutive, early trials in the mid-1990s at the Dana-Farber Cancer Institute assessing combinations of TPF in patients with potentially curable, locoregionally advanced HNSCC (22–25). The two initial phase I/II studies (TPFL-5 and TPFL-4) combined docetaxel with lower doses of an infusional PF regimen and leucovorin (L) followed by hyperfractionated (twice daily) radiation. The third phase I/II study in the series modified the TPFL regimen to fit an outpatient schedule, while the fourth study was a phase II trial of docetaxel (75 mg/m^2 day 1), cisplatin (75–100 mg/m^2 day 1), and infusional 5-FU (1,000 mg/m^2 days 1–4) without leucovorin. A total of 101 patients enrolled on the four studies and the results were reported collectively (26). ORRs to IC with TPF were greater than 90% in all four trials. At a median follow-up of 49 months, OS without evidence of disease was 64% among treated patients and the TPF combination therapies were generally well tolerated, despite two treatment-related deaths (one from sepsis and the other from delayed radionecrosis complicating laryngectomy). Despite these findings, locoregional recurrence (LRR) rates continued to be a major concern that affected 31 patients (30%) in these studies. Again distant failure rates remained low. Another initial phase II trial evaluated TPF as an IC regimen with granulocyte colony-stimulating factor (GCSF) support followed by radiation in untreated patients with locoregionally advanced HNSCC (27). Treatment consisted of docetaxel (80 mg/m^2 day 1), cisplatin (40 mg/m^2 days 2 and 3), and infusional 5-FU (1,000 mg/m^2 days 1–3) every 28 days for a maximum of four cycles. Radiation to the primary and involved neck sites occurred following IC. ORR after induction TPF was 90% and after radiation the ORR was 95% (CR rate of 73%). With a median follow-up of 36 months, median OS had not been reached, but 60% of treated patients were alive at 2 years. The median number of tolerated IC cycles was three and febrile neutropenia developed in two patients. Haddad and colleagues later reported the rate of pathologic CR with TPF IC at a single institution, with 89% of evaluable biopsies showing no residual cancer; 4% of patients with negative biopsy results succumbed to their head and neck cancer at 2 years compared with 25% of those with biopsy-positive disease post-TPF (28). These pathologic CR rates compared favorably with those reported using PF-based IC regimens. Finally, Schrijvers and colleagues reported their experience with two dosing schedules of TPF followed by radiation in unresectable patients with locoregionally advanced HNSCC (29). They used docetaxel (75 mg/m^2 day 1), cisplatin (70 mg/m^2 day 1), and infusional 5-FU (700 mg/m^2 days 1–5) every 21 days (level I) in one group and the same regimen with cisplatin at 100 mg/m^2 on day 1 (level II) in the other dose group. ORR was 78.3% in the level II group (95% CI: 56.3–92.5%) and all were PRs (with patients tolerating between two and four cycles of IC). Following these preliminary studies, a number of phase III trials in the United States and Europe sought to further clarify if adding taxanes to a PF-based regimen was the optimal IC combination. The aforementioned findings had also sparked an interest in investigating IC regimens followed by concurrent CRT (ST) given the increase in LRC offered by concurrent CRT strategies observed in prior studies and the desire to capitalize on improved distant failure rates by incorporating IC up front.

In the Spanish trial reported by Hitt and colleagues in 2005, a total of 382 patients were randomly assigned to three cycles of cisplatin (100 mg/m^2 day 1) and infusional 5-FU (1,000 mg/m^2 days 1–5) or a PF regimen (infusional 5-FU dosing was 500 mg/m^2 on days 2–6) plus paclitaxel (175 mg/m^2 day 1) every 21 days (30). Patients with any response (CR or PR) greater than 80% at the primary site went on to concurrent CRT (with bolus cisplatin 100 mg/m^2 on days 1, 22, and 43 of radiation to 70 Gy). The CR rate in the triple agent IC arm was 33% and there was a trend toward improved OS (43.0 vs. 37.0 months, p = .06) in the paclitaxel-containing IC arm. The difference in OS was more notable for those in the study with unresectable disease (36.0 vs. 26.0 months, p = .04). The triple agent IC regimen was better tolerated than PF with more mucositis in the latter arm. Another large, randomized phase III study performed by the EORTC/TAX 323 Study Group evaluated TPF versus PF as IC followed by radiation in stage III and IV patients with unresectable, locoregionally advanced HNSCC (31). Patients received three cycles of docetaxel (75 mg/m^2 day 1), cisplatin (75 mg/m^2 day 1), and infusional 5-FU (750 mg/m^2 days 1–5) versus a PF regimen consisting of cisplatin (100 mg/m^2 day 1) every 21 days. A total of 358 patients (80% with T3-4 disease, 71% with N2-3 nodal disease) were randomized and median progression-free survival (PFS) was 11.0 versus 8.2 months (p = .007) favoring the TPF arm. TPF resulted in a reduction in the risk of death of 27% (p = .02) and median OS was improved with TPF (18.8 vs. 14.5 months, p = .02). As expected, more grade 3 and 4 cytopenias were observed in the TPF arm but with only 2.3% of patients in this arm experiencing death from therapeutic toxicity. Rates of distant relapse were also significantly more frequent in the PF arm compared with TPF (22.9% vs. 13.5%). Published at the same time and in the same journal were the results of a large, multicenter phase III study performed in the United States by the TAX 324 Study Group (32). They randomized 501 patients with stage III and IV locoregionally advanced HNSCC (greater than 70% had T3-4 disease, greater than 60% had N2-3 nodal disease) to receive three cycles of TPF, docetaxel (75 mg/m^2 day 1), cisplatin (100 mg/m^2 day 1), and infusional 5-FU (1,000 mg/m^2 days 1–4) every 21 days versus PF (infusional 5-FU at 1,000 mg/m^2 days 1–5) at the same intervals both followed by concurrent CRT (weekly carboplatin infusion at an area under the curve [AUC] of 1.5 given for a maximum of seven weekly doses during radiation to 70–74 Gy). Median OS was improved with TPF compared with PF (71.0 vs. 30.0 months, p = .006), and the TPF arm demonstrated improved LRC (p = .04) without a difference in distant failure rates. Rates of febrile neutropenia were again higher in the TPF arm. Despite the improvement in LRC with TPF induction, locoregional failure remained the most important cause of treatment failure in TAX 324. Long-term results published from this study were reported in 2011 (33). At a median follow-up of 72.2 months, median OS remained significantly improved in those treated with TPF (70.6 vs. 34.8 months, p = .014). Estimated 5-year survival in the TPF arm was 52% versus 42% in the PF arm. No differences in long-term gastric feeding tube dependence or tracheostomies were observed between groups. Prophylactic antibiotic use was required in both TAX 323 and 324, but the use of GCSF support was optional and may have accounted for variations in infectious complications between the two studies. It became clear from these studies that the administration of TPF required aggressive supportive measures in the form of nursing, hydration, and oral care to optimize tolerability.

A follow-up study of the TAX 323 cohort evaluated the short-term health-related quality of life (HRQOL) and symptom control parameters in those treated with IC (34). HRQOL was assessed at baseline and at four additional time points including 9 months after radiation treatment. At the end of radiation therapy, global HRQOL was higher in the TPF arm with an added decrease in reported swallowing and coughing problems. While compliance with the HRQOL assessments diminished with time (compliance had dropped to 54% by 6 months), the authors concluded that TPF not only improved survival but it reduced patient-reported toxicity. Additionally, a cost–utility analysis was retrospectively performed from the TAX 323 and TAX 324 data that showed that TPF improved life expectancy by 0.33 and 0.41 quality-adjusted life-years (QALYs), respectively, when compared with PF and therefore was cost-effective (35). The conclusion drawn from both TAX 323 and 324 was that TPF improved survival compared with PF and the toxicity profile was manageable, thus establishing TPF as the preferred IC regimen when utilized in practice and for future investigations. In 2013, a meta-analysis including five randomized trials encompassing 1,772 patients treated with taxane–PF or PF IC regimens drew the same conclusion, showing improved survival with a taxane–PF combination (HR: 0.79, 95% CI: 0.70–0.89, $p < .001$) (36).

It was also around this time in the 2000s that a change in the demographics of patients with locoregionally advanced HNSCC was being reported with the recognition of human papillomavirus (HPV) infection. Several retrospective analyses were presented that demonstrated the significant impact of HPV on survival, regardless of therapeutic approach (37,38). This topic is covered extensively elsewhere and is not the focus of this discussion. However, Posner and colleagues retrospectively examined the impact of HPV-associated oropharyngeal carcinoma (OPC) and survival from the TAX 324 cohort (39). Of 264 patients with OPC, 42% had evaluable biopsies and half were HPV positive. HPV-positive patients were significantly younger, they had lower primary tumor staging, and indeed PFS and OS were more favorable in this subgroup (HR: 0.20, $p < .0001$). It soon became appreciated that HPV-associated OPC represented a distinct biologic entity in head and neck cancer. Specific trials aimed at tailoring treatment to those with more favorable HPV head and neck cancers would subsequently ensue.

With TPF accepted as the preferred IC regimen, a number of subsequent trials evaluated the use of TPF compared with the standard PF regimen utilized in early organ preservation trials for larynx and hypopharynx cancers. In the GORTEC 2000–01 study, Pointreau and colleagues randomized patients with resectable, locoregionally advanced HNSCC of the larynx and hypopharynx to three cycles of TPF or PF (40). Patients with a CR or PR to IC received radiotherapy with or without additional chemotherapy. Nonresponders went on to total laryngectomy followed by postoperative radiation. With a median follow-up of 36 months, 80% of patients in the TPF arm demonstrated a response after IC and the LPR rate was 70.3% with TPF versus 57.5% with PF ($p = .03$). Cytopenias were more frequently observed in the TPF arm, as expected. The TREMPLIN trial was a phase II study of previously untreated patients with stage III and IV larynx and hypopharynx HNSCC who received IC with TPF (docetaxel at 75 mg/m^2 day 1, cisplatin at 75 mg/m^2 day 1, and infusional 5-FU at 750 mg/m^2 days 1–5) (41). Poor responders went to salvage surgery whereas those with greater than or equal to 50% tumor response were then randomly assigned to one of two arms: concurrent CRT (with cisplatin 100 mg/m^2 on days 1, 22, and 43; radiation to 70 Gy) or concurrent cetuximab and radiation (400 mg/m^2 loading dose and 250 mg/m^2 weekly thereafter during radiation). Of 153 patients, 74% completed three cycles of TPF at the planned dosing. Toxicity was notable with four patients experiencing death during IC and 23.5% experiencing grade 3 or 4 toxicity (most commonly febrile neutropenia and nephrotoxicity). In line with prior studies, 85% of those receiving TPF had an adequate response to IC allowing for randomization to concurrent therapy. Toxicity in both the cisplatin- and cetuximab-containing arms was notable (57% of the cisplatin arm required protocol modification for toxicity), but treatment compliance was higher for the cetuximab arm. There was no difference in LPR at 3 months (95% vs. 93%, p = NS), larynx function preservation (87% vs. 82%), and OS at 18 months (92% vs. 89%) between arms—but only responders to TPF were included in the analysis. From this trial it became evident that bolus cisplatin following TPF induction yielded significant toxicity. Additionally, although outcomes for patients who were randomly assigned following TPF were favorable in this study, there was no advantage over the prior strategy of TPF followed by radiation—which remains the reference regimen in Europe. The long-term results of GORTEC 2000–01 were reported in 2015 with 213 patients treated and a median follow-up of 105 months; the 5-year and 10-year LPR rates were improved with TPF compared to PF (74.0% vs. 58.1% and 70.3% vs. 46.5%, respectively) (42). Ten-year larynx dysfunction-free survival, an end point designed to capture survival with an intact and functioning organ, was 63.7% favoring the TPF arm (p = .001). Fewer grade 3 and 4 toxicities of the larynx were observed in the TPF arm (9.3 vs. 17.1%, p = .038). The authors concluded that long-term follow-up confirmed the benefit of TPF as IC in improving LPRs and larynx dysfunction-free survival. These later laryngeal and hypopharyngeal trials support the role of TPF as the preferred regimen when an attempted organ preservation approach is utilized, recognizing that the risk of toxicity is not insignificant. Despite improved LPR rates with TPF noted earlier, OS may have been influenced by the option of surgical salvage unique to organ preservation trials. All together, these trials (Table 9.2) led to regulatory approval of TPF when used as IC in head and neck cancer.

SEQUENTIAL VERSUS CONCURRENT CHEMORADIOTHERAPY IN LOCOREGIONALLY ADVANCED HNSCC

While concurrent CRT remained the standard of care for the treatment of locoregionally advanced HNSCC, the optimal IC regimen appeared to be TPF and thus the next phase of large-scale trials focused on IC followed by concurrent CRT (ST) to optimize both LRC and establish early distant disease control. In a phase II trial, Paccagnella and colleagues (in the Gruppo di Studio Tumori della Testa e del Collo XRP 6976 F/2501 Study) randomly assigned patients with stage III and IV head and neck cancers to receive concurrent CRT alone (two cycles of cisplatin at 20 mg/m^2 on days 1–4, infusional 5-FU at 800 mg/m^2 on day 1 for 96 hours, both during weeks 1 and 6 of radiation) or TPF (three cycles of docetaxel at

TABLE 9.2

Key Induction Chemotherapy Trials Incorporating Taxanes in HNSCC

Trial	Enrollment	Regimens	cCR	LPR	OS*	DFR
Spanish trial (2005) (30)	n = 382 stage III, IV disease	PF → CRT vs. TPF → CRT (P)	14% 33%	–	37.0 43.0	14%[†]
TAX 323 (2007) (31)	n = 358 stage III, IV unresectable disease	PF → RT vs. TPF → RT	20% 33%	–	14.5 18.8	10% 13%
TAX 324 (2007) (32)	n = 501 stage III, IV disease	PF → CRT vs. TPF → CRT (C)	15% 17%	–	30.0 71.0	9% 5%
GORTEC 2000–01 (2009) (40)	n = 113 stage III, IV larynx, hypopharynx	PF → RT ± CT vs. TPF → RT ± CT, NR → TL + RT	30% 42%	58% 70%	60% 60% (3 y)	16% 11%
TREMPLIN (2013) (41)	n = 116 stage III, IV larynx, hypopharynx	TPF → CRT (P) vs. TPF → CTX-RT, NR → TL + RT	68% 64%	95% 93%	75% 73% (3 y)	8% 5%

*Median reported in months unless otherwise stated; [†]total distant failure rate for the overall trial reported.

C, carboplatin; cCR, clinical complete response; CRT, concurrent chemoradiation; CT, chemotherapy; CTX, cetuximab; DFR, distant failure rate; HNSCC, head and neck squamous cell carcinoma; LPR, larynx preservation rate; NR, nonresponders; OS, overall survival; P, cisplatin; PF, cisplatin + 5-fluorouracil; RT, radiation therapy; TL, total laryngectomy; TPF, taxane + cisplatin + 5-fluorouracil.

75 mg/m^2 day 1, cisplatin at 80 mg/m^2 day 1, and infusional 5-FU at 800 mg/m^2 on day 1 for 96 hours every 21 days) followed by the same concurrent CRT regimen in the control arm (43). Of 101 patients enrolled, the radiologic CR rate more than doubled in the TPF arm compared with the concurrent CRT alone arm (50.0% vs. 21.3%) following the completion of all therapy. Median OS was improved in the TPF-containing arm (39.6 vs. 33.3 months, respectively)—with 86% of patients alive at 2 years in the TPF treatment arm. Eight percent of patients in the TPF arm experienced febrile neutropenia, but no treatment-related deaths were reported. What followed these observations were series of large phase III trials attempting to clarify the role of ST as compared to concurrent CRT.

In 2013, the results of one of two large, randomized phase III studies performed in the United States investigating TPF-based ST versus concurrent CRT were reported (44). PARADIGM enrolled previously untreated patients with stage III and IV locoregionally advanced HNSCC who were unresectable or had a low likelihood of surgical curability (T3 and 4, N2 or 3, except T1N2), or were candidates for organ preservation. The ST arm consisted of TPF (three cycles of docetaxel at 75 mg/m^2 day 1, cisplatin at 100 mg/m^2 day 1, and infusional 5-FU at 1,000 mg/m^2 on days 1–4 every 21 days; GCSF prophylaxis was permitted) followed by concurrent CRT (weekly docetaxel 20 mg/m^2 for 4 weeks for poor responders or weekly carboplatin AUC 1.5 for 7 weeks in favorable responders during radiation) versus concurrent CRT alone (two doses of weekly cisplatin at 100 mg/m^2 on days 1 and 22 of radiation). Three-year PFS (67.0% vs. 69.0%) and OS (73.0% vs. 78.0%) between the two treatment arms were similar (HR: 1.07, 95% CI: 0.59–1.92, p = .82; HR: 1.09, 95% CI: 0.59–2.03, p = .77, respectively), while there was a nonsignificant trend in favor of the ST arm in patients with non-OPC cancers in terms of PFS. ST also seemed to benefit those with N2b/N2c and N3 nodal involvement in an unplanned subgroup analysis. Febrile neutropenia again was more often noted in the TPF arm, but global toxicity assessments were similar between groups. While the trial showed no survival difference between ST and concurrent CRT alone, it did close early owing to poor accrual, which may have blunted a measurable survival difference between arms. The other randomized phase III trial performed in the United States that completed around the same time was DeCIDE, which enrolled stage III and IV locoregionally advanced HNSCC patients (with N2 and N3 nodal disease) assigned to ST with TPF (two cycles of docetaxel at 75 mg/m^2 day 1, cisplatin at 75 mg/m^2 day 1, and infusional 5-FU at 750 mg/m^2 on days 1–5 every 21 days) followed by concurrent CRT (docetaxel, 5-FU, and hydroxyurea [DFHX] plus radiotherapy at 0.15 Gy twice daily every other week) versus the same concurrent CRT regimen alone (45). As in the PARADIGM study, no difference in OS was observed between arms (HR: 0.91, 95% CI: 0.59–1.41, p = .68). Although excellent rates of LRC were noted in the study with DFHX concurrent CRT (87%–90%), this study too failed to reach accrual (280 enrolled vs. 400 planned). Fewer distant failures were observed in the ST arm (19 vs. 29, p = .11). The Spanish Head and Neck Cancer Cooperative Group (TTCC) similarly published their results of a trial comparing TPF- and PF-based IC regimens as part of ST versus concurrent CRT alone showing no significant difference in survival between treatment arms (46). Two IC regimens were studied in this trial because it was designed before the superiority of TPF was known. Patients with unresectable, locoregionally advanced HNSCC were randomized to TPF (three cycles of docetaxel at 75 mg/m^2 day 1, cisplatin at 75 mg/m^2 day 1, and infusional 5-FU at 750 mg/m^2 on days 1–5 every 21 days) or PF (at the same dosing in the docetaxel-containing arm), both followed by concurrent CRT (cisplatin at 75 mg/m^2 on days 1, 22, and 43 of radiation to 70 Gy) versus the same concurrent CRT regimen alone. In the intention-to-treat population, median PFS was similar among all three arms (TPF: 14.6, PF: 14.3, and CRT alone: 13.8 months; p = .56). The median time to treatment failure (TTF) was also similar (TPF: 7.9, PF: 7.9, and CRT alone: 8.2 months; p = .90). There was no difference in median OS among all three treatment arms (35.6, 37.1, and 29.4 months, respectively). When considering these three trials together, it is important to consider that when they were designed and implemented in the early 2000s, our knowledge of HPV-associated OPC and its resulting favorable prognosis was not fully appreciated. HPV status was not considered in these studies, and these patients are now known to do very well regardless of treatment strategy. In addition, improvements in the delivery of radiotherapy and supportive care measures are important to consider. These factors combined may have muted any detectable survival difference that may have proved an ST approach superior. Our own institution sought to understand the impact of HPV in patients treated with an ST or a concurrent CRT approach by reviewing over 500 patients and 10 years of data, including those enrolled on aforementioned protocols (47). HPV status was known in 279 cases and was positive in 77% of those. Similar to observations from the aforementioned trials, OS was similar among those treated with ST versus concurrent CRT (HR: 0.90, $p = .66$) with 3-year OS above 80% in both groups. When separating outcomes by treatment and HPV status, HPV-positive patients enjoyed excellent survival outcomes regardless of treatment strategy (3-year OS 91% in both ST and concurrent CRT treated patients, $p = .81$). However, HPV-negative patients showed a trend toward improved survival when treated with ST (3-year OS 85% vs. 75%, $p = .32$) although it was not statistically significant. Even though this represents a single institution's experience and overall outcomes were excellent, it does raise the question of whether IC strategies may afford a survival advantage in those with HPV-negative, high-risk disease.

Adding to the complexity of these approaches, an Italian group recently published data from a phase II/III, multicenter 2 x 2 factorial study to evaluate TPF as IC followed by either concurrent CRT with platinum-based therapy or cetuximab with concurrent radiation with intriguing results (48). The choice of cetuximab plus radiation for definitive therapy was based on an earlier multicenter, randomized phase III study comparing cetuximab with radiation to radiotherapy alone for patients with locoregionally advanced HNSCC (49). Median duration of LRC was 24.4 months (vs. 14.9 months, $p = .005$) favoring the cetuximab-containing arm with a median OS of 49.0 months (vs. 29.3 months, $p = .03$) in the cetuximab-treated group. Acneiform rash and infusion reactions were notable in the cetuximab arm, but there was no difference in grade 3 or greater treatment-related toxicity. While studies comparing cetuximab plus radiation and platinum-based concurrent CRT have been designed and reached accrual, the results of these trials have not been reported. Returning to the Italian study, 421 patients were randomized to one of four treatments: concurrent CRT alone (two cycles of PF with standard radiation), cetuximab plus radiation, three cycles of TPF followed by the same concurrent CRT regimen, or three cycles of TPF followed by cetuximab plus radiation (the cetuximab arms being added later). With a median follow-up of 44.8 months, radiologic CR rates were 43.5% in the IC arms and 28% in the platinum- or cetuximab-based concurrent CRT arms. Median PFS was 29.7 months favoring the IC arms (vs. 18.5 months in the concurrent CRT arms) with a median OS of 53.7 months versus 30.3 months (HR: 0.72, 95% CI: 0.55–0.96, $p = .025$) in favor of the TPF-containing IC arms (3-year OS was 57.6% vs. 45.7%, respectively). Compliance to concurrent CRT or cetuximab radiation was not compromised in the patients receiving IC. This represents the first phase III study comparing ST and concurrent CRT using TPF to report a survival benefit for ST.

At the American Society of Clinical Oncology (ASCO) Annual Meeting in 2016, two additional trials reported preliminary results adding to the collective data surrounding the use of IC as part of ST in head and neck cancer. In GORTEC 2007–02, Geoffrois and colleagues investigated ST consisting of IC with TPF followed by cetuximab plus radiotherapy versus concurrent CRT alone in patients with T2-4, N2b-3 locoregionally advanced HNSCC (50). Three cycles of standard TPF dosing were used followed by standard cetuximab dosing, along with concurrent CRT (three cycles of carboplatin at 70 mg/m^2 plus infusional 5-FU at 600 mg/m^2 on days 1–4). With a median follow-up of 31.2 months, median PFS was similar between treatment groups (11.5 for ST vs. 12.5 months for concurrent CRT; HR: 0.95, 95% CI: 0.72–1.27, $p = .74$). Median OS was also similar (24.6 for ST vs. 22.8 months for concurrent CRT; HR: 1.10, 95% CI: 0.84–1.45, $p = .48$). LRC and rates of distant failure were also not significantly different. Of note, 5.5% of patients in the TPF arm experienced progressive disease during IC and therefore did not proceed with concurrent cetuximab therapy. The second study presented was from Hitt et al. comparing TPF IC as part of ST followed by either concurrent CRT or cetuximab with radiotherapy (51). Patients received two cycles of standard doses of TPF and those with any response or stable disease were randomized to concurrent CRT (cisplatin at 100 mg/m^2 on days 1, 22, and 43 with radiation) or cetuximab (400 mg/m^2 loading dose on day 1, 250 mg/m^2 weekly thereafter during radiation). With enrollment of 530 patients, the majority of patients had T3-4 and N2-3 nodal disease. Seventy-one percent of patients responded to IC, with end-of-treatment ORRs of 72% in the concurrent CRT arm and 78% in the cetuximab plus radiation arm. Toxicity from either platinum- or cetuximab-based radiation was similar. With a median follow-up of 36 months, LRC was 56% in the ST arm with concurrent CRT versus 52% in the ST arm with cetuximab plus radiation (HR: 1.13, 95% CI: 0.84–1.51, p = .40). We await final results of these additional studies, but the fact remains that these data are in line with the majority of phase III data comprising the IC literature showing no clear survival advantage with ST as compared to concurrent CRT in an unselected patient population (Table 9.3). Lastly, an Italian study of TPF induction followed by definitive radiation with either cetuximab or cisplatin (INTERCEPTOR) has reached accrual, with preliminary toxicity data (on 170 patients) suggesting notable rates of grade 3-4 neutropenia caused by the induction arm (NCT00999700) (52). Until further study data are available, IC should remain a therapeutic option in locoregionally advanced HNSCC, particularly in those patients at high risk for distant relapse.

Worth mentioning are the results of a recent open-label, phase III multicenter study performed in China, which randomized patients with newly diagnosed, stage III and IV nasopharyngeal carcinoma of the head and neck to receive IC consisting of TPF (three cycles of docetaxel at 60 mg/m^2 on day 1, cisplatin at 60 mg/m^2 on day 1, and infusional 5-FU at 600 mg/m^2 on days 1–5 every 21 days) followed by concurrent CRT with bolus cisplatin versus concurrent CRT with bolus cisplatin alone (53). A total of 480 patients were enrolled with a median follow-up of 45 months. Three-year failure-free survival was 80% in the ST arm versus 72% in the concurrent CRT alone arm (HR: 0.68, 95% CI: 0.48–0.97, p = .034). Neutropenia and mucositis were again common (42% and 41% in the ST arm, respectively). While trial data and management specific to nasopharyngeal carcinoma of the head and

TABLE 9.3

Sequential Therapy Trials Using Induction Chemotherapy in HNSCC

Trial	Enrollment	Regimens	PFS*	OS*	DFR
PARADIGM (2013) (44)	n = 145 stage III, IV disease	TPF → CRT vs. CRT (D or C)	67% 69%	73% 78% (3 y)	4% 4%
DeCIDE (2014) (45)	n = 285 stage III, IV disease (N2 or 3)	TPF → CRT vs. CRT (DFHX)	–	75% 73%	14% 21%
Spanish group (2014) (46)	n = 439 stage III, IV disease	PF or TPF → CRT (P) vs. CRT (P)	14.6 14.3 13.8	27.0 27.2 26.6	–
Italian group (2014) (48)	n = 421 stage III, IV disease	TPF → CRT or CTX-RT vs. CRT or CTX-RT	29.7 18.5	53.7 30.3	–
GORTEC 2007–02 (2016) (50)	n = 370 unresectable, stage III, IV disease	TPF → CTX-RT vs. CRT (CF)	12.5 11.5	22.8 24.6	7% 14%

*Median reported in months unless otherwise stated.
C, carboplatin; CRT, concurrent chemoradiation; CTX, cetuximab; D, docetaxel; DFHX, docetaxel, 5-fluorouracil, hydroxyurea; DFR, distant failure rate; F, 5-fluorouracil; OS, overall survival; P, cisplatin; PF, chemotherapy regimen comprised of cisplatin-5-FU; PFS, progression-free survival; RT, radiation therapy; TPF, taxane + cisplatin + 5-fluorouracil.

neck are discussed elsewhere, this represents an important study in the growing IC literature. Although long-term follow-up is needed, the addition of TPF induction to concomitant CRT significantly improved survival in this population with manageable toxicity.

PREOPERATIVE INDUCTION CHEMOTHERAPY IN RESECTABLE, ORAL CAVITY HNSCC

The approach to locoregional disease control in patients with oral cavity HNSCC has been improved as a result of optimized surgical approaches and advances in radiotherapy administration. It is widely accepted that surgical resection followed by postoperative concomitant CRT improves LRC and survival in patients who demonstrate evidence of pathologically high-risk features such as positive margins and extracapsular extension of involved lymph nodes (54,55). But similar to other sites of disease in the head and neck, long-term survival rates remain suboptimal in these patients and distant failure rates can be significant. In line with these observations, a series of trials have been designed to evaluate the role of IC in this specific population.

An Italian group published results of a randomized, multicenter phase III study comparing three cycles of IC with a standard PF-based regimen (cisplatin at 100 mg/m^2 on day 1 and 5-FU 1,000 mg/m^2 on day 1 as a 120-hour infusion every 21 days) followed by surgical resection versus surgery alone in 195 patients with resectable (T2-4, N0-2) and previously untreated oral cavity HNSCC (56). In both arms, patients with high-risk features were eligible for adjuvant radiation. In the PF arm, three deaths attributable to toxicity were noted. PF-based IC did not significantly improve OS prior to resection (5-year OS was 55% in both arms, p = NS). However, IC was able to reduce the number of patients who required mandibulectomy and/or radiation thereby improving some morbidity. Kies and colleagues reported the results of a phase II study of patients under the age of 50 with T2-3, N0-2 oral cavity HNSCC who underwent IC comprising paclitaxel, ifosfamide, and carboplatin followed by glossectomy and neck dissection with adjuvant radiation with or without additional chemotherapy (57). This IC regimen was selected by the investigators based on historical experience using IC in young adults with tongue cancers (58). Pathologic CR in the aforementioned study was noted in 39% of patients at the primary oral site and 39% had a pathologic CR in the neck or remained node negative. No treatment-related deaths were reported. At a median follow-up of 52 months, 10 patients (43%) had developed evidence of recurrent disease and all 10 succumbed to their disease. While cancer recurrence and death rates were suboptimal in the study, the majority of patients had adverse pathologic features following final surgical resection (33% with 1–2 poor risk features, 70% with 3–5 poor risk features). Recurrence rates were lower for those with a pathologic CR at the primary oral site (11.1 vs. 64.3%, p = .029) following IC, leading the authors to conclude that IC remained a viable option worth further exploration in oral cavity HNSCC management. A phase II trial at the University of Michigan (UMCC 9921) also evaluated the role of IC (cisplatin or carboplatin plus 5-FU) in patients with oral cavity HNSCC. Patients with at least a 50% response rate to IC underwent concurrent CRT (cisplatin or carboplatin) versus surgical resection followed by radiation in nonresponders. However, primary surgical management showed significantly better survival in a matched patient cohort analysis (59). A group of Chinese investigators evaluated the use of TPF as IC prior to surgery and postoperative radiation versus surgery and postoperative radiation in a prospective, open-label phase III randomized trial of patients with stage III or IVA, locoregionally advanced and resectable oral cavity HNSCC (60). Of 256 enrolled participants, there was no significant increase in perioperative complications in those receiving TPF (two cycles of docetaxel 75 mg/m^2 on day 1, cisplatin 100 mg/m^2 on day 1, and 5-FU 750 mg/m^2 on days 1–5). The clinical ORR to TPF was 80.6% in the study. With a median follow-up of 30 months, OS was similar between treatment arms (HR: 0.98, 95% CI: 0.63–1.50, p = .918). Subgroup analysis did reveal that those patients in the TPF IC arm who had a clinical response or favorable pathologic response (characterized as ≤10% viable tumor cells on biopsy) had improved OS as well as distant disease control. Long-term results of the Italian group study discussed earlier were reported with a median follow-up of 11.5 years (61). There remained no difference in LRC (p = .634), rates of distant recurrence (p = .153), or OS (p = .340) between PF-based IC and the surgery-alone arms. However, those patients with a pathologic CR to PF-based IC did have a greater likelihood of survival at 10 years (76.2% vs. 41.3%, $p = .0004$), and certain late toxicities (e.g., fibrosis and dysphagia) were less frequent in the PF-based IC arm. Despite the suggestion that a favorable response to IC prior to oral cavity tumor resection may improve OS, none of the aforementioned studies were powered to answer that question. However, a meta-analysis published in 2015 combined the results of the Italian and Chinese studies that used IC prior to surgical resection in oral cavity HNSCC and found that OS was significantly improved in those with clinical N2 disease at diagnosis (HR: 0.42, 95% CI: 0.18–0.98, $p = .04$) (62). A recent meta-analysis including 27 randomized trials (2,872 patients) with oral cavity HNSCC treated with IC regimens concluded there was no significant OS advantage (HR: 0.95, 95% CI: 0.85–1.05, $p = .318$) or decrease in distant recurrence (RR: 0.63, 95% CI: 0.36–1.09, $p = .096$) in this population (with the longest follow-up data of 11.5 years included) (63). These data suggest that while there may be some benefit in utilizing IC prior to surgical resection in high-risk oral cavity HNSCC patients, no clear survival benefit has been demonstrated and therefore further prospective data are needed.

ALTERNATIVES TO THE STANDARD INDUCTION CHEMOTHERAPY REGIMEN

ALTERNATIVE THREE-DRUG REGIMENS

While years of outcomes data in prospectively designed trials have confirmed that the TPF regimen as IC is preferable, other chemotherapy and targeted therapy combinations have been investigated to determine any survival signal and minimize potential toxicity. An early phase II study published in 2003 prospectively treated 64 patients with locoregionally advanced HNSCC with 6-weekly cycles of carboplatin (AUC 2 on day 1) and paclitaxel (135 mg/m^2 on day 1) followed by five cycles of concomitant TFHX (paclitaxel, infusional 5-FU, hydroxyurea, and twice-daily hyperfractionated radiation administered every other week) (64). The majority of patients had stage IV disease and the ORR to IC was 82% with a CR rate of 42%—while at the completion of all therapy clinical CR was reported at 100%. Three-year OS was 70% with excellent rates of LRC. While only supported by phase II data, the ORR to carboplatin and paclitaxel IC appeared on par with TPF-based regimens (31,32). Given favorable response rates with cetuximab in the definitive treatment setting (49), interest in adding the epidermal growth factor receptor (EGFR) antibody therapy to a platinum–taxane backbone became of interest. In a phase II study performed by Kies and colleagues, 47 previously untreated patients with locoregionally advanced HNSCC of all primary tumor sites (T1-4, N2b-3) were treated with IC consisting of 6-weekly cycles of paclitaxel 135 mg/m^2 on day 1, carboplatin AUC 2 on day 1, and cetuximab 400 mg/m^2 on day 1 (250 mg/m^2 thereafter; PCC) and evaluated for clinical and radiologic response (65). Following IC with PCC, patients proceeded to definitive local treatment with radiation, surgery, or concurrent CRT, as deemed appropriate by the investigators. Nine patients (19%) achieved a CR following PCC-based IC with an ORR of 96%. Toxicities were tolerable, comprising mainly skin rash and fever without neutropenia. At a median follow-up of 33 months, 3-year PFS and OS were 87% and 91%, respectively. HPV-associated disease was confirmed in 46% of patients in the study, and was associated with improved PFS ($p = .012$) and OS ($p = .046$), as anticipated. While HPV patients comprised nearly half of the trial population, excellent ORRs to PCC and its attenuated toxicity profile fueled interest in exploring this regimen further as IC. Another phase II study included 74 patients with operable, stage III and IV locoregionally advanced HNSCC, utilized weekly PCC followed by sequential biopsy, and showed pathologic CR rates of 65% following IC and 100% at the end of treatment—similar to the Kies trial (66). Last, Seiwert and colleagues (67) at the University of Chicago explored the use of PCC for two cycles followed by randomization to either CetuxFHX (cetuximab, infusional 5-FU, hydroxyurea, and hyperfractionated radiation every other week) or CetuxPX (cetuximab, cisplatin, and accelerated radiation with concomitant boost). The ORR to IC was 91.8% and 2-year OS was excellent in both treatment arms (CetuxFHX: 91.2%, CetuxPX: 94.3%). Of note, OPC patients comprised 49% to 66% of the treatment arms and a formal HPV analysis was not reported. Based on these data, some institutions have adopted a PCC regimen for IC supported by favorable ORR rates and a modest toxicity profile. Investigators at the University of Pennsylvania reported their experience with 30 patients with locoregionally advanced HNSCC treated with IC consisting of PCC and showed a 97% ORR rate—with HPV analysis demonstrating CRs in 80% of HPV-positive patients compared with only 33% in those with HPV-negative disease (68). While considered an alternative regimen to TPF by some institutions and clinicians, further prospective data in appropriately selected patients is warranted before definitive conclusions can be drawn regarding the use of PCC as IC.

STRATEGIES TARGETING HPV-POSITIVE PATIENTS

In light of the fact that HPV-positive patients exhibit improved outcomes, the head and neck community has also focused on de-escalation trials aimed at minimizing late toxicity without jeopardizing excellent clinical outcomes in this population—the details of which are reviewed elsewhere in this book. Cmelak et al. recently presented preliminary data from the Eastern Cooperative Oncology Group (ECOG) 1308 study, a phase II trial of patients with HPV-associated OPC with resectable, stage III and IV disease using IC consisting of three cycles of paclitaxel (90 mg/m^2 on days 1, 8, and 15), cisplatin (75 mg/m^2 on day 1), and standard weekly cetuximab followed by response determined intensity modulated radiotherapy (IMRT) (69). IMRT to a dose of 54 Gy in 27 fractions was given if the patient demonstrated a clinical CR to IC versus 69.3 Gy in 33 fractions for anything less than a CR. With 90 patients enrolled and a median follow-up of 23.3 months, the complete CR rate to IC was 71% with 78% receiving dose attenuated cetuximab with radiation. The combination of IC and dose attenuated cetuximab with radiation produced LRC rates of 94% and distant control rates of 92%. Late toxicity was minimal in all patients. Two-year OS was 95% among those patients who received lower dose radiation with cetuximab. We await the final results of this study in a favorable risk HPV population, but this provides initial data to support the use of a PCC-like regimen as an alternative to TPF in certain circumstances—perhaps in favorable risk HPV-positive patients, in those patients who decline infusional therapy with port access, and in those patients warranting an induction strategy but who have significant comorbid conditions or a poor performance status.

ALTERNATIVE FOUR-DRUG REGIMENS

Other alternative combinations building on the TPF backbone have also been considered in recent years. A phase I trial recently reported results of combining a maximum tolerated dose of 50 mg daily of erlotinib (an EGFR receptor tyrosine kinase inhibitor with significant activity in non–small-cell lung cancer) with TPF (TPF-E) followed by cisplatin, bevacizumab, and erlotinib with radiation in 11 patients with locoregionally advanced, stage IV HNSCC (70). While two patients had significant gastrointestinal complications (bleeding or perforation) and one had dose-limiting diarrhea, 38% of patients had no evidence of disease at a median follow-up of 23.4 months. The authors rightfully concluded the combination was active, but too toxic for further investigation. Similar in concept and principle, a phase I study evaluating the combination of carboplatin (AUC 6 mg/mL min on day 1) and paclitaxel (175 mg/m^2 on day 1) with the protein kinase inhibitor that irreversibly binds the human epidermal growth factor receptor 2 (HER-2) and EGFR kinases, afatinib, was recently reported (71). Afatinib was started at 20 mg daily and at dose escalation given as a lead-in and during IC. Former smokers with locoregionally advanced HNSCC (regardless of HPV status) received this IC regimen with afatinib followed by concurrent CRT (40 mg/m^2 on day 1 weekly during radiation). Only 7 of 9 patients completed the afatinib lead-in phase and treatment during IC. Five had a PR and two had stable disease with no CRs observed. Afatinib at 20 mg daily resulted in grade 2-3 liver function test elevations and neutropenia. Again, the toxicity observed with this combination of targeted therapy and IC likely limits its clinical utility moving forward.

The proven efficacy of cetuximab in combination with radiation therapy in the definitive treatment setting also prompted exploration of enhancing the existing TPF regimen with this active agent. Our own group reported single institutional experience in a phase I study of cetuximab combined with TPF (C-TPF) as IC in patients with locoregionally advanced HNSCC (72). Infusional 5-FU cohorts of 700, 850, and 1,000 mg/m^2 on days 1 to 4 of treatment were explored. Thirty patients were enrolled and a dose of 850 mg/m^2 of 5-FU was selected based on toxicity (mucositis and diarrhea), which became the recommended phase II dosing. A single-arm phase II study was performed by the TTCC in Europe and treated patients with unresectable, locoregionally advanced HNSCC with four cycles of TPF (docetaxel at 75 mg/m^2 on day 1, cisplatin at 75 mg/m^2 on day 1, and infusional 5-FU at 750 mg/m^2 on days 1–5 every 21 days) with cetuximab at standard dosing (C-TPF) with prophylactic antibiotics and GCSF support (73). Fifty patients were enrolled with 82% receiving four planned cycles of C-TPF, and 86% receiving ST comprising additional cetuximab with concurrent radiation. ORR to C-TPF was 86% with a CR rate of 24%. At a median follow-up of 40.7 months, median OS was 40.7 months and the 2-year LRC was 57%. Neutropenic fever remained a significant concern (occurred in 24% of treated patients) and there were three (6%) treatment-related deaths. C-TPF did yield favorable ORRs but again the toxicity profile of this combination was limiting. Vermorken and colleagues also used C-TPF induction but followed by radiation with either carboplatin or cisplatin in 47 patients with competing comorbid conditions and the trial was terminated early: grade 3-4 hematologic toxicity was a major concern, although 66% of patients went on to definitive CRT (74). An additional phase II study performed at the University of Pittsburgh investigated combining cetuximab with a modified TPF regimen, which omitted 5-FU (75). Patients with locoregionally advanced head and neck cancer were treated with three cycles of docetaxel at 75 mg/m^2 on day 1, cisplatin at 75 mg/m^2 on day 1, and cetuximab at standard dosing (TPE) every 21 days followed by concurrent cisplatin (30 mg/m^2 weekly) and weekly cetuximab with radiotherapy and maintenance cetuximab for 6 months. With 39 enrolled patients, grade 3 and 4 mucositis (54%) was the most notable toxicity. At a median follow-up of 36 months, 3-year OS was 74%, but treatment efficacy based on HPV status was not assessed in this study. Another phase II study combined induction PCC for 6 weeks or C-TPF for 9 weeks followed by risk-based definitive local therapy defined by HPV, initial staging, and smoking status (76). Response rates for both regimens exceeded 75% following induction and 2-year estimated PFS for intermediate- or high-risk patients was 72% to 75%. The toxicity profile was significant as expected, but preliminary outcomes were favorable.

The group from Washington University in St. Louis reported their phase II results of 30 patients with locoregionally advanced HNSCC treated with nab-paclitaxel (100 mg/m^2 on day 1), cetuximab at standard dosing, cisplatin (75 mg/m^2 on day 1), and infusional 5-FU (750 mg/m^2 on days 1–3; ACPF) followed by bolus cisplatin with radiation as definitive treatment (77). Patients were often smokers with advanced T stages (T3-4, 73%) and nodal disease (N2-3, 80%). The CR rate at the primary tumor site after two cycles of ACPF was the primary end point, with 53% achieving this outcome, and an ORR of 100% to the IC regimen. The majority of patients completed the three planned cycles of ACPF and 90% went on to complete concurrent CRT. Estimated 2-year OS was 84% in treated patients (94% in HPV-positive OPC patients, 83% in HPV-negative patients). The authors later reported results of a similar study evaluating APF without cetuximab (78). They again enrolled 30 patients to receive APF followed by concurrent CRT with bolus cisplatin. Former smokers and advanced T and N stage tumors composed the majority of the cohort. With a median follow-up of 21 months, 2-year OS was 93% (94% among HPV-positive OPC patients and 92% among HPV-negative patients), with 1 relapse recorded. While the PARADIGM and DeCIDE trials did not prospectively assess patients based on HPV status, the authors in this study note very favorable outcomes with the APF regimen as IC. While outcomes with APF followed by concurrent CRT in the HPV-positive patients are similar to those in which CRT is used alone, the outcomes in HPV-negative patients are improved compared to the aforementioned trial data—but longer follow-up time and randomized phase III data are needed.

CURRENT AND EMERGING ROLE

Thus far, we have attempted to summarize decades of work and clinical trials aimed at understanding the role of IC in the management of head and neck cancers. Concurrent CRT and TPF IC approaches are effective in managing locoregionally advanced HNSCC, with no clear superiority of one approach versus the other except in the case of larynx and hypopharynx cancers where an IC approach might improve OS based on the long-term results of RTOG 91-11 (16). In addition, it remains clear that IC improves rates of distant disease control. Interpreting the data from large-scale trials investigating IC has been complicated by variation in chemotherapy regimens and radiation schedules, poor accrual to key trials, and a lack of prospective stratification based on HPV status. In addition, the benefit of intense IC regimens like TPF is often overshadowed by toxicity rates that diminish treatment compliance. In 2018, we reserve IC as an option for treating patients with locoregionally advanced disease at high risk for distant failure. Our institutional approach is to consider TPF IC in those patients with N2b, N2c, or N3 disease or lower cervical neck disease, in patients with dermal metastases, or those with presumed locoregionally advanced disease with possible oligometastatic spread that cannot be pathologically confirmed. In addition, when patients present with profound symptoms and bulky cervical neck disease warranting treatment prior to radiation planning, IC should be considered. Long-term data have also suggested that HPV-positive patients may be at risk for late, distant recurrence and therefore IC may have a role in improving outcomes in this population.

The challenge with incorporating cetuximab into the standard TPF regimen and the difficulty of the 5-FU component of the traditional three-drug induction regimen must be acknowledged as potential barriers to many prior IC studies—and thus regimens with better tolerability and similar efficacy are needed. Building on years of prior work exploring the optimal IC regimen and the benefit of ST incorporating IC, contemporary clinical trials continue to modify the standard IC regimens. Early phase studies investigating the inclusion of various cytotoxic chemotherapeutic agents (e.g., pemetrexed [NCT 01172470], nab-paclitaxel [NCT 02573493], cabazitaxel [NCT 01379339], tegafur–gimeracil–oteracil or S-1 [NCT 01645748]), monoclonal antibodies against the vascular endothelial growth factor and EGFR receptors (bevacizumab [NCT 01588431], nimotuzumab [NCT 00910117]), and targeted therapies active against cellular signaling pathways implied in head and neck cancer (everolimus [NCT 00935961]) to an IC regimen in locoregionally advanced HNSCC are all currently at various stages of development, implementation, and completion. The challenge remains one of optimizing an existing platinum–5-FU–taxane backbone but with caution given the toxicity observed in other trials that sought to enhance this combination, or identifying novel combinations that may minimize toxicity and address the risk of distant disease spread while affording a survival benefit. Gemcitabine and cisplatin are also being combined as IC to treat patients with locoregionally advanced nasopharyngeal carcinoma on protocol, as this combination has shown significant disease activity in the advanced, metastatic setting (79). Further evaluations of IC in nasopharyngeal carcinoma will likely be propelled by recent data presented that have suggested a survival signal when using an IC regimen as part of ST (53).

While cytotoxic chemotherapies have traditionally been the main components of our drug arsenal in treating head and neck cancer, we are on the verge of a paradigm shift with the emergence of systemic immunotherapy. It has been appreciated that tumor progression is facilitated by the ability of cancer cells to escape immune detection. Immune checkpoint receptors exist to block normal T cell activation, moderating a normal immune response (80,81). Immune cell expression of programmed death-1 (PD-1), one of many immune checkpoint receptors, serves to bind the ligands of PD-1 (PD-L1 and PD-L2) expressed on tumor and other immune cells allowing for attenuation of a T cell response, thereby promoting tumor immune evasion (82,83). Blocking PD-1 or its ligands represents a novel mechanism to promote tumor detection by the immune system—facilitating T cell recognition and stimulation to promote tumor cell death. In a phase Ib study of 104 patients with advanced, metastatic HNSCC (KEYNOTE-012) with any level of PD-L1 tumor expression as measured by immunohistochemistry treated with the anti-PD-1 antibody, pembrolizumab, the drug was well tolerated with no treatment-related deaths (84). ORR by central imaging review was 18% in all patients and 25% in those with HPV-associated tumors. In the expansion phase of the study, which permitted an unselected PD-L1 population of advanced HNSCC patients, 132 patients received fixed dose pembrolizumab at 200 mg intravenously every 3 weeks with an ORR of 18% by central imaging review (85). Six-month PFS and OS rates were 23% and 59%, respectively. A significantly increased ORR was observed in those patients with tumors demonstrating PD-L1 positivity (22% vs. 4%, $p = .021$). This led to the U.S. Food and Drug Administration (FDA) accelerated approval of pembrolizumab in the advanced, metastatic setting on August 5, 2016 (86). Soon to follow, a phase III trial that randomized 361 patients with recurrent, metastatic HNSCC to the anti-PD-1 antibody nivolumab or standard chemotherapy (CheckMate-141) was reported in patients who had progressed within 6 months of receiving a platinum-containing regimen (87). ORR was 13.3% in the nivolumab-treated group (vs. 5.8% in those receiving standard chemotherapy), with an improvement in OS favoring immunotherapy (HR: 0.70, 95% CI: 0.51–0.96, $p = .01$) and a 1-year survival estimate of 36% in the nivolumab arm. These data highlight a new class of available therapies active in advanced head and neck cancer. While efforts are now focused on biomarker selection to identify those likely to respond to these agents, future studies will seek to integrate immunotherapy into an IC regimen. Their novel immune-based mechanism and unique side effect profile could facilitate the combination of immunotherapy with cytotoxic chemotherapy to enhance IC. The studies using anti-PD-1 therapies in head and neck cancer outlined earlier have demonstrated that those patients who do respond often enjoy a durable response. Capitalizing on this notion and lessons learned from traditional IC approaches in head and neck cancer, a combined chemoimmunotherapy approach to induction could potentially afford early treatment of micrometastatic disease and tumor shrinkage, while resulting in durable responses aimed at improving survival. Early studies incorporating immunotherapies into the definitive, concurrent treatment setting are under way [NCT 02764593, NCT 02759575], and studies exploring immunotherapy as part of IC in head and neck cancer are emerging [NCT 02919683].

We conclude that IC remains a viable option in the treatment of patients with locoregionally advanced HNSCC, including those with laryngeal and hypopharyngeal cancers desiring organ preservation. Some preliminary data have shown a potential survival signal favoring IC in more recent studies, but we await further data and long-term results before settling on any conclusions. IC continues to warrant investigation as part of a selection strategy for treatment de-intensification in favorable risk, HPV-positive patients and in HPV-positive patients at risk for distant disease relapse. TPF remains the standard IC regimen, with PCC as an acceptable alternative. Contemporary trials continue to modify and enhance IC using various antibody and targeted therapies with limited success attributed to toxicity—but perhaps the most exciting future trials are those that will focus on immunotherapy or chemoimmunotherapeutic approaches to an induction strategy.

REFERENCES

1. Pointreau Y, Atean I, Fayette J, et al. Induction chemotherapy in head and neck cancer: a new paradigm. *Anticancer Drugs.* 2011;22(7):613–620. doi:10.1097/CAD.0b013e3283425871
2. Pignon JP, Bourhis J, Domenge C, et al. Chemotherapy added to locoregional treatment for head and neck squamous-cell carcinoma: three meta-analyses of updated individual data. MACH-NC Collaborative Group. Meta-Analysis of Chemotherapy on Head and Neck Cancer. *Lancet.* 2000;355(9208): 949–955.
3. Pignon JP, le Maître A, Maillard E, et al. Meta-analysis of chemotherapy in head and neck cancer (MACH-NC): an update on 93 randomised trials and 17,346 patients. *Radiother Oncol.* 2009;92(1):4–14.
4. Amrein PC, Fingert H, Waitzman JA. Cis-platinum-vincristine-bleomycin therapy in squamous cell carcinoma of the head and neck. *J Clin Oncol.* 1983;1:421–427.
5. Kuten A, Zidan J, Cohen Y, et al. Multidrug chemotherapy using bleomycin, methotrexate and cis-platinum alone or combined with radiotherapy in advanced head and neck cancer. *Treat Rep.* 1983;67: 573–574.
6. Tamock I, Cummings B, Jorrenti V. Combination chemotherapy used prior to radiation therapy for locally advanced squamous cell carcinoma of the head and neck. *Cancer Treat Rep.* 1982;66:1421–127.
7. Rooney M, Kish J, Jacobs J, et al. Improved complete response rate and survival in advanced head and neck cancer after three-course induction therapy with 120-hour 5-FU infusion and cisplatin. *Cancer.* 1985;55(5):1123–1128.
8. Schuller DE, Metch B, Stein DW, et al. Preoperative chemotherapy in advanced resectable head and neck cancer: final report of the Southwest Oncology Group. *Laryngoscope.* 1988;98(11):1205–1211.
9. Institutions and contributors of the Head and Neck Contracts Program. Adjuvant chemotherapy for advanced head and neck squamous carcinoma. Final report of the Head and Neck Contracts Program. *Cancer.* 1987;60(3):301–311.
10. Paccagnella A, Orlando A, Marchiori C, et al. Phase III trial of initial chemotherapy in stage III or IV head and neck cancers: a study by the Gruppo di Studio sui Tumori della Testa e del Collo. *J Natl Cancer Inst.* 1994;86(4):265–272.
11. Domenge C, Hill C, Lefebvre JL, et al. Randomized trial of neoadjuvant chemotherapy in oropharyngeal carcinoma. *Br J Cancer.* 2000;83(12):1594–1598.
12. The Department of Veterans Affairs Laryngeal Cancer Study Group. Induction chemotherapy plus radiation compared with surgery plus radiation in patients with advanced laryngeal cancer. *N Engl J Med.* 1991;324(24):1685–1690.
13. Lefebvre JL, Chevalier D, Luboinski B, et al. Larynx preservation in pyriform sinus cancer: preliminary results of a European Organization for Research and Treatment of Cancer phase III trial. EORTC Head and Neck Cancer Cooperative Group. *J Natl Cancer Inst.* 1996;88(13):890–899.
14. Lefebvre JL, Andry G, Chevalier D, et al. Laryngeal preservation with induction chemotherapy for hypopharyngeal squamous cell carcinoma: 10-year results of EORTC trial 24891. *Ann Oncol.* 2012;23(10):2708–2714.

15. Forastiere AA, Goepfert H, Maor M, et al. Concurrent chemotherapy and radiotherapy for organ preservation in advanced laryngeal cancer. *N Engl J Med.* 2003;349(22):2091–2098.
16. Forastiere AA, Zhang Q, Weber RS, et al. Long-term results of RTOG 91-11: a comparison of three nonsurgical treatment strategies to preserve the larynx in patients with locally advanced larynx cancer. *J Clin Oncol.* 2013;31(7):845–852.
17. Vokes EE. Competing roads to larynx preservation. *J Clin Oncol.* 2013;31(7):833–835.
18. Lefebvre JL, Rolland F, Tesselaar M, et al. Phase 3 randomized trial on larynx preservation comparing sequential vs alternating chemotherapy and radiotherapy. *J Natl Cancer Inst.* 2009;101(3):142–152.
19. Forastiere AA, Shank D, Neuberg D, et al. Final report of a phase II evaluation of paclitaxel in patients with advanced squamous cell carcinoma of the head and neck: an Eastern Cooperative Oncology Group trial (PA390). *Cancer.* 1998;82(11):2270–2274.
20. Couteau C, Chouaki N, Leyvraz S, et al. A phase II study of docetaxel in patients with metastatic squamous cell carcinoma of the head and neck. *Br J Cancer.* 1999;81(3):457–592.
21. Dreyfuss AI, Clark JR, Norris CM, et al. Docetaxel: an active drug for squamous cell carcinoma of the head and neck. *J Clin Oncol.* 1996;14(5):1672–1678.
22. Colevas AD, Busse PM, Norris CM, et al. Induction chemotherapy with docetaxel, cisplatin, fluorouracil, and leucovorin for squamous cell carcinoma of the head and neck: a phase I/II trial. *J Clin Oncol.* 1998;16(4):1331–1339.
23. Colevas AD, Norris CM, Tishler RB, et al. Phase II trial of docetaxel, cisplatin, fluorouracil, and leucovorin as induction for squamous cell carcinoma of the head and neck. *J Clin Oncol.* 1999;17(11):3503–3511.
24. Colevas AD, Norris CM, Tishler RB, et al. Phase I/II trial of outpatient docetaxel, cisplatin, 5-fluorouracil, leucovorin (opTPFL) as induction for squamous cell carcinoma of the head and neck (SCCHN). *Am J Clin Oncol.* 2002;25(2):153–159.
25. Posner MR, Glisson B, Frenette G, et al. Multicenter phase I-II trial of docetaxel, cisplatin, and fluorouracil induction chemotherapy for patients with locally advanced squamous cell cancer of the head and neck. *J Clin Oncol.* 2001;19(4):1096–1104.
26. Haddad R, Colevas AD, Tishler R, et al. Docetaxel, cisplatin, and 5-fluorouracil-based induction chemotherapy in patients with locally advanced squamous cell carcinoma of the head and neck: the Dana Farber Cancer Institute experience. *Cancer.* 2003;97(2):412–418.
27. Janinis J, Papadakou M, Panagos G, et al. Sequential chemoradiotherapy with docetaxel, cisplatin, and 5-fluorouracil in patients with locally advanced head and neck cancer. *Am J Clin Oncol.* 2001;24(3):227–231.
28. Haddad R, Tishler R, Wirth L, et al. Rate of pathologic complete responses to docetaxel, cisplatin, and fluorouracil induction chemotherapy in patients with squamous cell carcinoma of the head and neck. *Arch Otolaryngol Head Neck Surg.* 2006;132(6):678–681.
29. Schrijvers D, Van Herpen C, Kerger J, et al. Docetaxel, cisplatin and 5-fluorouracil in patients with locally advanced unresectable head and neck cancer: a phase I-II feasibility study. *Ann Oncol.* 2004;15(4):638–645.
30. Hitt R, Lopez-Pousa A, Martínez-Trufero J, et al. Phase III study comparing cisplatin plus fluorouracil to paclitaxel, cisplatin, and fluorouracil induction chemotherapy followed by chemoradiotherapy in locally advanced head and neck cancer. *J Clin Oncol.* 2005;23(34):8636–8645.
31. Vermorken JB, Remenar E, van Herpen C, et al. Cisplatin, fluorouracil, and docetaxel in unresectable head and neck cancer. *N Engl J Med.* 2007;357(17):1695–1704.
32. Posner MR, Hershock DM, Blajman CR, et al. Cisplatin and fluorouracil alone or with docetaxel in head and neck cancer. *N Engl J Med.* 2007;357(17):1705–1715.
33. Lorch JH, Goloubeva O, Haddad RI, et al.Induction chemotherapy with cisplatin and fluorouracil alone or in combination with docetaxel in locally advanced squamous-cell cancer of the head and neck: long-term results of the TAX 324 randomised phase 3 trial. *Lancet.* 2011;12(2):153–159.
34. van Herpen CM, Mauer ME, Mesia R, et al. Short-term health-related quality of life and symptom control with docetaxel, cisplatin, 5-fluorouracil and cisplatin (TPF), 5-fluorouracil (PF) for induction in unresectable locoregionally advanced head and neck cancer patients (EORTC 24971/TAX 323). *Br J Cancer.* 2010;103(8):1173–1181.
35. Liberato NL, Rognoni C, Rubrichi S, et al. Adding docetaxel to cisplatin and fluorouracil in patients with unresectable head and neck cancer: a cost-utility analysis. *Ann Oncol.* 2012;23(7):1825–1832.
36. Blanchard P, Bourhis J, Lacas B, et al. Taxane-cisplatin-fluorouracil as induction chemotherapy in locally advanced head and neck cancers: an individual patient data meta-analysis of the meta-analysis of chemotherapy in head and neck cancer group. *J Clin Oncol.* 2013;31(23):2854–2860.
37. Ang KK, Harris J, Wheeler R, et al. Human papillomavirus and survival of patients with oropharyngeal cancer. *N Engl J Med.* 2010;363(1):24–35.
38. Rischin D, Young RJ, Fisher R, et al. Prognostic significance of p16INK4A and human papillomavirus in patients with oropharyngeal cancer treated on TROG 02.02 phase III trial. *J Clin Oncol.* 2010;28(27):4142–4148.
39. Posner MR, Lorch JH, Goloubeva O, et al. Survival and human papillomavirus in oropharynx cancer in TAX 324: a subset analysis from an international phase III trial. *Ann Oncol.* 2011;22(5):1071–1077.
40. Pointreau Y, Garaud P, Chapet S, et al. Randomized trial of induction chemotherapy with cisplatin and 5-fluorouracil with or without docetaxel for larynx preservation. *J Natl Cancer Inst.* 2009;101(7):498–506.
41. Lefebvre JL, Pointreau Y, Rolland F, et al. Induction chemotherapy followed by either chemoradiotherapy or bioradiotherapy for larynx preservation: the TREMPLIN randomized phase II study. *J Clin Oncol.* 2013;31(7):853–859.

42. Janoray G, Pointreau Y, Garaud P, et al. Long-term results of a multicenter randomized phase III trial of induction chemotherapy with cisplatin, 5-fluorouracil, ± docetaxel for larynx preservation. *J Natl Cancer Inst.* 2015;108(4):1–7.
43. Paccagnella A, Ghi MG, Loreggian L, et al. Gruppo di Studio Tumori della Testa e del Collo XRP 6976 F/2501 Study, Concomitant chemoradiotherapy versus induction docetaxel, cisplatin and 5 fluorouracil (TPF) followed by concomitant chemoradiotherapy in locally advanced head and neck cancer: a phase II randomized study. *Ann Oncol.* 2010;21(7):1515–1522.
44. Haddad R, O'Neill A, Rabinowits G, et al. Induction chemotherapy followed by concurrent chemoradiotherapy (sequential chemoradiotherapy) versus concurrent chemoradiotherapy alone in locally advanced head and neck cancer (PARADIGM): a randomised phase 3 trial. *Lancet Oncol.* 2013;14(3):257–264.
45. Cohen EE, Karrison TG, Kocherginsky M, et al. Phase III randomized trial of induction chemotherapy in patients with N2 or N3 locally advanced head and neck cancer. *J Clin Oncol.* 2014;32(25):2735–2743.
46. Hitt R, Grau JJ, López-Pousa A, et al. A randomized phase III trial comparing induction chemotherapy followed by chemoradiotherapy versus chemoradiotherapy alone as treatment of unresectable head and neck cancer. *Ann Oncol.* 2014;25(1):216–225.
47. Lorch JH, Hanna GJ, Posner MR, et al. Human papillomavirus and induction chemotherapy versus concurrent chemoradiotherapy in locally advanced oropharyngeal cancer: The Dana Farber Experience. *Head Neck.* 2016;38(1):E1618–E1624.
48. Ghi MG, Paccagnella A, Ferrari D, et al. Induction TPF followed by concomitant treatment versus concomitant treatment alone in locally advanced head and neck cancer. A phase II-III trial. *Ann Oncol.* 2017;28(9):2206–2212.
49. Bonner JA, Harari PM, Giralt J, et al. Radiotherapy plus cetuximab for squamous-cell carcinoma of the head and neck. *N Engl J Med.* 2006;354(6):567–578.
50. Geoffrois L, Martin L, Garaud P, et al. Induction docetaxel platinum 5-FU (TPF) followed by cetuximab-radiotherapy (cetux-RT) versus concurrent chemo-radiotherapy (CT/RT) in patients with N2b/c-N3 non operated stage III-IV squamous cell cancer of the head and neck (SCCHN): Results of the GORTEC 2007-02 phase III randomized trial. *J Clin Oncol.* 2016;34(suppl):6000.
51. Hitt R, Grau JJ, Lopez-Pousa A, et al. Final results of a randomized phase III trial comparing induction chemotherapy with cisplatin/5-FU or docetaxel/cisplatin/5-FU follow by chemoradiotherapy (CRT) versus CRT alone as first-line treatment of unresectable locally advanced head and neck cancer (LAHNC). *J Clin Oncol.* 2016;27:15s(suppl; abstr 6009).
52. Merlano M, Vecchio S, Bacigalupo A, et al. The phase III study: interceptor in locally advanced head and neck cancer (LA-HNC). Preliminary safety report. *Eur J Cancer.* 2015;51:S560.
53. Sun Y, Li WF, Chen NY, et al. Induction chemotherapy plus concurrent chemoradiotherapy versus concurrent chemoradiotherapy alone in locoregionally advanced nasopharyngeal carcinoma: a phase 3, multicentre, randomised controlled trial. *Lancet Oncol.* 2016;17(11):1509–1520.
54. Bernier J, Domenge C, Ozsahin M, et al. European Organization for research and treatment of cancer trial 22931. Postoperative irradiation with or without concomitant chemotherapy for locally advanced head and neck cancer. *N Engl J Med.* 2004;350(19):1945–1952.
55. Cooper JS, Pajak TF, Forastiere AA, et al. Postoperative concurrent radiotherapy and chemotherapy for high-risk squamous-cell carcinoma of the head and neck. *N Engl J Med.* 2004;350(19):1937–1944.
56. Licitra L, Grandi C, Guzzo M, et al. Primary chemotherapy in resectable oral cavity squamous cell cancer: a randomized controlled trial. *J Clin Oncol.* 2003;21(2):327–323.
57. Kies MS, Boatright DH, Li G, et al. Phase II trial of induction chemotherapy followed by surgery for squamous cell carcinoma of the oral tongue in young adults. *Head Neck.* 2012;34(9):1255–1262.
58. Sturgis EM, Moore BA, Glisson BS, et al. Neoadjuvant chemotherapy for the young adult with squamous cell carcinoma of the oral tongue: a case series. *Head Neck.* 2005;27(9):748–756.
59. Chinn SB, Spector ME, Bellile EL, et al. Efficacy of induction selection chemotherapy vs primary surgery for patients with advanced oral cavity carcinoma. *JAMA Otolaryngol Head Neck Surg.* 2014;140(2):134–142.
60. Zhong LP, Zhang CP, Ren GX, et al. Randomized phase III trial of induction chemotherapy with docetaxel, cisplatin, and fluorouracil followed by surgery versus up-front surgery in locally advanced resectable oral squamous cell carcinoma. *J Clin Oncol.* 2013;31(6):744–751.
61. Bossi P, Lo Vullo S, Guzzo M, et al. Preoperative chemotherapy in advanced resectable OCSCC: long-term results of a randomized phase III trial. *Ann Oncol.* 2014;25(2):462–466.
62. Marta GN, Riera R, Bossi P, et al. Induction chemotherapy prior to surgery with or without postoperative radiotherapy for oral cavity cancer patients: Systematic review and meta-analysis. *Eur J Cancer.* 2015;51(17):2596–2603.
63. Lau A, Li KY, Yang WF, et al. Induction chemotherapy for squamous cell carcinomas of the oral cavity: A cumulative meta-analysis. *Oral Oncol.* 2016;61:104–114.
64. Haraf DJ, Rosen FR, Stenson K, et al. Induction chemotherapy followed by concomitant TFHX chemoradiotherapy with reduced dose radiation in advanced head and neck cancer. *Clin Cancer Res.* 2003;9(16, Pt. 1):5936–5943.
65. Kies MS, Holsniger FC, Lee JJ, et al. Induction chemotherapy and cetuximab for locally advanced squamous cell carcinoma of the head and neck: results from a phase II prospective trial. *J Clin Oncol.* 2010;28(1):8–14.
66. Wanebo HJ, Ghebremichael M, Burtness B, et al. Phase II evaluation of cetuximab (C225) combined with induction paclitaxel and carboplatin followed by C225, paclitaxel, carboplatin, and radiation for stage III/IV operable squamous cancer of the head and neck (ECOG, E2303). *J Clin Oncol.* 2007;(18S):6015.

67. Seiwert TY, Melotek JM, Blair EA, et al. Final results of a randomized phase 2 trial investigating the addition of cetuximab to induction chemotherapy and accelerated or hyperfractionated chemoradiation for locoregionally advanced head and neck cancer. *Int J Radiat Oncol Biol Phys.* 2016;96(1):21–29. doi:10.1016/j.ijrobp.2016.04.030
68. Bauman J, Langer C, Quon H, et al. Induction chemotherapy with cetuximab, carboplatin and paclitaxel for the treatment of locally advanced squamous cell carcinoma of the head and neck. *Exp Ther Med.* 2013;5(4):1247–1253.
69. Cmelak A, Li S, Marur S, et al. E1308: Reduced-dose IMRT in human papilloma virus (HPV)-associated resectable oropharyngeal squamous carcinomas (OPSCC) after clinical complete response (cCR) to induction chemotherapy (IC). *J Clin Oncol.* 2014;32:(Suppl; abstr LBA6006).
70. Ahn PH, Machtay M, Anne PR, et al. Phase I trial using induction ciplatin, docetaxel, 5-FU and erlotinib followed by cisplatin, bevacizumab and erlotinib with concurrent radiotherapy for advanced head and neck cancer. *Am J Clin Oncol.* 2016. [Epub ahead of print]. doi:10.1097/COC.0000000000000317
71. Chung CH, Rudek MA, Kang H, et al. A phase I study afatinib/carboplatin/paclitaxel induction chemotherapy followed by standard chemoradiation in HPV-negative or high-risk HPV-positive locally advanced stage III/IVa/IVb head and neck squamous cell carcinoma. *Oral Oncol.* 2016;53:54–9.
72. Haddad RI, Tishler R, Norris C, et al. Phase I study of C-TPF in patients with locally advanced squamous cell carcinoma of the head and neck. *J Clin Oncol.* 2009;27(27):4448–4453.
73. Mesía R, Vazquez S, Grau JJ, et al. A Phase 2 open label, single-arm trial to evaluate the combination of cetuximab plus taxotere, cisplatin, and 5-flurouracil as an induction regimen in patients with unresectable squamous cell carcinoma of the head and neck. *Int J Radiat Oncol Biol Phys.* 2016;94(2):289–296.
74. Vermorken JB, Remenar E, van den Weyngaert D, et al. Feasibility of cetuximab plus sequential platinum-based therapy (TPF→CRT) in advanced squamous cell head and neck cancer (SCCHN): a randomized phase II study of the EORTC Head and Neck Cancer Group (EORTC-HNCG # 24061). *European Archives of Oto-Rhino Laryngology.* 2012;269:OP43.
75. Argiris A, Heron DE, Smith RP, et al. Induction docetaxel, cisplatin, and cetuximab followed by concurrent radiotherapy, cisplatin, and cetuximab and maintenance cetuximab in patients with locally advanced head and neck cancer. *J Clin Oncol.* 2010;28(36):5294–5300.
76. Massarelli E, Haddad RI, Lee JJ, et al. Weekly paclitaxel, carboplatin, cetuximab (PCC), and cetuximab, docetaxel, cisplatin, and fluorouracil (C-TPF), followed by risk-based local therapy in previously untreated, locally advanced head and neck squamous cell carcinoma (LAHNSCC). *J Clin Oncol.* 2015.33;2015(suppl;abstract 6001).
77. Adkins D, Ley J, Trinkaus K, et al. A phase 2 trial of induction nab-paclitaxel and cetuximab given with cisplatin and 5-fluorouracil followed by concurrent cisplatin and radiation for locally advanced squamous cell carcinoma of the head and neck. *Cancer.* 2013;119(4):766–773.
78. Adkins D, LeyJ, Michel L, et al. nab-Paclitaxel, cisplatin, and 5-fluorouracil followed by concurrent cisplatin and radiation for head and neck squamous cell carcinoma. *Oral Oncol.* 2016;61:1–7.
79. Zhang L, Yu G, Jia J, et al. Gemcitabine plus cisplatin (GP) versus 5-FU plus cisplatin (FP) as first-line treatment for recurrent or metastatic nasopharyngeal carcinoma (NPC): a randomized, open-label, multicenter, phase III trial. *J Clin Oncol.* 2016;34:(suppl; abstr 6007).
80. Ramsay AG. Immune checkpoint blockade immunotherapy to activate anti-tumour T-cell immunity. *Br J Haematol.* 2013;162(3):313–325.
81. Ferris RL. Immunology and immunotherapy of head and neck cancer. *J Clin Oncol.* 2015;33(29):3293–3304.
82. Leach DR, Krummel MF, Allison JP. Enhancement of antitumor immunity by CTLA-4 blockade. *Science.* 1996;271(5256):1734–1736.
83. Lyford-Pike S, Peng S, Young GD, et al. Evidence for a role of the PD-1:PD-L1 pathway in immune resistance of HPV-associated head and neck squamous cell carcinoma. *Cancer Res.* 2013;73(6):1733–1741.
84. Seiwert TY, Burtness B, Mehra R, et al. Safety and clinical activity of pembrolizumab for treatment of recurrent or metastatic squamous cell carcinoma of the head and neck (KEYNOTE-012): an open-label, multicentre, phase 1b trial. *Lancet Oncol.* 2016;17(7):956–965.
85. Chow LQ, Haddad R, Gupta S, et al. Antitumor activity of pembrolizumab in biomarker-unselected patients with recurrent and/or metastatic head and neck squamous cell carcinoma: results from the phase Ib KEYNOTE-012 expansion cohort. *J Clin Oncol.* 2016;34(32):3838–3845.
86. U.S.A. Food and Drug Administration. 2016. https://www.fda.gov/Drugs/InformationOnDrugs/ApprovedDrugs/ucm526430.htm
87. Ferris RL, Blumenschein G Jr, Fayette J, et al. Nivolumab for recurrent squamous-cell carcinoma of the head and neck. *N Engl J Med.* 2016;375:1856–1867.

10

Immunotherapy for HNSCC: Rationale and Clinical Applications

Jennifer Moy
Jennifer M. Johnson
Jessica Moskovitz
Robert L. Ferris
Athanassios Argiris

Despite advances in chemotherapy, radiotherapy, surgical techniques, and combined modality approaches, only modest improvements in the survival rate of head and neck squamous cell carcinoma (HNSCC) have been achieved over the past decade. Treatment failures remain unacceptably common, even among human papillomavirus (HPV)-associated cancers, calling for new paradigms to treat HNSCC (1).

Pioneering laboratory work has led to the recognition of the major role of the immune system in cancer, leading to the acceptance of immune-based treatment as a clinically applied treatment for cancer. With new immunotherapeutic approaches continuing to develop, the clinical trial arena for HNSCC has shifted greatly over the past decade. Previously, investigations were primarily focused on targeted therapies to block an oncogenic signaling pathway. Today, however, the majority of ongoing clinical trials in HNSCC are focusing on immunotherapies.

Cancer immunotherapy is a promising novel therapeutic strategy that may both reduce treatment-related toxicities and improve disease control rates. In tumors with a favorable prognosis, such as HPV-positive tumors, immunotherapy is being investigated as a de-intensification strategy in place of toxic chemotherapy or radiotherapy. Alternatively, in aggressive localized disease or in the setting of recurrent or metastatic HNSCC, immunotherapy may be used in combination with conventional treatments to improve tumor control. Today HNSCC immunotherapy encompasses a variety of diverse treatment approaches including tumor-specific and immune-modulating monoclonal antibodies, vaccines, oncolytic viruses, and adoptive cell transfer. In this chapter, we discuss immunology of cancer, biological mechanisms of immune escape, clinical implications for immunotherapy in HNSCC, current clinical trials, and future directions.

IMMUNOLOGY OF CANCER

IMMUNE SURVEILLANCE AND IMMUNOEDITING

The idea of immune surveillance was first introduced by Burnet in 1970, who suggested that premalignant cells frequently develop, but are quickly eradicated by the immune system before an invasive tumor can develop (2). Since then, mounting evidence has supported the role of the immune system in preventing malignant transformation in at least three different ways: (a) it provides protection against viral infection and subsequently suppresses virus-induced tumors, such as HPV; (b) it prevents the development of an inflammatory environment from which tumorigenesis flourishes by eliminating pathogens and promptly resolving inflammation; and (c) it eradicates tumor cells by the activation of innate and adaptive immune cells. However, there seems to be a breakdown in this system leading to clinically evident malignancies. This relationship between the immune system and malignancy can be seen clearly in immunocompromised patients who have an increased risk of HNSCC, such as solid organ and bone marrow transplant patients, as well as in HIV-positive patients (3–5). Furthermore, tumors in these patients tend to be poorly responsive (6). Most patients who develop HNSCC, however, are immunocompetent, and these tumors are therefore thought to evade the immune response through "cancer immunoediting" (7). This theory suggests that while the immune system can eradicate some transformed cells, others that are less immunogenic and have gained a survival advantage will allow immune evasion and subsequent tumor formation (8). Cancer immunoediting proceeds sequentially through three distinct phases termed "elimination," "equilibrium," and "escape."

Elimination

During this initial stage, the innate and adaptive immune systems recognize developing tumor cells and destroy them before they become a clinically apparent tumor. While activation of the immune system at this stage is not fully understood, possibilities include "danger signals," such as interferon (IFN) and other cytokines that are induced early in tumor development, or damage-associated molecular pattern (DAMP) molecules, which are released from dying tumor cells or damaged tissues from the invasive growth of the tumor. These danger signals lead to the activation of dendritic cells (DCs) and subsequent adaptive antitumor immune responses. If the tumor cells are completely eradicated, the cancer immunoediting process ends at this phase.

Equilibrium

If a rare cancer cell variant survives the elimination phase, the adaptive immune system keeps these residual cells in a state of dormancy (latent tumor cells), for up to many years. In this phase, immunity is specifically responsible for the prevention of tumor cell outgrowth. The immunogenicity of the tumor cells is also sculpted during this stage as the genetically unstable and rapidly mutating tumor cells undergo darwinian selection, providing new variants with increased resistance to immune attack. Evidence of an immunologically driven equilibrium phase came from primary tumorigenesis experiments showing that while immunocompetent mice harbored occult cancer cells for a prolonged time period without any apparent tumor development, when the immune system was ablated with T cell and IFN-γ depleting monoclonal antibodies (mAbs), tumors rapidly developed in the original injection site in half the mice and resembled unedited sarcoma cells (9). Furthermore, adaptive immunity—specifically, interleukin 12 (IL-12), IFN-γ, $CD4^+$, and $CD8^+$ T cells—but not innate immunity was responsible for maintaining the occult tumor cells in equilibrium. Thus, dormancy is maintained through growth inhibitory and cytocidal actions of immunity on the residual tumor cells, providing the selective pressure to promote tumor outgrowth in those cells that have acquired the most immunoevasive mutations.

Escape

These tumor cells that have acquired the mechanisms to thwart immune recognition and destruction are able to grow and develop into visible tumors. Progression to immune escape can be due to immune system deterioration or changes in the tumor cell population in response to increased cancer-induced immunosuppression.

MECHANISMS OF IMMUNE ESCAPE IN HNSCC AND RATIONALE FOR THERAPEUTIC TARGETS

As the majority of HNSCC patients are immunocompetent, understanding the mechanisms by which these tumor cells are able to evade immune attack is imperative to the development of successful immunotherapies. Tumor cell escape can occur by a number of mechanisms. At the tumor level, escape may result from reduced immune recognition or increased resistance to the cytotoxic effects of immunity. At the host level, escape may result from the establishment of an immunosuppressive state within the tumor microenvironment (TME). T cells have been the major focus of immune-modulating therapies due to their selective recognition of peptides in all cellular compartments (via major histocompatibility [MHC] presentation), their ability to directly recognize and kill antigen-expressing cells ($CD8^+$ killer T cells), and their capability of orchestrating diverse immune responses ($CD4^+$ helper T cells), integrating adaptive and innate immunity. T cell activation requires three simultaneous signals at the "immune synapse" in order to carry out its antitumor effects (Figure 10.1). Signal 1 comprises the T cell receptor (TCR) and human leukocyte antigen (HLA) interaction, with presentation of nonself-antigens from the tumor cell. Signal 2 is a summation of costimulatory and coinhibitory signals. These signals must occur in the presence of signal 3, made up of immune activating cytokines, such as IL-2 or IFN-γ. Immune evasion can occur at any of these signals, impairing the immune system from effectively eradicating malignant cells. As the receptors, ligands, and signaling pathways that facilitate immune tolerance are uncovered, these factors and pathways can be selectively inhibited in a way to shift the balance away from cancer promotion to antitumor immune responses.

ANTIGEN PRESENTATION AND PROCESSING

Genetic instability is a basic hallmark of cancer, and results in a distinct tumor antigen profile that identifies it as nonself, often products of aberrantly expressed normal genes (such as epidermal growth factor receptor [EGFR]), mutated cellular genes (such as TP53), or genes encoding viral proteins (such as HPV). These neoantigens can then be used to activate the innate and adaptive immune systems. Loss of tumor antigen recognition as an escape mechanism is well studied, and can occur in at least three ways: (a) through the loss of antigen expression, (b) through loss of antigen presentation by HLA proteins and associated molecules, or (c) through loss of antigen-processing function within the tumor cell. These changes are likely driven by a combination

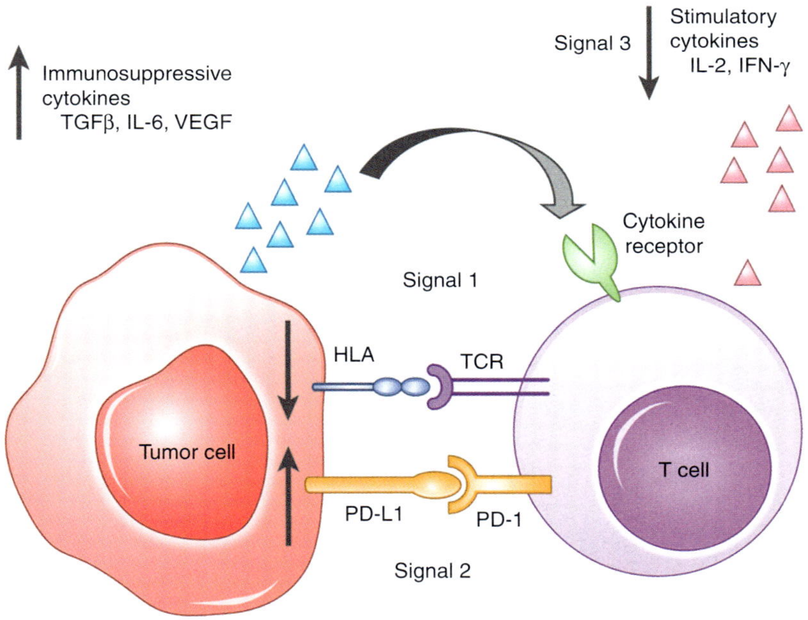

FIGURE 10.1 Immune surveillance and targets for evasion: T cell activation requires three simultaneous signals at the "immune synapse" in order to carry out its antitumor effects. Signal 1 involves the presentation of nonself-antigens from the tumor cell to the T cell through the human leukocyte antigen (HLA)–T cell receptor (TCR) interaction. Signal 2 is a summation of costimulatory and coinhibitory signals. Signal 3 is made up of immune activating cytokines, such as interleukin 2 (IL-2) or interferon (IFN-γ). Immune evasion can occur at any of these signals (arrows), impairing the immune system from effectively eradicating malignant cells.

HLA, human leukocyte antigen; PD-1, programmed cell death protein 1; PD-L1, programmed death-ligand 1; TCR, T cell receptor; TGF, transforming growth factor β; VEGF, vascular endothelial growth factor.

of genetic instability and immunoselection, ultimately leading to the establishment of poorly immunogenic tumor cell variants that become "invisible" to the immune system and thus gain the ability to proliferate (8,10).

The HLA complex, which presents captured tumor antigens (TAs) to T cells, is necessary to activate effector T cells, and highlights a potential evasion mechanism (Figure 10.2). While tumor cells could evade T cell recognition through the complete loss of HLA function, this however serves as a strong stimulus for NK-cell activation and subsequent tumor cell killing (11). Large-scale sequencing has revealed that HNSCC tumor cells have developed several mutations in HLA alleles and antigen-processing machinery (APM) components, allowing tumor cell mechanisms to evade antigen recognition without total loss of HLA expression (3,12–20). These abnormalities are present in 20% of HNSCC specimens, and correlate with lymph node metastasis and poor prognosis in HNSCC patients (17,21–23), and may impact the clinical response to T cell based immunotherapy. Although mechanisms behind APM component deficiency are still unclear, it has been suggested that signal transducer and activator of transcription (STAT) family of proteins controls defects in APM components and antigen-presenting cell (APC) function. For instance, STAT1 deficiency leads to reduced expression of APM components, while aberrant

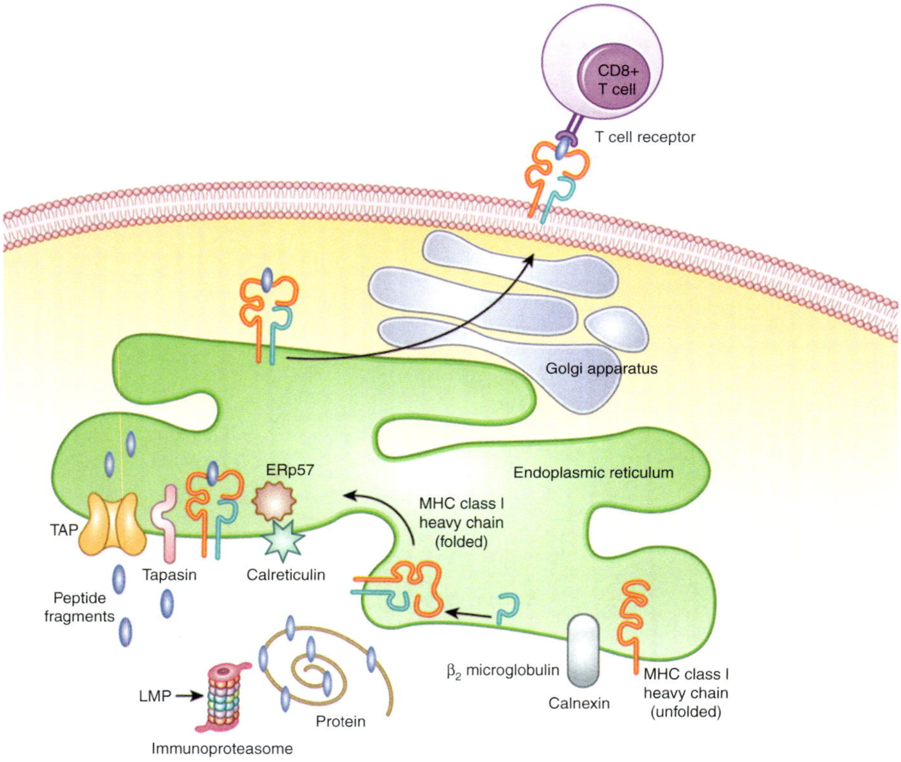

FIGURE 10.2 MHC class I antigen processing and presentation: Intracellular proteins are degraded via the ubiquitin–proteasome pathway. Once tagged by ubiquitin, the target protein is degraded by the proteasome. The proteasome is a multimeric protein complex formed by the 20S catalytic core and 2 regulatory 19S particles at each end. Importantly, 3 of the β-subunits of the 20S core are replaced by the IFN-γ inducible subunits, LMW proteins 2, 7, and 10 (LMP2, LMP7, and LMP10), forming the immunoproteasome. This structure generates different antigenic peptides with high affinity for HLA I alleles. The immunogenic peptides are then transported into the ER by the TAP 1/2 complex. With the assistance of chaperones (calnexin, tapasin, calreticulin, ERp57), the peptides are loaded onto the MHC class I heavy chain/β2 microglobulin complex. The trimeric complex then traverses through the Golgi apparatus and is incorporated into the cell membrane where the peptide can interact with $CD8^+$ T cells. Defects anywhere along this pathway can lead to impaired presentation and CTL activation.

CTL, cytotoxic T cell; ER, endoplasmic reticulum; LMW, low molecular weight; TAP, transporter of antigen processing.

expression of STAT3 promotes impaired tumor antigen presentation by DCs (18,24). Since EGFR is expressed in 80% of HNSCC tumors, EGFR-induced HLA downregulation may be an important mechanism in evading immune recognition. This escape mechanism is achieved through many oncogenic downstream pathways, including SHP2/STAT1 suppression, MAPK, and PI3K-AKT (25–28). Furthermore, HLA class I and APM component deficiency can be reversed in HNSCC by depleting SHP2, or by using the STAT1 agonist IFN-γ, both increasing peptide:HLA class I complexes and enhancing CTL-mediated lysis of tumor cells (13,15,16,18,29–32). Therefore, approaches that boost IFN-γ signaling and STAT1 activation, such as EGFR antagonism, may be significant in restoring antigen presentation through increased expression of HLA class I molecules and proinflammatory cytokines (30,33).

IMMUNE CHECKPOINTS

Some tumors contain cancer cells that express strong antigens and the adequate machinery to mount an immune response; however they can develop T cell tolerance to these antigens and escape immune activation under chronic antigen exposure (34). In addition to antigen recognition, T cell activation is functionally determined by the summation of many costimulatory and coinhibitory signals (Figure 10.3). The immune system employs these checkpoints to thwart an exaggerated immune response, preventing the development of autoimmune diseases, a process termed “adaptive immune resistance.” However, these inhibitory checkpoints can be dysregulated by tumors as an important mechanism to weaken effector immune responses, contributing to tumor-promoting immunosuppression and tolerance, and can even induce T cell apoptosis (35).

Tumors have developed mechanisms to take advantage of this mechanism by expressing the ligands necessary to activate these immune inhibiting signals and upregulate inhibitory receptors. The two best-studied checkpoint receptors are cytotoxic T lymphocyte antigen 4 (CTLA4) and programmed cell death protein 1 (PD-1), both of which are the targets of Food and Drug Administration (FDA) approved inhibitory antibodies (36). There is emerging data for the use of other novel checkpoint inhibitory receptors in the treatment of HNSCC, including lymphocyte activation gene 3 (LAG3), T cell membrane protein 3 (TIM3), and killer immunoglobulin-like receptor (KIR). In the presence of these coinhibitory signals, the stimulatory “signal 2” will fail, leading to the induction of T cell anergy or apoptosis (37). The classically described costimulatory pathway involves CD28/B7 interaction; however, other costimulatory interactions between TCRs and their corresponding APC ligands include CD137/CD137-L, OX40/OX40-L, and CD40/CD40-L. These costimulatory receptors are members of the tumor necrosis factor receptor superfamily, and a decrease in their expression has been observed on T cells of HNSCC specimens, correlating with poor outcomes (38). Therefore, blocking the coinhibitory signals and increasing the costimulatory signals may enhance tumor control through increased cytotoxic activity of T cells. Many mAbs targeting these signaling pathways have been developed in attempts to shift the immune system toward an antitumor function and are currently entering the therapeutic armamentarium for HNSCC.

CTLA4 is expressed primarily on T cells in response to TCR activation, and counteracts CD28-mediated costimulatory signals (39,40). This impairs the activation of T cells, thus limiting an exaggerated immune response (41). Although the transient expression of CTLA4 on $CD8^+$ T cells regulates effector/memory activity (42–44), the inhibitory function of CTLA4 appears to be more important on $CD4^+$ regulatory T cells (Tregs), where CTLA4 is constitutively expressed at high levels (45,46). CLTA4 and CD28 share B7 ligands, CD80, and CD86, whose expression is limited to APCs (47). Compared to CD28, CTLA4 binds these ligands with higher affinity and avidity, competitively inhibiting “signal 2” in the T cell activation cascade (47). Interestingly, activated $CTLA4^+$ T cells can deplete acquired B7 ligands from APCs by CTLA4-dependent endocytosis and degradation, further impairing the activation of T cells (48,49).

PD-1 is highly expressed on the surface of activated immune cells in the setting of chronic stimulation, with minimal expression on resting cells of the immune system (50). PD-1 binds two distinct ligands, programmed death-ligand 1 (PD-L1) and PD-L2, members of the B7 family. PD-L1 is expressed constitutively on a wide range of hematopoietic cells, inhibiting T cell cytokine production, as well as nonhematopoietic cells, including tumor cells (51). PD-L2 on the other hand, exhibits much more restricted expression, largely limited to APCs, restraining effector T cell function within inflamed sites and lymphoid organs (52,53). Both ligands are

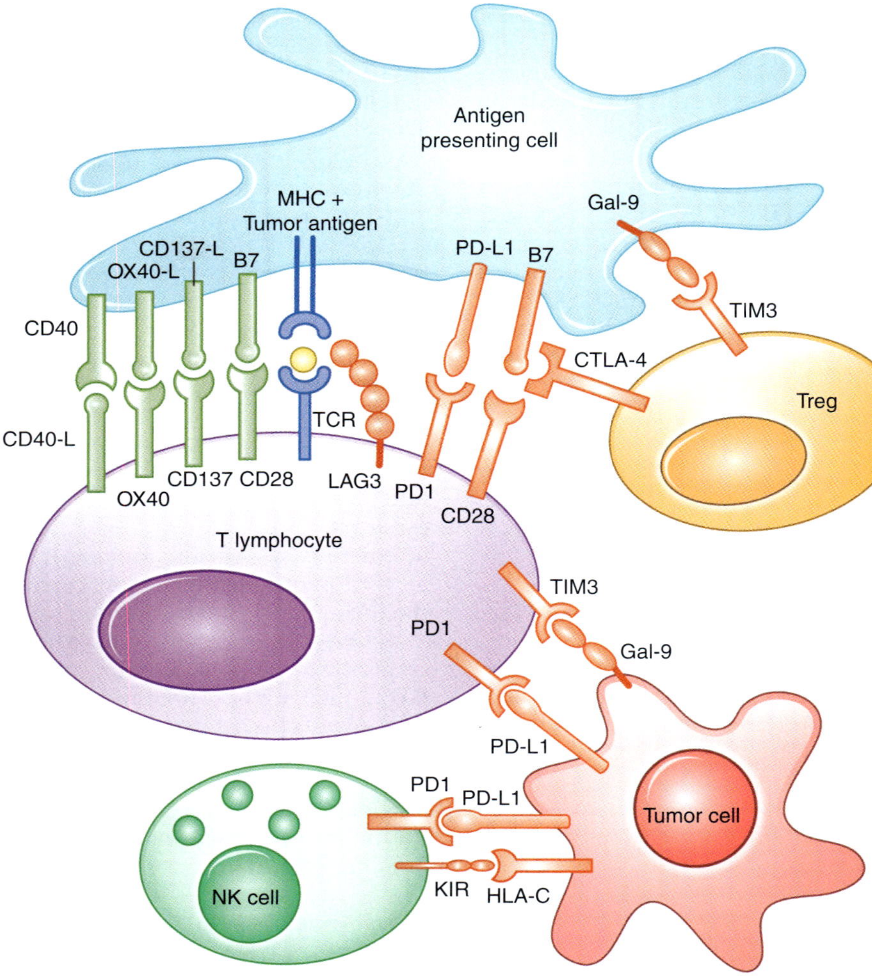

FIGURE 10.3 Monoclonal antibody targets. Multiple pathways, when summated, can trigger either immune recognition and killing, or immune tolerance and evasion. The goal of immunotherapy is to induce an immune stimulatory signal that activates effector T cells and NK cells, while inhibiting the immunosuppressive regulatory T cells (Treg).

Green, costimulatory signals; PD-1, programmed cell death protein 1; PD-L1, programmed death-ligand 1; red, coinhibitory signals.

induced by extrinsic proinflammatory signals, including IFN-γ, TNF-α, granulocyte macrophage colony stimulating factor (GM-CSF), and IL-4, suggesting that the inflammatory TME dictates tumor expression of PD-L1/2 in a feedback inhibitory loop frequently seen in chronic viral infection (54–56). Additionally, intrinsic signaling pathways may lead to PD-L1 overexpression in tumor cells, including the PI3K–AKT pathway (57), and the EGFR-mediated JAK2/STAT1 pathway (58).

In the setting of chronic antigenic stimulation during viral infection, increased PD-1 expression on $CD8^+$ T cells is a marker for an exhausted phenotype, indicating a loss of effector function, including proliferation and cytokine production (59). While PD-L1 expression by APCs has been shown to play a critical role in the induction of suppressive $PD1^+$ Tregs at the tumor periphery (60), the key function of tumor infiltrating Tregs expressing high PD-1 is not clear. In malignant glioma, these cells have impaired suppressive function, yet maintain high secretion of IFN-γ through increased PI3K/AKT activity (61). Blocking the PD-1 pathway with anti-PD-1 mAb drives differentiation toward a more dysfunctional state and increases IFN-γ to further enhance tumor clearance (61). In addition to the high expression of PD-1 on $CD8^+$ and $CD4^+$ T cells, PD-L1 is expressed on 50% to 60% of HNSCC tumors (58,62). PD-L1 is expressed in response to IFN-γ within the TME; therefore, even an immunogenic tumor with abundant IFN present will express PD-L1 and evade T cell mediated killing of tumor cells. While overexpression of PD-L1 inhibits tumor directed T cell cytotoxicity and permits immune evasion and tumor growth, the prognostic significance has been variable, correlating with worse outcomes in some cases (63–66) and improved outcomes in others (67).

LAG3 (also known as CD223), is an inhibitory checkpoint receptor that enhances the function of Tregs, and inhibits $CD8^+$ effector T cell function (68). MHC class II molecules are the only known LAG3 ligands, which are upregulated on some epithelial cancers in response to IFN-γ, but are also expressed on DCs (69). PD-1 and LAG3 are often coexpressed on exhausted or anergic T cells, and dual blockade synergistically reversed this anergy in tumor-specific $CD8^+$ T cells (70). Furthermore, *Pd1*$^{-/-}$*Lag3*$^{-/-}$ double knockout mice can completely reject even poorly immunogenic tumors in a T cell–dependent manner (71).

TIM3 (also known as HAVcr2) is selectively expressed on IFN-γ producing T cells, NK cells, and Tregs, and is closely involved in tumor-induced immune suppression. TIM3 marks the most exhausted or dysfunctional population of $CD8^+$ T cells and NK cells in both solid and hematologic malignancies (72,73), in which approximately 30% of patients with advanced melanoma, non–small cell lung cancer (NSCLC), and follicular B cell non-Hodgkin's lymphoma express TIM3 (74–76). Importantly, T cell exhaustion can be partially reversed with TIM3 blocking antibodies in vitro, restoring up to 30% to 65% of NK-cell function (77). In addition to regulating $CD8^+$ T cell and NK-cell function, TIM3 is expressed on up to 60% of Tregs in the TME in HNSCC patients, compared to less than 20% expression on Tregs of the peripheral blood lymphocytes (78). This is important as it leads to a more tumor-permissive environment, largely due to increased immunosuppressive cytokines and molecules (IL-10, perforin, and granzymes) (79). Interestingly, $TIM3^+$ $CD8^+$ T cells coexpress PD-1 and exhibit greater deficits in both effector cytokine production (IL-2, TNF, and IFN-γ) and cell cycle progression than with expression of either receptor alone (72).

KIR is expressed on NK cells and interacts with HLA molecules on target cells, playing a prominent role in modulating NK-cell immune surveillance and cytotoxicity (80). While most KIRs are inhibitory, there are a limited number of activating KIRs that bind HLA molecules with less affinity (81). Upon binding an autologous matched HLA-C molecule, the inhibitory KIRs recruit SHP-1 and SHP-2 phosphatases, leading to subsequent suppression of activation signals (82). However, when binding a mismatched HLA molecule, or blockade by anti-KIR Ab, the NK cell lyses as a result of the lack of an inhibitory signal. This inhibitory KIR/HLA relationship is overexpressed in patients with melanoma, breast cancer, and chronic leukemia (83). Activating KIRs are associated with better outcomes in leukemia and lymphoma (84,85). While there are limited studies in HNSCC, there seems to be an overexpression of KIR on the NK infiltration in HNSCC patients (86), suggesting this population is an excellent candidate for trials of anti-KIR Ab.

In addition to inhibitory receptors, tumors can manipulate the checkpoint system by downregulating costimulatory signals including CD137, OX40, and CD40. CD137 (also known as 4-1BB) is a costimulatory receptor expressed on the surface of activated T cells, DCs, and NK cells (87,88). When bound to its ligand (CD137-L), activated CD137 promotes antibody-dependent cell-mediated cytotoxicity (ADCC) by NK cells, differentiation of effector T cells, and inhibition of immunosuppressive Tregs (89). OX40 is expressed on the T cell surface, and when activated by its ligand, OX40-L, promotes T cell proliferation, antitumor cytokine secretion (IFN-γ), and enhanced memory T cell function (36). Thirty percent of activated Tregs isolated from HNSCC patients demonstrate OX40 expression in both tumors and tumor-draining lymph node samples, compared to none of the peripheral blood mononuclear cells (90). However, OX40-L expression is low in the tumor, and therefore fails to activate antitumor immune proliferation and cytokine production (91). CD40 is expressed on APCs, as well as nonimmunogenic cells and tumor cells (92,93). Upon binding with its trimeric ligand (CD40-L), the downstream effects are multifaceted and depend on the type of cell expressing CD40 and the TME in which it is expressed (93). Ligand binding on activated $CD40^+$ T cells causes the induction of adaptive immunity and cytokine release, whereas $CD40^+$ macrophages become tumoricidal, and

CD40⁺ tumor cells become apoptotic (92,94–97). Expression of both CD40 and CD40-L decreases with increasing HNSCC stage, and surgical resection results in increased APC expression of CD40 (98).

These immune checkpoint receptors and ligands are dysregulated in the infiltrated immune cells favoring anergy and immunosuppression. Therefore, if manipulated to favor immune activation through mAbs, they can lead to improved immune-mediated killing of cancer cells. However, in addition to poor antigen production, processing, and T cell activation, tolerance can be further enhanced through the immunosuppressive tumor environment, and may prove to be a key mechanism of immune resistance and low response to therapy.

TUMOR MICROENVIRONMENT

Cancers often arise at sites of chronic inflammation, whether from chronic toxin exposure, chronic infection, or inflammatory disease. As the uncontrolled growth of tumor cells invade through natural tissue barriers, the tissue disruption leads to cytokine and chemokine release and the infiltration of inflammatory mediators. While these signals are potentially capable of initiating immune responses, oncogenic pathways within the TME appear to organize the immunologic milieu in a tumor-promoting fashion by generating genotoxic stress, supporting cellular proliferation, increasing angiogenesis, and facilitating tumor cell invasiveness and metastasis (99). Additionally, many recent developments link this tumor-promoting microenvironment to the infiltration of suppressive immune cells including myeloid-derived suppressor cells (MDSCs), Tregs, and tumor-activated macrophages (TAMs), further dampening antitumor immune responses.

The HNSCC TME can support tumor growth through the production of an immunosuppressive environment via the production of various immunosuppressive cytokines (100). TGF-β blocks the function of NK and T cells and plays a key role in the differentiation of suppressive Tregs (101). IL-10 downregulates expression of costimulatory molecules and MHC, whereas IL-6 inhibits DC maturation and activation of NK cells, T cells, neutrophils, and macrophages (102,103), and has been correlated with recurrence and poor survival in HNSCC (104). PGE-2, a prostaglandin that promotes angiogenesis and is produced by many cancers, including HNSCC (105), has also been found to suppress TCR signaling. Vascular endothelial growth factor (VEGF), an inflammatory cytokine released from tumor cells, inhibits the maturation of DC, leading to T cell dysfunction and inactivation and is overexpressed in 90% of HNSCCs (106). EGFR, a tyrosine kinase receptor, also facilitates immunosuppressive effects, including downregulation of HLA and APM components, and the upregulation of suppressive cytokines and ligands on HNSCC cells (107). Indolamine-pyrrole 2,3-dioxygenase or IDO, produced by DC in tumors and tumor draining lymph nodes, as well as tumor cells themselves, induces apoptosis in locally activated T cells through the catabolism of tryptophan (108). These immunosuppressive cytokines and receptors are further driven by an imbalance of STAT proteins, leading toward increased levels of activated STAT3, promoting immunosuppressive pathways and cell survival, while decreased STAT1 impairs antigen presentation (109).

Additionally, the immunosuppressive cytokines and chemokines recruit a skewed cellular population of tumor-infiltrating lymphocytes (TILs), favoring immunosuppression. One of the major cellular components of the TME is the immunosuppressive CD4⁺ Foxp3+ Treg. Tregs have emerged as a central player in tolerance to tumor antigens as well as downregulation of immune responses (78). Through the production of IL-10 and TGF-β, and the consumption of IL-2, Tregs promote cancer progression by causing anergy, apoptosis, and cell cycle arrest of activated T cells and inhibit the action of DCs, NK cells, and B cells. High numbers of Tregs are seen in both the periphery and the tumor infiltration in head and neck cancer (HNC) patients (78,110), and this finding is correlated with poor survival (111,112). Tregs in the HNC TME also express the immune checkpoint inhibitors CTLA4, TIM-3, and PD-1, as well as the immunosuppressive molecules CD39 and TGF-β, collectively leading to an anergic state (78).

Another major cellular component of the TME is MDSCs, a group of immature myeloid cells with potent immunosuppressive potential. Recent reports show that HNSCC patients have elevated numbers of MDSCs in the blood, lymph nodes, and tumors, and can suppress effector T cell function through PD-L1 expression, TGF-β release, arginase and nitric oxide synthase activity, depletion of key amino acids, and Treg induction (113). Additionally, immature monocytes or macrophages have the ability to differentiate into various phenotypes depending on the interactions they make with various growth factors, cytokines, and chemokines within their particular environment, including the TAMs, with the antitumor M1-phenotype, and tumor-promoting M2-phenotype. However, within the HNSCC TME, the macrophage population is dominated by the M2-phenotype, which produces tumor-permissive cytokines EGF, IL-6, and IL-10; promotes angiogenesis, cell invasiveness, and metastasis; and correlates with worse clinical outcomes (114,115).

The composition of the TME has translation into prognostic ability, with improved prognosis with infiltration of IFN-γ producing $CD4^+$ T cells and $CD8^+$ T cells, and the presence of IFN-γ and TNF-α, all promoting tumor control (116). About 50% of carcinogen-associated HNSCCs, and a higher proportion of HPV-associated HNSCCs, demonstrated $CD8^+$ TIL infiltration (117,118). Analysis of TCGA supports that a significant subset of HNSCCs demonstrate a gene expression profile consistent with elevated $CD8^+$ TIL presence and activation (119). HNSCCs demonstrating a higher number of TILs respond better to definitive chemoradiotherapy (120), and have better outcomes following surgery with adjuvant therapy (121). That HPV-associated HNSCC demonstrates in general a higher degree of immunogenicity is not surprising; the observation that virally induced malignancies are more likely to induce deregulated immune responses than sporadic or carcinogen-induced cancer was made decades ago (122). The type and density of tumor infiltrate can even have more prognostic ability than tumor staging and oncogene expression in colon and lung cancers (123).

The physical barriers of immune attack cannot be ignored. Interstitial pressure within a solid tumor is created from cellular proliferation, permeable vasculature, and lack of lymphatic drainage (124), and can prevent lymphocyte infiltration and can lead to geographic variability in lymphocyte distribution. Additionally, the hypoxic TME can suppress immune cell function (125), and when vascularity is normalized, the tumors can become more sensitive to immune activating treatments (126).

TARGETS OF IMMUNOTHERAPY IN HNSCC

Understanding that the immune system is not only responsible for the recognition and destruction of cancer cells, but also to shape cancer immunogenicity, we can now attempt to control cancer through immunological means. Based on restoring key signaling pathways of the host immune system to counteract immune escape by malignant cells, cancer immunotherapy shows potential for durable responses with less adverse effects than conventional treatments. To be effective, immunotherapies will have to increase the quality or quantity of immune effector cells, increase antigen expression and effector cell activation, and/or eliminate cancer-induced immunosuppressive mechanisms and the environment in which they grow. There are many forms of immunotherapy available, including tumor-specific monoclonal antibodies, immune-modulating antibodies, vaccines, oncolytic viruses, and adoptive cell transfer.

TUMOR-TARGETED MONOCLONAL ANTIBODIES

Cetuximab, a chimeric murine/human IgG1 mAb blocking EGFR, can be viewed as an immunotherapeutic agent. Cetuximab activity largely lies within the activation of Fc gamma receptor (FcγR), leading to ADCC, and subsequent enhancement of antigen processing (127–130). This leads to DC maturation and activation of cytotoxic T lymphocytes (CTLs), linking innate and adaptive tumor immunity (36,131,132). Because EGFR is highly expressed in tumor cells, cetuximab could therefore overcome the immunosuppressive environment in HNSCC and increase clinical response to cancer treatment. However, patients treated with cetuximab have demonstrated an increase in suppressive regulatory T cells (Tregs) that impair ADCC, translating into modest 10% to 13% response rates when used as a monotherapy (131,133,134). When combined with the CTLA4 inhibitor ipilimumab, EGFR-antagonism was able to overcome this suppression and showed enhanced ADCC (134). This has stressed the need for further investigation into active immunomodulating agents, such as the inhibitory and costimulatory immune checkpoint receptors and their ligands and are the focus of the majority of clinical trials in HNSCC today.

IMMUNE CHECKPOINT RECEPTORS

It is now evident that tumors exploit certain immune checkpoint pathways as a major mechanism of immune evasion, particularly against tumor-specific T cells. Because many of these checkpoints are induced by ligand–receptor interactions, they can be blocked by antibodies or modulated by recombinant forms of ligands or receptors. The real breakthrough in immunotherapy came in 2010, with the development of immune checkpoint monoclonal antibodies. The first to be approved by the FDA in 2011 was ipilimumab, a CTLA4-blocking mAb, approved for metastatic melanoma. This has opened up new possibilities for anticancer immunotherapy in other malignancies, such as HNSCC.

Many of these agents have been developed and are being studied clinically in HNSCC, such as CTLA4, PD-1/PD-L1, LAG3, TIM3, CD137, and OX40 among others. In light of the mounting evidence in their effectiveness, the PD-1 blocking mAbs, pembrolizumab, and nivolumab were FDA approved for HNSCC in 2016 (Table 10.1).

VACCINES

Based on priming the adaptive immune system against pathogens, vaccines have received considerable interest for cancer treatment due to their capacity of inducing a robust immune response, satisfactory safety profile, low cost, and easy production (135). The viral oncogenes E6 and E7 responsible for HPV-positive cancers are ideal targets for vaccine mediated immune strategies. The primary goal of prophylactic vaccination is to induce high titers of tumor-specific neutralizing antibodies capable of preventing initial infections. In contrast, therapeutic vaccines focus on the generation of $CD8^+$ tumor-specific T cell immune response. Various vaccination techniques have been developed and are under preclinical investigations and clinical trials for both HPV-positive and -negative cancers. DNA vaccines produce nonliving antigens able to induce $CD4^+$ and $CD8^+$ T cell and B cell immunity. Peptide vaccines incorporate amino acid sequences that are synthesized to form an immunogenic peptide molecule representing the specific epitope of a tumor specific antigen that binds onto HLA, activating CTL (136). DC vaccines are produced from culturing ex vivo DCs and

TABLE 10.1

Immune Checkpoint Inhibitors in Development for HNSCC

Name	Sponsor	Isotype	Target	Status of Development in HNSCC
Atezolizumab	Genentech	IgG1	PD-L1	Phase I trials
Avelumab	Merck KGaA and Pfizer	IgG1	PD-L1	Phase III trials in locally advanced HNSCC
Durvalumab	AstraZeneca/ MedImmune	IgG1	PD-L1	Phase III trials in recurrent or metastatic HNSCC
Ipilimumab	Bristol-Myers Squibb	IgG1	CTLA4	Phase III trials in combination regimens in recurrent or metastatic HNSCC
Nivolumab	Bristol-Myers Squibb and Ono	IgG4	PD-1	FDA approved in recurrent or metastatic HNSCC in patients who have progressed after platinum Phase II and III trials in first-line recurrent or metastatic and locally advanced HNSCC
Pembrolizumab	Merck/MSD	IgG4	PD-1	FDA approved in recurrent or metastatic HNSCC in patients who have progressed after platinum. Phase II and III trials in first-line recurrent or metastatic and locally advanced HNSCC
Tremelimumab	AstraZeneca	IgG2	CTLA4	Phase III trials in combination regimens in recurrent or metastatic HNSCC

FDA, Food and Drug Administration; HNSCC, head and neck squamous cell carcinoma; PD-1, programmed cell death protein 1; PD-L1, programmed death-ligand 1.

loading with tumor-specific antigens, and they are injected back into the patient after maturation and activation, usually into the tumor or into lymphocytes (37). Several different vaccine approaches have shown promise in early clinical trials in patients with HNSCC, with evidence of induction of antitumor immunity and acceptable safety profiles.

ONCOLYTIC VIRAL THERAPY

Intratumoral oncolytic viral therapy uses naturally occurring or modified viruses to infect and kill tumor cells as well as stimulate the host antitumor immune response. Talimogene laherparepvec (T-VEC) is an attenuated herpes simplex virus engineered to express GM-CSF in replicating tumor cells to induce host immunity. T-VEC is the first oncolytic virus to be approved for melanoma in the United States, Europe, and Australia. With increased IFN-γ and TNF-α production, T-VEC can promote effector T cell influx and reduce Treg suppression, restoring the immunosuppressive TME (137). This has led to early phase trials in combination with pembrolizumab in HNSCC (NCT02626000; Table 10.2), and with ipilimumab in melanoma (NCT01740297).

ADOPTIVE T CELL THERAPY (ACT)

Another promising strategy to activate the immune system is through adoptive T cell transfer. This technique involves harvesting and in vitro expansion of the patient's own tumor antigen specific T cells, and subsequently reintroducing these cells back into the patient to enhance immunity and improve anticancer responses (138). Early phase trials are ongoing for ACT in both HPV-positive and -negative HNSCC with promising results thus far.

THE RATIONALE FOR COMBINATION THERAPIES

CYTOTOXIC-INDUCED IMMUNOGENIC CELL DEATH AND IMMUNOGENIC MODULATION

The traditional dogma of radiobiology states that cytotoxicity results from DNA double strand breaks, leading to cell death. The formative work by Zitvogel and Kroemer enhanced the understanding of radiation-induced cell death to include roles of the host immune system and the tumor microenvironment (139). Chemotherapy and radiotherapy not only lead to tumor cell death, but both induce "immunogenic cell death" of cancer cells. After exposure to certain cytotoxic agents, dying cancer cells release endogenous "danger signals," or DAMPs, that are then recognized by the APCs (such as DCs), followed by the activation of T cell mediated adaptive immunity (140). Released DAMPs that are hallmarks of immunogenic cell death include adenosine triphosphate (ATP) and high mobility group protein B1 (HMGB1), and molecules expressed on the surface of dying cells include calreticulin, heat-shock proteins (Hsp90 and HSP70), and endoplasmic reticulum (ER) sessile proteins (141). Calreticulin, released early in cell death, is a potent phagocytosis signal to DCs, thus facilitating their tumor antigen presentation and activation of cytotoxic T cells (139). HMGB1 release during the late stages of cell death initiates powerful inflammatory response by binding to different surface receptors on APCs, including TLR4, and TIM3, stimulating the production of proinflammatory cytokines (142). ATP binds the P2Y2 receptor on phagocytes and induces migration into inflamed sites (143). Furthermore, radiation triggers ATP release through the interaction with the P2X7 receptor, leading to the secretion of the proinflammatory IL-1β. Cytotoxic therapy thus increases antigen presentation from cancer cells as well as amplifying cytokine expression (102,144).

Additionally, accumulating evidence demonstrates that the surviving tumor cells recovering from conventional cytotoxic cancer therapies become more amenable to immune-mediated killing and induces a more immunostimulatory environment, termed "immunogenic modulation" (145,146). This encompasses a variety of molecular alterations to tumor cells, including the downregulation of antiapoptotic/survival genes, modulation of APM components, and upregulating immune relevant surface proteins. These phenotypic changes translated into increased tumor sensitivity to T cell mediated lysis after low doses of chemotherapy or radiation (147,148). Even though these antitumor immune responses are noncurative in themselves, they can, however, be used in synergistic regimens with immunotherapeutic agents to improve their efficacy.

The immunogenic properties induced by cytotoxic therapies have been shown in several preclinical models to act synergistically with such immune checkpoint receptor inhibitors such as anti-CTLA4 agents and anti-PD-1

TABLE 10.2

Ongoing and Completed Trials of Immune Checkpoint Inhibitors in Recurrent or Metastatic HNSCC

Trial	Agent(s)	Immune Target	Phase	Population
Second Line				
KEYNOTE-012 (NCT01848834)	Pembrolizumab	PD-1	Ib	Previously untreated recurrent or metastatic HNSCC, ≥6 months since last dose of platinum, or recurrent and metastatic, platinum failure
KEYNOTE-055 (NCT02255097)	Pembrolizumab	PD-1	II	Recurrent or metastatic, platinum failure
KEYNOTE-040 (NCT02252042)	Pembrolizumab vs. investigator's choice standard of care therapy (docetaxel, methotrexate, cetuximab)	PD-1	III	Recurrent or metastatic, platinum failure
CheckMate-141 (NCT02105636)	Nivolumab vs. investigator's choice standard of care therapy (docetaxel, methotrexate, cetuximab)	PD-1	III	Recurrent or metastatic, platinum failure
CheckMate-714 (NCT02823574)	Nivolumab vs. nivolumab and ipilimumab	PD-1 CTLA4	II	(a) recurrent or metastatic, platinum-refractory, (b) recurrent or metastatic, platinum-eligible
HAWK (NCT02207530)	Durvalumab	PD-L1	II	Recurrent or metastatic, platinum failure PD-L1 positive
CONDOR (NCT02319044)	Durvalumab vs. tremelimumab vs. durvalumab and tremelimumab	PD-1 CTLA4	II	Recurrent or metastatic, platinum failure PD-L1 negative
EAGLE (NCT02369874)	Durvalumab vs. durvalumab and tremelimumab vs. standard of care chemotherapy (taxane, methotrexate, cetuximab, fluoropyrimidine)	PD-L1 CTLA4	III	Recurrent or metastatic, platinum failure

(*continued*)

TABLE 10.2 (*continued*)

Ongoing and Completed Trials of Immune Checkpoint Inhibitors in Recurrent or Metastatic HNSCC

Trial	Agent(s)	Immune Target	Phase	Population
First Line				
KEYNOTE-048 (NCT02358031)	Pembrolizumab vs. pembrolizumab with carboplatin and 5-fluorouracil vs. EXTREME	PD-1	III	Previously untreated recurrent/ metastatic HNSCC, ≥6 months since last dose of platinum
CheckMate-651 (NCT02741570)	Nivolumab and ipilimumab vs. EXTREME	PD-1 CTLA4	III	Previously untreated recurrent/ metastatic HNSCC, ≥6 months since last dose of platinum
KESTREL (NCT02551159)	Durvalumab vs. durvalumab and tremelimumab vs. EXTREME	PDL-1 CTLA4	III	Previously untreated recurrent/ metastatic HNSCC, ≥6 months since last dose of platinum

HNSCC, head and neck squamous cell carcinoma; PD-1, programmed cell death protein 1; PD-L1, programmed death-ligand 1.

agents. In fact, these studies show in some cases an amplified clearance of tumor compared to cytotoxic chemotherapy and radiation alone (149). Studies are under way that investigate the optimal dosage and fractionation regimens that induce adaptive immune responses; however, tumors may also develop resistance mechanisms during this inflammatory response phase (150). Preclinical models have shown the induction of PD-L1 expression in tumors following radiotherapy, highlighting the possible resistance mechanisms to conventional treatments and how we can overcome this resistance by adding immune-modulating therapies, such as anti-PD-1 mAb to conventional cytotoxic regimens.

While conventional cytotoxic therapies have frequent and significant acute and lifelong side effects, immunotherapy has thus far shown to be safely tolerated with manageable side effects. Therefore, adding immunotherapy to our clinical repertoire may be a means to not only reduce the cytotoxic load and subsequent side effects, but also increase efficacy and durability compared to cytotoxic treatment alone. These findings have translated into promising clinical benefits for HNSCC patients and are the basis of many clinical trials under way as discussed in the following.

COMBINATION IMMUNOTHERAPY

Immunotherapy agents have rapidly been entering the oncologic treatment armamentarium with the success of agents such as nivolumab and ipilimumab. Currently, there are over 300 active trials using immunotherapy agents for carcinoma (clinicaltrials.gov queried 1/2/2017). Despite significant promise, clinical benefit of these immunomodulatory agents as a monotherapy has been limited thus far. As tumor cells have gained multiple layers of compensatory immune resistance, overcoming one is often not sufficient to eradicate the tumor. However, recent evidence suggests that targeted blockade of multiple immunosuppressive pathways can induce synergistic and effective antitumor responses.

T cell exhaustion leads to upregulation of multiple immune checkpoint inhibitory

receptors, including CTLA4, PD-1, TIM3, and many more. Blockade with monocolonal antibodies of just one pathway may effectively remove this inhibitory signal, only to have a separate but equally powerful inhibitory path unaffected, leaving the T cell just as dysfunctional. However, removal of multiple suppressive signals acting on unique resistant pathways may overcome the net inhibition and lead to T cell activation and immune attack. Many preclinical studies and clinical trials have looked into the combination of immunotherapy agents with clear differences between their therapeutic approaches, including CTLA4, an influencer of T cell activation and proliferation, with the PD-1/PDL1 axis, which is responsible for T cell function and cytolysis. Preclinical models support a role for reversing T cell exhaustion and increasing T cell stimulation through cell proliferation and chemokine production as a means to effectively activate the anticancer fighting properties of T cells (151). Indeed, this was translated to a triple-arm phase III trial in malignant melanoma, studying the combination regimen of anti-PD-1 antibody nivolumab and anti-CTLA4 antibody ipilimumab versus monotherapy. Combined therapy had a progression-free survival (PFS) of 11.5 months, compared to 6.9 months in the nivolumab-only arm and 2.9 months in the ipilimumab-only arm, leading to FDA approval for the treatment of malignant melanoma (152). Other combinations with inhibitory checkpoints, such as PD-1 with TIM3 or LAG3, may also provide increased antitumor activity. Additionally, improved efficacy is seen in combinations of PD-1 blockade with agonistic antibodies for OX40 or CD137, likely due to alterations in Treg cells and changes in the ratio of effector to regulatory T cells (153,154).

Other resistance mechanisms have been acquired by tumor cells to circumvent T cell killing that may render monotherapy ineffective, including cytokine signaling and the immunosuppressive TME. For example, the production of IFN-γ by activated T cells in the tumor microenvironment induces the upregulation of PD-L1 on tumor cells (155). The various signaling mechanisms and cells within the TME produce a variety of changes that argues for the need for combination immunotherapy agents, such as VEGF and IDO. Tumor vasculature is known to exert immunosuppressive effects through many different mechanisms, including expression of immunosuppressive ligands and downregulation of adhesion molecules. Therefore, when used in combination, VEGF inhibition could augment the activity of immunomodulatory antibodies. In a clinical trial combining ipilimumab with VEGF inhibitor bevacizumab, there was a 67% disease control rate and increased tumor lymphocyte infiltration (156). IDO, on the other hand, is expressed by many cancers and inhibits immune responses and promotes Treg differentiation and is a possible resistance mechanism to anti-CTLA4 immunotherapy. Preclinical studies of ipilimumab combined with IDO inhibitors show increased lymphocyte infiltration and increased response to therapy (157).

While the major focus in immunology today has been on T cell modulation and adaptive immunity, targeting the innate immune system, a population of cells that are much less suppressed in the TME, has become an attractive option for anticancer therapy. NK cells, a component of the innate immune system, are capable of spontaneously destroying cancer cells without prior sensitization in contrast to T cells of the adaptive immune system, and are garnering more attention as new agents are being developed. Targeting multiple lymphocyte populations, as well as tumor-targeted agents, can be an effective approach to increase both the innate and adaptive immune response. For instance, CD137 stimulates T cells as well as augments NK-cell activity and is upregulated on NK cells when exposed to cetuximab coated EGFR expressing HN cell lines (158). Therefore, CD137 may be used in combination with cetuximab to target both the tumor and the host immune system to enhance NK-mediated ADCC. Additionally, blocking KIR, which is heavily upregulated on infiltrating NK cells of HNSCC patients, is another approach to improve responsiveness to anti-EGFR treatments (86,159).

CLINICAL DATA WITH IMMUNE CHECKPOINT INHIBITORS IN RECURRENT OR METASTATIC HNSCC

Patients with recurrent or metastatic HNSCC have a poor prognosis. The cornerstone of therapy for these patients has traditionally been a platinum (cisplatin or carboplatin) based regimen. The current standard first-line treatment regimen is the combination of platinum, 5-fluorouracil (5-FU), and cetuximab followed

by maintenance cetuximab until progressive disease (the "EXTREME" regimen) (160). Patients who progress after a platinum-based regimen are usually treated with single-agent chemotherapy with response rates of less than 10% and median overall survival of about 5 to 6 months. Therefore, new treatment options for platinum-refractory disease are sorely needed. It is within this patient group that immunotherapies have garnered their first positive results and regulatory approvals. Initial clinical results have been encouraging and indicated that durable responses and even long-term survival are achievable for a small fraction of patients. Moreover, unique but rare treatment-related toxicities that relate to autoimmune phenomena have emerged. We review available efficacy and safety results with immune checkpoint inhibitors, namely, the anti-PD-1 monoclonal antibodies pembrolizumab and nivolumab as well as the anti-PD-L1 monoclonal antibody durvalumab, and planned clinical trials with immunotherapy in HNSCC.

PEMBROLIZUMAB

Pembrolizumab was initially tested in HNSCC in the context of KEYNOTE-012 trial, a phase Ib multicohort study of pembrolizumab in advanced solid tumor malignancies that enrolled a total of 192 patients with recurrent or metastatic HNSCC (161). The initial cohort of this study (n =60) selected patients for PD-L1 positivity (78% had PD-L1 positive tumors) and used a pembrolizumab dose of 10 mg/kg given intravenously every 2 weeks, whereas a subsequent expansion cohort (n = 132) enrolled patients irrespective of PD-L1 tumor status and employed a fixed dose of pembrolizumab at 200 mg administered intravenously every 3 weeks. Results from the first cohort of 60 patients showed an objective response rate of 18% by central review (162). HPV-driven disease appeared to have had a somewhat greater response rate of 25% versus 14%. Median time to response was 8 weeks with a median duration of response of 53 weeks. Although the median PFS was only 2 months, the median overall survival was 13 months, with 1-year overall survival of 51%. Therefore, pembrolizumab produced many durable responses and was associated with an encouraging overall survival. Similarly, in the expansion cohort of KEYNOTE-012 there was an objective response rate of 18% (by central review), median PFS of 2 months, 6-month PFS of 23%, median overall survival of 8 months, and 6-month overall survival of 59% (161). No cases of pseudoprogression were documented in patients treated in the expansion cohort.

Pembrolizumab was well-tolerated in recurrent or metastatic HNSCC with rare autoimmune toxicities. A combined analysis that included all 192 patients treated with pembrolizumab in KEYNOTE-012 (163) reported a 13% incidence of treatment-related grade 3-4 adverse events. These events included increased transaminases (2%), fatigue (1%), and pneumonitis (1%). This combined analysis showed an objective response rate of 18%, median overall survival of 8 months, and median PFS of 2 months. Data from the KEYNOTE-012 trial led to the accelerated FDA approval of pembrolizumab for patients with recurrent or metastatic HNSCC with disease progression on or after platinum-containing therapy in August 2016.

PD-L1 expression was evaluated as a predictor of pembrolizumab efficacy in KEYNOTE-012. In the expansion cohort as well the analysis of all 192 patients treated with pembrolizumab, PD-L1 expression in the tumor cells alone did not correlate with response or survival. However, increased PD-L1 expression in both tumor cells and immune cells (using a cutoff of 1% or more) was associated with better response and overall survival (161,164).

A subsequent single-arm phase II trial of pembrolizumab in the second-line treatment of HNSCC (KEYNOTE-055) enrolled 171 patients who had progression after receiving platinum and cetuximab. Patients received 200 mg intravenously every 3 weeks until progression or a maximum of 24 months (165). This study reported an objective response rate of 16% and median overall survival of 8 months with a 6-month overall survival of 65%. The median PFS was 2.1 months but the duration of response averaged at 8 months (with a range of 2 to 12+ months). Overall response rates were similar in HPV-positive and HPV-negative patients (16% vs. 15%).

In KEYNOTE-055 there was an analysis of outcomes by PD-L1 expression measured on both tumor and mononuclear inflammatory cells, as was done in the previous KEYNOTE-012 trial; the percentage of cells staining positively was reported as the combined positive score (CPS). In contrast with KEYNOTE-012 results, there wereno statistically significant differences in efficacy parameters between patients with PD-L1 positive and PD-L1 negative tumors. Overall response rates

for patients with a CPS of ≥1% was 18% versus a response rate of 12% for those whose CPS was <1%. When the CPS cutoff was moved to 50%, patients with CPS ≥50% had a response rate of 27% versus 13% for patients with CPS <50%. However, this difference also did not reach statistical significance.

A confirmatory phase III trial of pembrolizumab versus standard therapy in the second-line setting (KEYNOTE-040) recently reported results (166). This trial had a similar design to the phase III CheckMate 141 trial of nivolumab; it enrolled patients who had recurrent or metastatic disease with progression after a platinum-containing regimen for recurrent or metastatic HNSCC (no more than 2 prior regimens) or recurrence within 3 to 6 months of multimodal therapy using platinum. Patients were randomized in a 1:1 ratio to receive either flat dosing of pembrolizumab 200 mg intravenously for up to 2 years or the investigator's choice of methotrexate, docetaxel, or cetuximab. The overall survival in the intent-to-treat population was 8.4 months for pembrolizumab and 7.1 months for investigator choice therapy, with a hazard ratio (HR) of 0.81 (95% CI: 0.66–0.99; p = .0204) (166). This failed to meet the prespecified efficacy boundary. The objective response rate with pembrolizumab was 14.6% and standard of care treatment was 10.1% (p = .061). For patients with response, the median duration of response for pembrolizumab was 18.4 months as compared to only 5 months with standard of care. Adverse events were lower in the pembrolizumab arm with 13.4% of patients experiencing grade 3-5 treatment-related adverse events versus 36.3% in the control group. While the prespecified end point was not reached, the trend toward overall survival benefit and impressive duration of response with pembrolizumab as well as its favorable toxicity profile are supportive of the role of pembrolizumab in HNSCC. The inability to reach the prespecified end point could be due to various reasons, including the better than anticipated survival seen in the control arm, which may be related to the use of subsequent immunotherapy by 12.5% of patients in the control arm.

Of major interest was the analysis by PD-L1 expression using CPS and tumor proportion score (TPS), which were secondary study objectives. In patients with tumors with CPS ≥1%, pembrolizumab was associated in better overall survival than standard therapy with a HR of 0.75 (95% CI: 0.59–0.95; p = .0078); the 1-year survival was 40.1% versus 26.7% and the median overall survival 8.7 months versus 7.1 months. An even larger survival benefit with pembrolizumab was evident in the smaller subset of patients with TPS ≥50% (n = 129) with a HR of 0.54 (95% CI: 0.35–0.82; p = .00017), 1-year overall survival of 46.6% versus 25.8%, and median overall survival of 11.6 months versus 7.9 months. The response rate and the PFS was also better with pembrolizumab versus standard of care in the TPS 50% or above group. These results suggest that benefit with pembrolizumab is more pronounced in patients with strongly PD-L1 positive tumors. Nivolumab efficacy, on the other hand, was not as significantly dependent on PD-L1 expression in the CheckMate 141 trial, the results of which are reviewed in the following.

Pembrolizumab is being studied in the first-line treatment of recurrent or metastatic HNSCC (i.e., for previously untreated patients or for those who have relapsed 6 months or more after platinum-based chemotherapy in the setting of prior combined modality therapy for potentially curable HNSCC, and, therefore, are considered platinum sensitive). KEYNOTE-048, an international, phase III, randomized trial randomizes patients in three arms: (a) the standard combination of platinum, 5-FU, and cetuximab (EXTREME regimen), (b) platinum, 5-FU plus pembrolizumab, or (c) pembrolizumab alone (NCT02358031).

NIVOLUMAB

Nivolumab was evaluated in CheckMate 141, a randomized, controlled, phase III clinical trial in HNSCC (167). In this trial, 361 patients with recurrent or metastatic HNSCC who had failed platinum-based chemotherapy within the previous 6 months were assigned in a 2:1 ratio to receive either nivolumab at a dose of 3 mg/kg every 2 weeks or standard single-agent investigator's choice systemic therapy (methotrexate, docetaxel, or cetuximab). No minimum PD-L1 tumor expression level was required. The study met its primary end point, overall survival. Median overall survival was 7.5 months for the nivolumab arm versus 5.1 months for the investigator's choice group, with a HR of 0.70 (97.73% CI: 0.51–0.96; p = .01). Updated information with a median follow-up of 11.4 months for these groups confirmed the difference with an overall survival of 7.7 months versus 5.1 months (HR 0.71,

$p = .0048$ [168]). At 1 year, the overall survival rates were 36% and 16.6% with nivolumab and investigator's choice therapy, respectively, and at 18 months 21.5% and 8.3%, respectively. However, there were no statistically significant differences in PFS (median PFS was 2 months with nivolumab vs. 2.3 months with standard therapy) or the objective response rate (13.3% with nivolumab vs. 5.8% with standard therapy). Grade 3-4 treatment-related adverse events occurred in 13.1% of the nivolumab group versus 35.1% of the standard of care therapy group. Nivolumab preserved physical, role, and social functioning, whereas patients treated with standard of care therapy had decrements in these quality of life measures. CheckMate 141 showed survival benefit with nivolumab regardless of PD-L1 positivity or HPV status; however, the study was not powered to assess treatment effect in subgroups. In 260 of 361 patients who could be evaluated for PD-L1, 57% had a positive PD-L1 expression level (1% or more). In patients with tumors with a PD-L1 expression level of 1% or more, the HR for death among patients treated with nivolumab versus standard therapy was 0.55 (95% CI: 0.36–0.83), whereas in patients with tumors with a PD-L1 expression level of less than 1%, the HR was 0.89 (95% CI: 0.54–1.45; $p = .17$ for interaction). Further clinical studies will have to identify useful biomarkers for patient selection for nivolumab therapy. Based on the results of the CheckMate 141 trial, the FDA approved nivolumab monotherapy for patients with recurrent or metastatic HNSCC who have progressed after platinum-based therapy in November 2016.

Currently, nivolumab is under further investigation in several clinical trials in HNSCC, including CheckMate 651 (NCT02741570) and CheckMate 714 (NCT02823574), which are investigating the combination of nivolumab with the CTLA4 inhibitor ipilimumab. CheckMate 651 is an ongoing phase III trial in the first-line treatment of recurrent or metastatic HNSCC; patients are randomized to receive either standard of care EXTREME regimen, that is, platinum (cisplatin or carboplatin), 5-FU, and cetuximab or the combination of nivolumab and ipilimumab. In CheckMate 714, a phase II trial, patients with recurrent HNSCC are randomized to receive either nivolumab with ipilimumab or nivolumab with placebo. The target population is a cohort of platinum-refractory patients and a cohort of platinum-sensitive patients.

DURVALUMAB

Durvalumab is a monoclonal antibody directed against PD-L1. A phase I study of durvalumab monotherapy in patients with advanced solid tumors (NCT01693562) included a cohort of 62 HNSCC patients who had been treated with a median of three prior lines of therapy (169). The objective response rate was 11%, with a higher response of 18% in PD-L1 positive patients (8% in PD-L1 negative) and HPV-negative versus HPV-positive patients (16% vs. 4%). Survival results were promising with a median overall survival of 8.9 months, and a 6-month and 1-year overall survival of 62% and 42%, respectively. Grade 3 or more drug-related adverse events (AEs) were seen in only 8% of patients (169).

Several studies with durvalumab are ongoing in recurrent or metastatic HNSCC. A phase II trial (HAWK) has been conducted evaluating durvalumab monotherapy in platinum-refractory recurrent or metastatic disease, PD-L1 positive (170). Treatment continued until disease progression, intolerable toxicity, or a maximum of 12 months of therapy completed. The response rate for durvalumab was 18% with a median PFS of 2.1 months, and a median overall survival of 7.1 months. Grade 3/4 AEs occurred in only 8% of patients and there were no treatment-related deaths. This trial also explored the impact of HPV status on response to therapy, showing a response rate of 29.4% in HPV-positive disease versus 10.8% in negative, demonstrating a trend in the opposite direction compared with the data presented from the previous phase 1 trial of durvalumab.

Durvalumab is also under investigation in combination with the anti-CTLA4 antibody tremelimumab. CONDOR is a randomized, open-label, phase II study for patients with PD-L1 negative platinum-refractory recurrent or metastatic HNSCC. Patients are randomized 2:1:1 to durvalumab plus tremelimumab, durvalumab monotherapy, or tremelimumab monotherapy with a primary end point of objective response rate. EAGLE is a phase III trial (NCT02369874) in patients with HNSCC who have progressed after platinum therapy (both PD-L1 positive and negative). Patients are randomized (1:1:1) to one of three arms: durvalumab monotherapy, durvalumab plus tremelimumab, or investigator's choice standard

of care therapy. The coprimary end points are PFS and overall survival. Finally, KESTREL (NCT02551159) is a phase III trial in the first-line treatment of recurrent or metastatic HNSCC that is randomizing patients 2:1:1 to receive durvalumab plus tremelimumab, durvalumab monotherapy, or the EXTREME regimen. The primary end points are PFS and overall survival.

OTHER IMMUNE CHECKPOINT INHIBITORS

Avelumab is a monoclonal antibody directed against PD-L1 that is being investigated in several cancers, including HSNCC. A phase I dose-escalation trial of avelumab included a cohort of patients with HNSCC. Accrual to this cohort has completed and results are pending. A number of avelumab trials have been launched in locally advanced HNSCC (Table 10.3). Phase IA results have also been presented for the PD-L1 directed agent atezolizumab in which 32 patients with failure of their prior therapy were treated with either weight-based or flat dosing of the product. The initial 10 patients were enrolled without selection, but the remaining 22 required expression of PD-L1 on 5% or greater of the tumor-infiltration immune cells. For all patients in the trial, the objective response rate was 22%. A suggestion of a higher response rate for patients with 5% or greater PD-L1 on the immune cells was noted at 24% for patients above this cutoff and 14% for those below it. HPV status did not appear to be associated with this response. The progression free and overall survivals were 2.6 months and 6 months, respectively. The duration of response was 7.4 months for all HNC patients treated in this trial, but up to 26.2 months for those with PD-L1 in 5% or greater of the immune cells. Treatment-related grade 3/4 AEs were reported in 13% of patients.

CLINICAL APPLICATIONS OF IMMUNOTHERAPY IN LOCALLY ADVANCED HNSCC

The successful application of immunotherapy in the recurrent or metastatic setting has also spurred interest in the treatment of locally advanced HNSCC. Treatment for these patients is frequently multimodal and is based on the location and extent of disease; it may incorporate surgery, radiotherapy, and chemotherapy. Unlike the recurrent or metastatic setting, treatment is given with curative intent. The cornerstone of chemotherapy has been cisplatin. However, the gains achieved by cisplatin in both the definitive and adjuvant settings while statistically significant have been modest (171). Moreover, acute and late toxicities can be considerable. With respect to immunotherapies, strategies have focused on either the addition of checkpoint inhibitors to currently accepted regimens or the replacement of traditional chemotherapies with immunotherapy (Table 10.3).

THE COMBINATION OF IMMUNOTHERAPY WITH RADIATION

As discussed previously, radiation has been shown to have several immune-stimulating functions, such as release of tumor antigens, activation and maturation of antigen-presenting cells, redirection of macrophages from an immunosuppressive phenotype to an immune-stimulating phenotype, and recruitment of cytotoxic T cells by inducing expression of chemokines needed for T cell trafficking (172,173). These data suggest that radiation can function as an immune adjunct and may help reverse the immunosuppressive tumor environment. Thus, the combination of immune checkpoint inhibitors and radiotherapy is of major interest for the development of new treatment options in locally advanced HNSCC. Multiple clinical trials are under way looking at this combination in both the definitive and adjuvant setting (Table 10.3).

FUTURE THERAPEUTIC TARGETS OF IMMUNOTHERAPY

Strategies in immunotherapy have been primarily focused on targeting PD-1, PD-L1, and CTLA4. However, as noted previously, cancer immunotherapy has many potential targets beyond these immune checkpoints. Future strategies may include the use of oncolytic viruses, protein, or cells, combination T cell directed therapies, or other therapies (Table 10.4) to both overcome tumor-induced immune suppression and enhance recognition of noninfiltrated or "immunologically inert" tumors. Emerging challenges are the potential toxicities from combination therapies and the appropriate selection of patients and tumors for the optimal therapeutic approach.

TABLE 10.3

Selected Ongoing Clinical Trials of Immune Checkpoint Inhibitors in Locally Advanced HNSCC

Trial	Agent(s)	Targets	Phase	Population	Treatment
Induction/Neoadjuvant					
NCT03021993	Nivolumab	PD-1	II	Oral cavity (T stage 2-4), scheduled for surgical resection, may be recurrent	Nivolumab
IMCISION (NCT03003637)	Nivolumab and ipilimumab	PD-1, CTLA4	Ib/II	T3-4 N0-3 M0 HNSCC (with soft tissue infiltration depth of ≥1 cm) eligible for curative surgery as primary treatment or salvage surgery after failed (chemo)radiation	Nivolumab and ipilimumab
MEDINDUCTION (NCT02997332)	Durvalumab	PD-L1	I	HNSCC amenable to induction chemotherapy according to investigator	Durvalumab + docetaxel + cisplatin + 5-FU
NCT02827838	Durvalumab	PD-L1	Pilot	HNSCC amenable to resection	Durvalumab
Definitive					
NCT02764593, RTOG	Nivolumab	PD-1	I / III	Oropharynx: p16+, >10 pack-years of smoking, T1-2 N2b-N3 or ≤10 pack-years, stage T4 N0-N3 or T1-3N3, or oral cavity, larynx, hypopharynx, or p16-negative oropharynx cancer, stage T1-2 N2a-N3 or T3-4 N0-3	Nivolumab + weekly cisplatin + IMRT, nivolumab + high-dose cisplatin + IMRT, nivolumab + cetuximab + IMRT, nivolumab + IMRT
CA209-931	Nivolumab ipilimumab	PD-1 CTLA4	Pilot	Stage IVA-B disease of the oral cavity, oropharynx (p16-), hypopharynx, or larynx	Nivolumab + ipilimumab + IMRT
NCT02641093	Pembrolizumab	PD-1	II	HNSCC Any T with ≥N2 disease; T4 any N, or T3 oral cavity any N, or any evidence of extracapsular extension on scans	Pembrolizumab given prior to surgery and then with adjuvant therapy (IMRT +/– cisplatin)

(continued)

TABLE 10.3 (*continued*)

Selected Ongoing Clinical Trials of Immune Checkpoint Inhibitors in Locally Advanced HNSCC

Trial	Agent(s)	Targets	Phase	Population	Treatment
NCT02777385	Pembrolizumab	PD-1	II	Surgically unresectable oral cavity; larynx T4 any N, T2-3 and N ≥2a; oropharynx: p16(-) AND T3-4 or ≥ N2a; oropharynx: p16(+) AND one of the following T3 or ≥ N2a AND ≥ 10 pack-years tobacco T4 or N3 disease irrespective of tobacco exposure; unknown primary: p16(-) AND ≥N2a or p16(+) AND one of the following ≥N2a AND ≥10 pack-years tobacco exposure, N3 disease irrespective of tobacco exposure	Cisplatin and IMRT, randomized to receive pembrolizumab either with concurrent chemoradiation or after chemoradiation
NCT02586207	Pembrolizumab	PD-1	Ib	Stage III, IVA, or IVB HNSCC, eligible for curative intent chemoradiotherapy	Pembrolizumab + cisplatin + IMRT
NCT02609503	Pembrolizumab	PD-1	II	Stage III/IV HNSCC who are not eligible for high-dose cisplatin	IMRT + pembrolizumab
NCT02759575	Pembrolizumab	PD-1	I/II	Locally advanced laryngeal squamous cell, T2-3, N0-3	Cisplatin + IMRT + pembrolizumab
NCT01860430	Ipilimumab	CTLA4	Ib	Stage III/IV HNSCC, excluding T1 N1	Cetuximab + ipilimumab + IMRT
NCT03051906	Durvalumab	PD-L1	II	HPV-negative oropharynx and all hypopharynx and larynx: T1-2, N2a-N3 or T3-4, any N, HPV-positive oropharynx: T2-4, N2b-N3	Cetuximab + durvalumab + IMRT
JAVELIN HEAD AND NECK 100 (NCT02952586)	Avelumab	PD-L1	III	HPV-negative disease, stage III, IVa, IVb or nonoropharyngeal HPV-positive disease, stage III, IVa, IVb, or HPV-positive oropharyngeal disease T4, N2c, or N3	High-dose cisplatin + IMRT + avelumab
NCT02938273	Avelumab	PD-L1	I	Locally advanced stage III/IV HNSCC	Cetuximab + avelumab + IMRT
NCT02999087 (REACH)	Avelumab	PD-L1	III	Locally advanced stage III/VI HNSCC	Avelumab + cetuximab + IMRT vs. cisplatin + IMRT (fit patients) or cetuximab + IMRT (unfit patients)

(*continued*)

TABLE 10.3 (*continued*)

Selected Ongoing Clinical Trials of Immune Checkpoint Inhibitors in Locally Advanced HNSCC

Trial	Agent(s)	Targets	Phase	Population	Treatment
Adjuvant					
NCT02775812 (NCI- HN003)	Pembrolizumab	PD-1	I	Stage III/IV HNSCC being treated with definitive cisplatin and radiation	Pembrolizumab with concurrent chemoradiation
PATHWay (NCT02841748)	Pembrolizumab	PD-1	II	Stage III/IV who have completed curative intent therapy	Pembrolizumab *vs.* placebo

5-FU, 5-fluorouracil; HNSCC, head and neck squamous cell carcinoma; IMRT, intensity modulated radiotherapy; PD-1, programmed cell death protein 1; PD-L1, programmed death-ligand 1.

TABLE 10.4

Future Immune Strategies in HNSCC

Agent(s)	Targets	Phase	Being Studied in Combination With
Oncolytic			
ADXS11-001	*Listeria monocytogenes* therapeutic vaccine, E7	I/II	Durvalumab
Ankara vaccine	P53	I	Pembrolizumab
E7 TCR T cells	E7	I	Pembrolizumab
Enadenotucirev	Oncolytic virus	I	Nivolumab
HPVST cells	HPV16/18 E6/E7-specific T lymphocytes	I	Monotherapy Nivolumab
LTX-315	Oncolytic peptide	I	Pembrolizumab Ipilimumab
MAGE-A3/HPV16	Vaccine therapy	I	Montanide
P16_37-63 Peptide (VICORYX-2)	Vaccine therapy	I	
Talimogene Laherparevec	Oncolytic herpesvirus	Ib/III	Pembrolizumab
T Cell Directed			
ABBV-368	OX-40	I	Monotherapy Nivolumab
Urelumab	CD137	Ib	Cetuximab, Nivolumab
Utomilumab	CD137 (AKA 4-1 BB)	Ib	Pembrolizumab
Varlilumab	CD27	I/II	Nivolumab
B Cell Directed			
Acalabrutinib	Bruton's tyrosine kinase	II	Pembrolizumab
Itacitinib (INCB039110)	JAK1	I	Pembrolizumab
Other Immune Targets			
AZD5069	CXCR2	I	Durvalumab
AZD9150	STAT3	I	Durvalumab
Cabiralizumab (FPA008)	CSF1R	Ia/Ib	Nivolumab
Enoblituzumab (MGA271)	B7-H3	I	Pembrolizumab Ipilimumab

(*continued*)

TABLE 10.4 (*continued*)

Future Immune Strategies in HNSCC

Agent(s)	Targets	Phase	Being Studied in Combination With
INC050465	PI3K-delta	I	Pembrolizumab
IPI-549	PI3K-gamma	I/Ib	Monotherapy Nivolumab
Mogamulizumab	CCR4	I	Durvalumab, tremelimumab
Motolimob (VTX-2337)	Toll-like receptor 8 (TLR8)	Ib	Nivolumab
NSH-IL12	IL12	Ib	Avelumab
PLX3397	CSF1R	I/IIa	Pembrolizumab
SD 101	TLR9	I	Pembrolizumab
TAK-659	Dual inhibitor of SYK and FLT-3	Ib	Nivolumab
Microenvironment			
CB-1158	Arginase	I	Monotherapy Nivolumab
Epacadostat	Indoleamine 2,3-dioxygenase (IDO1)	I/II	Nivolumab (ECHO-204) Durvalumab (ECHO-203)
Other Targets			
Azacytidine	Epigenetic modifier	Ib/II	Durvalumab, tremelimumab
MGCD0103	Histone deacetylase inhibitor (epigenetic modifier)	I	Durvalumab

HNSCC, head and neck squamous cell carcinoma; TCR, T cell receptor.

REFERENCES

1. de Costa A-M, Young MR. Immunotherapy for head and neck cancer: advances and deficiencies. *Anti-cancer Drugs*. 2011;22(7):674–681. doi:10.1097/CAD.0b013e328340fd18
2. Burnet FM. The concept of immunological surveillance. *Prog Exp Tumor Res*. 1970;13:1–27.
3. Badoual C, Sandoval F, Pere H, et al. Better understanding tumor-host interaction in head and neck cancer to improve the design and development of immunotherapeutic strategies. *Head Neck*. 2010;32(7):58.
4. Bhatia S, Louie AD, Bhatia R, et al. Solid cancers after bone marrow transplantation. *J Clin Oncol*. 2001;19(2):464–471.
5. Haigentz M. Aerodigestive cancers in HIV infection. *Curr Opin Oncol*. 2005;17(5):474–478.
6. Deeb R, Sharma S, Mahan M, et al. Head and neck cancer in transplant recipients. *Laryngoscope*. 2012;122(7):1566–1569.
7. Schreiber RD, Old LJ, Smyth MJ. Cancer immunoediting: integrating immunity's roles in cancer suppression and promotion. *Science*. 2011;331(6024):1565–1570.
8. Dunn GP, Bruce AT, Ikeda H, et al. Cancer immunoediting: from immunosurveillance to tumor escape. *Nat Immunol*. 2002;3(11):991–998.
9. Koebel CM, Vermi W, Swann JB, et al. Adaptive immunity maintains occult cancer in an equilibrium state. *Nature*. 2007;450(7171):903–907.
10. Chatrchyan S, Khachatryan V, Sirunyan AM, et al. Evidence of *b*-jet quenching in PbPb collisions at $\sqrt{s_{NN}}$ = 2.76 TeV. *Phys Rev Lett*. 2014;113(13):132301.
11. Ljunggren HG, Kärre K. In search of the 'missing self': MHC molecules and NK cell recognition. *Immunol Today*. 1990;11(7):237–244.

12. Duray A, Demoulin S, Hubert P, et al. Immune suppression in head and neck cancers: a review. *Clin Dev Immunol.* 2010;2010:1–15.
13. Campoli M, Ferrone S. HLA antigen changes in malignant cells: epigenetic mechanisms and biologic significance. *Oncogene.* 2008;27(45):5869–5885.
14. Seliger B. Different regulation of MHC class I antigen processing components in human tumors. *J Immunotoxicol.* 2008;5(4):361–367.
15. López-Albaitero A, Nayak JV, Ogino T, et al. Role of antigen-processing machinery in the in vitro resistance of squamous cell carcinoma of the head and neck cells to recognition by CTL. *J Immunol.* 2006;176(6):3402–3409.
16. Ferris RL, Whiteside TL, Ferrone S. Immune escape associated with functional defects in antigen-processing machinery in head and neck cancer. *Clin Cancer Res.* 2006;12(13):3890–3895.
17. Concha-Benavente F, Srivastava R, Ferrone S, et al. Immunological and clinical significance of HLA class I antigen processing machinery component defects in malignant cells. *Oral Oncol.* 2016;58:52–58.
18. Leibowitz MS, Andrade Filho PA, Ferrone S, et al. Deficiency of activated STAT1 in head and neck cancer cells mediates TAP1-dependent escape from cytotoxic T lymphocytes. *Cancer Immunol Immunother.* 2011;60(4):525–535.
19. Ferris RL, Hunt JL, Ferrone S. Human leukocyte antigen (HLA) class I defects in head and neck cancer: molecular mechanisms and clinical significance. *Immunol Res.* 2005;33(2):113–134.
20. Matsui M, Ikeda M, Akatsuka T. High expression of HLA-A2 on an oral squamous cell carcinoma with down-regulated transporter for antigen presentation. *Biochem Biophys Res Commun.* 2001;280(4):1008–1014.
21. Meissner M, Reichert TE, Kunkel M, et al. Defects in the human leukocyte antigen class I antigen processing machinery in head and neck squamous cell carcinoma: association with clinical outcome. *Clin Cancer Res.* 2005;11(7):2552–2560.
22. Ogino T, Shigyo H, Ishii H, et al. HLA class I antigen down-regulation in primary laryngeal squamous cell carcinoma lesions as a poor prognostic marker. *Cancer Res.* 2006;66(18):9281–9289.
23. Ogino T, Bandoh N, Hayashi T, et al. Association of tapasin and HLA class I antigen down-regulation in primary maxillary sinus squamous cell carcinoma lesions with reduced survival of patients. *Clin Cancer Res.* 2003;9(11):4043–4051.
24. Wang T, Niu G, Kortylewski M, et al. Regulation of the innate and adaptive immune responses by Stat-3 signaling in tumor cells. *Nat Med.* 2004;10(1): 48–54.
25. Concha-Benavente F, Srivastava RM, Ferrone S, et al. EGFR-mediated tumor immunoescape: the imbalance between phosphorylated STAT1 and phosphorylated STAT3. *Oncoimmunology.* 2013;2(12):e27215.
26. Leibowitz MS, Srivastava RM, Andrade Filho PA, et al. SHP2 is overexpressed and inhibits pSTAT1-mediated APM component expression, T-cell attracting chemokine secretion, and CTL recognition in head and neck cancer cells. *Clin Cancer Res.* 2013;19(4):798–808.
27. Agazie YM, Hayman MJ. Molecular mechanism for a role of SHP2 in epidermal growth factor receptor signaling. *Mol Cell Biol.* 2003;23(21):7875–7886.
28. Mimura K, Shiraishi K, Mueller A, et al. The MAPK pathway is a predominant regulator of HLA-A expression in esophageal and gastric cancer. *J Immunol.* 2013;191(12):6261–6272.
29. Trivedi S, Concha-Benavente F, Srivastava RM, et al. Immune biomarkers of anti-EGFR monoclonal antibody therapy. *Ann Oncol.* 2015;26(1):40–47.
30. Pollack BP, Sapkota B, Cartee TV. Epidermal growth factor receptor inhibition augments the expression of MHC class I and II genes. *Clin Cancer Res.* 2011;17(13):4400–4413.
31. Srivastava RM, Trivedi S, Concha-Benavente F, et al. STAT1-Induced HLA Class I Upregulation Enhances Immunogenicity and Clinical Response to Anti-EGFR mAb Cetuximab Therapy in HNC Patients. *Cancer Immunol Res.* 2015;3(8):936–945.
32. Chang CC, Campoli M, Ferrone S. Classical and non-classical HLA class I antigen and NK cell-activating ligand changes in malignant cells: current challenges and future directions. *Adv Cancer Res.* 2005;93:189–234.
33. Fletcher EV, Love-Homan L, Sobhakumari A, et al. EGFR inhibition induces proinflammatory cytokines via NOX4 in HNSCC. *Mol Cancer Res.* 2013;11(12):1574–1584.
34. Chatrchyan S, Khachatryan V, Sirunyan AM, et al. Search for invisible decays of Higgs bosons in the vector boson fusion and associated ZH production modes. *Eur Phys J C Part Fields.* 2014;74(8):2980.
35. Chatrchyan S, Khachatryan V, Sirunyan AM, et al. Measurement of WZ and ZZ production in pp collisions at [Formula: see text] in final states with b-tagged jets. *Eur Phys J C Part Fields.* 2014;74(8):2973.
36. Bauman JE, Ferris RL. Integrating novel therapeutic monoclonal antibodies into the management of head and neck cancer. *Cancer.* 2014;120(5):624–632.
37. Ferris RL. Immunology and immunotherapy of head and neck cancer. *J Clin Oncol.* 2015;33(29):3293–3304.
38. Baruah P, Lee M, Odutoye T, et al. Decreased levels of alternative co-stimulatory receptors OX40 and 4-1BB characterise T cells from head and neck cancer patients. *Immunobiology.* 2012;217(7):669–675.
39. Rudd CE, Taylor A, Schneider H. CD28 and CTLA-4 coreceptor expression and signal transduction. *Immunol Rev.* 2009;229(1):12–26.
40. Schwartz RH. Costimulation of T lymphocytes: the role of CD28, CTLA-4, and B7/BB1 in interleukin-2 production and immunotherapy. *Cell.* 1992;71(7):1065–1068.
41. Honeychurch J, Cheadle EJ, Dovedi SJ, et al. Immuno-regulatory antibodies for the treatment of cancer. *Expert Opin Biol Ther.* 2015;15(6):787–801.

42. Alegre ML, Noel PJ, Eisfelder BJ, et al. Regulation of surface and intracellular expression of CTLA4 on mouse T cells. *J Immunol.* 1996;157(11):4762–4770.
43. Chambers CA, Kuhns MS, Allison JP. Cytotoxic T lymphocyte antigen-4 (CTLA-4) regulates primary and secondary peptide-specific CD4(+) T cell responses. *Proc Natl Acad Sci USA.* 1999;96(15):8603–8608.
44. Egen JG, Allison JP. Cytotoxic T lymphocyte antigen-4 accumulation in the immunological synapse is regulated by TCR signal strength. *Immunity.* 2002;16(1):23–35.
45. Takahashi T, Tagami T, Yamazaki S, et al. Immunologic self-tolerance maintained by CD25(+)CD4(+) regulatory T cells constitutively expressing cytotoxic T lymphocyte-associated antigen 4. *J Exp Med.* 2000;192(2):303–310.
46. Wing K, Onishi Y, Prieto-Martin P, et al. CTLA-4 control over Foxp3+ regulatory T cell function. *Science.* 2008;322(5899):271–275.
47. Linsley PS, Greene JL, Brady W, et al. Human B7-1 (CD80) and B7-2 (CD86) bind with similar avidities but distinct kinetics to CD28 and CTLA-4 receptors. *Immunity.* 1994;1. 1((9):793–801.
48. Qureshi OS, Zheng Y, Nakamura K, et al. Trans-endocytosis of CD80 and CD86: a molecular basis for the cell-extrinsic function of CTLA-4. *Science.* 2011;332(6029):600–603.
49. Oderup C, Cederbom L, Makowska A, et al. Cytotoxic T lymphocyte antigen-4-dependent down-modulation of costimulatory molecules on dendritic cells in CD4+ CD25+ regulatory T-cell-mediated suppression. *Immunology.* 2006;118(2):240–249.
50. Keir ME, Butte MJ, Freeman GJ, et al. PD-1 and its ligands in tolerance and immunity. *Annu Rev Immunol.* 2008;26:677–704.
51. Keir ME, Liang SC, Guleria I, et al. Tissue expression of PD-L1 mediates peripheral T cell tolerance. *J Exp Med.* 2006;203(4):883–895.
52. Liang SC, Latchman YE, Buhlmann JE, et al. Regulation of PD-1, PD-L1, and PD-L2 expression during normal and autoimmune responses. *Eur J Immunol.* 2003;33(10):2706–2716.
53. Latchman Y, Wood CR, Chernova T, et al. PD-L2 is a second ligand for PD-1 and inhibits T cell activation. *Nat Immunol.* 2001;2(3):261–268.
54. Freeman GJ, Long AJ, Iwai Y, et al. Engagement of the PD-1 immunoinhibitory receptor by a novel B7 family member leads to negative regulation of lymphocyte activation. *J Exp Med.* 2000;192(7):1027–1034.
55. Eppihimer MJ, Gunn J, Freeman GJ, et al. Expression and regulation of the PD-L1 immunoinhibitory molecule on microvascular endothelial cells. *Microcirculation.* 2002;9(2):133–145.
56. Butte MJ, Keir ME, Phamduy TB, et al. Programmed death-1 ligand 1 interacts specifically with the B7-1 costimulatory molecule to inhibit T cell responses. *Immunity.* 2007;27(1):111–122.
57. Parsa AT, Waldron JS, Panner A, et al. Loss of tumor suppressor PTEN function increases B7-H1 expression and immunoresistance in glioma. *Nat Med.* 2007;13(1):84–88.
58. Concha-Benavente F, Srivastava RM, Trivedi S, et al. Identification of the Cell-Intrinsic and -Extrinsic Pathways Downstream of EGFR and IFNγ That Induce PD-L1 Expression in Head and Neck Cancer. *Cancer Res.* 2016;76(5):1031–1043.
59. Wherry EJ. T cell exhaustion. *Nat Immunol.* 2011;12(6):492–499.
60. Francisco LM, Salinas VH, Brown KE, et al. PD-L1 regulates the development, maintenance, and function of induced regulatory T cells. *J Exp Med.* 2009;206(13):3015–3029.
61. Lowther DE, Goods BA, Lucca LE, et al. PD-1 marks dysfunctional regulatory T cells in malignant gliomas. *JCI Insight.* 2016;1(5)
62. Seiwert TY, Burtness B, Mehra R, et al. Safety and clinical activity of pembrolizumab for treatment of recurrent or metastatic squamous cell carcinoma of the head and neck (KEYNOTE-012): an open-label, multicentre, phase 1b trial. *Lancet Oncol.* 2016;17(7):956–965.
63. Hamanishi J, Mandai M, Iwasaki M, et al. Programmed cell death 1 ligand 1 and tumor-infiltrating CD8+ T lymphocytes are prognostic factors of human ovarian cancer. *Proc Natl Acad Sci USA.* 2007;104(9):3360–3365.
64. Inman BA, Sebo TJ, Frigola X, et al. PD-L1 (B7-H1) expression by urothelial carcinoma of the bladder and BCG-induced granulomata: associations with localized stage progression. *Cancer.* 2007;109(8):1499–1505.
65. Ohigashi Y, Sho M, Yamada Y, et al. Clinical significance of programmed death-1 ligand-1 and programmed death-1 ligand-2 expression in human esophageal cancer. *Clin Cancer Res.* 2005;11(8):2947–2953.
66. Iwai Y, Ishida M, Tanaka Y, et al. Involvement of PD-L1 on tumor cells in the escape from host immune system and tumor immunotherapy by PD-L1 blockade. *Proc Natl Acad Sci USA.* 2002;99(19):12293–12297.
67. Taube JM, Anders RA, Young GD, et al. Colocalization of inflammatory response with B7-h1 expression in human melanocytic lesions supports an adaptive resistance mechanism of immune escape. *Sci Transl Med.* 2012;4(127):127ra37.
68. Goldberg MV, Drake CG. LAG-3 in cancer immunotherapy. *Curr Top Microbiol Immunol.* 2011;344:269–278.
69. Camisaschi C, de Filippo A, Beretta V, et al. Alternative activation of human plasmacytoid DCs in vitro and in melanoma lesions: involvement of LAG-3. *J Invest Dermatol.* 2014;134(7):1893–1902.
70. Grosso JF, Goldberg MV, Getnet D, et al. Functionally distinct LAG-3 and PD-1 subsets on activated and chronically stimulated CD8 T cells. *J Immunol.* 2009;182(11):6659–6669.
71. Woo SR, Turnis ME, Goldberg MV, et al. Immune inhibitory molecules LAG-3 and PD-1 synergistically regulate T-cell function to promote tumoral immune escape. *Cancer Res.* 2012;72(4):917–927.
72. Sakuishi K, Apetoh L, Sullivan JM, et al. Targeting Tim-3 and PD-1 pathways to reverse T cell exhaustion and restore anti-tumor immunity. *J Exp Med.* 2010;207(10):2187–2194.

73. Zhou Q, Munger ME, Veenstra RG, et al. Coexpression of Tim-3 and PD-1 identifies a CD8+ T-cell exhaustion phenotype in mice with disseminated acute myelogenous leukemia. *Blood*. 2011;117(17):4501–4510.
74. Fourcade J, Sun Z, Benallaoua M, et al. Upregulation of Tim-3 and PD-1 expression is associated with tumor antigen-specific CD8+ T cell dysfunction in melanoma patients. *J Exp Med*. 2010;207(10):2175–2186.
75. Gao X, Zhu Y, Li G, et al. TIM-3 expression characterizes regulatory T cells in tumor tissues and is associated with lung cancer progression. *PLOS ONE*. 2012;7(2):e30676.
76. Yang ZZ, Grote DM, Ziesmer SC, et al. IL-12 upregulates TIM-3 expression and induces T cell exhaustion in patients with follicular B cell non-Hodgkin lymphoma. *J Clin Invest*. 2012;122(4):1271–1282.
77. da Silva IP, Gallois A, Jimenez-Baranda S, et al. Reversal of NK-cell exhaustion in advanced melanoma by Tim-3 blockade. *Cancer Immunol Res*. 2014;2(5):410–422.
78. Jie HB, Gildener-Leapman N, Li J, et al. Intratumoral regulatory T cells upregulate immunosuppressive molecules in head and neck cancer patients. *Br J Cancer*. 2013;109(10):2629–2635.
79. Sakuishi K, Ngiow SF, Sullivan JM, et al. TIM3+-FOXP3+ regulatory T cells are tissue-specific promoters of T-cell dysfunction in cancer. *Oncoimmunology*. 2013;2(4):e23849.
80. Thielens A, Vivier E, Romagné F. NK cell MHC class I specific receptors (KIR): from biology to clinical intervention. *Curr Opin Immunol*. 2012;24(2):239–245.
81. Moesta AK, Parham P. Diverse functionality among human NK cell receptors for the C1 epitope of HLA-C: KIR2DS2, KIR2DL2, and KIR2DL3. *Front Immunol*. 2012;3:336.
82. Yusa S, Campbell KS. Src homology region 2-containing protein tyrosine phosphatase-2 (SHP-2) can play a direct role in the inhibitory function of killer cell Ig-like receptors in human NK cells. *J Immunol*. 2003;170(9):4539–4547.
83. Purdy AK, Campbell KS. Natural killer cells and cancer: regulation by the killer cell Ig-like receptors (KIR). *Cancer Biol Ther*. 2009;8(23):2209–2218.
84. Besson C, Roetynck S, Williams F, et al. Association of killer cell immunoglobulin-like receptor genes with Hodgkin's lymphoma in a familial study. *PLOS ONE*. 2007;2(5):e406.
85. Verheyden S, Bernier M, Demanet C. Identification of natural killer cell receptor phenotypes associated with leukemia. *Leukemia*. 2004;18(12):2002–2007.
86. Chatrchyan S, Khachatryan V, Sirunyan AM, et al. Probing color coherence effects in pp collisions at [Formula: see text]. *Eur Phys J C Part Fields*. 2014;74(6):2901.
87. Pollok KE, Kim YJ, Zhou Z, et al. Inducible T cell antigen 4-1BB. Analysis of expression and function. *J Immunol*. 1993;150(3):771–781.
88. Melero I, Johnston JV, Shufford WW, et al. NK1.1 cells express 4-1BB (CDw137) costimulatory molecule and are required for tumor immunity elicited by anti-4-1BB monoclonal antibodies. *Cell Immunol*. 1998;190(2):167–172.
89. Lynch DH. The promise of 4-1BB (CD137)-mediated immunomodulation and the immunotherapy of cancer. *Immunol Rev*. 2008;222:277–286.
90. Vetto JT, Lum S, Morris A, et al. Presence of the T-cell activation marker OX-40 on tumor infiltrating lymphocytes and draining lymph node cells from patients with melanoma and head and neck cancers. *Am J Surg*. 1997;174(3):258–265.
91. Bell RB, Leidner RS, Crittenden MR, et al. OX40 signaling in head and neck squamous cell carcinoma: Overcoming immunosuppression in the tumor microenvironment. *Oral Oncol*. 2016;52:1–10.
92. Eliopoulos AG, Young LS. The role of the CD40 pathway in the pathogenesis and treatment of cancer. *Curr Opin Pharmacol*. 2004;4(4):360–367.
93. van Kooten C, Banchereau J. CD40-CD40 ligand. *J Leukoc Biol*. 2000;67(1):2–17.
94. Cao W, Cavacini LA, Tillman KC, et al. CD40 function in squamous cell cancer of the head and neck. *Oral Oncol*. 2005;41(5):462–469.
95. Posner MR, Cavacini LA, Upton MP, et al. Surface membrane-expressed CD40 is present on tumor cells from squamous cell cancer of the head and neck in vitro and in vivo and regulates cell growth in tumor cell lines. *Clin Cancer Res*. 1999;5(8):2261–2270.
96. Funakoshi S, Longo DL, Beckwith M, et al. Inhibition of human B-cell lymphoma growth by CD40 stimulation. *Blood*. 1994;83(10):2787–2794.
97. von Leoprechting A, van der Bruggen P, Pahl HL, et al. Stimulation of CD40 on immunogenic human malignant melanomas augments their cytotoxic T lymphocyte-mediated lysis and induces apoptosis. *Cancer Res*. 1999;59(6):1287–1294.
98. Sathawane D, Kharat RS, Halder S, et al. Monocyte CD40 expression in head and neck squamous cell carcinoma (HNSCC). *Hum Immunol*. 2013;74(1):1–5.
99. Grivennikov SI, Greten FR, Karin M. Immunity, inflammation, and cancer. *Cell*. 2010;140(6):883–899.
100. Jebreel A, Mistry D, Loke D, et al. Investigation of interleukin 10, 12 and 18 levels in patients with head and neck cancer. *J Laryngol Otol*. 2007;121(3):246–252.
101. Chatrchyan S, Khachatryan V, Sirunyan AM, et al. Study of the production of charged pions, kaons, and protons in pPb collisions at sqrt(sNN) = 5.02 TeV. *Eur Phys J C Part Fields*. 2014;74(6):2847.
102. Thompson RF, Maity A. Radiotherapy and the tumor microenvironment: mutual influence and clinical implications. *Adv Exp Med Biol*. 2014;772:147–165.
103. Chatrchyan S, Khachatryan V, Sirunyan AM, et al. Measurement of the top-quark mass in all-jets $t\bar{t}$ events in pp collisions at $\sqrt{s}$ = 7 TeV. *Eur Phys J C Part Fields*. 2014;74(4):2758.
104. Duffy SA, Taylor JM, Terrell JE, et al. Interleukin-6 predicts recurrence and survival among head and neck cancer patients. *Cancer*. 2008;113(4):750–757.
105. Snyderman CH, Milanovich M, Wagner RL, et al. Prognostic significance of prostaglandin E2 production in fresh tissues of head and neck cancer patients. *Head Neck*. 1995;17(2):108–113.

106. Seiwert TY, Cohen EE. Targeting angiogenesis in head and neck cancer. *Semin Oncol*. 2008;35(3):274–285.
107. Ciardiello F, Tortora G. Epidermal growth factor receptor (EGFR) as a target in cancer therapy: understanding the role of receptor expression and other molecular determinants that could influence the response to anti-EGFR drugs. *Eur J Cancer*. 2003;39(10):1348–1354.
108. Uyttenhove C, Pilotte L, Théate I, et al. Evidence for a tumoral immune resistance mechanism based on tryptophan degradation by indoleamine 2,3-dioxygenase. *Nat Med*. 2003;9(10):1269–1274.
109. Ho HH, Ivashkiv LB. Role of STAT3 in type I interferon responses. Negative regulation of STAT1-dependent inflammatory gene activation. *J Biol Chem*. 2006;281(20):14111–14118.
110. Schaefer C, Kim GG, Albers A, et al. Characteristics of CD4+CD25+ regulatory T cells in the peripheral circulation of patients with head and neck cancer. *Br J Cancer*. 2005;92(5):913–920.
111. Wansom D, Light E, Worden F, et al. Correlation of cellular immunity with human papillomavirus 16 status and outcome in patients with advanced oropharyngeal cancer. *Arch Otolaryngol Head Neck Surg*. 2010;136(12):1267–1273.
112. Green VL, Michno A, Stafford ND, et al. Increased prevalence of tumour infiltrating immune cells in oropharyngeal tumours in comparison to other subsites: relationship to peripheral immunity. *Cancer Immunol Immunother*. 2013;62(5):863–873.
113. Chikamatsu K, Sakakura K, Toyoda M, et al. Immunosuppressive activity of $CD14^+$ $HLA\text{-}DR^-$ cells in squamous cell carcinoma of the head and neck. *Cancer Sci*. 2012;103(6):976–983.
114. Costa NL, Valadares MC, Souza PP, et al. Tumor-associated macrophages and the profile of inflammatory cytokines in oral squamous cell carcinoma. *Oral Oncol*. 2013;49(3):216–223.
115. Fujii N, Shomori K, Shiomi T, et al. Cancer-associated fibroblasts and CD163-positive macrophages in oral squamous cell carcinoma: their clinicopathological and prognostic significance. *J Oral Pathol Med*. 2012;41(6):444–451.
116. Blankenstein T, Coulie PG, Gilboa E, et al. The determinants of tumour immunogenicity. *Nat Rev Cancer*. 2012;12(4):307–313.
117. Allen CT, Judd NP, Bui JD, et al. The clinical implications of antitumor immunity in head and neck cancer. *Laryngoscope*. 2012;122(1):144–157.
118. Wolf GT, Chepeha DB, Bellile E, et al. University of Michigan Head and Neck SPORE Program. Tumor infiltrating lymphocytes (TIL) and prognosis in oral cavity squamous carcinoma: a preliminary study. *Oral Oncol*. 2015;51(1):90–95.
119. Keck MK, Zuo Z, Khattri A, et al. Integrative analysis of head and neck cancer identifies two biologically distinct HPV and three non-HPV subtypes. *Clin Cancer Res*. 2015;21(4):870–881.
120. Balermpas P, Michel Y, Wagenblast J, et al. Tumour-infiltrating lymphocytes predict response to definitive chemoradiotherapy in head and neck cancer. *Br J Cancer*. 2014;110(2):501–509.
121. Balermpas P, Rödel F, Rödel C, et al. CD8+ tumour-infiltrating lymphocytes in relation to HPV status and clinical outcome in patients with head and neck cancer after postoperative chemoradiotherapy: a multicentre study of the German cancer consortium radiation oncology group (DKTK-ROG). *Int J Cancer*. 2016;138(1):171–181.
122. Klein G, Klein E. Immune surveillance against virus-induced tumors and nonrejectability of spontaneous tumors: contrasting consequences of host versus tumor evolution. *Proc Natl Acad Sci USA*. 1977;74(5):2121–2125.
123. Galon J, Costes A, Sanchez-Cabo F, et al. Type, density, and location of immune cells within human colorectal tumors predict clinical outcome. *Science*. 2006;313(5795):1960–1964.
124. Ariffin AB, Forde PF, Jahangeer S, et al. Releasing pressure in tumors: what do we know so far and where do we go from here? A review. *Cancer Res*. 2014;74(10):2655–2662.
125. Trédan O, Galmarini CM, Patel K, et al. Drug resistance and the solid tumor microenvironment. *J Natl Cancer Inst*. 2007;99(19):1441–1454.
126. Kwilas AR, Donahue RN, Tsang KY, et al. Immune consequences of tyrosine kinase inhibitors that synergize with cancer immunotherapy. *Cancer Cell Microenviron*. 2015;2(1)
127. Schoppy DW, Sunwoo JB. Immunotherapy for head and neck squamous cell carcinoma. *Hematol Oncol Clin North Am*. 2015;29(6):1033–1043.
128. Ferris RL, Jaffee EM, Ferrone S. Tumor antigen-targeted, monoclonal antibody-based immunotherapy: clinical response, cellular immunity, and immunoescape. *J Clin Oncol*. 2010;28(28):4390–4399.
129. Lee SC, Srivastava RM, López-Albaitero A, et al. Natural killer (NK): dendritic cell (DC) cross talk induced by therapeutic monoclonal antibody triggers tumor antigen-specific T cell immunity. *Immunol Res*. 2011;50(2-3):248–254.
130. Kondadasula SV, Roda JM, Parihar R, et al. Colocalization of the IL-12 receptor and FcgammaRIIIa to natural killer cell lipid rafts leads to activation of ERK and enhanced production of interferon-gamma. *Blood*. 2008;111(8):4173–4183.
131. Srivastava RM, Lee SC, Andrade Filho PA, et al. Cetuximab-activated natural killer and dendritic cells collaborate to trigger tumor antigen-specific T-cell immunity in head and neck cancer patients. *Clin Cancer Res*. 2013;19(7):1858–1872.
132. Trivedi S, Jie HB, Ferris RL. Tumor antigen-specific monoclonal antibodies and induction of T-cell immunity. *Semin Oncol*. 2014;41(5):678–684.
133. Vermorken JB, Herbst RS, Leon X, et al. Overview of the efficacy of cetuximab in recurrent and/or metastatic squamous cell carcinoma of the head and neck in patients who previously failed platinum-based therapies. *Cancer*. 2008;112(12):2710–2719.
134. Jie HB, Schuler PJ, Lee SC, et al. $CTLA\text{-}4^+$ Regulatory T cells increased in Cetuximab-treated head and neck cancer patients suppress NK cell cytotoxicity and correlate with poor prognosis. *Cancer Res*. 2015;75(11):2200–2210.

135. Gildener-Leapman N, Lee J, Ferris RL. Tailored immunotherapy for HPV positive head and neck squamous cell cancer. *Oral Oncol.* 2014;50(9):780–784.
136. Huppa JB, Davis MM. T-cell-antigen recognition and the immunological synapse. *Nat Rev Immunol.* 2003;3(12):973–983.
137. Curran MA, Montalvo W, Yagita H, et al. PD-1 and CTLA-4 combination blockade expands infiltrating T cells and reduces regulatory T and myeloid cells within B16 melanoma tumors. *Proc Natl Acad Sci U S A.* 2010;107(9):4275–4280.
138. June CH. Adoptive T cell therapy for cancer in the clinic. *J Clin Invest.* 2007;117(6):1466–1476.
139. Li L, Chang W, Yang G, et al. Targeting poly(ADP-ribose) polymerase and the c-Myb-regulated DNA damage response pathway in castration-resistant prostate cancer. *Sci Signal.* 2014;7(326):ra47.
140. Chatrchyan S, Khachatryan V, Sirunyan AM, et al. Observation of the associated production of a single top quark and a *W* boson in *pp* collisions at $\sqrt{s}$ = 8 TeV. *Phys Rev Lett.* 2014;112(23):231802.
141. Chatrchyan S, Khachatryan V, Sirunyan AM, et al. Measurement of inclusive *W* and *Z* boson production cross sections in *pp* collisions at $\sqrt{s}$ = 8 TeV. *Phys Rev Lett.* 2014;112(19):191802.
142. Chatrchyan S, Khachatryan V, Sirunyan AM, et al. Search for flavor-changing neutral currents in top-quark decays $t \rightarrow Zq$ in *pp* collisions at $\sqrt{s}$ = 8 TeV. *Phys Rev Lett.* 2014;112(17):171802.
143. Chatrchyan S, Khachatryan V, Sirunyan AM, et al. Search for top squark and Higgsino production using diphoton Higgs boson decays. *Phys Rev Lett.* 2014;112(16):161802.
144. Walunas TL, Lenschow DJ, Bakker CY, et al. CTLA-4 can function as a negative regulator of T cell activation. *Immunity.* 1994;1(5):405–413.
145. Hodge JW, Ardiani A, Farsaci B, et al. The tipping point for combination therapy: cancer vaccines with radiation, chemotherapy, or targeted small molecule inhibitors. *Semin Oncol.* 2012;39(3):323–339.
146. Hodge JW, Kwilas A, Ardiani A, et al. Attacking malignant cells that survive therapy: exploiting immunogenic modulation. *Oncoimmunology.* 2013;2(12):e26937.
147. Hodge JW, Garnett CT, Farsaci B, et al. Chemotherapy-induced immunogenic modulation of tumor cells enhances killing by cytotoxic T lymphocytes and is distinct from immunogenic cell death. *Int J Cancer.* 2013;133(3):624–636.
148. Gameiro SR, Jammeh ML, Wattenberg MM, et al. Radiation-induced immunogenic modulation of tumor enhances antigen processing and calreticulin exposure, resulting in enhanced T-cell killing. *Oncotarget.* 2014;5(2):403–416.
149. Golden EB, Frances D, Pellicciotta I, et al. Radiation fosters dose-dependent and chemotherapy-induced immunogenic cell death. *Oncoimmunology.* 2014;3:e28518.
150. Deng L, Liang H, Burnette B, et al. Irradiation and anti-PD-L1 treatment synergistically promote antitumor immunity in mice. *J Clin Invest.* 2014;124(2):687–695.
151. das R, Verma R, Sznol M, et al. Combination therapy with anti-CTLA-4 and anti-PD-1 leads to distinct immunologic changes in vivo. *J Immunol.* 2015;194(3):950–959.
152. Larkin J, Chiarion-Sileni V, Gonzalez R, et al. Combined nivolumab and ipilimumab or monotherapy in untreated melanoma. *N Engl J Med.* 2015;373(1):23–34.
153. Wei H, Zhao L, Li W, et al. Combinatorial PD-1 blockade and CD137 activation has therapeutic efficacy in murine cancer models and synergizes with cisplatin. *PLOS ONE.* 2013;8(12):e84927.
154. Guo Z, Wang X, Cheng D, et al. PD-1 blockade and OX40 triggering synergistically protects against tumor growth in a murine model of ovarian cancer. *PLOS ONE.* 2014;9(2):e89350.
155. Nguyen LT, Ohashi PS. Clinical blockade of PD1 and LAG3—potential mechanisms of action. *Nat Rev Immunol.* 2015;15(1):45–56.
156. Hodi FS, O'Day SJ, Mcdermott DF, et al. Improved survival with ipilimumab in patients with metastatic melanoma. *N Engl J Med.* 2010;363(8):711–723.
157. Holmgaard RB, Zamarin D, Munn DH, et al. Indoleamine 2,3-dioxygenase is a critical resistance mechanism in antitumor T cell immunotherapy targeting CTLA-4. *J Exp Med.* 2013;210(7):1389–1402.
158. Kohrt HE, Colevas AD, Houot R, et al. Targeting CD137 enhances the efficacy of cetuximab. *J Clin Invest.* 2014;124(6):2668–2682.
159. Morales-Estevez C, de La Haba-Rodriguez J, Manzanares-Martin B, et al. KIR genes and their ligands predict the response to anti-EGFR monoclonal antibodies in solid tumors. *Front Immunol.* 2016;7:561.
160. Vermorken JB, Mesia R, Rivera F, et al. Platinum-based chemotherapy plus cetuximab in head and neck cancer. *N Engl J Med.* 2008;359(11):1116–1127. doi:10.1056/NEJMoa0802656
161. Chow LQM, Haddad R, Gupta S, et al. Antitumor Activity of Pembrolizumab in Biomarker-Unselected Patients With Recurrent and/or Metastatic Head and Neck Squamous Cell Carcinoma: Results From the Phase Ib KEYNOTE-012 Expansion Cohort. *J Clin Oncol.* 2016;34(32):3838–3845. doi:10.1200/JCO.2016.68.1478
162. Seiwert TY, Burtness B, Mehra R, et al. Safety and clinical activity of pembrolizumab for treatment of recurrent or metastatic squamous cell carcinoma of the head and neck (KEYNOTE-012): an open-label, multicentre, phase 1b trial. *Lancet Oncol.* 2016;17(7):956–965. doi:10.1016/S1470-2045(16)30066-3
163. Mehra R, Seiwert TY, Mahipal A, et al. Efficacy and safety of pembrolizumab in recurrent/metastatic head and neck squamous cell carcinoma (R/M HNSCC): Pooled analyses after long-term follow-up in keynote-012. *J Clin Oncol.* 2016;34(15)(suppl) abstract 6012.
164. Chow L, Mehra R, Haddad RI. Biomarkers and response to pembrolizumab (pembro) in recurrent/metastatic head and neck squamous cell carcinoma (R/M HNSCC). *J Clin Oncol.* 2016;(suppl):abstr 6010.

165. Bauml J, Seiwert TY, Pfister DG, et al. Pembrolizumab for platinum- and Cetuximab-refractory head and neck cancer: results from a single-arm, phase II study. *J Clin Oncol.* 2017;35(14):1542–1549. doi:10.1200/JCO.2016.70.1524
166. Cohen EE, Harrington KJ, Le Tourneau C, et al. LBA45_PRPembrolizumab (pembro) vs standard of care (SOC) for recurrent or metastatic head and neck squamous cell carcinoma (R/M HNSCC): Phase 3 KEYNOTE-040 trial. *AnnOncol.* 2017;28(suppl 5). doi:10.1093/annonc/mdx440.040
167. Ferris RL, Blumenschein G, Fayette J, et al. Nivolumab for recurrent squamous-cell carcinoma of the head and neck. *N Engl J Med.* 2016;375(19):1856–1867. doi:10.1056/HEJMoa1602252
168. Gillison ML, Blumenschein G, Fayette J, et al. Nivolumab (nivo) vs investigator's choice (IC) for platinum-refractory (PR) recurrent or metastatic (R/M) squamous cell carcinoma of the head and neck (SCCHN; Checkmate 141): outcomes in first-line (Il) R/m patients and updated safety and efficacy. *J Clin Oncol.* 2017;35(suppl):abstr 6019.
169. Segal NH, Ou SI, Balmanoukian AS, et al. 949O—updated safety and efficacy of durvalumab (MEDI4736), an anti-PD-L 1 antibody, in patients from a squamous cell carcinoma of the head and neck. *Ann Oncol.* 2016;27(6):328–350. doi:10.1093/annonc/mdw376.01
170. Zandberg D, Algazi A, Jimeno A, et al. 1042O Durvalumab for recurrent/metastatic (R/M) head and neck squamous cell carcinoma (HNSCC): preliminary results from a single-arm, phase 2 study. *Ann Oncol.* 2017;28(suppl 5):v372–v394. doi:10.1093/annonc/mdx374
171. Pignon JP, Le Maître A, Maillard E, et al. Meta-analysis of chemotherapy in head and neck cancer (MACH-NC): an update on 93 randomised trials and 17,346 patients. *Radiother Oncol.* 2009;92(1):4–14. doi:10.1016/j.radonc.2009.04.014
172. Hellevik T, Martinez-Zubiaurre I. Radiotherapy and the tumor stroma: the importance of dose and fractionation. *Front Oncol.* 2014;4:1. doi:10.3389/fonc.2014.00001
173. Kershaw MH, Smyth MJ. Making macrophages eat cancer. *Science.* 2013;341(6141):41–42. doi:10.1126/science.1241716

11

Targeting the Human Epidermal Receptor Family in HNSCC

Emmanuel Seront
Sandra Schmitz
Jean-Pascal Machiels

Head and neck cancers represent the sixth most common cancer worldwide with approximately 630,000 new patients diagnosed annually resulting in more than 350,000 deaths every year (1). More than 90% of head and neck cancers are squamous cell carcinomas (HNSCC), arising from the epithelial cells that line the mucosal surfaces of oral cavity, pharynx, and larynx.

Patients with early-stage HNSCC are treated with a single modality, such as radiation therapy (RT) or surgery, whereas patients with locally advanced disease (LA-HNSCC), who represent approximately 60% of all patients, require a multimodal treatment approach that includes either definitive concurrent chemoradiation (CRT) or surgery followed by RT or CRT. Despite this aggressive strategy, more than 50% of these patients develop local or regional recurrences and approximately 20% develop distant metastases (2–4). In the recurrent or metastatic disease setting, a platinum agent remains the most active cytotoxic compound but offers modest benefit with a median overall survival (OS) that does not exceed 9 months (5). Identification of molecular alterations implicated in HNSCC carcinogenesis has led to the development of new therapeutic strategies. The aberrant functionality of the epidermal growth factor receptor (EGFR) pathway observed in HNSCC provides evidence for a relationship between EGFR and HNSCC development and progression, and suggests a role for EGFR as a promising target in the optimization of HNSCC treatment.

EGFR AND HNSCC

The EGFR family includes four tyrosine kinase receptors (ErbB1 or EGFR, ErbB2 or HER2, ErbB3 or HER3, and ErbB4 or HER4) that all have a glycosylated extracellular domain, a single hydrophobic transmembrane segment, and an intracellular portion with a protein kinase domain. Multiple natural ligands, including the epidermal growth factor (EGF) and the transforming growth factor-alpha (TGF-α) bind to EGFR, HER2, and HER4, leading to their homo- or heterodimerization. HER2 has no known soluble ligand but can form heterodimers with EGFR, HER3, and HER4. Upon dimerization, intracellular tyrosine residues undergo autophosphorylation, triggering a cascade of multiple important signaling pathways including the Ras/Raf/Mek/Erk, the phosphatidylinositol-3-kinase/protein kinase B/mammalian target of rapamycin (PI3K/Akt/mTOR), the Src tyrosine kinase, and the signal transducers and activators of transcription (STAT) pathways. These

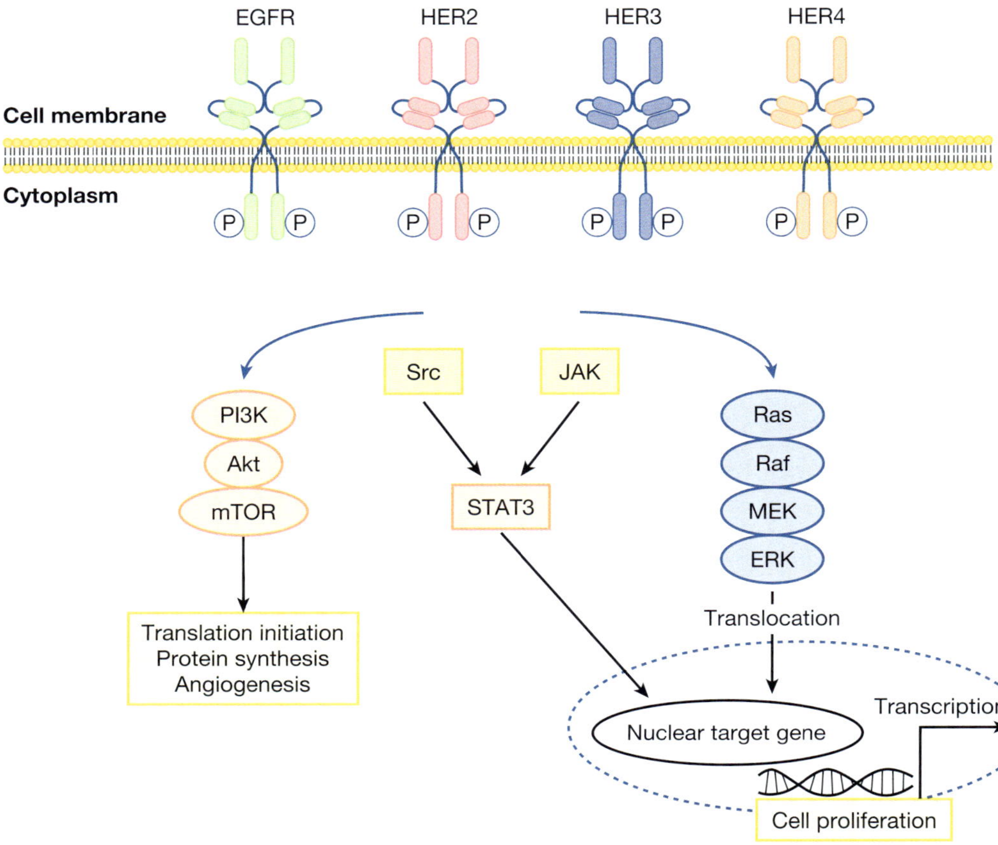

FIGURE 11.1 EGFR is a member of the HER tyrosine kinase receptor family composed of four different receptors (EGFR/c-erbB-1, c-erbB-2/HER-2/neu, c-erbB-3/HER-3, and c-erbB4/HER-4), all of which are transmembrane proteins with tyrosine kinase activity. The EGFR has an extracellular domain, which provides a ligand-binding site for multiple ligands. EGFR homodimerization or heterodimerization with another HER receptor occurs, which leads to the activation of the intracellular tyrosine kinase, resulting in stimulation of multiple signaling cascades. The PI3K/Akt/mTOR pathway stimulates protein synthesis, antiapoptotic signals, and angiogenesis. The Ras/Raf/MEK pathway stimulates gene transcription, cell cycle progression. Activation of other important kinases such as Src and JAK, also leads to stimulation of transcription factors including signal transducer and activator of transcription (STAT) proteins.

EGFR, epidermal growth factor receptor; HER, human epidermal receptor.

pathways play an important role in stimulating cellular proliferation, survival, and angiogenesis (6). EGFR can also act as a transcription factor itself. Stress factors such as radiation triggers translocation of EGFR to the nucleus where it takes part in a complex related to DNA damage repair (Figure 11.1).

EGFR is overexpressed in more than 90% of HNSCC (6,7). Interestingly, EGFR expression is also upregulated in normal mucosa from HNSCC patients, suggesting that increased EGFR expression could be an early event in the development of HNSCC. EGFR overexpression is mainly at the transcriptional level but amplification of the *EGFR* gene, reported in 10% to 58% of patients, could contribute to EGFR overexpression in malignant tissue. *EGFR* point mutations are reported in only 1% to 7% of patients with HNSCC (8–10). The most common mutated form of *EGFR* contains a six-exon deletion (in-frame deletion of exons 2–7) that encodes a 268–amino acid section of its extracellular domain (EGFRvIII) (11,12). This mutation results in a truncated extracellular EGF-binding domain that is constitutively activated. While earlier reports documented EGFRvIII in about 40% of HNSCC, EGFRvIII variant was identified in less than 0.5% of the samples analyzed by The Cancer Genome Atlas (TCGA) project (10). Therefore, the existence of EGFRvIII is controversial and requires further investigation. High levels of EGFR and TGF-α are poor prognostic factors, as well as *EGFR* amplification, and are correlated with advanced stage, increased tumor size, decreased survival, and decreased sensitivity to RT (13–20).

HER2 and HER3 expressions, both observed in 10% to 30% of HNSCC, are also linked to poor prognosis in HNSCC (21–25). HER2 overexpression was shown to be significantly associated with positive lymph node status and advanced stage as well as with reduced treatment response, increased recurrence, and decreased OS following CRT in HNSCC. Coexpression of HER2 with EGFR was associated in vitro and in vivo with resistance to therapeutic agents (24). HER3 overexpression was also found to be increased in metastatic tissues compared to primary tumors and was significantly correlated with worse survival.

The human papillomavirus (HPV) has emerged as an important cause of oropharyngeal cancer. HPV-positive oropharynx cancer demonstrates a more favorable prognosis and an improved response to CT and RT compared to HPV-negative patients. EGFR seems predominantly overexpressed in HPV-negative HNSCC. Conversely, HER2 and HER3 expression levels seem significantly higher in HPV-positive HNSCC than HPV-negative HNSCC. Although the contribution of EGFR family signaling pathway to HPV-related HNSCC remains unclear, HPV oncogenes have not been shown to modulate the anti-EGFR antibody responses in HNSCC (26–28).

The negative impact of EGFR family on survival and treatment sensitivity in HNSCC could be explained by downstream activation of several intracellular proliferative pathways resulting in cytoprotective mechanisms that increase tumor cell survival. It has been shown that ionizing RT triggers nuclear translocation of EGFR, inducing transcription of genes essential for cell proliferation and tumor cell repopulation after radiotherapy. Moreover, nuclear EGFR forms a complex with DNA-dependent protein kinase and is involved in removal of DNA damage. Finally, EGFR overexpression is implicated in fostering cancer stem cell survival, including expression of cancer stem cell genes (29–32).

All these observations make the human epidermal receptor (HER) family an attractive target for therapeutic strategies to improve HNSCC clinical outcome.

CETUXIMAB, THE ONLY APPROVED MONOCLONAL ANTIBODY TARGETING EGFR IN HNSCC (TABLE 11.1)

Cetuximab is a chimeric human/murine IgG1 monoclonal antibody (mAb) that specifically binds to the EGFR with high affinity and thereby blocks ligand-binding induced receptor activation. In addition to this direct effect on the EGFR, cetuximab could also activate antibody-dependent cell-mediated cytotoxicity (ADCC) through the binding of their Fc fraction to Fc gammaR (FcγR) on natural killer (NK) cells, monocytes, dendritic cells (DCs), and other granulocytes (33,34). Cetuximab also inhibits nuclear translocation of EGFR, impairing the DNA double strand-break repair that contributes to resistance to RT and CT (29–32). Although other antibodies have been developed, cetuximab has the most robust clinical data and is the only approved mAb routinely used for HNSCC treatment, both in locally advanced and metastatic settings (Figure 11.2).

CETUXIMAB FOR LA-HNSCC

A randomized phase III trial demonstrated that the addition of cetuximab to RT resulted in a significant clinical benefit over RT alone in patients with stage III-IV nonmetastatic HNSCC (35,36). Administration of intravenous cetuximab was initiated 1 week before RT at a loading dose of 400 mg/m^2 followed by weekly 250 mg/m^2 for the duration of RT. Approximately 60% of patients had oropharyngeal primary cancer. Patients receiving cetuximab-RT had a large and significant improvement in median duration of locoregional control (LRC; 24.4 months vs. 14.9 months; p = .005) and in median OS compared to those receiving RT alone (49.0 months vs. 29.3 months; p = .03). After 5 years of follow-up, OS rate was 45.6% for cetuximab–RT compared to 36.4% with RT alone (p = .018). Cetuximab had an acceptable toxicity profile, with the exception of acneiform rash and infusion-related events, which were more frequent with cetuximab. Subset analyses demonstrated that high performance status and age ≤65 years were associated with increased benefit from cetuximab–RT compared to RT. Interestingly, patients experiencing grade ≥2 acneiform rash presented median OS over 40 months longer than those with grade <2 (68.8 months vs. 25.6 months, p = .02), suggesting that rash could appear as

TABLE 11.1

Selected Trials With Cetuximab

Trial	Design	Disease Stage	*N*	Regimens	Response Rate or Duration	Median PFS	Median OS	Toxicity and Predictive factors
Definitive RT or CRT								
Bonner [36,37]	Randomized phase III	Stage III–IV Nonmetastatic Untreated HNSCC	213 211	RT + cetuximab RT	LRC 24.4 months* LRC 14.9 months	17.1 months* 12.4 months	49 months* (5-year 45.6%*) 29 months (5-year 36.4%)	Better OS in pts with skin rash
GSTTC Italian Study Group [40]	Randomized phase III	Stage III–IV Nonmetastatic Untreated HNSCC	161 260	RT + cetuximab CRT (cisplatin-5FU)	NA	20.7 months 21.6 months	44.7 mths 44.7 mths	Similar toxicities
RTOG 0522 [40]	Randomized phase III	Stage III–IV Nonmetastatic Untreated HNSCC	447 444	CRT (2 x HD cisplatin) CRT + cetuximab	NA	3-year PFS: 61.2% 3-year PFS: 58.9%	3-year OS: 72.9% 3-year OS: 75.8%	More frequent RT interruption with cetuximab; Better PFS and OS in P16+ pts
GORTEC 2007-01 [41]	Randomized phase III	Stage III–IV Nonmetastatic Untreated HNSCC	203 203	RT + cetuximab CRT (3 x carbo-5FU) + cetuximab	3-year LRC HR 0.54 (95% CI: 0.38–0.76)* in favor of CRT–cetuximab	3-year PFS: 40.5% 3-year PFS: 52 %*	3-year OS HR 0.80 (95% CI: 0.61–1.05)	Grade ≥3 mucositis and leucopenia more frequent with CRT–cetuximab
Induction chemotherapy followed by CRT								
TREMPLIN [42]	Randomized phase II	Resectable SCC of the larynx and hypopharynx	60 56	DPF → CRT (3 x HD cisplatin) DPF → RT+ cetuximab	3-month LFP: 87% Local failure: 13.3% 3-month LFP: 82%; Local failure: 21.4%	NA	18-month OS: 92% 18-month OS: 89%	More frequent grade ≥3 dermatitis with cetuximab

(continued)

TABLE 11.1 (*continued*)

Selected Trials With Cetuximab

Trial	Design	Disease Stage	*N*	Regimens	Response Rate or Duration	Median PFS	Median OS	Toxicity and Predictive factors
Adjuvant RT–CRT								
RTOG 0234 [43]	Randomized phase II	High risk Resected HNSCC	97 106	RT + cisplatin +cetuximab RT+ docetaxel + cetuximab	NA	2-year DFS: 57% 2-year DFS: 66%	2-year OS: 69% 2-year OS: 79%	Similar toxicities
Mesia [45]	Randomized phase II	Stage III/IV Nonmetastatic oropharynx SCC	45 46	RT + cetuximab RT + cetuximab → cetuximab	2-year LRC: 44% 2-year LRC: 44%	35.3 months 41 months	33.6 months 39.9 months	NA
R/M HNSCC								
EXTREME [47]	Randomized phase III	R/M HNSCC First-line setting	220 222	Platinum-5FU Platinum-5FU + cetuximab	NA	3.3 months* 5.6 months	7.4 months* 10.1 months	No effect of p16 expression
Baselga [48]	Single-arm phase II	R/M HNSCC Platinum-resistant	96	Platinum-based CT + cetuximab	ORR: 10%, SD: 43%	85 days	183 days	NA
Herbst [49]	Single-arm phase II	R/M HNSCC Pts progressing after first-line CT	25 54	2 x 3-week ciplatin CT in first line If PD: Cisplatin + cetuximab (n = 25) PD2 pts = PD pts within 90 days after CT (n = 54)	ORR PD1: 20% ORR PD2: 6%	PD1: 3 months PD2: 2 monhs	PD1: 6.1 months PD2: 4.3 months	NA
Vermorken [50]	Single-arm phase II	R/M HNSCC Platinum-resistant	103	Cetuximab	ORR: 13%	TTP: 70%	178 days	NA

*$p < .05$.

AE, adverse events; Carbo, carboplatin; DPF, induction chemotherapy with cisplatin, 5-fuorouracil, and docetaxel; EGFR, epidermal growth factor receptor; HD, high dose (100 mg/m^2, days 1, 22, and 43); HNSCC, head and neck squamous cell carcinoma; HR, hazard ratio; LFP, larynx function preservation; LRC, locoregional control; mAb, monoclonal antibody; NA, nonapplicable or not available; ORR, overall response rate; OS, overall survival; PD, progressive disease; PFS, progression-free survival; PR, partial response; pts, patients; R/M, recurrent and/or metastatic; SD, stable disease; TTP, time to progression.

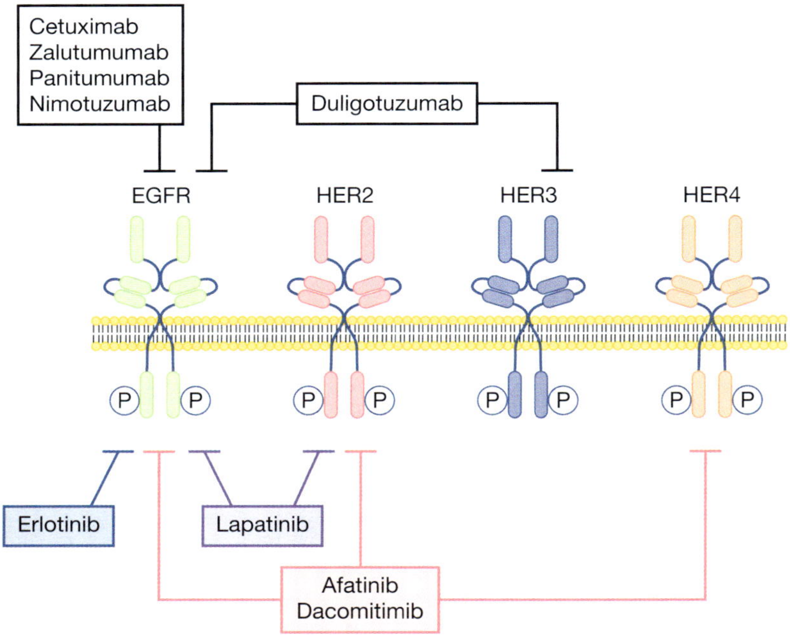

FIGURE 11.2 Monoclonal antibodies administered intravenously can specifically bind to the EGFR family. Cetuximab, panitumumab, zalutumumab, and nimotuzumab bind with high affinity to EGFR and thereby block ligand-binding-induced receptor activation. Duligotuzumab binds to both EGFR and HER3, inhibiting their mediated signaling. Oral tyrosine kinase competitive inhibitors reversibly or irreversibly inhibit the binding of ATP to the phosphate-binding loop of the ATP binding site in the intracellular domain of tyrosine kinase receptors. Erlotinib is a reversible TKI inhibiting EGFR. Lapatinib is an oral reversible dual TKI inhibiting activation of both EGFR and HER2. Afatinib and dacomitinib are newly developed irreversible small molecule pan-HER inhibitors targeting EGFR, HER2, and HER4.

ATP, adenosine 5′-triphosphate.

a surrogate clinical marker of treatment benefit. Retrospective analysis of tumor p16 expression (as a surrogate marker for HPV) did not demonstrate any significant interaction between p16 status and treatment, suggesting that the addition of cetuximab to RT improved clinical outcomes regardless of HPV status, although the magnitude of the benefit seemed higher in HPV oropharyngeal cancer (37). Despite significant benefit of cetuximab–RT over RT alone, this trial was criticized, as it did not include a control arm of platinum-based CRT. Indeed, CRT is still widely accepted as the standard treatment for patients with LA-HNSCC, based on an absolute 5-year survival benefit of 6.5% demonstrated in large meta-analysis (38). Cetuximab–RT combination should thus be only proposed in certain settings, such as patients in whom platinum-based CRT is not advisable (e.g., poor performance status, renal insufficiency, hematologic abnormalities).

The efficacy of the association cetuximab–RT was indirectly compared to CRT in the GSTTC Italian Study Group, which randomized 421 patients with unresectable stage III-IV nonmetastatic HNSCC according to a 2 x 2 factorial design: two cycles of cisplatin/5-fluorouracil (5-FU) concomitant to RT (arm A1), cetuximab–RT (arm A2), three cycles of induction docetaxel, cisplatin, and 5FU (DPF) followed by platinum-based CRT (arm B1), and three cycles of TPF followed by cetuximab-RT (arm B2). Induction chemotherapy followed by CRT or cetuximab–RT significantly improved median PFS (29.7 months vs. 18.5 months, p = .015) and median OS (53.7 months vs. 30.3 months, p = .025) compared to concomitant arm (CRT of cetuximab–RT). There was no difference between CRT and cetuximab–RT for median PFS (21.6 months vs. 20.7 months, respectively) and for median OS (44.7 months vs. 44.7 months, respectively). However, this study was not adequately powered to demonstrate that cetuximab plus RT was equivalent to cisplatin-based CRT. No significant differences for grade 3 and 4 in-field skin and mucositis toxicities were observed (39).

The addition of cetuximab to cisplatin-based CRT did not further improve survival. The phase III trial RTOG 0522 randomized 891 patients with stage III-IV nonmetastatic HNSCC to platinum-based (100 mg/m^2 per day on days 1, 22, and 43) CRT with or without weekly cetuximab. Cetuximab increased grade ≥3 toxicity rate including stomatitis (43% vs. 33% for CRT) and in-field dermatitis (25% vs. 15% for CRT) and resulted in more frequent RT interruption (26.9% vs. 15.1% for CRT alone). Addition of cetuximab to CRT compared to CRT did not improve the 3-year progression-free survival (PFS; 58.9% vs. 61.2%, respectively, p = .76) nor the 3-year OS (75.8% vs. 72.9%, respectively, p = .32). There was no difference in locoregional failure (25.9% vs. 19.9%, respectively, p = .97) or in distant metastases (9.7% vs. 13.0%, respectively, p = .08). Interestingly, subgroup analysis showed that patient with p16-positive oropharyngeal cancer, compared to p16-negative patients, had better 3-year PFS (72.8% vs. 49.2%, respectively, p < .001) and OS (85.6% vs. 60.1%, respectively, p < .001). EGFR expression was not correlated to cetuximab effect (40).

Cetuximab was evaluated in association with carboplatin-based CRT (three cycles of carboplatin–5FU) and compared with cetuximab–RT in a randomized phase III trial that enrolled 406 patients with LA-HNSCC. After a median follow-up of 4.4 years, the 3-year PFS rate was 52.3% in cetuximab–CRT arm versus 40.5% in cetuximab–RT arm A (p = .015). Even if there was also a benefit in terms of LRC with a hazard ratio of 0.54 (p = .0005) in favor of cetuximab–CRT, there was no significant OS difference (p = .11) (41).

In order to improve larynx preservation strategy, association of cetuximab to RT after induction chemotherapy did not seem to result in improved efficacy. The phase II TREMPLIN trial randomized 116 patients with stage III-IV laryngeal or hypopharyngeal SCC suitable for total laryngectomy. After three cycles of induction chemotherapy (DPF), further treatment was based on response to chemotherapy. Poor responders to induction chemotherapy (<50% response) underwent salvage surgery. Responders were randomly assigned to conventional RT (70 Gy) plus either cisplatin (100 mg/m^2 per day on days 1, 22, and 43) or cetuximab. In an intent-to-treat analysis (ITT), there was no significant difference between cisplatin–RT and cetuximab–RT in the rates of larynx preservation at 3 months (95% vs. 93%, respectively), larynx function preservation (87% vs. 82%, respectively), and OS at 18 months (92% vs. 89%, respectively). Even if there were fewer local failures in the CRT arm compared to cetuximab–RT (13.3% vs. 21.4%, respectively), salvage surgery was more successfully achieved in the cetuximab arm only, resulting in an ultimate similar disease control rate (DCR) and OS between the two arms. Treatment compliance was higher in the cetuximab-RT arm (71% completed all weekly doses) compared to cisplatin (42% received all three doses). Grade ≥3 in-field dermatitis was more common with cetuximab (57% vs. 26%) (42).

The association of cetuximab and ICT was tested in several induction studies. A phase II trial evaluated the combination of cetuximab plus six weekly cycles of paclitaxel and carboplatin in 47 LA-HNSCC patients. Induction treatment resulted in 19% of CR and 77% of PR. After induction regimen, patients underwent risk-based local therapy, including radiation, CRT, or surgery, based on tumor stage and site at diagnosis. The 3-year PFS and OS were 87% and 91%, respectively. The CR rate after completion of radiotherapy, with or without chemotherapy, was 70%. The most common grade 3 or 4 toxicity was skin rash (45%), followed by neutropenia (21%) (43).This study was however considered negative as the primary end point to increase the CR rate after induction from 30% (expected with paclitaxel/carboplatin [44]) to 50% was not met.

Another regimen including docetaxel and cisplatin every 3 weeks for three cycles incorporated cetuximab (TPE) as induction therapy, followed by RT with concurrent cisplatin 30 mg/m^2 and cetuximab weekly, and maintenance cetuximab for 6 months. In 39 LA-HNSCC patients, the 3-year PFS and OS were 70% and 74%, respectively. Acute toxicities during TPE included mostly neutropenic fever (10%) (45).

A phase II trial randomized 92 LA-HNSCC patients to receive three cycles of docetaxel and cisplatin (TP) with or without cetuximab (CTP) as induction chemotherapy. Patients in the TP arm received cisplatin-based CRT whereas patients in the CTP arm received RT with cisplatin–cetuximab. The primary end points ORR for induction chemotherapy in the CTP and TP arms were not different (81% vs.

82%). Adding cetuximab lowered the completion rate of induction chemotherapy. There was no statistically significant difference between CTP and TP in terms of 3-year PFS and OS (46). Adding cetuximab to induction regimens remains controversial, and further randomized clinical trials are required.

Administration of cetuximab in adjuvant setting has been evaluated in a randomized phase II trial (RTOG 0234) that investigated the addition of cetuximab to CRT in the postoperative treatment of 238 patients with HNSCC with high-risk pathologic features (47). Patients were randomly assigned to RT with cetuximab once per week plus either cisplatin 30 mg/m^2 or docetaxel 15 mg/m^2 once per week. Two-year OS was 69% for the cisplatin arm and 79% for the docetaxel arm; 2-year disease-free survival (DFS) was 57% and 66%, respectively. These results were compared to the historical control from the phase III RTOG 1216 trial (48) that compared RT alone versus cisplatin-based CRT in in the same high-risk HNSCC population. Addition of cetuximab resulted in a 24% reduction (p = .05) in the DFS failure rate in the cisplatin arm and in a 31% reduction (p = .01) in the docetaxel arm, corresponding to 2.5% and 11.1% improvements, respectively, in the 2-year DFS relative to the cisplatin-based CRT historical control of RTOG 1216. These results, particularly related to docetaxel efficacy, require confirmation in further randomized trials. Despite a greater grade 3-4 hematotoxicity with cisplatin (27.8% vs. 14.2%) compared to docetaxel, there was no difference in term of grade 3-4 mucositis (55.7% vs. 53.8%), dysphagia (38.1% vs. 36.8%), and skin rash (36.1% vs. 38.7%).

Another phase II trial evaluated the efficacy of maintenance cetuximab after definitive RT plus cetuximab. Ninety-one patients with stage III-IV nonmetastatic oropharyngeal cancer were randomized to receive cetuximab–RT or cetuximab–RT followed by 12 consecutive weeks of cetuximab maintenance therapy. Even if the primary end point of LRC at 1 year was superior in the cetuximab maintenance (59% vs. 47%), it became similar between both arms after 2 years of follow-up, as a result of increased locoregional recurrences after the first year in the maintenance group (49).

CETUXIMAB IN RECURRENT OR METASTATIC HNSCC

Approval of cetuximab in the metastatic setting was based on the EXTREME trial. The phase III EXTREME trial randomized 442 patients with recurrent or metastatic (R/M) HNSCC to receive 5-FU and platinum (cisplatin or carboplatin) alone or in combination with cetuximab as a first-line palliative regimen. In the experimental arm, patients who had at least stable disease (SD) after a maximum of six cycles of CT received weekly cetuximab monotherapy until the disease progressed or occurrence of unacceptable toxic effects. This study demonstrated a significant benefit of cetuximab with an improvement in median OS from 7.4 months to 10.1 months (p = .04). Addition of cetuximab prolonged also median PFS (from 3.3 to 5.6 months, p < .001) and the objective response rate (from 20% to 36%, p < .01). These benefits were not impaired by decreased quality of life and treatment with cetuximab was well tolerated. In a retrospective biomarker analysis, *EGFR* gene amplification was detected in 32% of tumors, but there was no predictive correlation between *EGFR* amplification and cetuximab efficacy (50). An unplanned retrospective analysis assessed the outcome by tumor p16 status and concluded that the survival benefit of adding cetuximab to chemotherapy was independent of tumor p16 or HPV status. However, this last analysis was limited by the low number of p16-positive patients (10% of the 416 available tumors) (51).

In the GORTEC phase II, cetuximab was associated with four cycles of docetaxel and with cisplatin (TPEx), followed by maintenance with cetuximab every 2 weeks in 54 patients with R/M HNSCC in first-line setting. The primary end point was met with an ORR of 44.4%. Median OS and PFS were 14 months and 6.2 months, respectively. The most common grade 3-4 adverse events (AEs) were skin rash (16.6%) and nonfebrile neutropenia (20.4%). The TPEx regimen showed promising activity as first-line treatment in fit patients. Further studies are needed to compare the TPEx versus EXTREME regimen in this population (52).

Cetuximab has also shown efficacy in second-line setting in R/M HNSCC in three phase II trials. These trials showed that cetuximab monotherapy or cetuximab in association with platinum agent could induce, after failure of first-line platinum-based CT, an ORR reaching 10% to 13%, and a median OS between 4.3 and 6.1 months (53–55). A pooled analysis of these three prospective trials (n = 278) (56) compared these results with retrospective studies evaluating various historical second-line agents (n = 151) (57) and showed that cetuximab monotherapy has the potential to improve overall survival in the platinum-refractory population. Based on these results, cetuximab was approved by the Food and Drug Administration (FDA) as monotherapy in R/M disease after failure of platinum-based CT.

All these studies demonstrated the efficacy of cetuximab in HNSCC in both the curative and in the R/M settings. In LA-HNSCC, cetuximab increased significantly the efficacy of RT; however, this association has not been proved to be equivalent to platinum-based CRT and should thus be only considered for patients for whom platinum-based chemotherapy is not feasible. In R/M HNSCC, cetuximab is considered as the standard of care in first-line setting in association with platinum-based CT and as monotherapy after failure of platinum-based chemotherapy. However, resistance occurs rapidly, explaining the rapid progression of cancer and the absence of long response duration. Thus, there is an urgent need to improve efficacy of cetuximab and to overcome treatment resistance to EGFR blocking.

ANTI-EGFR THERAPIES BEYOND CETUXIMAB

MAB TARGETING EGFR (TABLE 11.2)

Panitumumab

Panitumumab is a fully human IgG2 mAb with high affinity for EGFR. Unlike cetuximab, panitumumab's human structure results in minimal infusion-related reactions.

In patients with LA-HNSCC, the phase II CONCERT-2 trial randomized 151 patients to receive either panitumumab–RT (three cycles of panitumumab 9 mg/kg every 3 weeks administered with RT) or CRT (two cycles of cisplatin 100 mg/m^2 during RT). This trial demonstrated trends favoring CRT for the primary end point of 2-year LRC (51% with panitumumab–RT vs. 61% with CRT). Overall survival at 2 years in patients receiving CRT was 71% versus 63% (p = .10) in patients receiving panitumumab–RT. Even if rates of grade ≥3 AEs were similar in the two groups (85% vs. 81%), more toxic deaths occurred in the panitumumab–RT group (6% vs. 3%), as well as more RT interruptions ≥10days (7% vs. 0%), and more permanent discontinuations of study (16% vs. 5%). This study suggests that panitumumab cannot replace cisplatin-based CRT for LA-HNSCC (58).

The NCI Canadian group randomized 320 patients with LA-HNSCC between standard fractionated RT (70 Gy over 7 weeks) plus cisplatin (100 mg/m^2, three cycles) versus accelerated RT (70 Gy over 6 weeks) plus panitumumab (9 mg/kg for three doses). This trial failed to establish noninferiority for the primary end point of 2-year PFS (73% and 76%, respectively, p = .83). There was no statistically significant difference in the 2-year OS (85% in cisplatin–RT vs. 88% in panitumumab–RT; p = .66). Grade ≥3 nonhematological AE rates were similar (91% vs. 88%, p = .25) (59–60). A difference between the CONSERT-2 and the Canadian trial was the proportion of patients with p16-positive cancer that was higher in the Canadian trial (20% vs. 75%, respectively), supporting the hypothesis that anti-EGFR monoclonal antibody might be more active in HPV-positive disease when given in combination with RT.

The randomized phase II CONCERT-1 study compared panitumumab–CRT with CRT alone in patients with LAHNSCC. Addition of panitumumab to cisplatin-based CRT did not confer any benefit. The primary end point of 2-year LRC rate was 68% (95% CI: 54–78) in the CRT group and 61% (95% CI: 50–71) in the panitumumab–CRT group. Furthermore, serious AEs were also more common with panitumumab (32% with CRT vs. 43% with panitumumab–CRT). Treatment interruptions of ≥10 days were also more frequent with panitumumab–CRT compared to CRT alone (16% vs. 3%, respectively) (61).

The SPECTRUM trial randomized 657 patients with R/M HNSCC receiving cisplatin and 5-FU with or without panitumumab, every 3 weeks until disease progression or for a maximum of six cycles. Patients without disease progression could continue receiving panitumumab maintenance after the initial six cycles of chemotherapy (CT). Crossover was not allowed. Although the addition of panitumumab prolonged median PFS (5.8 vs 4.6 months, p = .004), it did not significantly improve the primary end point of OS compared to CT alone (11.1 months vs. 9.0 months, respectively; p = .14). Several grade ≥3 toxicities were more frequent with panitumumab, including skin or eye toxicity, diarrhea, hypomagnesemia, and cardiac arrhythmias. There were also more treatment-related deaths with panitumumab (4% vs. 2% with CT). An analysis of the results stratified by tumor p16 status suggested that panitumumab improved OS and PFS in p16-negative

TABLE 11.2

Selected Trials With Other mAb Targeting EGFR

Trial	Design	Disease Stage	*N*	Regimens	Response Rate or Duration	PFS	Median OS	Toxicity and Predictive Factors
Panitumumab								
CONCERT-2 [53]	Randomized phase II	Stage III–IV Nonmetastatic untreated HNSCC	90 61	RT + panitumumab CRT (2 x HD cisplatin)	2-year LRC: 61% 2-year LRC: 51%	2-year PFS: 41% 2-year PFS: 62%	2-year OS: 63% 2-year OS: 71%	RT interruption and toxic death more frequent with panitumumab
NCIC Clinical trial [54]	Randomized phase III	Stage III–IV Nonmetastatic untreated HNSCC	156 159	RT (70 Gy) + 3 x HD cisplatin Accelerated RT + panitumumab	NA	2-year PFS: 73% 2-year PFS 76%	2-year OS: 85% 2-year OS: 88%	Similar toxicities
CONCERT-1 [56]	Randomized phase II	Stage III–IV Nonmetastatic untreated HNSCC	63 87	CRT (3 x HD cisplatin) CRT + panitumumab	2-year LRC: 68% 2-year LRC: 61%	2-year PFS: 65% 2-year PFS: 61%	2-year OS: 78% 2-year OS: 69%	Grade ≥3 AEs and RT interruption more frequent with panitumumab
SPECTRUM [57]	Randomized phase III	R/M HNSCC First-line setting	330 327	Cisplatin-5-FU Cisplatin-5-FU + panitumumab	NA	4.6 months 5.8 months	9 months 11.1 months	Grade ≥3 AEs more frequent with panitumumab; Better OS and PFS in p16- pts
PARTNER [58]	Randomized phase II	R/M HNSCC First-line setting	51 52	Cisplatin + docetaxel Cisplatin+docetaxel+ panitumumab	NA	5.5 months 6 .9 months	13.8 months 12.9 months	Grade ≥3 AEs more frequent with panitumumab

(*continued*)

TABLE 11.2 (*continued*)

Selected Trials With Other mAb Targeting EGFR

Trial	Design	Disease Stage	*N*	Regimens	Response Rate or Duration	PFS	Median OS	Toxicity and Predictive Factors
Zalutumumab								
ZALUTE [59]	Randomized phase III	R/M HNSCC Platinum resistant	95 191	BSC or methotrexate Zalutumumab	NA	8 .4 weeks* 9.9 weeks*	5.2 months 6.7 months	Grade ≥ 3 rash more frequent with zalutumumab
Nimotuzumab								
Rodriguez [62]	Randomized phase II	Stage III–IV Nonmetastatic untreated HNSCC	44 42	RT + nimotuzumab RT + placebo	CR: 59.5%* CR: 34.2%	NA	12.5 months 9.4 months	No skin rash with nimotuzumab Better survival in EGFR+ pts
Babu [63]	Randomized phase II	Stage III–IV Nonmetastatic untreated HNSCC	46 46	(C)RT + nimotuzumab (C)RT + placebo	LRC: 100% (CRT) and 76% (RT) LRC: 70% (CRT) and 37% (RT)	NA	4-year OS: 47% (CRT)* and 34% (RT) 4-year OS:21% (CRT) and 13% (RT)	Better OS in EGFR+ pts treated with CRT + nimotuzumab
Bhatnagar [64]	Randomized phase II	Stage III–IV Nonmetastatic untreated HNSCC.	25 25	Nimotuzumab + CRT CRT	ORR 96%* ORR 72%	NA	NA	Similar toxicity

AE, adverse events; EGFR, epidermal growth factor receptor; HD, high dose; HNSCC, head and neck squamous cell carcinoma; LRC, locoregional control; mAb, monoclonal antibody; NA, nonapplicable or not available; ORR, overall response rate; OS, overall survival; PD, progressive disease; PFS, progression-free survival; PR, partial response; pts, patients; R/M, recurrent and/or metastatic; SD, stable disease.

patients but not in those who were p16-positive. These results should be interpreted with caution because of the low number of patients with p16-positive tumors and the low p16 cutoff threshold (≥10%) that was used, rendering difficult the direct comparison with other trials (i.e., in the EXTREME trial, the cutoff threshold was established at ≥70%, which is the standard definition). Furthermore, half of positive p16 tumors involved nonoropharyngeal primaries for which the importance of HPV status remains to be defined. This problem occurred also in EXTREME trial in which only 58% of p16-positive patients originated from the oropharynx. Therefore, further evaluation is needed to better understand the impact of HPV and p16 status on the activity of anti-EGFR such as panitumumab or cetuximab in the M/Rindications (62).

Despite similarities in the study designs of the SPECTRUM and EXTREME trials, these two phase III trials reported discordant survival results (50). Hypothetical explanations include the differences in the mechanisms of action of these two drugs (cetuximab activates ADCC while panitumumab does not), the population enrolled in both trials (most patients from Western Europe enrolled in the EXTREME trial compared to most patients from Eastern Europe enrolled in the SPECTRUM trial), or treatments prior to enrollment (38% received previous chemotherapy in the EXTREME trial, whereas 81% did so in the SPECTRUM trial).

The randomized phase II PARTNER trial investigated docetaxel and cisplatin with or without panitumumab in 103 patients in the first-line palliative treatment. The primary end point was PFS. Median PFS, median OS, and overall response rate (ORR) were 6.9 months, 12.9 months, and 44% in the panitumumab arm versus 5.5 months, 13.8 months, and 37% in the arm without panitumumab, suggesting a benefit to add panitumumab. Crossover to panitumumab monotherapy was allowed in the docetaxel/cisplatin arm and occurred in 57% of the patients, probably impairing the OS analysis. However, addition of panitumumab increased the grade ≥3 AEs compared to CT alone (73% vs. 56%, respectively) (63).

Panitumumab was also evaluated as second-line monotherapy (PRISM trial) in 51 patients with R/M HNSCC. Panitumumab showed limited activity with an ORR of only 4% and a disease control rate of 39%; median PFS was 1.4 months and median OS was 5.1 months (64).

Zalutumumab

Zalutumumab is a fully human IgG1 mAb that targets EGFR domain III, inhibiting the binding of EGF and TGF-α to EGFR and preventing conformational changes in EGFR that are necessary for its activation. Like cetuximab, zalutumumab is able to stimulate ADCC.

The ZALUTE trial randomized 286 patients with R/M HNSCC that progressed within 6 months of platinum-based therapy to receive either zalutumumab plus best supportive care (BSC) or BSC with optional methotrexate, in a 2:1 ratio. PFS was modestly better in the zalutumumab group compared to BSC (9.9 vs. 8.4 weeks; p = .0012), suggesting clinical activity of this agent. However, zalutumumab did not improve OS (primary end point) over BSC (6.7 months vs. 5.2 months, respectively; p = .06). The most common grade ≥3 AEs were rash (21% zalutumumab vs. 0% BSC), anemia (6% vs. 5%), and infections (15% vs. 9%) (65). Despite suspension of clinical development of zalutumumab, zalutumumab has also been evaluated in association with definitive RT or CRT in 619 patients with pharyngeal and laryngeal primaries. The phase III DAHANCA19 trial randomized patients to receive RT (platinum-based CRT in cases of stage 3-4) with or without zalutumumab. Treatment with zalutumumab was well tolerated but preliminary results showed absence of benefit with addition of zalutumumab, with a similar 4-year LCR rate compared to RT (or CRT; 71% vs. 73%, respectively) (66).

Nimotuzumab

The fully humanized IgG1 mAb nimotuzumab bivalently binds to the extracellular domain of the EGFR that overlaps with the binding site of cetuximab and EGF. Unlike zalutumumab, nimotuzumab prevents ligand binding, but not conformational receptor changes. Nimotuzumab has demonstrated less skin toxicity than cetuximab or panitumumab (67).

In a randomized phase II trial, the association RT–nimotuzumab was compared to RT–placebo in 106 patients with unresectable LA-HNSCC who were medically unfit for concurrent CRT. The primary end point of complete response (CR) was significantly higher in the nimotuzumab group compared to the placebo group (59.5% vs. 34.2%, respectively; p = .038). The ITT analysis demonstrated a nonsignificant trend toward improved median OS with nimotuzumab (12.5 vs. 9.47 months).

However, when analyzing outcome of 88 patients from a single recruiting center, nimotuzumab–RT was associated with significant increased in median OS compared to RT–placebo (median 14.0 vs. 8.8 months, respectively; $p = .02$), but these discrepancies have to be elucidated. Subgroup analyses showed a larger survival benefit with nimotuzumab–RT in patients whose tumors expressed EGFR when compared to RT–placebo (16.5 vs. 7.2 months, $p = .004$). No skin rash was reported and toxicities were limited to almost only grade 1-2. However, the radiation dose used in this study was 10% to 15% lower than what would be considered standard nowadays and could be questioned (68).

Another phase II study (69) randomized 92 patients with LA-HNSCC in two treatment groups (platinum-based CRT or RT for those with poor performance status), further stratified by whether they received nimotuzumab or placebo. Nimotuzumab improved locoregional response in both treatment group, 100% versus 70% in CRT arm and 76% versus 37% in RT arm. Nimotuzumab tended to improve the 4-year OS rate in RT arm (34% vs. 13%) and improved significantly OS in CRT (47% vs. 21%, $p = .01$). There was a significant correlation between EGFR expression and improved OS in the nimotuzumab–CRT arm ($p = .02$). Nimotuzumab was extremely well tolerated with absence of skin rash. Even if these results should be interpreted with caution due to the low number of patients included, this OS improvement with the addition of nimotuzumab CRT is promising.

Recently, preliminary results of a phase II trial of 56 patients with LA-HNSCC who were randomized to CRT with or without nimotuzumab demonstrated significantly higher ORR with nimotuzumab versus CRT alone (96% vs. 72%; $p = .02$). Furthermore, there was no potentiation of treatment-related toxicity, suggesting nimotuzumab could be safely added to standard CRT (70). Nimotuzumab appears thus as a promising agent and further studies are required to evaluate its role in HNSCC treatment.

mAb-806

The novel anti-EGFR mAb 806 selectively targets a unique epitope of the EGFR that is largely inaccessible when EGFR is expressed at normal physiologic levels. The targeted epitope is accessible in tumors with wild-type EGFR amplification or in tumors that express EGFRvIII that lacks the ligand-binding domain of exons 2 to 7 and retains constitutive kinase activity. As this mutation is expressed only in cancer cells, mAb806 should have tumor-specific binding properties and would not be expected to elicit the side effects of classical anti-EGFR. mAb-806 was shown to be effective in vitro and in vivo in HNSCC lines, and its efficacy was increased when combined with cytotoxic agents (71–72). A phase I trial of eight incurable and heavily pretreated patients whose solid tumors overexpressed EGFRvIII (including one with HNSCC) showed that mAb-806 was well tolerated and had promising clinical efficacy, inducing stable disease in five patients (73).

EGFR TYROSINE KINASE INHIBITORS (TKI; TABLE 11.3)

The second strategy for targeting EGFR is orally administered TKIs that reversibly or irreversibly inhibit the binding of ATP to the phosphate-binding loop of the ATP binding site in the intracellular domain of EGFR and thereby abrogate downstream signaling. Different oral small TKIs have been or are currently being evaluated (Figure 11.2).

Gefitinib

Gefitinib demonstrated modest efficacy in HNSCC. In a phase II trial, 226 patients with LA-HNSCC received either gefitinib or placebo in two phases: a concomitant phase (gefitinib or placebo with CRT), followed by a maintenance phase (gefitinib or placebo alone). Gefitinib did not improve the 2-year LRC compared with placebo, when given either concomitantly with CRT (32.7% vs. 33.6%, respectively, $p = .607$) or as maintenance therapy (28.8% vs. 37.4%, $p = .894$) (74). Gefitinib did not show better results in the metastatic setting. In a phase III trial, 186 patients with R/M HNSCC were randomly assigned to oral gefitinib at 250 mg/day, oral gefitinib at 500 mg/day, or weekly intravenous methotrexate at 40 mg/m^2 (75). No significant differences between gefitinib regimen and methotrexate were found in terms of median OS (5.6, 6.0, and 6.7 months, respectively). Furthermore, there was more tumor hemorrhage events in the gefitinib arms (8.9% in gefitinib 250 mg/day; 11.4% in gefitinib 500 mg/day, and 1.9% in methotrexate). Another phase III trial randomized 270 patients with R/M HNSCC with poor performance status

TABLE 11.3

Selected Trials With TKI

Trial	Design	Disease Stage	*N*	Regimens	Response Rate or Duration	PFS	Median OS	Toxicity and Predictive factors
Erlotinib								
Martins [71]	Randomized phase III	Stage III–IV Nonmetastatic untreated HNSCC	99 105	CRT (HD cisplatin) CRT (HD cisplatin) + erlotinib	CR: 40% CR: 52%	Hazard ratio: 0.9	Hazard ratio : 1.05	Better PFS in pts with rash No effect of p16
Soulières [73]	Single arm Phase II	R/M HNSCC Platinum resistant	115	Erlotinib	PR: 4.3%, SD: 38.3%	9.6 wks	6 mths	Better OS in pts with rash
Siu [74]	Single arm phase I/II	R/M HNSCC First-line setting	45	Cisplatin + erlotinib	ORR: 21%, SD: 49%	3.3 months	7.9 months	Better OS in pts with rash
Kim [75]	Single arm phase II	R/M HNSCC First-line setting	50	Cisplatin + docetaxel + erlotinib	ORR: 66%	6.01 months	11 months	NA
Lapatinib								
Del Campo [76]	Randomized phase III	Stage III–IV Nonmetastatic untreated HNSCC	36 71	Placebo (stage 1) → CRT (stage 2) Lapatinib (stage 1) → CRT (stage 2)	ORR: 17%(stage 1) and 86% (stage 2) ORR: 0% (stage 1) and 63% (stage 2)	NA	NA	EGFR expression in lapatinib responder pts
Harrington [77]	Randomized phase II	Stage III–IV Nonmetastatic untreated HNSCC	?	CRT + placebo → placebo CRT + lapatinib → lapatinib	CR: 36% CR: 53%	18-month DFS: 41% 18-month DFS: 55%	18-month OS: 57% 18-month OS: 68%	Better PFS in p16 pts Grade ≥ 3 rash and diarrhea with lapatinib

(continued)

TABLE 11.3 (*continued*)

Selected Trials With TKI

Trial	Design	Disease stage	N	Regimens	Response Rate or Duration	PFS	Median OS	Toxicity and Predictive factors
Harrington [78]	Randomized phase III	High risk Resected HNSCC	342	CRT (HD cisplatin) + placebo → placebo (12 months)	NA	3-year DFS 62%	3-year OS:66%	Similar toxicity
			346	CRT (HD cisplatin) + lapatinib → laptinib (12 monhs)		3-year DFS 61%	3-year OS 67% (estimate)	
De Souza [80]	Single arm phase II	R/M HNSCC Platinum failure	45	Lapatinib	ORR: 0%	52 days	288 days for pts with no prior anti-EGFR treatment 155 days for pts previously treated with anti-EGFR	
Seiwert [83]	Randomized phase II	R/M HNSCC Platinum failure	62	Afatinib (I) → cetuximab (II)	ORR (I): 8.1% and DCR 50%	13 weeks (I)–5.7 weeks (II)	35.9 weeks	NA
			62	Cetuximab (I) → afatinib (II)	ORR (I): 9.7% and DCR 56%	15 weeks (I)–9.3 weeks	47.1 weeks	
LUX-H&N 1 [84]	Randomized phase III	R/M HNSCC Platinum failure	161 322	Methotrexate Afatinib	ORR: 5.6% ORR: 10.2%	1.7 months* 2.6 months	6 months 6 .8 months	Better PFS in p16-, high PTEN expression, EGFR amplified, and low HER3 expression

(*continued*)

TABLE 11.3 (*continued*)

Selected Trials With TKI

Trial	Design	Disease stage	N	Regimens	Response Rate or Duration	PFS	Median OS	Toxicity and Predictive factors
Abdul Razak [88]	Single arm phase II	R/M HNSCC First-line setting	69	Dacomitinib	PR: 12.7% SD: 57.1%	12.1 weeks	34.6 weeks	NA
Vandetanib [90]	Randomized phase II	R/M HNSCC Platinum failure	15 14	Docetaxel + vandetanib Docetaxel	PR: 13% PR: 7%	9 weeks 3.2 weeks	24.1 weeks 26.8 weeks	NA

AE, adverse events; EGFR, epidermal growth factor receptor; HD, high dose; HNSCC, head and neck squamous cell carcinoma; LRC, locoregional control; mAb, monoclonal antibody; NA, nonapplicable or not available; ORR, overall response rate; OS, overall survival; PD, progressive disease; PFS, progression-free survival; PR, partial response; pts, patients; R/M, recurrent and/or metastatic; SD, stable disease.

or prior failure of platinum therapy to receive docetaxel with or without daily gefitinib 250 mg given orally until disease progression. The study was stopped at the interim analysis in November 2008 as there was no statistically significant difference between the placebo and gefitinib in the median OS (6 months vs. 7.3 months, respectively; p = .60) and in the ORR (6.2% vs. 12.5%, respectively; p = .13) (76). In regard to these results, there are no known plans to further evaluate gefitinib in HNSCC.

Erlotinib

Another reversible EGFR TKI, erlotinib, seems more promising in HNSCC than gefitinib. A phase II study evaluated erlotinib in 204 patients with LA-HNSCC; they were randomized to receive cisplatin-based CRT with or without erlotinib. The primary end point of CR was not significantly increased with erlotinib compared to CRT alone (CR 52% vs. 40%, respectively; p = .08) and there was no difference in PFS. Toxicity profile was similar in both arms except for rash that was more frequent (68% vs. 10%) and more severe (grade ≥3: 13% vs. 2%) with erlotinib plus CRT than with CRT alone. Even if p16-positive patients had a better outcome (higher CR rate and better PFS), there was no correlation between p16 expression and erlotinib efficacy. Interestingly, patients who developed rash had a better ORR and a superior PFS compared to patients who did not (77). An interesting phase II trial evaluated the feasibility and efficacy of adding bevacizumab and erlotinib to CRT in 60 patients with LA-HNSCC. They received induction chemotherapy (paclitaxel, carboplatin, 5-FU, and bevacizumab), followed by concurrent RT with weekly paclitaxel, bevacizumab, and erlotinib. Ninety-five percent of patients had either radiological partial response (PR) or CR. The estimated 3-year PFS and OS rates were 71% and 82%, respectively. This treatment was however associated with 88% of grade ≥3 mucositis during combined modality. The high level of efficacy suggests that incorporation of these targeted agents into first-line therapy should be further explored (78).

Erlotinib demonstrated antitumor activity with acceptable tolerability in R/M HNSCC. In a phase II trial, 115 heavily pretreated patients with R/M HNSCC received erlotinib, regardless of EGFR status. Even if the ORR was low (PR 4.3%), stabilization of the disease was maintained in 38.3% of patients for a median duration of 16.1 weeks. The median PFS was 9.6 weeks (95% CI: 8.1 –12.1 weeks), and the median OS was 6.0 months (95% CI: 4.8 –7.0 months). Subgroup analyses revealed a significant difference in OS favoring patients who developed grade ≥2 rash versus those who did not (p = .045), whereas no difference was detected based on EGFR expression. Rash and diarrhea were the most common drug-related toxicities, encountered in 79% and 37% of patients, respectively, though the severity was mild to moderate in most cases. This study showed that erlotinib was well tolerated and could induce clinical benefit in some patients in this heavily pretreated population (79).

Erlotinib efficacy was also evaluated in combination with cytotoxic agents. Association of erlotinib (100 mg PO daily) and cisplatin (75 mg/m^2 IV every 21 days) was evaluated in a phase I/II trial enrolling 45 patients with previously untreated R/M HNSCC. This combination was well tolerated. The ORR reached 21% and disease stabilization was achieved in 49%, resulting in a DCR of 70%. However, median PFS was only 3.3 months (95% CI: 2.7–4.8) months and median OS did not exceed 7.9 months (95% CI: 5.6–9.5), suggesting an absence of benefit compared to historical control subjects. Subgroup analysis suggested that patients who developed higher grade skin rashes had better survival outcomes; median survival durations of patients with no rash, grade 1 rash, and grade 2 rash were 4.2, 7.9, and 9.2 months, respectively (p = .034) (80).

A phase II trial of 50 patients receiving erlotinib in combination with cisplatin/docetaxel in first-line treatment for R/M HNSCC showed encouraging activity with an ORR of 66% and a DCR of 91%. Median PFS and OS were 6.01 months (95% CI: 4.37–8.25) and 11 months (95% CI: 8.61–22.5). This regimen was well tolerated with neutropenia as the most common grade ≥3 AE (13%) (81). This regimen was evaluated in a randomized phase 2 trial in 120 R/M HNSCC; adjunction of erlotinib to cisplatin and docetaxel as first-line regimen followed by maintenance erlotinib until progression improved PFS (primary end point) from 4.4 to 6.1 months compared to cisplatin–docetaxel + placebo (p = .026). The ORR was higher in erlotinib arm compared to placebo (56% vs. 44%) as was the median OS (17 vs. 13.7 months, p = .07). Benefits were more pronounced in oropharyngeal patients for PFS and OS (p ≤ .05 for interaction). Interestingly, grade 2-4 erlotinib-induced rash (34%) was associated with longer OS (p = .02). Erlotinib-treated patients experienced a higher incidence of grade 3-4 AE (53.3% vs. 33.9% for placebo) (82). This regimen may warrant further evaluation in randomized, phase 3 trials.

New studies are required to investigate the potential role of EGFR TKI in the treatment of HNSCC. However, the development of these agents is impaired due to the availabilities of more potent TKI. Interestingly, with these agents, skin rash appeared as a recurrent predictive positive factor of efficacy, although the rash frequency could have biased by a longer treatment duration.

TKI BLOCKING MULTIPLE HER RECEPTORS (TABLE 11.3)

Heterodimerization of EGFR with HER-2, HER-3, or HER-4 induced by ligand binding may be responsible for the limited activity of mAbs or TKI targeting only the EGFR. The ability to block more than just one HER receptor is therefore of interest (21–25) (Figure 11.2).

Lapatinib

Lapatinib is an oral reversible dual TKI inhibiting activation of both EGFR and HER2. Heterodimers of EGFR-HER2 have been shown to be more potent signaling complexes than EGFR homodimers.

In a phase II trial, 107 treatment-naive patients with LA-HNSCC were randomized (2:1) to receive lapatinib or placebo for 2 to 6 weeks before CRT. Single-agent lapatinib resulted in a higher ORR compared to placebo (17% vs. 0%, respectively). Among these lapatinib responding patients, all had EGFR overexpression, 50% had *EGFR* amplification, and 50% had HER2 expression. Following CRT, ORR reached 86% and 63% in the lapatinib and placebo arms, respectively. Paired biopsies allowed demonstrating that lapatinib reduced the level of phospho-EGFR in 63% of cases, versus 33% in the placebo group (p = .11). There was no clear correlation between changes in apoptosis or proliferation and response to CRT (83).

Lapatinib was evaluated in association with CRT in patients with unresected stage III-IV LA-HNSCC. Sixty-seven patients were randomized to three cycles of cisplatin-based CRT with or without concurrent and maintenance lapatinib. The CR rates at 6 months were 53% with lapatinib and 36% with placebo. There was no difference in the primary end point of 3-year DFS (61.1% vs. 62.2%, respectively). Lapatinib did not impair the completion of CRT (84).

A phase III trial evaluated the efficacy of lapatinib in adjuvant setting. Six hundred eighty-eight patients with high-risk surgically treated HNSCC were randomly assigned to CRT (66 Gy total radiation dose and cisplatin 100 mg/m^2 on days 1, 22, and 43) plus placebo or lapatinib (1,500 mg per day) before and during CRT followed by 12 months of maintenance monotherapy. Addition of lapatinib to CRT and its use as long-term maintenance therapy does not offer any efficacy benefit as median DFS was 53.6 months for lapatinib and not reached for placebo (hazard ratio, 1.10; 95% CI: 0.85 –to 1.43). The 3-year DFS rate was 62.2% (95% CI: 56.1%–67.7%) for placebo and 61.1% (95% CI: 55.0% –66.7%) for lapatinib. No treatment effect was observed for DFS by HPV and EGFR status. Lapatinib resulted in more serious AEs compared to placebo group (48% vs. 40%, respectively). The most commonly observed treatment-related toxicities were diarrhea and rash, both predominantly in the lapatinib arm (85).

Adding lapatinib to DPF induction chemotherapy followed by CRT in phase I study for locally advanced laryngeal and hypopharyngeal SCC was found to be too toxic (86).

In metastatic setting, efficacy of lapatinib was very modest; a phase II trial evaluating lapatinib monotherapy in 45 patients with R/M HNSCC demonstrated good tolerability but yielded no objective response, regardless of prior EGFR treatment (87).

Afatinib

Afatinib is an irreversible small molecule pan-HER inhibitor targeting EGFR, HER2, and HER4. Afatinib binds covalently and blocks irreversibly all heterodimers from the HER family, resulting in vitro and in vivo in a prolonged inhibition with the aim of improving clinical activity (88,89).

Seiwert et al. randomized 124 patients with R/M HNSCC who progressed following platinum-based chemotherapy to receive (1:1) afatinib (50 mg/day) or cetuximab until disease progression or intolerable AEs (stage I), with optional crossover (stage II). The ORR in stage I was the primary end point and was 8.1% for afanitib and 9.7% for cetuximab.

Median PFSs were 13 and 15 weeks in the afatinib and cetuximab arms, respectively. Sixty-eight patients crossed over to stage II. For the 32 patients crossing from afatinib to cetuximab, DCR was 19% with a median PFS of 5.7 weeks, whereas for the 36 patients switching from cetuximab to afatinib, the DCR was 33% and the median PFS was 9.3 weeks. Most common grade ≥3 AEs were skin rash (18% vs. 8.3%), diarrhea (14.8% vs. 0%), and mucositis (11.5% vs. 0%) with afatinib and cetuximab, respectively. This trial showed that sequential strategy with afatinib and cetuximab could provide sustained clinical benefit in patients after crossover, suggesting a lack of cross-resistance (90).

The phase III trial LUX-Head & Neck 1 randomized (2:1) 483 patients with R/M HNSCC progressing after first-line platinum regimens to oral afatinib (40 mg/day) or intravenous methotrexate (40 mg/m²/week). Afatinib statistically improved the primary end point of PFS versus methotrexate by 0.9 month (median 2.6 vs. 1.7 months; p = .030), without significant improvement in OS (p = .70) (67). The ORR was 10% with afatinib and 6% with methotrexate, with a DCR of 49% and 39%, respectively. Afatinib was associated with delayed deterioration of global health status. The most common 3-4 AEs with afatinib were skin rash (10%) and diarrhea (9%) (91). A biomarker analysis found a propensity for greater PFS benefit with afatinib than methotrexate in the settings of p16-negative (2.7 vs. 1.6 months; p = .029), PTEN-high (2.9 vs. 1.4 months; p = .014), HER3-low (2.9 vs. 2.0 months; p = .014), and *EGFR*-amplified (2.8 vs. 2.2 months; p = .162) disease (92). A subgroup analysis showed that advancing age (≥65 years) did not adversely affect clinical outcomes or safety with afatinib versus methotrexate in this trial (93). Afatinib is also evaluated in ongoing trials including in neoadjuvant setting.

Dacomitinib

Dacomitinib, another pan-HER TKI (94) demonstrated clinical activity in RM-HNSCC in a phase II study enrolling 69 previously untreated patients. Dacomitinib monotherapy resulted in DCR of 68% (12.7% PR and 57.1% SD). The median PFS was 12.1 weeks and the median OS was 34.6 weeks. Dacomitinib was well tolerated. The most common grade ≥3 AEs were diarrhea (15.9%), acneiform dermatitis (8.7%), and fatigue (8.7%) (95).

Vandetanib

Vandetanib is a multitargeted TKI targeting EGFR and vascular endothelial growth factor receptor 2 (VEGFR2) (96). Efficacy of vandetanib is evaluated in a phase II trial randomizing patients with R/M HNSCC to receive docetaxel alone or docetaxel plus vandetanib. Preliminary results demonstrated higher ORR with vandetanib plus docetaxel compared to docetaxel alone (PR of 13% vs. 7%, respectively) and a higher median PFS (9 vs. 3.2 weeks, respectively); serious AEs were comparable between arms (97). A phase II trial of vandetanib with adjuvant CRT in high-risk, stage III–IV HNSCC was terminated early because of withdrawal of the study drug; as only 34 of 170 planned patients were accrued, no analysis was performed (NCT00720083).

DUAL TARGETING MONOCLONAL ANTIBODIES OR MIXTURE OF MABS

A large variety of bispecific antibodies are under development. The goal of such antibodies is to simultaneously block two receptors or mediators in order to overcome resistance or to stimulate immune effector cells.

The IgG1 antibody duligotuzumab (MEHD7945A) inhibits both EGFR- and HER3-mediated signaling and mediates ADCC in vitro and in vivo. High tumor expression of neuregulin 1 (NRG1), a ligand to HER3, was shown to enhance sensitivity to duligotuzumab (98). A phase I study of 36 patients with advanced solid tumors showed an encouraging safety profile and evidence of antitumor activity, even in patients previously treated with anti-EGFR. A randomized phase II trial compared duligotuzumab (1,100 mg IV, biweekly) to cetuximab (400 mg/m² load, 250 mg/m² IV, weekly) in patients with R/M HNSCC that progressed during or shortly after platinum-based chemotherapy. There were no differences between duligotuzumab and cetuximab regarding PFS (4.2 vs. 4.0 months), OS (7.2 vs. 8.7 months), and ORR (12 vs. 14.5%) and there were no differences between the two groups for patients with *NRG1*-high tumors or HER3-low tumors. Grade ≥3 AEs were more frequent with duligotuzumab than with cetuximab, including infections (22 vs. 11.5%) and gastrointestinal disorders (17 vs. 7%); however, any grade cutaneous rash was less frequent with duligotuzumab (49 vs. 67%). These data indicate that inhibition of EGFR alone could be sufficient to block EGFR-HER3 signaling.

Extensive biomarker analyses showed that responses in both arms were confined to HPV-negative patients (99).

Finally, Sym004 is a drug mixture of two IgG1 mAbs targeting nonoverlapping epitopes on the EGFR. In preclinical models, Sym004 exhibited more pronounced EGFR internalization, degradation, and tumor growth inhibition than cetuximab. Sym004 was recently investigated as palliative monotherapy in patients with HNSCC and showed modest activity (100). Twenty-six patients (including 23 progressing while on anti-EGFR mAb treatment) were included. Median PFS and OS were 82 days and 156 days, respectively. Even if no objective response was observed, 50% of patients had SD as best response, including minor tumor shrinkages in 31% of patients. Interestingly, paired biopsies showed a significant downregulation of EGFR in both skin and tumors following exposure to Sym004. All patients had EGFR-related AEs, including 50% of grade 3 skin toxicities and 38% of grade ≥3 hypomagnesemia (101).

PERSPECTIVES

Cetuximab improves survival in combination with RT or chemotherapy. However, its efficacy remains modest in an unselected population and resistance generally occurs rapidly. This is probably explained by the fact that EGFR is not the unique pathway implicated in HNSCC pathogenesis. Multiple other pathways interact with EGFR network and could play a role in precipitating resistance to anti-EGFR agents. TCGA work characterized the molecular landscape of HNSCC (10). They found other potential actionable genetic alterations (i.e., *PIK3CA, PTEN, AKT, FGFR* family, *CCND1*). This led to a better understanding of HNSCC pathogenesis and to the development of novel treatment strategies. Clinical trials are currently investigating the efficacy of combined therapy, such as PI3K/mTOR inhibitor and cetuximab (NCT01816984), CDK4/6 inhibitor (palbociclib or ribociclib) and cetuximab (NCT02101034, NCT02429089), and ficlatuzumab (hepatocyte growth factor inhibitor) and cetuximab (NCT02277197). Other EGFR-related signaling networks appear also as interesting targets. STAT is a family of cytoplasmic transcription factors (STAT1-6) that are activated either by EGFR or by receptor associated tyrosine kinases like Janus kinases (JAKs) and that are also implicated in head and neck carcinogenesis. STAT inhibitor and JAK inhibitor are currently investigated in clinical trials (NCT02593929).

EGFR antisense (AS) therapy was evaluated in a phase I clinical trial in patients with advanced HNSCC who were refractory to standard therapies, and those who had at least one assessable and accessible lesion were enrolled. The EGFR AS dose was injected directly in the tumor escalated in successive cohorts (six dose levels; 60 to 1,920 mcg/injection). Among 17 patients, 5 patients (29%) achieved a clinical response, which included two cCRs and three PRs; two additional patients had stable disease (SD) as the best response. No grades 3 to 4 or dose-limiting toxicities were noted, and a maximum tolerated dose was not reached. Intratumoral EGFR AS was safe and resulted in antitumor activity in patients with advanced HNSCC. Baseline levels of high EGFR and low STAT3 may be associated with antitumor effects (102).

Reexamining the ideal cytotoxic agent to be combined with anti-EGFR should help also to increase efficacy. Cetuximab acts as a radiosensitizer by preventing translocation of EGFR to nucleus, limiting DNA damage repair, as does cisplatin by interfering with protein transcription and DNA damage repair. Benefit could be more important by combining EGFR targeting agents with cytotoxic agents that operate based on a different mechanism such as docetaxel. That was already suggested in the RTOG 0234 trial.

Immune checkpoint inhibitors such as nivolumab have recently been identified as effective antitumoral agents in HNSCC (103). Given the ADCC effect induced by cetuximab, combination of immunotherapy with cetuximab might represent a valuable option to improve HNSCC outcome, both in the curative and in palliative settings.

Better selection of patients is mandatory for designing future studies of EGFR targeting agents. Efforts should be placed to identify predictive biomarkers of resistance and treatment activity. While HPV association is a powerful prognostic factor in HNSCC, some questions remain regarding its predictive role. In this context, the results of the RTOG 1016 study that randomized p16-positive oropharyngeal cancer between accelerated CRT (high-dose cisplatin) and accelerated RT plus cetuximab are eagerly awaited (NCT01302834).

CONCLUSIONS

Among all anti-EGFR agents, cetuximab is the only approved mAb for the treatment of HNSCC. However, the modest efficacy observed in the different clinical trials illustrates the need for identifying potential resistance mechanisms. Because EGFR signaling involves an interplay of multiple oncogenic pathways, combination therapies including anti-EGFR and innovative agents have to be evaluated in further clinical trials.

REFERENCES

1. Ferlay J, Soerjomataram I, Dikshit R, et al. Cancer incidence and mortality worldwide: sources, methods and major patterns in GLOBOCAN 2012. *Int J Cancer*. 2015;136(5):E359–E386. doi:10.1002/ijc.29210
2. Seiwert TY, Cohen EE. State-of-the-art management of locally advanced head and neck cancer. *Br J Cancer*. 2005;92(8):1341–1348. doi:10.1038/sj.bjc.6602510
3. National Comprehensive Cancer Network. NCCN clinical practice guidelines in oncology (NCCN Guidelines®). Head and Neck Cancers. Version 1. NCCN; 2015.
4. Gibson MK, Li Y, Murphy B, et al. Randomized phase III evaluation of cisplatin plus fluorouracil versus cisplatin plus paclitaxel in advanced head and neck cancer (E1395): an intergroup trial of the Eastern Cooperative Oncology Group. *J Clin Oncol*. 2005;23(15):3562–3567. doi:10.1200/JCO.2005.01.057
5. Colevas AD. Chemotherapy options for patients with metastatic or recurrent squamous cell carcinoma of the head and neck. *J Clin Oncol*. 2006;24(17):2644–2652. doi:10.1200/JCO.2005.05.3348
6. Normanno N, De Luca A, Bianco C, et al. Epidermal growth factor receptor (EGFR) signaling in cancer. *Gene*. 2006;366(1):2–16. doi:10.1016/j.gene.2005.10.018
7. Kalyankrishna S, Grandis JR. Epidermal growth factor receptor biology in head and neck cancer. *J Clin Oncol*. 2006;24(17):2666–2672. doi:10.1200/JCO.2005.04.8306
8. Nagatsuka H, Ishiwari Y, Tsujigiwa H, et al. Quantitation of epidermal growth factor receptor gene amplification by competitive polymerase chain reaction in pre-malignant and malignant oral epithelial lesions. *Oral Oncol*. 2001;37(7):599–604. doi:10.1016/S1368-8375(01)00051-3
9. Mrhalova M, Plzak J, Betka J, et al. Epidermal growth factor receptor—its expression and copy numbers of EGFR gene in patients with head and neck squamous cell carcinomas. *Neoplasma*. 2005;52(4):338–343. PMID: 16059652
10. Cancer Genome Atlas Network. Comprehensive genomic characterization of head and neck squamous cell carcinomas. *Nature*. 2015;517(7536):576–582. doi:10.1038/nature14129
11. Sok JC, Coppelli FM, Thomas SM, et al. Mutant epidermal growth factor receptor (EGFRvIII) contributes to head and neck cancer growth and resistance to EGFR targeting. *Clin Cancer Res*. 2006;12(17):5064–5073. doi:10.1158/1078-0432.CCR-06-0913
12. Chau NG, Perez-Ordonez B, Zhang K, et al. The association between EGFR variant III, HPV, p16, c-MET, EGFR gene copy number and response to EGFR inhibitors in patients with recurrent or metastatic squamous cell carcinoma of the head and neck. *Head Neck Oncol*. 2011;3:11. doi:10.1186/1758-3284-3-11
13. Ang KK, Berkey BA, Tu X, et al. Impact of epidermal growth factor receptor expression on survival and pattern of relapse in patients with advanced head and neck carcinoma. *Cancer Res*. 2002;62(24):7350–7356. PMID: 12499279
14. Wheeler S, Siwak DR, Chai R, et al. Tumor epidermal growth factor receptor and EGFR PY1068 are independent prognostic indicators for head and neck squamous cell carcinoma. *Clin Cancer Res*. 2012;18(8):2278–2289. doi:10.1158/1078-0432.CCR-11-1593
15. Rubin Grandis J, Melhem MF, Gooding WE, et al. Levels of TGF-α and EGFR protein in head and neck squamous cell carcinoma and patient survival. *J Natl Cancer Inst*. 1998;90(11):824–832. PMID: 9625170
16. Jedlinski A, Ansell A, Johansson AC, et al. EGFR status and EGFR ligand expression influence the treatment response of head and neck cancer cell lines. *J Oral Pathol Med*. 2013;42(1):26–36. doi:10.1111/j.1600-0714.2012.01177.x
17. Bentzen SM, Atasoy BM, Daley FM, et al. Epidermal growth factor receptor expression in pretreatment biopsies from head and neck squamous cell carcinoma as a predictive factor for a benefit from accelerated radiation therapy in a randomized controlled trial. *J Clin Oncol*. 2005;23(24):5560–5567. doi:10.1200/JCO.2005.06.411
18. Temam S, Kawaguchi H, El-Naggar AK, et al. Epidermal growth factor receptor copy number alterations correlate with poor clinical outcome in patients with head and neck squamous cancer. *J Clin Oncol*. 2007;25(16):2164–2170. doi:10.1200/JCO.2006.06.6605
19. Chung CH, Ely K, McGavran L, et al. Increased epidermal growth factor receptor gene copy number is associated with poor prognosis in head and neck squamous cell carcinomas. *J Clin Oncol*. 2006;24(25):4170–476. doi:10.1200/JCO.2006.07.2587
20. Chiang W-F, Liu S-Y, Yen C-Y, et al. Association of epidermal growth factor receptor (EGFR) gene copy number amplification with neck lymph node metastasis in areca-associated oral carcinomas. *Oral Oncol*. 2008;44(3):270–276. doi:10.1016/j.oraloncology.2007.02.008
21. Wei Q, Sheng L, Shui Y, et al. EGFR, HER2, and HER3 expression in laryngeal primary tumors and corresponding metastases. *Ann Surg Oncol*. 2008;15(4):1193–1201. doi:10.1245/s10434-007-9771-3

22. Del Sordo R, Angiero F, Bellezza G, et al. HER family receptors expression in squamous cell carcinoma of the tongue: study of the possible prognostic and biological significance. *J Oral Pathol Med*. 2010;39(1):79–86. doi:10.1111/j.1600-0714.2009.00815.x
23. Cavalot A, Martone T, Roggero N, et al. Prognostic impact of *HER-2/neu* expression on squamous head and neck carcinomas. *Head Neck*. 2007;29(7):655–664. doi:10.1002/hed.20574
24. Wheeler D, Huang S, Kruser T, et al. Mechanisms of acquired resistance to cetuximab: role of HER (ErbB) family members. *Oncogene*. 2008;27(28):3944–3956. doi:10.1038/onc.2008.19
25. Takikita M, Xie R, Chung JY, et al. Membranous expression of Her3 is associated with a decreased survival in head and neck squamous cell carcinoma. *J Transl Med*. 2011;9:126. doi:10.1186/1479-5876-9-126
26. Marur S, D'Souza G, Westra W, et al. HPV-associated head and neck cancer: a virus-related cancer epidemic. *Lancet Oncol*. 2010;11(8):781–789. doi:10.1016/S1470-2045(10)70017-6
27. Troy J, Weissfeld J, Youk A, et al. Expression of EGFR, VEGF, and NOTCH1 suggest differences in tumor angiogenesis in HPV-positive and HPV-negative head and neck squamous cell carcinoma. *Head Neck Pathol*. 2013;7(4):344–355. doi:10.1007/s12105-013-0447-y
28. Pollock NI, Wang L, Wallweber G, et al. Increased expression of HER2, HER3 and HER2: HER3 heterodimers in HPV-positive HNSCC using a novel proximity based assy: implication for targeted therapies. *Clin Cancer Res*. 2015;21(20):4597–4606. doi:10.1158/1078-0432.CCR-14-3338
29. Dittmann K, Mayer C, Fehrenbacher B, et al. Radiation-induced epidermal growth factor receptor nuclear import is linked to activation of DNA-dependent protein kinase. *J Biol Chem*, 2005;280(35):31182–31189. doi:10.1074/jbc.M506591200
30. Dittmann K, Mayer C, Kehlbach R, et al. Radiation-induced caveolin-1 associated EGFR internalization is linked with nuclear EGFR transport and activation of DNA-PK. *Mol Cancer*. 2008;7:69. doi:10.1186/1476-4598-7-69
31. Kavanagh BD, Lin PS, Chen P, et al. Radiation-induced enhanced proliferation of human squamous cancer cells in vitro: a release from inhibition by epidermal growth factor. *Clin Cancer Res*. 1995;1(12):1557–1562. PubMed 9815956
32. Chen DJ, Nirodi CS. The epidermal growth factor receptor: a role in repair of radiation-induced DNA damage. *Clin Cancer Res*. 2007;13(22):6555–6560. doi:10.1158/1078-0432.CCR-07-1610
33. Torres S, Bartolomé RA, Mendes M, et al. Proteome profiling of cancer-associated fibroblasts identifies novel proinflammatory signatures and prognostic markers for colorectal cancer. *Clin Cancer Res*. 2013;19(21):6006–6019. doi:10.1158/1078-0432.CCR-13-1130
34. Ferris RL, Jaffee EM, Ferrone S. Tumor antigen-targeted, monoclonal antibody-based immunotherapy: clinical response, cellular immunity, and immunoescape. *J Clin Oncol*, 2010;28(28):4390–4399. doi:10.1200/JCO.2009.27.6360
35. Bonner JA, Harari PM, Giralt J, et al. Radiotherapy plus cetuximab for squamous-cell carcinoma of the head and neck. *N Engl J Med*. 2006;354(6):567–578. doi:10.1056/NEJMoa053422
36. Bonner JA, Harari PM, Giralt J, et al. Radiotherapy plus cetuximab for locoregionally advanced head and neck cancer: 5-year survival data from a phase 3 randomised trial, and relation between cetuximab-induced rash and survival. *Lancet Oncol*. 2010;11(1):21–28. doi:10.1016/S1470-2045(09)70311-0
37. Rosenthal DI, Harari PM, Giralt J, et al. Impact of p16 status on the results of the phase III cetuximab (cet)/radiotherapy (RT). *J Clin Oncol*. 2014;32:abst 6001. doi:10.1200/jco.2014.32.15_suppl.6001
38. Pignon JP, Bourhis J, Domenge C, et al. Chemotherapy added to locoregional treatment for head and neck squamous-cell carcinoma: three meta-analyses of updated individual data. *Lancet*. 2000; 355(9208):949–955. PMID: 10768432
39. Ghi MG, Paccagnella A, Ferrari D, et al. Concomitant chemoradiation (CRT) or cetuximab/RT (CET/RT) versus induction Docetaxel/ Cisplatin/5-Fluorouracil (TPF) followed by CRT or CET/RT in patients with Locally Advanced Squamous Cell Carcinoma of Head and Neck (LASCCHN). A randomized phase III factorial study (NCT01086826). *J Clin Oncol*, 2014;32:abst 6004. doi:10.1200/jco.2014.32.15_suppl.6004
40. Ang KK, Zhang Q, Rosenthal DI, et al. Randomized phase III trial of concurrent accelerated radiation plus cisplatin with or without cetuximab for stage III to IV head and neck carcinoma: RTOG 0522. *J Clin Oncol*. 2014;32(27):2940–2950. doi:10.1200/JCO.2013.53.5633
41. Bourhis J, Sun XS, Sire C, et al. Cetuximab-radiotherapy versus cetuximab-radiotherapy plus concurrent chemotherapy in patients with N0-N2a squamous cell carcinoma of the head and neck (SCCHN): results of the GORTEC 2007-01 phase III randomized trial. *J Clin Oncol*. 2016;34(suppl):abstr 6003. doi:10.1200/JCO.2016.34.15_suppl.6003
42. Lefebvre JL, Pointreau Y, Rolland F, et al. Induction chemotherapy followed by either chemoradiotherapy or bioradiotherapy for larynx preservation: the TREMPLIN randomized phase II study. *J Clin Oncol*. 2013;31(7):853–859. doi:10.1200/JCO.2012.42.3988
43. Kies MS, Holsinger FC, Lee JJ, et al. Induction chemotherapy and cetuximab for locally advanced squamous cell carcinoma of the head and neck: results from a phase II prospective trial. *J Clin Oncol*. 2010;28(1):8–14. doi:10.1200/JCO.2009.23.0425
44. Vokes EE, Stenson K, Rosen FR, et al. Weekly carboplatin and paclitaxel followed by concomitant paclitaxel, fluorouracil, and hydroxyurea chemoradiotherapy: curative and organ-preserving therapy for advanced head and neck cancer. *J Clin Oncol*. 2003;21:320–326. doi:10.1200/JCO.2003.06.006
45. Argiris A, Heron DE, Smith RP, et al. Induction docetaxel, cisplatin, and cetuximab followed by concurrent radiotherapy, cisplatin, and cetuximab and maintenance cetuximab in patients with locally advanced head and neck cancer. *J Clin Oncol*. 2010;28(36):5294–5300. doi:10.1200/JCO.2010.30.6423

46. Lee K-W, Koh Y, Kim S-B, et al. A randomized, multicenter, phase II study of cetuximab with docetaxel and cisplatin as induction chemotherapy in unresectable, locally advanced head and neck cancer. *Oncologist* 2015;20(10):1119–1120. doi:10.1634/theoncologist.2015-0208
47. Harari PM, Harris J, Kies MS, et al. Postoperative chemoradiotherapy and cetuximab for high-risk squamous cell carcinoma of the head and neck: Radiation Therapy Oncology Group RTOG-0234. *J Clin Oncol.* 2014;32(23):2486–2495. doi:10.1200/JCO.2013.53.9163
48. Bernier J, Domenge C, Ozsahin M, et al. Postoperative irradiation with or without concomitant chemotherapy for locally advanced head and neck cancer. *N Engl J Med.* 2004;350(19):1945–1952. doi:10.1056/NEJMoa032641
49. Mesia R, Rueda A, Vera R, et al. Adjuvant therapy with cetuximab for locally advanced squamous cell carcinoma of the oropharynx: results from a randomized, phase II prospective trial. *Ann Oncol.* 2013;24(2):448–453. doi:10.1093/annonc/mds291
50. Vermorken JB, Mesia R, Rivera F, et al. Platinum-based chemotherapy plus cetuximab in head and neck cancer. *N Engl J Med.* 2008;359(11):1116–1127. doi:10.1056/NEJMoa0802656
51. Vermorken JB, Psyrri A, Mesia R, et al. Impact of tumor HPV status on outcome in patients with recurrent and/or metastatic squamous cell carcinoma of the head and neck receiving chemotherapy with or without cetuximab: retrospective analysis of the phase III EXTREME trial. *Ann Oncol.* 2014;25(4):801–807. doi:10.1093/annonc/mdt574
52. Guigay J, Fayette J, Dillies AF, et al. Cetuximab, docetaxel, and cisplatin as first-line treatment in patients with recurrent or metastatic head and neck squamous cell carcinoma: a multicenter, phase II GORTEC study. *Ann Oncol.* 2015:26(9):1941. doi:10.1093/annonc/mdv268
53. Baselga J, Trigo JM, Bourhis J, et al. Phase II multicenter study of the antiepidermal growth factor receptor monoclonal antibody cetuximab in combination with platinum-based chemotherapy in patients with platinum-refractory metastatic and/or recurrent squamous cell carcinoma of the head and neck. *J Clin Oncol.* 2005;23(24):5568–5577. doi:10.1200/JCO.2005.07.119
54. Herbst RS, Arquette M, Shin DM, et al. Phase II multicenter study of the epidermal growth factor receptor antibody cetuximab and cisplatin for recurrent and refractory squamous cell carcinoma of the head and neck. *J Clin Oncol.* 2005;23(24):5578–5587. doi:10.1200/JCO.2005.07.120
55. Vermorken JB, Trigo J, Hitt R, et al. Open-label, uncontrolled, multicenter phase II study to evaluate the efficacy and toxicity of cetuximab as a single agent in patients with recurrent and/or metastatic squamous cell carcinoma of the head and neck who failed to respond to platinum-based therapy. *J Clin Oncol.* 2007;25(16):2171–2177. doi:10.1200/JCO.2006.06.7447
56. Vermorken JB, Herbst RS, Leon X, et al. Overview of the efficacy of cetuximab in recurrent and/or metastatic squamous cell carcinoma of the head and neck in patients who previously failed platinum-based therapies. *Cancer.* 2008;112(12):2710–2719. doi:10.1002/cncr.23442
57. Leon X, Hitt R, Constenla M, et al. A retrospective analysis of the outcome of patients with recurrent and/or metastatic squamous cell carcinoma of the head and neck refractory to a platinum-based chemotherapy. *Clin Oncol.* 2005;17(6):418–424. doi:10.1016/j.clon.2005.02.014
58. Giralt J, Trigo J, Nuyts S, et al. Panitumumab plus radiotherapy versus chemoradiotherapy in patients with unresected, locally advanced squamous-cell carcinoma of the head and neck (CONCERT-2): a randomised, controlled, open-label phase 2 trial. *Lancet Oncol.* 2015;16(2):221–232. doi:10.1016/S1470-2045(14)71200-8
59. Siu LL, Waldron JN, Chen BE, et al. Effect of standard radiotherapy with cisplatin vs accelerated radiotherapy with panitumumab in locoregionally advanced squamous cell head and neck carcinoma: a randomized clinical trial. *JAMA Oncol.* 2016. doi:10.1001/jamaoncol.2016.4510
60. Ringash J, Waldron JN, Siu LL, et al. Quality of life and swallowing with standard chemoradiotherapy versus accelerated radiotherapy and panitumumab in locoregionally advanced carcinoma of the head and neck: a phase III randomised trial from the Canadian Cancer Trials Group (HN.6). *Eur J Cancer.* 2016;72:192–199. doi:10.1016/j.ejca.2016.11.008
61. Mesia R, Henke M, Fortin A, et al. Chemoradiotherapy with or without panitumumab in patients with unresected, locally advanced squamous-cell carcinoma of the head and neck (CONCERT-1): a randomised, controlled, open-label phase 2 trial. *Lancet Oncol.* 2015;16(2): 208–220. doi:10.1016/S1470-2045(14)71198-2
62. Vermorken JB, Stohlmacher-Williams J, Davidenko I, et al. Cisplatin and fluorouracil with or without panitumumab in patients with recurrent or metastatic squamous-cell carcinoma of the head and neck (SPECTRUM): an open-label phase 3 randomised trial. *Lancet Oncol.* 2013;14(8):697–710. doi:10.1016/S1470-2045(13)70181-5
63. Wirth LJ, Dakhil SR, Kornek G, et al. A randomized phase II study of docetaxel/cisplatin (doc/cis) chemotherapy with or without panitumumab (pmab) as first-line treatment (tx) for recurrent or metastatic squamous cell carcinoma of the head and neck (R/M SCCHN). *J Clin Oncol.* 2013;31:abst 6029. doi:10.1200/jco.2013.31.15_suppl.6029
64. Rischin D, Spigel DR, Adkins D, et al. PRISM: Phase 2 trial with panitumumab monotherapy as second-line treatment in patients with recurrent or metastatic squamous cell carcinoma of the head and neck. *Head Neck.* 2016;38: E1756–E1761. doi:10.1002/hed.24311
65. Machiels JP, Subramanian S, Ruzsa A, et al. Zalutumumab plus best supportive care versus best supportive care alone in patients with recurrent or metastatic squamous-cell carcinoma of the head and neck after failure of platinum-based chemotherapy: an open-label, randomised phase 3 trial. *Lancet Oncol.* 2011;12(4):333–343. doi:10.1016/S1470-2045(11)70034-1

66. Eriksen JG, Maare C, Johansen J, et al. Four-year update of the randomized phase III trial DAHANCA 19: Primary C-RT or RT and zalutumumab for squamous cell carcinomas of the head and neck. Abstract presented at: The European Cancer Congress 2013, Amsterdam, Netherlands.
67. Crombet T, Torres L, Neninger E, et al. Pharmacological evaluation of humanized anti-epidermal growth factor receptor, monoclonal antibody h-R3, in patients with advanced epithelial-derived cancer. *J Immun.* 2003;2:139–148. PMID: 12616105
68. Rodriguez MO, Rivero TC, Del Castillo Bahi R, et al. Nimotuzumab plus radiotherapy for unresectable squamous-cell carcinoma of the head and neck. *Cancer Biol Ther.* 2010;9(5):343–349. PMID: 20448462
69. Reddy BKM, et al. Nimotuzumab provides survival benefit to patients with inoperable advanced squamous cell carcinoma of the head and neck: a randomized, open-label, phase IIb, 5-year study in Indian patients. *Oral Oncol.* 2014;50:498–505. doi:10.1016/j.oraloncology.2013.11.008
70. Bhatnagar AR, Singh DP, Sharma R, et al. A comparative study of monoclonal antibody against EGFR (nimotuzumab) used in combination with chemoradiationversus chemoradiation alone in the treatment of locally advanced inoperable squamous cell carcinoma of the head and neck. *J Clin Oncol.* 2012;30(suppl):abstract e16012. doi:10.1200/jco.2012.30.15_suppl.e16012
71. Jungbluth AA, Stockert E, Huang HJ, et al. A monoclonal antibody recognizing human cancers with amplification/ overexpression of the human epidermal growth factor receptor. *Proc Natl Acad Sci USA.* 2003;100(2):639–665. doi:10.1073/pnas.232686499
72. Gan HK, Burgess AW, Clayton AH, et al. Targeting of a conformationally exposed, tumor-specific epitope of EGFR as a strategy for cancer therapy. *Cancer Res.* 2012;72(12):2924–2930. doi:10.1158/0008-5472.CAN-11-3898
73. Reilly EB, Phillips AC, Buchanan FG, et al. Characterization of ABT-806, a humanized tumor-specific anti-EGFR monoclonal antibody. *Mol Cancer Ther.* 2015;14(5):1141–1151. doi:10.1158/1535-7163.MCT-14-0820
74. Gregoire V, Hamoir M, Chen C, et al. Gefitinib plus cisplatin and radiotherapy in previously untreated head and neck squamous cell carcinoma: a phase II, randomized, double-blind, placebo-controlled study. *Radiother Oncol.* 2011;100(1):62–69. doi:10.1016/j.radonc.2011.07.008
75. Stewart JS, Cohen EE, Licitra L, et al. Phase III study of gefitinib compared with intravenous methotrexate for recurrent squamous cell carcinoma of the head and neck. *J Clin Oncol.* 2009;27(11):1864–1871. doi:10.1200/JCO.2008.17.0530
76. Argiris A, Ghebremichael M, Gilbert J, et al. Phase III randomized, placebo-controlled trial of docetaxel with or without gefitinib in recurrent or metastatic head and neck cancer: an eastern cooperative oncology group trial. *J Clin Oncol.* 2013;31(11):1405–1414. doi:10.1200/JCO.2012.45.4272
77. Martins RG, Parvathaneni U, Bauman JE, et al. Cisplatin and radiotherapy with or without erlotinib in locally advanced squamous cell carcinoma of the head and neck: a randomized phase II trial. *J Clin Oncol.* 2013;31(11):1415–1421. doi:10.1200/JCO.2012.46.3299
78. Hainsworth JD, Spigel DR, Greco FA, et al. Combined modality treatment with chemotherapy, radiation therapy, bevacizumab, and erlotinib in patients with locally advanced squamous carcinoma of the head and neck: a phase II trial of the Sarah Cannon oncology research consortium. *Cancer J.* 2011;17(5):267–272. doi:10.1097/PPO.0b013e3182329791
79. Soulieres D, Senzer NN, Vokes EE, et al. Multicenter phase II study of erlotinib, an oral epidermal growth factor receptor tyrosine kinase inhibitor, in patients with recurrent or metastatic squamous cell cancer of the head and neck. *J Clin Oncol.* 2004;22(1):77–85. doi:10.1200/JCO.2004.06.075
80. Siu LL, Soulieres D, Chen EX, et al. Phase I/II trial of erlotinib and cisplatin in patients with recurrent or metastatic squamous cell carcinoma of the head and neck: a Princess Margaret Hospital phase II consortium and National Cancer Institute of Canada Clinical Trials Group Study. *J Clin Oncol.* 2007;25(16):2178–2183. doi:10.1200/JCO.2006.07.6547
81. Kim ES, Kies MS, Glisson BS, et al. Final results of a phase II study of erlotinib, docetaxel and cisplatin in patients with recurrent/metastatic head and neck cancer. *J Clin Oncol.* 2007;25(18S):abstract 6013. doi:10.1200/jco.2007.25.18_suppl.6013
82. William WN, Feng L, Kies MS, et al. Randomized, double-blind, placebo-controlled, phase II trial of first-line platinum/docetaxel with or without erlotinib (E) in patients (pts) with recurrent and/or metastatic (R/M) head and neck squamous cell carcinomas (HNSCCs). *J Clin Oncol.* 2017;35:(15, suppl):6017–6017. doi:10.1634/theoncologist.2017-0661
83. Del Campo JM, Hitt R, Sebastian P, et al. Effects of lapatinib monotherapy: results of a randomised phase II study in therapy-naive patients with locally advanced squamous cell carcinoma of the head and neck. *Br J Cancer.* 2011;105(5):618–627. doi:10.1038/bjc.2011.237
84. Harrington K, Berrier A, Robinson M, et al. Randomised Phase II study of oral lapatinib combined with chemoradiotherapy in patients with advanced squamous cell carcinoma of the head and neck: rationale for future randomised trials in human papilloma virus-negative disease. *Eur J Cancer.* 2013;49(7):1609–1618. doi:10.1016/j.ejca.2012.11.023
85. Harrington K, Temam S, Mehanna H, et al. Postoperative adjuvant lapatinib and concurrent chemoradiotherapy followed by maintenance lapatinib monotherapy in high-risk patients with resected squamous cell carcinoma of the head and neck: a Phase III, randomized, double-blind, placebo-controlled study. *J Clin Oncol.* 2015;33(35):4202–4209. doi:10.1200/JCO.2015.61.4370

86. Lalami Y, Specenier PM, Awada A, et al. EORTC 24051: unexpected side effects in a phase I study of TPF induction chemotherapy followed by chemoradiation with lapatinib, a dual EGFR/ErbB2 inhibitor, in patients with locally advanced resectable larynx and hypopharynx squamous cell carcinoma. *Radiother Oncol.* 2012;105(2): 238–240. doi:10.1016/j.radonc.2012.08.006
87. De Souza JA, Davis DW, Zhang Y, et al. A phase II study of lapatinib in recurrent/metastatic squamous cell carcinoma of the head and neck. *Clin Cancer Res.* 2012;18(8):2336–2343. doi:10.1158/1078-0432. CCR-11-2825
88. Li D, Ambrogio L, Shimamura T, et al. BIBW2992, an irreversible EGFR/HER2 inhibitor highly effective in preclinical lung cancer models. *Oncogene.* 2008;27(34):702–4711. doi:10.1038/onc.2008.109
89. Solca F, Dahl G, Zoephel A, et al. Target binding properties and cellular activity of afatinib (BIBW 2992), an irreversible ErbB family blocker. *J Pharmacol Exp Ther.* 2012;343(2):342–350. doi:10.1124/jpet.112.197756
90. Seiwert TY, Fayette J, Cupissol D, et al. A randomized, phase 2 study of afatinib versus cetuximab in metastatic or recurrent squamous cell carcinoma of the head and neck. *Ann Oncol.* 2014;25(9):1813–1820. doi:10.1093/annonc/mdu216
91. Machiels JP, Haddad RI, Fayette J, et al. Afatinib versus methotrexate (MTX) as second-line treatment for patients with recurrent and/or metastatic (R/M) head and neck squamous cell carcinoma. *Lancet Oncology.* 2015;16(5):583–594. doi:10.1016/S1470-2045(15)70124-5
92. Cohen EEW, Fayette LJ, Gauler TC, et al. Biomarker analysis in recurrent and/or metastatic head and neck squamous cell carcinoma (R/M HNSCC) patients (pts) treated with second-line afatinib versus methotrexate (MTX): LUX-Head & Neck 1 (LUX-H&N1). *J Clin Oncol.* 2015;33(suppl):abstract 6023. doi:10.1200/jco.2015.33.15_suppl.6023
93. Clement PM, Gauler T, Machiels JP, et al. Afatinib versus methotrexate in older patients with second-line recurrent and/or metastatic head and neck squamous cell carcinoma: subgroup analysis of the LUX-Head & Neck 1 trial. *Ann Oncol.* 2016;27(8):1585–1593. doi:10.1093/annonc/mdw151
94. Gonzales AJ, Hook KE, Althaus IW, et al. Antitumor activity and pharmacokinetic properties of PF-00299804, a second-generation irreversible pan-erbB receptor tyrosine kinase inhibitor. *Mol Cancer Ther.* 2008;7(7):1880–1889. doi:10.1158/1535-7163. MCT-07-2232
95. Abdul Razak AR, Soulieres D, Laurie SA, et al. A phase II trial of dacomitinib, an oral pan-human EGF receptor (HER) inhibitor, as first-line treatment in recurrent and/or metastatic squamous-cell carcinoma of the head and neck. *Ann Oncol.* 2013;24(3):761–769. doi:10.1093/annonc/mds503
96. Wedge SR, Ogilvie DJ, Dukes M, et al. ZD6474 inhibits vascular endothelial growth factor signaling, angiogenesis, and tumor growth following oral administration. *Cancer Res.* 2002;62(16):4645–4655.
97. Limaye S, Riley S, Zhao S, et al. A randomized phase II study of docetaxel with or without vandetanib in recurrent or metastatic squamous cell carcinoma of head and neck (SCCHN). *Oral Oncol.* 2013;49(8):835–841. doi:10.1016/j.oraloncology.2013.04.010
98. Cervantes-Ruiperez A, Juric D, Hidalgo M, et al. A phase I study of MEHD7945A (MEHD), a first-in-class HER3/EGFR dual-action antibody, in patients (pts) with refractory/recurrent epithelial tumors: expansion cohorts. *J Clin Oncol.* 2009;27:abst 2565.
99. Fayette J, Wirth L, Oprean C, et al. Randomized phase II study of duligotuzumab (MEHD7945A) vs. cetuximab in squamous cell carcinoma of the head and neck (MEHGAN Study). *Front Oncol.* 2016;6:232. doi:10.3389/fonc.2016.00232
100. Pedersen MW, Jacobsen HJ, Koefoed K, et al. Sym004: a novel synergistic anti-epidermal growth factor receptor antibody mixture with superior anticancer efficacy. *Cancer Res.* 2010;70(2):588–597. doi:10.1158/0008-5472.CAN-09-1417
101. Machiels JP, Specenier PM, Krauss J, et al. A proof of concept trial of the anti-EGFR antibody mixture Sym004 in patients with squamous cell carcinoma of the head and neck. *Cancer Chemother Pharmacol.* 2015;76(1):13–20. doi:10.1007/s00280-015-2761-4
102. Lai SY, Koppikar P, Thomas SM, et al. Intratumoral epidermal growth factor receptor antisense dna therapy in head and neck cancer: first human application and potential antitumor mechanisms. *J Clin Oncol.* 2009;27:1235–1242. doi:10.1200/JCO.2008.17.8251
103. Ferris RL, Blumenschein G Jr, Fayette J, et al. Nivolumab for recurrent squamous-cell carcinoma of the head and neck. *N Engl J Med.* 2016;375(19):1856–1867. doi:10.1056/NEJMoa1602252

eotaxin, granulocyte colony-stimulating factor, and stromal cell–derived factor-1α. Elevation in six to eight high-risk CAFs showed 100% sensitivity for disease progression. There was also a correlation between patients who had recurrence and an increase in levels of multiple CAFs, compared to baseline (22). Hence, initial VEGF measurement, in addition to other CAFs, might represent a marker for HNSCC recurrence. In 2005, a meta-analysis including 12 studies evaluated the correlation between VEGF and 2-year overall survival (OS) in patients with HNSCC. Patients with VEGF-positive tumors had a relative risk of almost twofold for mortality when compared to VEGF-negative patients. There was also a trend, although not statistically significant, toward the association between VEGF positivity and lymph node metastasis. This meta-analysis demonstrates that tumor VEGF overexpression has a prognostic significance in HNSCC (23). Another study assessed potential serum biomarkers in patients with locally advanced head and neck cancer treated with cisplatin, docetaxel, and cetuximab followed by radiotherapy, cisplatin, and cetuximab and maintenance cetuximab. Of the 31 biomarkers, including chemokines, cytokines, and growth factors, low baseline levels of VEGF and IL-6 were associated with better prognosis (24).

CLINICAL EVIDENCE

BEVACIZUMAB

Bevacizumab is a monoclonal antibody that binds and blocks VEGF. It represents the first Food and Drug Administration (FDA) approved agent to target angiogenesis. It was approved in the United States in 2004 for the treatment of metastatic colon cancer in addition to chemotherapy (25). In recurrent or metastatic HNSCC (R/M HNSCC), there have been several trials studying bevacizumab in combinations with other agents, such as chemotherapy and epidermal growth factor receptor (EGFR) inhibitors (Table 12.1).

Particular interest has been shown in combining bevacizumab with agents that target EGFR, because VEGF-mediated angiogenesis is believed to have a role in EGFR-resistant tumors (26,27). There exist also preclinical data that suggest increased antitumor activity when adding an anti-VEGF to an anti-EGFR molecule (28). In 2009, a phase I/II trial studied the combination of bevacizumab and erlotinib, an EGFR inhibitor in patients with R/M HNSCC who have had only up to one previous treatment regimen. It showed an objective response rate (ORR) of 15%, which was better when compared to ORR with erlotinib and sorafenib alone (4%) (29–31). However, the latter combination was globally inferior when compared to the combination of cetuximab, another EGFR inhibitor, cisplatin or carboplatin, and fluorouracil as first-line treatment in HNSCC, even though these two studies represent different designs (32). The bevacizumab and erlotinib combination was associated with a 6% rate of bleeding and 4% of infection grade 3 or higher. Cetuximab in combination with bevacizumab was also investigated in a phase II study (33). The ORR of 16% and median OS of 7.5 months were similar to the erlotinib and bevacizumab combination. Argiris et al. conducted a phase II study, which combined bevacizumab with pemetrexed. The rationale of using pemetrexed, an antifolate, was that methotrexate, also being an antifolate agent, has antitumor activity and is already approved in HNSCC treatment. The ORR was 30% and OS was 11.3 months. Moreover, a phase III trial compared chemotherapy (investigator's choice of one of four platinum doublets) with or without bevacizumab in the first-line treatment of R/M HNSCC. The primary end point was OS. There was a statistically significant benefit in median progression-free survival (PFS; 4.4 vs. 6.1 months) and ORR (25 vs. 36%) in favor of the combination group. However, there was no difference in median OS (34).

SUNITINIB

Sunitinib is an inhibitor of receptor tyrosine kinases (RTKs) such as VEGFR-1, -2, -3; platelet-derived growth factor receptor (PDGFR)–α and –β; c-KIT; and RET (35). As mentioned earlier, VEGFR and its ligand VEGF are expressed by head and neck cancer cells and are associated with worse clinical outcome. PDGFR is also significantly expressed in HNSCC (36). Preclinical data have shown that PDGFR stimulates VEGF expression, which promotes tumor vessel formation and tumor perfusion (37). Using a rat model, a study demonstrated that inhibiting PDGFR and VEGF simultaneously resulted in 40% reduction in tumor vasculature and in tumor hypoxia (38). Therefore, three phase II studies were completed (Table 12.1). They investigated sunitinib as a single agent in R/M HNSCC. Choong et al. showed that sunitinib had very

TABLE 12.1

Phase II Trials With Angiogenesis Targeting Agents in Recurrent or Metastatic Head and Neck Cancer

Anti-VEGF	Regimens	Population	Number of Patients	Clinical Outcomes	95% Confidence Intervals/ *p* values
Bevacizumab	Bevacizumab + erlotinib	Maximum of 1 prior line of treatment for R/M HNSCC	46	PFS 4.1 mos OS 7.1 mos	2·8–4·4 5·7–9·0
	Bevacizumab + cetuximab	Maximum of 1 prior line of treatment for R/M HNSCC	46	PFS 2.8 mos OS 7.5 mos	2.7–4.2 5.7–9.6
	Bevacizumab + pemetrexed	No prior chemotherapy or biologic therapy for R/M HNSCC	40	TTP 5.0 mos OS 11.3 mos	4.0–7.0* 8.7–16.8*
Sunitinib	Sunitinib	Maximum of 2 prior lines of treatment for R/M HNSCC Cohort A: PS 0-1 Cohort B: PS 2	Cohort A: 15 Cohort B: 7	Cohort A TTP: 8.4 wks OS: 21.0 wks Cohort B TTP: 10.5 wks OS: 19.0 wks	 N/A N/A N/A N/A
		No prior treatment for R/M HNSCC	17	TTP: 2.3 mos OS: 4.0 mos	1.0–3.6 3.2–4.9
		Maximum of 2 prior lines of treatment for R/M HNSCC	38	PFS: 60 days OS: 102 days	81.0–123.0 39.0–81.0
Sorafenib	Sorafenib	Maximum of 1 prior line of chemotherapy for R/M HNSCC	26	TTP: 1.8 mos OS: 4.2 mos	1.6–3.4 3.6–8.7
		No prior chemotherapy for R/M HNSCC	41	PFS: 4 mos OS: 9 mos	2.0–4.0 7.0–14.0
	Cetuximab + placebo (arm A) Sorafenib + cetuximab (arm B)	Maximum of 1 prior line of chemotherapy for R/M HNSCC	55 (27 in arm A and 28 in arm B)	Arm A PFS: 2 mos OS: 9 mos Arm B PFS: 3.2 mos OS: 5.7 mos	*p*-values PFS: 0.87 OS: 0.41
Axitinib	Axitinib	Any number of prior treatments for R/M HNSCC	30	PFS: 3.7 mos OS: 10.9 mos	3.5–5.7 6.4–17.8

(continued)

TABLE 12.1 (*continued*)

Phase II Trials With Angiogenesis Targeting Agents in Recurrent or Metastatic Head and Neck Cancer

Anti-VEGF	Regimens	Population	Number of Patients	Clinical Outcomes	95% Confidence Intervals/ *p* values
Vandetanib	Docetaxel alone (arm A) Docetaxel + vandetanib (arm B)	Progression on 1 prior line of platinum-based chemotherapy as definitive or palliative treatment	29 (14 in arm A and 15 in arm B)	Arm A PFS: 3.2 wks OS: 26.8 wks Arm B PFS: 9.0 wks OS: 24.1 wks	 3.0–22.0 17.7–100.7 5.9–18.1 16.4–171.1

N/A, not available; OS, overall survival; PFS, progression-free survival; R/M HNSCC, recurrent or metastatic head and neck squamous cell carcinoma; TTP, time to progression; .

little efficacy with median OS being 21 weeks in the group with better performance status (PS). Toxicity was not negligible with 18% of patients experiencing bleeding grades 3 or more (35). A second phase II study using sunitinib alone also demonstrated low efficacy with only 18% of patients presenting stable disease. Median OS was only 4 months (39). The last phase II trial investigating sunitinib as a single agent also had disappointing antitumor activity with a median OS of only 3.4 months. Adverse effects were significant. Approximately 40% of patients developed new or progressive tumor skin ulcers or fistulas (40). In brief, despite the scientific rationale of coinhibiting VEGF and PDFGR with sunitinib, poor clinical outcomes have resulted from phase II studies. Its use as a single agent in R/M HNSCC is thus not warranted.

SORAFENIB

Sorafenib also inhibits VEGF and its receptors VEGFR-2, -3, as well as FLT3 and c-kit. It is also an antagonist of serine/threonine kinases C-Raf and B-Raf. Hence, this agent was thought to have potential antitumor activity in R/M HNSCC because it targets two important signaling pathways involved in cancer, Ras-Raf-MEK-ERK and VEGF-VEGFR. They regulate cell growth/differentiation and angiogenesis, respectively (4–6,30,41). The first phase II trial was published in 2007 by Elser et al. and studied the tolerability and efficacy of sorafenib as a single oral agent in 26 patients with R/M HNSCC who had not received more than one line of chemotherapy in this setting. It was globally well tolerated with no grade 4 toxicities. Grade 3 adverse effects were mostly lymphopenias in 17% of patients. The efficacy was comparable to sunitinib, with a TTP of 1.8 months and a median OS of 4 months (30). Williamson et al. investigated the effect of sorafenib in another phase II trial, which was conducted on chemotherapy-naïve patients for R/M HNSCC. 14% of patients experienced grade 3 toxicity, such as nausea, hand–foot syndrome, and anorexia. The OS was 9 months, superior to what has been shown in a trial mentioned earlier. This can be partly explained by the difference in inclusion criteria. Williamson et al. included patients who had never received prior chemotherapy in the R/M setting, whereas Elser at al. included 30% of patients with prior palliative chemotherapy. Morever, Williamson et al.'s study included 9% more patients with ECOG 0 (39% versus 30%) (30,42). In 2015, a blinded, randomized phase II, placebo-controlled study compared a combination of cetuximab and placebo (arm A) versus sorafenib and cetuximab (arm B) in R/M HNSCC. The difference in OS between the combination and placebo groups was not statistically different. Furthermore, the combination was more toxic with 82% versus 11% grade 3 toxicities (43). In brief, even though there is scientific rationale for sorafenib efficacy in HNSCC, several studies have shown very modest antitumor activity as a single agent and when combined with an EGFR inhibitor (Table 12.1). There currently exists an ongoing phase I/II trial combining sorafenib with cisplatin and docetaxel in patients with R/M HNSCC. It will be interesting to know if a combination of sorafenib and chemotherapy brings any significant survival benefit.

AXITINIB

Axitinib, an oral tyrosine kinase inhibitor, has also been studied in a phase II trial in R/M HNSCC. Axitinib blocks VEGFR-1, -2, -3; PDGFR; and c-kit and has shown antitumor activity in renal cell carcinoma, medullary and differentiated thyroid cancers. Its use in patients with R/M HNSCC showed a median OS of 10.9 months. This clinical benefit still remains acceptable given that patients were heavily pretreated with 30% of them having received at least three prior lines of chemotherapy (Table 12.1) (44).

VANDETANIB

Vandetanib is similar to previously mentioned agents in that it inhibits VEGFR-2 and VEGF. Interestingly, it also antagonizes EGFR, and therefore targets two key signaling pathways in tumorigenesis. Vandetanib was first FDA-approved in 2012 for treatment of metastatic medullary thyroid cancer (45). It has shown antitumor activity in preclinical data, such as decreased survival, invasion, and tumor growth of HNSCC cell lines (46). In 2013, a randomized open-label phase II trial compared docetaxel alone or in combination with vandetanib in R/M HNSCC. There was no PFS or OS benefit in the combination group, even though 43% of patients had never received prior systemic treatment for their R/M disease (Table 12.1) (47). Furthermore, pazopanib, another multitargeted tyrosine kinase inhibitor, is being investigated in two ongoing trials, in a phase II as a single agent and in a phase I with cetuximab (NCT01377298, NCT01716416).

In brief, VEGF/VEGFR and multitargeted tyrosine kinase inhibitors have shown poor clinical efficacy as monotherapy or when combined with chemotherapy or other targeted therapies in R/M HNSCC. Some of these anti-VEGF/VEGFR agents, such as sunitinib or sorafenib, have shown stronger clinical activity in other types of cancers. An example is clear cell renal carcinoma (CCRC). This can mostly be explained by somatic genetic mutations or hypermethylation, which cause an inactivation of the von Hippel–Lindau (*VHL*) tumor suppressor gene and protein (pVHL). The frequency of *VHL* mutations in sporadic CCRC is at least 50%. *VHL* mutation then leads to HIF transcription factor accumulation followed by expression of VEGF (48). Thus, there is a clonal basis and rationale for use of VEGF-targeted therapy in CCRC. To our knowledge, no clonal event related to angiogenesis has been described in HNSCC. This possibly explains the poor clinical benefits mentioned earlier with anti-VEGF therapy.

VEGF INHIBITION AND RADIATION THERAPY

VEGF expression can be upregulated by different mechanisms, including hypoxic regulation and nonhypoxic regulation. Hypoxic tumor cells can increase the hypoxia-inducing factor-1 (HIF-1), which is a transcription factor that increases the expression of VEGF (49). Nonhypoxic regulation of VEGF involves a variety of effectors including growth factors, cytokines, and so on (50). Radiation exposure can activate EGFR, which in turn activates PI3K/AKT and STAT3 pathways, resulting in upregulation of VEGF (51). Combination of antiangiogenic therapies and radiation can help to overcome the radioresistance in tumor by normalizing tumor vasculature (52,53).

A phase I trial of 43 patients demonstrated the feasibility of adding bevacizumab (10 mg/kg every 2 weeks) to 5-fluorouracil plus hydroxyurea with radiation in patients with recurrent or poor prognostic HNSCC (54). In this study, approximately two thirds of patients had prior radiation for HNSCC. The doses of 5-fluorouracil and hydroxyurea were reduced (to 600 mg/m^2 and 500 mg, respectively) when bevacizumab was escalated to 10 mg/kg because of increased neutropenia associated with the addition of bevacizumab (54). Overall treatment was well tolerated without severe synergistic toxicities as possible bevacizumab-related toxicities (two deep venous thromboses, a fatal stroke, and two fatal bleeding events [54]) occurred at a similar rate as previously reported in this high-risk population treated without bevacizumab (55,56).

A subsequent phase II randomized trial explored the addition of bevacizumab to 5-fluorouracil, hydroxyurea, and twice-daily radiotherapy in patients with intermediate-stage and T4N0-1 HNSCC (57). Accrual was prematurely terminated because of a higher number of patients with locoregional progression in the bevacizumab arm. A total of 26 patients were enrolled, with 19 receiving bevacizumab (2:1 randomization). Locoregional progression was seen in four of five T4 patients in the bevacizumab arm versus zero of two patients in the comparison arm, with 2-year actuarial locoregional control of 67% (95% confidence interval [CI]: 34%–86%) versus 100%, respectively. Two-year survival was 58% (95% CI: 33%–78%) for patients in the bevacizumab arm, and 89% for patients in the comparison arm. Two patients in the bevacizumab arm died during therapy and one died shortly after therapy, but there was no catastrophic bleeding.

Another phase II study investigated the addition of bevacizumab to concurrent chemoradiation with cisplatin plus intensity modulated radiotherapy (IMRT) of 70 Gy in 42 patients with locally advanced HNSCC (58). This study reported 2-year OS of 88% (95% CI: 78.6%–98.4%) and PFS of 75.9% (95% CI: 63.9%–90.1%), and similar toxicity as described in prior studies with concurrent radiation and cisplatin (58).

Another phase II multiinstitutional trial, RTOG 0615, was designed to test the addition of bevacizumab to standard chemoradiation treatment in patients with locally advanced nasopharyngeal carcinoma (59). In this trial, bevacizumab was administered together with cisplatin during IMRT, and also with cisplatin and fluorouracil after completion of IMRT. The 2-year results with 46 patients reported the feasibility of addition of bevacizumab to standard chemoradiation, without major compromise in the delivery of chemoradiation (all but one patient received the prescribed radiation dose of 70 Gy, and nearly 70% of patients received all cycles of concurrent cisplatin) (59). The 2-year locoregional progression-free rate of this trial was 84%, lower than the expected 90% in other series (60,61), which might be due to major deviations in radiation target volume in almost a third of cases (59). The 2-year distant metastasis-free interval was 90.8%, showing the potential of bevacizumab to delay the progression of subclinical distant disease. The 2-year OS was 91%, higher than historical control groups (62–65), but the relevance of the historical comparison is limited because of changes in American Joint Committee on Cancer (AJCC) staging for nasopharyngeal carcinoma and improvements in cancer staging with MRI or PET scans.

A phase II trial of adding both a VEGF inhibitor (bevacizumab) and an EGFR inhibitor (erlotinib) to concurrent cheomoradiation in 60 patients with locally advanced head and neck cancer showed the feasibility of such a regimen (66). This study showed 95% of patients had complete or partial radiographic response, and OS of 82% at 3 years, which was much higher than the reported OS of 51% at 3 years in 123 patients treated with the identical chemotherapy and radiation therapy without bevacizumab or erlotinib (67). The combined modality therapy did not cause unexpected toxicity, and grade 3 or 4 mucositis was the most common side effect (66). Another noncomparative phase II randomized trial investigated the dual inhibition of EGFR and VEGF in 78 patients with locally advanced HNSCC, using the regimen of concurrent cetuximab, pemetrexed, radiation, with (arm A) or without bevacizumab (arm B) (68). Maintenance bevacizumab was administered for 24 weeks after chemoradiation in arm B. However, this part of the treatment was removed from the study protocol after a late fatal bleeding occurred in the first few patients enrolled. Patients receiving bevacizumab had significantly increased rate of hemorrhage, without apparent benefit in efficacy. Two-year PFS was 79% for arm A and 75% for arm B, both higher than historical control group (68).

There are also studies investigating combining other antiangiogenic agents with radiation therapy (Table 12.2), including phase I or II trials of sunitinib (70), and vandetanib (72) preclinical studies with sorafenib (73), motesanib (74), and linifanib (75). So far many phase I and II trials on combining VEGF inhibitors and radiation (or chemoradiation) have demonstrated acceptable toxicity and promising efficacy. However, currently there are no phase III randomized trials to evaluate the role of antiangiogenic agents combined with radiation in treating patients with locally advanced HNSCC.

NOVEL AGENTS IN HNSCC

PI3K INHIBITORS

PI3K signaling pathway is mutated or altered in 31% of HNSCC tumors. Up to 13% of these mutations involve the *PIK3CA* gene, which encodes a catalytic alpha class I PI3K. When activated, PI3K triggers the downstream target AKT, which then phosphorylates mammalian target of rapamycin (mTOR). The latter controls cellular proliferation, metabolism, and

TABLE 12.2

Studies With Angiogenesis Targeting Agents Combined With Radiation for HNSCC

Anti-VEGF	Regimens	Study Stage	Population	*N*	Clinical Outcomes	Reference
Bevacizumab	Bevacizumab + 5-FU + hydroxyurea + RT	Phase I	Recurrent, previously radiated, or poor prognosis, treatment-naive HNSCC	43	Bevacizumab was escalated to 10 mg/kg (with decreased chemotherapy) with acceptable toxicity	(54)
	Bevacizumab + cisplatin + RT	Phase II	Locally advanced, previously untreated HNSCC	42	Acceptable toxicity; OS 88% and PFS 76% at 2 years	(58)
	Bevacizumab + cisplatin + RT	Phase II	Locally advanced, previously untreated nasopharyngeal cancer	46	Feasible to add bevacizumab to CRT; LRC 83.7%, DC 90.8%, PFS 74.7%, OS 90.9% at 2 years	(59)
	Induction chemotherapy followed by bevacizumab + erlotinib + paclitaxel + T	Phase II	Locally advanced, previously untreated HNSCC	60	Feasible to administer such regimen; OS 82% at 3 years	(66)
	Pemetrexed + cetuximab + RT – -bevacizumab (arm A) + bevacizumab (arm B)	Phase II	Locally advanced, previously untreated HNSCC	78	Arm A: 2-year PFS 79% Arm B: 2-year PFS 75% Increased rate of hemorrhage in arm B	(68)
	Bevacizumab + docetaxel + RT	Phase II	Locally advanced, previously untreated HNSCC	30	Regimen was tolerable and effective, with PFS 61.7%, OS 68.2% at 3 years	(69)

(*continued*)

TABLE 12.2 (*continued*)

Studies With Angiogenesis Targeting Agents Combined With Radiation for HNSCC

Anti-VEGF	Regimens	Study Stage	Population	*N*	Clinical Outcomes	Reference
Sunitinib	Sunitinib + hypofractonated IGRT	Phase II	Oligometastatic HNSCC	25	LC 75%, DC 52%, PFS 56%, OS 71% at 18 months; 28% G3+ toxicities	(70)
	Sunitinib + cetuximab + RT	Phase I	Locally advanced or recurrent HNSCC	36	Trial terminated	(71)
Vandetanib	Vandetanib + RT +/-– cisplatin	Phase I	Locally advanced, previously untreated HNSCC	33	Feasible to combine vandetanib with CRT	(72)
Sorafenib	Sorafenib + cisplatin + RT	Preclinical	In vitro and in vivo models	na	Sorafenib enhances the antitumor effects of CRT	(73)
Motesanib	Motesanib + RT	Preclinical	In vivo models	NA	A favorable interaction between motesanib and RT	(74)
Linifanib	Linifanib + RT	Preclinical	In vitro models	NA	Enhanced inhibition of cell growth and apoptosis	(75)

CRT, chemoradiation; DC, distant control; HNSCC, head and neck squamous cell carcinoma; IGRT, image-guided radiation therapy; LR, local control; LRC, locoregional control; NA, not available; OS, overall survival; PFS, progression-free survival; RT, radiation therapy.

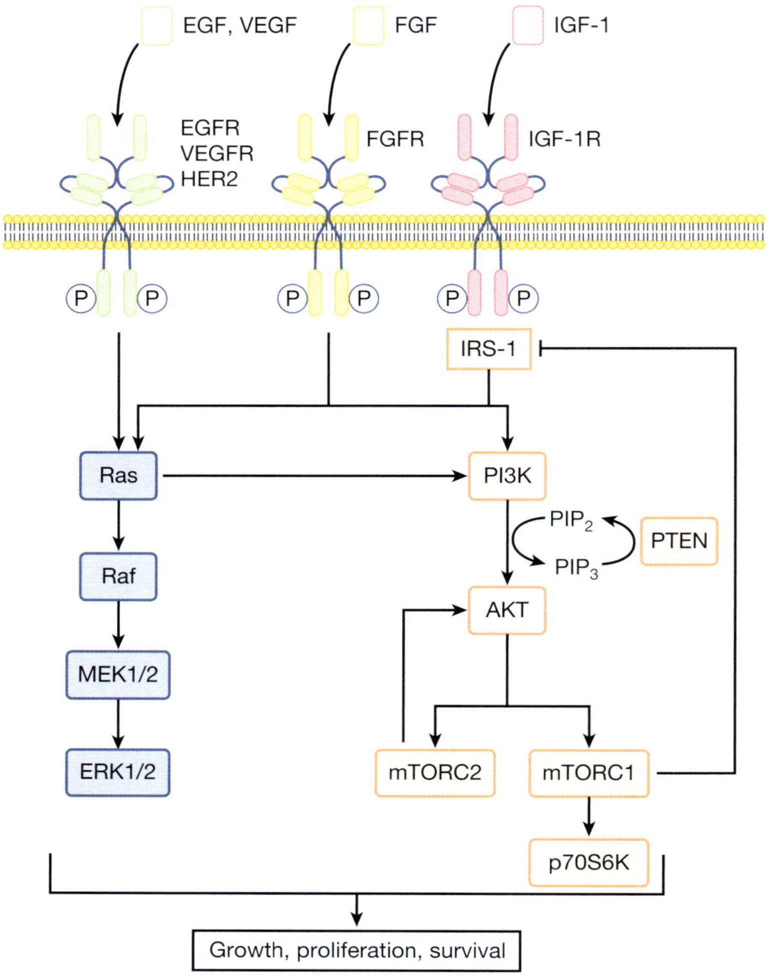

FIGURE 12.2 The PI3K/AKT/mTOR pathway.

mTOR, mammalian target of rapamycin.

Source: From Simpson DR, Mell LK, Cohen EEW. Targeting the PI3K/AKT/mTOR pathway in squamous cell carcinoma of the head and neck. *Oral Oncol.* 2015;51(4):291–298.

protein translation. Phosphatase and tensin homolog (PTEN) negatively regulate the PI3K pathway (Figure 12.2) (76). Inactivation of PTEN through mutations and gene copy loss has been reported in 4% and 8% of HNSCCs, respectively. This leads to uncontrolled PI3K cascade activation (77). Furthermore, several studies have shown that PI3K and EGFR pathways are necessary for cellular entry of human papillomavirus (HPV) (78,79). Analysis of HPV-positive HNSCCs demonstrated upregulation of PIK3CA, compared to HPV-negative tumors (80,81). Therefore, conceptually, HPV-positive patients with HNSCC might potentially have additional benefit from PI3K-targeted therapy.

Given the frequency of mutated PI3K signaling pathway in HNSCC, PI3K inhibitors are currently under investigation as monotherapy or combined with chemotherapy and/or radiation in patients with for the most part R/M HNSCC. Buparlisib (BKM120), a PI3K inhibitor, is being studied as a single agent in phase II trials and in combination with paclitaxel or cetuximab in R/M disease. Results from the randomized phase II study BERIL-1, which investigated the efficacy of buparlisib in addition to paclitaxel, were presented at ASCO 2016 (Table 12.3). Patients with platinum-pretreated R/M HNSCC were randomized to buparlisib and paclitaxel or placebo and paclitaxel. Patients had a favorable

TABLE 12.3

Completed Phase II Trials With Novel Agents in Recurrent or Metastatic HNSCC

Novel Agents	Regimens	Population	Number of Patients	Clinical Outcomes	95% Confidence Intervals/ *p* Values
Buparlisib	Paclitaxel + placebo (arm A) Paclitaxel + buparlisib (arm B)	Maximum of 1 prior line of chemotherapy, platinum-based, for R/M HNSCC	158	Arm A: PFS: 3.5 mos OS: 6.5 mos Arm B: PFS: 4.6 mos OS: 10.4 mos	 2.2–3.7 5.3–8.8 3.5–5.3 7.3–12.8
Temsirolimus	Temsirolimus	Failure on cetuximab or platinum-based chemotherapy in R/M HNSCC	40	PFS: 56 days OS: 152 days	36–113 76–256
	Temsirolimus + erlotinib	Progression during/after first line of platinum-based chemotherapy for R/M HNSCC	12	PFS: 1.9 mos OS: 4.0 mos	N/A N/A
Everolimus	Everolimus	At least 1 prior treatment for R/M HNSCC	9	PFS: 1.5 mos OS: 4.5 mos	N/A N/A
	Everolimus + erlotinib	Platinum-resistant R/M HNSCC with any number of prior treatments	35	PFS: 11.9 wks OS: 10.3 mos	N/A N/A

N/A, not available; OS, overall survival; PFS, progression-free survival; R/M HNSCC, recurrent or metastatic head and neck squamous cell carcinoma.

median OS of 10.4 versus 6.5 months in the combination and placebo groups, respectively. ORR was 39.2% in the buparlisib arm, compared to 14% in the placebo arm. Grade 3-4 adverse events were reported in 82% and 72% of patients in the combination and placebo arm, respectively. Interestingly, in BERIL-1, HPV-negative patients had higher clinical benefit from adding buparlisib to paclitaxel, which is opposite to what was theoretically expected. Moreover, a phase Ib is under way studying the combination of buparlisib, cisplatin, and radiotherapy in high-risk locally advanced disease. PX-866 and BYL719, other PI3K-blocking agents, are being investigated in phase II studies, combined with cetuximab or docetaxel and with cetuximab or paclitaxel, respectively (NCT01204099, NCT01252628, NCT02145312, NCT01602315, NCT012051751). In a randomized phase II trial, Jimeno et al. showed that combining PX-866 with cetuximab did not improve ORR, PFS, and OS, compared to cetuximab as a single agent in 83 patients with R/M HNSCC. Toxicities were significantly increased in the combination group (82). Given that HPV-positive tumors show upregulation of PIK3CA, Jimeno et al. subsequently compared clinical benefit from adding PX-866 in HPV-positive versus -negative patients. In spite of the aforementioned biologic rationale, there was no association between HPV-positivity and outcome when treating with PX-866 in this phase II study. In brief, there have been favorable clinical outcomes from adding buparlisib to a taxane as second-line treatment in R/M HNSCC. However, PX-866 combined with an anti-EGFR did not show any benefit. Other trials combining PX-866 with docetaxel and combining another PI3K inhibitor, BYL719, with paclitaxel and with cetuximab are ongoing.

mTOR INHIBITORS

The mTOR complexes represent downstream targets, which are activated via the PI3K signaling pathway through AKT/protein kinase B and the tuberous sclerosis complex (TSC1/2). When triggered, mTOR promotes messenger RNA translation and cell growth. Mutations in mTOR have been identified in 1.3% of HNSCC (77).

Temsirolimus

There have been two completed phase II trials studying temsirolimus, an mTOR inhibitor, in R/M HNSCC (Table 12.3). The TEMHEAD trial investigated the efficacy of temsirolimus as a single-arm treatment in heavily pretreated patients. The median OS was 152 days, which remains similar to the outcomes described in previous studies with multiple prior lines of treatment (83). Bauman et al. conducted a phase II trial studying the efficacy of combining temsirolimus and erlotinib. The latter combination was poorly tolerated with 6 out of 12 patients withdrawing, which terminated the study. Hence, efficacy analysis was limited and suboptimal (84).

Everolimus

Two recent completed phase II trials have studied efficacy of everolimus, another mTOR inhibitor (Table 12.3). Geiger et al. showed that everolimus as a single-arm treatment in patients with R/M HNSCC does not result in any clinical benefit. The small number of recruited patients can partly explain the lack of activity (85). Another phase II trial investigated the combination of everolimus and erlotinib in R/M HNSCC. Enrolled patients had platinum-resistant disease and were heavily pretreated, with 42% having received more than two lines of chemotherapy. The combination showed little clinical benefit (86).

In conclusion, mTOR inhibitors have demonstrated little clinical activity in R/M HNSCC. Other studies combining mTOR inhibitors with standard chemotherapy or other anti-EGFRs are under way or awaiting results.

COMBINATION OF OTHER NOVEL AGENTS WITH RADIATION

PI3K/AKT/MTOR INHIBITION AND RADIATION

Upregulation of PI3K/AKT/mTOR pathway, which is a downstream pathway of EGFR, is implicated in both EGFR resistance (87) and radiation resistance (88). Inhibition of PI3K/AKT/mTOR pathway has the potential to overcome such resistance and improve treatment efficacy.

Buparlisib (a PI3K inhibitor) was investigated in the preclinical experimental study combining it with cetuximab and radiation on an orthotopic xenograft model of HNSCC with *PIK3CA* mutation (89). This study found that adding buparlisib to cetuximab and radiation led to highest tumor inhibition ($p < .001$) compared to control, and the association of buparlisib and cetuximab with radiation inhibited radiation-induced activation of the MAPK pathway (89). Buparlisib is also investigated in an ongoing phase I trial (NCT02113878) where it is combined with standard chemoradiotherapy with weekly cisplatin in high-risk patients with locally advanced HNSCC (90).

Gedatolisib is a dual inhibitor of PI3K and mTOR. The preclinical study by Leiker et al. showed that gedatolisib resulted in significant radiosensitization of HNSCC cell lines both in vitro and in vivo (91). Another preclinical study by Ekshyyan et al. compared the radiosensitizing effects of temsirolimus (an mTOR inhibitor) to cisplatin in xenografts of HNSCC (92). This study found that temsirolimus combined with radiation had superior antitumor activity to chemoradiation with cisplatin (92).

MK2206 is an allosteric AKT inhibitor. It has been evaluated in a phase II study as a monotherapy in patients with recurrent and metastatic nasopharyngeal cancer where limited activity was observed in that heavily pretreated group of patients (93). To our knowledge, there is currently no study on the combination of AKT inhibitor and radiation in HNSCC.

HDAC INHIBITION AND RADIATION

Histone proteins facilitate the organization of DNA into compact structures of chromatin. Histone deacetylases (HDACs) regulate chromatin remodeling through epigenetic changes such as acetylation of histone proteins. Aberrant HDAC activity contributes to carcinogenesis, tumor progression, and treatment resistance (94). HDAC 1 and 2 expression is associated with worse outcomes in oral tongue cancers (95). HDAC inhibition provides a new way for anticancer therapy. Furthermore, HDAC inhibitors are thought to have synergy inhibition of ErbB, and upregulation of parallel receptor tyrosine kinases such as HER2 and HER3 (ErbB family) may play an important role in EGFR resistance (96). Therefore, HDAC inhibition has the potential to overcome EGFR resistance and to achieve better treatment efficacy.

Monotherapy with an HDAC inhibitor leads primarily to cytostasis of tumor cells in vitro (97,98), indicating its need to be combined to another therapy to achieve a cytotoxic effect. Laboratory studies have demonstrated that combination of an HDAC inhibitor and radiation resulted in prolonged expression of γH2AX, which is a sensitive indicator of DNA double-strand breaks (99). HDAC inhibition was also confirmed to have a synergy effect with EGFR inhibition in HNSCC cell lines, suggesting combination of HDAC and EGFR inhibition as a promising therapeutic strategy (100).

Clinical studies with HDAC inhibitor monotherapy were done in heavily pretreated patients with current or metastatic HNSCC, where no objective response was noted (101,102). This is consistent with the finding of in vitro studies in which cytostasis of tumor cells was observed. HDAC inhibitor was also investigated in combined therapy. CUDC-101 is a multitarget inhibitor of HDACs, EGFR, and HER2. The phase I study by Galloway et al. investigated CUDC-101 in combination with standard chemoradiation in patients with HNSCC (102). This study demonstrated the feasibility of combining CUDC-101, cisplatin, and radiation, with no unexpected adverse events reported (103). Further studies are still needed to assess the efficacy of combined therapy with HDAC inhibitors.

MET INHIBITION AND RADIATION

MET, also known as hepatocyte growth factor receptor (HGFR), is a tyrosine kinase receptor bound exclusively by the ligand hepatocyte growth factor (HGF). HGF-MET signaling is essential for normal processes such as embryogenesis, organ regeneration, and wound healing; abnormal MET expression is associated with tumor growth, invasion, and metastasis (104).

MET is overexpressed in roughly 80% of HNSCC and high expression is an independent marker of poor prognosis in HNSCC treated with chemoradiation (105,106). MET activation has been associated with cisplatin resistance (107), and it may also mediate recurrence and metastasis after cisplatin-based treatment in HNSCC (108). Treatment of HNSCC cell lines with cisplatin and a MET inhibitor was found to have a greater-than-additive inhibition of cell growth (105). The MET signaling converges with EGFR signaling on PI3K-AKT and RAS-MAPK (109), suggesting the ability for reciprocal compensation. Dual blockage of MET and EGFR resulted in an enhanced inhibition of tumor volumes accompanied by a decreased number of proliferating cells and increased apoptosis compared with single -agent treatment in HNSCC xenografts (109).

MET activation is also associated with radioresistance as radiation can induce overexpression and activity of MET oncogene and MET in turn prevents cell apoptosis and promotes cell invasion (110). In a cohort of 97 patients with radically irradiated oropharyngeal SCC, MET expression was a significant and independent predictor of worse local control, disease-free survival, and OS after radiation (111). However, in a study treating HNSCC xenografts with crizotinib (an MET inhibitor) and radiation, crizotinib failed to enhance the radiation response and failed to inhibit MET downstream signaling proteins in cell lines with MET expression (112). One possible reason for the failure is activation of an alternative pathway such as EGFR, which converges with MET pathway (109). Although MET remains a potential target in treating HNSCC, its role in combination with radiation therapy remains unclear.

CONCLUSIONS

The VEGF/VEGFR signaling pathway is a key regulator of angiogenesis and promotes tumorigenesis. It has also been shown to dampen antitumor immune response via several mechanisms such as enhanced Treg recruitment and inhibition of DC maturation. Promoting angiogenesis through VEGF/VEGFR signaling has been shown to mediate tumor resistance to chemotherapy (113–115). In HNSCC, both VEGF and VEGFR are overexpressed. Several studies have correlated the degree of VEGF positivity with worse outcomes, such as disease recurrence and mortality. Correlating VEGF positivity with predictive biomarker value needs to be further validated. In regard to VEGF-targeted therapy, agents used as monotherapy have shown modest clinical activity in the R/M disease setting and feasibility when combined with radiation in the definitive setting. The benefit from combining anti-VEGF molecules with chemotherapy, other targeted agents, and radiation remains to be demonstrated. Other signaling pathways of interest are PI3K-AKT and mTOR. The latter are mutated in HNSCC. PI3K inhibitor buparlisib in combination with paclitaxel has shown significant clinical benefit in R/M disease and warrants further investigation. However, with current data, mTOR inhibitors as monotherapy or combined with an anti-EGFR agent were not effective in HNSCC. Targeting of the PI3K/AKT/mTOR pathway, HDAC, and MET for treatment concurrently with (chemo)radiation is an area of active research.

REFERENCES

1. Folkman J, Merler E, Abernathy C, Williams G. Isolation of a tumor factor responsible for angiogenesis. *J Exp Med.* 1971;133(2):275–288. doi:10.1084/jem.133.2.275
2. Senger DR, Galli SJ, Dvorak AM, et al. Tumor cells secrete a vascular permeability factor that promotes accumulation of ascites fluid. *Science.* 1983;219(4587):983–985.
3. Senger DR, Brown LF, Claffey KP, Dvorak HF. Vascular permeability factor, tumor angiogenesis and stroma generation. *Invasion Metastasis.* 1994;14(1–6):385–394.
4. Shibuya M, Seetharam L, Ishii Y, et al. Possible involvement of VEGF-FLT tyrosine kinase receptor system in normal and tumor angiogenesis. *Princess Takamatsu Symp.* 1994;24:162–170.
5. Folkman J. The role of angiogenesis in tumor growth. *Semin Cancer Biol.* 1992;3(2):65–71.
6. Folkman J. Role of angiogenesis in tumor growth and metastasis. *Semin Oncol.* 2002;29(6, Suppl 16):15–18.
7. Christopoulos A, Ahn SM, Klein JD, Kim S. Biology of vascular endothelial growth factor and its receptors in head and neck cancer: beyond angiogenesis. *Head Neck.* 2011;33(8):1220–1229.
8. Vassilakopoulou M, Psyrri A, Argiris A. Targeting angiogenesis in head and neck cancer. *Oral Oncol.* 2015;51(5):409–415.
9. Hsu H-W, Wall NR, Hsueh C-T, et al. Combination antiangiogenic therapy and radiation in head and neck cancers. *Oral Oncol.* 2014;50(1):19–26.
10. Mimeault M, Batra SK. Hypoxia-inducing factors as master regulators of stemness properties and altered metabolism of cancer- and metastasis-initiating cells. *J Cell Mol Med.* 2013;17(1):30–54.
11. Cao Y, Wang G, Wang E, et al. VEGF exerts an angiogenesis-independent function in cancer cells to promote their malignant progression. *Cancer Res.* 2012;72(16):3912–3918.
12. Senger DR, Van De Water L. VEGF expression by epithelial and stromal cell compartments: resolving a controversy. *Am J Pathol.* 2000;157(1):1–3.
13. Mak P, Leav I, Pursell B, et al. ERβ impedes prostate cancer EMT by destabilizing HIF-1α and inhibiting VEGF-mediated snail nuclear localization: implications for Gleason grading. *Cancer Cell.* 2010;17(4):319–332.
14. Goel HL, Chang C, Pursell B, et al. VEGF/neuropilin-2 regulation of Bmi-1 and consequent repression of IGF-IR define a novel mechanism of aggressive prostate cancer. *Cancer Discov.* 2012;2(10):906–921.
15. Goel HL, Mercurio AM. VEGF targets the tumour cell. *Nat Rev Cancer.* 2013;13(12):871–882.
16. Hansen W, Hutzler M, Abel S, et al. Neuropilin 1 deficiency on CD4+Foxp3+ regulatory T cells impairs mouse melanoma growth. *J Exp Med.* 2012;209(11):2001–2016.
17. Gabrilovich DI, Chen HL, Girgis KR, et al. Production of vascular endothelial growth factor by human tumors inhibits the functional maturation of dendritic cells. *Nat Med.* 1996;2(10):1096–1103.
18. Karar J, Maity A. PI3K/AKT/mTOR Pathway in Angiogenesis. *Front Mol Neurosci.* 2011;4:51.
19. Neuchrist C, Erovic BM, Handisurya A, et al. Vascular endothelial growth factor C and vascular endothelial growth factor receptor 3 expression in squamous cell carcinomas of the head and neck. *Head Neck.* 2003;25(6):464–474.
20. Riedel F, Götte K, Schwalb J, et al. Serum levels of vascular endothelial growth factor in patients with head and neck cancer. *Eur Arch Oto-Rhino-Laryngol Off J Eur Fed Oto-Rhino-Laryngol Soc EUFOS Affil Ger Soc Oto-Rhino-Laryngol—Head Neck Surg.* 2000;257(6):332–336.
21. Lalla RV, Boisoneau DS, Spiro JD, Kreutzer DL. Expression of vascular endothelial growth factor receptors on tumor cells in head and neck squamous cell carcinoma. *Arch Otolaryngol Head Neck Surg.* 2003;129(8):882–888.
22. Byers LA, Holsinger FC, Kies MS, et al. Serum signature of hypoxia-regulated factors is associated with progression after induction therapy in head and neck squamous cell cancer. *Mol Cancer Ther.* 2010;9(6):1755–1763.
23. Kyzas PA, Cunha IW, Ioannidis JPA. Prognostic significance of vascular endothelial growth factor immunohistochemical expression in head and neck squamous cell carcinoma: a meta-analysis. *Clin Cancer Res.* 2005;11(4):1434–1440.

24. Argiris A, Lee SC, Feinstein T, et al. Serum biomarkers as potential predictors of antitumor activity of cetuximab-containing therapy for locally advanced head and neck cancer. *Oral Oncol.* 2011;47(10):961–966.
25. Shih T, Lindley C. Bevacizumab: an angiogenesis inhibitor for the treatment of solid malignancies. *Clin Ther.* 2006;28(11):1779–1802.
26. Viloria-Petit A, Crombet T, Jothy S, et al. Acquired resistance to the antitumor effect of epidermal growth factor receptor-blocking antibodies in vivo: a role for altered tumor angiogenesis. *Cancer Res.* 2001;61(13):5090–5101.
27. Ciardiello F, Bianco R, Caputo R, et al. Antitumor activity of ZD6474, a vascular endothelial growth factor receptor tyrosine kinase inhibitor, in human cancer cells with acquired resistance to antiepidermal growth factor receptor therapy. *Clin Cancer Res Off J Am Assoc Cancer Res.* 2004;10(2):784–793.
28. Ciardiello F, Bianco R, Damiano V, et al. Antiangiogenic and antitumor activity of anti-epidermal growth factor receptor C225 monoclonal antibody in combination with vascular endothelial growth factor antisense oligonucleotide in human GEO colon cancer cells. *Clin Cancer Res Off J Am Assoc Cancer Res.* 2000;6(9):3739–3747.
29. Soulieres D, Senzer NN, Vokes EE, et al. Multicenter phase II study of erlotinib, an oral epidermal growth factor receptor tyrosine kinase inhibitor, in patients with recurrent or metastatic squamous cell cancer of the head and neck. *J Clin Oncol Off J Am Soc Clin Oncol.* 2004;22(1):77–85.
30. Elser C, Siu LL, Winquist E, et al. Phase II trial of sorafenib in patients with recurrent or metastatic squamous cell carcinoma of the head and neck or nasopharyngeal carcinoma. *J Clin Oncol.* 2007;25(24):3766–3773.
31. Cohen EEW, Davis DW, Karrison TG, et al. Erlotinib and bevacizumab in patients with recurrent or metastatic squamous-cell carcinoma of the head and neck: a phase I/II study. *Lancet Oncol.* 2009;10(3):247–257.
32. Vermorken JB, Mesia R, Rivera F, et al. Platinum-based chemotherapy plus cetuximab in head and neck cancer. *N Engl J Med.* 2008;359(11):1116–1127.
33. Argiris A, Kotsakis AP, Hoang T, et al. Cetuximab and bevacizumab: preclinical data and phase II trial in recurrent or metastatic squamous cell carcinoma of the head and neck. *Ann Oncol Off J Eur Soc Med Oncol.* 2013;24(1):220–225.
34. Argiris A, Li S, Savvides P, et al. Phase III randomized trial of chemotherapy with or without bevacizumab (B) in patients (pts) with recurrent or metastatic squamous cell carcinoma of the head and neck (R/M SCCHN): Survival analysis of E1305, an ECOG-ACRIN Cancer Research Group trial. *J Clin Oncol.* 2017;35(15, suppl):6000–6000.
35. Choong NW, Kozloff M, Taber D, et al. Phase II study of sunitinib malate in head and neck squamous cell carcinoma. *Invest New Drugs.* 2010;28(5):677–683.
36. Ongkeko WM, Altuna X, Weisman RA, Wang-Rodriguez J. Expression of protein tyrosine kinases in head and neck squamous cell carcinomas. *Am J Clin Pathol.* 2005;124(1):71–76.
37. Guo P, Hu B, Gu W, et al. Platelet-derived growth factor-B enhances glioma angiogenesis by stimulating vascular endothelial growth factor expression in tumor endothelia and by promoting pericyte recruitment. *Am J Pathol.* 2003;162(4):1083–1093.
38. Erber R, Thurnher A, Katsen AD, et al. Combined inhibition of VEGF and PDGF signaling enforces tumor vessel regression by interfering with pericyte-mediated endothelial cell survival mechanisms. *FASEB J Off Publ Fed Am Soc Exp Biol.* 2004;18(2):338–340.
39. Fountzilas G, Fragkoulidi A, Kalogera-Fountzila A, et al. A phase II study of sunitinib in patients with recurrent and/or metastatic non-nasopharyngeal head and neck cancer. *Cancer Chemother Pharmacol.* 2010;65(4):649–660.
40. Machiels J-PH, Henry S, Zanetta S, et al. Phase II study of sunitinib in recurrent or metastatic squamous cell carcinoma of the head and neck: GORTEC 2006-01. *J Clin Oncol Off J Am Soc Clin Oncol.* 2010;28(1):21–28.
41. Beeram M, Patnaik A, Rowinsky EK. Raf: a strategic target for therapeutic development against cancer. *J Clin Oncol Off J Am Soc Clin Oncol.* 2005;23(27):6771–6790.
42. Williamson SK, Moon J, Huang CH, et al. Phase II evaluation of sorafenib in advanced and metastatic squamous cell carcinoma of the head and neck: Southwest Oncology Group Study S0420. *J Clin Oncol Off J Am Soc Clin Oncol.* 2010;28(20):3330–3335.
43. Gilbert J, Schell MJ, Zhao X, et al. A randomized phase II efficacy and correlative studies of cetuximab with or without sorafenib in recurrent and/or metastatic head and neck squamous cell carcinoma. *Oral Oncol.* 2015;51(4):376–382.
44. Swiecicki PL, Zhao L, Belile E, et al. A phase II study evaluating axitinib in patients with unresectable, recurrent or metastatic head and neck cancer. *Invest New Drugs.* 2015;33(6):1248–1256.
45. Leboulleux S, Bastholt L, Krause T, et al. Vandetanib in locally advanced or metastatic differentiated thyroid cancer: a randomised, double-blind, phase 2 trial. *Lancet Oncol.* 2012;13(9):897–905.
46. Klein JD, Christopoulos A, Ahn SM, et al. Antitumor effect of vandetanib through EGFR inhibition in head and neck squamous cell carcinoma. *Head Neck.* 2012;34(9):1269–1276.
47. Limaye S, Riley S, Zhao S, et al. A randomized phase II study of docetaxel with or without vandetanib in recurrent or metastatic squamous cell carcinoma of head and neck (SCCHN). *Oral Oncol.* 2013;49(8):835–841.
48. Shen C, Kaelin WG. The VHL/HIF axis in clear cell renal carcinoma. *Semin Cancer Biol.* 2013;23(1):18–25.
49. Richard DE, Berra E, Pouysségur J. Angiogenesis: how a tumor adapts to hypoxia. *Biochem Biophys Res Commun.* 1999;266(3):718–722.
50. Loureiro RMB, D'Amore PA. Transcriptional regulation of vascular endothelial growth factor in cancer. *Cytokine Growth Factor Rev.* 2005;16(1):77–89.

51. Bowers G, Reardon D, Hewitt T, et al. The relative role of ErbB1-4 receptor tyrosine kinases in radiation signal transduction responses of human carcinoma cells. *Oncogene*. 2001;20(11):1388–1397.
52. Tong RT, Boucher Y, Kozin SV, et al. Vascular normalization by vascular endothelial growth factor receptor 2 blockade induces a pressure gradient across the vasculature and improves drug penetration in tumors. *Cancer Res*. 2004;64(11):3731–3736.
53. Brieger J, Kattwinkel J, Berres M, et al. Impact of vascular endothelial growth factor release on radiation resistance. *Oncol Rep*. 2007;18(6):1597–1607.
54. Seiwert TY, Haraf DJ, Cohen EEW, et al. Phase I study of bevacizumab added to fluorouracil- and hydroxyurea-based concomitant chemoradiotherapy for poor-prognosis head and neck cancer. *J Clin Oncol*. 2008;26(10):1732–1741.
55. Salama JK, Vokes EE, Chmura SJ, et al. Long-term outcome of concurrent chemotherapy and reirradiation for recurrent and second primary head-and-neck squamous cell carcinoma. *Int J Radiat Oncol Biol Phys*. 2006;64(2):382–391.
56. Spencer SA, Harris J, Wheeler RH, et al. RTOG 96-10: reirradiation with concurrent hydroxyurea and 5-fluorouracil in patients with squamous cell cancer of the head and neck. *Int J Radiat Oncol Biol Phys*. 2001;51(5):1299–1304.
57. Salama JK, Haraf DJ, Stenson KM, et al. A randomized phase II study of 5-fluorouracil, hydroxyurea, and twice-daily radiotherapy compared with bevacizumab plus 5-fluorouracil, hydroxyurea, and twice-daily radiotherapy for intermediate-stage and T4N0-1 head and neck cancers. *Ann Oncol Off J Eur Soc Med Oncol*. 2011;22(10):2304–2309.
58. Fury MG, Lee NY, Sherman E, et al. A phase 2 study of bevacizumab with cisplatin plus intensity-modulated radiation therapy for stage III/IVB head and neck squamous cell cancer. *Cancer*. 2012;118(20):5008–5014.
59. Lee NY, Zhang Q, Pfister DG, et al. Addition of bevacizumab to standard chemoradiation for locoregionally advanced nasopharyngeal carcinoma (RTOG 0615): a phase 2 multi-institutional trial. *Lancet Oncol*. 2012;13(2):172–180.
60. Wolden SL, Chen WC, Pfister DG, Kraus DH, Berry SL, Zelefsky MJ. Intensity-modulated radiation therapy (IMRT) for nasopharynx cancer: update of the Memorial Sloan-Kettering experience. *Int J Radiat Oncol Biol Phys*. 2006;64(1):57–62.
61. Kwong DLW, Pow EHN, Sham JST, et al. Intensity-modulated radiotherapy for early-stage nasopharyngeal carcinoma: a prospective study on disease control and preservation of salivary function. *Cancer*. 2004;101(7):1584–1593.
62. Al-Sarraf M, LeBlanc M, Giri PG, et al. Chemoradiotherapy versus radiotherapy in patients with advanced nasopharyngeal cancer: phase III randomized Intergroup study 0099. *J Clin Oncol*. 1998;16(4):1310–1317.
63. Lee AWM, Tung SY, Chan ATC, et al. A randomized trial on addition of concurrent-adjuvant chemotherapy and/or accelerated fractionation for locally-advanced nasopharyngeal carcinoma. *Radiother Oncol*. 2011;98(1):15–22.
64. Lee AWM, Tung SY, Chua DTT, et al. Randomized trial of radiotherapy plus concurrent–adjuvant chemotherapy vs radiotherapy alone for regionally advanced nasopharyngeal carcinoma. *J Natl Cancer Inst*. 2010;102(15):1188–1198.
65. Chen L, Hu C-S, Chen X-Z, et al. Concurrent chemoradiotherapy plus adjuvant chemotherapy versus concurrent chemoradiotherapy alone in patients with locoregionally advanced nasopharyngeal carcinoma: a phase 3 multicentre randomised controlled trial. *Lancet Oncol*. 2012;13(2):163–171.
66. Hainsworth JD, Spigel DR, Greco FA, et al. Combined modality treatment with chemotherapy, radiation therapy, bevacizumab, and erlotinib in patients with locally advanced squamous carcinoma of the head and neck: a phase II trial of the Sarah Cannon oncology research consortium. *Cancer J*. 2011;17(5):267–272.
67. Hainsworth JD, Meluch AA, McClurkan S, et al. Induction paclitaxel, carboplatin, and Infusional 5-fu followed by concurrent radiation therapy and weekly paclitaxel/carboplatin in the treatment of locally advanced head and neck cancer: a phase II trial of the Minnie pearl cancer research network. *Cancer J*. 2002;8(4):311–321.
68. Argiris A, Bauman JE, Ohr J, et al. Phase II randomized trial of radiation therapy, cetuximab and pemetrexed with or without bevacizumab in patients with locoregionally-advanced head and neck cancer. *Ann Oncol*. 2016;27(8):1594–1600. doi:10.1093/annonc/mdw204
69. Yao M, Galanopoulos N, Lavertu P, et al. Phase II study of bevacizumab in combination with docetaxel and radiation in locally advanced squamous cell carcinoma of the head and neck. *Head Neck*. 2015;37(11):1665–1671.
70. Tong CCL, Ko EC, Sung MW, et al. Phase II trial of concurrent sunitinib and image-guided radiotherapy for Oligometastases. *PLOS ONE*. 2012;7(6):e36979.
71. National Cancer Institute. Sunitinib, cetuximab, and radiation therapy in treating patients with locally advanced or recurrent squamous cell carcinoma of the head and neck - tabular view. 2013. https://clinicaltrials.gov/ct2/show/NCT00906360?term=sunitinib&cond=Squamous+Cell+Carcinoma&rank=1.
72. Papadimitrakopoulou V, Frank S, Cohen E, et al. Phase I study of vandetanib with radiation therapy with or without cisplatin in locally advanced head and neck squamous cell carcinoma. *Head Neck*. 2016;38(3):439–447.
73. Yadav A, Kumar B, Teknos TN, Kumar P. Sorafenib enhances the antitumor effects of Chemoradiation treatment by downregulating ERCC-1 and XRCC-1 DNA repair proteins. *Mol Cancer Ther*. 2011;10(7):1241–1251.
74. Kruser TJ, Wheeler DL, Armstrong EA, et al. Augmentation of radiation response by motesanib, a multikinase inhibitor that targets vascular endothelial growth factor receptors. *Clin Cancer Res*. 2010;16(14):3639–3647.
75. Hsu H-W, Gridley DS, Kim PD, et al. Linifanib (ABT-869) enhances radiosensitivity of head and neck squamous cell carcinoma cells. *Oral Oncol*. 2013;49(6):591–597.

76. Simpson DR, Mell LK, Cohen EEW. Targeting the PI3K/AKT/mTOR pathway in squamous cell carcinoma of the head and neck. *Oral Oncol*. 2015;51(4):291–298.
77. Lui VWY, Hedberg ML, Li H, et al. Frequent mutation of the PI3K pathway in head and neck cancer defines predictive biomarkers. *Cancer Discov*. 2013;3(7):761–769.
78. Schelhaas M, Shah B, Holzer M, et al. Entry of human papillomavirus type 16 by actin-dependent, clathrin- and lipid raft-independent endocytosis. *PLOS Pathog*. 2012;8(4):e1002657.
79. Surviladze Z, Sterk RT, DeHaro SA, Ozbun MA. Cellular entry of human papillomavirus type 16 involves activation of the phosphatidylinositol 3-kinase/Akt/mTOR pathway and inhibition of autophagy. *J Virol*. 2013;87(5):2508–2517.
80. Slebos RJC, Yi Y, Ely K, et al. Gene expression differences associated with human papillomavirus status in head and neck squamous cell carcinoma. *Clin Cancer Res Off J Am Assoc Cancer Res*. 2006;12(3, Pt 1):701–709.
81. Sewell A, Brown B, Biktasova A, et al. Reverse-phase protein array profiling of oropharyngeal cancer and significance of PIK3CA mutations in HPV-associated head and neck cancer. *Clin Cancer Res Off J Am Assoc Cancer Res*. 2014;20(9):2300–2311.
82. Jimeno A, Shirai K, Choi M, et al. A randomized, phase II trial of cetuximab with or without PX-866, an irreversible oral phosphatidylinositol 3-kinase inhibitor, in patients with relapsed or metastatic head and neck squamous cell cancer. *Ann Oncol Off J Eur Soc Med Oncol*. 2015;26(3):556–561.
83. Grünwald V, Keilholz U, Boehm A, et al. TEMHEAD: a single-arm multicentre phase II study of temsirolimus in platin- and cetuximab refractory recurrent and/or metastatic squamous cell carcinoma of the head and neck (SCCHN) of the German SCCHN Group (AIO). *Ann Oncol Off J Eur Soc Med Oncol*. 2015;26(3):561–567.
84. Bauman JE, Arias-Pulido H, Lee S-J, et al. A phase II study of temsirolimus and erlotinib in patients with recurrent and/or metastatic, platinum-refractory head and neck squamous cell carcinoma. *Oral Oncol*. 2013;49(5):461–467.
85. Geiger JL, Bauman JE, Gibson MK, et al. Phase II trial of everolimus in patients with previously treated recurrent or metastatic head and neck squamous cell carcinoma. *Head Neck*. 2016;38(12):1759–1764.
86. Massarelli E, Lin H, Ginsberg LE, et al. Phase II trial of everolimus and erlotinib in patients with platinum-resistant recurrent and/or metastatic head and neck squamous cell carcinoma. *Ann Oncol Off J Eur Soc Med Oncol*. 2015;26(7):1476–1480.
87. Boeckx C, Baay M, Wouters A, et al. Anti-epidermal growth factor receptor therapy in head and neck squamous cell carcinoma: focus on potential molecular mechanisms of drug resistance. *Oncologist*. 2013;18(7):850–864.
88. Dent P, Yacoub A, Contessa J, et al. Stress and radiation-induced activation of multiple intracellular signaling pathways. *Radiat Res*. 2003;159(3):283–300.
89. Bozec A, Ebran N, Radosevic–Robin N, et al. Combination of phosphotidylinositol-3-kinase targeting with cetuximab and irradiation: a preclinical study on an orthotopic xenograft model of head and neck cancer. *Head Neck*. 2017;39(1):151–159.
90. Phase Ib study of BKM120 with cisplatin and XRT in high risk locally advanced squamous cell cancer of head and neck—full text view—ClinicalTrials.gov.
91. Leiker AJ, DeGraff W, Choudhuri R, et al. Radiation enhancement of head and neck squamous cell carcinoma by the dual PI3K/mTOR inhibitor PF-05212384. *Clin Cancer Res*. 2015;21(12):2792–2801.
92. Ekshyyan O, Rong Y, Rong X, et al. Comparison of radiosensitizing effects of the mammalian target of rapamycin inhibitor CCI-779 to cisplatin in experimental models of head and neck squamous cell carcinoma. *Mol Cancer Ther*. 2009;8(8):2255–2265.
93. Ma BBY, Goh BC, Lim WT, et al. Multicenter phase II study of the AKT inhibitor MK-2206 in recurrent or metastatic nasopharyngeal carcinoma from patients in the mayo phase II consortium and the cancer therapeutics research group (MC1079). *Invest New Drugs*. 2015;33(4):985–991.
94. Johnstone RW. Histone-deacetylase inhibitors: novel drugs for the treatment of cancer. *Nat Rev Drug Discov*. 2002;1(4):287–299.
95. Theocharis S, Klijanienko J, Giaginis C, et al. Histone deacetylase-1 and -2 expression in mobile tongue squamous cell carcinoma: associations with clinicopathological parameters and patients survival. *J Oral Pathol Med Off Publ Int Assoc Oral Pathol Am Acad Oral Pathol*. 2011;40(9):706–714.
96. Burtness B, Bauman JE, Galloway T. Novel targets in HPV-negative head and neck cancer: overcoming resistance to EGFR inhibition. *Lancet Oncol*. 2013;14(8):e302–e309.
97. Ogryzko VV, Hirai TH, Russanova VR, et al. Human fibroblast commitment to a senescence-like state in response to histone deacetylase inhibitors is cell cycle dependent. *Mol Cell Biol*. 1996;16(9):5210–5218.
98. Kim S, Benguria A, Lai CY, Jazwinski SM. Modulation of life-span by histone deacetylase genes in Saccharomyces cerevisiae. *Mol Biol Cell*. 1999;10(10):3125–3136.
99. Camphausen K, Burgan W, Cerra M, et al. Enhanced radiation-induced cell killing and prolongation of γH2AX foci expression by the histone deacetylase inhibitor MS-275. *Cancer Res*. 2004;64(1):316–321.
100. Bruzzese F, Leone A, Rocco M, et al. HDAC inhibitor vorinostat enhances the antitumor effect of gefitinib in squamous cell carcinoma of head and neck by modulating ErbB receptor expression and reverting EMT. *J Cell Physiol*. 2011;226(9):2378–2390.
101. Haigentz M, Kim M, Sarta C, et al. Phase II trial of the histone deacetylase inhibitor romidepsin in patients with recurrent/metastatic head and neck cancer. *Oral Oncol*. 2012;48(12):1281–1288.

102. Blumenschein GR, Kies MS, Papadimitrakopoulou VA, et al. Phase II trial of the histone deacetylase inhibitor vorinostat (Zolinza, suberoylanilide hydroxamic acid, SAHA) in patients with recurrent and/or metastatic head and neck cancer. *Invest New Drugs*. 2008;26(1):81–87.
103. Galloway TJ, Wirth LJ, Colevas AD, et al. A phase I study of CUDC-101, a multitarget inhibitor of HDACs, EGFR, and HER2, in combination with chemoradiation in patients with head and neck squamous cell carcinoma. *Clin Cancer Res*. 2015;21(7):1566–1573.
104. Appleman LJ. MET signaling pathway: a rational target for cancer therapy. *J Clin Oncol*. 2011;29(36):4837–4838.
105. Seiwert TY, Jagadeeswaran R, Faoro L, et al. The MET receptor tyrosine kinase is a potential novel therapeutic target for head and neck squamous cell carcinoma. *Cancer Res*. 2009;69(7):3021–3031.
106. Baschnagel AM, Williams L, Hanna A, et al. c-Met expression is a marker of poor prognosis in patients with locally advanced head and neck squamous cell carcinoma treated with chemoradiation. *Int J Radiat Oncol Biol Phys*. 2014;88(3):701–707.
107. Akervall J, Guo X, Qian C-N, et al. Genetic and expression profiles of squamous cell carcinoma of the head and neck correlate with cisplatin sensitivity and resistance in cell lines and patients. *Clin Cancer Res Off J Am Assoc Cancer Res*. 2004;10(24):8204–8213.
108. Sun S, Wang Z. Head neck squamous cell carcinoma c-Met$^+$ cells display cancer stem cell properties and are responsible for cisplatin-resistance and metastasis. *Int J Cancer*. 2011;129(10):2337–2348.
109. Xu H, Stabile LP, Gubish CT, et al. Dual blockade of EGFR and c-Met abrogates redundant signaling and proliferation in head and neck carcinoma cells. *Clin Cancer Res*. 2011;17(13):4425–4438.
110. Bacco FD, Luraghi P, Medico E, et al. Induction of MET by ionizing radiation and its role in radioresistance and invasive growth of cancer. *J Natl Cancer Inst*. 2011;103(8):645–661.
111. Aebersold DM, Kollar A, Beer KT, et al. Involvement of the hepatocyte growth factor/scatter factor receptor c–met and of Bcl–xL in the resistance of oropharyngeal cancer to ionizing radiation. *Int J Cancer*. 2001;96(1):41–54.
112. Baschnagel AM, Galoforo S, Thibodeau BJ, et al. Crizotinib fails to enhance the effect of radiation in head and neck squamous cell carcinoma xenografts. *Anticancer Res*. 2015;35(11):5973–5982.
113. Zhu H, Yun F, Shi X, Wang D. VEGF-C inhibition reverses resistance of bladder cancer cells to cisplatin via upregulating maspin. *Mol Med Rep*. 2015;12(2):3163–3169.
114. Shi S, Yuan C, Zhuang K, et al. Resistance of SMMC-7721 hepatoma cells to etoposide in hypoxia is reversed by VEGF inhibitor. *Mol Med Rep*. 2015;11(5):3842–3847.
115. Dias S, Choy M, Alitalo K, Rafii S. Vascular endothelial growth factor (VEGF)-C signaling through FLT-4 (VEGFR-3) mediates leukemic cell proliferation, survival, and resistance to chemotherapy. *Blood*. 2002;99(6):2179–2184.

SECTION III

Site-Specific Management

13

Oropharyngeal Cancer: HPV-Positive Disease

Christien A. Kluwe

Anthony J. Cmelak

Barbara A. Burtness

Traditionally arising in a population with significant alcohol and tobacco exposure, head and neck squamous cell carcinoma (HNSCC) has been notoriously difficult to cure—60% of patients have locally advanced disease at the time of diagnosis and current therapies with concurrent cisplatin yield a 3-year progression-free survival (PFS) rate of 50% and an overall survival (OS) rate of 60% (1). This has led to the development of intensified treatment regimens combining cytotoxic agents, both prior to and concurrent with high-dose radiation, accelerated regimens, trimodality therapies, and extensive prophylactic irradiation of lymph nodes. Severe toxicities have been noted and quantified but have largely driven less attention in treatment design than has tumor control to improve survival.

While the overall incidence of HNSCC has declined over the past several decades in the United States, that of oropharyngeal squamous cell carcinoma (OPSCC) has risen dramatically. From 1996 to 2016, new cases in the United States have increased from roughly 29,000 to 48,000 per year (2,3). Molecular analyses from patients over this period have shown a key driver to be infection with human papillomavirus (HPV)—more commonly associated with anogenital cancers but recently recognized as an important cause of OPSCC (4,5). Retrospective analyses indicate an improved prognosis in HPV-positive tumors, a finding that was later confirmed in the prospective Eastern Cooperative Oncology Group (ECOG) 2399 and Radiation Therapy Oncology Group (RTOG) 0129 trials, even when controlling for positive prognostic indicators such as age, performance status, and smoking (6,7).

PATIENT SELECTION FOR DE-INTENSIFICATION STRATEGIES

Given the improved treatment response and outcomes of patients with HPV-positive OPSCCs, considerable thought has been directed toward reevaluating historic treatment paradigms. Recent efforts pursue treatment de-intensification to reduce long-term toxicities associated with chemotherapy, radiation, and radical surgery while maintaining or improving cure rates. In addition, methods of early detection and surveillance after treatment are under reexamination.

An important step in studying treatment de-escalation is identification of patients who are suitable for each strategy under evaluation. This begins with sensitive and specific determination that a particular cancer is driven by HPV, with many competing methodologies having been proposed since the first demonstration of HPV 11 and 16 in head and neck carcinoma by zur Hausen in 1985 (8,9). The most widely used assay in current generation cooperative group head and neck cancer (HNC) trials is immunohistochemical staining for p16, seen as a surrogate for transcription of E7 because p16 is regulated by the tumor suppressor Rb and p16 levels rise when Rb levels are low (10). Specificity for HPV-driven cancer is increased when p16-positive cancers are also tested for HPV DNA with polymerase chain reaction (PCR) (9).

Accuracy in predicting patterns of failure, treatment responsiveness, and prognosis is required to conduct valid studies of novel treatment paradigms. For example, a group of patients in whom distant disease is the predominant mode of failure may not be appropriate for trials of radiation alone, while those with lesser treatment responsiveness may not be suitable for trials that explore the use of chemotherapy to reduce tumor burden, but may do well with minimally invasive surgery. Clinical characteristics of favorable outcome identified in a recursive partitioning analysis in R0129—a randomized phase III trial of chemoradiation—were minimal smoking history (defined as ≤10 pack-years) and lower N stage (7). Subsequently these data were extended in a joint analysis of the data from R0129 and an earlier trial, RTOG 9003. The risks of progression and death were both increased in a linear fashion as pack-years and years of smoking increased. In the older trial, which enrolled a higher proportion of active smokers, the risk of death doubled among those who smoked during radiotherapy after controlling for pack-years. Similar data have been reported by investigators at the University of Michigan, who observed that ever tobacco users with HPV-related oropharynx cancer had a 35% risk of recurrence compared with a 6% risk in never smokers. Among those with HPV-related cancers, current smokers were at fivefold higher risk of disease recurrence than never smokers ($p = .038$) (11). Retrospective analysis at the Princess Margaret Hospital of heterogeneously treated patients with HPV-related oropharynx cancer also identified advanced T stage (T4) as a predictor of worse outcome (12).

Ideally, correlation of biomolecular signatures to treatment outcome will lead to biomarker-based characterization of tumors at diagnosis into groups suitable or unsuitable for de-intensification, and will identify the optimal strategy to achieve cure and minimize long-term sequelae. An understanding of the biology of HPV-related squamous cell cancer and of treatment responsiveness will be necessary in refining such patient selection strategies.

HPV-ASSOCIATED OROPHARYNX CANCER BIOLOGY

HPVs immortalize keratinocytes via the actions of two dominantly acting oncoproteins, E6 and E7, on host gene products. E6 promotes degradation of the tumor suppressor p53 in an adenosine triphosphate (ATP) dependent fashion operating through ubiquitination (13). Similarly, the E7 oncoprotein segregates the tumor suppressor Rb, and efficiency of E7–Rb binding is correlated with oncogenicity of differing HPV types (14). For transformation by the high-risk HPV type 16, the HPV type responsible for more than 85% of HPV-driven oropharynx cancers in the United States, both E6 and E7 are required (15,16).

The best-studied manifestation of HPV-initiated transformation is human uterine cervical cancer. In cervical cancer, high-risk HPV DNA is integrated into the human genome and transcription of E6 and E7 immortalizes and transforms host epithelial cells. Studies of HNSCC cell lines demonstrate that HPV DNA integration can occur directly into cancer-relevant genes, including *TP53* (17). *TP53* is the most commonly mutated gene in HPV-negative HNSCC, and—as noted earlier—a gene whose product *p53* is an important target of degradation in HPV-related cancer. Integration of HPV DNA into cancer-relevant genes as opposed to intergenic regions has been associated with greater risk of disease recurrence following definitive therapy (18).

In contrast to the familiar model arising from studies in uterine cervical cancer, RNA-Seq and whole genome sequence data from HNSCC specimens analyzed in The Cancer Genome Atlas (TCGA) project demonstrate that HPV viral DNA in oropharyngeal cancer cells may be found in an integrated, an episomal, or a hybrid state, with roughly a third of cancers displaying each of the three states (19).

TCGA project initially profiled 279 HNSCCs, of which 33 (12%) arose in the oropharynx. The majority of oropharynx cancers profiled arose in smokers. The most common mutations in HPV-associated tumors were helical domain mutations of the oncogene *PIK3CA*. Novel observations from this study included the demonstration of loss of tumor necrosis factor receptor–associated factor 3 (TRAF3) via deletion (14%) or truncation mutation (8%) and amplification of the cell cycle gene *E2F1* (20) in HPV-associated cancers. Interestingly, TRAF3 alteration was not observed in HPV-negative cancers, raising the possibility that *TRAF3* mutation is associated with viral carcinogenesis. TRAF3 regulates NF-κB signaling as well as stimulates a potent type I interferon antiviral response. Thus, loss of TRAF3 may be associated with impaired anti-HPV immunity. Investigators at Yale University examined another regulator of NF-κB, the gene cylindromatosis lysine 63 deubiquitinase (*CYLD*), and found this is also mutated in a subset of HPV-positive HNSCC (21). The presence of *TRAF3* or *CYLD* mutation was strongly associated with episomal rather than integrated HPV DNA (p = .007) and with improved survival (p = .0318).

CpG methylation status has also been demonstrated to differ in HPV-positive compared with HPV-negative cancers. Specifically, HPV status significantly predicted DNA methylation of 12 genes in a cohort of HNSCC; these genes included the *CCNA1* promoter, *CASP8*, and *SYBL1*. Hypomethylation of cell cycle control genes was also found to differ between HPV-positive and -negative cancers. As with other cohorts, the majority (86%) of cases studied came from former or current smokers, potentially limiting applicability of these data to developing a biomarker of favorable prognosis.

Head and neck tumors are associated with inflammation and markers of immune exhaustion. Profiling of the tumor immune microenvironment demonstrates significantly greater numbers of CD4, CD8, FOXP3, and CD68 positive cells in HPV-positive compared with HPV-negative cancers (22). Though the field of immuno-oncology is relatively in its infancy, this may have implications for future trials examining immunomodulatory therapy.

RADIATION DOSE DE-ESCALATION

The current treatment approach to smoking-related HNSCC is the result of a multitude of rigorous prospective trials, ultimately determining that concurrent cisplatin-based chemoradiation with a dose approaching 70 Gy demonstrates the best therapeutic ratio between locoregional control (LRC) and toxicity (23,24). Unfortunately, this treatment paradigm is notable for its significant short- and long-term toxicities and has been advocated as a "one size fits all" regimen for stage III-IVb disease. In the acute phase fatigue, dermatitis, mucositis, dysgeusia/ageusia, and dysphagia (with concomitant risk of malnutrition) are common. Long-term sequelae include skin and muscle fibrosis, hypothyroidism, xerostomia, increased risk of stroke, and permanent swallowing difficulties. Radiation-induced microvascular changes can inhibit future wound healing as well, a particular concern in patients with poor dentition. In a historically elderly population with medical comorbidities driving patients' life spans, toxicity concerns have taken a back seat. As HPV-positive OPSCC is more common in younger populations, however, the morbidity and longevity of chronic toxicities are particularly burdensome and noteworthy.

The first prospective trial to evaluate the treatment responsiveness and outcome of 111 patients with HPV-positive OPSCC was ECOG 2399 (25). This large phase II study was designed as an organ-function preservation trial in resectable patients with both laryngeal and oropharyngeal primary tumors. Using induction chemotherapy with paclitaxel and carboplatin to evaluate tumor sensitivity, patients who obtained a partial clinical response (based on endoscopic examination) to two cycles then went on to concurrent 70 Gy with weekly paclitaxel. Tumor specimens were evaluated for HPV 16, 33, and 35 by in situ hybridization and PCR. Thirty-eight of 60 (63%, 95% confidence interval [CI]: 50%–75%) oropharyngeal versus 0 of 34 (0%, 95% CI: 0%–10%) laryngeal cancers were HPV positive ($p < .001$). Compared with patients with HPV-negative tumors, patients with HPV-positive tumors had higher response rates after induction chemotherapy (82% vs. 55%, difference = 27%, 95% CI: 9.3%–44.7%, p = .01) and after chemoradiation (84% vs. 57%, difference = 27%, 95% CI: 9.7%–44.3%, p = .007). After a median follow-up of 39.1 months, patients with HPV-positive tumors had improved OS (2-year OS = 95% [95% CI: 87%–100%] vs. 62% [95% CI: 49%–74%], difference = 33%, 95% CI: 18.6%–47.4%, p = .005, log-rank test) and, after adjustment for age, tumor stage, and ECOG performance status, lower risks of progression (hazard ratio [HR]: 0.27, 95% CI: 0.10–0.75) and death from any cause (HR = 0.36, 95% CI: 0.15–0.85) than those with HPV-negative tumors.

A follow-up prospective phase II trial of dose de-intensification assessed whether a triplet induction regimen could be used to cytoreduce stage III-IVb patients with HPV-OPSCC in order to effectively treat them with reduced-dose intensity modulated radiotherapy (IMRT) to 54 Gy (ECOG 1308, Figure 13.1). Patients received three cycles of cisplatin 75 mg/m^2 day 1, paclitaxel 90 mg/m^2 days 1, 8, and 15, and cetuximab 400 mg/m^2 day 1, cycle 1, followed by cetuximab 250 mg/m^2 weekly. Cycles were repeated every 21 days for three cycles. If cisplatin was not tolerated, substitution with carboplatin AUC (area under the curve) 5 was allowed after the first cycle. Patients were evaluated for clinical response by endoscopy and scored as a clinical complete response (cCR) or not (<cCR) before proceeding to IMRT-based radiation with concurrent weekly cetuximab 250 mg/m^2. Of the 90 patients enrolled on the trial, 70% achieved a cCR; of those, 78% then went on to receive reduced-dose IMRT; the incomplete responders received 69.3 Gy. After a median follow-up of 35.4 months, 2-year PFS and OS rates were 80% and 94%, respectively, for patients with primary-site cCR treated with 54 Gy of radiation (n = 51); 96% and 96%, respectively, for patients with <T4, <N2c, and <10 pack-year smoking history who were treated with ≤54 Gy of radiation (n = 27; Figures 13.2 and 13.3). Patient-reported symptoms were evaluated with a battery of instruments, including the Vanderbilt Head and Neck Symptom Survey Version 2 (26). At 12 months, significantly fewer patients treated with a radiation dose ≤54 Gy had difficulty swallowing solids (40% vs. 89%; p = .011) or had impaired nutrition (10% vs. 44%; p = .025). Only one late grade 3 toxicity was reported as an episode of hypomagnesemia almost 3 years out from treatment (27).

Another phase II trial of radiation de-intensification was reported by Chera et al. who enrolled 43 patients with favorable prognosis HPV-positive OPSCC or HNSCC of unknown primary (T0-T3, N0-N2c, M0 disease with limited or remote smoking history defined as ≤10 pack-years or ≤30 pack-years with abstinence in the past 5 years). Treatment consisted of concurrent weekly cisplatin and 60 Gy to the primary and gross nodal disease with 54 Gy delivered to regions at risk for subclinical disease as indicated (28). A posttreatment clinical and surgical investigation was performed to determine response rates. Four to eight weeks after completing CRT, patients were evaluated clinically by CT scan, fiberoptic laryngoscopy, and physical examination. Within 6 to 14 weeks after CRT all patients underwent a further surgical evaluation for pathologic response by resection or biopsy with neck dissection based on their primary disease state and clinical response. The overall cCR rate was 64%, with 98% in the primary site and 60% in the lymph nodes of the neck. At subsequent surgical evaluation, the pathologic complete response (pCR) rate was 86%, with 98% in the primary site and 84% in the neck. Though not directly comparable, their historic 3-year LRC for HPV-positive OPSCC

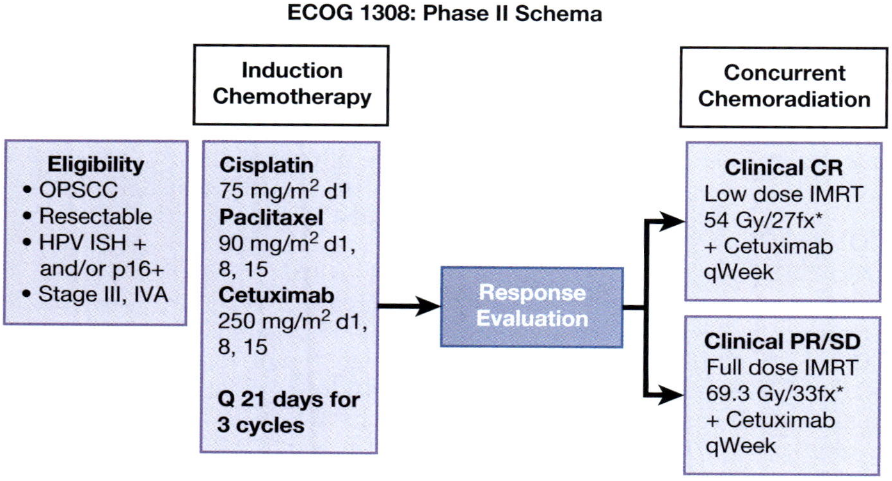

FIGURE 13.1 Treatment schema for E1308 for HPV-related oropharyngeal cancers.
HPV, human papillomavirus.

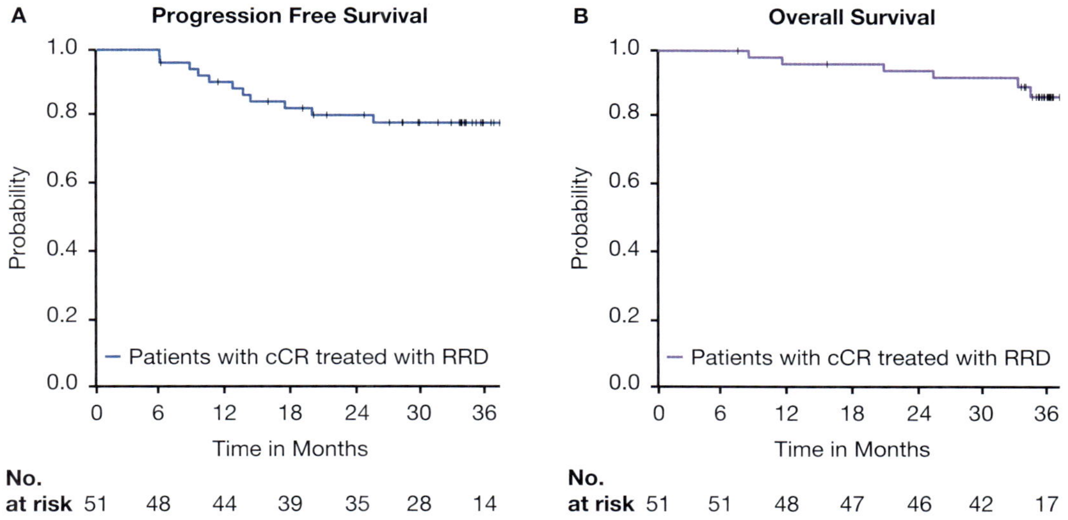

FIGURE 13.2 PFS and OS in cohort with cCR to ICT treated with low-dose radiation of 54 Gy (n = 51).

cCR, clinical complete response; ICT, induction chemotherapy; OS, overall survival; PFS, progression-free survival; RRD, reduced radiation dose.

patients with standard, more intensive therapy was 86.4% (7). This trial was also notable for thorough toxicity and quality of life assessments. In particular, study patients demonstrated a low rate of progression feeding tube dependence of 39% versus 85% in standard treatment regimens as per the PARADIGM trial (29), and none required a permanent feeding tube.

RESPONSE-ADAPTED VOLUME DE-ESCALATION

In conjunction with reduction in overall radiation dose, efforts have been directed to reduce the overall radiation volume. Conventional approaches for OPSCC involve extensive coverage of the bilateral cervical levels II to IV

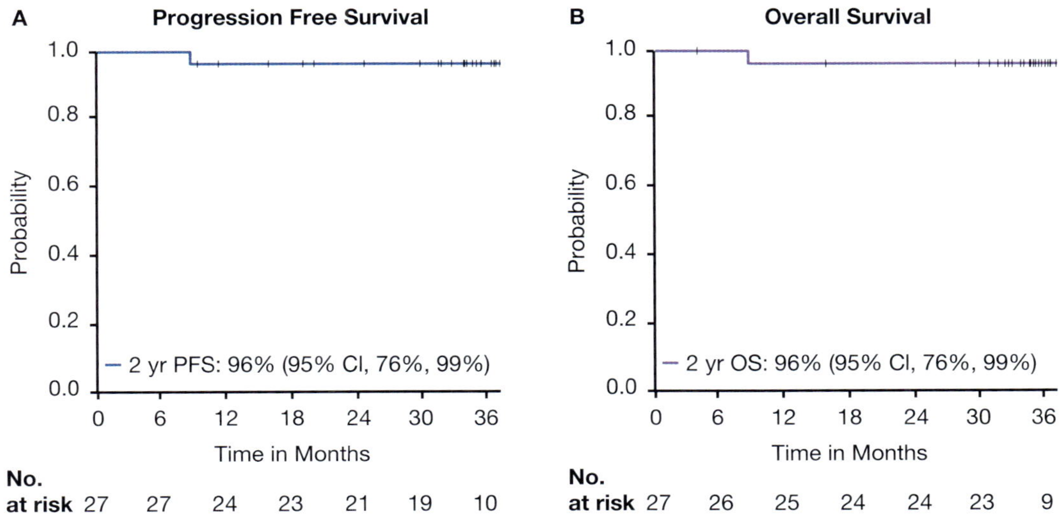

FIGURE 13.3 PFS and OS in favorable cohort (non-T4, non-N2c, ≤10 pack-year smokers) with cCR to ICT treated with low-dose radiation of 54 Gy (n = 27).

cCR, clinical complete response; ICT, induction chemotherapy; OS, overall survival; PFS, progression-free survival.

with 50 to 60 Gy for clinically negative regions, based on risk of involvement. Villaflor et al. recently incorporated a "response-adapted volume de-escalation" (RAVD) approach in a phase I/II trial examining the use of everolimus during induction (30). Ninety-four patients with stage IVa/b HNSCC were enrolled to receive induction chemotherapy ± everolimus. Radiographic response was determined in the 89 patients completing induction therapy as "good response" (GR, defined as ≥50% reduction in the sum of tumor diameters) or non-responsive (NR, <50% reduction). Patients with a GR to induction therapy were treated with IMRT to a single volume encompassing the gross disease (75 Gy in 1.5 Gy twice daily fractions given every other week). NR patients received additional radiation to the first uninvolved ipsilateral nodal bed (45 Gy to prophylactic volume) (see Figure 13.4). Both groups received concurrent multiagent chemotherapy. Of the HPV-positive OPSCC subset (59 total patients), 30 had GR to induction chemotherapy and underwent limited volume irradiation. The 2-year PFS and OS for this group were 93.1% and 92.1%, respectively. In comparison, NR patients had 2-year rates of 74.0% PFS and 95.2% OS. Though not statistically significant (p = .10 for PFS, too few deaths for OS), volume de-escalation did not appear to negatively impact disease outcomes.

For all HNSCC patients in the trial, a total of 13 patients failed locally within 2 years; 12 of these 13 (92.3%) occurred in-field, 11 of these in the high-dose treatment volume. The most common severe toxicities across all patients were ≥grade 3 mucositis and dermatitis. There was no significant difference between the treatment groups in these respects: 59.5% GR versus 59.6% NR, 27.0% GR versus 25.0% NR, respectively. NR patients with the enlarged treatment volume, however, were more likely to undergo feeding tube placement during treatment (73.5% vs. 50.0% for GR), and remain dependent at 3 months (57.1% vs. 22.9%) and 6-month follow-ups (32.6% vs. 5.7%). At 1 year after treatment, 8.6% of NR patients retained a feeding tube, whereas no GR patients remained dependent. This is in comparison to historical rates of approximately 25% (31).

CHEMOTHERAPY DE-ESCALATION

Randomized clinical trials and meta-analyses have shown a significant clinical benefit of combining chemotherapy with definitive radiation in locally advanced patients. An exhaustive review of OPSCC patients (n = 5,878) from the meta-analysis of chemotherapy in head and neck cancer (MACH-NC) demonstrated an overall 8.1% improvement in OS at 5 years for concurrent chemotherapy (32). The standard chemotherapeutic regimen is platinum-based and notorious for toxicities

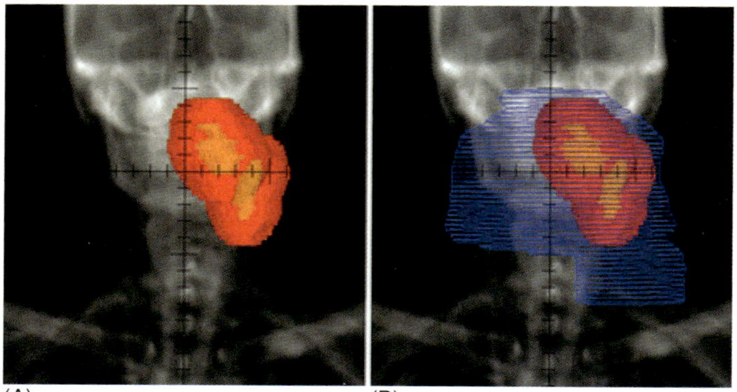

(A) (B)

FIGURE 13.4 IMRT volume differences with and without prophylactic nodal treatment (30). (A) A typical "involved field" only dose cloud covering gross tumor in the oropharynx as well as the involved node(s) with margin. (B) the same patient with a more standardized "extended field" dosimetry to cover distant lymph nodes historically felt to be at risk for harboring subclinical disease.

IMRT, intensity modulated radiotherapy.

Source: Villaflor VM, Melotek JM, Karrison TG, et al. Response-adapted volume de-escalation (RAVD) in locally advanced head and neck cancer. *Ann Oncol*. 2016;27(5):908–913. With permission of Oxford University Press.

including emesis, nephrotoxicity, ototoxicity, mucositis, and cytopenias (33). The substitution of a more tolerable agent such as cetuximab with radiotherapy was associated in retrospective studies with worse LRC, failure-free survival, and OS (34). These reports were, as noted, retrospective and plagued by significant differences in patient selection, as cetuximab is often favored in elderly patients or those with poor performance status. A prospective randomized trial by Magrini et al. directly compared the two therapeutic options and found no significant differences in LRC, OS, or metastasis-free survival. These patients were not evaluated for HPV status, however; additionally it should be noted that subset analysis of OPSCC (n = 43), LRC, and OS favored concurrent cisplatin over cetuximab (35). The discordant results of retrospective trials coupled with the conclusions of Magrini et al. would suggest that carefully selected patients may be safely treated with nonplatinum-based therapies in order to reduce acute and long-term toxicities.

Rosenthal et al. retrospectively evaluated 182 patients randomized on the IMCL-9815 study to receive definitive radiation alone or combined with weekly cetuximab. Forty-one percent were HPV related (36,37). HPV status was found to be strongly prognostic for patients with oropharyngeal carcinoma (OPC). In addition, data suggested that the addition of cetuximab to RT improved clinical outcomes regardless of p16 or HPV status versus RT alone. The study was not powered for the comparison of treatments in HPV-related or HPV-negative subgroups, but of note the HR for death with the addition of cetuximab was 0.38 among p16(+) and 0.72 among p16(−) cases.

Nolan et al. (38) also examined this relationship in a small retrospective review of HPV-positive OPSCC patients at the Ohio State Wexner Medical Center. Of 168 eligible patients including those treated postoperatively and definitively, 42 (25%) received concurrent cetuximab whereas 126 received concurrent cisplatin or carboplatin (n = 109, n = 17, respectively). The 2-year OS for cetuximab was 80% compared to 96% for platinum-based therapy; local relapse free survival was 74% versus 91%; distant metastasis free survival 74% versus 90% (16). A focused clinical trial comparing the two treatments in a prospective, randomized fashion has completed accrual in July 2014, with results anticipated in the near future (RTOG 1016) (31).

The Canadian Cancers Trial Group conducted a phase III randomized trial HN6 comparing standard chemoradiotherapy (70 Gy in 7 weeks/cisplatin 100 mg/m^2 every 3 weeks) versus accelerated radiotherapy (70 Gy in 6 weeks with EGFR inhibitor panitumumab 9 mg/kg x 3) in 320 locally advanced HNC patients. Quality of life was the primary end point with the Functional Assessment of Cancer Therapy Head and Neck (FACT-HN), MD Anderson Dysphagia Index (MDADI), and the SWAL-QOL instruments utilized. Although the study was underpowered for outcome, no clinically important differences in quality of life were seen aftertreatment between treatment regimens (39).

INTENSIFICATION WITH BIOLOGIC AGENTS

In light of these discordant results, and with the consideration that HPV-positive OPSCC typically arises in younger, healthier populations, some have postulated that *escalating* chemotherapy may produce better long-term control with good tolerability. A phase II randomized trial was recently published in which patients were assigned to cetuximab-enhanced chemotherapy protocols with comparison to historical controls (40). A total of 110 patients with stage III or IV nonmetastatic HNSCC were enrolled and received induction therapy with carboplatin, paclitaxel, and cetuximab. Patients were then treated on chemoradiation regimens including cetuximab, 5-fluorouracil (5-FU), and hydroxyurea ("Cetux-FHX," n = 57) or cetuximab and cisplatin ("Cetux-PX," n = 53). All patients were assessed at the completion of induction chemotherapy with an overall response rate of 91%; no significant differences were noted between the two arms prior to chemoradiation. At follow-up, the 2-year PFS for the entire cohort was 83.6%, a significant improvement over the historical control rate of 50%. A subgroup analysis was performed for outcomes according to HPV status (n = 47) with 5-year PFS and OS rates of 84.4% and 91.3%, versus the entire cohort rates of 74.1% and 80.3%. Although this is a limited dataset, the evidence indicates that properly selected patient populations such as those with HPV-positive tumors may benefit from combination chemotherapy and biologic agent regimens. Although this is a limited dataset and no toxicity data were included these results suggest that intensification may yield better outcomes, with properly selected patient populations such as those with HPV-positive tumors receiving an even greater benefit.

SURVEILLANCE FOLLOWING TREATMENT IN HPV DISEASE

Retrospective analysis of OPSCC patients suggests that HPV-positive patients have a distinct pattern of failure in comparison to their HPV-negative brethren. A review of the failure patterns of RTOG 0129 patients by Ang et al. showed a significant difference in the 3-year OS, PFS, and local–regional relapse rate (HPV-positive vs. HPV-negative: 82.4% vs. 57.1%, 37.7% vs. 43.4%, 13.6% vs. 35.1%); distant failure at 3 years was improved but did not achieve statistical significance: 8.7% versus 14.6%, $p = .23$, albeit the study was not powered for this end point (7). Trosman et al. evaluated 291 OPSCC patients with stage III-IVB disease treated with definitive chemoradiation at the Cleveland Clinic with known HPV status: 252 HPV related and 39 HPV negative (41). The 3-year distant control rate was significantly higher in HPV-positive patients (88% vs. 74%) with a longer time to distant failure as well (median 16.4 vs. 7.2 months). In addition, HPV-related patients who failed distantly had a longer OS (median 25.6 vs. 11.1 months). Interestingly, HPV-positive patients had a more diverse set of failure sites. While OPSCC has typically been associated with lung and brain metastases, the HPV-positive patients demonstrated metastases to sites including nonregional lymph nodes (axillary and intra-abdominal), kidney, skin, and skeletal muscle (41). This is in line with what Huang et al. (42) have termed a "disseminating" phenotype. Retrospective analysis of trials for recurrent or metastatic HNC conducted in the ECOG demonstrated longer median survival for HPV-associated disease treated with systemic therapy, and a retrospective analysis of RTOG trials demonstrated longer survival for HPV-associated than for HPV-negative disease whether patients were candidates for local or systemic therapy (43). These unique characteristics call to question the most appropriate form of surveillance, and whether patients should be managed on the historically accepted paradigm of planned neck dissections or CT imaging of the neck (see Table 13.1).

A retrospective review by Frakes et al. examined the posttreatment imaging of 246 patients with HPV-related OPSCC treated with definitive radiation or chemoradiation at Moffitt Cancer Center (44). All patients underwent a PET/CT scan 3 months after completing therapy as well as close follow-up with clinical examinations. At 3 years, local control was achieved in 239 of 245 patients (97.8%). All six local failures were identified on exam by direct visualization or flexible laryngoscopy. Nine patients failed regionally, with all but one identified by symptom progression or on PET/CT. Of the 21 patients who developed distant metastasis, 15 (71%) were identified by symptoms or on imaging. Overall, symptoms and/or 3-month follow-up PET/CT identified 92% of local–regional failures and 71% of distant failures. Thus, the authors suggest a 3-month PET/CT with close clinical follow-up would provide adequate surveillance.

The less invasive approach of PET/CT imaging has been directly compared with planned neck dissections as well. Mehanna et al. directed a prospective trial of 564 patients (84% OPSCC, 75% HPV related) with N2 or N3 HNSCC in the United Kingdom (45). Patients were randomized to undergo a planned neck dissection or PET/CT surveillance 3 months after the conclusion of chemoradiation. If the PET/CT patients showed an incomplete or equivocal response, salvage neck dissection was performed. Of the 270 patients who underwent PET/CT, 185 (69%) showed a complete response and an additional 19 showed incomplete response in the primary with a complete response in the neck. A total of 52 patients (19.3%) underwent neck dissection, with similar complication rates to the planned dissection group (42% vs. 38%). The 2-year OS rates between the two groups were similar (84.9% for PET/CT vs. 81.5% for planned dissection). The authors note that nodal disease in HPV-positive tumors may take longer to involute, suggesting a 3-month scan may be too early to assess response, but nonetheless indicate surveillance is a suitable approach associated with lower mortality and cost than planned posttreatment neck dissection.

With the success of prostate-specific antigen (PSA) monitoring for recurrence and response in prostate cancer, efforts have been directed

TABLE 13.1

Effect of Human Papillomavirus on Patterns of Distant Metastatic Failure in Oropharyngeal Squamous Cell Carcinoma Treated With Chemoradiotherapy

Site	No. of Patients With Metastatic Disease at Each Site		Metastatic Sites, No. (%)	
	HPV− Status	HPV+ Status	HPV− Status	HPV+ Status
Overall No.	9	28	12	57
Lung	7	23	7 (58.3)	23 (40.4)
Bone	2	12	2 (16.7)	12 (21.1)
Liver	1	7	1 (8.3)	7 (12.3)
Intra-abdominal lymph nodes	0	3	0	3 (5.3)
Axillary lymph nodes	0	2	0	2 (3.5)
Brain	2	2	2 (16.7)	2 (3.5)
Kidney	0	2	0	2 (3.5)
Muscle	0	2	0	2 (3.5)
Skin	0	2	0	2 (3.5)
Pericardium	0	1	0	1 (1.8)
Peritoneum	0	1	0	1 (1.8)

HPV, human papillomavirus.

Source: Reproduced with permission from Trosman SJ, Koyfman SA, Ward MC et al. Effect of human papillomavirus on patterns of distant metastatic failure in oropharyngeal squamous cell carcinoma treated with chemoradiotherapy. *JAMA Otolaryngol Head Neck Surg.* 2015May 1;141(5):457-462. Copyright©2015 American Medical Association. All rights reserved.

toward developing a biochemical surveillance test for oropharyngeal cancers. HPV DNA is an attractive target as it can be extracted from oral exfoliated cells in rinses. A prospective trial of 124 HPV-positive OPSCC patients by Rettig et al. examined the potential of HPV DNA in oral rinses as a prospective marker (46). Prior to treatment, 67 of the 124 patients (54%) tested positive for HPV16 DNA. After treatment, only six participants (5%) tested positive, including one who was not in the original 67. This patient subsequently cleared HPV DNA and did not develop recurrence. Of the five patients with persistent HPV DNA all recurred within 1 year, compared to a recurrence rate of 8% in the HPV DNA negative group. Though limited by small sample sizes, this trial suggests that persistent HPV DNA demonstrates high specificity and positive predictive value (PPV) for disease recurrence and could be a potentially useful tool in determining the need for adjuvant therapy or increased surveillance.

MINIMALLY INVASIVE SURGERY

The widespread adoption of radiation and—following the demonstration that concurrent chemoradiation is superior to radiation alone for locally advanced HNSCC—of the varieties of chemoradiation as definitive therapy for even resectable cancers arose in reaction to the risks and sequelae of open surgery with mandibulotomy and glossectomy. Contemporaneous with the rise in the incidence of HPV-related oropharynx cancers, often with small and well-lateralized tonsillar primary tumors, a radical change in the surgical approach to smaller oropharynx cancers was made possible through the use of transoral surgical robotic and laser approaches (47,48). Single and limited institution series have demonstrated excellent survival and suggested that long-term functional consequences of treatment may be limited because postoperative radiation therapy (PORT) can be given in lower doses or omitted altogether (49–51). The Eastern Cooperative Oncology Group-American College of Radiology Imaging Network (ECOG-ACRIN) has completed a multicenter randomized trial of radiation de-intensification in patients amenable to transoral resection (E3311, NCT01898494). Patients ($n = 575$) were eligible who had p16(+) T1 or T2 OPSCC and in whom radiographic and clinical assessment specifically note the absence of matted nodes. Patients underwent transoral resection of the primary and surgical neck dissection. Those with clear margins and either N0 or N1 disease were observed. Those with involved margins, evidence for extranodal extension, or involvement of five or more nodes, received postoperative radiation with weekly cisplatin. The remainder entered randomization between 50 and 60 Gy of postoperative radiation. Oncologic outcomes are expected to be reported in 2018.

ROLE OF IMMUNOTHERAPY

As noted previously, HNSCCs exhibit evidence of inflammation, as well as increases in markers of immune exhaustion and increased numbers of T regulatory cells, with these changes most marked in HPV-driven cancers. Trials of the PD-1 directed antibodies pembrolizumab and nivolumab have demonstrated activity in metastatic/recurrent HNSCC, with duration of response of 53 weeks with pembrolizumab, and a significant advantage of nivolumab over conventional systemic therapy for cisplatin-treated HNSCC (52,53). Activity is somewhat greater in HPV-associated than HPV-negative disease. These demonstrations of proof of principle for immunotherapy in HNSCC have led to numerous subsequent HNSCC trials exploring inhibition of the PD-1 immunoregulatory pathway with PD-1 or PD-L1 inhibitors alone, combined with CTLA-4 antagonists, or in combination with chemotherapy in the first-line treatment of metastatic/recurrent disease, as well as in combination with definitive chemoradiation, postoperatively, or as maintenance following definitive chemoradiation. Early phase trials explore the combination of PD-1 pathway directed therapy with HPV-specific therapeutic vaccines, oncolytic tumor virus, or other immune regulators such as IDO (indoleamine 2,3-dioxygenase). These approaches are not sufficiently mature for incorporation into de-intensification schemes at this time, but as biomolecular and clinical patient selection criteria are developed to identify patients with outstanding and durable responses to immunotherapy, as well as to exclude patients at high risk of serious autoimmune complications, appropriate incorporation of immunotherapy may permit substantial reductions in radiation and chemotherapy exposure.

CONCLUSIONS

HPV-associated oropharyngeal cancer has emerged as a unique subset of head and neck squamous cell carcinoma with a distinctive pathophysiology and patient population that necessitates reconsideration of our current treatment approach. While the tumor is more sensitive to treatment and has a better prognosis, these aspects present novel challenges with respect to minimizing long-term treatment-related morbidity and surveillance technique. Retrospective data indicate that HPV-positive patients stratify into a lower risk group that may benefit from de-intensification of chemotherapy and/or radiation, the incorporation of biologic therapies, and varying surveillance based on risk. The evolving data suggest that HPV-positive OPSCC patients could be a population that would significantly benefit from limited radiation fields and reduced doses, without sacrificing survival. Last, utilizing induction chemotherapy as a means to select for robust responders and to maximally cytoreduce HPV-associated tumors may warrant reconsideration as a viable treatment paradigm. Clinical trials evaluating these concepts are currently under way with highly anticipated results in the years to come.

CASE 13.1: LOW-VOLUME NEVER SMOKER HPV-POSITIVE (LOW RISK)

Pt DG is a 56-year-old man who presented with a small lump in the right neck he detected while shaving. The mass was nontender. Recent dental evaluation had been normal, and the patient had no history of recent upper respiratory illness. The patient was a lifetime never smoker, had used marijuana approximately twice a month for several years in the remote past, and he worked as a software engineer, with no discernable occupational exposures. He was seen at an urgent care center in a local mall, and referred for ear, nose, and throat (ENT) evaluation. Nasopharyngolaryngoscopy revealed minimal fullness and erythema of the right tonsil. CT scan was obtained and demonstrated a 1-cm enhancing mass in the right tonsil and a solitary 2.4-cm right lymph node at level II. This was surrounded by well-preserved fat planes with no evidence of fat stranding (Figure 13.5).

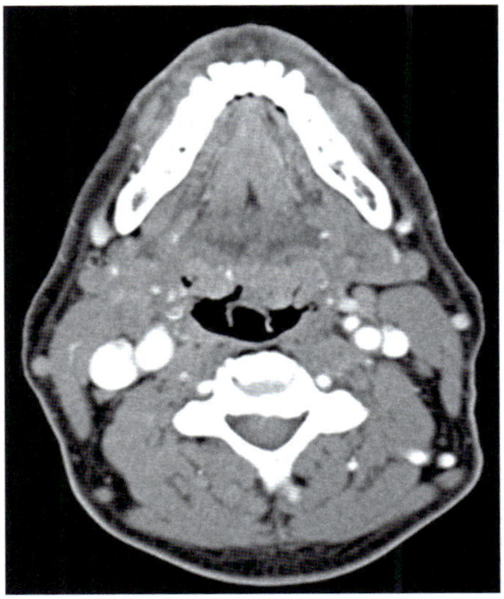

FIGURE 13.5 Contrast CT of "good prognosis" HPV patient with minimal smoking history and low-volume disease in the oropharynx and ipsilateral cervical nodes.

Fine needle aspiration (FNA) of the right lymph node was performed and demonstrated poorly differentiated squamous cell carcinoma. HPV 16 was detected by PCR. Biopsy of the tonsil lesion yielded poorly differentiated squamous cell carcinoma, which stained strongly and diffusely for p16 on immunohistochemistry. This was clinically staged as a T1N1 right tonsil cancer. The patient was referred to a high-volume head and neck surgeon skilled in transoral robotic surgery. He was discussed in a multidisciplinary tumor board and considered eligible for enrollment on E3311, a cooperative group study evaluating the use of minimally invasive surgery with dose-modified, risk-based postoperative therapy for early T stage HPV-related oropharynx cancer. Considerations for up-front use of transoral surgery and neck dissection include the likelihood of obtaining negative margins, and the functional outcome anticipated from the intervention, particularly with respect to swallowing solids. Function is impacted by the extent of local resection, whether the accompanying neck dissection will be ipsilateral only or bilateral, and the extent of postoperative radiation or chemoradiation that is required. In the case of extensive base of tongue lesions, resection may be less likely to achieve negative margins. Base of tongue lesions that cross or abut the midline will be managed with bilateral lymph node dissection, increasing morbidity. When matted nodes, nodes with frank radiographic evidence of extracapsular extension, or high node number (≥5 lymph nodes) are present, cisplatin will be added to postoperative radiation. Trimodality therapy is associated with higher rates of swallowing dysfunction, and the duration of the episode of care is increased for surgery followed by 6 weeks of chemoradiation compared with no surgery and 7 weeks of chemoradiation, as conventionally administered as definitive therapy.

The patient was enrolled on E3311 and taken to transoral resection with ipsilateral selective neck dissection. A 1.4-cm margin-negative, p16(+) right tonsil cancer was identified on pathologic examination. One of 22 lymph nodes was involved with a poorly differentiated squamous cell carcinoma, and there was no evidence of extranodal extension. The patient was observed, and has no evidence of recurrent disease at 20 months of follow-up.

CASE 13.2: HIGH-VOLUME DISEASE IN A SMOKER HPV-POSITIVE (INTERMEDIATE RISK)

The patient is a 69-year-old man with a 40 pack-year history of cigarette smoking who presented with a 6-month history of increasing odynophagia, right ear pain, and a 10-pound weight loss. His ECOG performance status was 1. Laboratory results were unremarkable and chest x-ray (CXR) showed mild hyperinflation consistent with his long smoking history. Physical exam showed mild bilateral level II fullness of the neck, and direct laryngoscopic exam in the office revealed a submucosal mass involving the right oropharyngeal structures, including the tongue base to midline and tonsil, with extension into the right soft palate. There was no involvement of the larynx or hypopharynx, with notable good airway and normally mobile vocal cords. CT of the neck with contrast was then performed. This corroborated the physical exam, showing a 4.1-cm right oropharyngeal mass involving most of the right-sided structures, with no extension over to the left tongue base. Bilateral level II nodes are seen up to 2.5 cm with necrotic center. Images through the lung apices confirm moderate emphysematous changes but no suspicious nodules nor mediastinal adenopathy. Triple endoscopy under anesthesia confirmed the extent of disease, and esophagoscopy and bronchoscopy were normal and without lesions. Biopsy of the mass demonstrated a nonkeratinizing invasive squamous cell carcinoma with intense staining for p16. (Figure 13.6). Whole body PET/CT showed no distant metastases. He was staged as T3N2cM0. His case was discussed at a comprehensive tumor board, where options of surgical resection, bilateral neck dissections, and postoperative radiation with or without chemotherapy, or definitive concurrent chemoradiation were reviewed. The latter was deemed a better option to avoid bilateral neck dissection and the risk of positive margins at the primary.

He completed 7 weeks of therapy with no interruptions but a percutaneous endoscopic gastrostomy (PEG) tube was placed at 4 weeks. The PEG tube was removed 4 months later, and he remains free of disease at 3 years.

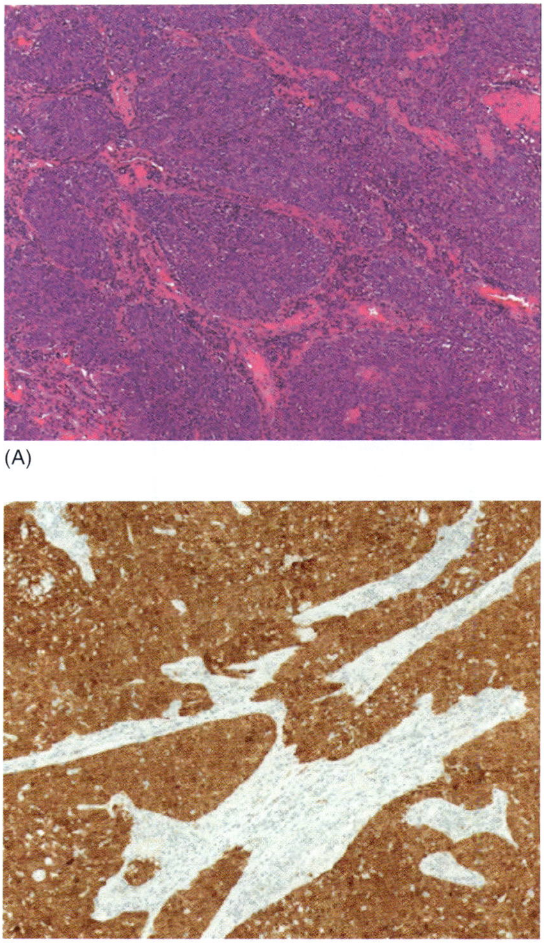

(A)

(B)

FIGURE 13.6 Nuclear and cytoplasmic staining of basaloid nonkeratinizing SCC (A). IHC staining for p16 is diffuse (B).

IHC, immunohistochemistry; SCC, squamous cell carcinoma.

REFERENCES

1. Ang KK, Zhang Q, Rosenthal DI, et al. Randomized phase III trial of concurrent accelerated radiation plus cisplatin with or without cetuximab for stage III to IV head and neck carcinoma: RTOG 0522. *J Clin Oncol*. 2014;32(27):2940–2950. doi:10.1200/JCO.2013.53.5633
2. Parker SL, Tong T, Bolden S, Wingo PA. Cancer statistics, 1996. *CA Cancer J Clin*. 1996;46(1):5–27. https://www.ncbi.nlm.nih.gov/pubmed/8548526
3. Seigel RL, Miller KD, Jemel A. Cancer statistics, 2016. *CA Cancer J Clin*. 2016;66(1):7–30. doi:10.3322/caac.21332
4. Gillison ML, Koch WM, Capone RB, et al. Evidence for a causal association between human papillomavirus and a subset of head and neck cancers. *J Natl Cancer Inst*. 2000;92(9):709–720. https://www.ncbi.nlm.nih.gov/pubmed/10793107
5. Stransky N, Egloff AM, Tward AD, et al. The mutational landscape of head and neck squamous cell carcinoma. *Science*. 2011;333(6046):1157–1160. doi:10.1126/science.1208130
6. Fahkry C, Zhang Q, Nguyen-Tan PF, et al. Human papillomavirus and overall survival after progression of oropharyngeal squamous cell carcinoma. *J Clin Oncol*. 2014;32(30):3365–3373. doi:10.1200/JCO.2014.55.1937
7. Ang KK, Harris J, Wheeler R, et al. Human papillomavirus and survival of patients with oropharyngeal cancer. *N Engl J Med*. 2010;363(1):24–35. doi:10.1056/NEJMoa0912217
8. Löning T, Ikenberg H, Becker J, et al. Analysis of oral papillomas, leukoplakias, and invasive carcinomas for human papillomavirus type related DNA. *J Invest Dermatol*. 1985;84(5):417–420. https://www.ncbi.nlm.nih.gov/pubmed/2987361
9. Boscolo-Rizzo P, Pawlita M, Holzinger D. From HPV-positive towards HPV-driven oropharyngeal squamous cell carcinomas. *Cancer Treat Rev*. 2016;42:24–29. doi:10.1016/j.ctrv.2015.10.009
10. Klussmann JP, Gültekin E, Weissenborn S, et al. Expression of p16 protein identifies a distinct entity of tonsillar carcinomas associated with human papillomavirus. *J Pathol*. 2003;162(3):747–753. doi:10.1016/S0002-9440(10)63871-0
11. Maxwell JH, Kumar B, Feng Y, et al. Tobacco use in human papillomavirus-positive advanced oropharynx cancer patients related to increased risk of distant metastases and tumor recurrence. *Clin Cancer Res*. 2010;16(4):1226–1235. doi:10.1158/1078-0432.CCR-09-2350
12. O'Sullivan B, Huang SH, Siu LL. Deintensification candidate subgroups in human papillomavirus-related oropharyngeal cancer according to minimal risk of distant metastasis. *J Clin Oncol*. 2013;31(5):543–550. doi:10.1200/JCO.2012.44.0164
13. Scheffner M, Werness BA, Huibregste JM, et al. The E6 oncoprotein encoded by human papillomavirus types 16 and 18 promotes the degradation of p53. *Cell*. 1990;63(6):1129–1136. https://www.ncbi.nlm.nih.gov/pubmed/2175676
14. Heck DV, Yee CL, Howley PM, et al. Efficiency of binding the retinoblastoma protein correlates with the transforming capacity of the E7 oncoproteins of the human papillomaviruses. *Proc Natl Acad Sci U S A*. 1992;89(10):4442–4446. https://www.ncbi.nlm.nih.gov/pubmed/1316608
15. Saraiya M, Unger ER, Thompson TD, et al. US assessment of HPV types in cancers: implications for current and 9-valent HPV vaccines. *J Natl Cancer Inst*. 2015;107(6):djv086. doi:10.1093/jnci/djv086
16. Munger K, Phelps WC, Bubb V, et al. The E6 and E7 genes of the human papillomavirus type 16 together are necessary and sufficient for transformation of primary human keratinocytes. *J Virol*. 1989;63(10):4417–4421. https://www.ncbi.nlm.nih.gov/pubmed/2476573
17. Walline HM, Goudsmit CM, McHugh JB, et al. Integration of high-risk human papillomavirus into cellular cancer-related genes in head and neck cancer cell lines. *Head Neck*. 2017;39(5):840–852. doi:10.1002/hed.24729
18. Walline HM, Komarck CM, McHugh JB, et al. Genomic integration of high-risk HPV alters gene expression in oropharyngeal squamous cell carcinoma. *Mol Cancer Res*. 2016;14(10):941–952. doi:10.1158/1541-7786.MCR-16-0105
19. Nulton TJ, Olex AL, Dozmorov M, et al. Analysis of the Cancer Genome Atlas sequencing data reveals novel properties of the human papillomavirus 16 genome in head and neck squamous cell carcinoma. *Oncotarget*. 2017;8(11):17684–17699. doi:10.18632/oncotarget.15179
20. Cancer Genome Atlas Network. Comprehensive genomic characterization of head and neck squamous cell carcinomas. *Nature*. 2015;517(7536):576–582. doi:10.1038/nature11404
21. Hajek M, Sewell A, Kaech S, et al. TRAF3/CYLD mutations identify a distinct subset of human papillomavirus-associated head and neck squamous cell carcinoma. *Cancer*. 2017;123(10):1778–1790. doi:10.1002/cncr.30570
22. Nguyen N, Bellile E, Thomas D, et al. Tumor infiltrating lymphocytes and survival in patients with head and neck squamous cell carcinoma. *Head Neck*. 2016;38(7):1074–1084. doi:10.1002/hed.24406
23. Budach W, Bolke E, Kammers K, et al. Induction chemotherapy followed by concurrent radio-chemotherapy versus concurrent radio-chemotherapy alone as treatment of locally advanced squamous cell carcinoma of the head and neck (HNSCC): A meta-analysis of randomized trials. *Radiother Oncol*. 2016;118(2):238–243. doi:10.1016/j.radonc.2015.10.014
24. Forasteire AA, Goepfert H, Maor M, et al. Concurrent chemotherapy and radiotherapy for organ preservation in advanced laryngeal cancer. *N Engl J Med*. 2003;349(22):2091–2098. doi:10.1056/NEJMoa031317
25. Fakhry C, Westra WH, Li S, et al. Improved survival of patients with human papillomavirus-positive head and neck squamous cell carcinoma in a prospective clinical trial. *J Natl Cancer Inst*. 2008;100(4):261–269. doi:10.1093/jnci/djn011

26. Cooperstein E, Gilbert J, Epstein JB, et al. Vanderbilt head and neck symptom survey version 2.0: report of the development and initial testing of a subscale for assessment of oral health. *Head Neck*. 2012;34(6):797–804. doi:10.1002/hed.21816
27. Marur S, Li S, Cmelak AJ, et al. E1308: phase II trial of induction chemotherapy followed by reduced-dose radiation and weekly cetuximab in patients with HPV-associated resectable squamous cell carcinoma of the oropharynx—ECOG-ACRIN Cancer Research Group. *J Clin Oncol*. 2017;35(5):490–497. doi:10.1200/JCO.2016.68.3300
28. Chera BS, Amdur RJ, Tepper J, et al. Phase 2 trial of de-intensified chemoradiation therapy for favorable-risk human papillomavirus-associated oropharyngeal squamous cell carcinoma. *Int J Radiat Oncol Biol Phys*. 2015;93(5):976–985. doi:10.1016/j.ijrobp.2015.08.033
29. Haddad R, O'Neill A, Rabinowitz G, et al. Induction chemotherapy followed by concurrent chemoradiotherapy (sequential chemoradiotherapy) versus concurrent chemoradiotherapy alone in locally advanced head and neck cancer (PARADIGM): a randomised phase 3 trial. *Lancet Oncol*. 2013;14(3):257–264. doi:10.1016/S1470-2045(13)70011-1
30. Villaflor VM, Melotek JM, Karrison TG, et al. Response-adapted volume de-escalation (RAVD) in locally advanced head and neck cancer. *Ann Oncol*. 2016;27(5):908–913. doi:10.1093/annonc/mdw051
31. Nguyen-Tan PF, Zhang Q, Ang KK, et al. Randomized phase III trial to test accelerated versus standard fractionation in combination with concurrent cisplatin for head and neck carcinomas in the Radiation Therapy Oncology Group 0129 trial: long-term report of efficacy and toxicity. *J Clin Oncol*. 2014;32(34):3858–3866. doi:10.1200/JCO.2014.55.3925
32. Blanchard P, Baujat B, Holostenco V, et al. Meta-analysis of chemotherapy in head and neck cancer (MACH-NC): a comprehensive analysis by tumour site. *Radiother Oncol*. 2011;100(1):33–40. doi:10.1016/j.radonc.2011.05.036
33. Guan J, Zhang Y, Li Q, et al. A meta-analysis of weekly cisplatin versus three weekly cisplatin chemotherapy plus concurrent radiotherapy (CRT) for advanced head and neck cancer (HNC). *Oncotarget*. 2016;7(43):70185–70193. doi:10.18632/oncotarget.11824
34. Robert F, Ezekiel MP, Spencer SA, et al. Phase I study of anti-epidermal growth factor receptor antibody cetuximab in combination with radiation therapy in patients with advanced head and neck cancer. *J Clin Oncol*. 2001;19:3234–3243. doi:10.1200/JCO.2001.19.13.3234
35. Magrini SM, Bugkione M, Corvo R, et al. Cetuximab and radiotherapy versus cisplatin and radiotherapy for locally advanced head and neck cancer: a randomized phase II trial. *J Clin Oncol*. 2016;34(5):427–435. doi:10.1200/JCO.2015.63.1671
36. Rosenthal DI, Harari PM, Giralt J, et al. Association of human papillomavirus and p16 status with outcomes in the IMCL-9815 phase III registration trial for patients with locoregionally advanced oropharyngeal squamous cell carcinoma of the head and neck treated with radiotherapy with or without cetuximab. *J Clin Oncol*. 2016;34(12):1300–1308. doi:10.1200/JCO.2015.62.5970
37. Bonner JA, Harari PM, Giralt J, et al. Radiotherapy plus cetuximab for squamous-cell carcinoma of the head and neck. *N Engl J Med*. 2006;354(6):567–578. doi:10.1056/NEJMoa053422
38. Nolan N, Diavolitsis VM, Blakaj D, et al Intensity modulated radiation therapy with cetuximab versus platinum chemotherapy in p16-positive oropharyngeal squamous cell carcinoma. *International Journal of Radiation Oncology Biology Physics*. 2015;93(3):E333. doi:10.1016/j.ijrobp.2015.07.1397
39. Ringash J, Waldron JN, Siu LL, et al. Quality of life and swallowing with standard chemoradiotherapy versus accelerated radiotherapy and panitumumab in locoregionally advanced carcinoma of the head and neck: a phase III randomised trial from the Canadian Cancer Trials Group (HN.6). *Eur J Cancer*. 2017;72:192–199. doi:10.1016/j.ejca.2016.11.008
40. Seiwert TY, Melotek JM, Blair EA, et al. Final results of a randomized phase 2 trial investigating the addition of cetuximab to induction chemotherapy and accelerated or hyperfractionated chemoradiation for locoregionally advanced head and neck cancer *Int J Radiat Oncol Biol Phys*. 2016;96(1):21–29. 10.1016/j.ijrobp.2016.04.030
41. Trosman SJ, Koyfman SA, Ward MC, et al. Effect of human papillomavirus on patterns of distant metastatic failure in oropharyngeal squamous cell carcinoma treated with chemoradiotherapy. *JAMA Otolaryngol Head Neck Surg*. 2015;141(5):457–462. doi:10.1001/jamaoto.2015.136
42. Huang SH, Perez-Ordonez B, Weinreb I, et al. Natural course of distant metastases following radiotherapy or chemoradiotherapy in HPV-related oropharyngeal cancer. *Oral Oncol*. 2013 Jan;49(1):79–85. doi:10.1016/j.oraloncology.2012.07.015
43. Argiris A, Li S, Ghebremichael M, et al. Prognostic significance of human papillomavirus in recurrent or metastatic head and neck cancer: an analysis of Eastern Cooperative Oncology Group trials. *Ann Oncol*. 2014;25(7):1410–1416. doi:10.1093/annonc/mdu167
44. Frakes JM, Naghavi AO, Demetriou SK, et al. Determining optimal follow-up in the management of human papillomavirus-positive oropharyngeal cancer. *Cancer*. 2016;122(4):634–641. doi:10.1002/cncr.29782
45. Mehanna H, Wong WL, McKonkey CC, et al. PET-CT Surveillance versus neck dissection in advanced head and neck cancer. *N Engl J Med*. 2016;374(15):1444–1454. doi:10.1056/NEJMoa1514493
46. Rettig EM, Wentz A, Posner MR, et al. Prognostic implication of persistent human papillomavirus type 16 DNA detection in oral rinses for human papillomavirus-related oropharyngeal carcinoma. *JAMA Oncol*. 2015;1(7):907–915. doi:10.1001/jamaoncol.2015.2524

47. O'Malley BW Jr, Weinstein GS, Snyder W, et al. Transoral robotic surgery (TORS) for base of tongue neoplasms. *Laryngoscope*. 2006;116(8):1465–1472. doi:10.1097/01.mlg.0000227184.90514.1a
48. Haughey BH, Hinni ML, Salassa JR, et al. Transoral laser microsurgery as primary treatment for advanced-stage oropharyngeal cancer: a United States multi-center study. *Head Neck*. 2011;33(12):1683–1694. doi:10.1002/hed.21669
49. Weinstein GS, Quon H, O'Malley BW Jr, et al. Selective neck dissection and deintensified postoperative radiation and chemotherapy for oropharyngeal cancer: a subset analysis of the University of Pennsylvania transoral robotic surgery trial. *Laryngoscope*. 2010;120(9):1749–1755. doi:10.1002/lary.21021
50. Weinstein GS, O'Malley BW Jr, Magnuson JS, et al. Transoral robotic surgery: a multicenter study to assess feasibility, safety, and surgical margins. *Laryngoscope*. 2012;122(8):1701–1707. doi:10.1002/lary.23294
51. Rich JT, Liu J, Haughey BH. Swallowing function after transoral laser microsurgery (TLM) ± adjuvant therapy for advanced-stage oropharyngeal cancer. *Laryngoscope*. 2011;121(11):2381–2390. doi:10.1002/lary.21406
52. Seiwart TY, Burtness B, Mehra R, et al. Safety and clinical activity of pembrolizumab for treatment of recurrent or metastatic squamous cell carcinoma of the head and neck (KEYNOTE-012): an open-label, multicentre, phase 1b trial. *Lancet Oncol*. 2016;17(7):956–965. doi:10.1016/S1470-2045(16)30066-3
53. Ferris RL, Gillison ML. Nivolumab for squamous-cell cancer of head and neck. *N Engl J Med*. 2017;376(6):596. doi:10.1056/NEJMc1615565

14

Non–HPV-Associated Oropharyngeal Cancer

Meghan T. Turner

Anirudh Saraswathula

F. Christopher Holsinger

BACKGROUND

Until the 1990s, oropharyngeal cancer was one of the many subsites of aerodigestive tract squamous cell carcinoma (SCC) caused by the synergistic carcinogenic effects of long-term tobacco and alcohol abuse. Since 2003, we understand that oropharyngeal squamous cell carcinoma (OPSCC) is actually two separate diseases with two disparate patient populations and two different clinical courses. The first is caused by the human papillomavirus (HPV positive) and is related to sexual practices (1,2). The second is caused by excessive smoking and drinking (HPV negative) (2,3). The HPV-negative patient is older, presents with a symptomatic (dysphagia/odynophagia), large, primary tumor (4), and has a history of tobacco and/or alcohol abuse (1), pathology showing a keratinized tumor, worse overall prognosis, and a high risk of second, primary cancers due to "field cancerization" (1,5). The HPV-positive patient is a younger, nonsmoker, nondrinker (6), with multiple oral sex partners (>five) (1), who presents with large, cystic lymph node metastases (4,6), and has a small, sometimes undetectable, primary tumor with nonkeratinizing, basaloid appearance on pathology (7), and substantially better survival outcomes (8).

The identification of these two different cancers has led to renewed interest in studying outcomes for OPSCC based on treatment (either with definitive chemoradiotherapy protocols or primary surgery) and risk stratification that incorporates HPV status (8–10). The landmark studies that originally established organ-sparing chemoradiotherapy protocols as the standard of care for OPSCC in the late 1990s were performed prior to the discovery of HPV-related OPSCC, and were not stratified by HPV status (11,12). Since then, the improved prognosis of HPV-positive OPSCC has been studied with rigor. Many studies have examined the impact of HPV status on survival and have found improved survival of HPV-positive patients (8,13–16). A meta-analysis revealed that HPV-positive OPSCC has a 28% reduced risk of death compared to HPV-negative OPSCC (17). Posner et al. reported an 80% reduction in mortality for highly selected HPV-positive versus HPV-negative OPSCC (14).

More recently, the improved survival in the HPV-positive patient population has spurred interest in treatment de-intensification following a landmark study by Machtay et al. that reported on the long-term toxicities of organ-sparing protocols for head and neck cancers (18). To date, there is a wealth of literature on treatment outcomes for HPV-positive OPSCC. However, very few studies have focused on the treatment and outcomes of the HPV-negative patient population using modern surgical approaches, intensity-modulated radiotherapy, and novel adjuvant systemic therapies.

EPIDEMIOLOGY OF HPV-NEGATIVE OPSCC

Chaturvedi et al. recently described the population-based estimated incidence of HPV-positive and HPV-negative oropharyngeal cancer in the United States using the Surveillance, Epidemiology, and End Results (SEER) database (2). From 1988 to 2004, the incidence of HPV-negative cancers significantly declined by 50% (from 2.0 per 100,000 to 1.0 per 100,000), while HPV-positive cancers increased by 225% (from 0.8 per 100,000 to 2.5 per 100,000). In a recent Radiation Therapy Oncology Group trial (RTOG 0129), the prevalence of HPV-negative tumors was approximately 40% of the total oropharyngeal study population (8). This is a robust estimate of the prevalence of HPV-negative oropharyngeal tumors in the United States, given the multi-institutional nature of the cooperative group and the geographic diversity of this study population. While the incidence of HPV-negative OPSCC may continue to decline along with tobacco use in the United States, the worldwide prevalence of is still 35.6% (17). In certain populations this remains a higher percentage. A recent study from Germany found 79% of its OPSCC patients to be HPV-negative (19).

THE DIAGNOSIS OF HPV-NEGATIVE OPSCC

Establishing a diagnosis of HPV-positive tumors has undergone considerable study and scrutiny. HPV-related tumors are characterized by the presence of active, high-risk HPV infection (either with HPV DNA, RNA, or mRNA in situ hybridization (ISH) (20). The most common high-risk HPV subtype found in oropharyngeal tumors is HPV 16 (17). In two separate meta-analyses, oropharyngeal tumors were associated with active high-risk HPV 16 infection (86.7%), p16 overexpression (86.7%), and viral E6/E7 mRNA (86.9%) (17,21). The presence of strong nuclear and cytoplasmic p16 staining in greater than 70% of the tumor is a pathologic, surrogate marker for HPV-induced cancer, and is currently the standard routine screening test (22).

However, p16 staining alone leads to some false negative results. The combination of p16 and HPV DNA polymerase chain reaction (PCR) testing provides 100% sensitivity and specificity compared with the gold standard HPV E6 or E7 mRNA (RT-PCR or RNA ISH) (20). When staining reveals a p16-negative oropharyngeal primary carcinoma or SCC of unknown primary origin, additional testing with PCR to look for HPV DNA and/or Epstein-Barr virus (EBV) DNA is necessary (23). This may lead to identification of an additional 6% to 8% of patients being diagnosed as HPV positive or a diagnosis of nasopharyngeal primary for cancer of the unknown primary (24).

NONSURGICAL TREATMENT FOR HPV-NEGATIVE OPSCC

Fakhry et al. (13) were the first to highlight the importance of HPV status on prognosis for SCC of multiple subsites with respect to overall survival (OS) and progression-free survival (PFS). This group reported on ECOG 2399 trial studying the use of induction paclitaxel and carboplatin to identify partial and complete responders versus nonresponders. Nonresponders were offered surgery. Patients refusing surgery were treated with concurrent chemoradiotherapy. HPV-negative tumors were less likely to respond to induction chemotherapy than HPV-positive tumors (55% vs. 82%). HPV-negative tumors were also less likely to respond to chemoradiotherapy compared to HPV-positive tumors (57% vs. 84%). Two-year OS and PFS for HPV-negative patients were 62% and 33% compared to 95% and 86% for HPV-positive patients. A study by Felice et al. (29) recently compared the use of standard chemoradiotherapy with cisplatin to induction cisplatin followed by standard chemoradiotherapy with cisplatin for the treatment of locally advanced oropharyngeal cancer. This group unfortunately found no significant difference in two-year OS or disease-free survival (DFS).

Next, the Danish Head and Neck Cancer (DAHANCA) Study Group 5 trial, performed in 2009, studied the effect of p16 status on outcomes of head and neck cancers of all subsites stratified and treated with conventional radiotherapy alone (25). HPV-negative patients had significantly worse 5-year OS, disease-specific survival (DSS), and locoregional control (LRC), 26%, 34%, and 28%, respectively. In contrast, HPV-positive patients had substantially improved 5-year OS, DSS, and LRC, 62%, 72%, and 58%, respectively. Later, the same group looked at survival outcomes comparing conventional and accelerated fraction radiation in oropharyngeal cancer of all subsites and found improved 5-year LRC for tumors treated with accelerated fractions, but no difference in 5-year OS. This was also true in the HPV-negative tumor oropharyngeal cancers (26).

RTOG 0129 attempted to examine the use of accelerated fraction radiation and cisplatin compared to standard chemoradiotherapy with cisplatin for the treatment of oropharyngeal cancer, specifically. There was no improvement in outcome with radiation intensification. However, Ang et al. examined outcomes in OPSCC and was the first to provide a risk stratification schema for oropharyngeal cancers that included HPV status as the strongest predictor of survival, followed by T-stage, nodal metastasis, and significant smoking history (>10 pack-years); see Figure 14.1 (8). It also highlighted the dismal survival of patients with HPV-negative OPSCC, who were treated with definitive chemoradiotherapy. Looking at OS in this study, patients with HPV-negative tumors had a 25.1% worse 3-year survival (57.1% vs. 82.4%) when compared with patients with HPV-positive tumors. Locoregional recurrence at 3 years was 21% higher in patients with HPV-negative tumors compared to HPV-positive tumors: 35.1% (95% confidence interval [CI]: 26.4–43.8) versus 13.6% (95% CI: 8.9%–18.3%), respectively ($p < .001$) (8). A subset analysis of OPSCC cases gathered from the Meta-Analysis of Radiotherapy in Carcinomas of the Head and neck (MARCH) project (which included the study by Ang et al.) looked at the combined impact of HPV status and smoking on impact on prognosis (see Figure 14.2). HPV-negative smokers and nonsmokers had 5-year PFS of 22.6% and 33.9%, respectively. HPV-positive smokers and nonsmokers in contrast had 5-year PFS of 55.2% and 73.9%, respectively.

Surprisingly, the use of definitive radiotherapy with and without chemotherapy for oropharyngeal cancer stratified by HPV status was only very recently studied by Hall et al. This population-based, retrospective study on all patients with OPSCC treated in Ontario cancer treatment centers and Princess Margaret Hospital in Canada during the preconcurrent chemoradiotherapy and postconcurrent chemoradiotherapy eras is the only study to date examining the efficacy of patients treated with conventional RT versus concurrent chemoradiotherapy stratified by retrospective collection of HPV status. Based on their study of 1,028 patients, there was no improvement in 5-year OS for either HPV-negative or HPV-positive patients with the addition of chemotherapy (27).

Posner et al. conducted a subset analysis of patients with OPSCC that participated in the TAX 324 trial using standard radiotherapy and compared outcomes with the following adjuvant chemotherapy regimens: doclitaxel, cisplatin, and 5-fluorouracil, or cisplatin and 5-fluorouracil. Results were stratified by HPV status. HPV-negative patients had significantly worse OS, PFS, and disease failure rates, 31%, 29%, and 49%, respectively. By contrast, HPV-positive rates of OS, PFS, and disease failure were 79%, 73%, and 16%. There was no significant difference in outcomes based on the treatment arm, because subset analysis was significantly underpowered for analyzing treatment effect based on the treatment arm when looking solely at oropharyngeal cancers (14).

The role of cetuximab as treatment intensification for patients who are not candidates for cisplatin-based therapy has been studied in large head and neck cancer trials. However, only two trials have looked at outcomes in OPSCC. The first by Rosenthal et al. conducted a subset analysis of the original IMCL-9815 Phase II trial looking at radiotherapy with or without cetuximab. Outcomes in the OPSCC patients were stratified by HPV status. HPV-negative patients had worse OS and PFS as expected. HPV-positive patients had nonsignificant improvement in 3-year OS rates with cetuximab and radiotherapy versus radiation alone, 41.9% versus 33.5%, respectively. Similarly, HPV-negative patients had nonsignificant 3-year PFS rates with the radiation and cetuximab versus the radiation alone, 29.1% versus 15.6%, respectively. The small numbers of the subset analysis may be the reason that these findings were insignificant, as the trial was not originally designed to study this question. Another more recent study by Mehta et al. examined outcomes based on definitive therapy with either radiation and concurrent cisplatin or radiation and concurrent cetuximab. Results were stratified by HPV status. On multivariate analysis, HPV-negative patients had significantly more favorable outcomes in the cetuximab arm (see Figure 14.3). By contrast, HPV-positive patients had significantly worse outcomes in the cetuximab arm (28). The second study was designed and powered to study

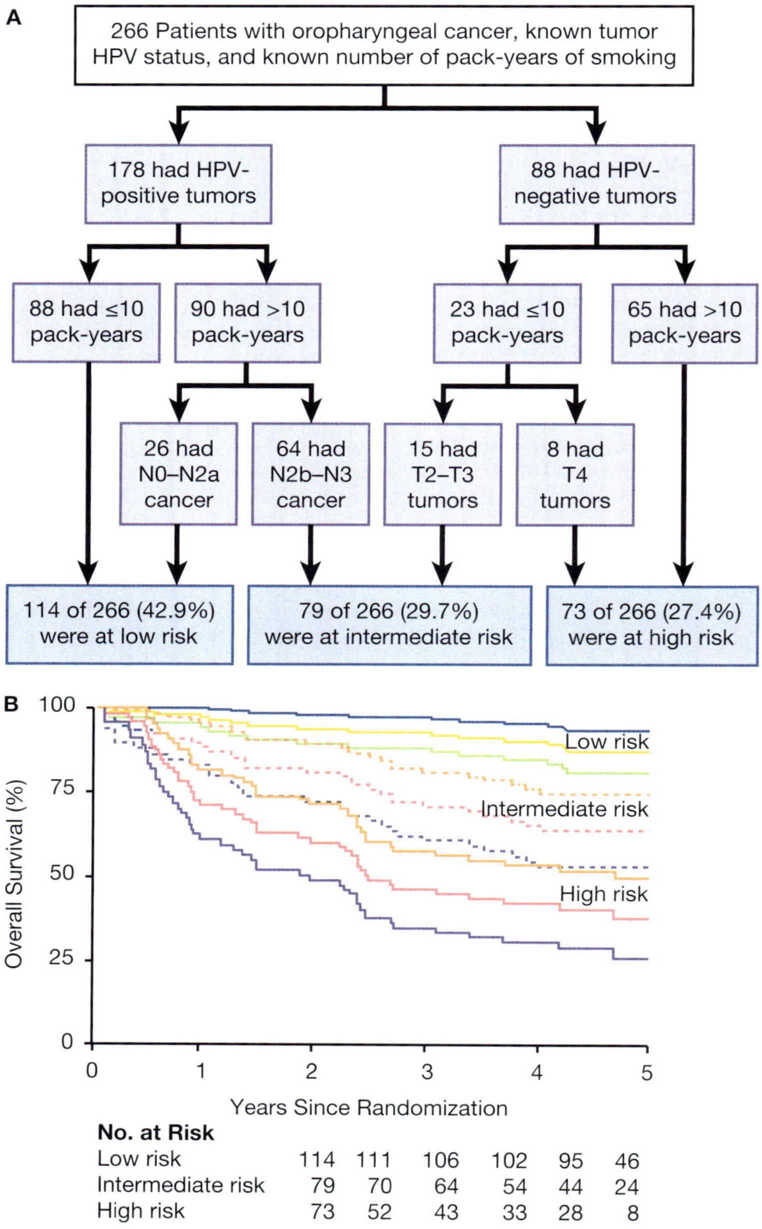

FIGURE 14.1 Langmark risk stratification schema established by Ang et al. with respect to HPV- and smoking status.

HPV, human papillomavirus.

outcomes based on the treatment arm and HPV status. From their results, it seems reasonable to conclude that HPV-negative tumors may respond more favorably to cetuximab.

Finally, several groups have begun looking at intensification of radiotherapy with the use of novel hypoxic cytotoxins. The DAHANCA Study Group examined the use of nimorazole added to radiation therapy for head and neck cancer and looked at outcomes stratified by HPV status. They found improved 5-year LRC when this drug was added to radiation in HPV-negative tumors. Next, Rischin et al. performed an open-label, randomized study of concurrent chemoradiotherapy with cisplatin versus cisplatin and tirapazimine, a hypoxic cytoxin for the

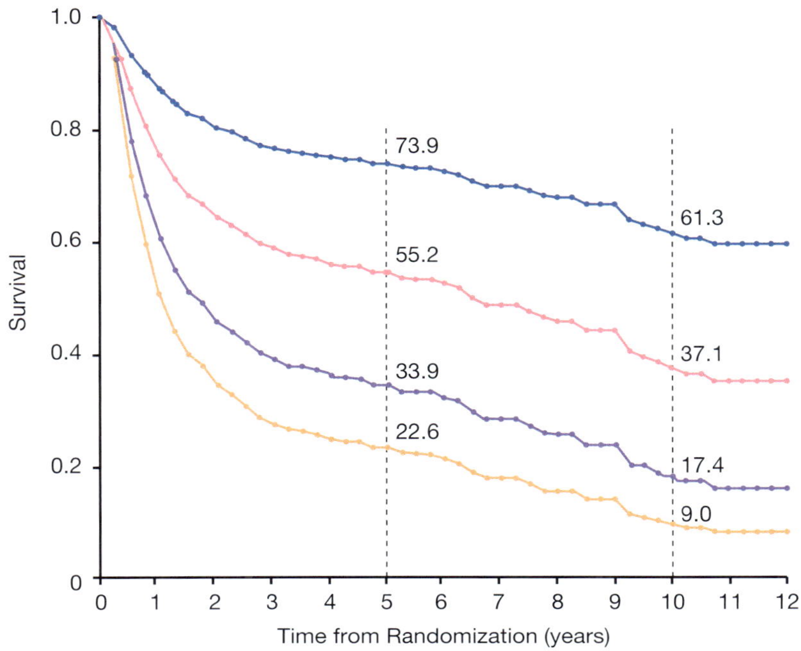

At Risk

— p16-positive	Never	86	76	70	60	34	10	8
— p16-positive	Former or current	252	170	145	126	78	38	34
— p16-negative	Never	21	10	9	9	3	3	1
— p16-negative	Former or current	290	99	68	55	30	14	12

FIGURE 14.2 MARCH study results. One of a few large studies to look at surivial base on p16 status and smoking status.

treatment of OPSCC as stratified by p16 status. This group found a trend toward improved 2-year LRC in p16-negative patients (15). Both studies reaffirm the still dismal outcome of HPV-negative patients compared to HPV-positive patients using novel agents and suggest that further use in HPV-negative OPSCC may be warranted.

HPV-negative OPSCC represents a significant and special subset of head and neck cancer patients, for whom there is dismal OS, PFS, and LRC in spite of maximal therapy. This fact remains in spite of intensified, modern-day, nonsurgical therapy protocols that include accelerated fractionation radiotherapy protocols, chemoradiotherapy protocols, induction protocols, and the use of novel agents (15,16,19,27–29). The treatment of HPV-negative OPSCC demands expert understanding of the outcomes using currently available treatments, so that patients can be properly counseled about their prognosis, options, and the opportunity to try novel therapy. It also demands special future study, because our understanding of nonsurgical therapy for HPV-negative OPSCC comes mostly from unplanned, underpowered subset analysis of larger, more inclusive studies on head and neck cancer, regardless of primary site or HPV status.

MODERN SURGICAL TREATMENT OF OPSCC

In the past, surgical resection of OPSCC required disfiguring incisions and functionally morbid procedures such as mandibular lingular release (30), pharyngotomy (lateral or suprahyoid) (31), and transmandibular approaches (midline labiomandibuloglossotomy or composite resection with lateral segmental mandibulectomy) (32). Recently, however, "endoscopic" head and neck surgery (eHNS) has emerged, which comprises minimally invasive approaches to the oropharynx with transoral laser microsurgery (TLM) and transoral robotic surgery (TORS) (33). Compared with traditional “open” head and neck surgery, TLM with endoscopic assistance and TORS for OPSCC, is performed

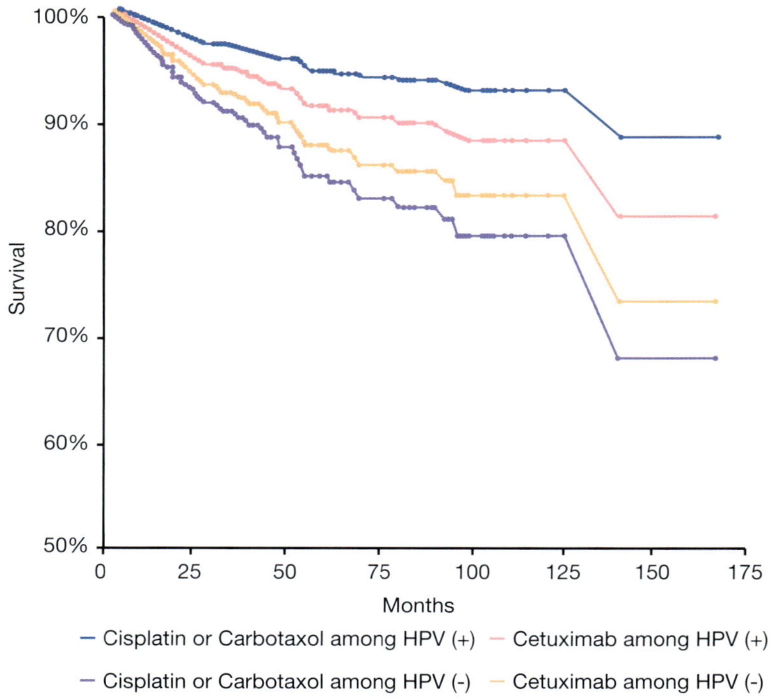

FIGURE 14.3 Rosenthal et al. conducted a subset analysis of the original IMCL-9815 Phase II trial looking at radiotherapy with or without cetuximab. Outcomes in the OPSCC patients were stratified by HPV status. Their results are shown above. HPV-negative patients had worse survival than HPV-positive patients. HPV-negative patients receiving cetuximab had improved survival compared to cisplatin. HPV-positive patients fared worse with cetuximab compared to cisplatin.

HPV, human papillomavirus

without external incisions and obviates the need for transmandibular access. This approach can be considered "inside-out" surgery, using incisions that start from the mucosal (inner) surface and extend into deep tissues, such as the tongue musculature or parapharyngeal space without connection to the neck dissection.

TLM is performed under direct vision with microsuspension laryngoscopy and is facilitated with an operating microscope, microsurgical instruments, and a carbon dioxide laser. First described by Steiner in 1972, TLM has since been proved to be oncologically sound (34,35). However, it is an adaptive surgical technique that relies on the surgeon's understanding of the three-dimensional anatomy and proper selection of "resectable tumors" for success. Standard surgical instruments, including tissue forceps, an electrocautery spatula, or CO_2 and thalium laser are then used to perform an en bloc resection of the oropharyngeal tumor. A few multicenter experiences have been published with excellent oncologic results, but this technique has not been widely adopted due to technical challenges in this approach and surgeons' fear of piecemeal resection as a cause of positive margins on final pathology. As such, TLM has only been reliably practiced in a few other high-volume centers (36,37).

Robotic surgery for the oropharynx was first described by Hockstein et al. in 2005 (60). After several reported series of successful treatments of OPSCC, the da Vinci Surgical System® (Intuitive Surgical Inc., Sunnyvale, California) was approved for TORS head and neck surgery by the Food and Drug Administration (FDA) in 2009. A retractor (several models may need to be considered to obtain ideal exposure) is positioned to retract the tongue and expose the posterior pharyngeal wall, tonsillar fossa, and base of tongue. The endoscope is then introduced into the pharynx, followed by two other arms carrying interchangeable 5-mm wide working instruments (e.g., grasping forceps and electrocautery). The two arms and endoscope are then controlled by the surgeon, who is sitting at a

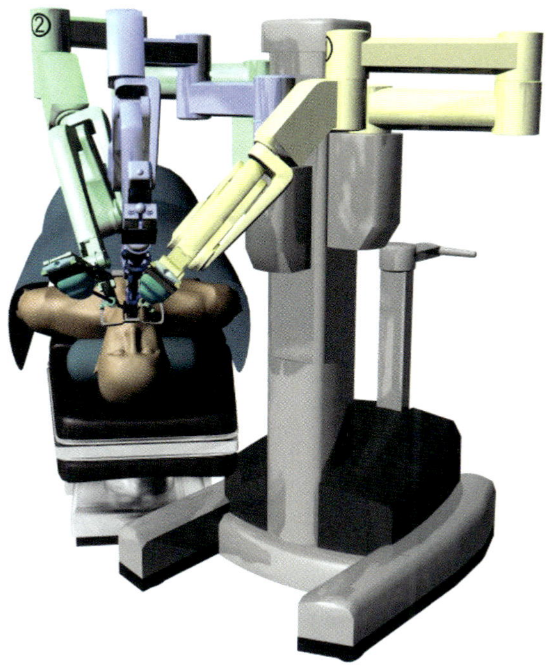

FIGURE 14.4 Positioning of the da Vinci system with mouth gag, trocars, and camera (diagrammatic). The camera is positioned centrally (blue arm). The working arms are positioned laterally at approximately 30 degrees (green and yellow arms).

remote console. The assistant sits at the head of the bed, and provides additional retraction and suction as necessary (see Figure 14.4 and 14.5). Recently, a novel robotic "snake" camera was approved by the FDA for transoral head and neck surgery in 2015. This monocular camera was combined with two-wristed, manual laparoscopic instruments and commercialized as the Medrobotics Flex Surgical System® (Raynham, MA). This system was specially designed to provide visualization and access for surgical procedures when nonlinear exposures and indirect insertion and use of surgical instruments are necessary in transoral surgery (38). Using either robotic system a complete resection of the oropharyngeal tumor can be achieved with negative oncologic margins.

Both TLM and TORS provide a highly magnified view of the tumor. This allows for confident resection of tumor margins, which are not often well visualized with standard open or transoral surgical techniques. The Flex Robot® is the only system that can work in patients with limited direct view of the tumor or cases in which trismus or cervical spine immobility may prevent exposure of the tumor (38). Numerous retrospective single-institution studies and a few retrospective multicenter trials have generated significant evidence in support of eHNS in the multidisciplinary treatment of OPSCC. However, prospective clinical evidence is limited.

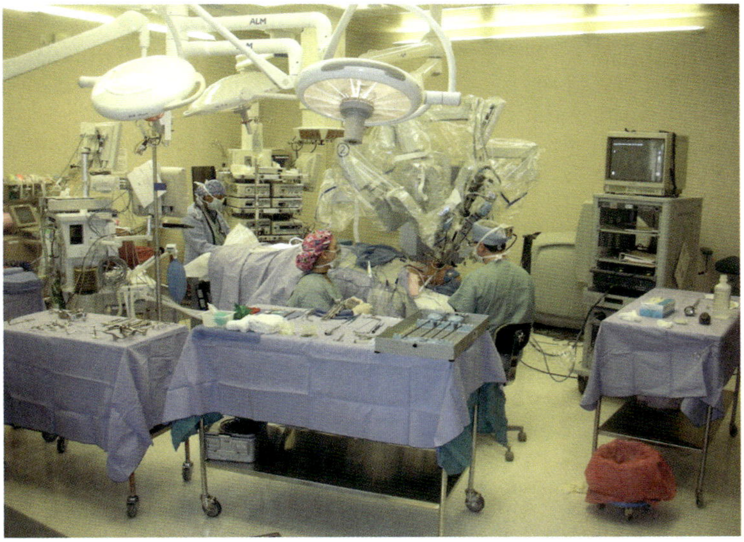

FIGURE 14.5 Intraoperative setup for da Vinci robot.

Compared with open surgery, eHNS is minimally invasive (33). Numerous publications demonstrate improved immediate postoperative outcomes including dysphagia scores, length of hospital stay, gastrostomy tube dependence, tracheostomy dependence, and recovery times (39–41). Advocates for surgery in the management of OPSCC (TLM or TORS) cite excellent functional results and argue that it may prevent the long-term toxicity that is sometimes associated with a primary radiation-based approach for OPSCC (18). Skeptics of surgical management of OPSCC cite the regular use of multimodality therapy and the possibility of close or positive margins.

SURGICAL TREATMENT OF HPV-NEGATIVE OPSCC

A relevant approach to the treatment of HPV-negative OPSCC would be to reinstitute surgery as the primary treatment modality and a form of treatment intensification. This would allow for pathologic staging, pathologic risk stratification using well-known adverse features, and identification of particular HPV-negative OPSCC using postoperative risk stratification to identify responders and appropriate trial candidates. There is little prospective literature examining the role of TORS in HPV-negative tumors within the multidisciplinary paradigm in the past 20 years, because of landmark organ-preservation therapy protocols that became the standard of care in the late 1990s and early 2000s. Recent understanding of the poor outcomes for HPV-negative cancer has led to a renewed interest in surgery as treatment intensification of HPV-negative OPSCC (10,19,42–45).

Kelly et al. recently studied the efficacy of upfront surgery versus definitive chemoradiotherapy for low-volume primary HPV-negative cT1-2 N1-2b patients with OPSCC. This was a retrospective study performed by a group at Yale University using cases logged in the National Cancer Data Base (NCDB); 1,044 cases were included. On multivariate analysis, upfront surgery was not associated with increased 4-year OS compared to concurrent chemoradiotherapy (CRT) (Hazard ratio [HR]: 1.01, 95% CI: 0.74–1.39, $p = .93$). Propensity score matching also showed equivalent OS between the two treatment methods, in spite of margin-negative resection (HR: 1.14, 95% CI: 0.81–1.62, $p = .46$) (43).

In another study using the NCDB, Kamran et al. examined the efficacy of primary surgery versus radiation only for the treatment of locally advanced OPSCC using the NCDB between 2004 and 2013. This group showed that HPV status and surgery with adjuvant treatment were predictive of outcome. In this study, which included 8,555 patients undergoing surgery with adjuvant treatment and 14,121 patients undergoing primary nonsurgical therapy, 3-year OS was significantly improved in the surgical treatment arm. On multivariate analysis, HPV-negative OPSCC had improved 3-year OS with surgery versus definitive CRT ($p = .0005$). Studies using the NCDB have significant limitations including the lack of HPV status in the NCDB until 2010, retrospective staging (meaning that surgical patients are often upstaged to stage III for small nodal metastases), lack of chemotherapy data (including type), and lack of information of surgical technique (including treatment of the primary and neck) (44). The NCDB, therefore, cannot be well applied to the study of efficacy of transoral (robotic or laser) surgery in the treatment of HPV-negative OPSCC or treatment intensification with definitive or adjuvant nonsurgical treatment.

Wagner et al. recently studied outcomes in surgically treated patients stratified by HPV status. This was a retrospective study by a German group on unselected OPSCC patients treated with curative intent between 2000 and 2009. Outcomes were stratified by HPV status. In this study, ECOG performance status was the most important factor affecting outcome in HPV-negative OPSCC. More importantly, surgical treatment led to improved 5-year OS in low- ($p = .002$), intermediate- ($p < .001$), and high-risk ($p = .035$) patients based primarily on unselected OPSCC treated with upfront surgery (10). Future trials on surgical management with similar patient population profiles (incidence of HPV-negative tumors and smoking) should consider risk stratification based on this schema. Wuerdemann et al. performed a very similar study and found that 5-year OS for HPV-negative patients was 39.7%. In this study, upfront surgery in HPV-negative patients resulted in significantly improved OS after 5 years; $p < .001$ (19).

Other recent studies using upfront surgery to stratify risk in OPSCC have examined prognostic factors that differ between HPV-negative and HPV-positive carcinoma. Meyer et al. recently looked at the relevance of lymph-node ratio (LNR), or the ratio of positive nodes to the total number of all resected lymph nodes, as a predictor of prognosis in OPSCC. They found that an LNR of 0.77 or greater was a significant predictor of worse OS in OPSCC regardless of

HPV status or presence of extracapsular spread. However, on multivariate analysis, LNR only remained predictive of OS and recurrence-free survival (RFS) in the HPV-negative population (p = .033 and p = .004, respectively) (46), which is reflected in the most recent staging guidelines for HPV-positive OPSCC.

SURGICAL SALVAGE FOR HPV-NEGATIVE OPSCC

Guo et al. examined salvage treatment for OPSCC in a retrospective analysis of patients treated at two institutions between 2000 and 2012. This was the first study to examine both surgical and nonsurgical salvage therapies for recurrent locoregional and distant metastatic OPSCC. Results were stratified by HPV status using p16 as a surrogate marker. This study found no difference in the distribution of recurrence (local, locoregional, or distant) between HPV-negative and HPV-positive tumors. The lung was the most common distant metastatic site regardless of HPV status. Recurrence was likely to occur in 89% (95% CI: 74.9–97.3) of HPV-negative patients within 2 years compared to 66.0% (95% CI: 55.4–76.3) of HPV-positive patients. HPV-negative patients had significantly worse 3-year OS after recurrence compared to HPV-positive patients (25.2% vs. 55.7%, $p < .001$). However, surgical salvage improved OS in HPV-negative patients as compared to nonsurgical treatment (p = .003) (47).

Outcomes of salvage surgery comparing TORS and open approaches for OPSCC have been studied by White et al. in 2013. This group conducted a retrospective, multi-institutional case–control study that matched 64 patients undergoing salvage TORS to 64 patients undergoing open salvage surgery between 2003 and 2011. This study found that patients undergoing TORS had significantly decreased incidence of positive margins, shorter overall hospital stays, decreased incidence of tracheostomy and feeding-tube use, and shorter operative times (48). Unfortunately, this study did not stratify by HPV status and patients with large-volume primary tumors were included in the open surgery arm. Given that HPV-negative cancers often have large-volume primaries and worse prognosis, no conclusions can be made about survival, because such patients are known to have worse outcomes and selection bias skews these results. However, given HPV-negative's poor response to nonsurgical protocols, TORS used in appropriately selected patients in the salvage setting can have favorable outcomes. Therefore, TORS should be considered as part of the salvage surgery treatment algorithm.

SURGICAL CLINICAL TRIALS FOR HPV-NEGATIVE OPSCC

Despite the recent surge in interest of transoral surgery as treatment intensification for HPV-negative OPSCC, there is no "level 1" evidence-based clinical data to support its use. Surgery, eHNS, represents a considerable advancement in surgical technique, similar to advancement in radiotherapy techniques between conventional three-dimensional radiation beam therapy versus intensity modulated radiation therapy. For this reason, surgical treatment of HPV-negative OPSCC warrants careful study going forward, including the impact of margins and the role of adjuvant therapies following TORS and TLM. Recently, Adelstein and Ridge hosted a National Cancer Institute (NCI) sponsored, R13-funded Clinical Trials Planning Meeting to discuss the role of transoral endoscopic surgery for the treatment of OPSCC (18). Since then, multiple surgical trials on HPV-positive OPSCC have been initiated. Few, however, on HPV-negative disease have been designed.

The RTOG 1221 trial was designed to test the efficacy of TORS for early T-stage, HPV-negative OPSCC. Though well-conceived and supported by multiple centers across the United States, the study was forced to close in February 2015 owing to failure to enroll any patients after 15 months. Participating surgeons noted that HPV-negative OPSCC patients often presented with advanced disease, which was not amenable to TORS (4,45). The efficacy of TORS for the treatment of HPV-negative disease remains an important question. However, the rarity of surgical candidates may mean that a large, retrospective, multi-institutional collaborative effort in the highest volume centers may be the only way to examine outcomes in this population.

The ORATOR trial, a phase II trial of patients with HPV-positive and -negative OPSCC, is under way comparing transoral surgery (TLM or TORS-based treatment) to definitive radiotherapy with or without chemotherapy for early-stage OPSCC. This is a single-institution, prospective trial in London, Ontario, that just completed its needed enrollment of 68 patients. Primary end points are 1-year quality-of-life outcomes at 1 year posttreatment, while secondary end points include 1-year and 5-year overall, PFS, toxicity, quality-of-life outcomes, and swallow outcomes posttreatment (49). This study will require more patients to make more meaningful conclusions for HPV-negative patients, which represent an increasing minority of OPSCC patients and will likely represent a very small percentage of enrolled patients based on the RTOG 1211 trial. Still, this will be one of the first prospective outcome studies using stratification by HPV status. The estimated completion date is June 2021.

MOLECULAR MARKERS AND NOVEL THERAPIES IN OPSCC

The different epidemiology, clinical behavior, and outcomes between the two types of OPSCC patients have led to interest in the differences in the molecular biology and oncologic pathogenesis between HPV-negative and HPV-positive tumors. A review by Dillon and Harrington provides a nice diagrammatic representation of the oncologic pathways in HPV-negative tumors (Figure 14.6). HPV-negative tumors have a higher mutational burden, multiple mutations affecting the *p53* tumor suppressor gene, as well as alterations in *EGFR*, *CCND1*, and *CDKN2A*. HPV-positive tumors are caused by viral proteins E6 and E7 that alter function of wild-type *p53* and *RB-1* and are associated with radiation sensitivity (50).

In 2015, The Cancer Genome Atlas (TCGA) performed a comprehensive multiplatform characterization of genomic alterations in 279 head and neck cancers. Thirty-three were oropharyngeal tumors. Only 5% of HPV-positive

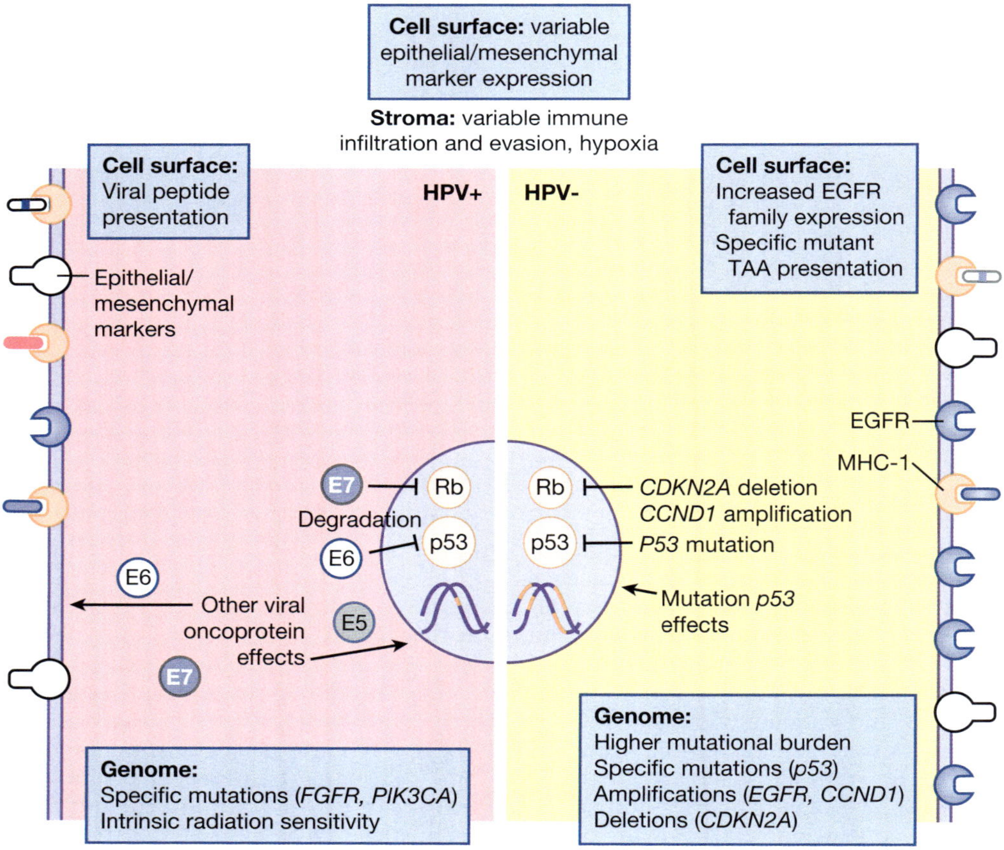

FIGURE 14.6 Mutational differences between HPV-negative and HPV-positive tumors. Diagrammatic representation based on Dillington and Harrington et al.

EGFR, epidermal growth factor receptor.

tumors were outside the oropharynx. Smoking-related, HPV-negative HNSCCs demonstrated near universal loss-of-function *TP53* mutations and *CDKN2A* inactivation. "Patients with HPV-positive and HPV-negative wild-type TP53 tumors had better outcomes compared to HPV-negative *TP53* mutant tumors and 11q13/CCND1-amplified tumors" (51). This study also found that the mutational burden is higher in HPV-negative tumors and in the smokers with HPV-positive tumors. This may explain the radioresistance of HPV-negative OPSCC and the poorer outcomes in intermediate-risk, HPV-positive OPSCC patients. Since then, groups have looked at outcomes based on specific molecular markers and targets. A study by Seiwert et al. examined HPV-negative tumors and found targetable genomic alterations in *FGFR1, DDR2, EGFR, FGFR2/3, EPHA2,* and *PIK3CA* (52). This supports the use of therapies targeting these receptors and pathways in future studies and trials.

With respect to epidermal growth factor receptor (EGFR), Nakano et al. found that expression is higher in HPV-negative cancers and lower in HPV-positive cancers in cell culture (53). This may have prognostic significance with respect to outcomes, particularly when treated with adjuvant cetuximab, a monoclonal antibody targeting EGFR. It has been shown to be beneficial in advanced/recurrent head and neck cancer patients, who are not candidates for cisplatin-based chemotherapy. However, in a study by Mehta et al., HPV-negative cancers had a better response following definitive therapy with radiation and adjuvant cetuximab therapy in terms of OS and PFS after 175 months of follow-up (28).

Ki67 is a marker of tumor proliferation and is an antigen expressed during the G1, S, and G2 phases of cell cycles. Ki67 positivity has been shown to be a marker of poorer prognosis of head and neck cancers of multiple subsites. With regard to pharyngeal tumors, a review of the literature showed conflicting results for Ki67 positivity as a marker of prognosis (OS and recurrence) (54). The first group to study the prognostic significance of this marker in oropharyngeal cancers as stratified by HPV status was Liu et al. In this study, HPV-negative tumors were more likely than HPV-positive tumors to be Ki67 negative (33% vs. 56%, respectively); $p = .015$. In multivariate analysis, Ki67-positive tumors had significantly increased risk of death (HR: 3.13, $p = .014$). In HPV-negative tumors, Ki67-positive tumors had a 5.6-fold increase in DSS and a 5.5-fold increase in OS compared with Ki67-negative tumors ($p = .002$ and .001, respectively; see Figure 14.7). Furthermore, HPV-negative/Ki67-positive patients had 33-fold higher risk of locoregional recurrence compared to HPV-positive/Ki67-positive patients (55).

Another multi-institutional group has looked at the immune checkpoint receptors on tumor-infiltrating lymphocytes (TILs) in HPV-positive and HPV-negative tumors. This study found that HPV-negative patients had TIL with high levels of expression of the immune checkpoint receptor, programmed death-1 receptor (PD-1), and CD8 positivity, which represents a more dysfunctional subset of TIL. These markers in head and neck cancers are associated with worse DFS and higher likelihood of recurrence. Kansy et al. also showed that higher expression of PD-1 and CD8 positivity in TIL may serve as a potential biomarker when selecting patients for anti-PD-1 based immunotherapy, such as nivolumab (56). In a groundbreaking clinical trial studying nivolumab for cisplatin resistant head and neck cancers, Ferris et al. performed a subset analysis of the effect on oropharyngeal tumors with p16 status and observed that tumors with PD-1 expression level of 1% or more or p16-positive tumors (or both) benefited from a greater treatment effect compared to standard therapy. A greater effect was also seen in HPV-negative tumors, but this was not significant (57).

Future studies that use biomarkers to select patients for therapy are needed. Furthermore, intensification/de-intensification of treatment with novel agents and immunotherapy should be specifically studied for OPSCC and examine efficacy as stratified by HPV status and marker positivity in oropharynx tumors. Given the dismal prognosis of the HPV-negative cohort, special consideration should be given to enrolling these patients in clinical trials and treatment at tertiary care facilities associated with cancer centers.

CONCLUSIONS

In recent years, considerable progress has been made in refining the treatment of OPSCC. However, the treatment of HPV-negative cancers needs considerable improvement. Surgical intensification with transoral surgery may play a role by providing more accurate staging and pathologic risk stratification that may help improve understanding the role of adjuvant therapies including radiation, chemotherapy,

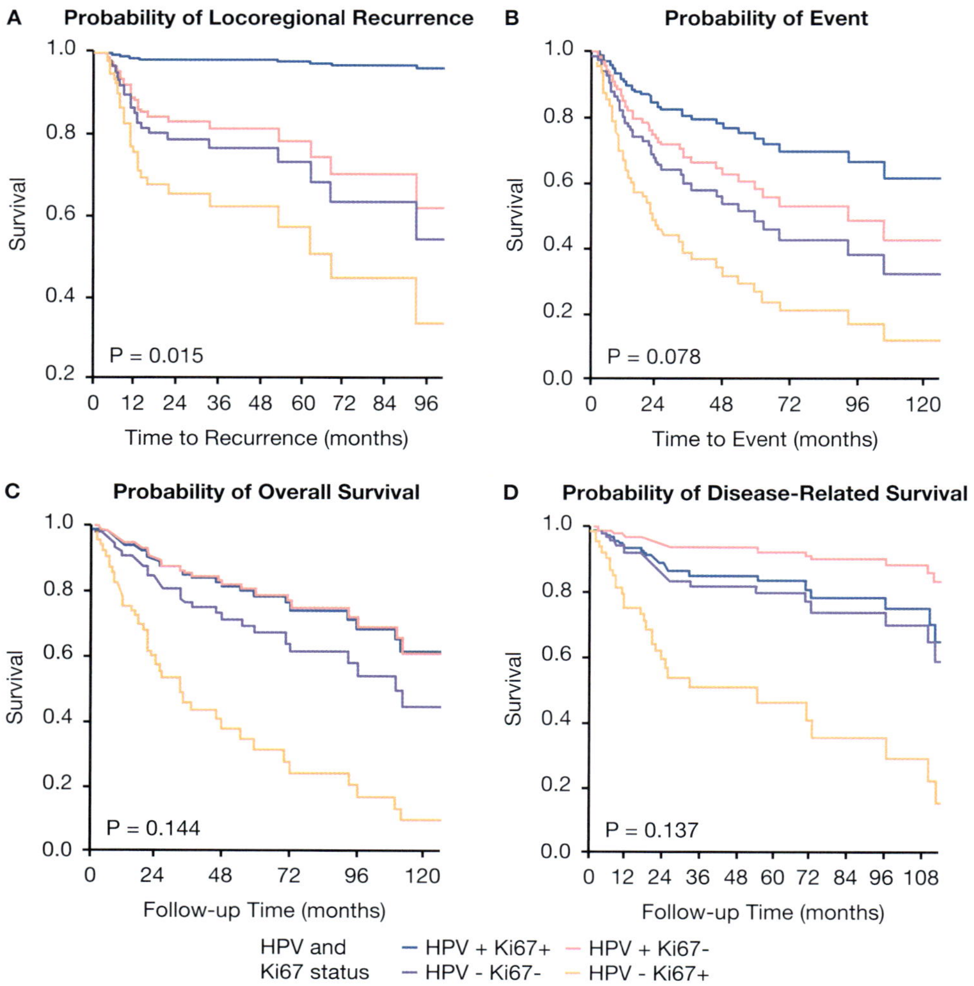

FIGURE 14.7 Results from Pich et al. Analyis of survival based on HPV status and Ki67 status. Ki67-positive tumors had increased survival compaired with Ki67-negative tumors.
HPV, human papillomavirus.

molecular therapy, and immunotherapy in the treatment of HPV-negative cancers. In the setting of salvage surgery for OPSCC, HPV-negative tumors are more likely to be large primary tumors requiring open approaches; however using a combined open and robotic approaches may play a role to improve surgical outcomes with regard to margin status, particularly regarding inferior and deep margins within the tongue base. Given the increasing rarity of HPV-negative OPSCC in the United States, its' grave prognosis, and the need for appropriate training in robotic surgery to ensure negative margins (58), HPV-negative OPSCC should be treated in high-volume centers, where access to cutting edge care is the standard (59).

In the future, we will be able to better evaluate the true clinical impact of these technical and scientific breakthroughs in terms of survival, quality-of-life, and functional outcomes in the treatment of HPV-negative OPSCC. Previous clinical trials on HPV-negative OPSCC have not been able to enroll enough patients. Given this reality, HPV-negative OPSCC may be best studied with nonrandomized, prospective, multi-institutional collaborative studies on HPV-negative disease. Future research focusing on HPV-negative OPSCC will be enlightening, because this is a unique disease with new treatment algorithms that include novel molecular and immunotherapy that have yet to be studied, and that may provide hope in the future (see Figure 14.8).

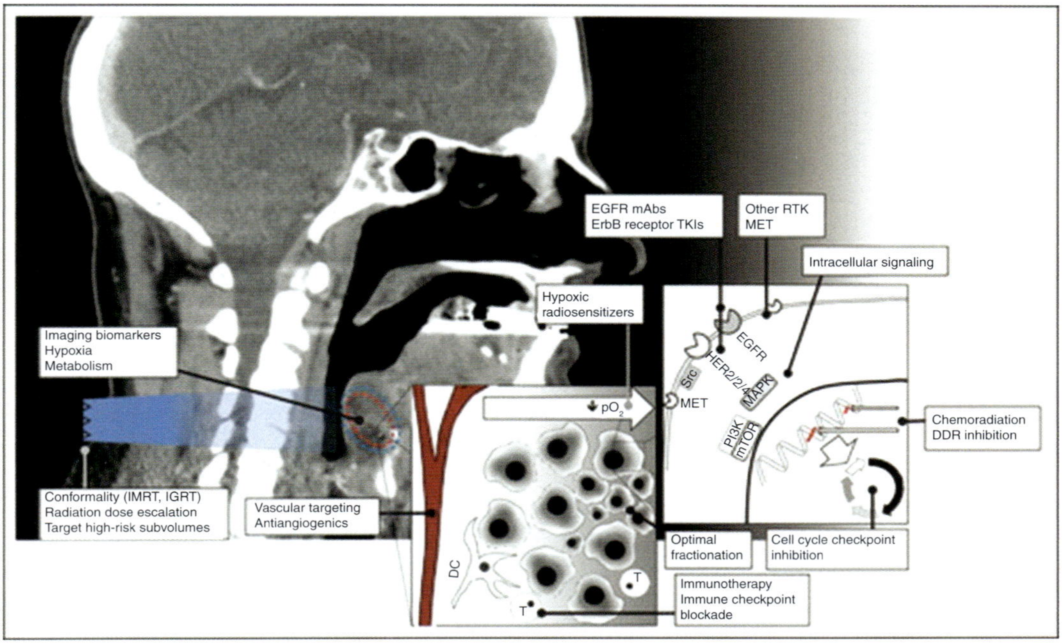

FIGURE 14.8 Diagrammatic representation of targets ammenable to novel treatments currently available for HPV-negative cancers.

CASE 14.1

A 52-year-old woman was referred for evaluation and treatment of a T2N0M0 HPV-negative (by p16 status) OPSCC originating from the left tonsillar fossa. She presented to her primary care physician following 2 weeks of dysphagia and left neck pain. Upon self-examination in the mirror, the patient noticed a "white spot" in the back of her throat. Her primary physician ordered a contrast-enhanced CT scan of her neck, which was radiographically negative for lymph node metastases. She was then referred to an otolaryngologist, who noted a left tonsillar fossa lesion with ulceration. Her local otolaryngologist referred her to a high-volume tertiary-care academic hospital for the treatment of head and neck cancer.

On initial presentation to our head and neck cancer center, flexible fiberoptic examination revealed a tonsillar mass with extension into the glossopharyngeal sulcus. There was no noted involvement of larynx or hypopharynx. An office-based biopsy was performed revealing a moderately differentiated keratinizing SCC on final pathologic analysis. A PET–CT scan was ordered and confirmed increased fluorodeoxyglucose (FDG) uptake in the left palatine tonsil. No pathologic cervical lymphatic nodules were identified. Further MRI of the lesion demonstrated asymmetric, enhancing soft tissue in the left lateral pharyngeal wall and tonsillar pillar (see Figure 14.9).

After case discussion at a multi-institutional tumor board treatment planning conference, surgical examination under anesthesia was recommended. Shortly thereafter, in the operating room, surgeons noted a 2.5-cm tumor centered in the left tonsillar fossa with minimal extension to the anterolateral tonsillar pillar and caudal soft palate. The uvula, ipsilateral hard palate, and intermaxillary mucosa were free of disease on examination. Careful palpation

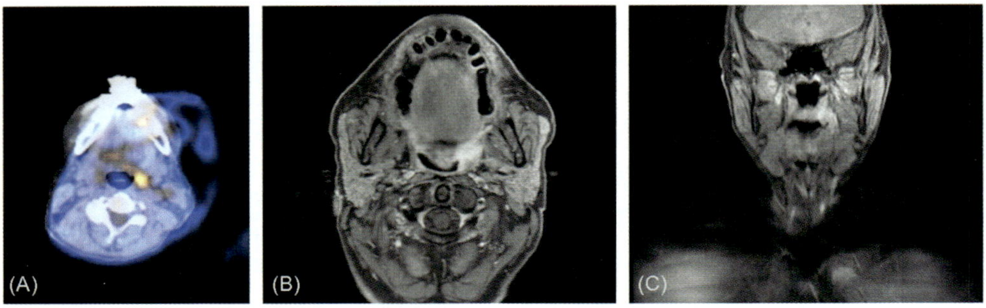

FIGURE 14.9 (A) PET/CT imaging demonstrating FDG avidity in the left lateral oropharyngeal wall. Corresponding axial (B) and coronal (C) MR imaging showing subtle extension onto the soft palate.

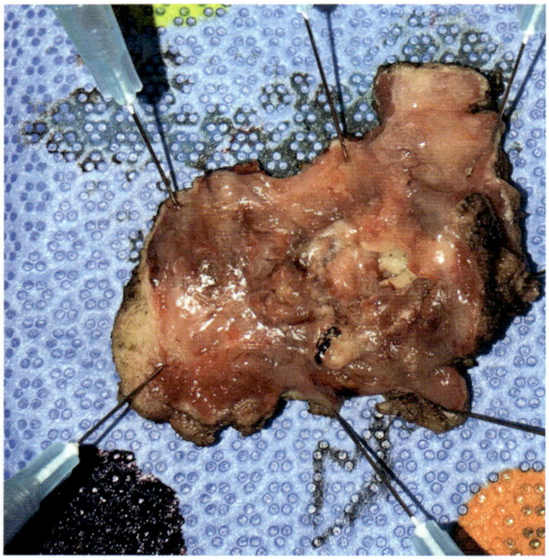

FIGURE 14.10 Final pathologic specimen after robotic oropharyngectomy.

revealed that the tumor moved relative to the underlying superior constrictor. Moreover, a tongue depressor could be placed lateral to the tumor and a plane between the mandible and tumor could be defined.

After examination under anesthesia, the patient's case was re-presented at the multidisciplinary head and neck cancer conference and could be described as having the following favorable features: size <4 cm, mobility of the mass relative to the constrictor, and the absence of metastatic adenopathy. The final recommendation for surgery included special consideration of the patient's age, comorbidity, performance status, need for therapeutic neck dissection, and the likelihood of adjuvant treatment modalities using primary surgical treatment. The potential for significant late side effects and poor quality-of-life outcomes for a 52-year-old treated with definitive radiation at a dose of 68 to 70 Gy for an HPV-negative tumor was also taken into consideration, as compared to these effects on a 65- to 70-year-old survivor.

Robotic-assisted transoral robotic oropharyngectomy (en bloc resection of the left lateral oropharynx from soft palate to tongue base) was performed using the da Vinci Surgical System. The specimen was sent for frozen section analysis to determine intraoperative margin status (see Figure 14.10). Four quadrant mucosal margins were negative for carcinoma. However, a small isolated focus of severe dysplasia was noted in the soft-palate margin, so an additional 1-cm margin of tissue was resected and was negative for severe dysplasia or carcinoma. Simultaneous neck dissection of levels II to IV was performed as well as intraoperative ligation of the lingual and facial arteries. The patient was discharged after routine postoperative hospital course and length of stay. The final pathologic analysis identified no additional cervical lymphadenopathy and no adverse pathologic features. These results were reviewed in the multidisciplinary tumor board and the decision was made to observe her without the addition of adjuvant treatment.

CASE 14.2

A 58-year-old woman was referred for evaluation of a T1N2bM0 p16-negative SCC of the left tongue base. Her initial symptom was a palpable lymph node in the left neck for 2 months, but she went on to also develop odynophagia, otalgia, and a 7- to 8-pound weight loss. PET–CT imaging at the time demonstrated FDG avidity in the left tongue base and in a single left neck level II, correlating with MRI findings of a left lateral tongue base tumor abutting the glossotonsillar sulcus.

She was evaluated by a multidisciplinary team including a head and neck surgeon, radiation oncologist, medical oncologist, and speech language pathologist. Transoral examination showed some subtle firmness in the left lateral tongue base near the glossotonsillar sulcus, but otherwise normal on inspection and palpation. On examination of her neck, multiple nodes were palpated in left neck level II. These were firm, nontender, and greater than 3 cm in size, but mobile. A small lesion of the left lateral tongue base and glossopharyngeal sulcus was apparent on fiberoptic examination.

The patient's case was discussed at the H&N multidisciplinary treatment planning conference, where the recommendation was made for definitive radiation with CRT with the possibility that she may require a neck dissection after completing CRT. Although the surgical team discussed the role of transoral endoscopic head and neck surgery, the majority of the tumor board felt that she should pursue a frontline approach with radiation and concurrent cisplatin chemotherapy. The rationale given for this treatment recommendation was that surgery would expose her to risk without clear benefit in terms of cancer outcome. Based on the interpretation of her MRI, the group felt that there was greater than 50% chance that after surgery she would require chemotherapy due to the potential for extracapsular extension in that single node. The patient completed definitive CRT and continued to receive regular tumor surveillance. Following treatment a baseline PET–CT showed a good metabolic response to treatment.

However, one year after she had finished CRT, surveillance PET–CT imaging showed increased activity in a 13-mm left upper neck node but no other disease elsewhere in the body. A modified radical neck dissection was performed with resection of the spinal accessory nerve (CN XI) and the superior aspect of the sternocleidomastoid muscle, which were directly involved with tumor.

Further surveillance imaging 9 months postoperatively (approximately 2 years postdiagnosis) demonstrated no evidence of local–regional recurrence, but the interval development of distant hepatic and pulmonary metastases. Despite additional systemic chemotherapy, she died from her disease 26 months after diagnosis at the age of 60.

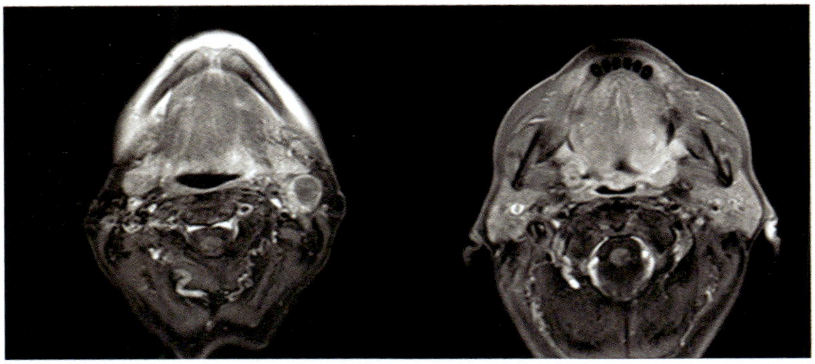

FIGURE 14.11 Postgadolinium IDEAL T1-weighted MR image demonstrating left lateral tongue base mass.

REFERENCES

1. Gillison ML, Koch WM, Capone RB, et al. Evidence for a causal association between human papillomavirus and a subset of head and neck cancers. *J Natl Cancer Inst.* 2000;92(9):709–720. doi:10.1093/jnci/92.9.709
2. Chaturvedi AK, Engels EA, Pfeiffer RM, et al. Human papillomavirus and rising oropharyngeal cancer incidence in the United States. *J Clin Oncol.* 2011;29(32):4294–4301.
3. Pytynia KB, Dahlstrom KR, Sturgis EM. Epidemiology of HPV-associated oropharyngeal cancer. *Oral Oncol.* 2014;50(5):380–386.
4. McIlwain WR, Sood AJ, Nguyen SA, Day TA. Initial symptoms in patients with HPV-positive and HPV-negative oropharyngeal cancer. *JAMA Otolaryngol Head Neck Surg.* 2014;140(5):441–447.
5. Slaughter DP, Southwick HW, Smejkal W. Field cancerization in oral stratified squamous epithelium; clinical implications of multicentric origin. *Cancer.* 1953;6(5):963–968.
6. Deschler DG, Richmon JD, Khariwala SS, et al. The "new" head and neck cancer patient-young, nonsmoker, nondrinker, and HPV positive: evaluation. *Otolaryngol Head Neck Surg.* 2014; 151(3):375–380.
7. El-Mofty SK, Patil S. Human papillomavirus (HPV)-related oropharyngeal nonkeratinizing squamous cell carcinoma: characterization of a distinct phenotype. *Oral Surg Oral Med Oral Pathol Oral Radiol Endod.* 2006;101(3):339–345.
8. Ang KK, Harris J, Wheeler R, et al. Human papillomavirus and survival of patients with oropharyngeal cancer. *N Engl J Med.* 2010;363(1):24–35.
9. Rietbergen MM, Witte BI, Velazquez ER, et al. Different prognostic models for different patient populations: validation of a new prognostic model for patients with oropharyngeal cancer in Western Europe. *Br J Cancer.* 2015;112(11):1733–1736.
10. Wagner S, Wittekindt C, Sharma SJ, et al. Human papillomavirus association is the most important predictor for surgically treated patients with oropharyngeal cancer. *Br J Cancer.* 2017;116(12):1604–1611.
11. Calais G, Alfonsi M, Bardet E, et al. Randomized trial of radiation therapy versus concomitant chemotherapy and radiation therapy for advanced-stage oropharynx carcinoma. *J Natl Cancer Inst.* 1999;91(24): 2081–2086.
12. Parsons JT, Mendenhall WM, Stringer SP, et al. Squamous cell carcinoma of the oropharynx: surgery, radiation therapy, or both. *Cancer.* 2002;94(11):2967–2980.
13. Fakhry C, Westra WH, Li S, et al. Improved survival of patients with human papillomavirus-positive head and neck squamous cell carcinoma in a prospective clinical trial. *J Natl Cancer Inst.* 2008;100(4):261–269.
14. Posner MR, Lorch JH, Goloubeva O, et al. Survival and human papillomavirus in oropharynx cancer in TAX 324: a subset analysis from an international phase III trial. *Ann Oncol.* 2011;22(5):1071–1077.
15. Rischin D, Young RJ, Fisher R, et al. Prognostic significance of $p^{16INK4A}$ and human papillomavirus in patients with oropharyngeal cancer treated on TROG 02.02 phase III trial. *J Clin Oncol.* 2010;28(27):4142–4148.
16. Rosenthal DI, Harari PM, Giralt J, et al. Association of human papillomavirus and p16 status with outcomes in the IMCL-9815 phase III registration trial for patients with locoregionally advanced oropharyngeal squamous cell carcinoma of the head and neck treated with radiotherapy with or without cetuximab. *J Clin Oncol.* 2016;34(12):1300–1308.
17. Ragin CC, Taioli E. Survival of squamous cell carcinoma of the head and neck in relation to human papillomavirus infection: review and meta-analysis. *Int J Cancer.* 2007;121(8):1813–1820.
18. Machtay M, Moughan J, Trotti A, et al. Factors associated with severe late toxicity after concurrent chemoradiation for locally advanced head and neck cancer: an RTOG analysis. *J Clin Oncol.* 2008;26(21):3582–3589.
19. Wuerdemann N, Wittekindt C, Sharma SJ, et al. Risk factors for overall survival outcome in surgically treated human papillomavirus-negative and positive patients with oropharyngeal cancer. *Oncol Res Treat.* 2017;40(6):320–327.
20. Wang H, Sun R, Lin H, Hu W. $P16^{INK4A}$ as a surrogate biomarker for human papillomavirus-associated oropharyngeal carcinoma: consideration of some aspects. *Cancer Sci.* 2013;104(12):1553–1559.
21. Ndiaye C, Mena M, Alemany L, et al. HPV DNA, E6/E7 mRNA, and $p16^{INK4a}$ detection in head and neck cancers: a systematic review and meta-analysis. *Lancet Oncol.* 2014;15(12):1319–1331.
22. Singhi AD, Westra WH. Comparison of human papillomavirus in situ hybridization and p16 immunohistochemistry in the detection of human papillomavirus-associated head and neck cancer based on a prospective clinical experience. *Cancer.* 2010;116(9):2166–2173.
23. Katabi N, Lewis JS. Update from the 4th edition of the World Health Organization classification of head and neck tumours: what is new in the 2017 WHO blue book for tumors and tumor-like lesions of the neck and lymph nodes. *Head Neck Pathol.* 2017;11(1):48–54.
24. Lewis JS, Jr., Chernock RD. Human papillomavirus and epstein barr virus in head and neck carcinomas: suggestions for the new WHO classification. *Head Neck Pathol.* 2014;8(1):50–58.
25. Lassen P, Lacas B, Pignon JP, et al. Prognostic impact of HPV-associated p16-expression and smoking status on outcomes following radiotherapy for oropharyngeal cancer: the MARCH-HPV project. *Radiother Oncol.* 2017.
26. Lassen P, Eriksen JG, Krogdahl A, et al. The influence of HPV-associated p16-expression on accelerated fractionated radiotherapy in head and neck cancer: evaluation of the randomised DAHANCA 6&7 trial. *Radiother Oncol.* 2011;100(1):49–55.
27. Hall SF, Liu F-F, O'Sullivan B, et al. Did the addition of concurrent chemotherapy to conventional radiotherapy improve survival for patients with HPV+ve and HPV-ve oropharynx cancer? A population-based study. *Br J Cancer.* 2017;117(8):1105–1112.

28. Mehta V, Moore-Medlin T, Flores JM, et al. Survival outcomes based on systemic agent used concurrently with radiation in human-papillomavirus associated oropharyngeal cancer. *Oncotarget.* 2017;8(41):70907–70915.
29. Felice DEF, Abate G, Galdieri A, et al. Impact of induction chemotherapy in locally advanced HPV-negative oropharyngeal cancer. A propensity score-matched analysis. *Anticancer Res.* 2016;36(12):6667–6672.
30. Stanley RB. Mandibular lingual releasing approach to oral and oropharyngeal carcinomas. *Laryngoscope.* 1984;94(5, Pt 1):596–600.
31. Zeitels SM, Vaughan CW, Ruh S. Suprahyoid pharyngotomy for oropharynx cancer including the tongue base. *Arch Otolaryngol Head Neck Surg.* 1991;117(7):757–760.
32. Christopoulos E, Carrau R, Segas J, et al. Transmandibular approaches to the oral cavity and oropharynx. A functional assessment. *Arch Otolaryngol Head Neck Surg.* 1992;118(11):1164–1167.
33. Holsinger FC, Ferris RL. Transoral endoscopic head and neck surgery and its role within the multidisciplinary treatment paradigm of oropharynx cancer: robotics, lasers, and clinical trials. *J Clin Oncol.* 2015;33(29):3285–3292.
34. Canis M, Martin A, Kron M, et al. Results of transoral laser microsurgery in 102 patients with squamous cell carcinoma of the tonsil. *Eur Arch Otorhinolaryngol.* 2013;270(8):2299–2306.
35. Canis M, Ihler F, Wolff HA, et al. Oncologic and functional results after transoral laser microsurgery of tongue base carcinoma. *Eur Arch Otorhinolaryngol.* 2013;270(3):1075–1083.
36. Rich JT, Milov S, Lewis JS, Jr., et al. Transoral laser microsurgery (TLM) +/– adjuvant therapy for advanced stage oropharyngeal cancer: outcomes and prognostic factors. *Laryngoscope.* 2009;119(9):1709–1719.
37. Haughey BH, Hinni ML, Salassa JR, et al. Transoral laser microsurgery as primary treatment for advanced-stage oropharyngeal cancer: a United States multicenter study. *Head Neck.* 2011;33(12):1683–1694.
38. Mandapathil M, Duvvuri U, Guldner C, et al. Transoral surgery for oropharyngeal tumors using the Medrobotics((R)) Flex((R)) System—a case report. *Int J Surg Case Rep.* 2015;10:173–175.
39. Weinstein GS, O'Malley BW, Jr., Cohen MA, Quon H. Transoral robotic surgery for advanced oropharyngeal carcinoma. *Arch Otolaryngol Head Neck Surg.* 2010;136(11):1079–1085.
40. Hurtuk AM, Marcinow A, Agrawal A, et al. Quality-of-life outcomes in transoral robotic surgery. *Otolaryngol Head Neck Surg.* 2012;146(1):68–73.
41. Moore EJ, Olsen SM, Laborde RR, et al. Long-term functional and oncologic results of transoral robotic surgery for oropharyngeal squamous cell carcinoma. *Mayo Clin Proc.* 2012;87(3):219–225.
42. Howard J, Masterson L, Dwivedi RC, et al. Minimally invasive surgery versus radiotherapy/chemoradiotherapy for small-volume primary oropharyngeal carcinoma. *Cochrane Database Syst Rev.* 2016;12: CD010963.
43. Kelly JR, Park HS, An Y, et al. Comparison of survival outcomes among human papillomavirus-negative cT1-2 N1-2b patients with oropharyngeal squamous cell cancer treated with upfront surgery vs definitive chemoradiation therapy: an observational study. *JAMA Oncol.* 2017;3(8):1107–1111.
44. Kamran SC, Qureshi MM, Jalisi S, et al. Primary surgery-versus primary radiation-based treatment for locally advanced oropharyngeal cancer. *Laryngoscope.* 2017. doi:10.1002/laryn.26903
45. Sload R, Silver N, Jawad BA, Gross ND. The role of transoral robotic surgery in the management of HPV negative oropharyngeal squamous cell carcinoma. *Curr Oncol Rep.* 2016;18(9):53.
46. Meyer MF, Meinrath J, Seehawer J, et al. The relevance of the lymph node ratio as predictor of prognosis is higher in HPV-negative than in HPV-positive oropharyngeal squamous cell carcinoma. *Clin Otolaryngol.* 2018;43(1):192–198.
47. Guo T, Qualliotine JR, Ha PK, et al. Surgical salvage improves overall survival for patients with HPV-positive and HPV-negative recurrent locoregional and distant metastatic oropharyngeal cancer. *Cancer.* 2015;121(12):1977–1984.
48. White H, Ford S, Bush B, et al. Salvage surgery for recurrent cancers of the oropharynx: comparing TORS with standard open surgical approaches. *JAMA Otolaryngol Head Neck Surg.* 2013;139(8):773–778.
49. Nichols AC, Yoo J, Hammond JA, et al. Early-stage squamous cell carcinoma of the oropharynx: radiotherapy vs. trans-oral robotic surgery (ORATOR)--study protocol for a randomized phase II trial. *BMC Cancer.* 2013;13:133.
50. Dillon MT, Harrington KJ. Human papillomavirus–negative pharyngeal cancer. *J Clin Oncol.* 2015;33(29):3251–3261.
51. Cancer Genome Atlas Network. Comprehensive genomic characterization of head and neck squamous cell carcinomas. *Nature.* 2015;517(7536):576–582.
52. Seiwert TY, Zuo Z, Keck MK, et al. Integrative and comparative genomic analysis of HPV-positive and HPV-negative head and neck squamous cell carcinomas. *Clin Cancer Res.* 2015;21(3):632–641.
53. Nakano T, Yamamoto H, Nakashima T, et al. Molecular subclassification determined by human papillomavirus and epidermal growth factor receptor status is associated with the prognosis of oropharyngeal squamous cell carcinoma. *Hum Pathol.* 2016;50:51–61.
54. Pich A, Chiusa L, Navone R. Prognostic relevance of cell proliferation in head and neck tumors. *Ann Oncol.* 2004;15(9):1319–1329.
55. Liu J, Zhang M, Rose B, et al. Ki67 expression has prognostic significance in relation to human papillomavirus status in oropharyngeal squamous cell carcinoma. *Ann Surg Oncol.* 2015;22(6):1893–1900.
56. Kansy BA, Concha-Benavente F, Srivastava RM, et al. PD-1 status in $CD8^+$ T cells associates with survival and anti-PD-1 therapeutic outcomes in head and neck cancer. *Cancer Res.* 2017.

57. Ferris RL, Blumenschein G, Jr., Fayette J, et al. Nivolumab for recurrent squamous-cell carcinoma of the head and neck. *N Engl J Med.* 2016;375(19):1856–1867.
58. Cracchiolo JR, Baxi SS, Morris LG, et al. Increase in primary surgical treatment of T1 and T2 oropharyngeal squamous cell carcinoma and rates of adverse pathologic features: National Cancer Data Base. *Cancer.* 2016;122(10):1523–1532.
59. Boero IJ, Paravati AJ, Xu B, et al. Importance of radiation oncologist experience among patients with head-and-neck cancer treated with intensity-modulated radiation therapy. *J Clin Oncol.* 2016;34(7): 684–690.
60. Hockstein NG, O'Malley BW, Jr., Weinstein GS. Assessment of intraoperative safety in transoral robotic surgery. *Laryngoscope.* 2006;116(2):165–168.

15

Oral Cavity Cancer: Surgical Approaches and Postoperative Treatment

Antoine Eskander

Jacques Bernier

Lisa Licitra

Paolo Bossi

Theodoros N. Teknos

Oral cavity cancer (OCC) is the 10th most common cause of cancer in the United States (1). However, the incidence is much higher in other parts of the world including Melanesia, South–Central Asia, and Central and Eastern Europe (2). The incidence of oral cavity cancer is strongly linked to the use of tobacco products and alcohol. Smoking and alcohol behave as synergistic risk factors in the development of OCC (3). The most common (>90%) pathologic cancer diagnosis in the oral cavity is squamous cell carcinoma (SCC), which is the focus of this chapter.

Cancers of the oral cavity have a detrimental impact on function including speech, swallowing, and sometimes airway and persistent reduction of quality of life after completion of treatment (4). The primary management of OCC is surgery, which, depending on the stage of the disease, can be followed with adjuvant radiotherapy with or without chemotherapy. A multidisciplinary approach is warranted in the management of OCC. A collaborative effort between the head and neck surgical oncologist, the radiation oncologist, the medical oncologist, dietitian, speech language pathologist, dentist, and other healthcare specialists is necessary to achieve optimal survival, functional, and cosmetic outcomes. Although the primary goal of treatment is to eradicate the disease providing the highest chance of cure, functional and cosmetic implications are also very important. Advances in reconstructive techniques have allowed for improvements in function and quality of life for patients with OCC.

EPIDEMIOLOGY

Oral cavity cancer is the 8th most common male cancer and the 10th most common cancer in the United States with an estimated 45,780 new cases and 8,650 deaths in 2015 (5). However, the rates are higher in the developing world (6), with the highest rates in Melanesia, South–Central Asia, Central and Eastern Europe (Figures 15.1 and 15.2) (2,7). Despite a relatively low incidence compared to other cancers, OCC continues to be associated with poor outcomes, and survival has not improved over the years with relatively high mortality rates compared to other cancers (8). Large variations exist in the survival rate of OCC patients

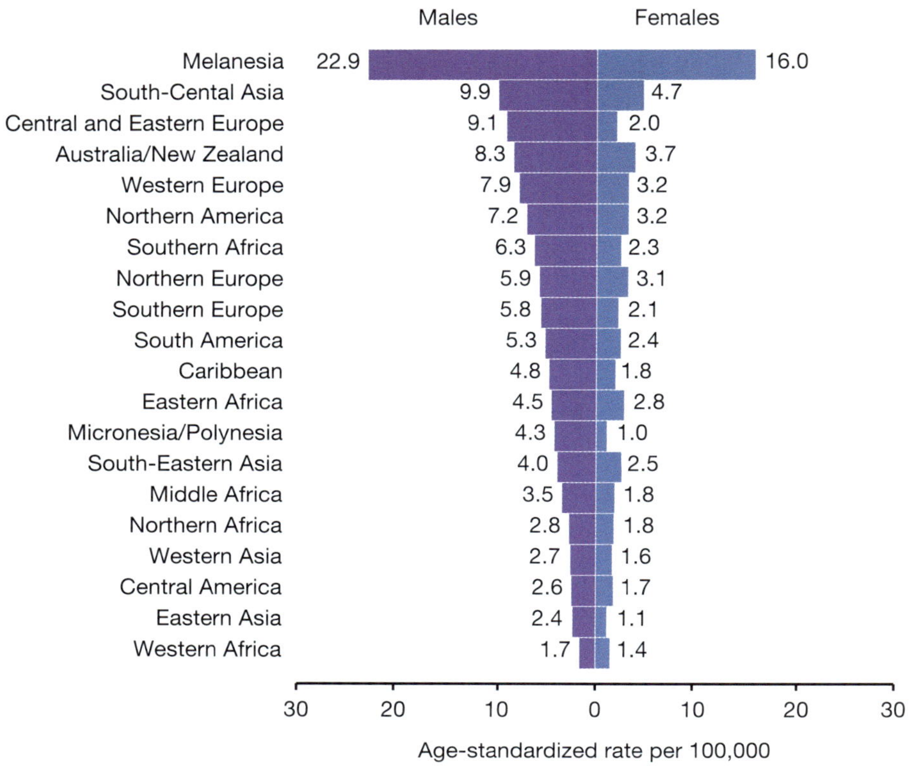

FIGURE 15.1 Variations in OCC incidence rates among men and women around the world.
OCC, oral cavity cancer.
Source: From Torre LA, Bray F, Siegel RL, et al. Global cancer statistics, 2012. *CA Cancer J Clin.* 2015;65(2):87–108.

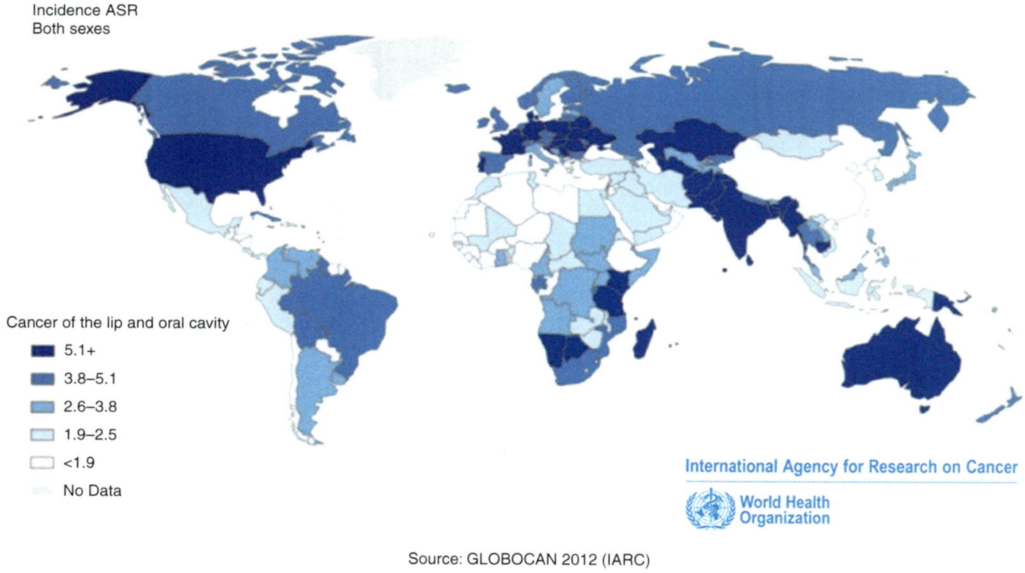

FIGURE 15.2 Worldwide OCC incidence map.
OCC, oral cavity cancer.
Source: From GLOBOCAN 2012: estimated cancer incidence, mortality and prevalence worldwide in 2012 [Internet]. Lyon, France: World Health Organization; 2013 [updated December 12, 2013; cited November 16, 2016]. http://globocan.iarc.fr.

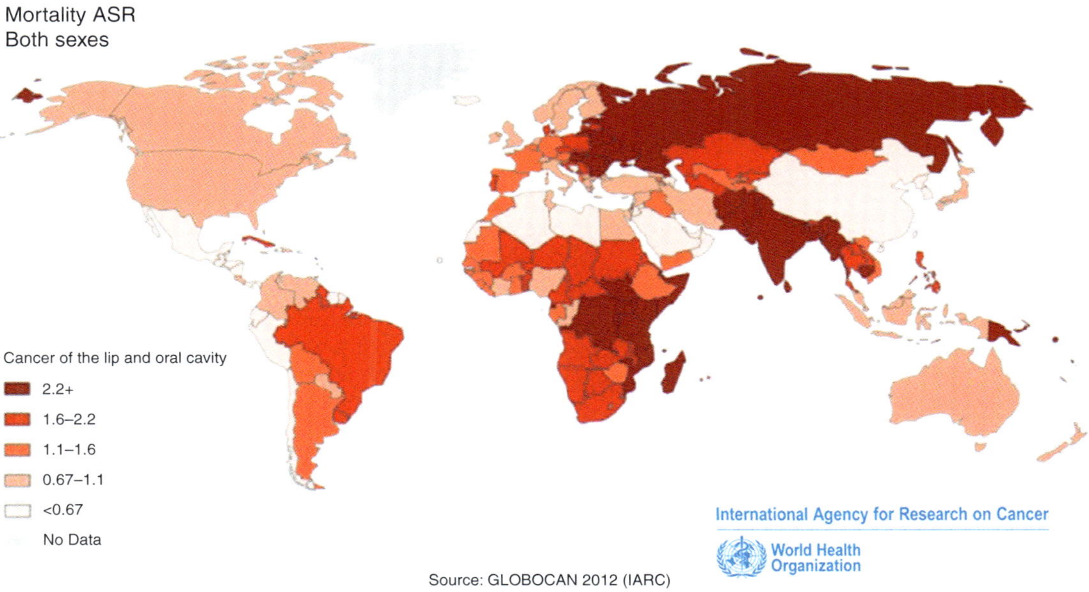

FIGURE 15.3 Worldwide OCC mortality map.
OCC, oral cavity cancer.
Source: From GLOBOCAN 2012: estimated cancer incidence, mortality and prevalence worldwide in 2012 [Internet]. Lyon, France: World Health Organization; 2013 [updated December 12, 2013; cited November 16, 2016]. http://globocan.iarc.fr.

depending on the country in which they are diagnosed (Figure 15.3), with countries in the developing world having both a higher incidence rate and a lower survival rate compared to the developed world (7). OCC also has a higher incidence rate in men, in older adults, in those with lower socioeconomic status, and in those who live in more rural communities (9).

ETIOLOGY

SMOKING AND ALCOHOL

The main etiologic factors associated with OCC are tobacco products, specifically smoking, and alcohol. Cigarette smoking triples the likelihood of developing OCC, while the addition of alcohol synergistically increases the likelihood by 10- to 15-fold (10). There has been an overall decline in incidence at this head and neck cancer site (11), likely related to public health campaigns and government taxation policies, as it relates to cigarette consumption (12). The variation in incidence between countries is also related to large differences in cigarette smoking. Despite an overall decline in incidence in the United States, a rise in incidence in young patients (age <45) who are nonsmokers of unknown etiology has been noted (13–15). Some have postulated that this may be, similar to oropharyngeal cancers, related to human papillomavirus (HPV); however, on molecular analysis, OCC is almost never HPV related (16). In North America, HPV incidence in OCC is less than 3% while in the Asian continent it has been reported as high as 19% and is associated with worse survival outcomes (17). Further study is required to understand the molecular and genetic basis for OCC in patients without known risk factors.

SMOKELESS TOBACCO PRODUCTS AND BETEL NUT

Other important etiologic factors exist and impact the worldwide incidence of OCC. Smokeless tobacco products (e.g., chewing tobacco) are strongly associated with OCC and have a higher propensity for oral cavity subsites with direct contact to these products (e.g., buccal mucosa) as well as subsites with dependent saliva drainage (e.g., floor of mouth, mandibular alveolus, and wet lip). Betel nut/quid chewing is endemic to some parts of Asia and India and in these parts of the world OCC is one of the most common cancers (18,19). Betel nut chewing is also associated with submucous fibrosis, which adds an additional challenge in the management of patients who present with a concurrent OCC (19).

OTHER ETIOLOGIC FACTORS

Marijuana

Marijuana is becoming increasingly common in North America and Europe with many districts decriminalizing this activity. There is a strong correlation between marijuana smoking and head and neck cancer (odds ratio, comparing ever users with never users, 2.6; 95% confidence interval [CI]: 1.1–6.6), including a dose–response relationship, with both relationships being stronger in patients who were 55 years of age and younger (20).

Diet

As with many other cancers, a diet high in red meats and salted meats (21) and low in fruits and vegetables is associated with a slightly increased risk of OCC (22). Although these associations exist, they are far weaker than the association between smoking and alcohol. Furthermore, these relationships are often confounded by socioeconomic status.

Chronic Irritation and Oral Hygiene

The International Head and Neck Cancer Epidemiology (INHANCE) consortium assessed the impact of oral hygiene on the incidence of OCC (23). Specifically, better oral hygiene quantified by <5 missing teeth, annual dentist visits, daily toothbrushing, no gum disease, and wearing dentures was assessed after pooling 17 case–control studies (23). Denture use was not associated with OCC. The remaining four factors were independent statistically significant inverse predictors of OCC. The attributable fraction for ≤2 out of 5 good oral hygiene indicators was 8.9% (95% CI: 3%–14%) for OCC (23). Therefore, poor oral hygiene is associated with a higher risk of OCC.

IMMUNOSUPPRESSION

Patients who are immunosuppressed are at an increased risk of cancer, and head and neck cancer is no different. Solid organ and bone marrow transplant patients are at increased risk of cutaneous malignancy and OCC (24). Patients with OCC with a past medical history of solid organ transplantation have poor treatment outcomes with high locoregional recurrence rates (24). Patients with HIV infection with or without AIDS have a higher rate of head and neck cancer with poorer results compared to patients who are HIV negative (25,26).

Genetic Conditions

Patients with certain genetic conditions are at a higher risk of developing OCC, specifically, dyskeratosis congenita (27,28), Bloom's syndrome (14,29), and Fanconi anemia (30). It is important to question the patient regarding these conditions, particularly in the absence of known risk factors for developing OCC.

Premalignant Lesions

A number of oral cavity premalignant lesions have been identified and are associated with potential transformation to OCC. This presents a subset of pathological features that can be identified early, which may lead to superior results. Such lesions are often identified by the primary care provider, dental hygienist, or dentist and may require biopsy to refute the diagnosis of cancer. This is often followed by close observation, given the risk of malignant transformation. The most important of these lesions are leukoplakia and erythroplakia, but these can also include oral lichen planus, oral submucous fibrosis, discoid lupus erythematosus, and ulceration secondary to reverse cigarette smoking. Oral lichen planus has a lifetime malignant transformation rate of approximately 1% (31). Patients who develop OCC arising from lichen planus appear to have better survival rates (97% 2-year disease-free survival), likely due to early detection of malignant transformation (32).

Leukoplakia is defined as a white patch or plaque that does not have any other clinical or pathologic diagnosis. It is therefore a diagnosis of exclusion. Given that these lesions have a 1% annual risk of malignant transformation, we recommend a biopsy to rule out malignancy followed by an excision with very narrow margins (33). The biopsy and excision are also helpful in determining whether dysplasia is present, which increases the likelihood of malignant transformation (34). Risk factors for malignant transformation include large lesions, erythroleukoplakia, or heterogeneous lesions, along the tongue or floor of mouth (35). Although female gender and nonsmoking status used to be considered risk factors, pooled analysis did not reveal these to be significant (35). When these lesions are multifocal, excision sometimes cannot be performed.

In these cases, smoking cessation and avoidance of betel nut can significantly decrease the malignant transformation rate and patients are often closely observed (36).

Erythroplakia is defined as a red patch or plaque that does not have any other clinical or pathologic diagnosis. These lesions have a higher propensity for dysplasia and carcinoma in situ than leukoplakia and therefore an excisional biopsy with wide margins (1 cm) is recommended.

Patients with submucous fibrosis have a 2% to 8% chance of malignant transformation to OCC SCC (37). This is usually secondary from chewing betel nut, which is a seed of a type of palm tree called the *Areca catechu*. Betel quid is a product of the *Areca* seed in which after being ground up it is wrapped in leaves from the same tree and coated with lime. It is the fourth most popular psychoactive substance in the world after nicotine, alcohol, and caffeine. It is commonly used in the Asian continent.

ANATOMY

SUBSITES AND BORDERS

The oral cavity is divided into multiple subsites including the (a) mucosal lip, (b) mandibular alveolus, (c) floor of mouth, (d) tongue (anterior two thirds), (e) buccal mucosa, (f) retromolar trigone, (g) maxillary alveolus, and (h) hard palate (Figure 15.4). Despite similarities in pathology, treatment, and survival, these subsites have some unique oncologic properties such as propensity for and levels of regional metastases. Here we discuss the borders, vascular supply, lymphatic drainage, and important characteristics of each subsite as it relates to the management of OCC.

The vermilion border defines the anterior limit of the oral cavity. The posterior border of the oral cavity is defined by the hard palate soft – palate junction superiorly and the circumvallate papillae on the tongue inferiorly. Laterally the junction between the retromolar trigone and the anterior tonsillar pillar defines the posterolateral junction of the oral cavity. Posterior to these borders is the oropharynx with important functional implications when tumors of the oral cavity extend to the oropharynx and require a partial oropharyngectomy for clear surgical margins.

LIP

The mucosal lip (or wet lip) is bordered externally by the vermilion border and internally by the opposed lips beyond which is the buccal mucosa before reaching the maxillary and mandibular gingiva. The vascular supply is from the superior and inferior labial arteries, which are branches of the facial artery and form a circular arcade. The upper lip is supplied by cranial nerve (CN) V2 (maxillary branch) whereas the lower lip is supplied by N V3 (mandibular

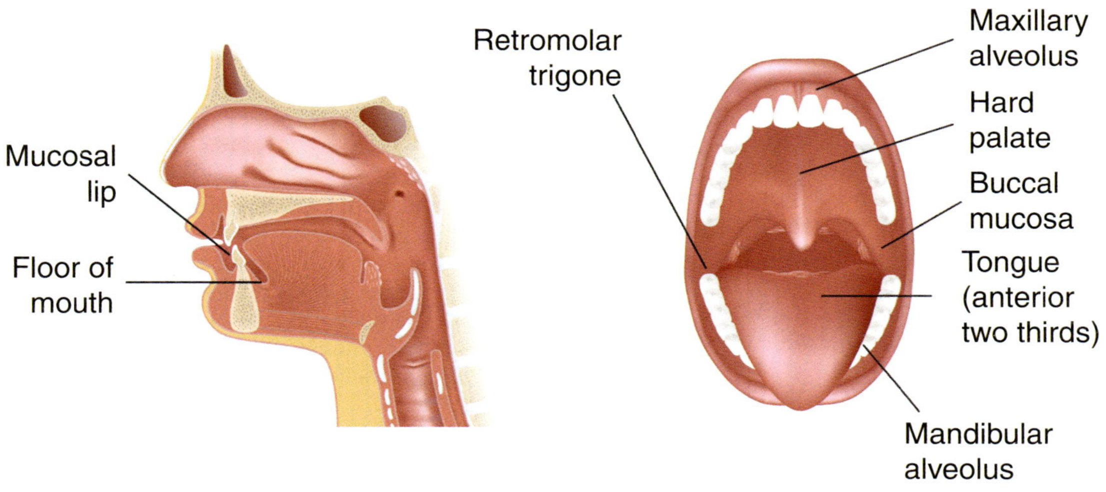

FIGURE 15.4 Oral cavity anatomic subsites.
Source: Alila Medical Media/Shutterstock.

branch) and the inferior alveolar nerve as it becomes the mental nerve. The lymphatic drainage is primarily to the submental (level IA) and submandibular triangle (level IB) followed by the upper cervical nodes (II), which ultimately drain into the middle cervical nodes (III).

MANDIBULAR ALVEOLUS

The mandibular alveolus is located posterior to the wet lip and extends to the floor of mouth posteriorly. Laterally it is bound by the buccal mucosa and posteriorly ends at the second/third molar, which is the anterior border of the retromolar trigone subsite. The neurovascular supply for the mandible is the inferior alveolus artery and nerve (branch of V3) until it exits from the mental foramen to become the mental nerve. Lymphatic drainage of this subsite is similar to the adjacent lip subsite with primary drainage to the submental (level IA) and submandibular triangles (IB) followed by level II/III.

FLOOR OF MOUTH

The floor of mouth begins just below the lingual surface of the mandibular alveolus and ends at the ventral tongue where the frenulum connects the floor of mouth to the tongue. Just deep to the floor of mouth mucosa is the submandibular (Wharton's) duct and sublingual minor salivary glands followed by the mylohyoid muscle and finally the hyoglossus muscle. The lingual nerve (a branch of V3) provides sensory innervation to this subsite. The lymphatic drainage of this subsite is rich and starts at the adjacent level IB but can also extend to levels IA, II, and III.

TONGUE (ANTERIOR TWO THIRDS)

The anterior two thirds of the tongue is bordered by the circumvallate papillae posteriorly and the floor of mouth anteriorly and can be divided into a ventral component adjacent to the floor of mouth and a dorsal component, which makes contact with the hard palate. The tongue is composed of intrinsic muscles (longitudinal, vertical, and transverse muscle fibers) and extrinsic muscles (genioglossus, hyoglossus, styloglossus, and palatoglossus). The motor innervation to all of these muscles is through the hypoglossal nerve (CN XII) except for the palatoglossus, which is innervated by the vagus nerve (CN X). Somatosensory innervation of this subsite is from the lingual nerve while special sensory (taste) function is provided by the chorda tympani (branch of CN VII), which runs with the lingual nerve. The arterial supply of the tongue is through the lingual artery, a branch of the external carotid artery, and the venous supply is through the vein, which drains directly into the internal jugular vein. The primary lymphatic drainage basin for the tongue is the submandibular triangle (level IB) followed by the submental triangle (level IA), particularly for cancers of the tip of the tongue. Skip metastases to levels II and III are not uncommon; however, there is relatively rare extension to levels IV and V (38,39). Contralateral drainage is not uncommon particularly for tumors that abut the midline raphe of the tongue. The oral tongue has significant implications for speech (articulation) and swallowing including the oral preparatory and oral phases of swallowing. The tongue needs to be able to protrude 0.8 cm or more after resection and reconstruction for better swallowing results (40). Premaxillary contact is also important for speech and articulation.

BUCCAL MUCOSA

The buccal mucosa is bounded anteriorly by the junction of the upper and lower wet lips opposing each other and posteriorly/laterally by the maxillary and mandibular gingiva. The buccal mucosa contains the parotid (Stensen's) duct opening adjacent to the first/second maxillary molar. The layers of the cheek from medial to lateral are (a) buccal mucosa, (b) pharyngobasilar fascia, (c) buccinator muscle, (d) buccopharyngeal fascia, (e) buccinator fat pad, (f) masseter muscle, (g) muscles of facial expression and the superficial muscular aponeurotic system (SMAS), (h) subcutaneous tissue, and (i) facial skin. These layers are important in that they are very closely adherent, and therefore, cancers of the buccal mucosa have a propensity for deep invasion and early lymphatic spread. It is not uncommon for advanced cancers at this subsite to require a resection to the skin/subcutaneous tissue to achieve a clear margin. The lymphatic drainage is to the submandibular triangle (level IB) but depending on the depth of invasion of the tumor can also spread to perifacial nodes (41). From these levels it then spreads to levels II and III. The neurovascular supply to this subsite is through branches of the facial artery, facial vein, and branches of CN V3.

HARD PALATE AND MAXILLARY ALVEOLUS

Although these have classically been considered two separate subsites, because of their anatomic contiguity and the similarities in their oncologic outcomes they are often discussed together (42). The posterior border of this subsite is the hard palate–soft palate junction. The posterolateral border is the maxillary tuberosity, which separates the retromolar trigone from the maxillary alveolus. The mucosa at this subsite is strongly adherent to the periosteum, and as such, even with the most superficial of lesions, a resection of the bone is required to achieve a clear margin. The neurovascular supply is from the greater palatine artery (a branch of the internal maxillary artery, which runs in the pterygopalatine canal) and branches from V2, namely the nasopalatine nerves through the incisive foramen anteriorly and the greater palatine nerves posteriorly. This subsite typically drains to level II followed by levels IB, III, and IV.

RETROMOLAR TRIGONE

The retromolar trigone (RMT) is bordered laterally by the buccal mucosa, medially by the anterior tonsillar pillar, anteriorly by the second or third molar, posteriorly by the maxillary tuberosity, inferiorly by the posterior mandibular alveolus, and superiorly by the coronoid process of the mandible. To achieve a negative margin at this subsite, even if there is no radiologic evidence of mandibular cortical invasion, a marginal shave mandibulectomy is often required. To do so, through a transoral approach, requires that the lips and cheek be carefully retracted to avoid injury to these subsites. It is also common for tumors at this subsite to extend to its borders including the maxillary tuberosity, buccal mucosa, floor of mouth, and posterolateral ventral tongue. The vascular and lymphatic drainage of this subsite is the same as that for the mandibular alveolus and buccal mucosa.

RISK FACTORS BY SUBSITE

Different subsites also have a different propensity for different etiologic risk factors. Cancers of the buccal mucosa are strongly associated with betel nut and tobacco chewing. The dependent portions of the oral cavity, namely the floor of mouth and the lingual surface of the mandibular alveolus, are associated with smoking carcinogens from pooling of saliva. The hard palate is associated with cancers related to reverse smoking.

The most commonly performed OCC surgery was a tongue resection (48.5%), followed in frequency by floor of mouth resection (15.3%), buccal resection (6.8%), mandibular alveolus resection (3.4%), and lip resection (1.2%). Mandibular resection was performed in 18.7% of the cohort and maxilla resection in 5.5%. With increasing age, patients were more likely to have a maxilla or mandibular alveolus resection and less likely to have a tongue resection.

PATHOLOGY

Table 15.1 lists the histologic classification of tumors of the oral cavity. The vast majority of tumors (>90%) are epithelial SCCs, which are the focus of this chapter. However, a brief discussion of the nonepithelial (<10%) tumors is warranted given the unique subsite distribution and treatment/outcome implications (43).

EPITHELIAL TUMORS

Epithelial tumors are the most common tumor type in the oral cavity, with classical SCC being the most common subtype (>90%). SCC is invasive with nests, sheets, or strands of squamous cells seen in the submucosa. Keratin pearls in the submucosa are diagnostic but their absence does not rule out this pathology. The degree of differentiation—well, moderately, and poorly differentiated—is based on the relative absence of normal tissue replaced by invasive tumor.

Of the subtypes two need to be discussed for their unique outcomes. The spindle cell variant of SCC is notoriously hard to treat with a higher propensity for regional and distant metastases, and worse prognosis secondary to a high mitotic rate and poorly differentiated histologic appearance (44,45). Verrucous carcinoma is on the opposite end of the spectrum. These cancers are typically exophytic, present early, and have excellent cure rates (46). This correlates well with their histologic appearance, which is typically well differentiated with low mitotic rates, and pushing borders along the lamina propria with invaginations without true invasion. There is a strong association (>50%) with human papillomavirus in this oral cavity pathology (47). It is however not clear whether this is an HPV-driven cancer despite a number of high-risk HPV subtypes identified in oral verrucous carcinoma including HPV-16 and -18 but also HPV-19, -24, and -36 (48,49). Verrucous carcinomas rarely if ever metastasize to the regional basis, and a local resection alone is often all that is needed to achieve high cure rates (46).

TABLE 15.1

Histologic Classification of Tumors of the Oral Cavity

Epithelial Tumors

SCC
  SCC, conventional
  Acantholytic SCC
  Adenosquamous carcinoma
  Basaloid SCC
  Papillary SCC
  Spindle cell SCC
  Verrucous carcinoma

Giant cell carcinoma
Lymphoepithelial carcinoma (non-nasopharyngeal)
Nonepithelial Tumors

Carcinomas of minor salivary glands
  Acinic cell carcinoma
  Adenoid cystic carcinoma (low, intermediate, or high grade)
  Adenocarcinoma, not otherwise specified (low, intermediate, or high grade)
  Basal cell adenocarcinoma
  Carcinoma ex pleomorphic adenoma (malignant mixed tumor; low grade, high grade, invasive, or noninvasive/ intracapsular)
  Carcinoma, type cannot be determined
  Carcinosarcoma
  Clear cell adenocarcinoma
  Cystadenocarcinoma
  Epithelial–myoepithelial carcinoma
  Mucoepidermoid carcinoma (low, intermediate, or high grade)
  Mucinous adenocarcinoma (colloid carcinoma)
  Myoepithelial carcinoma (malignant myoepithelioma)
  Oncocytic carcinoma
  Polymorphous low-grade adenocarcinoma
  Salivary duct carcinoma

Adenocarcinoma, nonsalivary gland type   Adenocarcinoma, not otherwise specified (low, intermediate, or high grade)

Neuroendocrine carcinoma
  Typical carcinoid tumor (well-differentiated neuroendocrine carcinoma)
  Atypical carcinoid tumor (moderately differentiated neuroendocrine carcinoma)
  Large cell carcinoma, neuroendocrine type (poorly differentiated neuroendocrine carcinoma)
  Small cell carcinoma, neuroendocrine type (poorly differentiated neuroendocrine carcinoma)
  Combined (or composite) small cell carcinoma, neuroendocrine type

Mucosal Malignant Melanoma
Secondary or Metastatic Tumors

SCC, squamous cell carcinoma.

Source: Adapted from the College of American Pathologists Cancer Protocol Templates. Protocol for the Examination of Specimens From Patients With Carcinomas of the Lip and Oral Cavity [Internet]. Washington, DC: College of American Pathologists; 2013 [updated October 1, 2013; cited November 16, 2017]. http://www.cap.org/ShowProperty?nodePath=/UCMCon/Contribution%20Folders/WebContent/pdf/liporalcaversion-13protocol.pdf.

NONEPITHELIAL TUMORS

It is uncommon (<10%) for nonepithelial malignant tumors to present in the oral cavity (Table 15.1). These are most commonly minor salivary gland cancers presenting in the sublingual space or on the hard palate. Salivary gland tumors in this region are more likely to be malignant (>80%) compared to the major salivary gland tumors (submandibular and parotid gland) (50). The vast majority of these are adenoid cystic and mucoepidermoid carcinomas (>85%) and present with an advanced stage (III/IV) (50,51). Local excision continues to be the recommended primary approach while adjuvant radiotherapy is associated with improved survival particularly in patients with advanced local or regional disease, adenoid cystic histology, and high-grade tumors (52).

EVALUATION

HISTORY AND PHYSICAL EXAMINATION

The evaluation of a patient with a suspected or confirmed OCC SCC begins with a thorough history and physical examination. History should assess onset of symptoms, progression, and pain. Otalgia is common. Changes in speech (articulation), swallowing (odynophagia), and tongue mobility may indicate extrinsic tongue muscle invasion or involvement of the hypoglossal nerve, both of which are signs of advanced disease. Trismus can indicate pterygoid and masticator space invasion. Poorly fitting dentures or loose teeth may indicate a mandibular or maxillary alveolar ridge invasion. Patients may complain of tongue or facial skin numbness along the V3 distribution indicating invasion of the lingual or inferior alveolar nerve.

It is very important to assess and treat pain in patients with OCC, as this is often their chief presenting symptom and impacts their ability to continue tolerating oral intake. Higher pain scores are associated with perineural invasion (PNI) and advanced stage disease (53). Rarely, patients will complain of difficulty breathing, particularly when lying down if they present with a bulky tumor in the posterior oral cavity extending to the oropharynx.

The history should also include past medical history, medications, and review of systems. Many patients with oral cavity cancer are heavy smokers, and alcoholism is not uncommon in this group. Furthermore, patients are more likely to be of lower socioeconomic status and may not have access to good primary care (9). Therefore, they may have a number of undiagnosed cardiopulmonary, renal, and hepatic diseases, which may require intervention and optimization prior to management of their cancer. These problems can often be picked up on a brief review of systems at initial assessment.

A thorough head and neck examination is critical in assessing the stage of disease and can impact surgical approach. A full cranial nerve examination is warranted in all patients with head and neck cancer. Inspection and palpation of the oral cavity is important. Palpation provides information regarding depth of invasion and can inform posterior extent of the tumor toward the base of tongue or tonsillar fossa. Tumors can be endo- or exophytic, usually start as a granular friable growth, which then results in necrosis. Halitosis is common. Trigeminal (V2 and V3 distributions), facial (marginal mandibular and buccal branches), accessory, and hypoglossal nerve examination is important. "Field cancerization" postulates that the same carcinogens that have caused a cancer at one upper aerodigestive tract site have likely started similar epigenetic and genetic alterations at adjacent sites (54). It is therefore important to examine the entire upper aerodigestive tract to rule out any synchronous second primary tumors using fiberoptic nasolaryngoscopy. In-office, transnasal esophagoscopy has increased in popularity and can also be used to examine the esophageal mucosa in a clinic setting. Finally, a thorough neck examination can provide information about metastatic disease to the regional basin.

INVESTIGATIONS

Locoregional

If a biopsy has not been performed, this is the first step in confirming the diagnosis. This can usually be performed in the clinic after appropriate local anesthetic administration. Staging is of the utmost importance. A CT scan of the head and neck with intravenous contrast agent is the best initial investigation because it is fast, cheap, and tolerated by most patients. CT scan is useful in determining the extent of the tumor and is the best imaging modality for assessing bony invasion. It is also more sensitive and specific than physical examination in assessing cervical lymphadenopathy. However, the key images used to assess tumor extent can be obscured by dental artifact. In such cases, MRI can be employed as it provides better soft tissue delineation and is a more reliable way of assessing for PNI. In some head and neck oncologists' practice, all oral tongue cancers are imaged with an MRI prior to resection to assess for submucosal and posterior extent of the mass, which is not well assessed on CT scan.

Increasingly, PET with CT fusion (PET–CT) is being used to assess the locoregional extent of the tumor and to assess for distant metastases and second primary cancers. There are no randomized trials comparing CT alone versus PET–CT in the preoperative assessment of patients with OCC. PET scan alone does not provide additional information at the primary site, whereas it is twice as likely as CT or MRI to identify occult regional disease in the clinically node negative setting (55,56). However, PET–CT is generally not recommended in the preoperative assessment of patients with OCC as it has not been shown to change the management plan yet.

Neck imaging can also provide information regarding lymphatic extracapsular extension (ECE), which is a key and important prognostic factor impacting treatment. Unfortunately, this is not accurately diagnosed on contrast enhanced neck CT by expert neuroradiologists, making surgery the primary and best method of diagnosing ECE (57).

Distant Metastatic Workup

One added benefit of PET–CT scanning is that it provides whole body imaging and can pick up distant metastases, although this is fraught with a very high false positive rate and has thus not been recommended by the National Comprehensive Cancer Network (NCCN) guidelines for this reason (58). There is no difference between CT chest and PET–CT in the ability to identify intrathoracic metastases (59). Chest imaging is however recommended (58). This can be in the form of a chest x-ray in patients with small localized disease and a clinically negative neck; however, we recommend a CT scan with contrast for all patients. Among all head and neck cancer patients, the detection rate of lung metastasis or synchronous lung primary tumors by CT is 11% with a higher rate noted in patients with large primary tumors or multiple lymph nodes (60). In OCC, the discovery rate of thoracic lesions is however lower than that found in hypopharyngeal, supraglottic, and oropharyngeal cancer (60).

STAGING

Staging OCC is based on the American Joint Committee on Cancer (AJCC) staging system, which assesses the primary tumor extent (T), nodal metastases (N), and distant metastasis (M), also known as the TNM system (Table 15.2) (61). The overall stage is then based on the different combinations of the T, N, and M categories in this classification system.The AJCC staging manual's eighth edition, updated in 2016, did not make significant changes to the OCC chapter (62).

Mandibular and maxillary alveolus tumors originating from the gingiva that are immediately adjacent to a tooth socket or bone are not considered T4a with superficial erosion of the bone. As it relates to bony invasion, a T4a tumor has to invade through cortical bone into the medullary space. Floor of mouth and hard palate tumors have a propensity toward cortical invasion given the thin mucosa and proximity to bone. Last, midline nodes in the submental triangle are considered ipsilateral nodes as this triangle is not divided into right and left sides.

MANAGEMENT

MULTIDISCIPLINARY CARE

Speech Language Therapists and Dietitians

The evaluation and management of head and neck cancer patients require the collaboration and care of a large multidisciplinary team. At the time of initial consultation, and throughout treatment, the NCCN guidelines recommend assessment by a registered dietitian and speech language pathologist because patients with head and neck cancers often present with weight loss and poor nutritional habits. Furthermore, weight loss during treatment is independently associated with deterioration in quality of life (63).

Dentistry

Dental evaluation is also warranted for many patients who have ongoing periodontal disease and dental conditions, which may need to be addressed preoperatively. Intra- and perioperatively, collaboration with dentists can be helpful in the reconstruction and rehabilitation of patients who require obturators and dental implants including osseointegrated implants.

TABLE 15.2

AJCC TNM Staging System for Oral Cavity Cancer

<table>
<tr><th colspan="2">T/M \ N</th><th>cN0</th><th>cN1</th><th>cN2a</th><th>cN2b</th><th>cN2c</th><th>cN3a</th><th>cN3b</th></tr>
<tr><td>T1</td><td>• ≤2 cm
• DOI ≤5 mm</td><td>I</td><td rowspan="2">III</td><td colspan="4" rowspan="5">IVA</td><td rowspan="5"></td></tr>
<tr><td>T2</td><td>• ≤2cm and DOI (5.1–10 mm)
• 2.1–4 cm and DOI ≤10 mm</td><td>II</td></tr>
<tr><td>T3</td><td>• >4 cm
• DOI >10 mm but ≤20 mm</td><td colspan="2"></td></tr>
<tr><td>T4a lip</td><td>• Invasion[1]</td><td colspan="2"></td></tr>
<tr><td>T4a oral cavity</td><td>• Invasion[2] or DOI >20 mm</td><td colspan="2"></td></tr>
<tr><td>T4b oral cavity</td><td>• Invasion[3]</td><td colspan="7">IVB</td></tr>
<tr><td>M1</td><td>• Distant metastasis</td><td colspan="7">IVC</td></tr>
</table>

*Major changes compared to seventh edition include use of depth of invasion, removal of deep intrinsic tongue muscle invasion as T4 (included in DOI), introduction of pN classification and use of ENE in nodal classification.

Notes: Invasion[1], invasion into cortical bone or involves inferior alveolar nerve, floor of mouth, or skin of face; Invasion[2], invasion through cortical bone or mandible/maxilla, into maxillary sinus, or skin of face; Invasion[3], invasion into masticator space, pterygoid plates, or skull base, and/or encases internal carotid artery.

AJCC, American Joint Committee on Cancer; cN1, single ipsilateral LN (≤3 cm) and -ENE; cN2a, single ipsilateral LN (3.1–6 cm) and –ENE; cN2b, multiple ipsilateral LN (≤6 cm) and –ENE; cN2c, bilateral or contralateral LN (≤6 cm) and –ENE; cN3a, LN (>6 cm) and –ENE; cN3b, clinically overt ENE; DOI, depth of invasion; pN1, single LN (≤3 cm) and –ENE; pN2a, single ipsilateral or contralateral LN (≤3 cm) and +ENE or single ipsilateral LN (3.1–6 cm) and – ENE; pN2b, multiple ipsilateral LN (≤6 cm) and – ENE; pN2c, bilateral or contralateral LN (≤6 cm) and –ENE; pN3a, LN (>6 cm) and –ENE; pN3b, LN (>3 cm) and + ENE; TNM, tumor, node, and metastasis.

Source: Adapted from Amin EB, Edge S, Greene F, et al., eds. *AJCC Cancer Staging Manual.* 8th ed. New York, NY: Springer; 2017.

Certainly, postoperatively in those patients whom radiotherapy is recommended, dental evaluation is critical in preventing treatment complications.

Smoking Cessation Program

The preoperative and perioperative periods are ideally situated for smoking cessation intervention. Patients who continue to smoke after treatment are at a three- to fourfold increased risk of developing a recurrent or second primary tumor (64–66). Smoking can also worsen the side effect profile of treatment and lead to poor treatment adherence and hence reduced efficacy (67). A study by Chan et al. looked at patients diagnosed with head and neck cancers, and showed that of the patients who were smoking at diagnosis, only 54% were able to quit (68). This suggests that smoking cessation is particularly difficult in this subpopulation. A number of studies have shown that disease extent, location, and heavy alcohol use are predictors of continued smoking (69–71). A nursing-led intensive smoking cessation program can be integrated into the treatment algorithm for patients with head and neck cancer. However, successful cessation rates have not been higher than the standard of care, which involves discussion at the point of care regarding the risks of continued smoking and the benefits of cessation (72). Smoking cessation programs are expensive for head and neck oncology programs, and to date, there have not been any randomized trials comparing an intensive program with the standard of care.

Volume-Outcome Associations and Process Measures

Strong evidence suggests that patients treated by high case volume surgeons, radiation oncologists, and centers have superior survival outcomes compared to those treated by lower volume physicians and centers (73). This may be because higher volume centers follow NCCN guideline process measures at a higher rate (74). Higher adherence to these process measures, providing higher quality care, has been strongly associated with improved survival outcomes (75). Both the Graboyes and Eskander et al. studies examining process-related quality metrics identified multidisciplinary consultation with radiation and medical oncology to be important quality metrics (74,75). This is often performed through an organized tumor board with surgical oncology, medical oncology, and radiation oncology present to discuss cases. In addition, some cancer centers have simultaneous clinics where the patient is assessed by both radiation and surgical oncology simultaneously before treatment recommendations are made.

MANAGEMENT OVERVIEW

The management of oral cavity cancer is primarily surgical with adjuvant radiotherapy or chemoradiotherapy based on select pathologic factors. As with most head and neck cancers, early-stage disease (I/II) can be treated with unimodality whereas advanced-stage disease (III/IV) requires multimodality treatment. Although surgery provides the best chance of cure and is recommended by the NCCN guidelines (58), it may not be possible in all patients because the risk of surgery may be prohibitively high in certain populations. Also, patients with incurable disease (T4b or M1) are often not surgical candidates.

SURGICAL MANAGEMENT OF THE PRIMARY SITE

Approaches to the Oral Cavity

Regardless of the approach, achieving negative surgical margins is of the utmost importance for optimal survival outcomes (76). Intraoperative tumor cut through, producing positive frozen section margins, which are revised to negative frozen section margins, adversely affects cancer control and survival rates in patients with OCC, but this effect is minimal in patients with no regional disease (77,78). Regardless of the surgical approach, the surgical oncologist should feel comfortable removing the tumor on-bloc. An excellent meta-analysis demonstrated that a minimum margin on final pathological examination of 5 mm is required to achieve optimal disease-free and overall survival results in OCC (79).

Most of the surgical decision making regarding approach can be made during clinic physical examination. In some cases, patients' trismus can be overcome in the operating room after administration of muscle relaxing agents. In our practice, most oral cavity cancers can be excised ***transorally*** even when there is minimal extension to the oropharynx.

A ***visor flap*** can be used to achieve improved access, especially in those with microstomia. Here, a midneck incision is made and then carried above the mandibular periosteum with anterior and lateral releasing intraoral mucosal incisions along the gingivobuccal sulcus. This allows the neck and lower lip skin to be retracted superiorly toward the upper lip, bypassing the lips and overcoming poor visualization due to limited mouth opening.

A ***lingual release*** approach can also be used to improve access. With this approach the lingual surface of the floor of mouth mucosa and musculature attached to the mandible is incised and connected to bilateral neck dissections allowing the contents of the oral cavity to be dropped into the neck. This allows for improved access to the posterior oral tongue when it extends to the oropharynx.

A ***lower cheek flap*** and ***mandibulotomy*** have similar incisions where the lip is split extending into the submental region and ultimately connecting to the neck skin incision. In the lower cheek flap this is then carried into the gingivobuccal sulcus on one side while raising the cheek skin off of the mandible over the periosteum. With this approach the mental nerve on the ipsilateral side is often sacrificed for access. With a mandibulotomy approach, the mental nerve does not need to be sacrificed. Here the lip is split, with minimal elevation of the mandibular periosteum to allow for preplating with mandibular reconstruction plates prior to dividing the mandible. This is followed by floor of mouth incisions allowing the mandible to swing toward the ipsilateral side and providing excellent visualization of the OCC. An excellent matched study compared the lip-split mandibulotomy approach to the transoral approach and found no difference in aesthetic appearance as judged by the patients, and no differences in lower-lip sensation or movement, nor were there any differences in oral continence as assessed by videofluoroscopic swallowing studies (80). Complication rates between median and paramedian mandibulotomy are the same. However, a paramedian mandibulotomy (between lateral incisor and canine) is favored because it allows for preservation of the geniohyoid and genioglossus muscles, and is therefore associated with better functional outcomes (81,82). There is more room between teeth for a paramedian mandibulotomy as opposed to a midline mandibulotomy; however, the paramedian approach is associated with a slightly increased rate of plate complications (83). Following radiotherapy, there is increased incidence of nonunion, malunion, hardware exposure, and osteoradionecrosis of the mandible after mandibulotomy regardless of where the mandibulotomy is placed (83).

Midface resection as might be required for hard palate and maxillary alveolus cancers are often approached through a ***Caldwell–Luc*** upper gingivobuccal sulcus incision. This is often adequate for an infrastructure maxillectomy. However, if the disease extends cephalad toward the orbital floor or laterally toward the lateral maxilla and the zygoma, as can occur in advanced cancers, an extended incision is required. This is often through a ***lateral rhinotomy*** incision along the upper lip through the vermilion border, then along the filtrum of the lip, extending along the nasal base at the nare then along the nasofacial groove. This incision can be extended in an infraorbital crease 4 to 6 mm below the lower lid, which in combination with the lateral rhinotomy and lip split is called a ***Weber–Ferguson*** incision.

For bilateral tumors or tumors that are slightly more cephalad than can be approached with a Caldwell–Luc incision alone but not extending to the orbital floor and therefore not requiring a lateral rhinotomy and Weber–Ferguson incision, a ***midfacial degloving*** approach can be used. This approach involves bilateral Caldwell–Luc incisions. These incisions are ultimately connected at the pyriform aperture through intranasal incisions, which include a full transfixion incision connected to bilateral intercartilaginous incisions and bilateral nasal vestibular floor incisions. This allows the upper lip and nasal skin to be completed elevated off of the nasal dorsum up to the infraorbital nerves bilaterally after significant periosteal and perichondrial dissection over nasal and maxillary bones.

Segmental Versus Marginal Mandibulectomy

No single imaging modality is consistent in capturing early mandibular cortical invasion, although the CT scan is the standard of care. Nonetheless, physical examination and intraoperative judgment often drive the final decision regarding mandibular invasion.

OCC, specifically of the gingivobuccal region, floor of mouth, and ventral tongue, has a propensity for mandibular invasion. This initially begins with mucosal and submucosal spread. The periosteum is a robust barrier from the mandibular cortical bone; however, with advanced tumors invasion does occur. The process by which OCC invades the mandible is well established and depends on the dental status of the patient. In edentulous patients, mandibular invasion is increased owing to a thinner and weaker periosteum. After periosteal invasion, dental pores of the alveolar process are the entry point into the bone (84,85). In dentate patients, cancer cells invade through the tooth socket into cortical bone (84,85).

Mandibular invasion is a negative prognostic factor and is associated with advanced T stage (T4a). It can, however, in some patients with minimal invasion, be managed with a marginal mandibulectomy. The combination of appropriate preoperative imaging and good clinical intraoperative judgement helps with this decision. When there is uncertainty but the tumor is thought to be superficial, intraoperative assessment involves exposing the mandible by raising the periosteum adjacent to the tumor and assessing the periosteal–cortical bone junction. With a marginal mandibulectomy, often used in cases of superficial or questionable invasion, a small portion of bone is removed with the specimen, without having to perform a segmental resection. This approach has been demonstrated to be equivalent to segmental mandibulectomy in oncologic outcomes in small tumors with periosteal invasion (86).

However, this is not always possible in advanced tumors. Imaging can help identify some factors that may require a segmental mandibulectomy: (a) through and through mandibular invasion, (b) mental nerve or foramen invasion, and (c) medullary space and inferior alveolar nerve invasion. Intraoperative assessment is critical to assess whether the tumor is adjacent to a tooth socket or caried tooth in the dentate patient. In our practice, these patients receive a segmental mandibulectomy because of the increased risk of medullary space invasion. Edentulous patients may not be good candidates for marginal mandibulectomy if there is no adequate vertical height of the mandible. In our practice we will perform a segmental mandibulectomy with appropriate reconstruction if less than 1.5 cm of vertical height will remain with a marginal mandibulectomy. In heavily radiated patients, as may occur in the second primary or recurrent setting, intraoperative assessment of trismus and mandibular fixation may also lead to improved outcomes with a segmental mandibulectomy.

In the RMT region, careful intraoperative assessment of the inferior alveolar nerve as it enters the mandibular foramen just posterior the mandibular lingula may identify gross perineural invasion. In these cases the nerve should be followed and resected superiorly toward the skull base until a negative margin is achieved. This can often be assessed preoperatively with an MRI.

SURGICAL MANAGEMENT OF THE NECK

Neck Levels

The neck is divided into levels using anatomic boundaries. The submental triangle and submandbular triangles are level Ia and Ib, respectively. The upper, middle, and lower jugular lymph nodes are levels II, III, and IV, respectively. Level II is divided into IIa below the accessory nerve (CN XI) and IIb above the nerve. The posterior triangle (level V) is posterior to the sternocleidomastoid muscle, anterior to the trapezius muscle, and superior to the clavicle. The neck dissection levels are demonstrated in Figure 15.5 (87).

Extent of Neck Dissection

In general, a neck dissection is recommended for upper aerodigestive tract malignancies, when the risk of occult disease is greater than 20% (88). Approximately 80% of patients with oral cavity cancer present as clinically node negative (cN0); however, the rate of occult metastatic disease is approximately 30% and differs by subsite (89). Historically, all patients with oral cavity cancer received a radical neck dissection with sacrifice of the internal jugular vein, sternocleidomastoid muscle, and accessory nerve including dissection of levels I to V.

However, in the late 1980s as pathology reports were reviewed, the true incidence of neck disease in OCC became evident, and more importantly, the neck levels with a predilection

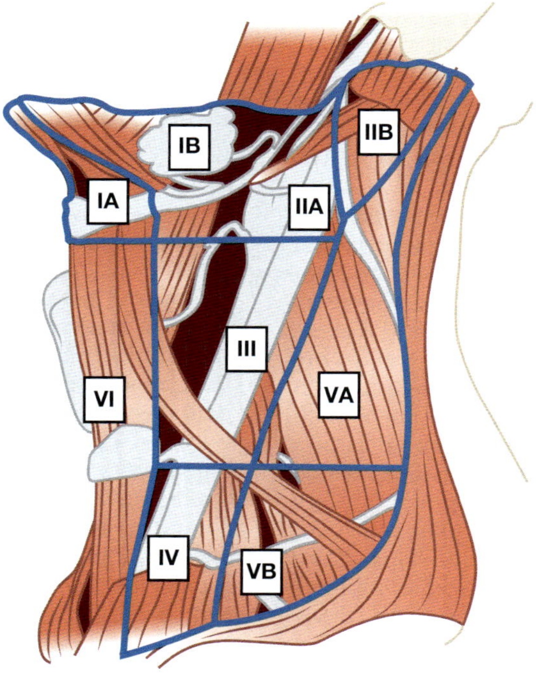

FIGURE 15.5 Neck levels.

for nodal metastases were narrowed. OCC tends to metastasize to the ipsilateral neck levels I to III (89). One of the landmark studies on this topic identified only 3% prevalence of disease in level IV in patients who were cN0 (89). Those who received a therapeutic neck dissection (for clinically node positive disease; cN+) had a 17% prevalence of disease in level IV. The prevalence of metastases to level V was extremely rare at less than 1%.

The role of the supraomohyoid neck dissection (levels I–III; including level IIb) was then investigated in this setting for both cN0 and cN+ patients. It was found to be an oncologically safe diagnostic procedure with far less morbidity than the radical neck dissection (90,91).

The management of level IIb continues to be controversial. Dissecting level IIb is associated with added shoulder morbidity due to the additional manipulation of the accessory nerve (CN XI) required to clean this level. A pooled analysis revealed that metastases to this level are relatively uncommon (6%) (92). Less than 1% of patients in this analysis had an isolated level IIb metastasis. Most patients (85%; 95% CI: 64%–95%) had a metastasis at another level, with nearly all patients with a level IIb metastasis having a level IIa metastasis. Although other large series have demonstrated similar results (3.3% level IIb) with no isolated level IIb nodes (93), the current recommendation continues to be a supraomohyoid neck dissection including level IIb because a regional recurrence, particularly after surgery and radiotherapy, is associated with very poor outcomes.

Isolated contralateral metastases on patients with lateralized tumors are extremely rare and therefore a contralateral neck dissection is not recommended in OCC unless the tumor abuts or crosses the midline (94,95).

Clinically and Radiographically Negative Neck

Risk factors for occult nodal metastases in OCC include an advanced T stage, PNI, and lymphovascular invasion (LVI) (96). One of the most important predictors that has been well studied is tumor thickness (96,97). Table 15.3 demonstrates the results of a well-performed meta-analysis on the topic of tumor thickness as it relates to occult metastatic rate in OCC, demonstrating a high rate in patients with a greater than or equal to 5 mm thick tumor on final pathological examination ($p = .007$) (97).

There is only a single randomized trial on the topic of elective neck dissection versus observation in the cN0 OCC (98). The study focused on patients with T1 and T2 OCC because it is commonly accepted that patients with a higher stage of disease, despite being cN0, have a sufficiently high enough occult metastatic disease rate so that an elective neck dissection is warranted. The vast majority of patients in the study had tongue cancer (85%), with very few buccal mucosa and floor of mouth cancers. The study did not include any RMT, hard palate/maxillary alveolus, or mandibular alveolus cancers. After randomizing 245 patients to the elective surgery group and 255 to the therapeutic surgery group, at 3 years, elective neck dissection resulted in

TABLE 15.3

Tumor Thickness in cN0 OCC Patients: Negative Predictive Value for Occult Regional Disease

Tumor Thickness Cutoff	Number of Studies	Negative Predicted Value
3 mm	4	94.7
4 mm	9	95.5
5 mm	6	83.4
6 mm	4	87.0

OCC, oral cavity cancer.

Source: Adapted from Huang SH, Hwang D, Lockwood G, et al. Predictive value of tumor thickness for cervical lymph-node involvement in squamous cell carcinoma of the oral cavity: a meta-analysis of reported studies. *Cancer*. 2009;115(7):1489–1497.

better (p = .01) overall survival (80%; 95% CI: 74%–86%) compared to therapeutic neck dissection (68%; 95% CI: 61%–74%). Similar results were reported for disease-free survival (70% elective vs. 46% therapeutic, p < .001). Even after looking for interactions on other important variables such as PNI, LVI, histologic grade, and tumor depth, the results were unchanged. Therefore, many have changed their practices to include elective neck dissection in cN0 patients with tongue, floor of mouth, and buccal cancers, even small T1 cancers.

The RMT and buccal subsites are associated with high rates of occult metastatic disease, even in early tumors, and portend worse prognosis than other OCC subsites; therefore elective neck dissection is also performed in these patients (99,100).

The maxillary alveolus and hard palate subsites have recently had a resurgence of data demonstrating high rates of occult disease even in patients with early T-stage (T1/T2) tumors. Occult metastasis in patients with maxillary alveolus and hard palate OCC range from 26% to 29% (42,101). Patients with regional recurrences had lower overall survival (101). Elective neck dissection in this population was associated with lower rates of recurrence and improved survival, even though patients who received elective neck dissection had a higher rate of advanced tumors (T3/T4) and high positive margin rates (42). Patients who did not undergo elective neck dissection were at a twofold increased risk of recurrence.

In summary, elective neck dissection (supraomohyoid; levels I–III including IIb) is recommended for all patients with cN0 OCC. This provides diagnostic information and can help stratify patients to adjuvant treatment. Furthermore, it is therapeutic in many patients given the high occult metastatic disease rate even in early-stage tumors. Elective neck dissection should also be considered in patients who are noncompliant, who are difficult to follow on clinical examination alone due to their neck girth, and who would otherwise require surgical violation of the neck for donor vessels during free flap reconstruction. Last, elective neck dissection in T1/T2 cN0 OCC patients reduces costs and improves health outcomes, making it an extremely cost-effective treatment strategy (102).

Sentinel Lymph Node Biopsy

Sentinel lymph node biopsy (SLNB) is a technique that has recently been studied in both the United States and Europe for early T-stage clinically node negative OCCs. This technique identifies the first echelon of lymph nodes draining a tumor followed by a very thorough pathologic analysis (submitted in toto), which is far more thorough than the usual analysis lymph nodes from a comprehensive neck dissection undergo, as they are usually cut through at only a single point. The technique affords the surgeon and patient additional information while avoiding the morbidity associated with a comprehensive neck dissection. A European trial found the technique to be reliable with the SLN identified in 99.5% of cases, a high rate of occult disease at 23%, a sensitivity of 86%, and negative predictive value of 95% in cT1-T2N0 OCC SCC (103). The negative predictive value was higher in the tongue than in the floor of mouth. Similar results were reported in a U.S. clinical trial demonstrating a negative predictive value of 96% (104). This technique has been largely adopted in Europe but not in North America owing to the inconvenience of the preoperative workup required, the difficulty in booking second operations for those who have positive SLNB, and the steep learning curve involved in the technique. Furthermore, there are no head-to-head comparisons between SLNB and elective neck dissection in early-stage OCC comparing survival outcomes.

CLINICALLY POSITIVE NECK

A recent meta-analysis has corroborated that supraomohyoid neck dissection is effective and oncologically sound in patients with cN+ OCC (105). In a pooled analysis of 443 patients, no significant difference was found regarding regional recurrence, disease-specific survival, or overall survival between the supraomohyoid neck dissection and a comprehensive neck dissection including levels IV and V (105). Therefore, in the cN+ setting, a therapeutic supraomohyoid neck dissection is recommended and should include level IIb.

However, the management of level IV continues to be controversial. Dissecting level IV is associated with increased risk of injury to the phrenic nerve, the brachial plexus, and chylous fistula. In the cN0 patient, occult metastases to this level are extremely rare (6%) and most surgical oncologists would not peform a level IV neck dissection (106). However, when level III is positive, there is an increased risk of occult disease in level IV and many surgical oncologists would perform an extended supraomohyoid dissection including level IV in the therapeutic (cN+) setting while others would perform a supraomohyoid neck dissection only with the expectation that postoperative radiotherapy will treat level IV (107). Part of the controversy relates to there being a small proportion of patients who are cN+ who do not have disease in level III with disease in level IV, described as skip metastases (94). However, no study has demonstrated any oncologic benefit to dissecting level IV. The 3-year neck recurrence-free survival and disease-specific survival were not different among patients who received a supraomohyoid neck dissection, extended supraomohyoid neck dissection (including a portion of level IV), or modified radical neck dissection (107). In our practice, level IV is not routinely dissected unless there is evidence of disease in level III or IV.

In patients with bulky nodal disease (N3), the internal jugular vein (IJV), sternocleidomastoid muscle (SCM), and/or the accessory nerve (CN XI) may need to be sacrificed. A radical neck dissection (levels I–V; sacrificing all three of these structures) is rarely indicated, typically in the setting of multiple matted nodes. With bulky nodal disease, particularly with ECE involving the IJV and the SCM, resection using a modified radical neck dissection (MRND; level I–V) type I (preservation of CN XI) is often required. Preoperative imaging with loss of fat planes between the tumor mass and these structures can help identify the need for their sacrifice preoperatively. However, intraoperative assessment provides the most accurate information regarding the necessity to sacrifice these structures.

The extent of the neck dissection can be tailored to the extent of the disease using intraoperative findings. MRND type II (preserving the SCM and CN XI) or type III (preserving all three structures: SCM, CN XI, IJV) can be performed for patients with bulky disease so long as these structures are not invaded. It is rare to have to sacrifice CN XI in the management of patients with OCC as there are usually multiple small nodes in different levels that can be addressed with an MRND type III.

The extent of dissection in level V can be tailored to the extent of disease. It is rare to have to perform a formal level V neck dissection including the entire posterior triangle for OCC. However, in the setting of bulky nodal disease at multiple levels, at least removing the anterior portion of level V while dissecting levels II to IV from an anterior approach is recommended.

RECONSTRUCTION OF THE SURGICAL DEFECT

One of the major advances in the management of head and neck cancers in the past several decades has been the increasing use of microvascular free flap reconstruction. This has resulted in improved oncologic outcomes likely due to the ablative surgeons' increased willingness to achieve wide negative margins knowing that free flap reconstruction will provide cosmetic and functional benefits (108). Despite a higher proportion of advanced tumors in a head-to-head comparison between those that did and did not receive free flaps, free flap reconstruction was associated with lower positive margin rates and comparable survival and recurrence rates (108).

The oral cavity is a complex structure vital to normal speech, articulation, and swallowing (oral phase). The goals of reconstruction are multiple including functional and aesthetic. The goals of reconstruction and ideal reconstructive techniques differ by oral cavity subsite. After the introduction of free flaps, the fistula and tracheotomy dependence rates have significantly decreased and intelligible speech increased (108). However, the reconstructive ladder should be considered in all patients because free flap reconstruction is not always required.

Tongue reconstruction is critical to achieve good speech, articulation, and swallowing through bolus manipulation. The goals of tongue reconstruction include obliterating the oral cavity to minimize dead space by recreating the bulk of the tongue, achieve premaxillary contact for articulation and intelligibility, and to allow tongue mobility for bolus manipulation (oral phase of swallowing). Superficial or small tongue cancers without significant loss of bulk can be reconstructed with primary closure, skin grafts, or local flaps including the submental island flap and the facial artery musculomucosal flap, among other techniques. A landmark study by Chepeha et al. demonstrated that tongue protrusion of at least 0.8 cm achieves improved speech and swallowing outcomes (40). Tongue elevation was also found to be important. This is usually achieved with a radial forearm free flap (RFFF) reconstruction. When the tumor resection necessitates that a portion of the base of tongue is resected, one can achieve additional bulk in this region using the beavertail modification of the forearm flap (109). When a subtotal or total glossectomy is performed, the anterolateral thigh (ALT) is often used to recreate the bulk of the tongue (i.e., mound shaped), with particular attention paid to recreation of the tip with excisional and suture techniques (110). Sensory reinnervation of flaps used for glossectomy defects achieves sensory recovery but this has not translated into any functional benefits and has been largely abandoned (111).

Mandible reconstruction is important for cosmesis, mandibular continuity (facial height and contour), mastication with symmetric temporomandibular joint displacement while avoiding trismus, speech, and swallowing impairment. Segmental defects can be reconstructed with plate only, plate and soft tissue free flap, or osteocutaneous free flap. Without mandibular bony continuity, the forces of mastication, particularly in a dentate patient, will inevitably lead to plate fracture. For this reason, most patients receive a bony reconstruction. Options include the fibular flap, iliac crest flap, scapular flap, or osteocutaneous RFFF. These flaps have varying utilities depending on the defect. Iliac crest reconstruction has been largely abandoned due to the extremely high rate of hernias despite primary mesh reconstruction. The osteocutaneous RFFF is excellent for small mandibular alveolus defects with a short segment of bone. Through and through defects often benefit from the independently mobile soft tissue components afforded in a scapular flap, which includes the lattissimus dorsi skin paddle, a scapular/parascapular skin paddle, and up to 14 cm of scapular bone (112). The scapular tip free flap bases the bony vascular supply on the angular branch of the thoracodorsal artery and allows for increased pedicle length with an easier harvest (113). The fibular flap provides the longest bone and is best suited for long segment mandibular defects.

The goals of hard palate and maxillary alveolus reconstruction include achieving oronasal separation, cosmetic (facial projection), and providing an appropriate premaxillary contact point for the tongue to assist with articulation and swallowing. Dental rehabilitation is a secondary goal. Reconstruction is based on the size of the defect, the number of remaining teeth, and can include a prosthesis/obturator, soft tissue reconstruction, or bony free flap reconstruction. For soft tissue only reconstruction, usually for small defects not involving the maxillary alveolus, the RFFF is an excellent flap option but often an obturator can be used as well. For very short anterior segment maxillary alveolus defects, the osteocutaneous RFFF is an excellent option. For larger infrastructure maxillectomy and total maxillectomy defects the layered fibular free flap or the scapular free flap are both excellent options (114). The scapula tip based on the angular branch of the thoracodorsal artery offers the added advantage of a longer pedicle, thereby not requiring vein grafts and excellent morphology matching the shape of the hard palate (115,116). Furthermore, osseointegrated dental implants' success rate is comparable between scapular and fibular free flaps (117).

The RMT, buccal mucosa, and floor of mouth are often reconstructed with RFFF when a free flap is required because it is thin and pliable. Very small defects can be reconstructed with primary closure or skin grafts. The goal with the former two subsites includes avoiding circumferential scar and trismus. The floor of mouth, even with small defects, often requires reconstruction to avoid ventral tongue tethering on the mandibular alveolus, which would affect speech and swallowing. With larger defects, a flap is used to separate the oral cavity from the neck and to provide a base for the intrinsic and remaining extrinsic tongue musculature to produce protrusion and elevation.

ROLE OF INDUCTION CHEMOTHERAPY

The role of induction chemotherapy prior to surgery with or without postoperative radiotherapy (PORT) for OCC has been recently assessed in two excellent prospective phase III clinical trials (118–120). The results of these studies have been recently studied in a meta-analysis, which demonstrated no significant overall benefit in favor of induction chemotherapy regarding locoregional recurrence, disease-free survival, and overall survival despite 89% of patients being stage III/IV (121). A subgroup analysis of patients who were clinically N2 showed an improvement in overall survival in favor of induction chemotherapy. Toxicity and safety outcomes could not be compared between the two groups.

Interestingly, in these two trials, 27% of the patients after chemotherapy obtained a favorable pathologic complete response (defined as absence of viable cells at whole pathologic surgical examination or minimal residual disease with less than 10% of viable tumor cells), that translated into a substantial survival benefit, both in disease-free and overall survival. A pathologic complete response (pCR) has been associated with the presence of "functional" p53 protein status, defined as the finding in pretreatment biopsy of a *TP53* wild type gene or a mutation having partial or full transactivation activity (122). In this context, 86% of pCR was obtained in p53 functional tumor; conversely, 40% of the patients harboring a p53 functional protein status achieved a pCR. So, a better molecular identification of patients achieving a favorable response to induction chemotherapy and the clinical evaluation of a molecularly profiled induction approach could constitute the next research step. However, currently, no routine application of such a strategy could be suggested in clinical practice.

ROLE OF ADJUVANT RADIOTHERAPY AND CHEMOTHERAPY

As in most patients with stage II-III head and neck SCCs, postoperative radiation therapy (PORT) is the mainstay treatment for locally advanced OCCs. In particular, PORT is known to improve both local–regional control and overall survival for lymph node–positive patients (123–125). Even in patients with pathologically staged N1 disease, PORT is associated with improved survival, especially in those younger than 70 years and those with T2 disease (126).

RADIOTHERAPY TECHNIQUES

Nowadays, it is highly recommended to use high-precision techniques to optimize the distribution of irradiation doses between tumor target volumes and normal organs at risk. The use of *intensity modulated radiotherapy* (IMRT) and its more recent derivates (*volumetric arc therapy* [VMAT] and *helical tomotherapy*) allows indeed a much better sparing of normal tissues as salivary glands, spinal cord, pharyngeal constrictors, or bony structures. Another innovative technology, called *image-guided radiation therapy* (IGRT), significantly improves the treatment precision by reducing markedly the interfractional uncertainties in organ and patient motion. Finally, *adaptive radiotherapy*, an approach recently introduced into routine clinical practice in head and neck cancer radiotherapy, helps radio-oncologists and physicists ensure adequate dose coverage within the target volumes. Using deformable image coregistration and side-by-side reconstruction, its application compensates the changes in the applied dose distribution caused by the geometrical variations occurring all along the treatment, in particular as regards anatomic deformations (127).

IRRADIATION VOLUMES

An adequate definition of target volume has to integrate both host- and tumor-related factors (127). It includes decision-making processes as whether or not to cover postoperatively the primary tumor site, and encompass neck node levels, either positive at the pathology report or at the risk of microscopic infiltration. Guidelines have been published regarding the delineation of nodal target volumes in postoperative setting (129). Together with host-related parameters, such as patients' age, performance status, and comorbidities, the oral cavity subsite(s), tumor stage laterality, extension through midline structures, and burden of lymph node disease are the main criteria leading to the appropriate definition of neck irradiation volumes. Still, treatment outcomes after PORT are reported as somewhat unpredictable, in terms of both in-field and out-of-field failures (128,130–133).

A number of reports have highlighted the risks of too selective approaches to adjuvant radiotherapy (123,128,130,134,135). These uncertainties led some institutions to favor rather systematically bilateral neck irradiation for anatomic sites such as oral tongue (128). For example, Spaulding et al. reported, in a retrospective study on 84 N0 oral tongue carcinoma patients, 3-year neck control rates of 38% and 95% (123), after unilateral/partial bilateral or comprehensive bilateral radiation, respectively. A systematic coverage of the bilateral neck has nevertheless to be weighted in function of the estimated risk of contralateral extension: in a cohort of 129 patients with a lateralized OCC, Kurita et al. reported that, while the presence of contralateral neck node infiltration was independently predicted by

T stage, number of involved ipsilateral lymph nodes and histopathologic grading, this presence was observed only in patients with ipsilateral lymph node metastasis (136).

RADIOTHERAPY DOSES

Using conventional fractionation, doses of 66 Gy, in 33 fractions of 2 Gy each, are delivered over 6.5 weeks to high-risk areas, namely the site of the primary tumor, especially in the presence of very close margins <2 mm or positive margin, and the neck levels where adenopathies are infiltrated. Anatomic areas at intermediate of risk of recurrence, located in close vicinity to the areas mentioned perviously, are given 60 Gy in 30 fractions over 6 weeks. Finally, elective irradiation to neck node levels with only potential microscopic infiltration delivers 50 Gy in 25 fractions over 5 weeks.

RADIOTHERAPY TOXICITY

During the last 3 weeks of treatment and immediately after postoperative radiotherapy, a majority of OCCs develop grade 3 mucositis and epidermitis. Following PORT, late side effects include fibrosis, reduced salivary function, trismus, compromised dental health, and a risk of osteoradionecrosis, all with potential unfavorable impact on patient's quality of life (137). With respect to xerostomia, the use of IMRT-based techniques is known to reduce irradiation dose levels to the parotid glands. In a randomized trial assessing the incidence of severe xerostomia after conventional techniques of irradiation or parotid-sparing IMRT, Nutting et al. showed that this latter technique significantly reduced the incidence of xerostomia and led to faster salivary flow recovery, translating into better patient's quality of life (138).

RADIOTHERAPY INDICATIONS

Due to the usually low number of patients accrued to prospective studies, there is until now no clear evidence based on randomized trials that would help teams identify those patients with OCC who clearly benefit from PORT. Indeed the fact that, in the literature, overall survival is found to be consistently poorer in the PORT group undoubtedly reflects the statistical biases known to result from analyses on retrospective studies and the fact that patients treated with PORT were considered to have a high risk of recurrence (139,140). Regarding the primary site, PORT should be delivered in patients with bulky disease, or in the presence of very close margins <2 mm or positive margin, whatever the pathologic stage (133). As for neck nodes, the role of PORT in pN1 patients is still a matter of debate, while the addition of radiotherapy is systematically recommended in the presence of three nodes or extracapsular spread.

OUTCOME FOLLOWING PORT

Outcomes can be analyzed in terms of local–regional recurrences and survival indices. In 2012, a systematic review of essentially nonrandomized studies by Brown et al. compared surgery alone and surgery followed by PORT (140). Overall local recurrence rates were found to be 11% and 17%, for stages I-II and stages III-IV, respectively, after surgery alone, compared with 13% and 19% in patients treated with PORT. The corresponding figures for regional recurrence rates were 13% and 12% after surgery alone compared with 6% and 11% after PORT. In terms of overall survival, the rates were 76% and 74% for surgery alone compared with 65% and 62%, respectively. It is acknowledged that this is a weak level of evidence as patients who have PORT probably have a high pathologic stage of disease. Interestingly, the only prospective trial comparing surgery alone with surgery followed by PORT for 122 patients with stages III-IV disease yielded a significantly higher disease-free survival rate in the PORT arm (68 vs. 38%, $p = .005$) (141). Finally, Shrime et al. showed that, for pT1-2 pN1, PORT improved overall survival at 5 years (41 vs. 54.2%; $p < .001$) (142).

Concomitant Chemoradiotherapy

In 2004, the Radiation Therapy Oncology Group (RTOG) and European Organisation for Research and Treatment of Cancer (EORTC) published their results on two randomized trials of adjuvant radiotherapy and concurrent chemotherapy (RTOG 9501 and EORTC 22931), in which about 25% of the cases were presenting with OCC. These trials as well as the pooled analysis of their results clearly showed that the addition of chemotherapy to PORT yielded a significant survival benefit in those patients with either close or positive margins and/or extracapsular spread (Figure 15.6) (137,143,144). It is also recommended to deliver concomitant chemoradiotherapy in OCC patients presenting with extensive neck disease and in those with infiltrated supraclavicular adenopathies (137).

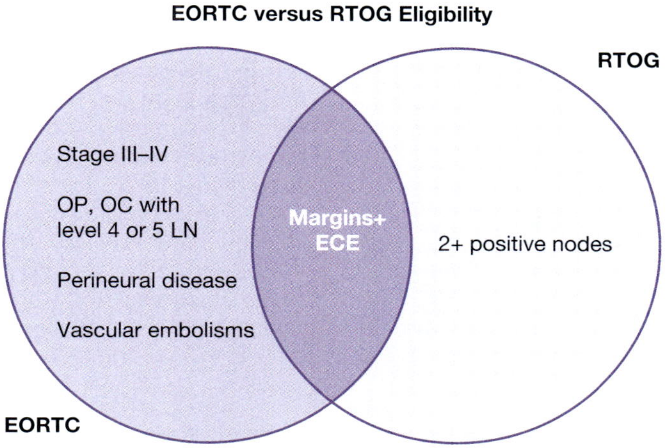

FIGURE 15.6 Indications for chemoradiotherapy in RTOG 9501 and EORTC 22931.

ECE, extracapsular extension; EORTC, European Organisation for Research and Treatment of Cancer; LN, lymph node; OC, oral cavity; OP, oropharynx; RTOG, Radiation Therapy Oncology GroupECE extracapsular extensionLN, lymph node.

Source: Adapted from Bernier J, Cooper JS, Pajak TF, et al. Defining risk levels in locally advanced head and neck cancers: a comparative analysis of concurrent postoperative radiation plus chemotherapy trials of the EORTC (#22931) and RTOG (# 9501). *Head Neck.* 2005;27(10):843–850.

TIMING OF ADJUVANT TREATMENT

Patients who are candidates for adjuvant treatment should receive this treatment within 6 to 8 weeks after surgery. The time interval between surgery and adjuvant treatment has an important statistically significant impact on survival. In one study, this time interval had the strongest influence on the incidence of first locoregional recurrence after controlling for stage and other important patient and tumor variables (145). The longer the wait (>143 days vs. 56–143 days vs. 55 days or less) the worse the disease-free survival outcomes.

OUTCOMES AND SURVEILLANCE

Patients with OCC have worse outcomes with advanced stage disease (67% 5-year disease-free survival for advanced stage and 87% for early stage) (146). Survival has improved over the past three decades due to increasing use of neck dissection, PORT, and postoperative chemoradiotherapy (147). Beyond the usual staging criteria, which are good prognosticators, a number of additional pathologic factors have been identified that predict outcomes.

FURTHER N-STAGE PROGNOSTICATION

ECE has always been demonstrated to be a negative prognostic factor benefiting from postoperative chemoradiotherapy; however, recent evidence suggests that the extent of ECE is also important. Disease-specific survival is lower for patients with major ECE (>1.7 mm) compared to patients with minor ECE (1.7 mm or less) but not significantly different between patients with minor ECE and those without ECE (148).

In OCC, the number of lymph nodes removed during elective neck dissection in patients who were ultimately pathologically staged as N0 has a strong impact on overall survival regardless of whether this was analyzed using lymph node yield quartiles or as a continuous variable (149). The exact mechanism for this is unknown and may be related to removal of a larger burden of microscopic metastatic disease given a 15% false negative rate on final pathologic analysis of oral cavity neck dissection specimens (150). It can also be a surrogate for the quality of surgery being performed, similar to surgeon case volume-outcome associations previously discussed. A minimum lymph node yield per neck dissection in OCC should include at least 18 lymph nodes (151).

Nodal ratio, the number of positive lymph nodes divided by the total number of lymph nodes resected, is also an independent predictor of regional recurrence, disease-specific survival, and overall survival in OCC SCC (152–155). There is a ratio–response relationship, with higher values, typically above 10% having the worse outcomes. Furthermore, nodal level distribution is also important as disease in level IV and V is associated with worse disease-specific survival (156).

SURVEILLANCE

Patients require close follow-up after treatment; every 3 months for the first year, every 4 months during the second year, and every 6 months after that for up to 5 years (58). This is to assess the primary and regional sites for recurrence. The vast majority of locoregional recurrences happen during the first 2 years and these are associated with poor outcomes despite salvage treatment (157,158). Also, it gives the multidisciplinary team, including dietitian, speech language pathologist, and dentists, an opportunity to assist with rehabilitation. Last, surveillance provides an opportunity to detect second primary cancers, which occur at a rate of approximately 4% to 7% per year (159). Follow-up visits also give the team an opportunity to discuss tobacco product and alcohol cessation, given that these increase locoregional failure and second primary cancer rates (64).

CASE 15.1: ADVANCED TONGUE RECONSTRUCTION

A 45-year-old man presented with a clinical endophytic left lateral tongue and floor of mouth SCC, which was clinically T2N1. After an appropriate resection he had a defect involving the lateral dorsal and ventral tongue, extending to the floor of mouth and onto the posterior mandibular alveolus, which was removed using a marginal mandibulectomy. His defect also extended minimally posterior to the retromolar trigone onto the tonsils.

A left radial forearm free flap (Figure 15.7A) was designed to incorporate all of those subsites. Furthermore the radial aspect of the flap along the floor of mouth and mandibular alveolus was designed for the most radial aspect of the flap because this provides thinner and more pliable mucosa whereas the more ulnar aspect of the flap is thicker and is best used to recreate the bulk of the tongue.

He had an uncomplicated hospital course. His tracheotomy tube was exchanged on postoperative day 5, corked, and he was successfully decannulated on day 6. On postoperative day 7, he worked with a speech language pathologist and initiated oral intake. He was discharged on postoperative day 8 after his nasogastric tube was removed. His postoperative speech and swallowing function are excellent (Figure 15.7B).

His pathology report demonstrated a moderately differentiated T2 (3.8 cm) N2b (2/42) SCC of the tongue with lymphovascular invasion but no perineural invasion. His margins were negative. He received postoperative radiotherapy.

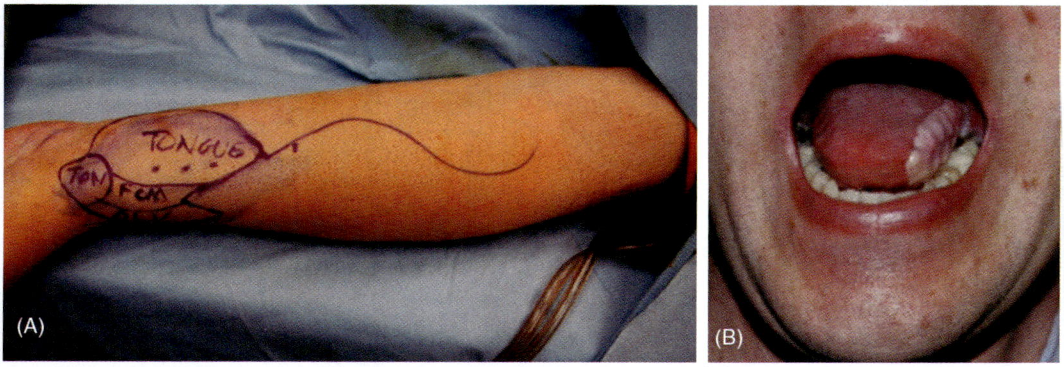

FIGURE 15.7 (A) A radial forearm flap design. (B) Postoperative intraoral flap.

CASE 15.2: ANTERIOR COMPOSITE DEFECT—SCAPULA SYSTEM FLAPS

A 72-year-old man presented with a clinically T4aN2b SCC of the left anterior floor of mouth extending through the mandible and into the left chin skin and subcutaneous tissue (Figure 15.8A).

Surgical extirpation with appropriate margins required reconstruction of composite anterior through and through defect. Internally the defect included a portion of the left ventral tongue as well as the entire anterior and left floor of mouth. Mandible was taken from the midline to the left mid ramus (Figure 15.8B). The external defect included the left hemilower lip, the entire chin subunit, and a significant portion of the left cheek extending into the neck (Figure 15.8C). The patient was placed into maxillomandibular fixation at the beginning of the procedure and a heavy locking reconstruction plate was used to preplate the mandible prior to extirpation of the tumor.

He had an uncomplicated hospital course. His tracheotomy tube was exchanged on postoperative day 5, he was corked on day 9, and he was successfully decannulated on day 10. He was discharged on postoperative day 11 with a nasogastric tube. He followed up in clinic at 1 week after discharge and oral diet was initiated after a speech language pathology assessment. His nasogastric tube was removed at the following visit (2 weeks after discharge). His postoperative speech and swallowing function are excellent.

His pathology report demonstrated a poorly differentiated T4aN2c (bilateral; 2/31 on the right and 6/42 on the left) SCC of the floor of mouth with mandibular and cutaneous involvement. The tumor demonstrated both lymphovascular invasion and perineural invasion. His margins were negative. One of the lymph nodes had evidence of extracapsular extension. He thus received postoperative chemoradiotherapy with cisplatin.

A 59-year-old woman presented with a clinically T2 (~2.5 cm) lesion on the lingual surface of the right mandibular alveolus abutting the teeth and extending inferiorly into the floor of mouth. Her neck was staged clinically and radiographically as N0.

She underwent a resection involving the dorsal tongue, floor of mouth, mandibular alveolus, both lingual and buccal regions, through a marginal mandibulectomy, and a small amount of buccal mucosa. She also underwent a right supraomohyoid neck dissection. This was reconstructed with a radial forearm free flap.

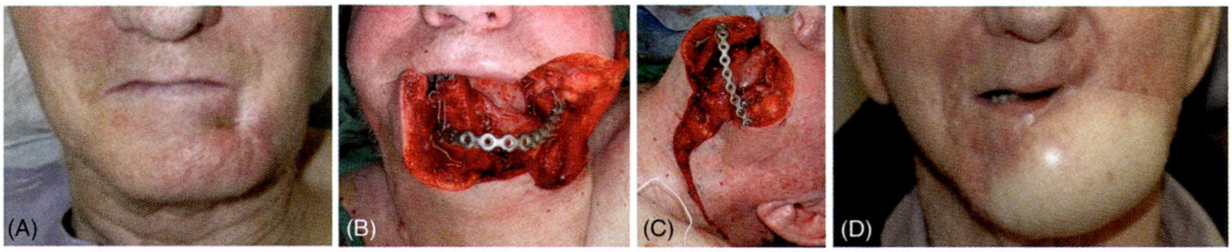

FIGURE 15.8 (A) Cutaneous involvement from oral cavity cancer. (B) Defect with plate application (frontal view). (C) Defect with plate application (oblique view). (D) Postoperative appearance.

CASE 15.3: MANDIBULAR ALVEOLUS DEFECT

She had an uncomplicated hospital course. Her tracheotomy tube was exchanged on postoperative day 5, corked, and she was successfully decannulated on day 7. She was assessed by speech language pathology on day 6 and started an oral diet on day 7. On day 8 her nasogastric tube was removed and she was discharged home. Her postoperative flap resurfaced the dorsal tongue, floor of mouth, mandibular alveolus, and buccal mucosa (Figure 15.9A and 15.9B). Her speech and swallowing function are excellent.

Her pathology report demonstrated a T2N0 (0/22) SCC of the mandibular alveolus with minimal bony invasion. There were no adverse pathologic features; margins were negative, there was no lymphovascular or perineural invasion, and the tumor was well differentiated.

She underwent dental rehabilitation with a partial denture (Figure 15.9C).

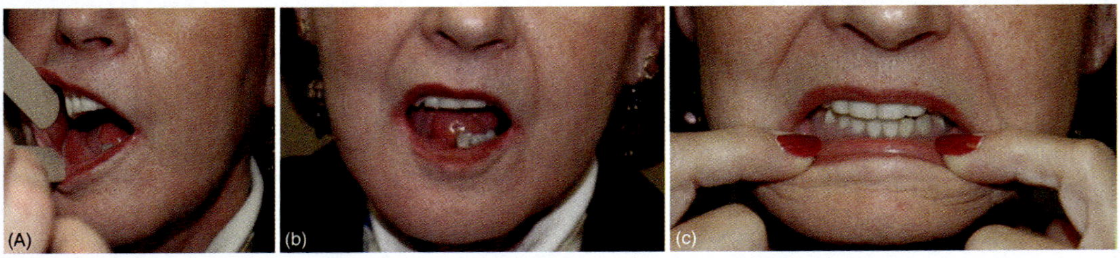

FIGURE 15.9 (A) Intraoral mucosalization of radial forearm free flap (oblique view). (B) Intraoral mucosalization of radial forearm free flap (frontal view). (C) Frontal view of oral cavity with partial denture.

CASE 15.4: LOCALLY ADVANCED INDUCTION CHEMOTHERAPY

A 36-year-old nonsmoking man with an unremarkable medical history presented for a physician consult with oral pain and right reflex otalgia. After an otolaryngologist evaluation, a biopsy of a mucosal lesion of the right side of tongue was performed. Histologic examination revealed a keratinizing SCC. Head and neck staging MRI revealed a solid nodular lesion on the right side of tongue body measuring 37 x 21 x 25 mm (anteroposterior x medioateral x craniocaudal diameters, respectively). Such mass involved the transverse muscle of tongue, the genioglossus, hyoglossus, and styloglossus muscles. Imaging did not show pathologic neck lymph nodes (Figure 15.10A). According to the eighth edition of AJCC cancer staging system, disease stage was IVA (cT4aN0).

Because of the disease stage and patient's good performance status (0 according to ECOG), after a multidisciplinary discussion the patient was proposed a clinical trial with induction chemotherapy in OCC SCC bearing wild type TP53 gene.

After informed consent signature, the histologic specimen was screened for the presence of TP53 mutations in the most frequently affected exons (5 to 8). No mutation was found, so the patient was enrolled in the trial. In light of adequate blood tests and in the absence of significant

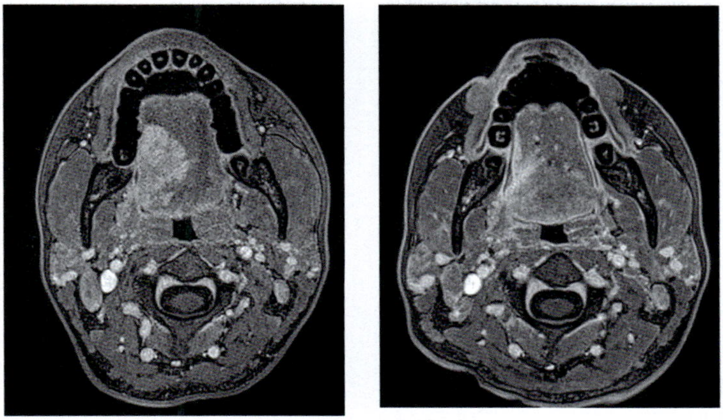

(A) (B)

FIGURE 15.10 (A) Preinduction axial MRI. (B) Postinduction axial MRI.

comorbid conditions, the patient was offered an induction chemotherapy with TPF. Such regimen, administered once every 21 days, consisted in docetaxel 75 mg/m^2 and cisplatin 75 mg/m^2 on day 1, followed by 5-fluorouracil 750 mg/m^2 in 120-hour continuous infusion (160).

Chemotherapy was followed by grade (G) 3 neutropenia, G2 nausea, and G2 oral mucositis in the first intercycle. Owing to the worsening of mucositis (G3) after the second cycle, total 5-fluorouracil dose was reduced by 20%.

After three courses of TPF chemotherapy, a head and neck MRI showed a significant partial response, with a definite dimensional reduction (90%–95% from baseline) of the tongue neoplasm (Figure 15.10B).

Therefore, in April 2012, the patient underwent surgical intervention consisting of right hemiglossectomy, bilateral neck node dissection (levels Ia, Ib, II, III), and reconstruction with revascularized anterolateral thigh myocutaneous free flap from right thigh. A temporary tracheotomy was performed. The feeding tube was removed after 15 days from the intervention; then the patient progressively restarted an autonomous and regular diet and speech.

The definitive histologic examination showed a pCR on the tongue and the presence of SCC foci in one node of the right neck (level IIa); all the remaining 57 bilaterally excised lymph nodes were negative. After a multidisciplinary consultation, the patient was given postoperative radiotherapy at a dose of 60 Gy. Such treatment was complicated by G3 oral mucositis requiring opioids and by G1 radiation dermatitis.

Thereafter, a clinical and radiologic follow-up was started. After about 5 years, the patient is still alive and disease free. Long-term toxicities observed consist in G1 neck fibrosis and G1 xerostomia.

Induction chemotherapy followed by surgery is not a standard of care in head and neck SCC, being reserved to clinical trials. In this case, the patient was offered an induction TPF trial based on a wild type TP53 bearing disease. This trial was based on the premise of a better responsiveness to chemotherapy of such diseases, due to the maintenance of the TP53 apoptotic machinery. The patient achieved an almost complete pathologic response (minimal residual foci in one node). pCR or minimal residual disease after induction chemotherapy represents a strong prognostic factor for outcome.

REFERENCES

1. Miller KD, Siegel RL, Lin CC, et al. Cancer treatment and survivorship statistics, 2016. *CA Cancer J Clin.* 2016;66(4):271–289. doi:10.3322/caac.21349
2. Torre LA, Bray F, Siegel RL, et al. Global cancer statistics, 2012. *CA Cancer J Clin.* 2015;65(2):87–108.
3. Blot WJ, McLaughlin JK, Winn DM, et al. Smoking and drinking in relation to oral and pharyngeal cancer. *Cancer Res.* 1988;48(11):3282–3287.
4. Smith GI, Yeo D, Clark J, et al. Measures of health-related quality of life and functional status in survivors of oral cavity cancer who have had defects reconstructed with radial forearm free flaps. *Br J Oral Maxillofac Surg.* 2006;44(3):187–192.
5. Siegel RL, Miller KD, Jemal A. Cancer statistics, 2015. *CA Cancer J Clin.* 2015;65(1):5–29.
6. Gupta B, Johnson NW, Kumar N. Global epidemiology of head and neck cancers: a continuing challenge. *Oncology.* 2016;91(1):13–23.
7. GLOBOCAN 2012: estimated cancer incidence, mortality and prevalence worldwide in 2012 [Internet]. Lyon, France: World Health Organization; 2013 [updated December 12, 2013; cited November 16, 2016]. http://globocan.iarc.fr
8. Pulte D, Brenner H. Changes in survival in head and neck cancers in the late 20th and early 21st century: a period analysis. *Oncologist.* 2010;15(9):994–1001.
9. Eskander A, Irish J, Gullane P, et al. Overview of surgery for oral cavity cancer in Ontario. *Head Neck.* 2016;38(7):1113–1118.
10. Hashibe M, Brennan P, Chuang SC, et al. Interaction between tobacco and alcohol use and the risk of head and neck cancer: pooled analysis in the International Head and Neck Cancer Epidemiology Consortium. *Cancer Epidemiol Biomarkers Prev.* 2009;18(2):541–550.
11. Eskander A, Irish JC, Urbach DR, Goldstein DP, eds. *Head and Neck Cancer Surgery in Ontario, 2003–2010: An ICES Atlas.* Toronto, Ontario, Canada: Institute for Clinical Evaluative Sciences; 2015.
12. Jha P, MacLennan M, Chaloupka FJ, et al. Global hazards of tobacco and the benefits of smoking cessation and tobacco taxes. In: Gelband H, Jha P, Sankaranarayanan R, Horton S, eds. *Cancer: Disease Control Priorities.* 3rd ed. vol 3. Washington, DC: International Bank for Reconstruction and Development/The World Bank; 2015.
13. Patel SC, Carpenter WR, Tyree S, et al. Increasing incidence of oral tongue squamous cell carcinoma in young white women, age 18 to 44 years. *J Clin Oncol.* 2011;29(11):1488–1494.
14. van Monsjou HS, Wreesmann VB, van den Brekel MW, Balm AJ. Head and neck squamous cell carcinoma in young patients. *Oral Oncol.* 2013;49(12):1097–1102.
15. van Monsjou HS, Lopez-Yurda MI, Hauptmann M, et al. Oral and oropharyngeal squamous cell carcinoma in young patients: the Netherlands Cancer Institute experience. *Head Neck.* 2013;35(1):94–102.
16. Zafereo ME, Xu L, Dahlstrom KR, et al. Squamous cell carcinoma of the oral cavity often overexpresses p16 but is rarely driven by human papillomavirus. *Oral Oncol.* 2016;56:47–53.
17. Lee LA, Huang CG, Tsao KC, et al. Human papillomavirus infections are common and predict mortality in a retrospective cohort study of Taiwanese patients with oral cavity cancer. *Medicine (Baltimore).* 2015;94(47):e2069.
18. Lin YS, Jen YM, Wang BB, et al. Epidemiology of oral cavity cancer in Taiwan with emphasis on the role of betel nut chewing. *ORL J Otorhinolaryngol Relat Spec.* 2005;67(4):230–236.
19. Chourasia NR, Borle RM, Vastani A. Concomitant association of oral submucous fibrosis and oral squamous cell carcinoma and incidence of malignant transformation of oral submucous fibrosis in a population of central India: a retrospective study. *J Maxillofac Oral Surg.* 2015;14(4):902–906.
20. Zhang ZF, Morgenstern H, Spitz MR, et al. Marijuana use and increased risk of squamous cell carcinoma of the head and neck. *Cancer Epidemiol Biomarkers Prev.* 1999;8(12):1071–1078.
21. De Stefani E, Boffetta P, Ronco AL, et al. Processed meat consumption and risk of cancer: a multisite case-control study in Uruguay. *Br J Cancer.* 2012;107(9):1584–1588.
22. La Vecchia C, Tavani A. Fruit and vegetables, and human cancer. *Eur J Cancer Prev.* 1998;7(1):3–8.
23. Hashim D, Sartori S, Brennan P, et al. The role of oral hygiene in head and neck cancer: results from International Head and Neck Cancer Epidemiology (INHANCE) consortium. *Ann Oncol.* 2016;27(8):1619–1625.
24. Nelissen C, Lambrecht M, Nevens F, et al. Noncutaneous head and neck cancer in solid organ transplant patients: single center experience. *Oral Oncol.* 2014;50(4):263–268.
25. (S008) The Impact of HPV, HIV, and smoking on oncologic and functional outcomes in patients with head and neck cancer. *Oncology (Williston Park).* 2015;29(4, Suppl 1):204954.
26. D'souza G, Carey TE, William WN, Jr, et al. Epidemiology of head and neck squamous cell cancer among HIV-infected patients. *J Acquir Immune Defic Syndr.* 2014;65(5):603–610.
27. Alter BP, Giri N, Savage SA, et al. Squamous cell carcinomas in patients with Fanconi anemia and dyskeratosis congenita: a search for human papillomavirus. *Int J Cancer.* 2013;133(6):1513–1515.
28. Ray JG, Swain N, Ghosh R, et al. Dyskeratosis congenita with malignant transformation. *BMJ Case Rep.* 2011;2011. doi::10.1136/bcr.03.2010.2848
29. Berkower AS, Biller HF. Head and neck cancer associated with Bloom's syndrome. *Laryngoscope.* 1988;98(7):746–748.
30. Kutler DI, Auerbach AD, Satagopan J, et al. High incidence of head and neck squamous cell carcinoma in patients with Fanconi anemia. *Arch Otolaryngol Head Neck Surg.* 2003;129(1):106–112.

31. Fitzpatrick SG, Hirsch SA, Gordon SC. The malignant transformation of oral lichen planus and oral lichenoid lesions: a systematic review. *J Am Dent Assoc.* 2014;145(1):45–56.
32. Bombeccari GP, Guzzi G, Tettamanti M, et al. Oral lichen planus and malignant transformation: a longitudinal cohort study. *Oral Surg Oral Med Oral Pathol Oral Radiol Endod.* 2011;112(3):328–334.
33. Silverman S, Jr, Gorsky M, Lozada F. Oral leukoplakia and malignant transformation. A follow-up study of 257 patients. *Cancer.* 1984;53(3):563–568.
34. Holmstrup P, Vedtofte P, Reibel J, Stoltze K. Long-term treatment outcome of oral premalignant lesions. *Oral Oncol.* 2006;42(5):461–474.
35. Narayan TV, Shilpashree S. Meta-analysis on clinicopathologic risk factors of leukoplakias undergoing malignant transformation. *J Oral Maxillofac Pathol.* 2016;20(3):354–361.
36. Shiu MN, Chen TH, Chang SH, Hahn LJ. Risk factors for leukoplakia and malignant transformation to oral carcinoma: a leukoplakia cohort in Taiwan. *Br J Cancer.* 2000;82(11):1871–1874.
37. Ray JG, Ranganathan K, Chattopadhyay A. Malignant transformation of oral submucous fibrosis: overview of histopathological aspects. *Oral Surg Oral Med Oral Pathol Oral Radiol.* 2016;122(2):200–209.
38. Feng Z, Li JN, Niu LX, Guo CB. Supraomohyoid neck dissection in the management of oral squamous cell carcinoma: special consideration for skip metastases at level IV or V. *J Oral Maxillofac Surg.* 2014;72(6):1203–211.
39. Khafif A, Lopez-Garza JR, Medina JE. Is dissection of level IV necessary in patients with T1-T3 N0 tongue cancer? *Laryngoscope.* 2001;111(6):1088–1090.
40. Chepeha DB, Teknos TN, Shargorodsky J, et al. Rectangle tongue template for reconstruction of the hemiglossectomy defect. *Arch Otolaryngol Head Neck Surg.* 2008;134(9):993–998.
41. Agarwal SK, Arora SK, Kumar G, Sarin D. Isolated perifacial lymph node metastasis in oral squamous cell carcinoma with clinically node-negative neck. *Laryngoscope.* 2016;126(10):2252–2256.
42. Givi B, Eskander A, Awad MI, et al. Impact of elective neck dissection on the outcome of oral squamous cell carcinomas arising in the maxillary alveolus and hard palate. *Head Neck.* 2016;38(Suppl 1):E1688–E1694.
43. Seethala RR, Weinreb I, Carlson DL. Protocol for the examination of specimens from patients with carcinomas of the lip and oral cavity [Internet]. Washington, DC: College of American Pathologists; 2013 [updated October 1, 2013; cited November 16, 2017]. http://www.cap.org/ShowProperty?nodePath=/UCMCon/Contribution%20Folders/WebContent/pdf/liporalcaversion-13protocol.pdf
44. Bice TC, Tran V, Merkley MA, et al. Disease-specific survival with spindle cell carcinoma of the head and neck. *Otolaryngol Head Neck Surg.* 2015;153(6):973–980.
45. Shigeta T, Minamikawa T, Matsui T, et al. Spindle cell carcinoma of the oral cavity: the impact of chemotherapy on pulmonary metastatic tumor doubling time. *Kobe J Med Sci.* 2015;61(3):E64–E70.
46. Candau-Alvarez A, Dean-Ferrer A, Alamillos-Granados FJ, et al. Verrucous carcinoma of the oral mucosa: an epidemiological and follow-up study of patients treated with surgery in 5 last years. *Med Oral Patol Oral Cir Bucal.* 2014;19(5):e506–e511.
47. Sonalika WG, Anand T. Oral verrucous carcinoma: a retrospective analysis for clinicopathologic features. *J Cancer Res Ther.* 2016;12(1):142–145.
48. Odar K, Kocjan BJ, Hosnjak L, et al. Verrucous carcinoma of the head and neck—not a human papillomavirus-related tumour? *J Cell Mol Med.* 2014;18(4):635–645.
49. Patel KR, Chernock RD, Zhang TR, et al. Verrucous carcinomas of the head and neck, including those with associated squamous cell carcinoma, lack transcriptionally active high-risk human papillomavirus. *Hum Pathol.* 2013;44(11):2385–2392.
50. Bradley PJ, Ferris RL. Surgery for malignant sublingual and minor salivary gland neoplasms. *Adv Otorhinolaryngol.* 2016;78:113–119.
51. Dalgic A, Karakoc O, Aydin U, et al. Minor salivary gland neoplasms. *J Craniofac Surg.* 2014;25(3):e289–e291.
52. Zeidan YH, Pekelis L, An Y, et al. Survival benefit for adjuvant radiation therapy in minor salivary gland cancers. *Oral Oncol.* 2015;51(5):438–445.
53. Yeh C-F, Li W-Y, Chu P-Y, et al. Pretreatment pain predicts perineural invasion in oral squamous cell carcinoma: a prospective study. *Oral Oncol.* 2016;61:115–119.
54. Jaiswal G, Jaiswal S, Kumar R, Sharma A. Field cancerization: concept and clinical implications in head and neck squamous cell carcinoma. *J Exp Ther Oncol.* 2013;10(3):209–214.
55. Ng S-H, Yen T-C, Liao C-T, et al. 18F-FDG PET and CT/MRI in oral cavity squamous cell carcinoma: a prospective study of 124 patients with histologic correlation. *J Nucl Med.* 2005;46(7):1136–1143.
56. Ng S-H, Yen T-C, Chang JT-C, et al. Prospective study of [^{18}F]fluorodeoxyglucose positron emission tomography and computed tomography and magnetic resonance imaging in oral cavity squamous cell carcinoma with palpably negative neck. *J Clin Oncol.* 2006;24(27):4371–4376.
57. Chai RL, Rath TJ, Johnson JT, et al. Accuracy of computed tomography in the prediction of extracapsular spread of lymph node metastases in squamous cell carcinoma of the head and neck. *JAMA Otolaryngol Head Neck Surg.* 2013;139(11):1187–1194.
58. National Comprehensive Cancer Network. *NCCN Clinical Practice Guidelines in Oncology (NCCN Guidelines®: Head and Neck Cancers.* United States: NCCN; 2016 June 5, 2016. Report No.: V1.2016.
59. Krabbe CA, Pruim J, van der Laan BF, et al. FDG-PET and detection of distant metastases and simultaneous tumors in head and neck squamous cell carcinoma: a comparison with chest radiography and chest CT. *Oral Oncol.* 2009;45(3):234–240.

60. Loh KS, Brown DH, Baker JT, et al. A rational approach to pulmonary screening in newly diagnosed head and neck cancer. *Head Neck.* 2005;27(11):990–994.
61. Edge S, Byrd D, Compton C, et al, eds. *AJCC Cancer Staging Manual.* 7th ed. New York, NY: Springer; 2010.
62. Amin EB, Edge S, Greene F, et al., eds. *AJCC Cancer Staging Manual.* 8th ed. New York, NY: Springer; 2017.
63. Langius JA, van Dijk AM, Doornaert P, et al. More than 10% weight loss in head and neck cancer patients during radiotherapy is independently associated with deterioration in quality of life. *Nutr Cancer.* 2013;65(1):76–83.
64. Leon X, del Prado Venegas M, Orus C, et al. Influence of the persistence of tobacco and alcohol use in the appearance of second neoplasm in patients with a head and neck cancer. A case-control study. *Cancer Causes Control.* 2009;20(5):645–652.
65. Day GL, Blot WJ, Shore RE, et al. Second cancers following oral and pharyngeal cancers: role of tobacco and alcohol. *J Natl Cancer Inst.* 1994;86(2): 131–137.
66. Do KA, Johnson MM, Doherty DA, et al. Second primary tumors in patients with upper aerodigestive tract cancers: joint effects of smoking and alcohol (United States). *Cancer Causes Control.* 2003;14(2): 131–138.
67. Chen AM, Chen LM, Vaughan A, et al. Tobacco smoking during radiation therapy for head-and-neck cancer is associated with unfavorable outcome. *Int J Radiat Oncol Biol Phys.* 2011;79(2):414–419.
68. Chan Y, Irish JC, Wood SJ, et al. Smoking cessation in patients diagnosed with head and neck cancer. *J Otolaryngol.* 2004;33(2):75–81.
69. Vander Ark W, DiNardo LJ, Oliver DS. Factors affecting smoking cessation in patients with head and neck cancer. *Laryngoscope.* 1997;107(7):888–892.
70. Ostroff JS, Jacobsen PB, Moadel AB, et al. Prevalence and predictors of continued tobacco use after treatment of patients with head and neck cancer. *Cancer.* 1995;75(2):569–576.
71. Gritz ER, Carr CR, Rapkin DA, et al. A smoking cessation intervention for head and neck cancer patients: trial design, patient accrual, and characteristics. *Cancer Epidemiol Biomarkers Prev.* 1991;1(1):67–73.
72. de Bruin-Visser JC, Ackerstaff AH, Rehorst H, et al. Integration of a smoking cessation program in the treatment protocol for patients with head and neck and lung cancer. *Eur Arch Otorhinolaryngol.* 2012;269(2):659–665.
73. Eskander A, Merdad M, Irish JC, et al. Volume-outcome associations in head and neck cancer treatment: a systematic review and meta-analysis. *Head Neck.* 2014;36(12):1820–1834.
74. Eskander A, Monteiro E, Irish J, et al. Adherence to guideline-recommended process measures for squamous cell carcinoma of the head and neck in Ontario: impact of surgeon and hospital volume. *Head Neck.* 2016;38(suppl 1):E1987–E1992.
75. Graboyes EM, Gross J, Kallogjeri D, et al. Association of compliance with process-related quality metrics and improved survival in oral cavity squamous cell carcinoma. *JAMA Otolaryngol Head Neck Surg.* 2016;142(5):430–437.
76. Loree TR, Strong EW. Significance of positive margins in oral cavity squamous carcinoma. *Am J Surg.* 1990;160(4):410–414.
77. Patel RS, Goldstein DP, Guillemaud J, et al. Impact of positive frozen section microscopic tumor cut-through revised to negative on oral carcinoma control and survival rates. *Head Neck.* 2010;32(11):1444–1451.
78. Guillemaud JP, Patel RS, Goldstein DP, et al. Prognostic impact of intraoperative microscopic cut-through on frozen section in oral cavity squamous cell carcinoma. *J Otolaryngol Head Neck Surg.* 2010;39(4):370–377.
79. Anderson CR, Sisson K, Moncrieff M. A meta-analysis of margin size and local recurrence in oral squamous cell carcinoma. *Oral Oncol.* 2015;51(5):464–469.
80. Dziegielewski PT, O'Connell DA, Rieger J, et al. The lip-splitting mandibulotomy: aesthetic and functional outcomes. *Oral Oncol.* 2010;46(8):612–617.
81. Dai TS, Hao SP, Chang KP, et al. Complications of mandibulotomy: midline versus paramidline. *Otolaryngol Head Neck Surg.* 2003;128(1):137–141.
82. Pan WL, Hao SP, Lin YS, et al. The anatomical basis for mandibulotomy: midline versus paramidline. *Laryngoscope.* 2003;113(2):377–380.
83. McCann KJ, Irish JC, Gullane PJ, et al. Complications associated with rigid fixation of mandibulotomies. *J Otolaryngol.* 1994;23(3):210–215.
84. Brown JS, Lowe D, Kalavrezos N, et al. Patterns of invasion and routes of tumor entry into the mandible by oral squamous cell carcinoma. *Head Neck.* 2002;24(4):370–383.
85. McGregor AD, MacDonald DG. Patterns of spread of squamous cell carcinoma within the mandible. *Head Neck.* 1989;11(5):457–461.
86. Wax MK, Bascom DA, Myers LL. Marginal mandibulectomy vs segmental mandibulectomy: indications and controversies. *Arch Otolaryngol Head Neck Surg.* 2002;128(5):600–603.
87. Robbins KT, Clayman G, Levine PA, et al. Neck dissection classification update: revisions proposed by the American Head and Neck Society and the American Academy of Otolaryngology-Head and Neck Surgery. *Arch Otolaryngol Head Neck Surg.* 2002;128(7):751–758.
88. Weiss MH, Harrison LB, Isaacs RS. Use of decision analysis in planning a management strategy for the stage N0 neck. *Arch Otolaryngol Head Neck Surg.* 1994;120(7):699–702.
89. Shah JP. Patterns of cervical lymph node metastasis from squamous carcinomas of the upper aerodigestive tract. *Am J Surg.* 1990;160(4):405–409.
90. Medina JE, Byers RM. Supraomohyoid neck dissection: rationale, indications, and surgical technique. *Head Neck.* 1989;11(2):111–122.
91. Spiro JD, Spiro RH, Shah JP, et al. Critical assessment of supraomohyoid neck dissection. *Am J Surg.* 1988;156(4):286–289.

92. Lea J, Bachar G, Sawka AM, et al. Metastases to level IIb in squamous cell carcinoma of the oral cavity: a systematic review and meta-analysis. *Head Neck.* 2010;32(2):184–190.
93. Bartella AK, Kloss-Brandstatter A, Kamal M, et al. "IIb or not IIb"—the necessity of dissection in patients with oral squamous cell carcinoma. *J Craniomaxillofac Surg.* 2016;44(10):1733–1736.
94. Woolgar JA. The topography of cervical lymph node metastases revisited: the histological findings in 526 sides of neck dissection from 439 previously untreated patients. *Int J Oral Maxillofac Surg.* 2007;36(3):219–25.
95. Lim YC, Lee JS, Koo BS, et al. Treatment of contralateral N0 neck in early squamous cell carcinoma of the oral tongue: elective neck dissection versus observation. *Laryngoscope.* 2006;116(3):461–465.
96. d'Alessandro AF, Pinto FR, Lin CS, et al. Oral cavity squamous cell carcinoma: factors related to occult lymph node metastasis. *Braz J Otorhinolaryngol.* 2015;81(3):248–254.
97. Huang SH, Hwang D, Lockwood G, et al. Predictive value of tumor thickness for cervical lymph-node involvement in squamous cell carcinoma of the oral cavity: a meta-analysis of reported studies. *Cancer.* 2009;115(7):1489–1497.
98. D'Cruz AK, Vaish R, Kapre N, et al. Elective versus therapeutic neck dissection in node-negative oral cancer. *N Engl J Med.* 2015;373(6):521–529.
99. Antoniades K, Lazaridis N, Vahtsevanos K, et al. Treatment of squamous cell carcinoma of the anterior faucial pillar-retromolar trigone. *Oral Oncol.* 2003;39(7):680–686.
100. Bachar G, Goldstein DP, Barker E, et al. Squamous cell carcinoma of the buccal mucosa: outcomes of treatment in the modern era. *Laryngoscope.* 2012;122(7): 1552–1557.
101. Os AD, Karakullukcu B, Leemans CR, et al. Management of the clinically N0 neck in squamous cell carcinoma of the maxillary alveolus and hard palate. *Head Neck.* 2016;38(12):1794–1798.
102. Acevedo JR, Fero KE, Wilson B, et al. Cost-effectiveness analysis of elective neck dissection in patients with clinically node-negative oral cavity cancer. *J Clin Oncol.* 2016;34(32):3886–3891.
103. Schilling C, Stoeckli SJ, Haerle SK, et al. Sentinel European Node Trial (SENT): 3-year results of sentinel node biopsy in oral cancer. *Eur J Cancer.* 2015;51(18):2777–2784.
104. Civantos FJ, Zitsch RP, Schuller DE, et al. Sentinel lymph node biopsy accurately stages the regional lymph nodes for T1-T2 oral squamous cell carcinomas: results of a prospective multi-institutional trial. *J Clin Oncol.* 2010;28(8):1395–1400.
105. Liang L, Zhang T, Kong Q, et al. A meta-analysis on selective versus comprehensive neck dissection in oral squamous cell carcinoma patients with clinically node-positive neck. *Oral Oncol.* 2015;51(12):1076–1081.
106. Motiee-Langroudi M, Amali A, Saedi B, et al. Occult level IV metastases in clinically node-negative patients with oral tongue squamous cell carcinoma. *J Laryngol Otol.* 2016;130(5):474–477.
107. Dogan E, Cetinayak HO, Sarioglu S, et al. Patterns of cervical lymph node metastases in oral tongue squamous cell carcinoma: implications for elective and therapeutic neck dissection. *J Laryngol Otol.* 2014;128(3):268–273.
108. Hanasono MM, Friel MT, Klem C, et al. Impact of reconstructive microsurgery in patients with advanced oral cavity cancers. *Head Neck.* 2009;31(10):1289–1296.
109. Seikaly H, Rieger J, O'Connell D, et al. Beavertail modification of the radial forearm free flap in base of tongue reconstruction: technique and functional outcomes. *Head Neck.* 2009;31(2):213–219.
110. Kimata Y, Sakuraba M, Hishinuma S, et al. Analysis of the relations between the shape of the reconstructed tongue and postoperative functions after subtotal or total glossectomy. *Laryngoscope.* 2003;113(5):905–909.
111. Baas M, Duraku LS, Corten EM, Mureau MA. A systematic review on the sensory reinnervation of free flaps for tongue reconstruction: does improved sensibility imply functional benefits? *J Plast Reconstr Aesthet Surg.* 2015;68(8):1025–1035.
112. Gibber MJ, Clain JB, Jacobson AS, et al. Subscapular system of flaps: an 8-year experience with 105 patients. *Head Neck.* 2015;37(8):1200–1206.
113. Usami S, Okazaki M, Tanaka K, et al. Lengthening the pedicle of a scapular osseous free flap by angular branch reconnection within the subscapular artery system. *Microsurgery.* 2014;34(8):662–665.
114. Shipchandler TZ, Waters HH, Knott PD, Fritz MA. Orbitomaxillary reconstruction using the layered fibula osteocutaneous flap. *Arch Facial Plast Surg.* 2012;14(2):110–115.
115. Miles BA, Gilbert RW. Maxillary reconstruction with the scapular angle osteomyogenous free flap. *Arch Otolaryngol Head Neck Surg.* 2011;137(11):1130–1135.
116. Pagedar NA, Gilbert RW, Chan H, et al. Maxillary reconstruction using the scapular tip free flap: a radiologic comparison of 3D morphology. *Head Neck.* 2012;34(10):1377–1382.
117. Burgess M, Leung M, Chellapah A, et al. Osseointegrated implants into a variety of composite free flaps: a comparative analysis. *Head Neck.* 2017;39(3):443–447.
118. Bossi P, Lo Vullo S, Guzzo M, et al. Preoperative chemotherapy in advanced resectable OCSCC: long-term results of a randomized phase III trial. *Ann Oncol.* 2014;25(2):462–466.
119. Licitra L, Grandi C, Guzzo M, et al. Primary chemotherapy in resectable oral cavity squamous cell cancer: a randomized controlled trial. *J Clin Oncol.* 2003;21(2):327–333.
120. Zhong LP, Zhang CP, Ren GX, et al. Randomized phase III trial of induction chemotherapy with docetaxel, cisplatin, and fluorouracil followed by surgery versus up-front surgery in locally advanced resectable oral squamous cell carcinoma. *J Clin Oncol.* 2013;31(6):744–751.

121. Marta GN, Riera R, Bossi P, et al. Induction chemotherapy prior to surgery with or without postoperative radiotherapy for oral cavity cancer patients: systematic review and meta-analysis. *Eur J Cancer.* 2015;51(17):2596–2603.
122. Perrone F, Bossi P, Cortelazzi B, et al. TP53 mutations and pathologic complete response to neoadjuvant cisplatin and fluorouracil chemotherapy in resected oral cavity squamous cell carcinoma. *J Clin Oncol.* 2010;28(5):761–766.
123. Spaulding CA, Korb LJ, Constable WC, et al. The influence of extent of neck treatment upon control of cervical lymphadenopathy in cancers of the oral tongue. *Int J Radiat Oncol Biol Phys.* 1991;21(3):577–581.
124. Chen TC, Wang CT, Ko JY, et al. Postoperative radiotherapy for primary early oral tongue cancer with pathologic N1 neck. *Head Neck.* 2010;32(5):555–561.
125. Lavaf A, Genden EM, Cesaretti JA, et al. Adjuvant radiotherapy improves overall survival for patients with lymph node-positive head and neck squamous cell carcinoma. *Cancer.* 2008;112(3):535–543.
126. Chen MM, Harris JP, Hara W, et al. Association of postoperative radiotherapy with survival in patients with N1 oral cavity and oropharyngeal squamous cell carcinoma. *JAMA Otolaryngol Head Neck Surg.* 2016;142(12):1224–1230.
127. Dawson LA, Anzai Y, Marsh L, et al. Patterns of local-regional recurrence following parotid-sparing conformal and segmental intensity-modulated radiotherapy for head and neck cancer. *Int J Radiat Oncol Biol Phys.* 2000;46(5):1117–1126.
128. Damast S, Wolden S, Lee N. Marginal recurrences after selective targeting with intensity-modulated radiotherapy for oral tongue cancer. *Head Neck.* 2012;34(6):900–906.
129. Gregoire V, Eisbruch A, Hamoir M, Levendag P. Proposal for the delineation of the nodal CTV in the node-positive and the post-operative neck. *Radiother Oncol.* 2006;79(1):15–20.
130. Chan AK, Huang SH, Le LW, et al. Postoperative intensity-modulated radiotherapy following surgery for oral cavity squamous cell carcinoma: patterns of failure. *Oral Oncol.* 2013;49(3):255–260.
131. Geretschlager A, Bojaxhiu B, Crowe S, et al. Outcome and patterns of failure after postoperative intensity modulated radiotherapy for locally advanced or high-risk oral cavity squamous cell carcinoma. *Radiat Oncol.* 2012;7:175,717X-7-175.
132. Inhestern J, Oertel K, Stemmann V, et al. Prognostic role of circulating tumor cells during induction chemotherapy followed by curative surgery combined with postoperative radiotherapy in patients with locally advanced oral and oropharyngeal squamous cell cancer. *PLOS ONE.* 2015;10(7):e0132901.
133. Metcalfe E, Aspin L, Speight R, et al. Postoperative (chemo)radiotherapy for oral cavity squamous cell carcinomas: outcomes and patterns of failure. *Clin Oncol (R Coll Radiol).* 2017;29(1):51–59.
134. Yao M, Chang K, Funk GF, et al. The failure patterns of oral cavity squamous cell carcinoma after intensity-modulated radiotherapy-the university of iowa experience. *Int J Radiat Oncol Biol Phys.* 2007;67(5):1332–1341.
135. Chen AM, Farwell DG, Luu Q, et al. Marginal misses after postoperative intensity-modulated radiotherapy for head and neck cancer. *Int J Radiat Oncol Biol Phys.* 2011;80(5):1423–1429.
136. Kurita H, Koike T, Narikawa JN, et al. Clinical predictors for contralateral neck lymph node metastasis from unilateral squamous cell carcinoma in the oral cavity. *Oral Oncol.* 2004;40(9):898–903.
137. Bernier J, Domenge C, Ozsahin M, et al. Postoperative irradiation with or without concomitant chemotherapy for locally advanced head and neck cancer. *N Engl J Med.* 2004;350(19):1945–1952.
138. Nutting CM, Morden JP, Harrington KJ, et al. Parotid-sparing intensity modulated versus conventional radiotherapy in head and neck cancer (PARSPORT): a phase 3 multicentre randomised controlled trial. *Lancet Oncol.* 2011;12(2):127–136.
139. Dixit S, Vyas RK, Toparani RB, et al. Surgery versus surgery and postoperative radiotherapy in squamous cell carcinoma of the buccal mucosa: a comparative study. *Ann Surg Oncol.* 1998;5(6):502–510.
140. Brown JS, Shaw RJ, Bekiroglu F, Rogers SN. Systematic review of the current evidence in the use of postoperative radiotherapy for oral squamous cell carcinoma. *Br J Oral Maxillofac Surg.* 2012;50(6):481–489.
141. Mishra RC, Singh DN, Mishra TK. Post-operative radiotherapy in carcinoma of buccal mucosa, a prospective randomized trial. *Eur J Surg Oncol.* 1996;22(5):502–504.
142. Shrime MG, Gullane PJ, Dawson L, et al. The impact of adjuvant radiotherapy on survival in T1-2N1 squamous cell carcinoma of the oral cavity. *Arch Otolaryngol Head Neck Surg.* 2010;136(3):225–228.
143. Cooper JS, Zhang Q, Pajak TF, et al. Long-term follow-up of the RTOG 9501/intergroup phase III trial: postoperative concurrent radiation therapy and chemotherapy in high-risk squamous cell carcinoma of the head and neck. *Int J Radiat Oncol Biol Phys.* 2012;84(5):1198–1205.
144. Bernier J, Cooper JS, Pajak TF, et al. Defining risk levels in locally advanced head and neck cancers: a comparative analysis of concurrent postoperative radiation plus chemotherapy trials of the EORTC (#22931) and RTOG (# 9501). *Head Neck.* 2005;27(10):843–850.
145. Brockmeyer P, Hemmerlein B, Kruppa J, et al. The time interval between primary surgery and adjuvant therapy determines prognosis of oral squamous cell carcinomas. *Oral Oncol.* 2015;51(11):e82–e85.
146. Noble AR, Greskovich JF, Han J, et al. Risk factors associated with disease recurrence in patients with Stage III/IV squamous cell carcinoma of the oral cavity treated with surgery and postoperative radiotherapy. *Anticancer Res.* 2016;36(2):785–792.

147. Schwam ZG, Judson BL. Improved prognosis for patients with oral cavity squamous cell carcinoma: Analysis of the National Cancer Database 1998–2006. *Oral Oncol.* 2016;52:45–51.
148. Wreesmann VB, Katabi N, Palmer FL, et al. Influence of extracapsular nodal spread extent on prognosis of oral squamous cell carcinoma. *Head Neck.* 2016;38(suppl 1):E1192–E1199.
149. Lemieux A, Kedarisetty S, Raju S, et al. Lymph node yield as a predictor of survival in pathologically node negative oral cavity carcinoma. *Otolaryngol Head Neck Surg.* 2016;154(3):465–472.
150. Amit M, Yen TC, Liao CT, et al. The origin of regional failure in oral cavity squamous cell carcinoma with pathologically negative neck metastases. *JAMA Otolaryngol Head Neck Surg.* 2014;140(12):1130–1137.
151. Ebrahimi A, Clark JR, Amit M, et al. Minimum nodal yield in oral squamous cell carcinoma: defining the standard of care in a multicenter international pooled validation study. *Ann Surg Oncol.* 2014;21(9):3049–3055.
152. Shrime MG, Ma C, Gullane PJ, et al. Impact of nodal ratio on survival in squamous cell carcinoma of the oral cavity. *Head Neck.* 2009;31(9):1129–1136.
153. Shrime MG, Bachar G, Lea J, et al. Nodal ratio as an independent predictor of survival in squamous cell carcinoma of the oral cavity. *Head Neck.* 2009;31(11):1482–1488.
154. Urban D, Gluck I, Pfeffer MR, et al. Lymph node ratio predicts the benefit of post-operative radiotherapy in oral cavity cancer. *Radiother Oncol.* 2013;106(1):74–79.
155. Ebrahimi A, Clark JR, Zhang WJ, et al. Lymph node ratio as an independent prognostic factor in oral squamous cell carcinoma. *Head Neck.* 2011;33(9):1245–1251.
156. Marchiano E, Patel TD, Eloy JA, et al. Impact of nodal level distribution on survival in oral cavity squamous cell carcinoma: a population-based study. *Otolaryngol Head Neck Surg.* 2016;155(1):99–105.
157. Goodwin WJ, Jr. Salvage surgery for patients with recurrent squamous cell carcinoma of the upper aerodigestive tract: when do the ends justify the means? *Laryngoscope.* 2000;110(3, Pt 2, Suppl 93):1–18.
158. Yuen AP, Wei WI, Lam LK, et al. Results of surgical salvage of locoregional recurrence of carcinoma of the tongue after radiotherapy failure. *Ann Otol Rhinol Laryngol.* 1997;106(9):779–782.
159. Leon X, Martinez V, Lopez M, et al. Second, third, and fourth head and neck tumors. A progressive decrease in survival. *Head Neck.* 2012;34(12):1716–1719.
160. Vermorken JB, Remenar E, van Herpen C, et al. Cisplatin, fluorouracil, and docetaxel in unresectable head and neck cancer. *N Engl J Med.* 2007;357(17):1695–1704.

16

Nasopharyngeal Cancer

Wai Tong Ng
Oscar S. H. Chan
Henry C. K. Sze
Ka On Lam
Anne W. M. Lee

In 2012, there were 87,000 new cases of nasopharyngeal carcinoma (NPC) worldwide (1). While NPC is rare at most parts of the world, this disease is highly prevalent in Southern China, Eskimos, and certain regions in North Africa. Epidemiological studies suggest that the etiology of NPC is multifactorial; major factors include genetic susceptibility, chemical carcinogen (particularly volatile nitrosamine in Cantonese salted fish), and latent Epstein–Barr virus (EBV) infection. Virtually all nonkeratinizing type NPC cancer cells are associated with EBV latent infection. An interplay of these etiological factors on susceptible individuals has been proposed (2).

The current pathologic classification by the World Health Organization (WHO) includes: keratinizing squamous cell carcinoma (formerly, WHO type I), nonkeratinizing squamous cell carcinoma including differentiated (formerly, WHO type II) and undifferentiated (formerly, WHO type III) subtypes, and basaloid squamous cell carcinoma. In endemic areas, the nonkeratinizing subtypes account for more than 95% of all cases (3).

NPC most commonly arises from the fossa of Rosenmüller. It is notorious for its aggressive natural behavior with extensive local infiltration, early lymphatic spread, and predilection for hematogenous dissemination. The most common presenting symptom is cervical lymphadenopathy, followed by nasal symptoms, such as postnasal drip and bleeding, and aural symptoms, such as tinnitus, hearing impairment, and discharge. Patients with advanced local disease may also suffer from headache and symptoms related to cranial nerve damage (facial numbness, diplopia).

Clinical evaluation for NPC includes examination of the neck and cranial nerves, nasopharyngoscopy, and MRI of the nasopharynx and neck. PET–CT is indicated especially for patients with N2-3 or T3-4 diseases, symptoms or signs suggestive of distant metastasis, abnormal liver function tests, and/or high copies of plasma EBV DNA.

The American Joint Committee on Cancer (AJCC)/Union for International Cancer Control (UICC) has recently revised the staging system to better reflect the treatment outcomes in the era of intensity modulated radiotherapy (IMRT; Table 16.1) (4–6). Changes in the new 8th edition include:

T category:

- Adjacent muscles' involvement (including medial pterygoid, lateral pterygoid, and prevertebral muscles) is now designated as T2. Medial and lateral pterygoid muscle involvement was staged as T4 as part of the "masticator space," and prevertebral muscle involvement was not included in previous staging systems.

TABLE 16.1

AJCC 8th ed. (2017) Staging for Nasopharynx Cancer*

<table>
<tr><th colspan="2">T/M \ N</th><th>cN0</th><th>cN1</th><th>cN2</th><th>cN3</th></tr>
<tr><td>T0</td><td>• No primary tumor, but EBV-positive cervical node(s)</td><td></td><td rowspan="3">II</td><td rowspan="4">III</td><td rowspan="5">IVA</td></tr>
<tr><td>T1</td><td>• Confined to nasopharynx or extension to oropharynx/nasal cavity</td><td>I</td></tr>
<tr><td>T2</td><td>• Extension to parapharyngeal space and/or medial pterygoid, lateral pterygoid, prevertebral muscles</td><td></td></tr>
<tr><td>T3</td><td>• Infiltration of bony structures[1]</td><td colspan="2"></td></tr>
<tr><td>T4</td><td>• Extension[2]</td><td colspan="3"></td></tr>
<tr><td>M1</td><td>• Distant metastasis</td><td colspan="4">IVB</td></tr>
</table>

**Major changes from AJCC 7th edition include adjacent muscle involvement (pterygoid/prevertebral) T2 classification, collapse of N3a-b into single N3 category, and grouped stage IVA and IVB merged into IVA, with IVC becoming IVB.*

[1]Skull base, cervical vertebrae, pterygoid plates, paranasal sinuses. [2]Intracranial extension and/or involvement of cranial nerves, hypopharynx, orbit, parotid gland, soft tissue beyond lateral surface of lateral pterygoid muscle.

AJCC, American Joint Committee on Cancer; cN0, no regional lymph node metastasis; cN1, unilateral LNs and/or unilateral or bilateral metastasis in RPNs (≤6 cm), above caudal border of cricoid; cN2, bilateral LNs (≤6 cm), above caudal border of cricoid; cN3, unilateral or bilateral LNs (>6 cm) and/or LNs below caudal border of cricoid cartilage; EBV, Epstein–Barr virus; LN, lymph node; RPN, retropharyngeal lymph node.

- The previous T4 criteria "masticator space" and "infratemporal fossa" are now replaced by specific description of soft tissue involvement to avoid ambiguity.

N category:

- The previous N3b criterion of supraclavicular fossa is now changed to lower neck (as defined by nodal extension below the caudal border of the cricoid cartilage).
- N3a and N3b are merged into a single N3 category, which is now defined as unilateral or bilateral metastasis in cervical lymph node(s), larger than 6 cm in greatest dimension, and/or extension below the caudal border of cricoid cartilage.

Stage group:

- The previous substages IVA (T4 N0-2 M0) and IVB (any T N3 M0) are now merged to form IVA.
- The previous IVC (any T any N M1) is now classified as IVB.

In addition to tumor, node, and metastasis (TNM) parameters, further refinement of prognostication has been proposed using nomogram incorporating other independent prognostic factors including tumor volume, lactate dehydrogenase, and age (7). Plasma EBV DNA is also a promising factor for predicting prognosis as well as disease monitoring. However, standardization of assay method is needed in order to allow valid comparisons between different series (8).

Definitive radiation therapy (RT) by IMRT is the primary treatment modality for NPC because it is a radiosensitive tumor and its anatomical location makes surgical resection technically challenging. Early cancers (stage I) are treated with RT alone with excellent outcome. Combined modality treatment with the addition of concurrent chemotherapy using cisplatin is recommended for locoregionally advanced diseases. There are variations in major guidelines regarding whether adjuvant or induction chemotherapy using cisplatin-based combinations should be further added (9–11). Concurrent chemoradiation (CRT) has been recommended for stage II based on past series treated with two-dimensional (2D) RT, but there is increasing retrospective evidence that excellent outcome can be achieved by IMRT alone; low-risk patients can be safely spared of unnecessary chemotherapy. Treatment for metastatic disease should be individualized: radical treatment could be attempted for those with oligometastasis and good performance status. All patients should be closely monitored because early detection of recurrence significantly affects the chance of survival. Aggressive salvage therapy should be considered for patients with local/regional recurrence or oligometastasis as far as possible. Patients should be followed up for life to ensure proper management of late toxicities.

CASE SUMMARIES

CASE 16.1

Mr. CKC was first diagnosed with NPC in 2006 when he was 46 years old. Nasopharyngoscopy showed a tumor over the nasopharynx and biopsy confirmed undifferentiated carcinoma. Staging evaluation by MRI and PET–CT showed stage II NPC (T2N0M0) with parapharyngeal space involvement. He was treated with RT alone using IMRT technique.

He was found to have local recurrence of NPC, stage rT3N0 disease in 2011 (i.e., 5 years later). Plasma level of EBV DNA was 0 copy/mL. He was recruited into a clinical trial and was treated with induction chemotherapy using docetaxel, cisplatin, and 5-fluorouracil for three cycles, followed by reirradiation concurrent with weekly cetuximab and docetaxel (12). He developed grade 2 soft tissue necrosis in 2012. In 2014, he had local recurrence again. He was given palliative chemotherapy using carboplatin and gemcitabine for 6 cycles (13); but disease progressed, and he was treated with capecitabine for 17 cycles. In 2016, he showed further disease progression together with asymptomatic temporal lobe necrosis (TLN); he was treated with pembrolizumab, a monoclonal antibody against programmed cell death 1 (PD-1) receptor (14). Stable disease was achieved and he remained progression free up to the latest assessment, 9 months following commencement of immunotherapy.

CASE 16.2

Mr. PWY, a 55-year-old gentleman, presented with throat discomfort and headache for 1 month in 2009. Nasopharyngoscopy revealed a large irregular growth occupying the whole nasopharynx, with bilateral nasal cavity extension. Biopsy of the tumor confirmed undifferentiated carcinoma. The plasma EBV DNA level was 2,338 copies/mL. MRI showed that the tumor had infiltrated into the left prevertebral muscle and clivus, but there was no regional lymphadenopathy. PET–CT did not show distant metastases. His clinical stage was T3N0M0, stage III NPC. The initial plan was RT concurrent with cisplatin, followed by three more cycles of adjuvant cisplatin and fluorouracil. The primary tumor and bilateral neck was irradiated using IMRT technique. However, the patient developed grade 3 mucositis and odynophagia requiring short-term tube feeding, accompanied by mild transient renal impairment after 50 Gy of IMRT. Adjuvant therapy was omitted because of the toxicities in concurrent phase treatment and patient's preference. The posttreatment assessment by MRI scan showed complete remission and the plasma EBV DNA returned to 0 copy/mL.

However, 18 months after initial therapy, plasma EBV DNA level became detectable (70 copies/mL); PET–CT scan was performed and a solitary right lower lung mass was detected. Biopsy confirmed metastatic undifferentiated carcinoma. This solitary lung metastasis was treated with stereotactic ablative RT to a total dose of 54 Gy in 3 weekly fraction (15), followed by six cycles of systemic chemotherapy using cisplatin and gemcitabine. His disease remains in remission after salvage treatment.

EVIDENCE-BASED CASE DISCUSSION

RADIATION THERAPY

Definitive RT is the primary treatment modality for NPC. Although NPC is a radiosensitive tumor, retrospective studies showed that high-dose RT of at least 70 Gy is needed even for T1-2 diseases. A recent study by Ng et al. (16) using IMRT showed that patients with gross tumor volume (GTV) receiving dose <66.5 Gy had significantly higher incidence of recurrence even with combined modality treatment using concurrent ± sequential chemotherapy.

With conventional 2D technique, the RT field arrangement typically included two lateral facial–cervical fields ± one anterior facial field, together with a matched low anterior cervical field. The whole RT course was split into two to three phases in order to deliver a radical dose of 66 to 70 Gy to the gross tumor and a lower elective dose to subclinical high-risk regions. With anatomical proximity of critical structures, the therapeutic margin is notoriously narrow. In addition to acute toxicities including mucositis, dysphagia, and skin reaction, there is substantial risk of late toxicities such as xerostomia, hearing impairment, soft tissue fibrosis, TLN, endocrine dysfunction, swallowing disorder, and second malignancy among long-term survivors (17). Additional boost dose by brachytherapy or stereotactic radiotherapy (SRT) has been advocated for improving local control (18–20). Brachytherapy was most commonly done with customized nasopharyngeal applicators and high-dose rate afterloading system. It is highly dependent on operator skill and the size and location of tumor to attain a satisfactory dose distribution. SRT allowed dose optimization with inverse planning technique and could be used even for eccentric and bulky tumors. However, such dose escalation was rarely needed in the modern era using IMRT.

Today, IMRT has become the standard of care because of its superior RT dose distribution, which allows better coverage of the complex concave-shaped target volumes and minimizing the dose to adjacent normal organs. Typically, multiple intensity modulated coplanar fields or volumetric modulated arcs are used to achieve the best dose conformity. Multiple retrospective and randomized studies on IMRT versus 2D-RT (21–25) have demonstrated that IMRT could achieve better disease control (22), fewer RT-related late complications (21,22,25), lower RT dose to the parotid glands (23,24), significant reduction of xerostomia-related symptoms (23), and better quality of life (24,25).

While IMRT has achieved excellent treatment outcomes in general, advanced local diseases are still difficult to tackle. In fact, the 5-year local control for T4 disease in multiple studies ranges from 74% to 80% (16,22,26,27), compared to the 90% for earlier diseases. Late toxicities, especially neurological damage, are also more common after treatments of T3-4 diseases (22). This is due to lesion abutting to critical structures, and studies have shown that both tumor volume and the degree of underdosing (in order to spare the organ at risk [OAR]) significantly affected the overall survival (OS). Various strategies (28) have been proposed including induction therapy, lessening of dose constraint for OARs, image-guided radiotherapy, and more recently, intensity modulated proton therapy (29).

Owing to the tight margin with IMRT, variations in body contour and volumes of tumor, as well as normal organs, which occur during the course of RT could alter the resultant dose distribution significantly, leading to suboptimal target dose coverage or excessive dose to the OARs (30,31). One strategy that has been proposed to tackle this problem is adaptive RT. CT, or less commonly MRI, is performed within the course of RT to assess the anatomical variation, and if necessary, treatment is replanned accordingly. Improvement in locoregional control and quality of life has been observed (32). Further studies are warranted to confirm the best timing and the benefit of such an adaptive approach.

Many recent studies have also looked at elective nodal irradiation. Although level II and retropharyngeal nodes are found to be the most common sites of lymph node metastasis, there is increasing evidence to support the omission of prophylactic RT to lower neck for N0 disease. For example, Gao et al. (33) found that RT to level II, III, and Va produced very favorable treatment outcomes for patients with N0 diseases. Li et al. (34) showed that prophylactic upper neck irradiation achieved similar survival outcomes as with whole neck irradiation. Furthermore, there is preliminary evidence showing a low incidence of level IB nodal metastasis; omission of level IB and sparing of submandibular gland to reduce xerostomia has also been suggested (35).

ROLE OF CHEMOTHERAPY FOR STAGE II DISEASE

Early-stage NPC has an excellent chance of cure by RT alone. Even in the era of conventional 2D-RT, favorable results with 5-year local failure-free (LFF) rates ranging from 84% to 93% and OS rates ranging from 71% to 95% have been reported (36–41). However, in some of the initial pivotal clinical trials (42,43) studying the effect of chemotherapy in combination with RT in locally advanced NPC, some of the patients were actually stage II by the current staging system due to changes in staging criteria; hence the recommendation of adding chemotherapy was extended to include stage II patients.

The only phase III randomized study comparing CRT versus RT alone was reported by Chen et al. (44). In this study, 230 patients with stage II disease by the Chinese 1992 staging system (90% stage II and 10% stage III by the AJCC/UICC system, 7th edition) were recruited and randomized to radical RT with or without concurrent weekly cisplatin 30 mg/m^2. Significant improvement in the 5-year rates of OS (95% vs. 86%, p = .007), progression-free survival (PFS; 88% vs. 78%, p = .017), and distant metastasis-free survival (MFS; 95% vs. 84%, p = .007) was achieved by CRT. The use of CRT also incurred significantly higher incidence of grade 3 to 4 acute toxicities (64% vs. 40%), but without excessive increase in late toxicity. However, all the patients in this trial were treated by conventional 2D-RT and it is uncertain whether the result could still be applicable when IMRT is commonly used nowadays.

It is noteworthy that in the update of individual patient data meta-analysis by the Meta-Analysis of Chemotherapy in Nasopharynx Carcinoma (MAC-NPC) collaborative group (45), a study of the variation of the chemotherapy effect according to stage (I–II [mostly stage II] vs. III vs. IV) was possible among the 10 trials (1,622 patients): the corresponding hazard ratios (HRs; 95% confidence interval [CI]) were 0.95 (0.65–1.44), 0.75 (0.59–0.94), and 0.72 (0.58–0.89), respectively (test for trend p = .24). The corresponding absolute benefits at 5-year OS were: 3.6%, 6.0%, and 8.1%, respectively. These results showed that the beneficial effect of adding chemotherapy was small in early-stage disease even in an era when the majority of the patients were treated with 2D technique.

With further improvement of local control by IMRT, the reported treatment outcomes for early-stage NPC were excellent: 5-year LFF and OS rates being 94% to 100% and 91% to 100%, respectively (46–48). Substantial improvement by the addition of concurrent chemotherapy would be limited. Several recently published retrospective studies showed that when IMRT was used, adding concurrent chemotherapy did not achieve additional benefit in tumor control, but incurred increase in toxicities (49–51).

It has been suggested that a more personalized approach for the use of chemotherapy in early-stage NPC according to individual risk should be adopted (52). Factors including the volume of the primary tumor (53,54), pretreatment level of plasma EBV DNA (55), and the extent of node positivity (36,41) are promising candidates to be considered. Trials exploring the benefit of concurrent chemotherapy in high-risk population of early-stage disease treated with modern RT technique are warranted.

COMBINED MODALITY THERAPY FOR LOCOREGIONALLY ADVANCED DISEASE

Chemoradiotherapy

Chemotherapy helps to further improve local control by potentiating RT effect and reduce distant failure by eradicating subclinical microscopic disease. It has been extensively studied in various combinations with RT and achieved great success. The Intergroup-0099 Study was the first randomized trial that achieved significant benefit by the addition of chemotherapy to RT (42). The regimen consisted of cisplatin (100 mg/m^2) every 3 weeks for three cycles given concurrently with conventionally fractionated RT followed by adjuvant chemotherapy using cisplatin (80 mg/m^2) and fluorouracil (4,000 mg/m^2 in 96 hours) every 4 weeks for three cycles. An unprecedented survival gain was demonstrated: the 3-year OS rates significantly improved from 47% by RT alone to 78% (p = .005) by the use of CRT. However, the result of the RT alone group was substantially poorer than that achieved by major centers. Four confirmatory randomized trials were then conducted in endemic regions (56–59). Although the magnitude of benefit was smaller, improvement in event-free survival (EFS) was consistently demonstrated.

In the first individual patient data MAC-NPC (60) over eight randomized trials and 1,753 patients, a significant absolute OS benefit of 6% (56% vs. 62%) and EFS benefit of 10% (42% vs. 52%) at 5 years by adding chemotherapy to RT was demonstrated. This benefit was found to have strong interaction with timing of chemotherapy when the HR was lowest for concomitant ± adjuvant trials (HR: 0.60, 95% CI: 0.48–0.76), compared with induction (HR: 0.99, 95% CI: 0.80–1.12) and adjuvant (HR: 0.97, 95% CI: 0.69–1.38) trials. It led to the conclusion that the magnitude of benefit is greatest when chemotherapy was administered concomitantly with RT.

Attempts have been made to replace cisplatin with less toxic platinum agents for concurrent CRT. In the studies by Zhang et al. and Wu et al. (61,62), oxaliplatin 70 mg/m^2 weekly concurrent with RT was compared with RT alone. Compliance with chemotherapy was excellent, with 97% of patients completing all planned doses of oxaliplatin and RT. The 5-year OS and MFS rates in the concurrent CRT group were significantly higher than those observed in the RT-alone group (OS, 73.2% vs. 60.2%; MFS, 74.7% vs. 63.0%). The survival benefit was demonstrated by the concurrent arm. Unfortunately there is no head-to-head comparison of oxaliplatin with cisplatin and further validation of its role is necessary. A randomized noninferiority trial in Thailand (63) consisting of 206 patients compared weekly carboplatin 100 mg/m^2 concurrently with RT followed by three more cycles of adjuvant carboplatin/fluorouracil versus cisplatin 100 mg/m^2 every 3 weeks for three cycles concurrent with RT followed by three more cycles of adjuvant cisplatin/fluorouracil. Carboplatin was shown to be better tolerated with a higher rate of completion of the planned CRT (73% vs. 59%) and adjuvant chemotherapy (70% vs. 42%). Carboplatin was associated with less renal toxicity, leucopenia, and anemia than cisplatin, but more thrombocytopenia. The 3-year disease-free survival (DFS) rates were similar (63% vs. 61%). However, in view of short follow-up (median: 26 months), a large number of patients being excluded for per protocol analysis and lack of confirmatory study, carboplatin is yet to be the standard option but can be considered for those who cannot tolerate cisplatin. Finally, the use of weekly cisplatin to ameliorate cisplatin toxicities is common among Asian centers. While randomized trial has shown the superiority of weekly concurrent cisplatin over RT alone for stage II disease based on the Chinese 1992 staging system (44), the benefit on locoregional advanced NPC is far less certain as a study by Chan et al. (43,64) showed only borderline statistically significant difference in OS in favor of the concurrent arm (p = .065) on unadjusted analysis. In a Korean phase II study (65), 109 stage II-IVB patients were randomly assigned to a regimen of either 7 weekly doses of cisplatin (40 mg/m^2) or 3 doses of cisplatin (100 mg/m^2) given every 3 weeks concurrently with RT. The mean total cisplatin dose was similar between the two arms. There were no significant differences in the 3-year PFS (65% vs. 64%) as well as the occurrence of grade 3-4 toxicities (47% vs. 39%) between the two regimens. Quality of life related to functional outcomes was better for the weekly regimen. Furthermore, in a recent phase III study, which compared cisplatin 100 mg/m^2 every 3 weeks for two cycles with cisplatin 40 mg/m^2 weekly up to six cycles concurrently with IMRT in 526 patients with stage II-IVB NPC (66), the estimated 2-year failure-free survival rates were not statistically different: 92% in the weekly arm and 88.3% in the every-3-week arm (HR: 1.056, 95% CI: 0.58–1.92). Despite similar grade 3 or 4 toxicities in both treatment arms, leucopenia and thrombocytopenia were in fact more common in the weekly cisplatin arm. Longer follow-up is needed to fully assess the treatment outcome and late toxicities.

Attempts have also been made to replace concurrent CRT with concurrent cetuximab-RT. In a study by Xu et al. (67), patients with stage III-IVb NPC were treated with IMRT and were randomized to concurrent weekly cisplatin 30 mg/m^2 or weekly cetuximab (loading dose of 400 mg/m^2 followed by weekly doses of 250 mg/m^2) after two cycles of induction chemotherapy (docetaxel 75 mg/m^2 and cisplatin 80 mg/m^2). The study was closed prematurely because of unexpectedly high rates of grade 3/4 mucositis observed in the cetuximab arm. Only 44 patients were enrolled. Oral mucositis, acneiform rash, and dysphagia were all increased in the cetuximab arm. No significant difference was observed for the 3-year DFS. The recommended treatment modality was still concurrent cisplatin–IMRT.

Concurrent Chemoradiation Followed by Adjuvant Chemotherapy

Because adjuvant chemotherapy is difficult to tolerate due to acute residual side effects from CRT and all randomized clinical trials examining RT with adjuvant chemotherapy versus RT alone have not shown any survival benefit (68,69), the effect of adjuvant chemotherapy in addition to concurrent CRT has been questioned. Chen et al. (70) reported a phase III randomized trial that randomized 508 patients with stage III-IVB disease to concurrent or concurrent–adjuvant CRT. Concurrent CRT consisted of cisplatin 40 mg/m^2 weekly and those allocated to concurrent–adjuvant CRT were given additional three cycles of cisplatin (80 mg/m^2) and fluorouracil (4,000 mg/m^2 in 120 hours) after RT. After a median follow-up of 38 months, there was no significant difference in the 2-year failure-free survival rates: 86% in the concurrent–adjuvant group versus 84% in the concurrent-only group. However, the compliance to treatment was poor. Long-term results are still awaited.

The updated individual patient data based MAC-NPC has shed further insights (45). In this update, 19 trials performed up to 2010 with 4,806 patients were included for analysis. Separate analyses were performed for the concurrent CRT alone and the concurrent–adjuvant CRT groups. With a median follow-up of 7.7 years, the study confirmed a small, but significant benefit in OS by adding chemotherapy: the absolute gain for OS was 6% at 5 years and 8% at 10 years (57% vs. 49%). A significant interaction between treatment effect on OS and the timing of chemotherapy was again observed. The HR for the use of concurrent–adjuvant CRT was the lowest (HR 0.65 [0.56;0.76]) compared to concurrent CRT alone (HR 0.79 [0.68;0.92]), induction chemotherapy (HR 0.96 [0.80;1.16]), and adjuvant chemotherapy alone (HR 0.93 [0.70;1.24]). Furthermore, in the individual patient data network meta-analysis by the MAC-NPC Collaborative Group (71), the three treatments with the highest probability of benefit on OS were concurrent–adjuvant CRT, followed by concurrent CRT alone and induction–concurrent CRT, with their respective *p* scores (higher score meaning a higher probability of being the best treatment) of 96%, 70%, and 63%. These translated into 5 years absolute benefit of 12%, 8%, and 6%, respectively, when compared with RT alone.

The use of post-RT EBV DNA has been studied as a biomarker to select patients to undergo further adjuvant chemotherapy. In a study by Chan et al. (72), among 789 patients with stage IIB-IVB NPC undergoing EBV DNA screening at 6 to 8 weeks after RT, 218 (27.6%) patients had detectable EBV DNA (>0 copy/mL), and 104 (13.2%) were randomized to adjuvant cisplatin 40 mg/m^2 and gemcitabine 1,000 mg/m^2, both given on days 1 and 8, every 3 weeks for six cycles, or observation alone. After median follow-up of 6.5 years, the 5-year rates of OS, locoregional, and distant failure-free survival were comparable for the two arms. The NRG [NSABP (National Surgical Adjuvant Breast and Bowel Project)—N, RTOG (Radiation Therapy Oncology Group)—R, GOG (Gynecologic Oncology Group)—G] is conducting a randomized study for stage III-IVB NPC to further explore the use of EBV DNA as a biomarker to select patients for adjuvant chemotherapy (NCT02135042). Those with undetectable EBV DNA after standard concurrent CRT will be randomized to either standard adjuvant chemotherapy with cisplatin and fluorouracil or observation, and those with detectable EBV DNA will be randomized to adjuvant chemotherapy with cisplatin and fluorouracil versus gemcitabine–paclitaxel. The results will help to define more clearly the role of adjuvant chemotherapy and whether EBV DNA is a useful tool for patient selection.

INDUCTION CHEMOTHERAPY FOLLOWED BY CONCURRENT CHEMORADIATION

In view of the poor tolerance to adjuvant chemotherapy, the use of induction chemotherapy has been studied as an alternative approach. It has most commonly been used for advanced local disease in order to improve the subsequent tumor coverage by high-dose RT. In a randomized phase II study (73), induction chemotherapy with docetaxel (75 mg/m^2) and cisplatin (75 mg/m^2) was given every 3 weeks for two cycles followed by weekly cisplatin (40 mg/m^2) concurrent with RT as compared with concurrent CRT alone. The OS rates for induction versus control arm were 94.1% vs. 67.7% (HR: 0.24, 95% CI: 0.078–0.73, p = .012), respectively, favoring the induction arm. However, the 3-year PFS was insignificant despite favorable trend: 88.2% versus 59.5% (HR: 0.49, 95% CI: 0.20–1.19, p = .12); furthermore, both end points became negative with longer follow-up (45). In addition, two other trials were negative. The randomized phase II study using epirubicin (75 mg/m^2), paclitaxel (175 mg/m^2), and cisplatin (75 mg/m^2) given every 3 weeks for three cycles as induction chemotherapy followed by concurrent CRT did not show any significant improvement in PFS and OS compared with concurrent CRT alone (74). A randomized phase III trial of induction therapy with paclitaxel (70 mg/m^2), carboplatin (area under the curve [AUC] 2.5), and gemcitabine (1,000 mg/m^2, day 1 and day 8) given every 3 weeks for three cycles followed by concurrent CRT with weekly cisplatin (40 mg/m^2) again failed to demonstrate any benefit by induction chemotherapy (75).

The preliminary results from several recent phase III randomized studies provided more encouraging results. In the study conducted in China (76), 480 patients with stage III-IVB NPC were randomized to induction chemotherapy with three cycles of docetaxel (60 mg/m^2), cisplatin (60 mg/m^2), and 5-fluorouracil (600 mg/m^2 per day, days 1–5) every 3 weeks followed by concurrent CRT (three cycles of cisplatin 100 mg/m^2 every 3 weeks) or concurrent CRT alone. Patients were all treated with IMRT. The 3-year rates of failure-free survival for induction–concurrent versus concurrent-alone arms were 80% versus 72% (HR: 0.68, 95% CI: 0·48–0·97, p = .034), OS 92% versus 86% (HR: 0.59, 95% CI: 0.36–0.95, p = .029); higher rates of neutropenia, leucopenia, and stomatitis were observed for induction–concurrent chemotherapy. Another study by the French Head and Neck Oncology and Radiotherapy Group (GORTEC) on stage II-IVB patients has stopped prematurely due to slow accrual (77). Among the 83 randomized patients, induction chemotherapy showed significant improvement in survival. Longer follow-up is necessary to evaluate the efficacy and late toxicity. In the study by Chen et al. (78), 476 patients with stage III-IVB (excluding T3N0-1) NPC were randomly assigned to receive induction chemotherapy using cisplatin (80 mg/m^2) and fluorouracil (800 mg/m^2 per day, days 1–5) every 3 weeks for two cycles followed by CRT or CRT alone. The induction chemotherapy arm achieved higher 3-year rates of DFS (82.0% vs. 74.1%; p = .028), though there were no statistically significant differences in OS or locoregional relapse-free survival.

The NPC-0501 trial by the Hong Kong Nasopharyngeal Cancer Study Group tested the sequencing of induction–concurrent CRT versus concurrent–adjuvant CRT, with the best studied Intergroup 0099 regimen as the control arm (79). It also evaluated the role of oral capecitabine in replacing 5-fluorouracil and accelerated RT fractionation. A total of 803 patients were randomized. Preliminary results showed that changing the sequence alone did not achieve significant improvement in PFS, but in the stratum irradiated with conventionally fractionated RT, the arm treated with induction chemotherapy using cisplatin–capecitabine (PX) versus adjuvant cisplatin–fluorouracil (PF), showed a better 3-year rate of PFS (81% vs. 75%; p = .045). Changing the fractionation from conventional to accelerated did not demonstrate any benefit. Longer follow-up is needed to confirm the findings.

MANAGEMENT OF LOCAL RELAPSE

Management of local relapse should be individualized based on recurrent tumor extent, availability of surgical expertise, time to recurrence from the first course of treatment, medical condition of the patient, and degree of previous RT-related late complications (80).

For patients with resectable local relapse, it is difficult to compare the efficacy of surgery versus reirradiation as patients from the surgical series generally have more favorable clinical factors such as low disease volume, early r-T categories, good performance status, and minimal comorbidity. Retrospective studies suggested that the local salvage rates by either modality were very similar (80). However, in view of the high incidence of serious late toxicities incurred by reirradiation, surgical salvage should be considered if expertise is available. Depending on the disease extent, various surgical techniques have been developed ranging from endoscopic resection and transoral robotic resection to open nasopharyngectomy. Excellent long-term local control rates up to 70% have been reported with no significant negative impact on patients' quality of life.

For the majority of patients with recurrent T3-4 disease, reirradiation with or without chemotherapy remains the cornerstone of treatment. Doses ≥60 Gy are usually recommended for effective salvage, but significant morbidities are often incurred. Various methods of radiation delivery have been attempted, reflecting the evolving technological advances in the field of RT. Currently IMRT represents the most commonly used method with the most promising treatment results (12,81–89). As shown in Table 16.2, durable local control of greater than 40% could be achieved even for rT3-4 disease. However, massive bleeding due to vascular damage and mucosal necrosis is not an uncommon cause of death. Although higher reirradiation dose can improve local salvage, it may not necessarily translate into longer survival because of excessive fatal late complications; an optimal balance is needed.

Despite the lack of randomized data, induction and concurrent chemotherapy is being used increasingly for reirradiation. While induction chemotherapy could reduce the recurrent tumor bulk leading to better sparing of adjacent OARs especially for rT3-4 disease, and possibly eradicate micrometastasis, concurrent chemotherapy may be more potent for improving local tumor control based on the experience in the treatment of primary NPC. However, the main concern is whether concurrent treatment would further aggravate the cumulative risk of late RT complications.

TABLE 16.2

Efficacy and Late Toxicities of Reirradiation by Intensity Modulated Radiotherapy

Author	Pt. no.	rT1-2 (%)	Dose (Gy)	Chemo.	Year	L-FFR (%)	OS (%)	Brain Necrosis (%)	Massive Bleeding (%)	RT Related Death (%)
Chua (81)	31	25	50–60	68%	1	56	63	7	NR	NR
Karam (82)	27	78	40–60 (1.1–1.4 Gy/fr BID)	85%	3	53	57	0	0	0
Koutcher (83)	29	45	45–59	93%	5	52	60	22	NR	NR
Ngan (12)	32	0	60	100%	2	75	68	35	13	13
Qiu (84)	70	53	Median 70	44% (I) +/– 18% (C)	3	49	52	NR	9	9
Han (85)	239	25	61.7–78.7	49%	5	86	45	28	NR	35
Chen (86)	54	20	49.8–76.6	52%	2	64	44	19	11	24
Tian (87)	117	21	65.4–73.1	0%	5	64–71	37	21	25	32
Kong (88)	77	49	46.2–70	71%	3	67	52	9%	NR	53
Chan (89)	38	0	50–64.8	92%	3	44	47	11	16	8

C, concurrent; I, induction; L-FFR, local failure-free rate; NR, not reported; OS, overall survival.

Cetuximab, an anti-epidermal growth factor receptor (EGFR) monoclonal antibody, has also been evaluated in the reirradiation setting. When it is combined with concurrent CRT as reirradiation, cetuximab appeared to be well tolerated (12,90). Further studies are necessary to confirm its efficacy in locally recurrent NPC in combination with reirradiation.

MANAGEMENT OF METASTATIC DISEASE

Distant metastasis is the main hurdle in the management of NPC. Despite the increasing incorporation of systemic chemotherapy in the primary treatment, the rate of distant failure remains at a range of 20% to 30% (91).

Currently, chemotherapy is the mainstay of treatment in the metastatic setting. Combination chemotherapy can achieve a higher response rate compared with a single agent, and cisplatin is the backbone. The most popular partnering agent to cisplatin is fluorouracil, but other drugs like gemcitabine, docetaxel, capecitabine, and paclitaxel have also been tested in various phase II trials (92–100). Response rates at a range of 50% to 75% are usually seen. The relatively favorable response in platinum doublets renders polychemotherapy less attractive, due to a higher toxicity rate and unproven superiority (101–104). Recently, there has been a large phase III randomized trial comparing two commonly used platinum doublet regimens: gemcitabine plus cisplatin (GP) versus fluorouracil plus cisplatin (PF) (13). GP outperformed PF in terms of objective response rate (64% vs. 42%), median PFS (7.0 vs. 5.6 months), and preliminary median OS (29.1 vs. 20.9 months) at the expense of more hematological toxicities but less mucositis. In addition, the shorter drug administration time is another advantage of GP.

Upon progression after first-line therapy, the efficacy of nonplatinum monotherapy (like capecitabine, docetaxel, and gemcitabine) or doublets (like gemcitabine–vinorelbine, ifosfamide–fluorouracil, ifosfamide–doxorubicin) was tested in multiple small phase II trials. The majority of them demonstrated response rates of 30% to 40% (105–110), except two small single-arm series reported response rates of 56% to 68% but the PFS was similar (110,111). Unfortunately, the lack of a comparator arm, variation in inclusion criteria, and baseline demographics make it impossible to recommend the most suitable therapy in the second-line setting. In a situation that the progression-free period is long, reintroduction of platinum-based therapy can also be considered. Further randomized trials are warranted to establish the standard therapy in the second-line setting.

Multiple target therapies have been tested but so far none of them have been approved for metastatic NPC at present. EGFR is abundantly expressed in NPC and it is rational to test the efficacy of EGFR tyrosine kinase inhibitor (TKI) in such a clinical scenario. However, no clinical response was seen in three different series testing EGFR TKIs in metastatic NPC (112–114). EGFR monoclonal antibodies like cetuximab have also been tested in combination with carboplatin. Again the response was modest and the PFS was short (115). Other TKIs like sunitinib and pazopanib were tested and modest clinical activity was again observed (116,117). However, fatal hemorrhagic complication was noted in previously irradiated sites, limiting its further development. Target therapies should only be considered in the context of clinical trials.

Immunotherapy by checkpoint inhibitors is novel, and this is a rapidly evolving entity in the field of oncology. A few reports have illustrated the relatively high programmed death-ligand 1 (PD-L1) and/or PD-1 expression in NPC. Some have suggested the prognostic role of PD-L1 expression but the current data are conflicting (118–120). Similar to other malignancies, much endeavor has been made to explore the possible activities of PD-L1/PD-1 inhibitors in NPC. A recent phase IB trial demonstrated encouraging antitumor activities of pembrolizumab in locally recurrent or metastatic NPC (14). The objective response rate was 26%. Of note, the median duration of response was 17 months, and the side effects were tolerable. More exciting data are anticipated in the near future.

Finally, it should be noted that stage IVC disease is a catch-all category ranging from solitary metastatic focus, oligometastases, to extensive dissemination. Retrospective reports have indicated the great variation in survival outcome in patients with different number and anatomical sites of metastases (121,122). Aggressive local therapies including surgery, radiofrequency ablation, and RT for treating limited lung and liver metastases have been reported (123–126). Superior survival outcomes were observed in this group of patients, compared to those being managed with systemic therapy alone. Selection bias was a potential confounder in these reports but nevertheless these results suggested that some patients are amenable to aggressive local therapy with prolonged survival. With the

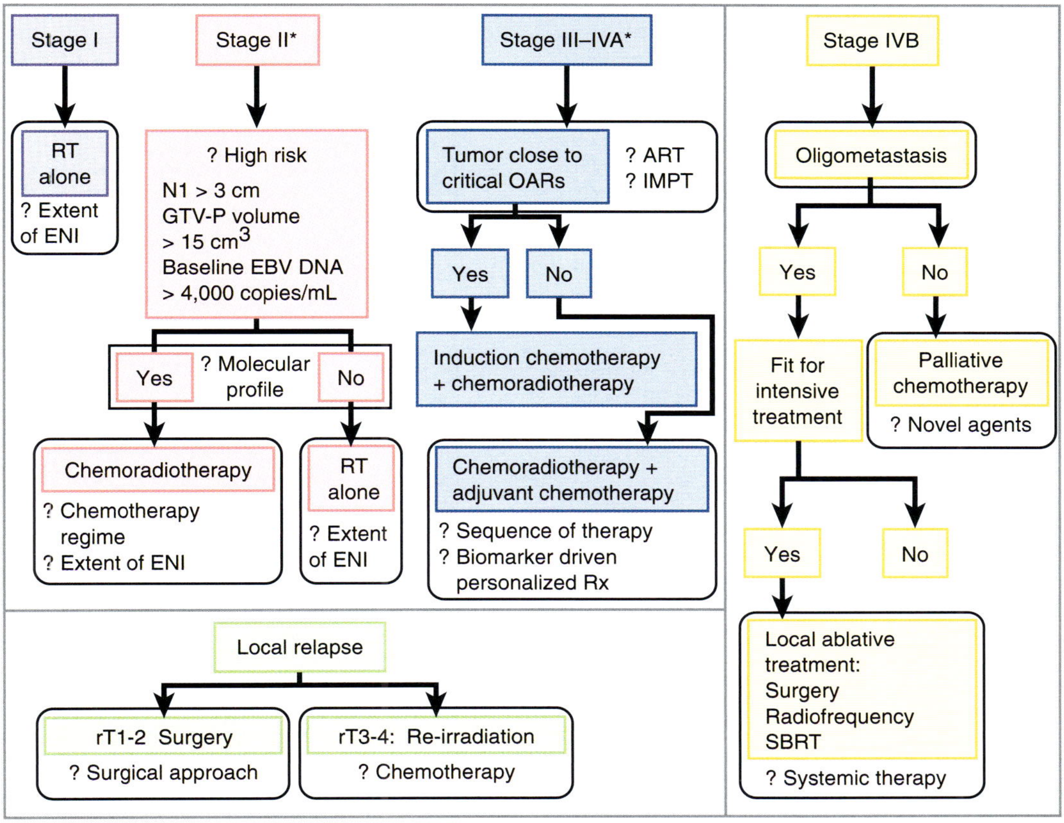

FIGURE 16.1 Treatment algorithm according to AJCC/UICC 8th edition.

*current NCCN guideline (version 2.2017) recommends concurrent chemoradiotherapy followed by adjuvant chemotherapy, concurrent chemoradiotherapy alone or induction chemotherapy followed by concurrent chemoradiotherapy.

AJCC/UICC, American Joint Committee on Cancer/Union for International Cancer Control; ART, adaptive RT; ENI, elective nodal irradiation; GTV_P, primary gross tumor volume; IMPT, intensity modulated proton therapy; OARs, organs at risk; RT, radiotherapy; RT, potential research area; Rx, treatment; SBRT, stereotactic body.

advent of technology, stereotactic ablative RT is another useful technique to tackle oligometastatic disease noninvasively, especially in surgically inaccessible sites or in patients who are medically inoperable (91).

CONCLUSIONS

NPC is a significant healthcare burden in endemic areas and EBV infection plays a crucial role in pathogenesis. The management has evolved in the past decades to transform this once very deadly cancer to a highly treatable one. Advances in RT technique and systemic treatment have substantially improved the treatment outcome. Although the prognosis of early NPC is favorable, long-term toxicity and quality of life issues continue to be the major problems of survivorship. On the other hand, patients with locoregionally advanced disease still suffer from a considerable rate of treatment failure and the prognosis is extremely poor for those with distant metastasis. Future research should focus on risk-adapted treatment strategies in order to achieve the ultimate goal of personalized medicine. Immunotherapy is an exciting area to explore and the results of ongoing studies are eagerly awaited (14). A practical treatment algorithm is proposed with the best level of evidence and important research questions raised (Figure 16.1).

REFERENCES

1. Ferlay J, Soerjomataram I, Dikshit R, et al. Cancer incidence and mortality worldwide: sources, methods and major patterns in GLOBOCAN 2012. *Int J Cancer*. 2015;136(5):E359–E386. doi:10.1002/ijc.29210
2. Young LS, Dawson CW. Epstein-Barr virus and nasopharyngeal carcinoma. *Chin J Cancer*. 2014;33(12):581–590. doi:10.5732/cjc.014.10197
3. Cheung F, Chan O, Ng WT, et al. The prognostic value of histological typing in nasopharyngeal carcinoma. *Oral Oncol*. 2012;48(5):429–433. doi:10.1016/j.oraloncology.2011.11.017
4. Pan JJ, Ng WT, Zong JF, et al. Proposal for the 8th edition of the AJCC/UICC staging system for nasopharyngeal cancer in the era of intensity-modulated radiotherapy. *Cancer*. 2016;122(4):546–558. doi:10.1002/cncr.29795
5. Amin MB, Edge S, Greene F. *AJCC Cancer Staging Manual*. 8th ed. New York, NY: Springer; 2017.
6. Brierley JD, Gospodarowicz MK, Wittekind C. *TNM Classification of Malignant Tumours*. 8th ed. Oxford: Wiley-Blackwell; 2017.
7. Pan JJ, Ng WT, Zong JF, et al. Prognostic nomogram for refining the prognostication of the proposed 8th edition of the AJCC/UICC staging system for nasopharyngeal cancer in the era of intensity-modulated radiotherapy. *Cancer*. 2016;122(21):3307–3315. doi:10.1002/cncr.30198
8. Le Q-T, Zhang Q, Cao H, et al. An international collaboration to harmonize the quantitative plasma Epstein-Barr virus DNA assay for future biomarker-guided trials in nasopharyngeal carcinoma. *Clin Cancer Res*. 2013;19(8):2208–2215. doi:10.1158/1078-0432.CCR-12-3702
9. Gooi Z, Richmon J, Agrawal N, et al. AHNS Series - Do you know your guidelines? Principles of treatment for nasopharyngeal cancer: A review of the National Comprehensive Cancer Network guidelines. *Head Neck*. 2017;39(2):201–205. doi:10.1002/hed.24635
10. Saba NF, Salama JK, Beitler JJ, et al. ACR Appropriateness criteria(R) for nasopharyngeal carcinoma. *Head Neck*. 2016;38(7):979–986. doi:10.1002/hed.24423
11. Chan AT, Gregoire V, Lefebvre JL, et al. Nasopharyngeal cancer: EHNS-ESMO-ESTRO clinical practice guidelines for diagnosis, treatment and follow-up. *Ann Oncol*. 2012;23(suppl. 7):vii83–vii85. doi:10.1093/annonc/mds266
12. Ngan RK NW, Kwong D, Tung S, et al. Preliminary results of HKNPC-1001 trial to evaluate the role of induction TPF followed by weekly docetaxel and cetuximab in combination with intensity modulated radiotherapy for locally advanced nasopharygeal carcinoma. *Annals Oncol*. 2015;26(suppl 9):ix93–ix102. doi:10.1093/annonc/mdv527.21
13. Zhang L, Huang Y, Hong S, et al. Gemcitabine plus cisplatin versus fluorouracil plus cisplatin in recurrent or metastatic nasopharyngeal carcinoma: a multicentre, randomised, open-label, phase 3 trial. *Lancet*. 2016;388(10054):1883–1892. doi:10.1016/S0140-6736(16)31388-5
14. Hsu C, Lee SH, Ejadi S, et al. Safety and antitumor activity of pembrolizumab in patients with programmed death-ligand 1-positive nasopharyngeal carcinoma: Results of the KEYNOTE-028 Study. *J Clin Oncol*. 2017:Jco2017733675. doi:10.1200/JCO.2017.73.3675
15. Helou J, Thibault I, Poon I, et al. Stereotactic ablative radiation therapy for pulmonary metastases: histology, dose, and indication matter. *Int J Radiat Oncol Biol Phys*. 2017;98(2):419–427. doi:10.1016/j.ijrobp.2017.02.093
16. Ng WT, Lee MC, Chang AT, et al. The impact of dosimetric inadequacy on treatment outcome of nasopharyngeal carcinoma with IMRT. *Oral Oncol*. 2014;50(5):506–512. doi:10.1016/j.oraloncology.2014.01.017
17. Tuan JK, Ha TC, Ong WS, et al. Late toxicities after conventional radiation therapy alone for nasopharyngeal carcinoma. *Radiother Oncol*. 2012;104(3):305–311. doi:10.1016/j.radonc.2011.12.028
18. Teo PM, Leung SF, Lee WY, Zee B. Intracavitary brachytherapy significantly enhances local control of early T-stage nasopharyngeal carcinoma: the existence of a dose-tumor-control relationship above conventional tumoricidal dose. *Int J Radiat Oncol Biol Phys*. 2000;46(2):445–458. doi:10.1016/S0360-3016(99)00326-0
19. Leung T-W, Wong VY, Sze W-K, et al. High-dose-rate intracavitary brachytherapy boost for early T stage nasopharyngeal carcinoma{private}. *Int J Radiat Oncol Biol Phys*. 2008;70(2):361–367. doi:10.1016/j.ijrobp.2007.06.078
20. Hara W, Loo BW, Jr., Goffinet DR, et al. Excellent local control with stereotactic radiotherapy boost after external beam radiotherapy in patients with nasopharyngeal carcinoma. *Int J Radiat Oncol Biol Phys*. 2008;71(2):393–400. doi:10.1016/j.ijrobp.2007.10.027
21. Lee AW, Ng WT, Chan LL, et al. Evolution of treatment for nasopharyngeal cancer—success and setback in the intensity-modulated radiotherapy era. *Radiother Oncol*. 2014;110(3):377–384. doi:10.1016/j.radonc.2014.02.003
22. Peng G, Wang T, Yang KY, et al. A prospective, randomized study comparing outcomes and toxicities of intensity-modulated radiotherapy vs. conventional two-dimensional radiotherapy for the treatment of nasopharyngeal carcinoma. *Radiother Oncol*. 2012;104(3):286–293. doi:10.1016/j.radonc.2012.08.013
23. Kam MK, Leung S-F, Zee B, et al. Prospective randomized study of intensity-modulated radiotherapy on salivary gland function in early-stage nasopharyngeal carcinoma patients. *J Clin Oncol*. 2007;25(31):4873–4879. doi:10.1200/JCO.2007.11.5501
24. Pow EH, Kwong DL, McMillan AS, et al. Xerostomia and quality of life after intensity-modulated radiotherapy vs. conventional radiotherapy for early-stage nasopharyngeal carcinoma: initial report on a randomized controlled clinical trial. *Int J Radiat Oncol Biol Phys*. 2006;66(4):981–991. doi:10.1016/j.ijrobp.2006.06.013

25. Huang TL, Chien CY, Tsai WL, et al. Long-term late toxicities and quality of life for survivors of nasopharyngeal carcinoma treated with intensity-modulated radiotherapy versus non-intensity-modulated radiotherapy. *Head Neck.* 2016;38(suppl 1):E1026–E1032. doi:10.1002/hed.24150
26. Wu F, Wang R, Lu H, et al. Concurrent chemoradiotherapy in locoregionally advanced nasopharyngeal carcinoma: treatment outcomes of a prospective, multicentric clinical study. *Radiother Oncol.* 2014;112(1):106–111. doi:10.1016/j.radonc.2014.05.005
27. Sun X, Su S, Chen C, et al. Long-term outcomes of intensity-modulated radiotherapy for 868 patients with nasopharyngeal carcinoma: an analysis of survival and treatment toxicities. *Radiother Oncol.* 2014;110(3):398–403. doi:10.1016/j.radonc.2013.10.020
28. Lee AW, Ma BB, Ng WT, Chan AT. Management of nasopharyngeal carcinoma: current practice and future perspective. *J Clin Oncol.* 2015;33(29):3356–3364. doi:10.1200/JCO.2015.60.9347
29. Chan A, Adams JA, Weyman E, et al. A phase II trial of proton radiation therapy with chemotherapy for nasopharyngeal carcinoma. *Int J Radiat Oncol Biol Phys.* 2012;84:S151–S152. doi:10.1016/j.ijrobp.2012.07.391
30. Cheng HC, Wu VW, Ngan RK, et al. A prospective study on volumetric and dosimetric changes during intensity-modulated radiotherapy for nasopharyngeal carcinoma patients. *Radiother Oncol.* 2012;104(3):317–323. doi:10.1016/j.radonc.2012.03.013
31. Wang X, Lu J, Xiong X, et al. Anatomic and dosimetric changes during the treatment course of intensity-modulated radiotherapy for locally advanced nasopharyngeal carcinoma. *Med Dosim.* 2010;35(2):151–157. doi:10.1016/j.meddos.2009.06.007
32. Yang H, Hu W, Wang W, et al. Replanning during intensity modulated radiation therapy improved quality of life in patients with nasopharyngeal carcinoma. *Int J Radiat Oncol Biol Phys.* 2013;85(1):e47–e54. doi:10.1016/j.ijrobp.2012.09.033
33. Gao Y, Zhu G, Lu J, et al. Is elective irradiation to the lower neck necessary for N0 nasopharyngeal carcinoma? *Int J Radiat Oncol Biol Phys.* 2010;77(5):1397–1402. doi:10.1016/j.ijrobp.2009.06.062
34. Li J-G, Yuan X, Zhang L-L, et al. A randomized clinical trial comparing prophylactic upper versus whole-neck irradiation in the treatment of patients with node-negative nasopharyngeal carcinoma. *Cancer.* 2013;119(17):3170–3176. doi:10.1002/cncr.28201
35. Lee AW, Sze H, Ng WT. Is selective neck irradiation safe for node-negative nasopharyngeal carcinoma? *Int J Radiat Oncol Biol Phys.* 2013;85(4):902–903. doi:10.1016/j.ijrobp.2012.09.010
36. Chua DT, Sham JS, Kwong DL, Au GK. Treatment outcome after radiotherapy alone for patients with Stage I-II nasopharyngeal carcinoma. *Cancer.* 2003;98(1):74–80. doi:10.1002/cncr.11485
37. Yeh S-A, Tang Y, Lui C-C, et al. Treatment outcomes and late complications of 849 patients with nasopharyngeal carcinoma treated with radiotherapy alone. *Int J Radiat Oncol Biol Phys.* 2005;62(3):672–679. doi:10.1016/j.ijrobp.2004.11.002
38. Leung T-W, Tung SY, Sze W-K, et al. Treatment results of 1070 patients with nasopharyngeal carcinoma: an analysis of survival and failure patterns. *Head Neck.* 2005;27(7):555–565. doi:10.1002/hed.20189
39. Lee AW, Sze WM, Au JS, et al. Treatment results for nasopharyngeal carcinoma in the modern era: the Hong Kong experience. *Int J Radiat Oncol Biol Phys.* 2005;61(4):1107–1116. doi:10.1016/j.ijrobp.2004.07.702
40. Song CH, Wu H-G, Heo DS, et al. Treatment outcomes for radiotherapy alone are comparable with neoadjuvant chemotherapy followed by radiotherapy in early-stage nasopharyngeal carcinoma. *Laryngoscope.* 2008;118(4):663–670. doi:10.1097/MLG.0b013e3181626cfe
41. Xiao WW, Han F, Lu TX, et al. Treatment outcomes after radiotherapy alone for patients with early-stage nasopharyngeal carcinoma. *Int J Radiat Oncol Biol Phys.* 2009;74(4):1070–1076. doi:10.1016/j.ijrobp.2008.09.008
42. Al-Sarraf M, LeBlanc M, Giri PG, et al. Chemoradiotherapy versus radiotherapy in patients with advanced nasopharyngeal cancer: phase III randomized Intergroup study 0099. *J Clin Oncol.* 1998;16(4):1310–1317. doi:10.1200/JCO.1998.16.4.1310
43. Chan AT, Leung SF, Ngan RK, et al. Overall survival after concurrent cisplatin-radiotherapy compared with radiotherapy alone in locoregionally advanced nasopharyngeal carcinoma. *J Natl Cancer Inst.* 2005;97(7):536–539. doi:10.1093/jnci/dji084
44. Chen QY, Wen YF, Guo L, et al. Concurrent chemoradiotherapy vs radiotherapy alone in stage II nasopharyngeal carcinoma: phase III randomized trial. *J Natl Cancer Inst.* 2011;103(23):1761–1770. doi:10.1093/jnci/djr432
45. Blanchard P, Lee A, Marguet S, et al. Chemotherapy and radiotherapy in nasopharyngeal carcinoma: an update of the MAC-NPC meta-analysis. *Lancet Oncol.* 2015;16(6):645–655. doi:10.1016/S1470-2045(15)70126-9
46. Wong FC, Ng AW, Lee VH, et al. Whole-field simultaneous integrated-boost intensity-modulated radiotherapy for patients with nasopharyngeal carcinoma. *Int J Radiat Oncol Biol Phys.* 2010;76(1):138–145. doi:10.1016/j.ijrobp.2009.01.084
47. Su SF, Han F, Zhao C, et al. Long-term outcomes of early-stage nasopharyngeal carcinoma patients treated with intensity-modulated radiotherapy alone. *Int J Radiat Oncol Biol Phys.* 2012;82(1):327–333. doi:10.1016/j.ijrobp.2010.09.011
48. Ng WT, Lee MC, Hung WM, et al. Clinical outcomes and patterns of failure after intensity-modulated radiotherapy for nasopharyngeal carcinoma. *Int J Radiat Oncol Biol Phys.* 2011;79(2):420–428. doi:10.1016/j.ijrobp.2009.11.024
49. Tham IW, Lin S, Pan J, et al. Intensity-modulated radiation therapy without concurrent chemotherapy for stage IIb nasopharyngeal cancer. *Am J Clin Oncol.* 2010;33(3):294–299. doi:10.1097/COC.0b013e3181d2edab

50. Xu T, Shen C, Zhu G, Hu C. Omission of chemotherapy in early stage nasopharyngeal carcinoma treated with IMRT: a paired cohort study. *Medicine*. 2015;94(39):e1457. doi:10.1097/MD.0000000000001457
51. Chen KH, Zhu XD, Li L, et al. Comparison of the efficacy between concurrent chemoradiotherapy with or without adjuvant chemotherapy and intensity-modulated radiotherapy alone for stage II nasopharyngeal carcinoma. *Oncotarget*. 2016;7(42):69041–69050. doi:10.18632/oncotarget.11978
52. Sze H, Blanchard P, Ng WT, et al. Chemotherapy for nasopharyngeal carcinoma—current recommendation and controversies. *Hematol Oncol Clin North Am*. 2015;29(6):1107–1122. doi:10.1016/j.hoc.2015.07.004
53. Sze WM, Lee AW, Yau TK, et al. Primary tumor volume of nasopharyngeal carcinoma: prognostic significance for local control. *Int J Radiat Oncol Biol Phys*. 2004;59(1):21–27. doi:10.1016/j.ijrobp.2003.10.027
54. Chua DT, Sham JS, Leung LH, et al. Tumor volume is not an independent prognostic factor in early-stage nasopharyngeal carcinoma treated by radiotherapy alone. *Int J Radiat Oncol Biol Phys*. 2004;58(5):1437–1444. doi:10.1016/j.ijrobp.2003.09.075
55. Leung SF, Chan AT, Zee B, et al. Pretherapy quantitative measurement of circulating Epstein-Barr virus DNA is predictive of posttherapy distant failure in patients with early-stage nasopharyngeal carcinoma of undifferentiated type. *Cancer*. 2003;98(2):288–291. doi:10.1002/cncr.11496
56. Wee J, Tan EH, Tai BC, et al. Randomized trial of radiotherapy versus concurrent chemoradiotherapy followed by adjuvant chemotherapy in patients with American Joint Committee on Cancer/International Union against cancer stage III and IV nasopharyngeal cancer of the endemic variety. *J Clin Oncol*. 2005;23(27):6730–6738. doi:10.1200/JCO.2005.16.790
57. Chen Y, Liu MZ, Liang SB, et al. Preliminary results of a prospective randomized trial comparing concurrent chemoradiotherapy plus adjuvant chemotherapy with radiotherapy alone in patients with locoregionally advanced nasopharyngeal carcinoma in endemic regions of china. *Int J Radiat Oncol Biol Phys*. 2008;71(5):1356–1364. doi:10.1016/j.ijrobp.2007.12.028
58. Lee AW, Lau WH, Tung SY, et al. Preliminary results of a randomized study on therapeutic gain by concurrent chemotherapy for regionally-advanced nasopharyngeal carcinoma: NPC-9901 Trial by the Hong Kong Nasopharyngeal Cancer Study Group. *J Clin Oncol*. 2005;23(28):6966–6975. doi:10.1200/JCO.2004.00.7542
59. Lee AW, Tung SY, Chan AT, et al. Preliminary results of a randomized study (NPC-9902 Trial) on therapeutic gain by concurrent chemotherapy and/or accelerated fractionation for locally advanced nasopharyngeal carcinoma. *Int J Radiat Oncol Biol Phys*. 2006;66(1):142–151. doi:10.1016/j.ijrobp.2006.03.054
60. Baujat B, Audry H, Bourhis J, et al. Chemotherapy in locally advanced nasopharyngeal carcinoma: an individual patient data meta-analysis of eight randomized trials and 1753 patients. *Int J Radiat Oncol Biol Phys*. 2006;64(1):47–56. doi:10.1016/j.ijrobp.2005.06.037
61. Zhang L, Zhao C, Peng PJ, et al. Phase III study comparing standard radiotherapy with or without weekly oxaliplatin in treatment of locoregionally advanced nasopharyngeal carcinoma: preliminary results. *J Clin Oncol*. 2005;23(33):8461–8468. doi:10.1200/JCO.2004.00.3863
62. Wu X, Huang PY, Peng PJ, et al. Long-term follow-up of a phase III study comparing radiotherapy with or without weekly oxaliplatin for locoregionally advanced nasopharyngeal carcinoma. *Ann Oncol*. 2013;24(8):2131–2136. doi:10.1093/annonc/mdt163
63. Chitapanarux I, Lorvidhaya V, Kamnerdsupaphon P, et al. Chemoradiation comparing cisplatin versus carboplatin in locally advanced nasopharyngeal cancer: randomised, non-inferiority, open trial. *Eur J Cancer*. 2007;43(9):1399–1406. doi:10.1016/j.ejca.2007.03.022
64. Chan AT, Teo PM, Ngan RK, et al. Concurrent chemotherapy-radiotherapy compared with radiotherapy alone in locoregionally advanced nasopharyngeal carcinoma: progression-free survival analysis of a phase III randomized trial. *J Clin Oncol*. 2002;20(8):2038–2044. doi:10.1200/JCO.2002.08.149
65. Lee JY, Sun JM, Oh DR, et al. Comparison of weekly versus triweekly cisplatin delivered concurrently with radiation therapy in patients with locally advanced nasopharyngeal cancer: a multicenter randomized phase II trial (KCSG-HN10-02). *Radiother Oncol*. 2016;118(2):244–250. doi:10.1016/j.radonc.2015.11.030
66. Liang H, Xia W-X, Lv X, et al. Concurrent chemoradiotherapy with 3-weekly versus weekly cisplatin in patients with locoregionally advanced nasopharyngeal carcinoma: a phase 3 multicentre randomised controlled trial (ChiCTR-TRC-12001979). *J Clin Oncol*. 2017;35:6006–6006. doi:10.1200/JCO.2017.35.15_suppl.6006
67. Xu T, Liu Y, Dou S, et al. Weekly cetuximab concurrent with IMRT aggravated radiation-induced oral mucositis in locally advanced nasopharyngeal carcinoma: results of a randomized phase II study. *Oral Oncol*. 2015;51(9):875–879. doi:10.1016/j.oraloncology.2015.06.008
68. Chi KH, Chang YC, Guo WY, et al. A phase III study of adjuvant chemotherapy in advanced nasopharyngeal carcinoma patients. *Int J Radiat Oncol Biol Phys*. 2002;52(5):1238–1244. doi:10.1016/S0360-3016(01)02781-X
69. Rossi A, Molinari R, Boracchi P, et al. Adjuvant chemotherapy with vincristine, cyclophosphamide, and doxorubicin after radiotherapy in local-regional nasopharyngeal cancer: results of a 4-year multicenter randomized study. *J Clin Oncol*. 1988;6(9):1401–1410. doi:10.1200/JCO.1988.6.9.1401

70. Chen L, Hu CS, Chen XZ, et al. Concurrent chemoradiotherapy plus adjuvant chemotherapy versus concurrent chemoradiotherapy alone in patients with locoregionally advanced nasopharyngeal carcinoma: a phase 3 multicentre randomised controlled trial. *Lancet Oncol.* 2012;13(2):163–171. doi:10.1016/S1470-2045(11)70320-5
71. Ribassin-Majed L, Marguet S, Lee AW, et al. What is the best treatment of locally advanced nasopharyngeal carcinoma? An individual patient data network meta-analysis. *J Clin Oncol.* 2017;35(5):498–505. doi:10.1200/JCO.2016.67.4119
72. Chan ATC, Hui EP, Ngan RKC, et al. A multicenter randomized controlled trial (RCT) of adjuvant chemotherapy (CT) in nasopharyngeal carcinoma (NPC) with residual plasma EBV DNA (EBV DNA) following primary radiotherapy (RT) or chemoradiation (CRT). *J Clin Oncol.* 2017;35:abstr 6002. doi:10.1200/JCO.2017.35.15_suppl.6002
73. Hui EP, Ma BB, Leung SF, et al. Randomized phase II trial of concurrent cisplatin-radiotherapy with or without neoadjuvant docetaxel and cisplatin in advanced nasopharyngeal carcinoma. *J Clin Oncol.* 2009;27(2):242–249. doi:10.1200/JCO.2008.18.1545
74. Fountzilas G, Ciuleanu E, Bobos M, et al. Induction chemotherapy followed by concomitant radiotherapy and weekly cisplatin versus the same concomitant chemoradiotherapy in patients with nasopharyngeal carcinoma: a randomized phase II study conducted by the Hellenic Cooperative Oncology Group (HeCOG) with biomarker evaluation. *Ann Oncol.* 2012;23(2):427–435. doi:10.1093/annonc/mdr116
75. Tan T, Lim WT, Fong KW, et al. Concurrent chemo-radiation with or without induction gemcitabine, Carboplatin, and Paclitaxel: a randomized, phase 2/3 trial in locally advanced nasopharyngeal carcinoma. *Int J Radiat Oncol Biol Phys.* 2015;91(5):952–960. doi:10.1016/j.ijrobp.2015.01.002
76. Sun Y, Li WF, Chen NY, et al. Induction chemotherapy plus concurrent chemoradiotherapy versus concurrent chemoradiotherapy alone in locoregionally advanced nasopharyngeal carcinoma: a phase 3, multicentre, randomised controlled trial. *Lancet Oncol.* 2016;17(11):1509–1520. doi:10.1016/S1470-2045(16)30410-7
77. Daoud J, Aupérin A, Tao YG, et al. A randomized trial of concomitant cisplatin-RT +/- induction TPF in locally advanced nasopharyngeal carcinomas. *Radiother Oncol.* 2015:114(supp 1):abstract: OC-004. doi:10.1016/S0167-8140(15)34764-2
78. Chen M-Y, Cao S-M, Yang Q, et al. Neoadjuvant chemotherapy followed by concurrent chemoradiotherapy versus concurrent chemoradiotherapy alone in locoregionally advanced nasopharyngeal carcinoma: a phase III multicentre randomised controlled trial. *J Clin Oncol.* 2017;35:abstract: 6005-6005. doi:10.1200/JCO.2017.35.15_suppl.6005
79. Lee AW, Ngan RK, Tung SY, et al. Preliminary results of trial NPC-0501 evaluating the therapeutic gain by changing from concurrent-adjuvant to induction-concurrent chemoradiotherapy, changing from fluorouracil to capecitabine, and changing from conventional to accelerated radiotherapy fractionation in patients with locoregionally advanced nasopharyngeal carcinoma. *Cancer.* 2015;121(8):1328–1338. doi:10.1002/cncr.29208
80. Lee AW, Fee WE, Jr., Ng WT, Chan LK. Nasopharyngeal carcinoma: salvage of local recurrence. *Oral Oncol.* 2012;48(9):768–774. doi:10.1016/j.oraloncology.2012.02.017
81. Chua DT, Sham JS, Leung LH, Au GK. Re-irradiation of nasopharyngeal carcinoma with intensity-modulated radiotherapy. *Radiother Oncol.* 2005;77(3):290–294. doi:10.1016/j.radonc.2005.10.010
82. Karam I, Huang SH, McNiven A, et al. Outcomes after reirradiation for recurrent nasopharyngeal carcinoma: North American experience. *Head Neck.* 2016;38(suppl 1):E1102–E1109. doi:10.1002/hed.24166
83. Koutcher L, Lee N, Zelefsky M, et al. Reirradiation of locally recurrent nasopharynx cancer with external beam radiotherapy with or without brachytherapy. *Int J Radiat Oncol Biol Phys.* 2010;76(1):130–137. doi:10.1016/j.ijrobp.2009.01.055
84. Qiu S, Lin S, Tham IW, et al. Intensity-modulated radiation therapy in the salvage of locally recurrent nasopharyngeal carcinoma. *Int J Radiat Oncol Biol Phys.* 2012;83(2):676–683. doi:10.1016/j.ijrobp.2011.07.006
85. Han F, Zhao C, Huang SM, et al. Long-term outcomes and prognostic factors of re-irradiation for locally recurrent nasopharyngeal carcinoma using intensity-modulated radiotherapy. *Clin Oncol (R Coll Radiol).* 2012;24(8):569–576. doi:10.1016/j.clon.2011.11.010
86. Chen H-Y, Ma X-M, Ye M, et al. Effectiveness and toxicities of intensity-modulated radiotherapy for patients with locally recurrent nasopharyngeal carcinoma. *PLOS ONE.* 2013;8(9):e73918. doi:10.1371/journal.pone.0073918
87. Tian YM, Zhao C, Guo Y, et al. Effect of total dose and fraction size on survival of patients with locally recurrent nasopharyngeal carcinoma treated with intensity-modulated radiotherapy: a phase 2, single-center, randomized controlled trial. *Cancer.* 2014;120(22):3502–3509. doi:10.1002/cncr.28934
88. Kong L, Wang L, Shen C, et al. Salvage Intensity-Modulated Radiation Therapy (IMRT) for locally recurrent nasopharyngeal cancer after definitive IMRT: a novel scenario of the modern era. *Scientific Reports.* 2016;6:32883. doi:10.1038/srep32883
89. Chan OS, Sze HC, Lee MC, et al. Reirradiation with intensity-modulated radiotherapy for locally recurrent T3 to T4 nasopharyngeal carcinoma. *Head Neck.* 2017;39(3):533–540. doi:10.1002/hed.24645
90. Xu T, Ou X, Shen C, Hu C. Cetuximab in combination with chemoradiotherapy in the treatment of recurrent and/or metastatic nasopharyngeal carcinoma. *Anticancer Drugs.* 2016;27(1):66–70. doi:10.1097/CAD.0000000000000294
91. Chan OS, Ngan RK. Individualized treatment in stage IVC nasopharyngeal carcinoma. *Oral Oncol.* 2014;50(9):791–797. doi:10.1016/j.oraloncology.2014.01.004

92. Wang TL, Tan YO. Cisplatin and 5-fluorouracil continuous infusion for metastatic nasopharyngeal carcinoma. *Ann Acad Med Singapore.* 1991;20(5):601–603. https://www.ncbi.nlm.nih.gov/pubmed/1781642
93. Au E, Ang PT. A phase II trial of 5-fluorouracil and cisplatinum in recurrent or metastatic nasopharyngeal carcinoma. *Ann Oncol.* 1994;5(1):87–89. doi:10.1093/oxfordjournals.annonc.a058703
94. Chi KH, Chan WK, Cooper DL, et al. A phase II study of outpatient chemotherapy with cisplatin, 5-fluorouracil, and leucovorin in nasopharyngeal carcinoma. *Cancer.* 1994;73(2):247–252. doi:10.1002/1097-0142(19940115)73:2<247::AID-CNCR2820730203>3.0.CO;2-7
95. Yeo W, Leung TW, Chan AT, et al. A phase II study of combination paclitaxel and carboplatin in advanced nasopharyngeal carcinoma. *Eur J Cancer.* 1998;34(13):2027–2031. doi:10.1016/S0959-8049(98)00280-9
96. Tan EH, Khoo KS, Wee J, et al. Phase II trial of a paclitaxel and carboplatin combination in Asian patients with metastatic nasopharyngeal carcinoma. *Ann Oncol.* 1999;10(2):235–237. doi:10.1023/A:1008390929826
97. Ngan RK, Yiu HH, Lau WH, et al. Combination gemcitabine and cisplatin chemotherapy for metastatic or recurrent nasopharyngeal carcinoma: report of a phase II study. *Ann Oncol.* 2002;13(8):1252–1258. doi:10.1093/annonc/mdf200
98. Chua DT, Sham JS, Au GK. A phase II study of docetaxel and cisplatin as first-line chemotherapy in patients with metastatic nasopharyngeal carcinoma. *Oral Oncol.* 2005;41(6):589–595. doi:10.1016/j.oraloncology.2005.01.008
99. Li Y-H, Wang F-H, Jiang W-Q, et al. Phase II study of capecitabine and cisplatin combination as first-line chemotherapy in Chinese patients with metastatic nasopharyngeal carcinoma. *Cancer Chemother Pharmacol.* 2008;62(3):539–544. doi:10.1007/s00280-007-0641-2
100. Chua DT, Yiu HH, Seetalarom K, et al. Phase II trial of capecitabine plus cisplatin as first-line therapy in patients with metastatic nasopharyngeal cancer. *Head Neck.* 2012;34(9):1225–1230. doi:10.1002/hed.21884
101. Siu LL, Czaykowski PM, Tannock IF. Phase I/II study of the CAPABLE regimen for patients with poorly differentiated carcinoma of the nasopharynx. *J Clin Oncol.* 1998;16(7):2514–2521. doi:10.1200/JCO.1998.16.7.2514
102. Hasbini A, Mahjoubi R, Fandi A, et al. Phase II trial combining mitomycin with 5-fluorouracil, epirubicin, and cisplatin in recurrent and metastatic undifferentiated carcinoma of nasopharyngeal type. *Ann Oncol.* 1999;10(4):421–425. doi:10.1023/A:1008342828496
103. Leong SS, Wee J, Rajan S, et al. Triplet combination of gemcitabine, paclitaxel, and carboplatin followed by maintenance 5-fluorouracil and folinic acid in patients with metastatic nasopharyngeal carcinoma. *Cancer.* 2008;113(6):1332–1337. doi:10.1002/cncr.23687
104. Huang H-Q, Cai Q-Q, Lin X-B, et al. [Preliminary result of multi-center clinical trial on the docetaxel, 5-Fu and DDP in the treatment of advanced, recurrent or metastatic nasopharyngeal carcinoma]. *Zhonghua Zhong Liu Za Zhi.* 2008;30(4):314–316. doi:10.3321/j.issn:0253-3766.2008.04.019
105. Chua DT, Sham JS, Au GK. A phase II study of capecitabine in patients with recurrent and metastatic nasopharyngeal carcinoma pretreated with platinum-based chemotherapy. *Oral Oncol.* 2003;39(4):361–366. doi:10.1016/S1368-8375(02)00120-3
106. Zhang L, Zhang Y, Huang PY, et al. Phase II clinical study of gemcitabine in the treatment of patients with advanced nasopharyngeal carcinoma after the failure of platinum-based chemotherapy. *Cancer Chemother Pharmacol.* 2008;61(1):33–38. doi:10.1007/s00280-007-0441-8
107. Chen C, Wang FH, Wang Z-Q, et al. Salvage gemcitabine-vinorelbine chemotherapy in patients with metastatic nasopharyngeal carcinoma pretreated with platinum-based chemotherapy. *Oral Oncol.* 2012;48(11):1146–1151. doi:10.1016/j.oraloncology.2012.05.021
108. Ngeow J, Lim WT, Leong SS, et al. Docetaxel is effective in heavily pretreated patients with disseminated nasopharyngeal carcinoma. *Ann Oncol.* 2011;22(3):718–722. doi:10.1093/annonc/mdq425
109. Wang C-C, Chang J-Y, Liu T-W, et al. Phase II study of gemcitabine plus vinorelbine in the treatment of cisplatin-resistant nasopharyngeal carcinoma. *Head Neck.* 2006;28(1):74–80. doi:10.1002/hed.20310
110. Chua DT, Kwong DL, Sham JS, et al. A phase II study of ifosfamide, 5-fluorouracil and leucovorin in patients with recurrent nasopharyngeal carcinoma previously treated with platinum chemotherapy. *Eur J Cancer.* 2000;36(6):736–741. doi:10.1016/S0959-8049(00)00008-3
111. Huang HQ, Zhou ZM, Li YH, et al. [Preliminary results of ifosfamide and doxorubicin regimen in treatment of patients with recurrent and metastatic nasopharyngeal carcinoma]. *Ai Zheng.* 2002;21(4):409–411. doi:10.3969/j.issn.1000-467X.2002.04.017
112. Ma B, Hui EP, King A, et al. A phase II study of patients with metastatic or locoregionally recurrent nasopharyngeal carcinoma and evaluation of plasma Epstein-Barr virus DNA as a biomarker of efficacy. *Cancer Chemother Pharmacol.* 2008;62(1):59–64. doi:10.1007/s00280-007-0575-8
113. Chua DT, Wei WI, et al. Phase II study of gefitinib for the treatment of recurrent and metastatic nasopharyngeal carcinoma. *Head Neck.* 2008;30(7):863–867. doi:10.1002/hed.20792
114. You B, Le Tourneau C, Chen EX, et al. A Phase II trial of erlotinib as maintenance treatment after gemcitabine plus platinum-based chemotherapy in patients with recurrent and/or metastatic nasopharyngeal carcinoma. *Am J Clin Oncol.* 2012;35(3):255–260. doi:10.1097/COC.0b013e31820dbdcc

115. Chan AT, Hsu MM, Goh BC, et al. Multicenter, phase II study of cetuximab in combination with carboplatin in patients with recurrent or metastatic nasopharyngeal carcinoma. *J Clin Oncol.* 2005;23(15):3568–3576. doi:10.1200/JCO.2005.02.147
116. Hui EP, Ma BB, King AD, et al. Hemorrhagic complications in a phase II study of sunitinib in patients of nasopharyngeal carcinoma who has previously received high-dose radiation. *Ann Oncol.* 2011;22(6):1280–1287. doi:10.1093/annonc/mdq629
117. Lim WT, Ng QS, Ivy P, et al. A phase II study of pazopanib in Asian patients with recurrent/metastatic nasopharyngeal carcinoma. *Clin Cancer Res.* 2011;17(16):5481–5489. doi:10.1158/1078-0432.CCR-10-3409
118. Chen BJ, Chapuy B, Ouyang J, et al. PD-L1 expression is characteristic of a subset of aggressive B-cell lymphomas and virus-associated malignancies. *Clin Cancer Res.* 2013;19(13):3462–3473. doi:10.1158/1078-0432.CCR-13-0855
119. Fang W, Zhang J, Hong S, et al. EBV-driven LMP1 and IFN-gamma up-regulate PD-L1 in nasopharyngeal carcinoma: Implications for oncotargeted therapy. *Oncotarget.* 2014;5(23):12189–12202. doi:10.18632/oncotarget.2608
120. Hsu MC, Hsiao JR, Chang KC, et al. Increase of programmed death-1-expressing intratumoral CD8 T cells predicts a poor prognosis for nasopharyngeal carcinoma. *Mod Pathol.* 2010;23(10):1393–1403. doi:10.1038/modpathol.2010.130
121. Pan CC, Lu J, Yu JR, et al. Challenges in the modification of the M1 stage of the TNM staging system for nasopharyngeal carcinoma: a study of 1027 cases and review of the literature. *Experimental and Therapeutic Medicine.* 2012;4(2):334–338. doi:10.3892/etm.2012.584
122. Hui EP, Leung SF, Au JS, et al. Lung metastasis alone in nasopharyngeal carcinoma: a relatively favorable prognostic group. A study by the Hong Kong Nasopharyngeal Carcinoma Study Group. *Cancer.* 2004;101(2):300–306. doi:10.1002/cncr.20358
123. Ma J, Wen Z-S, Lin P, et al. [The results and prognosis of different treatment modalities for solitary metastatic lung tumor from nasopharyngeal carcinoma: a retrospective study of 105 cases]. *Chin J Cancer.* 2010;29(9):787–795. http://www.cjcsysu.com/ENpdf/2010/9/787.pdf
124. Cheng LC, Sham JS, Chiu CS, et al. Surgical resection of pulmonary metastases from nasopharyngeal carcinoma. *Aust NZ J Surg.* 1996;66(2):71–73. doi:10.1111/j.1445-2197.1996.tb01114.x
125. Pan C, Wu P, Yu J, et al. CT-guided radiofrequency ablation prolonged metastatic survival in patients with liver metastases from nasopharyngeal carcinoma. *Int J Hyperthermia.* 2011;27(6):549–554. doi:10.3109/02656736.2011.593019
126. Pan CC, Wu PH, Yu JR, et al. Comparative survival analysis in patients with pulmonary metastases from nasopharyngeal carcinoma treated with radiofrequency ablation. *Eur J Radiol.* 2012;81(4):e473–e477. doi:10.1016/j.ejrad.2011.05.037

17

Hypopharyngeal Cancer: A Multidisciplinary Approach

Moran Amit
Loren K. Mell
Cristina P. Rodriguez
Neil D. Gross

Hypopharyngeal squamous cell carcinoma (SCC) represents approximately 7% to 9% of all cancers of the upper aerodigestive tract (1). Most of these cancers are localized in the pyriform sinus (75%) whereas the remaining cancers involve the posterior pharyngeal wall (20%) and the postcricoid region (5%) (2). Most patients with hypopharyngeal SCC are male and upper middle-aged (55–70 years) with a history of excessive smoking and alcohol consumption. Unlike oropharyngeal cancer, human papillomavirus (HPV) is rarely implicated in the pathophysiology of hypopharyngeal SCC.

The hypopharynx is more than a simple structural connection between the oropharynx and the larynx. It is a separate embryonal organ divided into three subsites: the pyriform sinus (bilateral), the posterior pharyngeal wall, and the postcricoid region. The lateral wall of the pyriform sinus communicates with the oropharynx while its medial wall is in close continuity with the aryepiglottic fold of the larynx. The posterior pharyngeal wall is in direct contact with the prevertebral fascia posteriorly. The close proximity of the pyriform sinus to the paraglottic space results in early fixation of the hemilarynx in many hypopharyngeal SCC cases. This can make cancers of the pyriform sinus difficult to separate from supraglottic primary cancers.

Hypopharyngeal cancers are characterized by submucosal extension that frequently results in thyroid and cricoid cartilage involvement. Furthermore, direct extension to the thyroid gland or soft tissue of the neck is common. Submucosal extension to the esophagus is also common and may mimic the presentation of a primary esophageal cancer.

Hypopharynx cancers drain to multiple levels of the neck with frequent bilateral and mediastinal involvement. This portends a relatively poor prognosis for most hypopharyngeal cancers. In cases of pyriform apex or esophageal involvement, level VI is frequently positive for regional metastasis. Distant metastasis, most commonly to the lungs, occurs in up to 60% of hypopharyngeal SCC patients during the course of the disease (3).

The lifetime occurrence of second primary upper aerodigestive tract cancer after treatment of a tobacco-related head and neck squamous cell cancer (HNSCC) is as high as 25% (4), suggesting a field cancerization effect. This is true of hypopharyngeal SCC. Epidermal growth factor receptor (EGFR) is an HER/erbB family tyrosine kinase receptor overexpressed in up to 90% of HNSCC (5). Overexpression of EGFR and EGFR high copy number are associated with poor prognosis and radioresistance (6). In hypopharyngeal SCC an 11q13 amplification (cyclin D1) and loss of p53 are found in 78% and 70% respectively (7). Furthermore, mutations in *p53* have been reported in 75% of hypopharynx SCC, which is significantly more frequent than in other subsites (8).

PRESENTATION AND STAGING

Early hypopharyngeal SCC is often asymptomatic. The most common symptom is chronic sore throat with or without unilateral referred otalgia. Laryngeal extension will often result in hoarseness. Other symptoms include foreign body sensation and dysphagia leading to weight loss. Most hypopharyngeal SCC patients are diagnosed at an advanced stage with resulting poor nutritional status. Nodal involvement is common at the time of presentation both in early (60%–70%) and advanced (75%–80%) primary tumors (9).

Workup includes assessment of nutritional and performance status (e.g., Karnofsky, Eastern Cooperative Oncology Group–World Health Organization [ECOG–WHO]). Full flexible fiberoptic endoscopy should be performed to assess tumor extent and vocal cord movement and to look for synchronous second primary cancers. Of note, visualization of pyriform sinus can be enhanced with the Valsalva maneuver. Neck examination should be performed to identify enlarged cervical nodes and possible anterolateral extent of advanced cancers.

Imaging is essential to assess the primary site, regional spread, and distant metastasis. In many cases, cross-sectional imaging results in an upstaging of the tumor due to submucosal spread or cartilage invasion. Contrast-enhanced CT is the workhorse imaging modality for the majority of HNSCCs including hypopharyngeal SCC. Some clinicians and radiologists prefer MRI for assessing possible cartilage invasion (10). However, motion artifact from respirations can often limit the utility of MRI in many hypopharyngeal SCC cases.

The most common site of distant metastasis from hypopharyngeal SCC is the pulmonary parenchyma. Chest CT is routinely used to screen for pulmonary metastases and second primary cancers. Fluorodeoxyglucose PET (FDG PET) is also frequently used in patients with hypopharyngeal SCC, given the increased risk of distant metastases (11).

All patients should be assessed by a dentist experienced in oncology. This is particularly important for patients whose primary treatment includes radiation therapy (RT). Radiation-induced xerostomia and mandibular devascularization can lead to accelerated dental decay and osteoradionecrosis. So any needed dental work should be completed prior to RT. Nutritional assessment is also critical to address any nutritional deficit via an enteral or hyperalimentary route. Percutaneous gastrostomy should be used liberally as enteral support for nutritionally marginal hypopharyngeal SCC patients.

Liver function tests are advisable for hypopharyngeal SCC patients at risk of underlying hepatic disease due to alcohol abuse. Renal function testing and a hearing assessment should be assessed before initiation of platinum-based chemotherapy. Finally, baseline thyroid function tests are advised before treatment, given the proximity of pathology to the thyroid.

Fine needle aspiration (FNA) biopsy is most commonly used to establish the diagnosis because the majority of hypopharyngeal SCC patients present with cervical lymph node metastases. Direct examination of the primary tumor in the operating room can be helpful for staging and is sometimes required to establish the diagnosis via direct biopsy. However, airway management can be hazardous in hypopharyngeal SCC patients undergoing a general anesthetic and therefore is not routinely required. In patients who present with airway obstruction, tracheotomy may be required.

TREATMENT CONSIDERATIONS

The management of hypopharyngeal SCC requires consideration of primary tumor location and extension, the status of regional lymph nodes, age, performance status, and perhaps most importantly, the anticipated functional outcome and long-term toxicity.

Advanced patient age is not a contraindication to treatment. However, the 5-year site-specific survival for patients older than 75 years is less than 10%, with many patients restricted from curative treatment because of comorbid conditions (12). A palliative approach may be the best option in hypopharyngeal SCC patients with comorbid conditions that limit treatment, regardless of age.

When surgery is planned, preoperative assessment of anesthetic risk should be done.

Patients with poor pulmonary status are not candidates for conservation surgery because of the increased likelihood of aspiration and pneumonia.

Prior radiation treatment to the head and neck can further limit the options for treatment. These patients represent a challenging clinical scenario with no high level evidence to guide decision making. In general, treatment regimens considered involve surgery with or without chemotherapy. Reirradiation is typically limited to select cases owing to the increased toxicity and risk of complications.

Elective treatment of the neck is warranted for all patients with hypopharyngeal SCC. Bilateral levels II to IV should be addressed by neck dissection (ND) and RT in most cases. Rarely, patients with early lateral wall pyriform sinus disease are suitable for unilateral treatment of the neck. Of note, prior neck treatment (ND or RT) alters lymphatic drainage and should be considered during treatment planning.

Functional deficits associated with treatment of hypopharyngeal SCC are a significant factor in decision making when equivalent treatment modalities are considered. For instance, either surgery or RT would be equally expected to control early local disease. In these rare cases, surgery resulting in minimal functional deficit may be preferred over RT. Conversely, when surgery requires sacrifice of the larynx or laryngopharyngeal complex, consideration must be given to an organ-sparing nonsurgical approach. So patient preference, the ability and willingness to adhere to treatment, and the functional consequences of treatment may significantly influence decisions regarding treatment. Logistic concerns (e.g., travel, family support) are also critically important in many cases and should be evaluated with the patient and family.

TREATMENT MODALITIES

The emergence of organ preservation treatment strategies has supplanted the role of primary surgery for many patients with hypopharyngeal SCC. Surgery, which usually includes a laryngectomy, is typically performed as primary treatment in patients who are not candidates for an organ preservation strategy either because of prior radiotherapy, comorbid conditions, baseline functional compromise, or other factors. Surgery is also used as salvage therapy after failed nonsurgical treatment. So, patient selection remains paramount.

Laryngeal conservation surgery is rarely considered for hypopharyngeal SCC since the emergence of advanced radiation techniques with similar outcomes for early tumor (T) class 1-2 disease. Conservation surgery is considered suitable in patients with good pulmonary function and functional status and a primary tumor that allows voice preservation with clear margins and a low likelihood of requiring adjuvant radiation. This is exceedingly uncommon. Multiple studies have demonstrated the limited ability to assess margins in hypopharyngeal cancer due to submucosal spread (13). Therefore, the risk for positive margins is high. Hypopharyngeal SCCs that may be considered for conservation surgery include cancers limited to the lateral pyriform sinus wall that do not involve the pyriform apex, postcricoid area, or larynx (e.g., vocal fold impaired movement). Superficial well-localized cancers of the posterior hypopharyngeal wall without submucosal spread or fixation to the prevertebral structures may also present an opportunity for transoral excision. In cases with a mucosal defect too large for primary closure, closure with myocutaneous flap or free flap is preferred. With any treatment approach to hypopharyngeal SCC, possible severe swallowing and speech dysfunction should be discussed with the patient. A thorough speech and swallowing evaluation is necessary before treatment.

Most patients with hypopharyngeal SCC are not suitable for conservation surgery and require total laryngectomy with or without pharyngectomy. Cervical esophagectomy may also be required in some cases. Primary total laryngectomy is advised for all T4a hypopharyngeal SCC and those in which laryngeal function is expected to be poor after primary nonsurgical treatment. In contrast, T2-T3 hypopharyngeal SCCs involving the pyriform sinus apex or postcricoid region with good laryngeal function are good candidates for organ preservation protocols.

Total laryngopharyngectomy requires reconstruction of the hypopharynx. The method of reconstruction is largely determined by the size of the defect, the availability of microvascular expertise, and the medical condition of the patient. Most advanced hypopharyngeal SCC treated with surgery will require a pedicled myocutaneous flap or free tissue transfer to restore swallowing function. Reconstruction varies between pedicled myocutaneous flaps, tubular fascicutaneous flap, or jejunal transposition. Surgery with curative intent is contraindicated in patients with T4b hypopharyngeal SCC because of prevertebral muscle involvement, extensive mediastinal nodal involvement, or carotid artery encasement. Of these, prevertebral muscle involvement can be the most difficult to assess on preoperative imaging. This may be best evaluated as the first step during surgery for hypopharyngeal SCC when fixation of the tumor to the prevertebral musculature could be recognized in time to abort the procedure.

Management of the neck is important for all patients with hypopharyngeal SCC. If surgery is planned as initial treatment, then all involved nodal basins should be addressed. At a minimum, a unilateral neck dissection should be performed in most cases of hypopharyngeal SCC treated surgically. Early consideration for bilateral neck dissection is advised given the propensity for bilateral neck involvement. Level VI nodes should also be included for hypopharyngeal SCC with pyriform apex or esophageal invasion.

Management of the neck is frequently influenced by management of the primary tumor in hypopharyngeal SCC. One general goal in treatment is to minimize the number of modalities utilized. For instance, for a T1N0 pyriform sinus cancer, surgery including ND or RT to the primary and the neck is considered equally oncologically effective. Conversely, a patient with T1N2b hypopharyngeal SCC should be treated with multimodality therapy.

In patients treated with primary RT, the therapeutic clinical target volume (CTV) for hypopharyngeal SCC is recommended to include between 10 and 15 mm of mucosa from the gross tumor volume (GTV) to cover potential submucosal infiltration. For pyriform sinus SCC, it is recommended for RT to include the ipsilateral thyroid cartilage. Radiation dose depends on multiple factors. For early T1-T2 hypopharyngeal SCC the therapeutic dose is typically 66 to 70 Gy in 2 Gy per fraction delivered over 6.5 to 7.0 weeks. For locally advanced hypopharyngeal SCC, a therapeutic dose of 70 to 72 Gy delivered in 2 Gy fractions over 7 weeks is usually prescribed with concomitant chemotherapy or targeted therapy. For postoperative RT with or without chemotherapy dosage will range from 60 to 66 Gy in 2 Gy fractions over 6.0 to 6.5 weeks. Low-risk areas are irradiated with 50 to 56 Gy, either sequentially or concurrently with an integrated boost. In patients for whom concurrent chemotherapy is not feasible, altered fractionation (e.g., acceleration using 6 fractions per week, or hyperfractionation using BID fractions of 1.2 Gy) should be considered (14).

Cytotoxic systemic agents (both single or in combination) have been extensively described in head and neck SCC. Most prospective studies include hypopharynx primary tumors as a subset. These trials have led to established roles for the use of systemic therapy in both the curative and palliative setting.

Perhaps the most widely adopted approach for curative intent treatment of locally advanced head and neck SCC has been the concurrent administration of systemic therapy with radiation therapy. This approach is supported by the MACH-NC meta-analysis that observed a survival benefit in favor of concurrent chemoradiation (14). The use of chemotherapy is also supported by the Intergroup trial (15), a three-arm randomized phase III trial that compared radiation alone to concurrent cisplatin-based radiation therapy, and to concurrent multiagent chemotherapy with split course radiation therapy among patients with unresectable head and neck SCC. Eighteen percent of the patients enrolled in that trial had hypopharyngeal primary tumors, and these were well balanced among the three study arms. Overall survival and disease-free survival were superior in the concurrent cisplatin-based radiation therapy arm, establishing this as a therapeutic standard in unresectable head and neck SCC including hypopharyngeal SCC. This Intergroup study used a bolus cisplatin regimen of 100 mg/m^2, a widely utilized regimen in chemoradiation studies. It must be noted that the toxicities observed in the concurrent chemoradiation arm were significantly higher compared to radiation alone, with grade 3-4 mucositis occurring in the majority of patients. Nausea, vomiting, renal insufficiency, and bone marrow failure are typical adverse events. This underscores the importance of patient selection and the necessity for aggressive supportive care for patients undergoing this treatment. There is an increasing trend for the use of low-dose weekly cisplatin given with radiation therapy. This has been prospectively studied among nasopharyngeal SCC (16) and found to be noninferior to the high-dose bolus regimen. There is continued controversy regarding the adoption of this low-dose regimen for non-nasopharyngeal primary sites, especially in light of registry and prospective data predominantly in the adjuvant postoperative setting for oral cavity cancer (17), associating weekly administration with less optimal oncologic outcomes. Multiple ongoing chemoradiation studies for head and neck SCC are exploring this weekly regimen. So, prospective data are forthcoming that may shed more light onto this clinical dilemma.

Another therapeutic approach in the curative intent setting has been the upfront administration of chemotherapy prior to local therapy, also referred to as induction, neoadjuvant, or sequential chemotherapy. The MACH-NC meta-analysis found a reduction in the rates of distant metastasis in patients treated with induction chemotherapy in earlier clinical trials, making it an attractive therapeutic approach to add to concurrent chemoradiation. The TAX 324 study compared induction chemotherapy with cisplatin, 5-fluorouracil, and docetaxel (TPF) to cisplatin and 5-fluorouracil alone, both followed by carboplatin concurrent with radiation therapy. An overall survival benefit was observed in the triplet induction chemotherapy arm, and is currently the standard for induction chemotherapy (18). However, induction strategies compared to standard concurrent chemoradiation approaches have not been found to improve overall survival in several randomized trials (19,20). Antibiotic (ciprofloxacin 500 mg BID days 5–15) and granulocyte colony-stimulating factor (G-CSF) prophylaxis is recommended during induction chemotherapy.

Among patients with recurrent or metastatic hypopharyngeal SCC who are not candidates for curative intent therapy, systemic therapy as a single modality is often employed to achieve palliation of symptoms. Single and combination cytotoxic regimens have been studied with most combinations containing a platinum agent.

In the past decade, the identification of novel targeted agents with activity in SCC has transformed the landscape of therapy for these patients. The epidermal growth factor receptor (EGRr) is almost universally overexpressed among SCC, and cetuximab, an EGFr targeting monoclonal antibody, has been extensively studied. A randomized phase III trial compared platinum, 5-fluorouracil, and cetuximab (the EXTREME regimen) to the platinum and 5-fluorouracil doublet, and demonstrated a statistically significant improvement in survival in patients receiving the triplet combination (21). This led to the Food and Drug Administration (FDA) approval of cetuximab in combination with platinum and 5-fluorouracil for patients with recurrent/metastatic head and neck SCC.

Immune checkpoint inhibitors also have activity in head and neck SCC, attributed to the high mutational burden of these tobacco- and alcohol-induced tumors. Nivolumab, a programmed cell death 1 (PD)-1 inhibitor, was compared to second-line systemic therapy in patients with recurrent, metastatic head and neck SCC who have progressed on a prior platinum-based therapy. There was a statistically significant overall survival benefit in favor of nivolumab leading to recent FDA approval (22). Pembrolizumab, a biosimilar agent, has also been shown to have encouraging activity in a phase I trial for recurrent, metastatic head and neck SCC patients (23).

The introduction of active novel targeted therapies for head and neck SCC has resulted in tremendous enthusiasm in studying these agents in both the curative and palliative setting. Multiple pharmaceutical-sponsored, and federally funded studies are currently examining the integration of these agents into definitive or adjuvant chemoradiation approaches. Similarly, in the palliative setting, scientific inquiry into optimizing responses to immune checkpoint inhibitors is ongoing, many combining PD-1 inhibitors with synergistic immunotherapy agents, therapeutic vaccines, radiation therapy, or cytotoxic chemotherapy.

TREATMENT SELECTION

The treatment of hypopharyngeal SCC has evolved considerably over the last half century. Traditionally, primary surgery was followed by postoperative radiotherapy for most cases of hypopharygeal SCC. This approach yielded a 5-year survival rate of 40%, underscoring the need for improved treatment strategies (24). A randomized phase III trial comparing the results of surgical versus nonsurgical treatment for hypopharyngeal SCC was conducted by the European Organisation for Research and Treatment of Cancer (EORTC) (25). One hundred and ninety-four patients were randomized between surgery followed by postoperative adjuvant radiotherapy versus induction chemotherapy (cisplatin followed by fluorouracil) and chemoradiotherapy. There was no statistically significant difference between the two groups with regard to local or regional recurrence and disease-free survival rates at 5 years. The 5-year estimate of retaining a functional larynx was 35%.

In 2004, the EORTC and Radiation Therapy Oncology Group (RTOG) published the results of two randomized trials (EORTC trial 22931 and RTOG trial 9501) that evaluated the role of concomitant CRT in the postoperative setting for this group of patients (26,27). Level I evidence was reached with the publication of the results of these two studies, which, except for the primary end points chosen and definition of high risk, had been designed similarly. Both trials demonstrated that, compared with postoperative radiation alone, adjuvant CRT was more efficacious in terms of locoregional control and disease-free survival. For patients with locoregionally advanced hypopharyngeal SCC, the addition of cetuximab to radiotherapy significantly improves the overall survival at 5 years when compared to radiation alone (45.6% vs. 36.4%, respectively) (28).

Despite general advances in treatment for HNSCC, hypopharyngeal SCC remains highly lethal. Overall poor outcomes are related to the rich lymphatic drainage of the hypopharynx and early opportunity for distant spread. At presentation, 60% of hypopharyngeal SCC patients have locoregional disease and 10% present with distant metastases. Five-year overall survival is roughly 50% for stage I-IV hypopharyngeal SCC. The survival for patients with locoregionally advanced hypopharyngeal SCC able to tolerate aggressive treatment is only 30%. Here we offer selected cases of hypopharyngeal SCC to highlight the nuances of treatment selection.

CASE 17.1

A 60-year-old man presented with a history of sarcoidosis and Hodgkin's lymphoma treated with radiation therapy to include the neck. The patient was found incidentally during PET/CT imaging to have an isolated FDG-avid lesion of the left pyriform sinus (Figure 17.1A). The patient denied pain, hoarseness, shortness of breath, dysphagia, weight loss, and hemoptysis. His functional status was excellent.

Physical examination including office laryngoscopy revealed an exophytic tumor arising from the left piriform sinus along the edge of the aryepiglottic fold and medial wall of the pyriform sinus (Figure 17.1B) with Valsalva maneuver (Figure 17.1C). There was no evidence of lymphadenopathy (Figure 17.1D). The patient was taken to the operating room for direct laryngoscopy and biopsy, which confirmed the diagnosis of moderately differentiated invasive SCC. The patient was assessed by head and neck surgery, radiation oncology, medical oncology, speech, and dental. His case was reviewed at a multidisciplinary tumor board.

IMPRESSION: T1N0M0, STAGE I HYPOPHARYNGEAL SCC

Single modality treatment may be considered in early-stage hypopharyngeal SCC (25,29). In this case, the options of surgery and RT were discussed. RT is preferred for most cases of early-stage hypopharyngeal SCC to optimize function. However, in this case the patient has a history of prior RT to the neck. The mantle received 30.6 Gy with a larynx block after 15 Gy and then there was a boost to the mediastinum in the supraclavicular area to 38.1 Gy. Reirradiation as primary treatment would be possible given the lower dose and long interval from prior treatment. However, any form of reirradiation carries the risk for serious complications. So, a primary surgical approach was preferred if feasible with minimal functional morbidity.

The patient was dispositioned to transoral laser microsurgical resection of the primary and staged ipsilateral ND. Final pathology demonstrated a 2.4

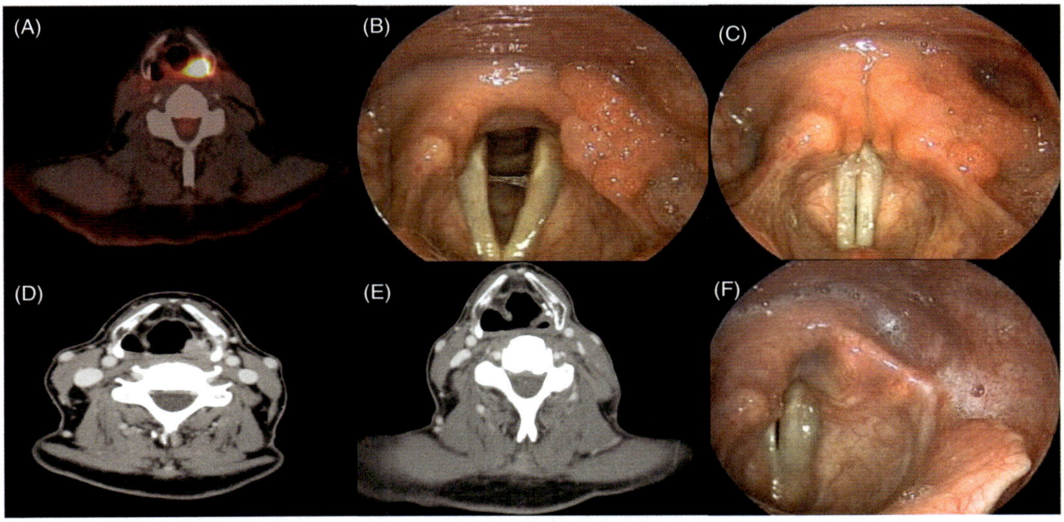

FIGURE 17.1 Pre and posttreatment left pyriform sinus squamous cell carcinoma. (A) positron emission tomography/CT demonstrating hypermetabolic lesion in the left pyriform sinus, (B) flexible nasal endoscopy view at the level of the glottis, note the exophytic fungating mass, filling the left pyriform sinus and limiting visualization of laryngeal structures (e.g., left arythenoid, AE fold). (C) endoscopic view of the hypopharynx during valsalva maneuver, note the pyriform sinus apex bilaterally. The tumor is lateral to the aryepiglottic fold and does not involve the larynx. (D) Axial, contrast enhanced, computed tomography image at the level of the AE folds demonstrating a mass filling, but limited to the left pyriform sinus. (E) posttreatment axial, contrast enhanced, computed tomography image at the level of the AE folds demonstrating the left pyriform sinus. (F) 6 months post-treatment flexible nasal endoscopy demonstrated no mass at the left pyriform sinus.

cm exophytic moderately differentiated invasive SCC with 4 mm depth of invasion and pushing borders. There was no perineural or vascular invasion and all margins were negative. None of the lymph nodes were positive for carcinoma (0/21). His postoperative course was unremarkable. At 4 years after surgery he has excellent function and remains free of disease (Figure 17.1E and 17.1F).

CASE 17.2

A 75-year-old male nonsmoker presented with complaints of a globus sensation, dysphagia, and hoarseness for 4 months. More recently, he has noted shortness of breath when lying flat and reports an unintentional 20 lb weight loss over 6 months. He is a retired painter with no previous diagnosis of cancer or radiation exposure.

On physical examination including endoscopic evaluation, there was exophytic mass of the left piriform sinus with extension onto the aryepiglottic fold and false vocal cord (Figure 17.2A). The true vocal cords were not visualized owing to the obstructing mass. Neck examination revealed a palpable enlarged lymph node in left level II.

Neck CT demonstrated a left hypopharyngeal tumor with extralaryngeal extension (Figure 17.2B). Multiple enlarged cervical nodes were present. Chest CT showed no evidence of pulmonary metastases. The diagnosis of

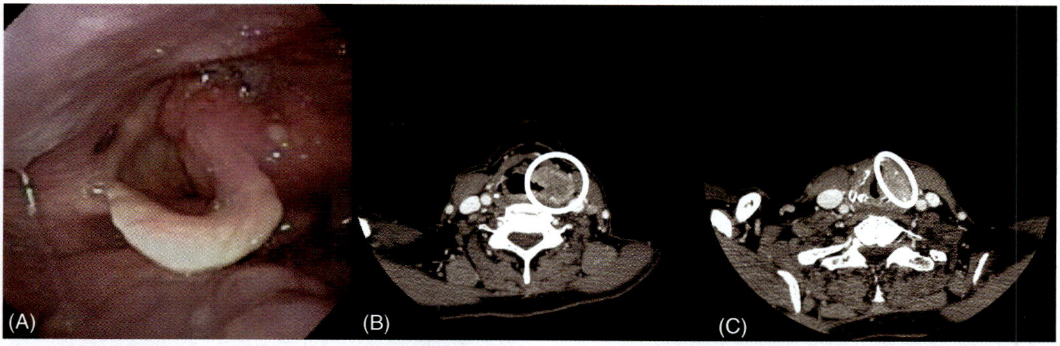

FIGURE 17.2 Advanced hypopharyngeal squamous cell carcinoma. (A) flexible nasal endoscopy view at the level of the supraglottis. Note the submucosal fullness obliterating the left pyriform sinus, pushing the epiglottis. (B) Axial, contrast enhanced, computed tomography image at the level of the epiglottis demonstrating a horseshoe mass filling the left pyriform sinus abbuting the lateral wall of the pyriform sinus. (C) Axial, contrast enhanced, computed tomography image at the level of the glottis demonstrating the left pyriform sinus tumor with destruction of the left ala of the thyroid cartilage.

hypopharyngeal SCC was confirmed by ultrasound-guided FNA of an abnormal cervical lymph node. The patient was assessed by head and neck surgery, radiation oncology, medical oncology, speech, and dental. His case was reviewed by a multidisciplinary tumor board.

IMPRESSION: T4AN2BM0, STAGE IV HYPOPHARYNGEAL SCC

In this case, imaging confirmed that the cancer involved the left supraglottic larynx and hypopharynx. The patient's airway was restricted but stable. Given evidence of extralaryngeal involvement, he was recommended a primary surgical approach followed by RT or CRT (25). However, the patient was reluctant to undergo primary laryngectomy and strongly desired a nonsurgical approach. Definitive concurrent CRT, which was favored as an alternative, would have required the placement of a tracheostomy tube to secure the airway during treatment (26,30). The patient requested an alternative strategy in hopes of avoiding a tracheostomy if possible. He was offered induction chemotherapy as chemoselection for possible nonsurgical management (31).

The patient had baseline hearing loss and was treated with induction chemotherapy using carboplatin, docetaxel, and cetuximab. He was revaluated after three cycles of induction chemotherapy and confirmed radiographically and clinically to have a partial response. Repeat imaging showed overall decreased bulkiness of the tumor but interval increase in glottic and subglottic extension with persistent laryngeal framework involvement (Figure 17.2C). Swallowing function was reevaluated and noted to have declined. He was found to have consistent penetration with thin liquids due to poor supraglottic closure.

Taken together, these factors made him a very poor candidate for a nonsurgical approach and he was advised surgery followed by radiation therapy. He subsequently underwent total laryngectomy, ipsilateral partial pharyngectomy, hemithyroidectomy, level II-IV selective neck dissection, and bilateral level VI neck dissection with microvascular free tissue transfer reconstruction.

Final pathology demonstrated a 5.5 cm poorly differentiated SCC with 25 mm depth of invasion and cartilage Invasion. The margins were negative and there was no perineural invasion. He had 5 positive lymph nodes out of 22 resected with extracapsular extension present. He was treated with postoperative RT without chemotherapy. He is currently free of disease in early surveillance.

CASE 17.3

A 72-year-old male nonsmoker presented with a right neck mass, which was confirmed SCC on FNA. The patient was otherwise asymptomatic with excellent performance status. Fiberoptic endoscopy (Figure 17.3A) showed the mass obliterating the pyriform sinus. The mass extended to the mucosa overlying the arytenoid cartilage, the false cord, lateral pharyngeal wall, and the laryngeal and lingual surfaces of the epiglottis. However, the true vocal cords were uninvolved and fully mobile.

PET–CT confirmed a bulky primary tumor with numerous ipsilateral enlarged lymph nodes. There was no evidence of contralateral neck disease or distant metastases.

CT imaging (Figures 17.3B and 17.3C) redemonstrated the hypopharyngeal SCC without extralaryngeal involvement and enlarged necrotic lymph nodes. The patient was assessed by head and neck surgery, radiation oncology, medical oncology, speech, and dental. His case was reviewed by a multidisciplinary tumor board.

IMPRESSION: T3N2BM0, STAGE IV HYPOPHARYNGEAL SCC

After a thorough discussion with the patient, an organ preservation strategy was selected. The patient was dispositioned for concurrent CRT using weekly carboplatin because of baseline hearing loss. The pretreatment tumor and nodal volumes were treated to 69.3 Gy in 33 fractions using an intensity modulated radiotherapy (IMRT) technique. The margins and at-risk portions of the neck were treated with 57 to 65 Gy.

An early posttreatment CT showed radiographic resolution of the primary tumor and improving right cervical adenopathy with residual nodes present at

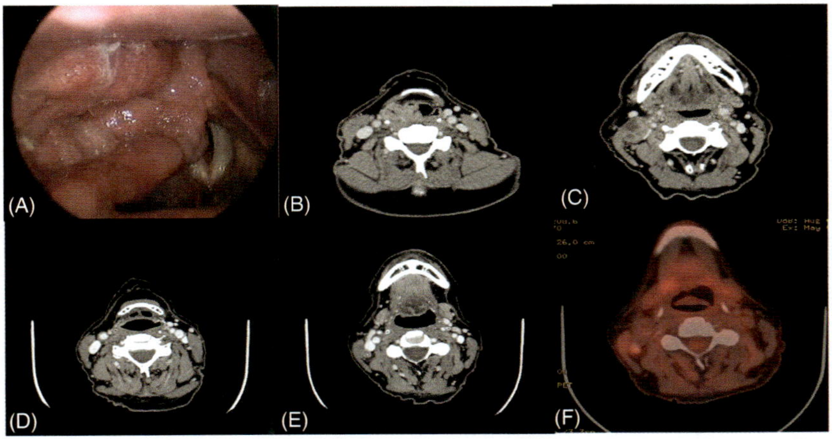

FIGURE 17.3 Pre and posttreatment right hypopharyngeal squamous cell carcinoma with nodal metastases. (A) flexible nasal endoscopic view at the level of the aryepiglottic folds. Submucosal mass, filling the right pyriform sinus and extending to the posterior pharyngeal wall. (B) Axial, contrast enhanced, computed tomography image at the level of the hyoid bone demonstrating the lateral extent of the tumor and the extensive posterior pharyngeal wall involvement. (C) Axial, contrast enhanced, computed tomography image at the level of the body of mandible demonstrating pathologically enlarged level 2 lymph node. Note the focal hypodensity of the lymph node, reflecting necrosis of the involved lymph node. Posttreatment axial, contrast enhanced, computed tomography image at the level of the (D) hyoid bone and (E) level 2 demonstrating complete resolution of the mass. AE folds demonstrating the left pyriform sinus. (F) 12 months posttreatment positron emission tomography/CT demonstrating normal metabolic activity in the right hypopharynx and neck.

right levels IIA, IIB, and III, (Figures 17.3D and 17.3E).

Metabolically active residual adenopathy was confirmed on PET/CT 3 months after treatment (Figure 17.3F). He then underwent selective neck dissection. Final pathology demonstrated 3 out of 13 metastatic lymph nodes with extracapsular extension. Tumor viability was estimated to be <20%. Currently, the patient remains free of disease 12 months after surgery with good functional and swallowing status.

CONCLUSIONS

- SCC of the hypopharynx represents a distinct clinical entity among other cancers of the head and neck region.
- These patients usually present late, commonly with nodal metastasis.
- Distant metastasis is reported to occur in up to 60% of the patients, either at presentation or during follow-up.
- The overall survival is relatively poor with high rates of regional and distant metastases early in the course of the disease.
- With the global trend toward organ-preserving therapy, CRT has gained increasing popularity over primary surgical therapies for early-stage hypopharyngeal SCC.
- Surgery is an excellent therapeutic option for those with locally advanced disease as well as salvage for failure after CRT.
- Reconstruction is often required in order to restore the swallowing function after surgery.

REFERENCES

1. Ries Lag EM, Kosary CL. *SEER Cancer Statistics Review, 1997–2002*. Bethesda, MD: National Cancer Institute; 2005.
2. Barnes L, Johnson JT. Pathologic and clinical considerations in the evaluation of major head and neck specimens resected for cancer. Part I. *Pathol Annu*. 1986;21(Pt 1):173–250.
3. Kotwall C, Sako K, Razack MS, et al. Metastatic patterns in squamous cell cancer of the head and neck. *Am J Surg*. 1987;154(4):439–442. doi:10.1016/0002-9610(89)90020-2
4. Argiris A, Brockstein BE, Haraf DJ, et al. Competing causes of death and second primary tumors in patients with locoregionally advanced head and neck cancer treated with chemoradiotherapy. *Clin Cancer Res*. 2004;10(6):1956–1962.
5. Kalyankrishna S, Grandis JR. Epidermal growth factor receptor biology in head and neck cancer. *J Clin Oncol*. 2006;24(17):2666–2672. doi:10.1200/JCO.2005.04.8306
6. Chung CH, Ely K, Mcgavran L, et al. Increased epidermal growth factor receptor gene copy number is associated with poor prognosis in head and neck squamous cell carcinomas. *J Clin Oncol*. 2006;24(25):4170–4176. doi:10.1200/JCO.2006.07.2587
7. Rodrigo JP, González MV, Lazo PS, et al. Genetic alterations in squamous cell carcinomas of the hypopharynx with correlations to clinicopathological features. *Oral Oncol*. 2002;38(4):357–363.
8. Poeta ML, Manola J, Goldwasser MA, et al. TP53 mutations and survival in squamous-cell carcinoma of the head and neck. *N Engl J Med*. 2007;357(25):2552–2561. doi:10.1056/NEJMoa073770
9. Houck JR, Medina JE. Management of cervical lymph nodes in squamous carcinomas of the head and neck. *Semin Surg Oncol*. 1995;11(3):228–239.
10. Becker M, Zbären P, Casselman JW, et al. Neoplastic invasion of laryngeal cartilage: reassessment of criteria for diagnosis at MR imaging. *Radiology*. 2008;249(2):551–559. doi:10.1148/radiol.2492072183
11. Senft A, de Bree R, Hoekstra OS, et al. Screening for distant metastases in head and neck cancer patients by chest CT or whole body FDG-PET: a prospective multicenter trial. *Radiother Oncol*. 2008;87(2):221–229. doi:10.1016/j.radonc.2008.03.008
12. Jones AS, Houghton DJ, Beasley NJ, Husband DJ. Improved survival in patients with head and neck cancer in the 1990s. *Clin Otolaryngol Allied Sci*. 1998;23(4):319–325.
13. Hirano M, Kurita S, Tanaka H. Histopathologic study of carcinoma of the hypopharynx: implications for conservation surgery. *Ann Otol Rhinol Laryngol*. 1987;96(6):625–629.
14. Pignon JP, Le Maître A, Maillard E, Bourhis J. Meta-analysis of chemotherapy in head and neck cancer (MACH-NC): an update on 93 randomised trials and 17,346 patients. *Radiother Oncol*. 2009;92(1):4–14. doi:10.1016/j.radonc.2009.04.014
15. Adelstein DJ, Li Y, Adams GL, et al. An intergroup phase III comparison of standard radiation therapy and two schedules of concurrent chemoradiotherapy in patients with unresectable squamous cell head and neck cancer. *J Clin Oncol*. 2003;21(1):92–98. doi:10.1200/JCO.2003.01.008
16. Hu Liang W-XX, Lv X, Sun R, et al. Concurrent chemoradiotherapy with 3-weekly versus weekly cisplatin in patients with locoregionally advanced nasopharyngeal carcinoma: a phase 3 multicentre ran-

domised controlled trial (ChiCTR-TRC-12001979). *J Clin Oncol.* 2017;35(suppl; abstr 6006). 2017 ASCO Annual Meeting.
17. Vanita Noronha AJ, Patil VM, Agarwal J, et al. Phase III randomized trial comparing weekly versus three-weekly (W3W) cisplatin in patients receiving chemoradiation for locally advanced head and neck cancer. *J Clin Oncol* 2017;35(suppl; abstr 6007). 2017 ASCO Annual Meeting.
18. Lorch JH, Goloubeva O, Haddad RI, et al. Induction chemotherapy with cisplatin and fluorouracil alone or in combination with docetaxel in locally advanced squamous-cell cancer of the head and neck: long-term results of the TAX 324 randomised phase 3 trial. *Lancet Oncol.* 2011;12(2):153–159. doi:10.1016/S1470-2045(10)70279-5
19. Haddad R, O'Neill A, Rabinowits G, et al. Induction chemotherapy followed by concurrent chemoradiotherapy (sequential chemoradiotherapy) versus concurrent chemoradiotherapy alone in locally advanced head and neck cancer (PARADIGM): a randomised phase 3 trial. *Lancet Oncol.* 2013;14(3):257–264. doi:10.1016/S1470-2045(13)70011-1
20. Cohen EEW, Karrison T, Kocherginsky M, et al. DeCIDE: A phase III randomized trial of docetaxel (D), cisplatin (P), 5-fluorouracil (F) (TPF) induction chemotherapy (IC) in patients with N2/N3 locally advanced squamous cell carcinoma of the head and neck (SCCHN). *J Clin Oncol.* 2012;30:5500.
21. Vermorken JB, Mesia R, Rivera F, et al. Platinum-based chemotherapy plus cetuximab in head and neck cancer. *N Engl J Med.* 2008;359(11):1116–1127. doi:10.1056/NEJMoa0802656
22. Ferris RL, Blumenschein G, Fayette J, et al. Nivolumab for recurrent squamous-cell carcinoma of the head and neck. *N Engl J Med.* 2016;375(19):1856–1867. doi:10.1056/NEJMoa1602252
23. Seiwert TY, Burtness B, Mehra R, et al. Safety and clinical activity of pembrolizumab for treatment of recurrent or metastatic squamous cell carcinoma of the head and neck (KEYNOTE-012): an open-label, multicentre, phase 1b trial. *Lancet Oncol.* 2016;17(7):956–965. doi:10.1016/S1470-2045(16)30066-3
24. Laramore GE, Scott CB, al-Sarraf M, et al. Adjuvant chemotherapy for resectable squamous cell carcinomas of the head and neck: report on Intergroup Study 0034. *Int J Radiat Oncol Bio Phys.* 1992;23:705–713.
25. Lefebvre JL, Chevalier D, Luboinski B, et al. Larynx preservation in pyriform sinus cancer: preliminary results of a European Organization for Research and Treatment of Cancer phase III trial. EORTC Head and Neck Cancer Cooperative Group. *J Natl Cancer Inst.* 1996;88(13):890–899.
26. Cooper JS, Pajak TF, Forastiere AA, et al. Postoperative concurrent radiotherapy and chemotherapy for high-risk squamous-cell carcinoma of the head and neck. *N Engl J Med.* 2004;350(19):1937–1944. doi:10.1056/NEJMoa032646
27. Bernier J, Domenge C, Ozsahin M, et al. Postoperative irradiation with or without concomitant chemotherapy for locally advanced head and neck cancer. *N Engl J Med.* 2004;350(19):1945–1952. doi:10.1056/NEJMoa032641
28. Bonner JA, Harari PM, Giralt J, et al. Radiotherapy plus cetuximab for locoregionally advanced head and neck cancer: 5-year survival data from a phase 3 randomised trial, and relation between cetuximab-induced rash and survival. *Lancet Oncol.* 2010;11(1):21–28. doi:10.1016/S1470-2045(09)70311-0
29. Nakajima A, et al. Definitive radiotherapy for T1-2 hypopharyngeal cancer: a single-institution experience. *Inter J Rad Oncol Bio Phy.* 2012;82:e129–135. doi:10.1016/j.ijrobp.2011.03.040
30. Pignon JP, Bourhis J, Domenge C, Designé L. Chemotherapy added to locoregional treatment for head and neck squamous-cell carcinoma: three meta-analyses of updated individual data. MACH-NC Collaborative Group. Meta-Analysis of Chemotherapy on Head and Neck Cancer. *Lancet.* 2000;355(9208):949–955.
31. Worden FP, Moyer J, Lee JS, et al. Chemoselection as a strategy for organ preservation in patients with T4 laryngeal squamous cell carcinoma with cartilage invasion. *Laryngoscope.* 2009;119(8):1510–1517. doi:10.1002/lary.20294

18

Laryngeal Cancer: Organ Preservation Strategies

Arlene A. Forastiere
Jae Lee
Steven B. Chinn
Karim Boudadi
Avraham Eisbruch
Randal S. Weber

In 2017, the estimated number of new cases of larynx cancer in the United States was 13,360 (10,570 men, 2,790 women) and the estimated number of deaths was 3,660. Mortality trends for the years 2000 to 2014 show a significant reduction in larynx cancer mortality rate with an average annual percentage change of −2.5%, $p < .001$ (1). Approximately 45% of newly diagnosed patients have locally advanced disease (stage III/IV) and because of the etiologic association with tobacco use, medical comorbidity is common. An analysis of Surveillance, Epidemiology, and End Results (SEER) data of patient cohorts with stage III or IV larynx cancer diagnosed in three time periods—1992 to 1997, 1998 to 2003, and 2004 to 2009—shows increasing use of nonsurgical (larynx preservation) treatment with each cohort, 32%, 45%, and 62%, respectively, coincident with significantly better disease-specific survival (DSS) and overall survival (OS) rates over time, $p < .001$ (2). Comparing surgical and nonsurgical treatment (radiation ± chemotherapy), 2- and 5-year OS was significantly better with surgical treatment (64% vs. 57% and 44% vs. 39%, $p <.001$, respectively). The difference in survival narrowed with each diagnosis year cohort suggesting a potential effect of improvements in radiation, more use of chemoradiation, and better clinical staging with the use of advanced imaging. While this SEER analysis and other large population-based data (3,4) support the concept that no larynx preservation approach results in better survival than total laryngectomy and postoperative radiation, these analyses are limited by selection bias and the absence of clinical information on medical comorbidity and operability, volume of disease, and pretreatment function. These clinical factors play a critical role in management decisions and underscore the importance of multidisciplinary evaluation including assessment of airway, speech, and swallowing function. Randomized controlled trial data from nearly three decades of research presented in this chapter and published retrospective single institution chart review cohort studies from centers of excellence (5–7) support the conclusion that for stage III disease, the survival outcomes with a combined chemotherapy and radiation approach are not inferior to treatment with total laryngectomy, while quality of life (QOL) and function are better with a preserved larynx. The results of retrospective single institution cohort studies indicate that only selected patients with low-volume T4a cancers treated with chemoradiation for larynx preservation can achieve survival results that are similar to treatment with laryngectomy. The risk of local–regional failure and salvage laryngectomy is high. Thus, guidelines recommend laryngectomy for most patients with T4a cancers and specifically for those with high-volume disease and poor baseline function.

The indications and results of conservation laryngeal surgery (CLS), single modality radiation therapy (RT), and integrated chemotherapy in combined modality approaches for operable larynx cancer of the glottis and supraglottis are reviewed, as applicable, to all stages of larynx cancer. Integral to the success of management is appropriate patient selection, follow-up care including timely salvage laryngectomy, and pre- and posttreatment function assessment/rehabilitation and toxicity management.

RADIATION THERAPY

DEFINITIVE RADIATION FOR GLOTTIC CANCER

Carcinoma In Situ

In patients with carcinoma in situ of the true vocal cords, watchful waiting strategies may result in about two thirds of patients progressing to develop invasive cancer (8). The preferred management for carcinoma in situ of the glottic larynx includes conservative surgical approaches such as vocal cord stripping; however, voice quality can deteriorate with multiple strippings and definitive radiation can provide excellent control for recurrences or diffuse lesions not amenable to limited surgery. Modern series have demonstrated local control rates of approximately 90% 5 years after therapy, and these rates appear comparable to rates for invasive T1 disease (9,10). The disease-free interval to recurrence appears longer (generally over 2 years) for patients with carcinoma in situ as compared to patients with invasive disease (11,12).

T1 to T2 Glottic Cancer

As hoarseness manifests early in disease, most glottic cancers are diagnosed at an early stage. Patients with T1 squamous cell carcinoma (SCC) of the glottic larynx have been successfully treated with multiple treatment options including definitive radiation or voice-preserving partial laryngectomy. Although no phase III trials comparing radiation with surgery have been completed, numerous large published series are consistent with equivalent tumor control between the two treatment modalities. Definitive radiotherapy series demonstrate rates of local control ranging from approximately 85% to 95% with an ultimate control rate of 95% when salvage surgery is included (13–15). Voice quality preservation rates appear equal or slightly in favor of radiation as compared to laser excision. These findings have been largely consistent across objective and subjective measures such as incomplete glottic closure and hoarseness, as well as patient-reported or physician-reported voice assessments (16,17). A large meta-analysis of transoral laser excision versus radiation suggested a trend toward improved voice quality with radiation (18). T2 SCC outcomes after radiotherapy are less favorable with local control rates ranging from 65% to 80% with an ultimate control rate, following salvage surgery, of approximately 90% (14,19,20). Risk factors for failure after definitive radiotherapy for early-stage glottic carcinoma are largely based on retrospective studies with a recent systematic review highlighting patient-related factors such as male gender, low hemoglobin, and smoking during treatment as well as tumor characteristics such as T2 disease, tumor size, and possibly poor differentiation (21).

Classical Fields for Early-Stage Glottic Cancer

Owing to the near absence of lymphatic drainage of the true glottis, the classical fields for definitive radiation have omitted regional lymph nodes. For T1-2 N0 glottic SCC, an opposing pair of lateral photon fields is most commonly used. The superior border extends to the top of the thyroid notch with the inferior border at the lower edge of the cricoid cartilage. The anterior aspect of the vertebral bodies defines the posterior border and the anterior border is flashed beyond the skin surface. These borders are adjusted depending on extension beyond the glottis for T2 disease. Typically, the field sizes for simple opposed lateral beams have been 5 × 5 cm to 6 × 6 cm, and for T1 SCC, a randomized trial showed no difference in tumor control between the two field sizes (22).

Several anatomic considerations must be made that impact dose distribution using opposed lateral fields. First, the relatively tapered shape of the neck anteriorly results in less beam attenuation that can result in higher doses being deposited in the anterior aspect of the glottis as compared to the posterior aspect. This often necessitates wedging techniques to homogenize the dose throughout the glottis, which is critical for mid-glottic and posteriorly located lesions. However, in many patients with T1 glottic SCC the tumor is confined to the anterior third of the vocal cord. In these patients, especially if the anterior commissure is involved, wedges can be omitted, or "under-wedged," producing higher doses anteriorly and lower doses posteriorly, reducing doses to the arytenoids. Second, in patients with very thin necks, particularly with anteriorly located lesions, there is often inadequate tissue for dose buildup. Tissue equivalent bolus is often required in these situations to provide sufficient material for dose buildup (23). Finally, in patients with a short neck, an inferior tilt or anterior wedge paired beams are often necessary to avoid radiation through the shoulders.

A Japanese trial randomized patients with T1 glottic carcinomas to a total of 60 to 66 Gy in standard 2 Gy fractions versus a slightly hypofractionated approach of 56.25 to 63 Gy in 2.25 Gy fractions, with the higher dose delivered to tumors spanning more than two thirds of the glottis (24). A local control benefit was demonstrated in favor of hypofractionation. For T2 glottic carcinoma, dose escalation with hyperfractionation to 79.2 Gy in 1.2 Gy twice-daily fractions versus standard fractionation to 70 Gy in 2 Gy daily fractions was tested in a randomized trial by the Radiation Therapy Oncology Group (RTOG) 9512, with 5-year local control being modestly higher with hyperfractionation (25). However, because of cost and inconvenience, twice-daily fractions have not been adopted in routine clinical practice.

Intensity Modulated Radiation Therapy Techniques for Early-Stage Glottic Cancer

Given the generally excellent tumor control rates associated with definitive radiation for early-stage glottic cancer, attempts to minimize treatment-related toxicity have been sought with techniques such as intensity modulated radiotherapy (IMRT). With opposed lateral beams, a stretch of the bilateral carotid arteries within the field receives approximately the prescription dose. The data have been mixed with respect to whether this increases the rate of cerebrovascular events. In an earlier SEER database study (26), definitive radiation for head and neck cancer was associated with excess cerebrovascular events compared with primary surgical management. However, this study did not include patients with laryngeal cancer, whose radiation fields and lengths of irradiated carotid arteries are smaller than in typical head and neck cancer patients. A more recent SEER-Medicare study of early stage (T1-T2) glottic larynx cancer found that the 10-year risk of cerebrovascular events in patients over age 65 treated with primary radiation was high, 56.5% [95%CI 51.5–61.5] but not statistically different from patients treated with primary surgery, 48.7% [95%CI 41.1–56.3] (27).

Zumsteg et al. reported on a consecutive series of early glottic cancer patients treated with conventional radiation or carotid-sparing IMRT with no difference in local control (28). Within the study, the entire larynx plus a 1 cm circumferential margin was treated; therefore, a modest reduction in dose to the bilateral carotid arteries was seen with approximately 48 Gy still delivered to the bilateral carotid arteries. Whether or not this modest carotid dose reduction is likely to reduce cerebrovascular events is unknown. Moving beyond carotid-sparing IMRT, the Dutch experience of treating a single cord rather than the entire larynx for patients with T1a true glottis carcinoma was recently reported with a median follow-up of 30 months. The rationale was to exclude the noninvolved arytenoid from the irradiated fields, with the anticipation that this would improve voice quality. Treatment was delivered with a slightly more hypofractionated regimen of 58.08 Gy in 16 fractions, and special attention was paid to prevent swallowing (causing laryngeal movement) during treatment, resulting in a 2-year local control of 100% and significantly improved voice QOL as compared to their baseline, as well as that achieved by historical control groups with conventional radiation fields.

Role of Definitive Radiotherapy for Locally Advanced Glottic Cancer

Locally advanced glottic carcinoma is managed often with total laryngectomy with or without adjuvant radiation. There is no randomized phase III data comparing definitive radiation approaches with primary surgery.

Several small retrospective series have demonstrated control rates generally ranging from 44% to 68% for T3 glottic cancers with definitive radiation, albeit in highly selected populations (29). In nonrandomized comparisons of patients undergoing primary surgery followed by postoperative radiation as indicated or primary radiotherapy with surgical salvage, rates of DSS are not significantly different, though selection bias issues persist (30). Laryngeal preservation (LP) options tested in RTOG 9111 using either induction chemotherapy followed by radiotherapy or concurrent chemoradiation are discussed in a subsequent section on multimodality approaches. Overall, the role of definitive radiotherapy alone for locally advanced glottic cancers is limited though concurrent chemoradiation improves treatment efficacy.

DEFINITIVE RADIATION FOR SUPRAGLOTTIC CANCER

Supraglottic SCC can be managed with multiple treatment modalities including voice-preserving supraglottic laryngectomy or primary radiation. Combined modality approaches with chemoradiation are covered in a subsequent section. In contrast to the lack of lymphatic drainage in the glottis, up to a third of early-to-intermediate supraglottic primary tumors harbor subclinical nodal disease in series of elective neck dissections (31). Therefore, elective nodal coverage is usually indicated in supraglottic carcinoma patients managed nonsurgically. Pure treatment modality comparisons are difficult owing to the lack of randomized data but a large retrospective study from the University of Florida generally supports the notion that supraglottic laryngectomy produces a slightly higher rate of initial tumor control than radiation when matched stage for stage, though complications such as aspiration are greater postoperatively. T1 supraglottic carcinoma treated with primary radiation has reported rates of tumor control around 84% to 100% (32). A series from MD Anderson Cancer Center for T2 and selected T3 supraglottic tumors has reported control rates of 76% with once-daily radiation treatment, and up to 80% with twice-daily radiation treatments (33). One common selection criterion for T3 supraglottic tumors amenable for definitive radiotherapy is tumor size, with studies identifying that size cutoffs of primary tumors larger than 6 cm^3 or 8 cm^3 result in lower rates of tumor control (34,35).

SURGERY

Laryngeal SCC was historically treated with surgery followed by adjuvant radiation. It was not until the Department of Veterans Affairs (VA) larynx trial in 1991 that organ preservation became widely accepted and the preferred method for treating advanced laryngeal SCC (36,37). Although organ preservation has been proved effective for T1-3 tumors, T4 tumors or patients with a dysfunctional larynx are typically often treated with total laryngectomy. CLS for T1, T2, and some select T3 disease has a wide breadth of applicability for properly selected patients, ranging from transoral endoscopic resection to open conservative laryngeal surgery. The overarching goal of therapy, regardless of modality is the appropriate use of efficacious treatments to maximize disease control while maintaining the functions of the larynx: speech, swallowing, and protection of the airway.

Primary surgical management can be further divided into conservation of the larynx versus total laryngectomy/laryngopharyngectomy. CLS can further be divided into transoral versus open laryngeal surgery; however, there has been a shift toward transoral approaches over the past decade. Open CLS is often reserved for limited disease in a select group of patients, often in the salvage setting. Options for transoral CLS include transoral endoscopic microsurgery via cold steel or via transoral laser microsurgery (TLM). Recently transoral robotic surgery (TORS) has been used with excellent results for supraglottic cancers.

CONSERVATION OF THE LARYNX

Transoral Endoscopic Laryngeal Surgery

Transoral endoscopic laryngeal surgery can be performed using cold instruments, laser, or cautery. The extent of resection is dependent on the size and extent of the laryngeal malignancy. Very localized and superficial lesions can be managed with simple cordectomy, whereas larger tumors may require a more extensive resection. Thus, it is impossible to provide precise procedural methods. Based on this, the European Laryngological Society (ELS) developed a classification system for endoscopic surgical management of glottic and supraglottic tumors to allow for a universal description of the extent of resection (Table 18.1) (38,39).

TABLE 18.1

European Laryngological Society Classification of Endoscopic Glottis Cordectomy and Supraglottic Laryngectomy

Classification of Endoscopic Cordectomy	
I	Subepithelial cordectomy
II	Subligamental cordectomy
III	Transmuscular cordectomy
IV	Total cordectomy
V	Extended cordectomy Va including contralateral vocal fold Vb including the arytenoids Vc including the ventricular fold Vd including the subglottis
VI	Anterior commissurectomy with bilateral anterior cordectomy
Classification of Endoscopic Supraglottic Laryngectomy	
I	Excision of small, superficial lesions confined to a single subsite within the supraglottis
II	Medial supraglottic laryngectomy with preservation of the preepiglottic space IIa with superior hemi-epiglottectomy IIb with total epiglottectomy
III	Medial supraglottic laryngectomy including the preepiglottic space IIIa with preservation of the ventricular fold IIIb with resection of the ventricular fold
IV	Lateral supraglottic laryngectomy IVa with resection of the ventricular fold IVb with resection of the arytenoid

Source: From Remacle M, Eckel HE, Antonelli A, et al. Endoscopic cordectomy. A proposal for a classification by the Working Committee, European Laryngological Society. *Eur Arch Otorhinolaryngol.* 2000;257(4):227–231; (39). Remacle M, Hantzakos A, Eckel H, et al. Endoscopic supraglottic laryngectomy: a proposal for a classification by the working committee on nomenclature, European Laryngological Society. *Eur Arch Otorhinolaryngol.* 2009;266(7):993–998.

The benefits of transoral endoscopic laryngeal surgery (TOELS) are the avoidance of tracheostomy, immediate resumption of oral intake, and limited hospitalization. It can also be repeated if necessary for reinspection of the surgical site or further excision of tumor. Because the lymphatic drainage of the glottis larynx is sparse and many patients present with early T stage disease the risk of regional metastasis is low and single modality therapy to manage the primary is appropriate. Oncologic and functional outcomes after TOELS are excellent and comparable to radiation for early T-classification tumors and LP has been reported to be superior. Two meta-analyses comparing radiotherapy to TLM surgery for early-stage glottic lesions found local control rates and overall and disease-specific survival rates equal between the two treatment groups. In Abdurehim et al. the local control rates, OS, and DSS rates ranged from 71% to 96% (local control, compared to RT; p = .83, odds ratio [OR]: 0.94, 95% confidence interval [CI]: 0.57–1.57), 74% to 100% (OS, compared to RT; p = .21, OR: 1.22, 95% CI: 0.89–1.66), and 95% to 100% (DSS, compared to RT; p = .19, OR: 1.60, 95% CI: 0.79–3.26), respectively. Larynx preservation rates for surgery were significantly better compared to radiation with LP rates of 82% to 100% for surgery versus 77% to 100% for radiation (p = .02, OR: 3.11, 95% CI: 1.16–8.34) (40). Similarly Higgins et al. found no difference for local control or laryngectomy-free survival with a significant improvement in OS (18). Analysis of functionality and voice quality evaluated maximum phonation time, voice perturbation, airflow rate and fundamental frequency, and the voice handicap index, all of which were not significant, but in both studies RT was slightly favored (18,40).

Despite excellent outcomes, endoscopic resection has its limitations. These include adequate endoscopic exposure to allow complete visualization and access for resection. Preoperative evaluation of neck extension, mouth opening, tongue size, and dentition can mitigate some of these variables to help predict success for endoscopic resection. Complications of endoscopic resection include infection, bleeding, granuloma formation, anterior glottis web, airway fire, aspiration, dysphagia, pharyngocutaneous fistula, cervical emphysema, airway compromise, pharyngeal bruising, pneumothorax, and perichondritis. Bleeding is the most common complication with catastrophic bleeds often occurring after supraglottic or hypopharyngeal resections due to the close proximity of the lingual and superior laryngeal artery (41).

The recent advances of TORS in head and neck cancer therapy have been applied to CLS.

Several studies have shown feasibility of TORS for laryngeal cancer with enhanced techniques and the application of the CO_2 laser fiber to the robotic arms. TORS supraglottic laryngectomy is the most common application of the robot for CLS, but it has been applied to glottic and hypopharyngeal tumors (42–44). Despite the enthusiasm regarding TORS, substantive outcomes and cost data are still lacking for TORS CLS.

Whether cold steel, TLM, or TORS, it is critical to appropriately select patients and tailor treatment modalities to the tumor extent, access, and feasibility to maximize their oncologic and functional outcomes. The central goal of transoral laryngeal surgery is to offer a single modality as the definitive oncologic therapy while maintaining optimal posttreatment function. It has been well established that the addition of radiation to attempted transoral resection will increase the morbidity and negatively affect functional capacity (45). Surgeons must critically evaluate potential transoral candidates to allow for en bloc resection with tumor-free margins, thus avoiding the need for adjuvant therapy. These concepts are critical because one third of patients who undergo laser surgery for upper aerodigestive tract malignancies, especially for more advanced T stage cancers, require revision for positive margins. While initial positive margins subsequently converted to negative by further resection did not impact OS, it does have an adverse impact on local–regional control and functional outcome (46). Additionally, the surgeon must assess the patient's physiologic ability to tolerate silent aspiration after transoral laryngeal surgery, as poor patient selection may leave the patient at risk for chronic aspiration requiring permanent percutaneous endoscopic gastrostomy (PEG) tube placement or laryngectomy.

Open Conservation Laryngeal Surgery

Open CLS encompasses a wide range of procedures from simple open/laryngofissure approach for cordectomy to more advanced supracricoid laryngectomy. Pooled outcomes for all open partial laryngectomies demonstrate local control rates of 89.8% (69%–100%), OS rates of 80% (46%–100%), and larynx preservation rates of 91% (80%–100%) (47). However, prior to consideration of open CLS, one must adhere to four oncologic and functional principles to maximize success: (a) appropriate access for resection to maintain local control, (b) thorough preoperative imaging and endoscopic evaluation to fully evaluate tumor extent, (c) preservation of at least one functional cricoarytenoid unit (contralateral arytenoid, cricoid cartilage associated muscles, and the contralateral superior and recurrent laryngeal nerve), and (d) potential necessity for resection of normal tissue to improve functional outcomes. Indications and contraindications for CLS are outlined in Table 18.2 (48-50).

Laryngofissure with cordectomy is indicated for T1 midcord lesions without vocal cord mobility impairment where endoscopic exposure is inadequate (51). Local control rates have been reported to be 93% to 100% with 97% 5-year OS (52,53).

Vertical partial laryngectomy is indicated for T1 to T3 tumors with limited paraglottic extension and vocal cord hypomobility. For T1 tumors, local control is excellent, in excess of 90%. However, anterior commissure involvement drops local control to 75%. In T2 tumors, 74% to 96% local control has been described; with subglottic extension and vocal cord mobility impairment, either by involvement of the cricoarytenoid unit or thyroarytenoid muscle in the paraglottic space, leading to lower rates of local control. For T3 lesions, local control rates range from 54% to 100% and may represent an understaging bias; thus, vertical partial laryngectomies for T3 tumors should be utilized only in select cases when the full extent of tumor invasion can be identified (48,54). Unfortunately, direct comparisons of outcomes for definitive radiation to partial laryngectomy lack comparative homogeneous patient populations, making assessments invalid. From a functional standpoint, almost all patients will experience some degree of permanent hoarseness and greater than 90% are taking a normal oral diet. Vertical partial laryngectomy for T3 glottic carcinomas may require resection of the arytenoid resulting in poor voice quality and chronic aspiration. In this setting, a supracricoid laryngectomy with cricohyoidoepiglottopexy is preferable.

Horizontal procedures can be divided into supraglottic and supracricoid laryngectomy with the former used for supraglottic malignancies and the latter for anterior commissure, transglottic, and paraglottic malignancies. The local control rates are quite high; for supraglottic laryngectomy local control was 78% to 94%. In supracricoid laryngectomy, local control was 85% to 96%. While the majority (59%) can achieve normal speech and swallow,

TABLE 18.2

Indications and Contraindications for Open Conservation Laryngeal Surgery

Procedure	Indications	Contraindications
Vertical laryngectomy	T1 glottic cancer (midcord)	Cricoarytenoid joint invasion
	Small T2 glottic cancer with minimal extension into supraglottis/subglottis	Thyroid cartilage invasion
	Any early glottic cancer that cannot be accessed transorally	Involvement of >1/3 of the contralateral vocal cord
	Salvage for radiotherapy failure of T1-T2 glottic cancer	
Supraglottic laryngectomy	Tumors limited to the supraglottic larynx with minimal base of tongue invasion	Involvement of thyroid or cricoid cartilage
	Involvement of preepiglottic or paraglottic space	Vocal fold immobility or fixation
		Invasion into extrinsic base of tongue musculature
		Bilateral arytenoid invasion
		Glottic invasion
Supracricoid laryngectomy	T1b, T2, and/or select T3 glottic, transglottic, or supraglottic cancers	Posterior commissure involvement
	Thyroid invasion without outer cortex invasion	Bilateral arytenoid involvement
	Salvage after radiation failure	Fixation of arytenoids
		Subglottic extension (>10 mm anteriorly or >5 mm posteriorly)
		Extralaryngeal spread
		Hyoid invasion

Source: From Peretti G, Piazza C, Mora F, et al. Reasonable limits for transoral laser microsurgery in laryngeal cancer. *Curr Opin Otolaryngol Head Neck Surg*. 2016;24(2):135–139; . Tomeh C, Holsinger FC. Laryngeal cancer. *Curr Opin Otolaryngol Head Neck Surg*. 2014;22(2):147–153; Succo G, Peretti G, Piazza C, et al. Open partial horizontal laryngectomies: a proposal for classification by the working committee on nomenclature of the European Laryngological Society. *Eur Arch Otorhinolaryngol*. 2014;271(9):2489–2496.

over 20% will have severe grade 2 or 3 aspiration. Tracheostomy decannulation rates are 96% while gastrostomy tube dependency is only 2% (47).

MANAGEMENT OF T4 LARYNX CANCER

The management of T4 laryngeal cancer remains controversial. In the VA larynx trial, 26% of patients in the chemotherapy arm had T4 tumors; however, the T4 tumors required a higher rate of salvage laryngectomy compared to T3 tumors (56% vs. 28%, respectively) (36,55). The RTOG 91-11 trial only included minimal select T4a tumors (minimal cartilage erosion or minimal extension to the tongue base, based on the American Joint Committee on Cancer [AJCC] staging system in effect at the time of the trial) (37). The Michigan group looked at their experience using induction selection with T4 laryngeal cancer with cartilage invasion and extralaryngeal spread. Among 36

TABLE 18.3

Comparison of Survival Rates of the T4 Study Patients With the T3 Patients Treated With Chemoradiation From UMCC 9520 and UMCC 0056

At 3 y	UMCC 9520/0056 T4 Patients n = 36	UMCC 9520/0056 T3 Patients n = 73
Median follow-up, months	69 (44–74)	74 (60–83)
Laryngectomy-free survival	58 (40–73)	62 (49–72)
Disease-free survival	58 (41–72)	72 (60–81)
Disease-specific survival	80 (62–90)	88 (78–94)
Overall survival	78 (60–88)	83 (72–90)

UMCC, University of Michigan Comprehensive Cancer Center.

Source: From Worden FP, Moyer J, Lee JS, et al. Chemoselection as a strategy for organ preservation in patients with T4 laryngeal squamous cell carcinoma with cartilage invasion. *Laryngoscope.* 2009;119(8):1510–1517. Reprinted with permission from Wiley & Sons.

patients treated in two phase II trials, 81% were found to be responders to one cycle of cisplatin (100 mg/m^2) and 5-fluorouracil (5-FU). Of those who responded and underwent definitive chemoradiation, 85% obtained a complete histologic response and a 58% LP rate. The 3-year OS and DSS rates were 78% and 80%, respectively. Survival comparisons to T3 tumors are demonstrated in Table 18.3 (55).

From a functional standpoint, more T4 patients were gastrostomy tube dependent compared to a historical cohort of T3 tumors (17% vs. 4% respectively) yet tracheostomy tube dependency was equivalent (55). However, there is a lack of level I evidence comparing treatment modalities for T4 larynx cancer. For T4 cancer of the larynx, organ preservation is typically not offered owing to concerns over loss of function based on the destructive nature of T4 lesions, improved survival outcomes, and lower response rates to induction chemotherapy in T4 tumors. Two large population database analyses were done comparing organ preservation versus total laryngectomy for T4a tumors. Both found that surgery was associated with significantly improved 5-year OS and DSS compared to nonsurgical approaches (OS 69% vs. 56%, respectively; DSS 56% vs. 38%, respectively) (2,4). Based on this, surgery followed by radiation with pathology directed chemotherapy is the recommendation of the National Comprehensive Cancer Network (NCCN) for T4a tumors of the larynx. In these cases, total laryngectomy with bilateral selective neck dissections is indicated. Despite the laryngeal end organ being completely removed, 90% of patients can generally tolerate a regular diet and 83% can have intelligible voice after tracheal esophageal puncture (56). While tracheal esophageal puncture is the most commonly used speech rehabilitation method to date, other options for voicing include electrolarynx or esophageal speech.

MANAGEMENT OF THE NECK

The role of neck dissection at the time of primary laryngeal surgery is dependent on two main variables: (a) presence of clinically evident disease in the neck and (b) location of the primary. In the setting of clinically positive neck disease, therapeutic neck dissection is warranted at the time of laryngeal surgery. However, the choice to proceed with CLS in the setting of nodal disease must be weighed heavily against the need for adjuvant therapy independent of the stage of the laryngeal primary. We recommend avoiding surgery and proceeding with definitive radiation or concurrent chemoradiation in the setting of clinically positive neck disease as this will decrease the need for trimodality treatment to the primary, thus maximizing posttreatment function while maintaining equivalent survival. In the elective setting, the decision to address the neck is based on the location of the primary tumor. For early glottic tumors, the risk of having occult disease is very low, 0%, and 19% in early- and late-stage disease, respectively (57). Buckley and MacLennan prospectively performed elective neck dissections in patients with laryngeal and hypopharyngeal malignancies and found occult disease in 64% of supraglottic cancers, 50% of multiregional cancers, 36% of hypopharyngeal cancers, and 10% of glottic cancers (58). Based on these studies, observation is recommended for early-stage disease glottic cancers and elective neck dissection for all other subsites.

COMBINED MODALITY APPROACHES

INDUCTION CHEMOTHERAPY

LP through a combined modality approach was first established by the landmark Veterans Affairs Laryngeal Cancer Study Group (VALCSG) trial (59). This phase III trial randomized 332 patients with stages III and IV larynx cancer to total laryngectomy followed by RT, or to chemotherapy (ICT) with cisplatin and fluorouracil (PF) followed by RT in chemotherapy responders (Table 18.4). The study tested the hypothesis that a favorable response to ICT with no gross or small-volume residual disease would facilitate tumor eradication by RT and enable preservation of laryngeal function. Importantly, the trial design mandated that patients with a poor response after two cycles of PF or with persistent tumor after completion of RT undergo early salvage laryngectomy. This required the collaborative efforts of a multidisciplinary team for evaluation of response during the course of treatment, follow-up monitoring, and assessment of speech and swallowing function (60,61). At 3 years, 62% of surviving patients who had been randomized to induction PF had a preserved larynx. In addition, after 10 years of follow-up, there was no statistically significant difference in OS between the two groups (62). This trial demonstrated that LP through ICT was feasible and would not jeopardize survival. Other key study findings included the pattern of recurrence that showed a significantly lower rate of metastases in the ICT group but more local recurrences. In addition, 56% of patients with T4 cancers ultimately required salvage laryngectomy and these cancers were associated more frequently with glottic than supraglottic subsite, and gross cartilage invasion than no cartilage involvement. One important criticism of the trial was that the control rate for T3 cancers (which accounted for 65% of enrolled patients) was similar to historical published results with radiation alone (63,64), and that a comparator RT-only arm was needed. This led to the design of the Intergroup RTOG 91-11 trial (see Concurrent Chemoradiation).

Another randomized study of ICT as an organ preservation strategy was the Groupe d'Oncologie Radiothérapie Tête et Cou (GORTEC) 2000–2001 trial. This phase III study compared ICT with PF versus taxane (docetaxel), cisplatin, and fluorouracil (TPF) in 213 patients with stages III and IV larynx and hypopharynx cancers (Table 18.4) (65). The results demonstrated a significantly higher response rate with induction TPF compared to PF (80% vs. 59%, p = .002), which enabled more patients to undergo definitive RT. This in turn translated to a significantly higher rate of LP in the TPF group at 5 years (74% vs. 57.5%, p = .03) and at 10 years (70% vs. 46.5%, p = .01). However, other outcomes including the rates of local recurrence, late salvage surgery, distant metastases, and OS were not improved with TPF compared to PF. The small sample size precluded analysis according to primary site; thus, while providing support for induction TPF on the basis of response rate, it did not break new ground in the search for a more efficacious organ preservation approach specific to larynx cancer.

The European Organisation for Research and Treatment of Cancer (EORTC) conducted a trial that established ICT as the evidence-based standard for larynx preservation for patients with hypopharynx cancer (66). EORTC 24891 compared induction PF followed by RT with surgery (total laryngectomy and partial pharyngectomy) in 202 patients with cancer of the pyriform sinus (Table 18.4). LP rate, which was reported as a composite end point of DSS with larynx and no g-tube or tracheostomy, approached 42% at 3 years. The response to ICT correlated with T stage with rates of 82%, 48%, and 0% for T2, T3, and T4 disease, respectively. The feasibility of LP was demonstrated in patients who achieved a complete response of the primary, as was required to proceed with RT. In addition, a long-term follow-up report confirmed the initial observed results of equivalence of the two approaches for OS and pattern of failure (67). After a median follow-up of 10.5 years, there was no significant difference in OS for patients treated with ICT for three cycles compared with initial surgery and radiation.

TABLE 18.4

Combined Modality Larynx Preservation Randomized Trial Designs and Outcomes

Therapy	Study	Years	No. of Patients	Site	Stage	Treatment Sequence	Larynx Preservation*	Overall Survival
Induction chemotherapy	VALCSG Phase III (59)	1985–1988	332	Larynx SG (63%) G (37%)	III (57%) IV (43%)	a) TL → RT b) PF x 3 → RT	a) NA b) 62% (3 y)	a) 56% (3 y), 45% (5 y) b) 53% (3 y), 42% (5 y)
	GORTEC 2000–01 Phase III (65)	2000–2005	213	Larynx (46%) Hypopharynx (54%)	III, IV	a) PF x 3 → RT b) TPF x 3 → RT	a) 57.5% (3-y) b) 70.3% (3-y)	a) 60% (3 y) b) 60% (3 y)
	EORTC 24891 Phase III (66,67)	1986–1993	202	Hypopharynx	II (7%) III (57%) IV (37%)	a) TLP → RT b) PF x 3 → RT	a) NA b) 42% (3 y), 27% (10 y)	a) 43% (3 y), 14% (10 y) b) 57% (3 y), 13% (10 y)
Concurrent chemo radiation	RTOG 91-11 Phase III (37,68)	1992–2000	547	Larynx SG (69%) G (31%)	III (64%) IV (36%)	a) PF x 3 → RT b) RT + P c) RT	a) 71% (5 y), 68% (10 y) b) 84% (5 y), 82% (10 y) c) 66% (5 y), 64% (10 y)	a) 58% (5 y), 39% (10 y) b) 55% (5 y), 28% (10 y) c) 54% (5 y), 32% (10 y)
	EORTC 24954-22950 Phase III (69)	1996–2004	450	Larynx (48%) Hypopharynx (54%)	II (4%) III (39%) IV (58%)	a) PF x 4 → RT (70 Gy) b) PF alternating/RT (60 Gy)	a) 40% (3 y) b) 45% (3 y)	a) 62.2% (3 y) b) 64.8% (3 y)
Sequential therapy	TREMPLIN Phase II (70)	2006–2008	153	Larynx (41%) Hypopharynx (59%)	II (11%) III (56%) IV (33%)	a) TPF x 3 → RT + P b) TPF x 3 → RT + C	a) 79% (2 y) b) 72% (2 y)	a) 75% (3 y) b) 73% (3 y)

*The definition of larynx preservation varies with the study; refer to cited work and discussion in the text of this chapter.

C, cetuximab; EORTC, European Organisation for Research and Treatment of Cancer; G, glottic; GORTEC, Groupe d'Oncologie Radiothérapie Tête et Cou; NA, not applicable; P, cisplatin; PF, cisplatin plus fluorouracil; RT, radiation therapy; RTOG, Radiation Therapy Oncology Group; SG, supraglottic; TL, total laryngectomy; TLP, total laryngectomy with partial pharyngectomy; TPF, docetaxel plus cisplatin plus fluorouracil; VALCSG, Veterans Affairs Laryngeal Cancer Study Group.

CONCURRENT CHEMORADIATION

While ICT for the treatment of locally advanced operable larynx cancers evolved as the favored organ preservation approach in Europe, concomitant cisplatin and RT (CCR) using standard fractionation is the recommended standard of care in North America. This is based on significantly higher rates of larynx preservation and local control achieved for T3 and low-volume T4 cancers treated with concurrent cisplatin and RT demonstrated in direct comparison to the induction approach and to treatment with RT alone. The landmark Intergroup RTOG 91-11 trial was a critical study in establishing this standard. This phase III trial separately compared concomitant cisplatin (100 mg/m^2 on days 1, 22, and 43) plus RT and RT alone with induction PF followed by RT (Table 18.4) (37). A total of 547 patients with stages III and IV larynx cancer were enrolled; high-volume T4 cancers penetrating through cartilage or extending more than 1 cm into the base of the tongue were excluded. Because of this eligibility criterion, only 10% of patients enrolled had T4 disease and this precluded subset analysis by T stage. The primary end point was a composite end point of laryngectomy-free survival (laryngectomy or death as events). However, because this composite end point did not account for patients dying from noncancer-related causes with a retained larynx, all end points were reported separately for clarity. Both LP and local control rates were significantly higher in the CCR group with a 54% relative risk reduction (hazard ratio [HR]: 0.46, 95% CI: 0.30–0.71, p = .001) for undergoing laryngectomy for CCR compared with RT alone, and a 42% risk reduction (HR: 0.58, 95% CI: 0.37–0.89, p = .005) compared with induction PF followed by RT. At 2- and 5-year follow-up, there was no significant difference in OS between treatment groups. At 10 years of follow-up, this continued to be the case (68), although there was a trend favoring the ICT group with separation of the curves beginning around the 5-year mark. With long-term follow-up, the composite end point of laryngectomy-free survival changed from nonsignificant to significant for ICT versus RT (28.9% vs. 17.2%; p = .02) while laryngectomy-free survival was statistically significant for CCR versus RT at 2, 5, and 10-year analyses. The CCR group had the lowest rate of larynx cancer–related deaths while also having the highest rate of noncancer-related deaths. The reason for this finding remains unclear. It is speculated that late toxicity affecting swallowing function could have occurred and contributed to the higher rate of noncancer-related deaths although no difference in late effects, or speech and swallowing function was found. It should be noted that most patients in RTOG 91-11 were treated with two-dimensional RT plans in contrast to the modern RT techniques (IMRT, three-dimensional) of today.

Another trial of combined chemotherapy and radiation as a larynx preservation strategy was the EORTC 24954-22950 study (69). This phase III trial enrolled 450 patients with stages II to IV larynx (48%) or hypopharynx (52%) cancers, and compared induction PF followed by RT (the control arm) with a regimen of PF alternating with 2-week courses of RT (Table 18.4). The design and goal of alternating cycles of chemotherapy and RT rather than concurrent administration was to improve local control through the close timing of chemotherapy and RT but to reduce the greater potential for late effects of concurrent administration. All nonresponders underwent salvage laryngectomy and postoperative RT. LP was a composite end point defined as survival with a retained larynx without a tracheostomy or gastrostomy tube in place for more than 3 months. The initial results were reported in 2009 with a median follow-up of 6.5 years (69), and updated in 2016 after a median follow-up of 10.2 years (71). There was no statistically significant difference between the two groups in the primary end point of survival with a functional larynx (local control, no tracheotomy or feeding tube) or the secondary end points of larynx preservation, progression-free survival (PFS), and OS. The median survival time with a functional larynx was 1.6 years versus 2.3 years, and median OS 5.1 years versus 5.0 years for the induction PF and alternating groups, respectively. Analysis of LP rates showed a trend for a higher rate in the alternating treatment group, as 25.2% required salvage laryngectomy compared with 31.7% in the induction group. In addition, there was a trend for better laryngeal function in the alternating treatment group at 1 and 5 years after treatment. Acute mucosal and skin toxicities were significantly worse in the induction group, presumably due to the higher RT dose, but late toxicities were similar between the two groups. Because the alternating treatment did not significantly improve outcomes, this approach was not pursued further.

SEQUENTIAL THERAPY

Sequential therapy, or ICT followed by CCR, is another combined modality approach that has been studied in randomized mixed-site trials, but as yet, there are no data to demonstrate improved survival compared to CCR and the approach is investigational. Currently, there are no data from phase III randomized, controlled trials in larynx cancer. Based on the results of the GORTEC 2000–2001 trial (65), and the pivotal radiotherapy plus cetuximab trial (72,73), the TREMPLIN study (Radiotherapy with Cisplatin versus Radiotherapy with Cetuximab after Induction Chemotherapy for Larynx Preservation) evaluated the feasibility of a sequential approach for LP (70). This randomized phase II trial enrolled 153 patients with larynx or hypopharynx cancer (T2-3 and N0-3) to receive three cycles of induction TPF followed by either cetuximab or cisplatin concurrent with RT (Table 18.4). The primary end point of the study was LP 3 months after treatment completion. As a result of a high dropout rate (24%) from TPF toxicity and insufficient tumor response, the study did not meet the prespecified LP end point of 80%. In addition, concurrent RT plus cetuximab proved as toxic as RT plus cisplatin, causing similar rates of grade 3-4 acute mucositis with worse in-field skin toxicity. More local failures were seen in the RT plus cetuximab group, which raised the possibility that cetuximab may be inferior to cisplatin for concurrent treatment with RT for achieving local control in larynx cancer. This feasibility study demonstrated that both RT plus cetuximab and RT plus cisplatin were difficult to administer after induction TPF. Furthermore, the LP rate was no better than that seen with TPF followed by RT alone in the GORTEC 2000–2001 study (65).

Other feasibility data specific to larynx cancer come from a retrospective, unplanned subset analysis of operable larynx and hypopharynx cancers (n = 123) in the phase III multisite TAX-324 trial that was published in 2009 (74). This small cohort analysis compared two sequential regimens (three cycles of cisplatin and 5-FU with or without docetaxel followed by RT with concurrent carboplatin), and suggested that the addition of docetaxel improved laryngectomy-free survival and PFS but did not improve OS. The rate of LP was not specifically addressed in this report.

Another approach comes from a single institution, single-arm phase II trial conducted at the University of Michigan. These investigators used the response to a single cycle of induction platinum/5-FU as a predictive biomarker for selecting patients for LP with definitive CCR, in contrast to administering multiple cycles of ICT (75). A total of 97 patients with stages III and IV larynx cancer were enrolled in this prospective trial, including one third with T4 high-volume or deeply invasive cancers. After one cycle of platinum/5-FU, 75% of patients achieved at least a partial response. The LP rate was estimated at 70%. At 2 and 3 years, respectively, OS was 88% and 85%, disease-free survival was 80% and 78%, and laryngectomy-free survival was 63% and 61%. The excellent OS estimates reported for this advanced population may be explained by early patient selection and timely integration of surgery. It is important to note that while two cycles of adjuvant cisplatin/5-FU were planned, this was feasible in only 28% of 68 patients eligible for adjuvant chemotherapy.

This neoadjuvant "bioselection" experience was recently expanded by the same investigators in a retrospective case series of 153 patients with stage III/IV larynx cancer, of which 71 patients were treated with the neoadjuvant bioselection approach, 45 with chemoradiation (without induction), 32 with primary laryngectomy, and 5 with RT alone. All patients were evaluated in a multidisciplinary clinic and included function assessments and comorbidity scoring (76). The ultimate treatment was based on individual physician recommendation and patient preferences. For those treated with the bioselection approach, including 32 (45%) patients with T4a cancer, a DSS of 79%, and an OS rate of 76% at 5 years was reported. Only 9% of patients required total laryngectomy after poor response to ICT, while 18% of patients required salvage surgery after completion of definitive CCR. The overall LP rate was 66%, decreased to 48% for functional preservation when the presence of tracheostomy or feeding tube at 1 year after treatment was considered.

Using response to ICT as a surrogate predictive biomarker for successful organ preservation, followed by RT plus cisplatin to maximize local control, is an appealing concept. However, intensifying treatment by adding multiple cycles of ICT to CCR has yet to show a benefit in survival or organ preservation rate compared to a control group of CCR alone. The bioselection approach using a single cycle of ICT is intriguing and a broader evaluation appears warranted. Sequential therapy remains experimental; randomized controlled trials that are adequately powered for site-specific analyses are needed.

FOLLOW-UP CARE AND SALVAGE SURGERY

FOLLOW-UP CARE

After nonsurgical organ preservation or CLS of laryngeal cancer, follow-up is critical to identify recurrence and continued functional assessments. Despite high recurrence rates, salvage surgery has a higher rate of success and long-term survival than other subsites in the head and neck; thus early identification of recurrence and salvage is critical to improving outcomes. Control rates from the RTOG 91-11 trial are described in Table 18.5 (77). At 5 years, local failure rates are 41.8%, 28.9%, and 46.4% for induction chemotherapy, definitive concurrent chemoradiotherapy, and radiation alone, respectively. Locoregional failure rates range from 28% in the definitive concurrent chemoradiotherapy group and 48% in radiation alone. Based on this, close follow-up is warranted to identify any local, regional, or distant failures to allow for salvage.

The NCCN guideline recommends follow-up with a head and neck examination and flexible laryngoscopy every 1 to 3 months for the first year, then every 2 to 6 months for the second year, then every 4 to 8 months for years 3 to 5, and then annually after year 5 posttreatment. In the setting of organ preservation, a 3-month posttreatment PET–CT is our preferred method to evaluate for persistent disease and PET–CT response can serve as a mortality risk assessment tool (78). PET–CT imaging earlier than 3 months will yield higher rates of false positive results and unnecessary interventions. In salvage patients or those who received adjuvant therapy, it is imperative to monitor thyroid function. The rate of radiation-induced hypothyroidism is 20% to 30% with half occurring in the first 5 years after completion of radiation. Clinical risk factors for developing postradiation hypothyroidism are female gender (OR 1.6), neck surgery (independent of thyroidectomy; OR 1.7), Caucasian descent (OR 4.8), and a radiation dose response (although absolute dose amounts could not be determined) (79). We recommend thyroid-stimulating hormone (TSH) to be monitored every 6 months for the first 3 years and then annually thereafter.

An important point in laryngeal cancer is the high rate of former or current smokers. During follow-up it is important to screen for second primary lung cancers. The U.S. Preventive Services Task Force recommends an annual low-dose CT chest screening for all current and former smokers (former smokers must have quit smoking within 15 years) between the ages of 55 and 80 years with at least 30 pack-years of cigarette smoking (80,81). This screening strategy reduced lung cancer related mortality rate by 20% (81).

RECURRENCE AND SALVAGE SURGERY

In the RTOG 91-11 trial and VA larynx trial, 25% and 36% of patients required a total laryngectomy, predominantly for persistent or recurrent disease; 5% required total laryngectomy for a dysfunctional larynx (36,37). Disease control rates after salvage are excellent, with disease-free status reaching up to 82% and local–regional control ranging from 74% to 90% (82). Functionally, patients do quite well after salvage total laryngectomy with 80% to 84% taking an oral diet and 77% to 87% utilizing tracheoesophageal speech (83,84). Salvage surgery after organ preservation therapy often warrants total laryngectomy; however, in select cases open partial laryngectomy may have a role. Paleri and colleagues performed a systematic review of oncologic outcomes after open conservation salvage laryngectomy. They found that local control rates at 24 months were 86.9%, the OS rate was 83.1%, and the larynx preservation rates were 83.9%. Functional outcomes were limited with tracheostomy decannulation rates at 95%, and voice and swallow outcomes were vaguely reported as "satisfactory speech and swallow" in 76% of patients, while 13% reported no usable speech. There was significant heterogeneity in the swallowing function analysis, with only three studies reporting gastrostomy tube dependence in one patient, making interpretation of functional outcomes difficult (85). Ganly et al. compared salvage partial laryngectomy with salvage total laryngectomy. They found that salvage partial laryngectomy was associated with improved OS (89% vs. 50%) and improved DSS (93% vs. 51%). However, the age and clinical T stage were predictors of poor outcome. They did not report functional outcomes (86). There is inherent bias in this analysis as those who had more

TABLE 18.5

RTOG 91-11 5- and 10-Year Estimates of Efficacy End Points

End Point	RT + Induction Chemotherapy		RT + Concomitant Chemotherapy		RT Alone	
	Estimate (%)	95% CI (%)	Estimate (%)	95% CI (%)	Estimate (%)	95% CI (%)
Laryngectomy-free survival						
5 years	44.1	36.6 to 51.6	47.0	39.5 to 54.5	34.0	26.8 to 41.3
10 years	28.9	21.9 to 36.0	23.5	16.8 to 30.3	17.2	11.2 to 23.3
Larynx preservation						
5 years	70.8	63.9 to 77.6	83.6	78.1 to 89.2	65.8	58.7 to 73.0
10 years	67.5	60.4 to 74.6	81.7	75.9 to 87.6	63.8	56.5 to 71.1
Local control						
5 years	58.2	50.8 to 65.6	71.1	64.3 to 77.9	53.6	46.1 to 61.1
10 years	53.7	46.1 to 61.2	69.2	62.3 to 76.1	50.1	42.5 to 57.7
Locoregional control						
5 years	54.8	47.3 to 62.3	67.7	60.7 to 74.7	51.2	43.7 to 58.8
10 years	48.9	41.3 to 56.5	65.3	58.1 to 72.4	47.2	39.6 to 54.8
Distant control						
5 years	85.3	79.9 to 90.6	86.4	81.2 to 91.6	78.0	71.7 to 84.3
10 years	83.4	77.7 to 89.0	83.9	78.2 to 89.5	76.0	69.4 to 82.5
Disease-free survival						
5 years	37.7	30.4 to 45.0	38.0	30.8 to 45.3	28.0	21.1 to 34.8
10 years	20.4	14.0 to 26.7	21.6	15.2 to 28.0	14.8	9.2 to 20.3
Overall survival						
5 years	58.1	50.6 to 65.5	55.1	47.6 to 62.6	53.8	46.1 to 61.4
10 years	38.8	31.2 to 46.3	27.5	20.4 to 34.5	31.5	24.1 to 39.0

CI, confidence interval; RT, radiation therapy; RTOG, Radiation Therapy Oncology Group.
Source: From Duprez F, Madani I, De Potter B, et al. Systematic review of dose—volume correlates for structures related to late swallowing disturbances after radiotherapy for head and neck cancer. *Dysphagia*. 2013;28(3):337–349. Reprinted with permission from American Society of Clinical Oncology.

advanced disease were more likely to undergo salvage total laryngectomy. While survival may be similar, the dearth of quality data for functional outcomes requires further comparative study to determine CLS's overall efficacy in the salvage setting.

The role of elective neck dissection at the time of salvage laryngectomy is a point of contention among head and neck surgeons, particularly for early-stage glottic tumors. Some argue that the neck has been treated by the definitive radiation, while others argue that in early-stage glottis tumors, the rate of occult disease is low and the standard narrow field radiation is satisfactory. Recently, the prevalence and distribution of occult disease in the salvage setting were analyzed. Birkeland et al. retrospectively evaluated 233 patients who underwent salvage laryngectomy and neck dissection. Eighty-eight percent were clinically N0 and underwent elective neck dissection. Within this group, 17% had occult nodal disease. Advanced stage and supraglottic recurrence were the primary predictors of occult nodal metastasis. Supraglottic tumors were more likely to metastasize to levels II, III, and VI (17%, 16%, and 15% respectively) while glottis tumors were more likely to metastasize to paratracheal nodes (20%). Across other studies, the rate of occult metastasis is 17% with a range of 0% to 30% (87). We recommend elective neck dissection for all advanced stage tumors (independent of laryngeal subsite) and all supraglottic malignancies.

One of the challenges after salvage laryngectomy is the higher rates of postoperative complications. Subset analysis of the RTOG 91-11 trial found that in patients undergoing salvage laryngectomy, nearly 60% had a major or minor complication with fistula rates ranging from 15% to 30% (82). Goodwin reviewed complications following salvage total laryngectomy for upper aerodigestive tract cancer, and found the operative mortality rate to be 5% and the major complication rate was 27% (88). When looking at the type of radiation, Metson et al. found a threefold increase in the incidence of minor postoperative complications and an increased hospitalization following twice-a-day RT as opposed to conventional fractionation. The authors concluded that the increased rate of minor complications was justified for increased tumor control obtained with altered fraction radiation schedules (89).

Within the complications associated with salvage surgery, pharyngocutaneous fistula is one of the major and more challenging complications following salvage total laryngectomy; associated with delayed oral intake, increased hospitalization and costs, poor wound healing leading to increased risk of losing the remaining native neck skin, pharynx, and tracheostoma, ultimately leading to carotid artery or jugular vein blowout. Prolonged fistulas cause chronic inflammation that promotes scar formation ultimately leading to pharyngeal stricture and reduced survival (90). In the salvage setting, pharyngocutaneous fistula rates range from 14% to 80% with a 2.3-fold increase in risk due to prior radiation or chemoradiation (91,92). The literature is replete with single institutional retrospective analyses of the etiology of fistula formation with the goal to alter those variables. Several studies have investigated the use of out-of-field, vascularized tissue (free flap or pedicled flaps) as a method to minimize wound complications. Some studies have found that using nonirradiated, vascularized flaps reduced the incidence and severity of fistula. Sharaf and colleagues found that free flap reconstruction was associated with lower fistula rates compared to primary closure (5% vs. 11%, respectively) (93–95). While there are no randomized control trials, a recent systematic review concluded that flap reconstruction has a protective effect against fistula with a pooled relative risk of 0.63; thus the risk of fistula formation was 50% higher in primary closure (96). Based on this, we recommend flap reconstruction for all salvage total laryngectomies.

FUNCTIONAL LARYNX PRESERVATION AND QUALITY OF LIFE

For most cancers, survival is usually the top patient concern. However, laryngeal cancer patients are unique in that a subset who prioritize organ function over survival has been consistently identified, fueling the development of LP approaches for locally advanced tumors (97). Herein, we carefully define quality of life (QOL), challenges associated with its measurement, and the impact of dysphagia on laryngeal cancer patients.

TOXICITY VERSUS QUALITY OF LIFE

Numerous instruments to standardize the lexicon and grading of toxicity end points have been developed. The World Health Organization

(WHO) grading system developed in 1979 was the first, followed by the National Cancer Institute (NCI) Common Toxicity Criteria (CTC v1.0) system in 1983. Both scales were originally designed for chemotherapy-related acute toxicity but in 1984 the RTOG and the EORTC started developing specific systems for acute and late adverse effects following RT (98). Modern revisions of the NCI CTC scale incorporate elements of the RTOG criteria and grade both acute and late toxicities attributable to surgery, radiation, and chemotherapy (99).

QOL is multidimensional and defined by the WHO as an "individual's perception of their position in life in the context of the culture and value systems in which they live and in relation to their goals, standards and concerns" (100). Unlike toxicity, QOL is by definition a subjective outcome, necessitating patient-reported end points. Accurately capturing QOL is a considerable challenge, requiring instruments that are reliable, valid, responsive to change, and clinically practical (101,102).

Measuring Quality of Life in Head and Neck Cancer Patients

Several head and neck cancer specific QOL instruments have been developed, and are generally patient-administered and multidimensional yet with retention of an assessment of global QOL. One of the most commonly used instruments is the H&N-35 module, usually administered with the full EORTC Quality of Life Questionnaire (QLQ-C30). The University of Washington Quality Of Life Questionnaire (UW-QOL) is another validated head and neck cancer specific instrument and currently comprises 12 domain-specific questions and 3 global questions (103,104). The Functional Assessment of Cancer Therapy-Head and Neck (FACT-HN) Subscale is an 11-item instrument often administered with the 28-item generalized version (Functional Assessment of Cancer Therapy-General [FACT-G]) that describe patient functioning in six areas: physical well-being, social and family well-being, relationship with doctor, emotional well-being, functional well-being, and head and neck related symptoms (105,106). The University of Michigan Head and Neck Quality of Life (HN-QOL) instrument is a 20-item validated questionnaire grouped into four domains: communication, pain, eating, and emotion and also includes several global questions regarding overall bother and satisfaction (102). The NCI's Patient-Reported Outcomes Version of the Common Terminology Criteria for Adverse Events (PRO-CTCAE) has recently been developed and is under active investigation to become the standard for QOL data collection (107,108).

Notable Biases in Quality of Life Questionnaires

Patient-reported QOL questionnaires are more accurate than observer-rated reports as QOL is inherently subjective. However, these reports have limitations and biases stemming from several sources. First, pretreatment baseline QOL assessments are somewhat artificial because QOL data are usually obtained after the patient is under emotional or physical distress of having been diagnosed with cancer. This artificial baseline may not be truly reflective of the patient's status prior to diagnosis (109). Cancer patients may also change their health-related QOL assessments as they try to accommodate to their new status and life. Second, patients may exhibit response shift wherein their QOL assessments change as they adopt new internal standards in response to external factors, such as the disease itself or the associated treatment. Changes in patient-reported QOL scores over time are partially attributable to the patient's evolving standards of well-being (110,111). Third, as patients recover from acute treatment–related side effects, they may think more positively about the future (112). This change in attitude may result in a rise of QOL scores that are reflective of their optimism, though in an all-encompassing definition of QOL, this increase may be considered to be genuine. Finally, healthier patients are more compliant with QOL questionnaires, which may jeopardize the generalizability of QOL assessments for all patients (113). None of these issues pose insurmountable problems, but an awareness of such biases can help inform the interpretation of published QOL outcomes.

Impact of Concurrent Chemotherapy on Quality of Life

Quantitative models that aim to separate the effect of concurrent chemotherapy on tumor control versus treatment-related mucositis have been described (114). Using the biological effective dose (BED) formalism, the addition of concurrent chemotherapy was estimated to contribute an equivalent excess toxicity attributable to an additional 3.5 fractions of 2

Gy per fraction. An early phase I trial testing definitive radiotherapy concurrently with gemcitabine helped define the more severe end of the spectrum in terms of treatment-related toxicity. Patients with unresectable head and neck cancer treated with 70 Gy concurrently with weekly gemcitabine suffered from significant dysphagia and up to 65% of patients experienced aspiration (115). Beyond dysphagia and xerostomia decreasing QOL, Langendijk et al. showed that treatment with concurrent chemoradiation or surgery with adjuvant radiation was a significant factor in diminishing QOL compared to radiotherapy alone (116). The UW-QOL was used to show that patients treated with chemoradiation displayed a trend toward worse speech and swallowing related outcomes as compared to patients treated with radiation alone (117,118). Increased toxicity with concurrent chemotherapy does not appear to be mitigated by the use of targeted agents. Comparisons of concurrent cetuximab versus concurrent chemotherapy suggest that acute toxicity is worse and treatment compliance is lower with cetuximab, but that this does not translate into a significant difference in QOL between the two concurrent systemic therapies (119).

DYSPHAGIA

Organs at Risk for Dysphagia

Efficient swallowing involves a complex coordination of many structures including the superior, middle, and inferior pharyngeal constrictor muscles, the base of tongue, supraglottic and glottic larynx, and the upper esophageal sphincter (77). The ability to swallow strongly impacts QOL, and late dysphagia is often considered to be the main dose-limiting toxicity of radiotherapy (120). Eisbruch et al. first demonstrated that radiation-induced dysphagia could be mitigated by sparing dose to the pharyngeal constrictor muscles, glottis, and supraglottic larynx (121). Subsequent multivariable normal tissue complication probability (NTCP) models showed that mean dose to the superior constrictors and supraglottic larynx was the most predictive factor for the development of grade 2 or higher dysphagia at 6 months (122). In fact, the mean dose to pharyngeal constrictors and larynx has been consistently identified as being correlated with the prevalence of radiation-induced dysphagia (121,123,124). As a result, limiting the radiation dose to these structures has become an important goal in radiation treatment planning to minimize long-term radiation-induced dysphagia.

Impact of Dysphagia on Quality of Life

In a prospective Dutch study of 458 patients who were disease free 6 months after completion of definitive radiation to the head and neck, only xerostomia and dysphagia scores had a meaningful impact on self-reported QOL (116). Although xerostomia was the most frequent, QOL was most affected by dysphagia, especially during the first 18 months after treatment (116). Hunter et al. similarly demonstrated that despite the absence of or mild degree of observer-rated dysphagia, QOL scores correlated most with dysphagia (125). Preventing dysphagia is generally felt to be most consequential in head and neck cancer patients in general, and particularly in laryngeal cancer patients.

Dysphagia can be devastating for patient QOL, with 18% to 50% of patients reporting dysphagia as their main concern after treatment (125). The consequences of dysphagia can range from requiring mild diet changes to being completely feeding tube dependent and can also lead to life-threatening consequences, such as aspiration pneumonia (115). Even minor grade 1 dysphagia can adversely affect patient QOL (116). Furthermore, while acute treatment-related dysphagia usually improves after radiation in most patients, 20% of patients experience increasing severity of dysphagia, and many patients still suffer from grade 2 or higher dysphagia 2 years after treatment (126,127).

Management and Prevention of Radiation-Induced Dysphagia

Many studies have illustrated the dose–volume relationship for pharyngeal constrictors and dysphagia (121,123,124,128). Mean dose to pharyngeal constrictors has emerged as being most strongly correlated to dysphagia to solid and liquid foods. The proximity of the pharyngeal constrictors to tumors can be problematic, as the sparing of swallowing structures is mainly limited by the degree of overlap between planning target volumes and constrictor muscles. Some investigators have recommended limiting the volume receiving doses of 50 to 60 Gy within the pharyngeal constrictor muscles and larynx (129). However, more studies are needed to further refine dose and volume constraints. Currently, the recommendation is to keep the radiation dose to these structures as low as possible (120). Importantly, although reducing the severity of dysphagia is of great concern, the top priority is still treating and avoiding underdosing of target volumes.

Numerous studies have also investigated the benefits of swallowing exercises both before and after treatment to mitigate the impact of postradiotherapy dysphagia. In general, post-treatment swallowing rehabilitation, such as supraglottic swallowing and the Mendelsohn maneuver, have shown limited success (130), but prophylactic exercise with the Shaker method significantly improved preservation of swallowing motion. Kulbersh et al. also showed that a pretreatment swallowing therapy markedly improved QOL specifically by affecting the emotional response to swallowing difficulties as well as perception of difficulty associated with swallowing (131). However, despite intense swallowing rehabilitation and exercise programs, many patients are unable to regain pretreatment swallowing function, reinforcing the importance of sparing swallowing structures as much as possible rather than relying solely on rehabilitation (132,133).

QUALITY OF LIFE OUTCOMES AFTER LARYNGEAL PRESERVATION APPROACHES FOR LOCALLY ADVANCED LARYNGEAL CANCER

The VA Laryngeal Cancer Study first demonstrated that organ preservation can be accomplished on two of three patients with advanced laryngeal carcinoma with similar OS outcomes to total laryngectomy followed by adjuvant radiation (59). Speech communication was better at 2 years in patients who underwent LP versus those who underwent laryngectomy (60). However, this difference was not detectable 10 years after treatment with similar speech scores in organ preservation patients and laryngectomy patients, illustrating that as laryngectomy patients adjust to and practice using an artificial voice, favorable speech-related QOL can be attained (61). Beyond speech, QOL scores after 10 years were significantly better in larynx preservation patients, related to more freedom from pain, better emotional well-being, and lower levels of depression (61). Similar long-term 8-year QOL follow-up in the RTOG 91-11 study showed no differences in speech or voice quality between patients undergoing induction chemotherapy followed by radiation, concurrent chemoradiation, or radiation alone. Furthermore, no differences were noted with respect to swallowing function or diet alterations (68).

CONCLUSIONS

For patients with laryngeal carcinoma, QOL is of tremendous importance with some patients prioritizing laryngeal function over survival. The measurement of QOL is complicated by the fact that it is a highly subjective construct influenced by many factors and requires the use of standardized, patient-reported, validated instruments. Of all LP treatment-related toxicities, dysphagia appears consequential in impacting QOL. Retaining functional speech is also an important consideration but appears similar with long-term follow-up between LP patients and laryngectomy patients.

CASE 18.1 EARLY STAGE GLOTTIC CARCINOMA TREATED WITH IMRT

TH was a 57-year-old man at the time of diagnosis with no significant past medical history but a 30 pack year smoking history who developed dysphonia following an episode of influenza that failed to resolve after 2 months. Physical exam was unremarkable with no palpable cervical lymph nodes, fiberoptic nasopharyngoscopy revealed a whitish ulcerative lesion involving the entire right true vocal cord with extension to the anterior commissure. No lesions were present on the left, and vocal cords were mobile bilaterally. Videostroboscopy however revealed a loss of mucosal vibratory motion on the right. Biopsy of the site was positive for invasive keratinizing squamous cell carcinoma, well to moderately differentiated. CT of the neck demonstrated a soft tissue thickening measuring 8 mm in thickness involving the anterior commissure and right true vocal cord. No cervical lymphadenopathy was present. He was staged T1aN0M0 with anterior commissure involvement and was evaluated in multidisciplinary fashion. Given the extent and depth of his disease, definitive radiation was favored over transoral laser resection, particularly for voice preservation. The patient agreed with these recommendations and inquired about methods to maximally preserve his voice. In order to minimize dose to his arytenoids and carotid arteries, he was treated with IMRT using a slightly hypofractionated regimen as described in the Dutch experience with 16 fractions of 3.63 Gy (Figure 18.1).

During simulation, scans were obtained before and after swallowing to rule out any significant repositioning of the larynx. The patient was instructed to avoid swallowing during simulation and during treatments. The targets within the clinical target volume included the entire right true vocal cord, and given anterior commissure involvement, the anterior third of the contralateral left cord was also included. The contralateral arytenoid complex and bilateral carotid arteries were contoured as avoidance structures. The patient's pre-treatment Voice Handicap Index score was 17 which improved to a score of 0 only 1 month after completing treatment. Mucosal vibratory motion was improved 3 months after treatment, and he remains disease free.

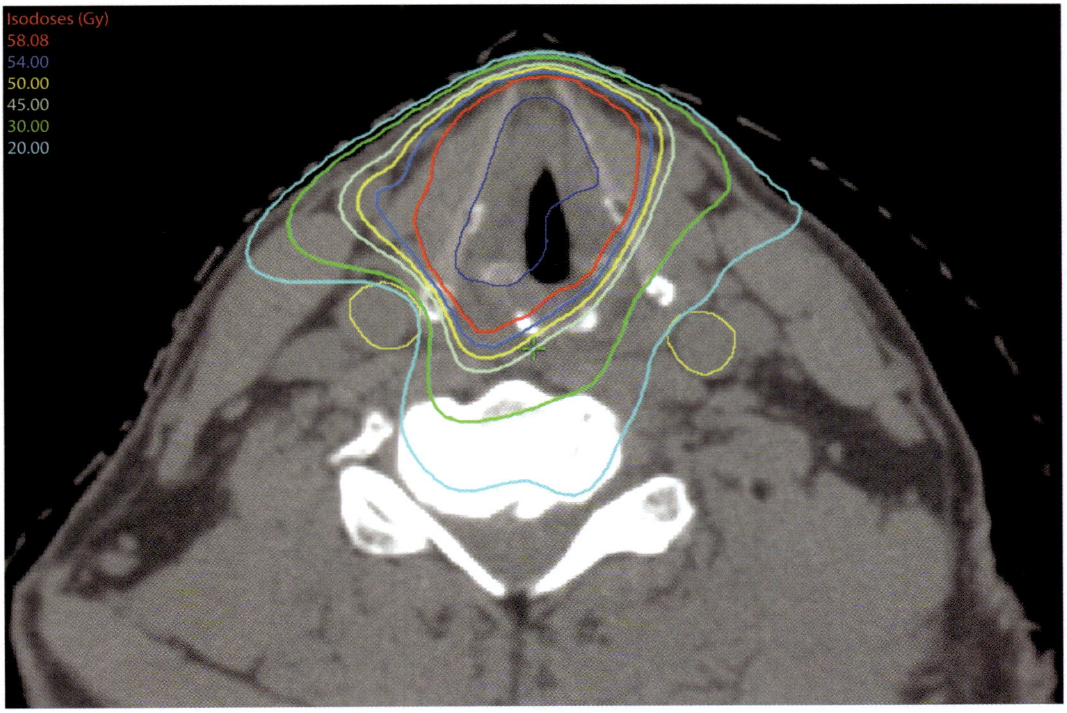

FIGURE 18.1. Axial slice of a CT simulation scan without contrast showing the definitive radiation plan for T1aN0M0 squamous cell carcinoma of the right true vocal cord with extension to the anterior commissure. The thin blue line represents the clinical target volume including the rt TVC and anterior lt TVC, and prescription dose (58.08 Gy in 16 fractions) is noted in red. The bilateral carotid arteries (yellow) were mostly spared outside of the 20 Gy isodose line (light blue), and dose was also reduced to the contalateral (lt) arytenoid.

CASE 18.2 LOCALLY ADVANCED SUPRAGLOTTIC CARCINOMA TREATED WITH DEFINITIVE CHEMORADIATION AFTER FAVORABLE RESPONSE WITH CHEMOSELECTION

TF was a 71-year-old healthy man with no significant past medical history and no personal smoking history but significant exposure to second hand smoke who presented with a 3-month history of dysphonia and odynophagia. Physical exam was unremarkable with no cervical lymphadenopathy. Flexible nasopharyngoscopy revealed a 2.5 cm tumor centered on the right arytenoid with extension past midline and laterally, there was submucosal spread into the right medial pyriform sinus. The right true vocal cord was paralyzed. CT of the neck showed a peripherally enhancing soft tissue mass arising from the right aryepiglottic fold with occupation of the right pyriform sinus up to the lateral wall with possible involvement of the hypopharynx, involvement of the contralateral left arytenoid, and a prominent right level III lymph node measuring 1.2 cm. PET/CT showed the primary right supraglottic mass to be FDG-avid as well as the right level III lymph node, no distant metastases were noted. Biopsy of the primary mass was positive for nonkeratinizing invasive squamous cell carcinoma, poorly differentiated. He was staged T3N1M0 and after multidisciplinary clinical evaluation, the patient wished to pursue laryngeal preservation over primary surgery which would have required a total laryngectomy given the extent of disease. He was treated under an institutional protocol using a chemoselection approach similar to that of the VA Larynx Study but with the goal of selecting responders (>50% response) to complete definitive concurrent chemoradiation versus total laryngectomy for nonresponders. After 1 cycle of carboplatin, taxotere, and a Bcl-xL inhibitor AT-101, the patient underwent a repeat CT neck which showed a 75% reduction in the size of the supraglottic primary mass, and on repeat nasopharyngoscopy, there was a near complete clinical response (Figure 18.2).

He continued on to receive concurrent chemoradiation with 70 Gy delivered to the areas of gross disease noted on his pre-chemotherapy scans, and 56 to 59.5 Gy to a margin around gross disease, and the bilateral neck, delivered concurrently with carboplatin (Figure 18.3).

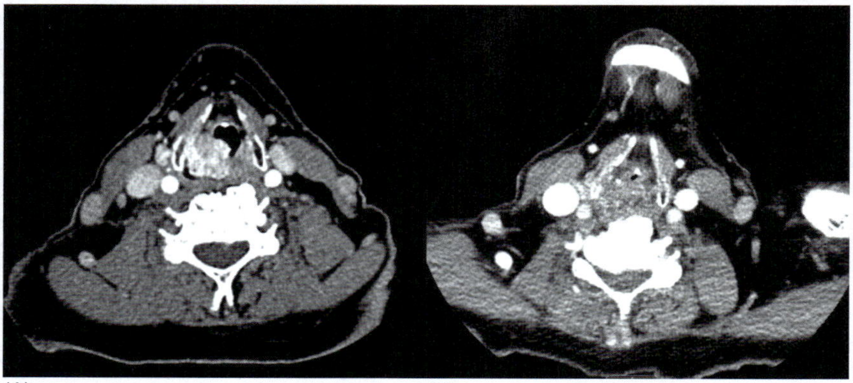

(A) (B)

FIGURE 18.2. Axial slices of diagnostic CT scans with intravenous contrast demonstrating an enhancing right supraglottic mass (A) before chemotherapy and (B) after chemotherapy. Given the favorable response to chemotherapy, the patient continued on to receive definitive concurrent chemoradiation.

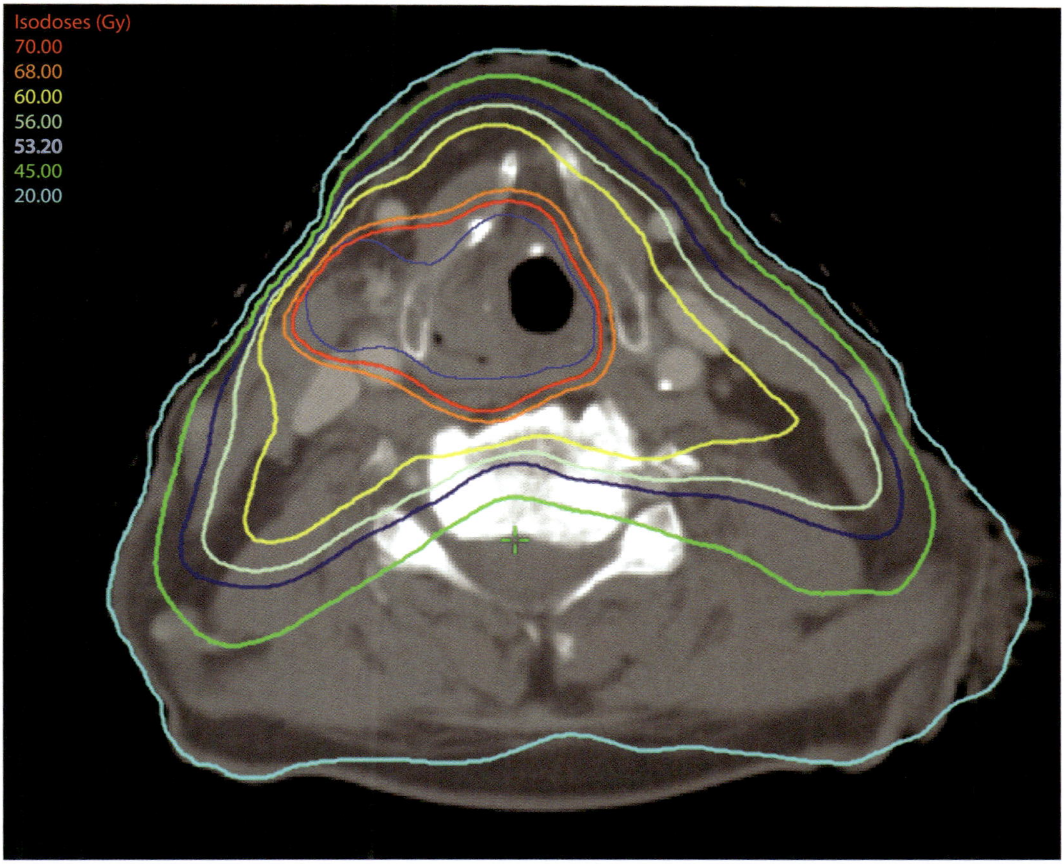

FIGURE 18.3. Axial slice of a CT simulation scan with intravenous contrast showing the definitive radiation plan for a right supraglottic squamous cell carcinoma T3N1M0. The thin blue line represents the clinical target volume encompassing the primary tumor and lymph node prior to chemoselection, and prescription dose (70 Gy in 35 fractions) is noted in red.

REFERENCES

1. Jemal A, Ward EM, Johnson CJ, et al. Annual Report to the Nation on the Status of Cancer, 1975–2014, Featuring Survival. *J Natl Cancer Inst*. 2017;109(9). doi:10.1093/jnci/djx030
2. Megwalu UC, Sikora AG. Survival outcomes in advanced laryngeal cancer. *JAMA Otolaryngol Head Neck Surg*. 2014;140(9):855–860. doi:10.1001/jamaoto.2014.1671
3. Chen AY, Halpern M. Factors predictive of survival in advanced laryngeal cancer. *Arch Otolaryngol Head Neck Surg*. 2007;133(12):1270–1276. doi:10.1001/archotol.133.12.1270
4. Grover S, Swisher-McClure S, Mitra N, et al. Total laryngectomy versus larynx preservation for t4a larynx cancer: Patterns of care and survival outcomes. *Int J Radiat Oncol Biol Phys*. 2015;92(3):594–601. doi:10.1016/j.ijrobp.2015.03.004
5. Fuller CD, Mohamed AS, Garden AS, et al. Long-term outcomes after multidisciplinary management of T3 laryngeal squamous cell carcinomas: Improved functional outcomes and survival with modern therapeutic approaches. *Head Neck*. 2016;38(12):1739–1751. doi:10.1002/hed.24532
6. Rosenthal DI, Mohamed AS, Weber RS, et al. Long-term outcomes after surgical or nonsurgical initial therapy for patients with T4 squamous cell carcinoma of the larynx: a 3-decade survey. *Cancer*. 2015;121(10):1608–1619. doi:10.1002/cncr.29241
7. Vengalil S, Giuliani ME, Huang SH, et al. Clinical outcomes in patients with T4 laryngeal cancer treated with primary radiotherapy versus primary laryngectomy. *Head Neck*. 2016;38(suppl 1):E2035–E2040. doi:10.1002/hed.24374

8. Hintz BL, Kagan AR, Nussbaum H, et al. A 'watchful waiting' policy for in situ carcinoma of the vocal cords. *Arch Otolaryngol.* 1981;107(12):746–751.
9. Sengupta N, Morris CG, Kirwan J, et al. Definitive radiotherapy for carcinoma in situ of the true vocal cords. *Am J Clin Oncol.* 2010;33(1):94–95. doi:10.1097/COC.0b013e3181a3194f
10. Spayne JA, Warde P, O'Sullivan B, et al. Carcinoma-in-situ of the glottic larynx: results of treatment with radiation therapy. *Int J Radiat Oncol Biol Phys.* 2001;49(5):1235–1238.
11. MacLeod PM, Daniel F. The role of radiotherapy in in-situ carcinoma of the larynx. *Int J Radiat Oncol Biol Phys.* 1990;18(1):113–117.
12. Pene F, Fletcher GH. Results in irradiation of the in situ carcinomas of the vocal cords. *Cancer.* 1976;37(6):2586–2590.
13. Cellai E, Frata P, Magrini SM, et al. Radical radiotherapy for early glottic cancer: results in a series of 1087 patients from two Italian radiation oncology centers. I. The case of T1N0 disease. *Int J Radiat Oncol Biol Phys.* 2005;63(5):1378–1386. doi:10.1016/j.ijrobp.2005.05.018
14. Chera BS, Amdur RJ, Morris CG, et al. T1N0 to T2N0 squamous cell carcinoma of the glottic larynx treated with definitive radiotherapy. *Int J Radiat Oncol Biol Phys.* 2010;78(2):461–466. doi:10.1016/j.ijrobp.2009.08.066
15. Le QT, Fu KK, Kroll S, et al. Influence of fraction size, total dose, and overall time on local control of T1-T2 glottic carcinoma. *Int J Radiat Oncol Biol Phys.* 1997;39(1):115–126.
16. Hirano M, Hirade Y, Kawasaki H. Vocal function following carbon dioxide laser surgery for glottic carcinoma. *Ann Otol Rhinol Laryngol.* 1985;94(3):232–235.
17. McGuirt WF, Blalock D, Koufman JA, et al. Comparative voice results after laser resection or irradiation of T1 vocal cord carcinoma. *Arch Otolaryngol Head Neck Surg.* 1994;120(9):951–955.
18. Higgins KM, Shah MD, Ogaick MJ, Enepekides D. Treatment of early-stage glottic cancer: meta-analysis comparison of laser excision versus radiotherapy. *J Otolaryngol Head Neck Surg.* 2009;38(6):603–612.
19. Frata P, Cellai E, Magrini SM, et al. Radical radiotherapy for early glottic cancer: results in a series of 1087 patients from two Italian radiation oncology centers. II. The case of T2N0 disease. *Int J Radiat Oncol Biol Phys.* 2005;63(5):1387–1394. doi:10.1016/j.ijrobp.2005.05.013
20. Groome PA, O'Sullivan B, Mackillop WJ, et al. Compromised local control due to treatment interruptions and late treatment breaks in early glottic cancer: population-based outcomes study supporting need for intensified treatment schedules. *Int J Radiat Oncol Biol Phys.* 2006;64(4):1002–1012. doi:10.1016/j.ijrobp.2005.10.010
21. Eskiizmir G, Baskin Y, Yalcin F, et al. Risk factors for radiation failure in early-stage glottic carcinoma: a systematic review and meta-analysis. *Oral Oncol.* 2016;62:90–100. doi:10.1016/j.oraloncology.2016.10.013
22. Teshima T, Chatani M, Inoue T. Radiation therapy for early glottic cancer (T1N0M0): II. Prospective randomized study concerning radiation field. *Int J Radiat Oncol Biol Phys.* 1990;18(1):119–123.
23. Foote RL, Grado GL, Buskirk SJ, et al. Radiation therapy for glottic cancer using 6-MV photons. *Cancer.* 1996;77(2):381–386. doi:10.1002/(SICI)1097-0142(19960115)77:2<381::AID-CNCR22>3.0.CO:2-x
24. Yamazaki H, Nishiyama K, Tanaka E, et al. Radiotherapy for early glottic carcinoma (T1N0M0): results of prospective randomized study of radiation fraction size and overall treatment time. *Int J Radiat Oncol Biol Phys.* 2006;64(1):77–82. doi:10.1016/j.ijrobp.2005.06.014
25. Trotti A, 3rd, Zhang Q, Bentzen SM, et al. Randomized trial of hyperfractionation versus conventional fractionation in T2 squamous cell carcinoma of the vocal cord (RTOG 9512). *Int J Radiat Oncol Biol Phys.* 2014;89(5):958–963. doi:10.1016/j.ijrobp.2014.04.041
26. Smith GL, Smith BD, Buchholz TA, et al. Cerebrovascular disease risk in older head and neck cancer patients after radiotherapy. *J Clin Oncol.* 2008;26(31):5119–5125. doi:10.1200/JCO.2008.16.6546
27. Hong JC, Kruser TJ, Gondi V, et al. Risk of cerebrovascular events in elderly patients after radiation therapy versus surgery for early-stage glottic cancer. *Int J Radiat Oncol Biol Phys.* 2013;87(2):290–296. doi:10.1016/j.ijrobp.2013.06.009
28. Zumsteg ZS, Riaz N, Jaffery S, et al. Carotid sparing intensity-modulated radiation therapy achieves comparable locoregional control to conventional radiotherapy in T1-2N0 laryngeal carcinoma. *Oral Oncol.* 2015;51(7):716–723. doi:10.1016/j.oraloncolgy.2015.02.003
29. Lundgren JA, Gilbert RW, van Nostrand AW, et al. T3N0M0 glottic carcinoma—a failure analysis. *Clin Otolaryngol Allied Sci.* 1988;13(6):455–465.
30. Bryant GP, Poulsen MG, Tripcony L, Dickie GJ. Treatment decisions in T3N0M0 glottic carcinoma. *Int J Radiat Oncol Biol Phys.* 1995;31(2):285–293. doi:10.1016/0360-3016(94)E0172-G
31. Wendt CD, Peters LJ, Ang KK, et al. Hyperfractionated radiotherapy in the treatment of squamous cell carcinomas of the supraglottic larynx. *Int J Radiat Oncol Biol Phys.* 1989;17(5):1057–1062.
32. Mendenhall WM, Parsons JT, Mancuso AA, et al. Radiotherapy for squamous cell carcinoma of the supraglottic larynx: an alternative to surgery. *Head Neck.* 1996;18(1):24–35. doi:10.1002/(SICI)1097-0347(199601/02)18:1<24::AID-HED4>3.0.CO:2-0
33. Garden AS, Forster K, Wong PF, et al. Results of radiotherapy for T2N0 glottic carcinoma: does the "2" stand for twice-daily treatment? *Int J Radiat Oncol Biol Phys.* 2003;55(2):322–328.
34. Freeman DE, Mancuso AA, Parsons JT, et al. Irradiation alone for supraglottic larynx carcinoma: can CT findings predict treatment results? *Int J Radiat Oncol Biol Phys.* 1990;19(2):485–490.
35. Kraas JR, Underhill TE, D'Agostino RB, Jr, et al. Quantitative analysis from CT is prognostic for local control of supraglottic carcinoma. *Head Neck.* 2001;23(12):1031–1036.

36. Department of Veterans Affairs Laryngeal Cancer Study Group. Treatment of advanced laryngeal carcinoma. *N Engl J Med.* 1991;325(23):1656–1657.
37. Forastiere AA, Goepfert H, Maor M, et al. Concurrent chemotherapy and radiotherapy for organ preservation in advanced laryngeal cancer. *N Engl J Med.* 2003;349(22):2091–2098. doi:10.1056/NEJMoa031317
38. Remacle M, Eckel HE, Antonelli A, et al. Endoscopic cordectomy. A proposal for a classification by the Working Committee, European Laryngological Society. *Eur Arch Otorhinolaryngol.* 2000;257(4):227–231.
39. Remacle M, Hantzakos A, Eckel H, et al. Endoscopic supraglottic laryngectomy: a proposal for a classification by the working committee on nomenclature, European Laryngological Society. *Eur Arch Otorhinolaryngol.* 2009;266(7):993–998. doi:10.1007/s00405-008-0901-8
40. Abdurehim Y, Hua Z, Yasin Y, et al. Transoral laser surgery versus radiotherapy: systematic review and meta-analysis for treatment options of T1a glottic cancer. *Head Neck.* 2012;34(1):23–33. doi:10.1002/hed.21686
41. Lee M, Buchanan MA, Riffat F, Palme CE. Complications after CO_2 laser surgery for early glottic cancer: An institutional experience. *Head Neck.* 2016;38(suppl 1):E987–E990. doi:10.1002/hed.24142
42. Dziegielewski PT, Kang SY, Ozer E. Transoral robotic surgery (TORS) for laryngeal and hypopharyngeal cancers. *J Surg Oncol.* 2015;112(7):702–706. doi:10.1002/jso.24002
43. Ozer E, Alvarez B, Kakarala K, et al. Clinical outcomes of transoral robotic supraglottic laryngectomy. *Head Neck.* 2013;35(8):1158–1161. doi:10.1002/he.23101
44. Mendelsohn AH, Remacle M. Transoral robotic surgery for laryngeal cancer. *Curr Opin Otolaryngol Head Neck Surg.* 2015;23(2):148–152. doi:10.1097/MOO.0000000000000144
45. Hinni ML, Salassa JR, Grant DG, et al. Transoral laser microsurgery for advanced laryngeal cancer. *Arch Otolaryngol Head Neck Surg.* 2007;133(12):1198–1204. doi:10.1001/archotol.133.12.1198
46. Jackel MC, Ambrosch P, Martin A, Steiner W. Impact of re-resection for inadequate margins on the prognosis of upper aerodigestive tract cancer treated by laser microsurgery. *Laryngoscope.* 2007;117(2):350–356. doi:10.1097/01.mlq.0000251165.48830.89
47. Thomas L, Drinnan M, Natesh B, et al. Open conservation partial laryngectomy for laryngeal cancer: a systematic review of English language literature. *Cancer Treat Rev.* 2012;38(3):203–211. doi:10.1016/j.ctrv.2011.05.010
48. Peretti G, Piazza C, Mora F, et al. Reasonable limits for transoral laser microsurgery in laryngeal cancer. *Curr Opin Otolaryngol Head Neck Surg.* 2016;24(2):135–139. doi:10.1097/MOO.0000000000000240
49. Tomeh C, Holsinger FC. Laryngeal cancer. *Curr Opin Otolaryngol Head Neck Surg.* 2014;22(2):147–153. doi:10.1097/MOO.0000000000000032
50. Succo G, Peretti G, Piazza C, et al. Open partial horizontal laryngectomies: a proposal for classification by the working committee on nomenclature of the European Laryngological Society. *Eur Arch Otorhinolaryngol.* 2014;271(9):2489–2496. doi:10.1007/s00405-014-3024-4
51. Flint PW. Minimally invasive techniques for management of early glottic cancer. *Otolaryngol Clin North Am.* 2002;35(5):1055–1066, vi–vii.
52. Muscatello L, Laccourreye O, Biacabe B, et al. Laryngofissure and cordectomy for glottic carcinoma limited to the mid third of the mobile true vocal cord. *Laryngoscope.* 1997;107(11, Pt 1):1507–1510.
53. Hoffman HT, McCulloch TM, Bulatti J, Funk G. Management of early glottic cancer. In Richardson MA, Robbins KT, Schuller DE, et al. eds. *Cummings: Otolaryngology Head and Neck Surgery.* Vol 3. 4th ed. Philadelphia, PA: Elsevier Mosby; 2005.
54. Riga M, Chelis L, Danielides V, et al. Systematic review on T3 laryngeal squamous cell carcinoma; still far from a consensus on the optimal organ preserving treatment. *Eur J Surg Oncol.* 2017;43(1):20–31. doi:10.1016/j.ejso.2016.05.030
55. Worden FP, Moyer J, Lee JS, et al. Chemoselection as a strategy for organ preservation in patients with T4 laryngeal squamous cell carcinoma with cartilage invasion. *Laryngoscope.* 2009;119(8):1510–1517. doi:10.1002/lary.20294
56. Roux M, Dassonville O, Ettaiche M, et al. Primary total laryngectomy and pharyngolaryngectomy in T4 pharyngolaryngeal cancers: Oncologic and functional results and prognostic factors. *Eur Ann Otorhinolaryngol Head Neck Dis.* 2017;134(3):151–154. doi:10.1016/j.anorl.2016.11.009
57. Yang CY, Andersen PE, Everts EC, Cohen JI. Nodal disease in purely glottic carcinoma: is elective neck treatment worthwhile? *Laryngoscope.* 1998;108(7):1006–1008.
58. Buckley JG, MacLennan K. Cervical node metastases in laryngeal and hypopharyngeal cancer: a prospective analysis of prevalence and distribution. *Head Neck.* 2000;22(4):380–385.
59. Department of Veterans Affairs Laryngeal Cancer Study Group. Induction chemotherapy plus radiation compared with surgery plus radiation in patients with advanced laryngeal cancer. *N Engl J Med.* 1991;324(24):1685–1690.
60. Hillman RE, Walsh MJ, Wolf GT, et al. Functional outcomes following treatment for advanced laryngeal cancer. Part I—Voice preservation in advanced laryngeal cancer. Part II—Laryngectomy rehabilitation: the state of the art in the VA System. Research Speech-Language Pathologists. Department of Veterans Affairs Laryngeal Cancer Study Group. *Ann Otol Rhinol Laryngol Suppl.* 1998;172:1–27.
61. Terrell JE, Fisher SG, Wolf GT. Long-term quality of life after treatment of laryngeal cancer. The Veterans Affairs Laryngeal Cancer Study Group. *Arch Otolaryngol Head Neck Surg.* 1998;124(9):964–971.
62. Wolf GT, Forastiere A, Ang K, et al. Workshop report: organ preservation strategies in advanced head and neck cancer--current status and future directions. *Head Neck.* 1999;21(8):689–693.

63. Harwood AR, Hawkins NV, Beale FA, et al. Management of advanced glottic cancer. A 10 year review of the Toronto experience. *Int J Radiat Oncol Biol Phys.* 1979;5(6):899–904.
64. Harwood AR, Beale FA, Cummings BJ, et al. Supraglottic laryngeal carcinoma: an analysis of dose-time-volume factors in 410 patients. *Int J Radiat Oncol Biol Phys.* 1983;9(3):311–319.
65. Pointreau Y, Garaud P, Chapet S, et al. Randomized trial of induction chemotherapy with cisplatin and 5-fluorouracil with or without docetaxel for larynx preservation. *J Natl Cancer Inst.* 2009;101(7):498–506. doi:10.1093/jnci/dip007
66. Lefebvre JL, Chevalier D, Luboinski B, et al. Larynx preservation in pyriform sinus cancer: preliminary results of a European Organization for Research and Treatment of Cancer phase III trial. EORTC Head and Neck Cancer Cooperative Group. *J Natl Cancer Inst.* 1996;88(13):890–899.
67. Lefebvre JL, Andry G, Chevalier D, et al. Laryngeal preservation with induction chemotherapy for hypopharyngeal squamous cell carcinoma: 10-year results of EORTC trial 24891. *Ann Oncol.* 2012;23(10):2708–2714. doi:10.1093/annonc/mds065
68. Forastiere AA, Zhang Q, Weber RS, et al. Long-term results of RTOG 91-11: a comparison of three nonsurgical treatment strategies to preserve the larynx in patients with locally advanced larynx cancer. *J Clin Oncol.* 2013;31(7):845–852. doi:10.1200/JCO.2012.43.6097
69. Lefebvre JL, Rolland F, Tesselaar M, et al. Phase 3 randomized trial on larynx preservation comparing sequential vs alternating chemotherapy and radiotherapy. *J Natl Cancer Inst.* 2009;101(3):142–152. doi:10.1093/jnci/djn460
70. Lefebvre JL, Pointreau Y, Rolland F, et al. Induction chemotherapy followed by either chemoradiotherapy or bioradiotherapy for larynx preservation: the TREMPLIN randomized phase II study. *J Clin Oncol.* 2013;31(7):853–859. doi:10.1200/JCO.2012.42.3988
71. Henriques De Figueiredo B, Fortpied C, Menis J, et al. Long-term update of the 24954 EORTC phase III trial on larynx preservation. *Eur J Cancer.* 2016;65:109–112. doi:10.1016/j.ejca 2016.06.024
72. Bonner JA, Harari PM, Giralt J, et al. Radiotherapy plus cetuximab for squamous-cell carcinoma of the head and neck. *N Engl J Med.* 2006;354(6):567–578. doi 10.1056/NEJMoa053422
73. Bonner JA, Harari PM, Giralt J, et al. Radiotherapy plus cetuximab for locoregionally advanced head and neck cancer: 5-year survival data from a phase 3 randomised trial, and relation between cetuximab-induced rash and survival. *Lancet Oncol.* 2010;11(1):21–28. doi:10.1016/S1470-2045(09)70311-0
74. Posner MR, Norris CM, Wirth LJ, et al. Sequential therapy for the locally advanced larynx and hypopharynx cancer subgroup in TAX 324: survival, surgery, and organ preservation. *Ann Oncol.* 2009;20(5):921–927. doi:10.1093/annonc/mdn752
75. Urba S, Wolf G, Eisbruch A, et al. Single-cycle induction chemotherapy selects patients with advanced laryngeal cancer for combined chemoradiation: a new treatment paradigm. *J Clin Oncol.* 2006 24(4):593–598. doi:10.1200/JCO2005.01.2047
76. Wolf GT, Bellile E, Eisbruch A, et al. Survival rates using individualized bioselection treatment methods in patients with advanced laryngeal cancer. *JAMA Otolaryngol Head Neck Surg.* 2017;143(4):355–366. doi:10.1001/jamaoto.2016.3669
77. Duprez F, Madani I, De Potter B, et al. Systematic review of dose—volume correlates for structures related to late swallowing disturbances after radiotherapy for head and neck cancer. *Dysphagia.* 2013;28(3):337–349. doi:10.1007/s00455-013-9452-2
78. Moeller BJ, Rana V, Cannon BA, et al. Prospective imaging assessment of mortality risk after head-and-neck radiotherapy. *Int J Radiat Oncol Biol Phys.* 2010;78(3):667–674. doi:10.1016/j.ijrobp.2009.08.063
79. Vogelius IR, Bentzen SM, Maraldo MV, et al. Risk factors for radiation-induced hypothyroidism: a literature-based meta-analysis. *Cancer.* 2011;117(23):5250–5260. doi:10.1002/cncr.26186
80. Moyer VA, Force USPST. Screening for lung cancer: U.S. Preventive Services Task Force recommendation statement. *Ann Intern Med.* 2014;160(5):330–338. doi:10.7326/M13-2771
81. Aberle DR, Adams AM, Berg CD, et al. Reduced lung-cancer mortality with low-dose computed tomographic screening. *N Engl J Med.* 2011;365(5):395–409. doi:10.1056/NEJMoa1102873
82. Weber RS, Berkey BA, Forastiere A, et al. Outcome of salvage total laryngectomy following organ preservation therapy: the Radiation Therapy Oncology Group trial 91-11. *Arch Otolaryngol Head Neck Surg.* 2003;129(1):44–49.
83. Sandulache VC, Vandelaar LJ, Skinner HD, et al. Salvage total laryngectomy after external-beam radiotherapy: a 20-year experience. *Head Neck.* 2016;38(suppl 1):E1962–1968. doi:10.1002/hed.24355
84. van der Putten L, de Bree R, Kuik DJ, et al. Salvage laryngectomy: oncological and functional outcome. *Oral Oncol.* 2011;47(4):296–301. doi:10.1016/j.oraloncology.2011.02.002
85. Paleri V, Thomas L, Basavaiah N, et al. Oncologic outcomes of open conservation laryngectomy for radiorecurrent laryngeal carcinoma: a systematic review and meta-analysis of English-language literature. *Cancer.* 2011;117(12):2668–2676. doi:10.1002/cncr.25831
86. Ganly I, Patel SG, Matsuo J, et al. Results of surgical salvage after failure of definitive radiation therapy for early-stage squamous cell carcinoma of the glottic larynx. *Arch Otolaryngol Head Neck Surg.* 2006;132(1):59–66. doi:10.1001/archotol.132.1.59
87. Birkeland AC, Rosko AJ, Issa MR, et al. Occult nodal disease prevalence and distribution in recurrent laryngeal cancer requiring salvage laryngectomy. *Otolaryngol Head Neck Surg.* 2016;154(3):473–479. doi:1177/0194599815627811
88. Goodwin WJ, Jr. Salvage surgery for patients with recurrent squamous cell carcinoma of the upper aerodigestive tract: when do the ends justify the means? *Laryngoscope.* 2000;110(3, Pt 2, suppl 93):1–18.

89. Metson R, Freehling DJ, Wang CC. Surgical complications following twice-a-day versus once-a-day radiation therapy. *Laryngoscope.* 1988;98(1):30–34. doi:10.1288/00005537-198801000-00008
90. Iteld L, Yu P. Pharyngocutaneous fistula repair after radiotherapy and salvage total laryngectomy. *J Reconstr Microsurg.* 2007;23(6):339–345. doi:10.1055/s-2007-992343
91. Gendreau-Lefevre AK, Audet N, Maltais S, Thuot F. Prophylactic pectoralis major muscle flap in prevention of pharyngocutaneous fistula in total laryngectomy after radiotherapy. *Head Neck.* 2015;37(9):1233–1238. doi:10.1002/hed.23742
92. Paydarfar JA, Birkmeyer NJ. Complications in head and neck surgery: a meta-analysis of postlaryngectomy pharyngocutaneous fistula. *Arch Otolaryngol Head Neck Surg.* 2006;132(1):67–72. doi:10.1001/archotol.132.1.67
93. Fung K, Teknos TN, Vandenberg CD, et al. Prevention of wound complications following salvage laryngectomy using free vascularized tissue. *Head Neck.* 2007;29(5):425–430. doi:10.1002/hed.20492
94. Patel UA, Moore BA, Wax M, et al. Impact of pharyngeal closure technique on fistula after salvage laryngectomy. *JAMA Otolaryngol Head Neck Surg.* 2013;139(11):1156–1162. doi:10.1001/jamaoto.2013.2761
95. Sharaf B, Xue A, Solari MG, et al. Optimizing outcomes in pharyngoesophageal reconstruction and neck resurfacing: 10-year experience of 294 cases. *Plast Reconstr Surg.* 2017;139(1):105e–119e. doi:10.1097/PRS.0000000000000002915
96. Paleri V, Drinnan M, van den Brekel MW, et al. Vascularized tissue to reduce fistula following salvage total laryngectomy: a systematic review. *Laryngoscope.* 2014;124(8):1848–1853. doi:10.1002/lary.25018
97. Blanchard P, Volk RJ, Ringash J, et al. Assessing head and neck cancer patient preferences and expectations: a systematic review. *Oral Oncol.* 2016;62:44–53. doi:10.1016/j.oraloncology.2016.09.08
98. Cox JD, Stetz J, Pajak TF. Toxicity criteria of the Radiation Therapy Oncology Group (RTOG) and the European Organization for Research and Treatment of Cancer (EORTC). *Int J Radiat Oncol Biol Phys.* 1995;31(5):1341–1346. doi:10.1016/0360-3016(95)00060-c
99. Trotti A, Colevas AD, Setser A, et al. CTCAE v3.0: development of a comprehensive grading system for the adverse effects of cancer treatment. *Semin Radiat Oncol.* 2003;13(3):176–181. doi:10.1016/S1053-4296(03)00031-6
100. The World Health Organization Quality of Life assessment (WHOQOL): position paper from the World Health Organization. *Soc Sci Med.* 1995;41(10):1403–1409.
101. Jensen K, Bonde Jensen A, Grau C. The relationship between observer-based toxicity scoring and patient assessed symptom severity after treatment for head and neck cancer. A correlative cross sectional study of the DAHANCA toxicity scoring system and the EORTC quality of life questionnaires. *Radiother Oncol.* 2006;78(3):298–305. doi:10.1016/j.radonc.2006.02.005
102. Terrell JE, Nanavati KA, Esclamado RM, et al. Head and neck cancer-specific quality of life: instrument validation. *Arch Otolaryngol Head Neck Surg.* 1997;123(10):1125–1132.
103. Hassan SJ, Weymuller EA, Jr. Assessment of quality of life in head and neck cancer patients. *Head Neck.* 1993;15(6):485–496.
104. Weymuller EA, Jr, Alsarraf R, Yueh B, et al. Analysis of the performance characteristics of the University of Washington Quality of Life instrument and its modification (UW-QOL-R). *Arch Otolaryngol Head Neck Surg.* 2001;127(5):489–493.
105. Cella DF, Tulsky DS, Gray G, et al. The functional assessment of cancer therapy scale: development and validation of the general measure. *J Clin Oncol.* 1993;11(3):570–579. doi:10.1200/JCO.1993.11.3.570
106. List MA, D'Antonio LL, Cella DF, et al. The performance status scale for head and neck cancer patients and the functional assessment of cancer therapy-head and neck scale. A study of utility and validity. *Cancer.* 1996;77(11):2294–2301. doi:10.1002/(SICI)1097-0142(19960601)77:11<2294:AID-CNCR17>3.0.co:2-S
107. Basch E, Reeve BB, Mitchell SA, et al. Development of the National Cancer Institute's patient-reported outcomes version of the common terminology criteria for adverse events (PRO-CTCAE). *J Natl Cancer Inst.* 2014;106(9). doi:10.1093/jnci/dju244
108. Dueck AC, Mendoza TR, Mitchell SA, et al. Validity and reliability of the US National Cancer Institute's patient-reported outcomes version of the common terminology criteria for adverse events (PRO-CTCAE). *JAMA Oncol.* 2015;1(8):1051–1059. doi:10.1001/jamaoncol.2015.2639
109. Ringash J. Survivorship and quality of life in head and neck cancer. *J Clin Oncol.* 2015;33(29):3322–3327. doi:10.1200/JCO.2015.61.4115
110. Ring L, Hofer S, Heuston F, et al. Response shift masks the treatment impact on patient reported outcomes (PROs): the example of individual quality of life in edentulous patients. *Health Qual Life Outcomes.* 2005;3:55. doi:10.1186/1477-7525-3-55
111. Sprangers MA, Schwartz CE. Integrating response shift into health-related quality of life research: a theoretical model. *Soc Sci Med.* 1999;48(11):1507–1515.
112. Sharot T, Riccardi AM, Raio CM, Phelps EA. Neural mechanisms mediating optimism bias. *Nature.* 2007;450(7166):102–105. doi:10.1038/nature06280
113. Guren MG, Dueland S, Skovlund E, et al. Quality of life during radiotherapy for rectal cancer. *Eur J Cancer.* 2003;39(5):587–594.
114. Lee IH, Eisbruch A. Mucositis versus tumor control: the therapeutic index of adding chemotherapy to irradiation of head and neck cancer. *Int J Radiat Oncol Biol Phys.* 2009;75(4):1060–1063. doi:10.1016/j.ijrobp.2008.12.011

115. Eisbruch A, Lyden T, Bradford CR, et al. Objective assessment of swallowing dysfunction and aspiration after radiation concurrent with chemotherapy for head-and-neck cancer. *Int J Radiat Oncol Biol Phys.* 2002;53(1):23–28.
116. Langendijk JA, Doornaert P, Verdonck-de Leeuw IM, et al. Impact of late treatment-related toxicity on quality of life among patients with head and neck cancer treated with radiotherapy. *J Clin Oncol.* 2008;26(22):3770–3776. doi:10.1200/JCO.2007.14.6647
117. Thomas L, Jones TM, Tandon S, et al. Speech and voice outcomes in oropharyngeal cancer and evaluation of the University of Washington Quality of Life speech domain. *Clin Otolaryngol.* 2009;34(1):34–42. doi:10.1111/j.1749-4486.2008.01830x
118. Thomas L, Jones TM, Tandon S, et al. An evaluation of the University of Washington Quality of Life swallowing domain following oropharyngeal cancer. *Eur Arch Otorhinolaryngol.* 2008;265(suppl 1):S29–S37. doi:10.1007/s00405-007-0470-2
119. Curran D, Giralt J, Harari PM, et al. Quality of life in head and neck cancer patients after treatment with high-dose radiotherapy alone or in combination with cetuximab. *J Clin Oncol.* 2007;25(16):2191–2197. doi:10.1200/JCO.2006.08.8005
120. Dirix P, Nuyts S. Evidence-based organ-sparing radiotherapy in head and neck cancer. *Lancet Oncol.* 2010;11(1):85–91. doi:10.1016/S1470-2045(09)70231-1
121. Eisbruch A, Schwartz M, Rasch C, et al. Dysphagia and aspiration after chemoradiotherapy for head-and-neck cancer: which anatomic structures are affected and can they be spared by IMRT? *Int J Radiat Oncol Biol Phys.* 2004;60(5):1425–1439. doi:10.1016/j.ijrobp.2005.05.050
122. Christianen ME, Schilstra C, Beetz I, et al. Predictive modelling for swallowing dysfunction after primary (chemo)radiation: results of a prospective observational study. *Radiother Oncol.* 2012;105(1):107–114. doi:10.1016/j.radonc.2011.08.009
123. Feng FY, Kim HM, Lyden TH, et al. Intensity-modulated chemoradiotherapy aiming to reduce dysphagia in patients with oropharyngeal cancer: clinical and functional results. *J Clin Oncol.* 2010;28(16):2732–2738. doi:10.1200/JCO.2009.24.6199
124. Jensen K, Lambertsen K, Grau C. Late swallowing dysfunction and dysphagia after radiotherapy for pharynx cancer: frequency, intensity and correlation with dose and volume parameters. *Radiother Oncol.* 2007;85(1):74–82. doi:10.1016/j.radonc.2007.06.004
125. Hunter KU, Schipper M, Feng FY, et al. Toxicities affecting quality of life after chemo-IMRT of oropharyngeal cancer: prospective study of patient-reported, observer-rated, and objective outcomes. *Int J Radiat Oncol Biol Phys.* 2013;85(4):935–940. doi:10.1016/j.ijrobp.2012.08.030
126. Hutcheson KA, Lewin JS, Barringer DA, et al. Late dysphagia after radiotherapy-based treatment of head and neck cancer. *Cancer.* 2012;118(23):5793–5799. doi:10.1002/cncr.27631
127. Nguyen NP, Moltz CC, Frank C, et al. Evolution of chronic dysphagia following treatment for head and neck cancer. *Oral Oncol.* 2006;42(4):374–380. doi 10.1016/j.oraloncology.2005.09.003
128. Levendag PC, Teguh DN, Voet P, et al. Dysphagia disorders in patients with cancer of the oropharynx are significantly affected by the radiation therapy dose to the superior and middle constrictor muscle: a dose-effect relationship. *Radiother Oncol.* 2007;85(1):64–73. doi:10.1016/j.radonc.2007.07.009
129. van der Laan HP, Christianen ME, Bijl HP, et al. The potential benefit of swallowing sparing intensity modulated radiotherapy to reduce swallowing dysfunction: an in silico planning comparative study. *Radiother Oncol.* 2012;103(1):76–81. doi:10.1016/j.radonc.2011.11.001
130. Ohba S, Yokoyama J, Kojima M, et al. Significant preservation of swallowing function in chemoradiotherapy for advanced head and neck cancer by prophylactic swallowing exercise. *Head Neck.* 2016;38(4):517–521. doi:10.1002/hed.23913
131. Kulbersh BD, Rosenthal EL, McGrew BM, et al. Pretreatment, preoperative swallowing exercises may improve dysphagia quality of life. *Laryngoscope.* 2006;116(6):883–886. doi:10.1097/01.mlq.0000217278.96901.fc
132. Kendall KA, Kosek SR, Tanner K. Quality-of-life scores compared to objective measures of swallowing after oropharyngeal chemoradiation. *Laryngoscope.* 2014;124(3):682–687. doi:10.1002/lary.24344
133. Vainshtein JM, Moon DH, Feng FY, et al. Long-term quality of life after swallowing and salivary-sparing chemo-intensity modulated radiation therapy in survivors of human papillomavirus-related oropharyngeal cancer. *Int J Radiat Oncol Biol Phys.* 2015;91(5):925–933. doi:10.1016/j.ijrobp.2014.12.045

19

Malignancies of the Paranasal Sinuses and Skull Base

Heather A. Osborn
Jong Chul Park
Nabil F. Saba
Pierre Blanchard
Derrick T. Lin

Sinonasal malignancies include a diverse group of uncommon tumors and present challenges in both diagnosis and management. They comprise approximately 3% of head and neck malignancies and 3.6% of tumors of the upper aerodigestive tract. The overall incidence is reported at 0.83 per 100,000 people, with a slight male predominance (1–6). Histologic subtypes include squamous cell carcinoma and malignancies of secretory cell origin such as adenocarcinoma and adenoid cystic carcinoma, as well as mucosal melanoma. Malignancies of neuroendocrine origin occur less frequently (7–11).

Dutta et al. assessed 13,295 cases of sinonasal malignancies using the Surveillance, Epidemiology and End Results (SEER) database from 1973–2011. Males (58.6%) outnumbered females at every subsite. The average age at diagnosis was 62.3 years. The three most common subsites in which sinonasal cancer occurred were the nasal cavity, the maxillary sinuses, and the ethmoid sinuses (3).

The initial diagnosis of sinonasal malignancies can be difficult, as early symptoms often mimic inflammatory sinus disease. Patients typically present with symptoms such as nasal obstruction, nasal discharge, headache, and facial pain. Combined with an insidious onset, these nonspecific symptoms often result in a delayed diagnosis and advanced local disease at initial diagnosis (1,4,12). According to Dutta et al., tumors that develop in the nasal cavity are more likely to be discovered at stage I, while 49.3% of tumors of the maxillary and 54.1% of tumors of the ethmoid sinuses are discovered at stage IV (3).

A multidisciplinary approach is essential in the diagnosis and workup of sinonasal malignancies. Multidisciplinary teams typically include an otolaryngologist—head and neck surgeon, a neuroradiologist, a specialized head and neck pathologist, a medical oncologist, and a radiation oncologist. Depending on the case, ophthalmology, neurosurgery, social work, and advanced-practice nursing may also be included (4). While prognosis varies according to stage and specific histopathology, sinonasal malignancies overall carry a poor prognosis, and both the disease and its treatment may impact surrounding structures resulting in significant morbidity (4).

PERSPECTIVES

SURGERY

The treatment options were discussed in detail, both with the patient, and at the multidisciplinary tumor board. Based on the localized nature of the tumor, our recommendation was that the best probability of cure would be obtained by surgical resection followed by adjuvant therapy radiation with or without chemotherapy in view of his advanced local disease (8,13). Obtaining a clear margin would be important to maximize his prognosis, and the possible extraocular muscle invasion seen on the MRI suggested that orbital exenteration may be required to obtain a clear margin. Neurosurgery was consulted, and together we planned an open craniofacial resection with a lateral rhinotomy incision, frozen margin control, and possible orbital exenteration depending on the intraoperative findings. The risk of subtotal resection was discussed. Although the objective was to obtain clear surgical margins, if possible, there is some evidence that gross total resection would result in an improved overall survival when compared to primary chemoradiation, even if the microscopic disease could not be cleared (14).

ONCOLOGY

Because of the rarity of the disease, there are no randomized controlled trials to guide the management of sinonasal carcinoma, and the role of systemic chemotherapy has not been established in nonmetastatic sinonasal carcinomas. Because the main pattern of failure in sinonasal cancer is locoregional, aggressive local therapy is warranted. Surgical resection remains a cornerstone primary treatment modality of sinonasal carcinomas, but achieving the clear surgical margin is often challenging because of anatomical restraints. Definitive radiation with or without chemotherapy can be an alternative primary treatment and is used when surgical resection is not feasible, either because the tumor involves critical surrounding structures or the patient is not medically fit for surgery. Upfront chemotherapy prior to surgery should only be considered in a selected subset of patients in whom unacceptable surgery-related morbidity is anticipated because the tumor involves critical surrounding structures and a reduction of primary tumor size is warranted to achieve adequate surgical margins (15).

The group consensus was to recommend surgery as the initial treatment modality, and the patient underwent anterior craniofacial resection with intraoperative frozen sections. His postoperative course was complicated by a cerebrospinal fluid (CSF) leak requiring a return to the operating room for repair.

His final pathologic test revealed schneiderian carcinoma invasive to bone and left orbit, with lymphovascular invasion and perineural invasion, p16 and human papillomavirus (HPV) 18 positive.

Given the high rate of local failure after surgery alone, adjuvant radiation is recommended in most cases of sinonasal carcinomas except for patients with a very early stage tumor (T1). A few small retrospective case series have demonstrated the improved locoregional control with adjuvant radiation in locally advanced sinonasal carcinomas (16). Although no prospective data exist to support the concurrent use of chemotherapy with radiation, adjuvant chemoradiation can be justified in patients with high-risk features based upon extrapolation from data of other head and neck mucosal disease sites wherein concurrent chemoradiation is associated with superior locoregional control and overall survival compared with radiation alone in patients with adverse features (17,18). Because this patient had several adverse risk features including a large primary tumor with extension into the surrounding structures and lymphovascular and perineural invasion, concurrent cisplatin with adjuvant radiation was recommended.

He subsequently commenced adjuvant radiation therapy with concurrent chemotherapy.

ETIOLOGY

The etiology of sinonasal cancer is complex, with multiple reported risk factors. (5,9,19,20). These include exposure to tobacco smoke, solvents, wood dust, leather dust, formaldehyde, or aerosolized chromium and nickel compounds. Other risk factors include a history of benign sinonasal papilloma and high-risk subtypes of HPV. Occupations at an increased risk of sinonasal cancer include machinists, bakers, and pastry confectioners, as well as employment in the textile industry, farming, construction, mining, or plumbing. Binazzi et al. performed a systematic review examining risk factors for sinonasal adenocarcinoma and squamous cell cancer. They included 28 studies from 1968 to 2013, and found that the occurrence of sinonasal cancer had a significant association with exposures to wood dust, leather dust, formaldehyde, nickel/chromium compounds, organic solvents, welding fumes, and arsenic (20).

Wood dust, in particular, showed a dose-dependent relationship, with longer durations of exposure resulting in a statistically significant increase in the relative risk of sinonasal cancer.

Adenocarcinomas, in particular, have a strong association with occupational wood dust exposure and exposure to mastic, solvents, or leather dust in footwear manufacturing (5). Wood furniture and cabinet makers appear to have the highest occupational exposure, particularly during machine sanding and similar procedures (20). According to Emanuelli and colleagues, respiratory protective equipment and exhaust ventilation reduces the risk of sinonasal cancer in patients with occupational wood dust exposure, with an odds ratio of 22.5 in patients with a low degree of protection compared with 9.37 in patients with a high degree of protection against wood dust (5).

DIAGNOSIS

Evaluation of any patient with a suspected sinonasal neoplasm should begin with a thorough history and physical examination. The history should address nasal symptoms, such as congestion, obstruction, rhinnorhea, epistaxis, foul odors, dysguesia, and anosmia or hyposmia. Specific attention should be paid to visual complaints, such as decreased acuity, diplopia, impaired extraocular movements or blurred vision, and to any areas of facial numbness. Red flags that should incite concern include unilateral symptoms, visual changes, or any symptoms suggestive of cranial neuropathies (12).

Initial physical examination should include a full head and neck review, including intraoral inspection to assess for lesions eroding through or distorting the palate, otoscopic assessment for middle ear effusions stemming from eustachian tube obstruction, and a careful neurological assessment for cranial neuropathies. The neck should be palpated to assess for cervical adenopathy. Nasal endoscopy should always be performed to delineate the extent of disease and to assess how the anatomy and tumor will impact endoscopic access (4). A mixture of topical anesthetic and decongestant can improve visualization and minimize discomfort for the patient during endoscopy.

In cases of large or invasive tumors, the involvement of other surgical specialties should be considered. Ophthalmalogic evaluation may be appropriate in cases of orbital involvement or tumor abutting the orbit, and neurosurgery should be consulted for assessment in cases of intracranial involvement (4).

IMAGING

Full radiographic evaluation of sinonasal tumors requires the use of two complementary imaging modalities (2). CT is often performed first owing to wide availability and minimal cost (2,12). It is particularly effective at examining osseous structures, identifying bony erosion, and remodeling of lytic destruction from high-grade malignancies. Moreover, it provides essential information regarding skull base and orbital invasion (2). MRI is more effective at distinguishing tumor bulk from inspissated secretions or mucosal inflammation. MRI also has the capacity to detect subtle signal abnormalities in osseous marrow that may suggest tumor invasion not visible on CT. Finally, it can more effectively delineate the extent of dural invasion and periorbital invasion (12). In some cases it can be difficult to differentiate periorbital edema from direct tumor invasion on imaging, and in such cases intraoperative frozen section may be helpful (12).

Specific attention should be paid to signs of perineural extension on MRI. Typical sites of extension include the pterygopalatine fossa, pterygomaxillary fissure, vidian canal, inferior orbital fissure, orbital apex, or foramen rotundum (2). On CT, this can be visualized as expansion of the neural foramina. On MRI, altered signal intensity and enhancement are of concern.

If there is concern regarding vascular invasion, such as involvement of the carotid or vertebral arteries, CT angiography or MR angiography can be used to assess the integrity of major vascular structures (4).

In most cases, imaging should be performed prior to biopsy. This will allow delineation of the lesion and identification of vascular lesions. Although masses that are easily visible in the nasal cavity can be biopsied in the clinic, vascular lesions should be biopsied in the operating room in view of the risk of uncontrolled bleeding (12).

Following pathologic confirmation of malignancy, positron emission tomography (PET) scan be be used to assess for occult regional or distant metastates (4). If PET is not used, CT assessment of the neck and chest is recommended.

PATHOLOGY

Sinonasal malignancies include a wide variety of histopathologic diagnoses (4). In broad terms, these lesions are classified based on their tissue of origin, including epithelial tumors, tumors of bone and cartilage, hematolymphoid, neuroendocrine, germ cell, and secondary tumors (4,9).

The most common sinonasal malignancy is squamous cell carcinoma (SCC). This comprises approximately 65% to 70% of sinonasal carcinomas (9,10). SCC is further subclassified into keratinizing or nonkeratinizing, with nonkeratinizing lesions significantly more likely to be secondary to HPV infection (9). Other variants of SCC include basaloid SCC, papillary SCC, spindle cell carcinoma, and lymphoepithelial carcinoma. Both papillary and basaloid SCC may also be associated with high-risk HPV subtypes, while lymphoepithelial carcinoma is associated with Epstein–Barr virus (EBV) (9).

The second major pathologic subgroup is sinonasal adenocarcinomas, which comprise approximately 10% to 20% of primary sinonasal malignancies (8). These are subclassified into intestinal-type adenocarcinomas (ITACs) and nonintestinal sinonasal adenocarcinomas (SNACs). ITACs have a strong association with wood and other dust exposure, but SNACs are a histologically diverse group of tumors with low- and high-grade forms (8,9). Sinonasal adenocarcinomas most frequently occur in the ethmoid sinuses, followed by the nasal cavity and maxillary sinus. Wood-dust associated adenocarcinomas, in particular, show a strong predilection for the ethmoid sinuses (8,21). Local recurrence is a significant risk after treatment, and occurs in roughly 50% of patients. Regional lymphatic metastases are uncommon, seen in approximately 10% of patients, and distant metastatic disease occurs in 10% to 20% (8,22).

Adenoid cystic carcinoma (ACC) is another neoplasm of secretory cells that occurs in the sinonasal complex (23). This tumor progresses slowly and often presents in an advanced stage with perineural invasion causing symptoms such as facial hypesthesia or trigeminal neuralgia. Treatment is typically surgical resection followed by adjuvant radiation therapy. Unfortunately, complete resection is difficult because of the perineural involvement and skull base invasion, and 5-year recurrence rates have been reported to be as high as 30% (23,24).

Neuroendocrine neoplasms of the sinonasal tract include neuroendocrine carcinomas (NECs) and olfactory neuroblastomas (ONBs), alternately called esthesioneuroblastomas. NECs comprise approximately 5% of all sinonasal malignancies (11). They most frequently present with nonspecific symptoms of nasal obstruction, facial pain, or epistaxis. However, paraneoplastic syndrome, in particular, a syndrome of inappropriate antidiuretic hormone (SIADH), may be due to small cell neuroendocrine carcinoma (11). ONBs arise from olfactory stem cells (basal reserve cells) in the olfactory mucosa (11). ONBs represent 3% to 6% of sinonasal malignancies (11,25). They most frequently present with anosmia, nasal obstruction, and bleeding, although patients rarely do present with ectopic production of adrenocorticotropic hormone (ACTH) or SIADH (11).

Sinonasal undifferentiated carcinoma (SNUC) is a rare, aggressive malignancy thought to be a part of the spectrum of neuroendocrine carcinomas (26). Histologically, SNUC has been a diagnosis of exclusion, when a lesion reveals neither identifiable squamous or glandular features (9). SNUC is usually locally advanced at the time of initial diagnosis, with clinically appreciable adenopathy in up to 30% of patients (26). Even with surgical resection and adjuvant radiation, the prognosis is poor (26).

Mucosal melanoma is a rare malignancy arising from melanocytes found in mucosal surfaces and comprises approximately 1% of melanoma cases (27). Approximately 0.3% to 2% of malignant melanomas are primary sinonasal melanomas, making it the most common location for mucosal melanoma in the head and neck region (27). These lesions are typically diagnosed at an advanced stage but display aggressive oncologic behavior, resulting in a poor prognosis.

Other sinonasal neoplasms include extranodal NK/T cell lymphoma, biphenotypic sinonasal sarcoma, and glomangiopericytoma. Specific discussion about these tumor types is beyond the scope of this chapter. In view of the diversity of potential diagnoses, it is essential that biopsy specimens be evaluated by an experienced head and neck pathologist, as histopathologic misdiagnoses are not uncommon (4,28).

MANAGEMENT

Sinonasal cancer presents a therapeutic challenge because of the close proximity of vital structures. In view of the variable histology, complex local anatomy, and high locoregional recurrence rates, involvement of a multidisciplinary team is essential in treatment planning. This usually occurs in the setting of a multidisciplinary clinic or tumor board (4).

Surgical resection is generally considered first-line therapy, with the objective of obtaining a negative surgical margin (4,8,29). This is typically followed by adjuvant radiation therapy or concurrent chemotherapy and radiation in patients with locally advanced disease (29). However, therapeutic approaches have expanded substantially over the past several decades, owing to the expansion of minimally invasive surgical techniques and development of targeted nonsurgical treatments (12).

Surgical access may be obtained via an endoscopic, open, or combined approach. Traditional open approaches include lateral rhinotomy or the Caldwell-Luc approach or craniofacial resection. The most appropriate approach is whichever provides adequate access to allow total resection with clear margins (8).

An endoscopic-assisted approach is most appropriate when the sinonasal extent of the tumor is well defined and endoscopically resectable, but a craniotomy is required to address the superior or anterior aspects of the tumor (4).

Endoscopic approaches are most ideal for small, well-defined lesions without skull base or orbital invasion. However, as evidence of good oncologic outcomes continues to accrue, the indications for endoscopic resection have expanded, and lesions with skull base invasion are now frequently resected with an endoscopic approach. Although endoscopic resection does not respect the traditional oncologic model of en bloc resection (4,12), it appears to offer comparatively good outcomes (30,31). Lund et al. reported on a prospective cohort of 49 patients who underwent endoscopic resection of various sinonasal malignancies and obtained an overall survival of 88% at 5 years (31). Although these relatively good outcomes are clearly biased by the accessibility of smaller, lower grade tumors to endoscopic resection, endoscopic resection has overall exhibited oncologic results comparable to those of traditional external approaches (32). In such cases, accurate intraoperative frozen sections are essential to ensure clearance of all microscopic disease (4).

MANAGEMENT OF THE SKULL BASE

Surgical approaches to the skull base can be broken into three categories: open craniofacial approaches, endonasal endoscopic approaches, and endoscopic-assisted approaches, which combines an endoscopic transnasal approach with a craniotomy (4).

Open craniofacial approaches to skull base masses were initially described in the 1960s and have become well established as the primary surgical approach to many advanced skull base tumors (4). However, beginning in the 1990s, surgeons began to apply new endoscopic techniques to the resection of skull base tumors. As these minimally invasive approaches advanced, it became clear that they provide an option that may reduce surgical morbidity and mortality in selected cases (4). In general, endoscopic approaches have been shown to provide excellent access to masses involving the anterior, middle, and posterior cranial fossa as well as the craniocervical junction (4). Moreover, as endoscopic approaches have expanded over the past decade, "expanded endonasal approaches" have been developed to access the entire ventral skull base (30). The limits of endoscopic approaches to the skull base and the optimal patient selection criteria continue to be elucidated.

Contraindications to an exclusively endoscopic approach include significant intracranial involvement; significant involvement of the orbit, lateral maxilla, or palate; lateral extension above the orbit; involvement of the anterior table or lateral recesses of the frontal sinus; involvement of the nasal bones; or any extension into the subcutaneous soft tissues that would mandate cutaneous resection in order to obtain clear surgical margins (4). However, an endoscopic approach can be used to address any tumor that is limited to the anterior cranial skull base from the posterior table of the frontal sinus to the planum sphenoidale and bilaterally up to the lamina papyracea. If the intraoperative tumor extent prevents the surgeon from obtaining clear margins, conversion to an endoscopic-assisted or open approach is appropriate.

An endonasal approach is described in detail by Roxbury and colleagues (4). In brief, access is optimized by addressing septal deflection and inferior turbinates as needed. Tumor debulking is performed in order to define the tumor margins. A nasoseptal flap may be raised if this is expected to be used in reconstruction of the skull base. The ablation is then completed via bilateral middle turbinectomies, maxillary antrostomies, ethmoidectomies, sphenoidotomies, and modified Lothrop procedures as appropriate. The septal incisions are performed, with removal of the spenoid rostrum and septae, if appropriate. At that point, circumferential margins are taken for frozen section analysis. The skull base portion of the tumor, if present, is then resected. The anterior and posterior ethmoid arteries are controlled and lateral osteotomies are performed lateral to the cribriform plate. The anterior and posterior osteotomies are then performed to encompass the entirety of the tumor. The crista galli is dissected from the surrounding dura and separated from its attachment to the posterior table. The cribriform plate is thus separated from the remainder of the skull base. At that point, the dural cuts are performed and the olfactory nerves are divided. The cribriform plate and tumor are then removed through the nasal cavity. Dural margins are then taken for frozen section analysis. Further resection is performed if the margins are positive on intraoperative pathologic assessment.

In most cases, when the tumor extends laterally above the orbit, into the facial soft tissues, skin, or nasal bones, or where there is significant intracranial or intraorbital invasion, an open craniofacial resection is most appropriate (4).

SKULL BASE RECONSTRUCTION

The primary goals of skull base reconstruction is to separate the sinonasal cavity from the intradural space, and to obtain a water-tight closure in order to prevent bacterial contamination and leakage of CSF. Open surgical techniques provide excellent access for reconstruction using pericranial or temporoparietal fascia flaps. When performing endoscopic resections, the limited access prevents the use of these flaps, and the pedicled nasoseptal flap has become a common reconstructive choice. If it can be harvested while obtaining clear septal margins, such a flap provides a robust vascularized reconstructive option, particularly appropriate for larger defects (4). In cases in which tumor involvement precludes the use of a nasoseptal flap, other options must be considered, such as other pedicled flaps, autograft, or allografts (4).

Despite these options, the reconstruction of large dural defects has remained a challenge of endonasal skull base surgery (30). In cases of high-flow leaks or recurrent or persistent leaks despite initial endoscopic surgical repair, a lumbar spinal drain may be required (30). Packing is typically placed to bolster the reconstruction against the skull base defect (12).

UNRESECTABLE LESIONS

Traditional indications of unresectability include encasement of the internal carotid artery, significant intracranial involvement, and any lesion in which it is not possible or feasible to obtain negative margins (12). However, some authors have suggested that even in the setting of microscopic positive margins, surgical resection carries benefit (33). Obtaining standard oncologic negative margins in this area of critical functional anatomy may cause excessive morbidity, particularly when the tumor is a high-grade pathologic type for which postoperative radiation and chemotherapy will be recommended regardless of margin status, and in such cases, gross total resection may be a more appropriate management option (33).

MANAGEMENT OF THE NECK

Management of the neck is essential in cases of clinical or radiographic evidence of cervical adenopathy or tumor stage or histology suggestive of a high rate of regional metastases. Options include neck dissection at the time of primary resection, postoperative radiation therapy, or both.

COMPLICATIONS

Infectious complications of endonasal skull base surgery are relatively rare. CSF leaks are estimated to occur in 3% to 5% of expanded endoscopic resections, when the surgery is performed in centers with a high level of expertise (4,34). Rates of meningitis appear to be low, with a rate of less than 1% obtained in a recent study of 120 patients who underwent endoscopic resection of sinonasal cancer with or without craniotomy (34). This low rate is likely because of prophylactic antibiotic therapy, the use of vascularized flaps, and aggressive management of postoperative CSF leaks. Snyderman et al. recommend against the use of nonvascularized materials, such as bone cement or titanium plates, because of an increased risk of infectious complications (30).

Other complications include pneumocephalus, neurovascular complications and ocular complications including loss of vision (4). Overall, the complication rate of expanded endoscopic approaches is estimated at 9% to 11% (4,34,35).

NONSURGICAL THERAPIES

RADIATION THERAPY

In general, the first line treatment for sinonasal malignancies is surgical. Radiation therapy is used as the primary modality in patients who are unable to undergo general anesthesia or surgical resection because of medical comorbid conditions, in patients with lesions considered grossly unresectable, or in select histologic types that are considered to be highly radiosensitive. In such cases, intensity-modulated radiation therapy (IMRT) is considered the standard of care. Other options include proton therapy and stereotactic radiation therapy (gamma knife).

As an adjuvant treatment modality, radiation is used for locally advanced disease, close or positive margins, or if the pathologic examination reveals aggressive features such as perineural invasion (8).

Radiation is a critical adjunct in advanced sinonasal cancer and has shown significant benefit in the adjuvant setting (33). Outcomes have been shown to be improved by higher radiation doses, but this must be balanced against the increased morbidity (33). Late radiation effects include severe morbidities, such as blindness, brain necrosis, and osteoradionecrosis, and these factors have limited the dosages of standard radiation (33).

PROTON BEAM RADIATION

The introduction of proton beam therapy has allowed for dose intensification to the targeted area with relative sparing of adjacent uninvolved tissues (36). As Russo et al. note, this is essential because the predominant failure pattern in sinonasal cancer is local (36). These authors recently examined a homogeneous population of 54 patients with sinonasal SCC treated with proton therapy (37 underwent surgical resection first) and obtained a locoregional control rate of 76% at 2 years and 73% at 5 years, while obtaining an overall survival rate of 67% at 2 years and 47% at 5 years. Patients had inferior outcomes if a gross total resection could not be obtained prior to proton therapy (36). Overall, the relative benefits of proton radiation therapy for sinonasal malignancy as compared to IMRT continue to be elucidated, and are the focus of ongoing research, including a currently accruing clinical trial (NCT01586767).

CHEMOTHERAPY

The traditional role of chemotherapy in sinonasal cancer was for palliative care in advanced unresectable disease (37,38). However, it has been explored in other settings including neoadjuvant and adjuvant use and is now most commonly used concurrently with radiation therapy in the adjuvant setting (17,18).

In resectable disease, surgery is generally considered a first-line treatment modality and may be followed by adjuvant concurrent chemotherapy and radiation based on the extent of tumor, stage, subsite, and other prognostic factors (12,38–40). Although prospective trials are lacking, platinum-based agents are most commonly used in epithelial tumors, often combined with either 5-fluorouracil, taxane, ifosfamide, or vincristine (41).

No prospective randomized trials have examined the role of neoadjuvant chemotherapy in sinonasal cancer. However, several smaller single-center studies have obtained promising results (15,38,41–44). In one of the earliest studies on this topic, LoRusso et al. reported on 16 previously untreated patients with advanced sinonasal cancer who were treated with platinum-based chemotherapy followed by surgery and/or radiation therapy. A complete response to chemotherapy was obtained in 44% and a partial response rate was found in 38% of these patients (41,44). In a more recent study, Hanna et al examined 46 patients with previously untreated sinonasal SCC treated with induction chemotherapy followed by surgery and/or radiation or concurrent chemoradiation. A response to induction chemotherapy was obtained in 67% of patients and was predictive of prognosis. Patients who experienced at least a partial response or stable disease during induction chemotherapy obtained a 2-year survival rate of 77%, compared to 36% in those patients who experienced progressive disease during induction chemotherapy (42). The potential role of induction chemotherapy in the management of sinonasal cancer continues to be elucidated and the potential benefits must be balanced against the risk of delaying multimodal treatment in view of the toxicity of chemotherapy (38,45). A currently ongoing clinical trial (NCT02099175) is attempting to improve our understanding of optimal multimodal treatment in resectable sinonasal cancer.

There is limited data regarding chemotherapy for the treatment of ONB, although it is used in both neoadjuvant and concurrent settings in patients with advanced disease (46). However, several case series suggest that induction chemotherapy has a high response rate (47,48). Modesto and colleagues retrospectively reviewed 43 patients with ONB, including 23 who underwent neoadjuvant chemotherapy with an overall response rate of 74%, including 6 complete responses and 11 partial responses (48). Similarly, Su et al. examined 15 patients with advanced ONB who were treated with induction chemotherapy, with the choice of agent at the discretion of the medical oncologist (47). After two cycles they were assessed for response using MRI. Patients with complete or partial response could then receive up to two additional cycles of chemotherapy. This was followed by definitive treatment, including surgery and postoperative radiation therapy, or radiotherapy with or without chemotherapy in patients with either complete response or unresectable disease. The majority of patients (80%) were treated with cisplatin and etoposide. Overall, they found a 68% response to chemotherapy, with 47% of patients showing complete response, and 20% showing partial response. The response to chemotherapy was higher (78%) in the Hyams high-grade patients. Gay and colleagues recently performed comprehensive genomic profiling of 41 stage III and IV ONBs and detected genomic alterations in 28 ONBs, with a mean of 1.5 genomic alterations per sample. In 51% of evaluations, ONBs had genetic alterations that could be linked to drugs either currently available or under evaluation in clinical trials, suggesting potential future use of targeted therapies (49).

Other neuroendocrine carcinomas carry a worse prognosis and are often treated in a multimodal fashion. Chemotherapy has variably been used in the neoadjuvant, concurrent, and adjuvant settings, with drug regimens including cisplatin with etoposide or 5-FU or carboplatin with etoposide or docetaxel (41). One of the larger case series available looked at 41 patients treated for neuroendocrine carcinoma of the paranasal sinuses at MD Anderson between 1992 and 2008. Multimodal treatment including surgery, chemotherapy, and radiation was used in most patients. Chemotherapy was administered variably as neoadjuvant, concurrent, and adjuvant therapy, and drug regimens included cisplatin with etoposide, carboplatin with etoposide, cisplatin with 5-FU, and taxotere. Median overall disease-free survival was 23.6 months and overall survival was 58.6 months (50).

SNUC has shown itself to be a chemosensitive disease in a number of small studies (41). A meta-analysis by Reiersen et al., published in 2012, examined a total of 167 patients and showed improved survival with the addition of chemotherapy to surgical resection. Chemotherapeutic regimens varied, but the most common agents were cyclophosphamide, doxorubicin, and vincristine (CAV) (40). Small study sizes and variability in published treatment regimens continue to make determination of the optimal regimen difficult.

Unlike other sinonasal malignancies, the role of adjuvant chemotherapy in primary mucosal melanoma was examined in a randomized phase II clinical trial. This trial randomized patients into three groups: (a) observation alone; (b) temozolomide plus cisplatinum; and (c) high-dose interferon. The authors obtained a significant improvement in relapse-free survival in the temozolomide and cisplatinum group (20.8 months compared to 5.4 months in the observation group and 9.4 months in the interferon group) (51).

PROGNOSIS

Although prognosis varies significantly according to stage and specific histopathology, sinonasal malignancies overall carry a poor prognosis (4). Unfortunately, because of the nonspecific nature of early symptoms, sinonasal malignancies are typically identified once they have already reached an advanced stage (12). Predictably, orbital involvement is associated with a dramatic reduction in survival (12). The ability to obtain a clear surgical margin is of great prognostic significance, as positive surgical margins result in decreased local control and decreased survival (8).

CONCLUSIONS

Endoscopic approaches have revolutionized the treatment of sinonasal cancers, and in appropriate selected patients they result in decreased surgical morbidity without compromising oncologic outcomes. Nonsurgical management approaches, such as chemotherapeutic regimens, are continuing to be developed. Therapeutic management remains a challenging and continuously evolving area.

CASE 19.1

A 64-year-old man initially presented to an otolaryngology clinic for assessment of nasal obstruction and nasal congestion. At that time, he reported a 12-week history of progressive nasal obstruction, which progressed to near-complete left unilateral obstruction. He had undergone three courses of antibiotics and two courses of prednisone without improvement in his symptoms. He also reported a recent onset of intermittent epistaxis and headaches. He did not report any visual disturbances, including no diplopia, and no facial pain, numbness, or tingling. A review of systems was otherwise negative.

His past medical history was significant only for a remote colectomy.

On initial physical examination, pertinent findings included proptosis, a hyponasal voice, and bilateral rhinorrhea. Flexible nasal endoscopy revealed a large papillomatous lesion filling the left nasal cavity and bowing the septum rightward. The oral cavity and oropharynx did not show any concerning features and there was no palpable adenopathy. Cranial nerve examination did not reveal any deficits and extraocular movements were normal.

A CT scan was obtained, which can be seen in Figure 19.1.

The patient returned to the clinic and an in-office biopsy was performed under endoscopic visualization. The biopsy revealed fragments of papillary squamous cell carcinoma and he was subsequently referred to a large tertiary head and neck oncology group for multidisciplinary assessment.

An MRI of the sinuses and a chest CT were performed to better elucidate the extent of disease and to complete pretreatment staging. Select images from

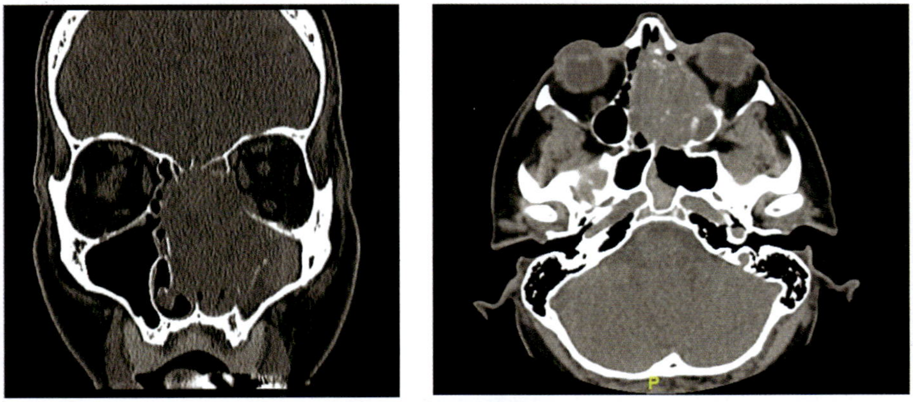

FIGURE 19.1 CT revealed a large mass in the left nasal cavity with extension into the left maxillary sinus, the ethmoids, and the left frontal sinus. Loss of the left lamina papyracea and extension into the left orbit with displacement of the medial rectus was noted. No cervical adenopathy was detected.

the MRI can be seen in Figure 19.2. The CT of the chest did not reveal any distant metastatic disease.

In addition to otolaryngology, the patient was assessed by a neurosurgeon, medical oncologist, and radiation oncologist and was discussed at the weekly head and neck tumor board. The mass was clinically staged as cT4aN0M0.

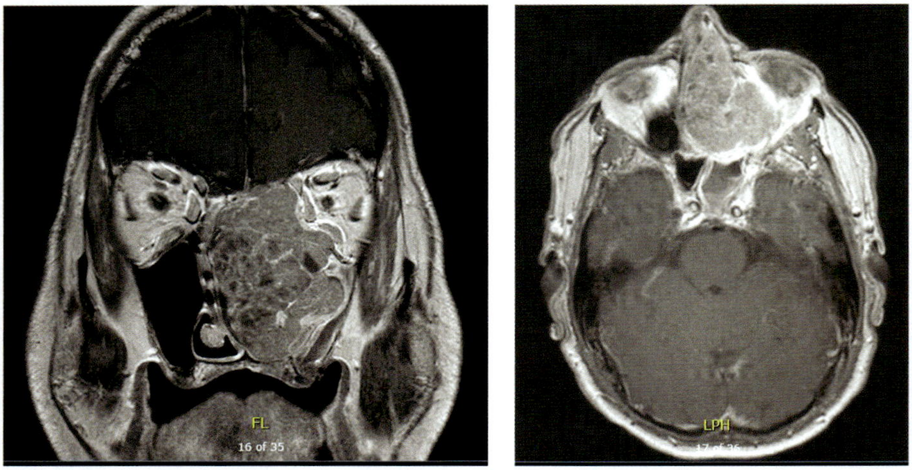

FIGURE 19.2 MRI revealed a large heterogeneously enhancing mass that entirely occupied and expanded the left nasal cavity, and invaded through the left lamina papyracea and bony orbital floor into the left orbit extraconal space. It was inseparable from the superior oblique muscle and contacted the medical rectus and inferior rectus muscles. There was mass effect on the left eye resulting in left proptosis. Superiorly, the mass was inseparable from the left ethmoid roof and crista galli, suggesting that these structures may be eroded or invaded.

REFERENCES

1. Johnson JT, Rosen CA. *Bailey's Head and Neck Surgery: Otolaryngology*. 5th ed. Vols 1 and 2. Philadelphia, PA: Lippincott Williams & Wilkins; 2014:3016.
2. Koeller KK. Radiologic features of sinonasal tumors. *Head Neck Pathol*. 2016;10(1):1–12. doi:10.1007/s12105-016-0686-9
3. Dutta R, Dubal PM, Svider PF, et al. Sinonasal malignancies: a population-based analysis of site-specific incidence and survival. *Laryngoscope*. 2015;125(11):2491–2417.
4. Roxbury CR, Ishii M, Richmon JD, et al. Endonasal endoscopic surgery in the management of sinonasal and anterior skull base malignancies. *Head Neck Pathol*. 2016;10(1):13–22.
5. Emanuelli E, Alexandre E, Cazzador D, et al. A case-case study on sinonasal cancer prevention: effect from dust reduction in woodworking and risk of mastic/solvents in shoemaking. *J Occup Med Toxicol Lond Engl*. 2016;11:35.
6. Ansa B, Goodman M, Ward K, et al. Paranasal sinus squamous cell carcinoma incidence and survival based on Surveillance, Epidemiology, and End Results data, 1973 to 2009. *Cancer*. 2013;119(14):2602–2610.
7. Poursadegh M, Poursadegh F, Esmaeili M, Bakhshaee M. Epidemiological survey of sinonasal malignancy in north-east Iran. *Iran J Otorhinolaryngol*. 2015;27(80):225–229.
8. Lund VJ, Chisholm EJ, Takes RP, et al. Evidence for treatment strategies in sinonasal adenocarcinoma. *Head Neck*. 2012;34(8):1168–1178.
9. Stelow EB, Bishop JA. Update from the 4th edition of the World Health Organization classification of head and neck tumours: tumors of the nasal cavity, paranasal sinuses and skull base. *Head Neck Pathol*. 2017;11(1):3–15.
10. Lewis JS. Sinonasal squamous cell carcinoma: a review with emphasis on emerging histologic subtypes and the role of human papillomavirus. *Head Neck Pathol*. 2016;10(1):60–67.
11. Shah K, Perez-Ordóñez B. Neuroendocrine neoplasms of the sinonasal tract: neuroendocrine carcinomas

and olfactory neuroblastoma. *Head Neck Pathol.* 2016;10(1):85–94.

12. Svider PF, Setzen M, Baredes S, et al. Overview of sinonasal and ventral skull base malignancy management. *Otolaryngol Clin North Am.* 2017.
13. Airoldi M, Garzaro M, Valente G, et al. Clinical and biological prognostic factors in 179 cases with sinonasal carcinoma treated in the Italian Piedmont region. *Oncology.* 2009;76(4):262–269.
14. Resto VA, Deschler DG. Sinonasal malignancies. *Otolaryngol Clin North Am.* 2004;37(2):473–487.
15. Licitra L, Locati LD, Cavina R, et al. Primary chemotherapy followed by anterior craniofacial resection and radiotherapy for paranasal cancer. *Ann Oncol Off J Eur Soc Med Oncol.* 2003;14(3):367–372.
16. Duru Birgi S, Teo M, Dyker KE, et al. Definitive and adjuvant radiotherapy for sinonasal squamous cell carcinomas: a single institutional experience. *Radiat Oncol Lond Engl.* 2015;10:190. http://www.ncbi.nlm.nih.gov/pmc/articles/PMC4574072
17. Cooper JS, Pajak TF, Forastiere AA, et al. Postoperative concurrent radiotherapy and chemotherapy for high-risk squamous-cell carcinoma of the head and neck. *N Engl J Med.* 2004;350(19):1937–1944.
18. Bernier J, Domenge C, Ozsahin M, et al. Postoperative Irradiation with or without concomitant chemotherapy for locally advanced head and neck cancer. *N Engl J Med.* 2004;350(19):1945–1952.
19. Celakovsky P, Kalfert D, Tucek L, et al. Deep neck infections: risk factors for mediastinal extension. *Eur Arch Oto-Rhino-Laryngol Off J Eur Fed Oto-Rhino-Laryngol Soc EUFOS Affil Ger Soc Oto-Rhino-Laryngol - Head Neck Surg.* 2014;271(6):1679–1683.
20. Binazzi A, Ferrante P, Marinaccio A. Occupational exposure and sinonasal cancer: a systematic review and meta-analysis. *BMC Cancer.* 2015;13(15):49.
21. Leivo I. Update on sinonasal adenocarcinoma: classification and advances in immunophenotype and molecular genetic make-up. *Head Neck Pathol.* 2007;1(1):38.
22. Barnes L. Intestinal-type adenocarcinoma of the nasal cavity and paranasal sinuses. *Am J Surg Pathol.* 1986;10(3):192–202.
23. Unsal AA, Chung SY, Zhou AH, et al. Sinonasal adenoid cystic carcinoma: a population-based analysis of 694 cases. *Int Forum Allergy Rhinol.* 2017;7(3):312–320.
24. Rhee C-S, Won T-B, Lee CH, et al. Adenoid cystic carcinoma of the sinonasal tract: treatment results. *Laryngoscope.* 2006;116(6):982–986.
25. Jethanamest D, Morris LG, Sikora AG, Kutler DI. Esthesioneuroblastoma: a population-based analysis of survival and prognostic factors. *Arch Otolaryngol Neck Surg.* 2007;133(3):276–280.
26. Tanzler ED, Morris CG, Orlando CA, et al. Management of sinonasal undifferentiated carcinoma. *Head Neck.* 2008;30(5):595–599.
27. Göde S, Turhal G, Tarhan C, et al. Primary sinonasal malignant melanoma: effect of clinical and histopathologic prognostic factors on survival. *Balk Med J.* 2017;34(3):255–262.
28. Cohen ZR, Marmor E, Fuller GN, DeMonte F. Misdiagnosis of olfactory neuroblastoma. *Neurosurg Focus.* 2002;12(5):e3.
29. Kasemsiri P, Prevedello DMS, Otto BA, et al. Endoscopic endonasal technique: treatment of paranasal and anterior skull base malignancies. *Braz J Otorhinolaryngol.* 2013;79(6):760–779.
30. Snyderman CH, Pant H, Carrau RL, et al. What are the limits of endoscopic sinus surgery? The expanded endonasal approach to the skull base. *Keio J Med.* 2009;58(3):152–160.
31. Lund V, Howard DJ, Wei WI. Endoscopic resection of malignant tumors of the nose and sinuses. *Am J Rhinol.* 2007;21(1):89–94.
32. Bogaerts S, Vander Poorten V, Nuyts S, et al. Results of endoscopic resection followed by radiotherapy for primarily diagnosed adenocarcinomas of the paranasal sinuses. *Head Neck.* 2008;30(6):728–736.
33. Resto VA, Chan AW, Deschler DG, Lin DT. Extent of surgery in the management of locally advanced sinonasal malignancies. *Head Neck.* 2008;30(2):222–229.
34. Hanna E, DeMonte F, Ibrahim S, et al. Endoscopic resection of sinonasal cancers with and without craniotomy: oncologic results. *Arch Otolaryngol Head Neck Surg.* 2009;135(12):1219–1224.
35. Nicolai P, Battaglia P, Bignami M, et al. Endoscopic surgery for malignant tumors of the sinonasal tract and adjacent skull base: a 10-year experience. *Am J Rhinol.* 2008;22(3):308–316.
36. Russo AL, Adams JA, Weyman EA, et al. Long-term outcomes after proton beam therapy for sinonasal squamous cell carcinoma. *Int J Radiat Oncol.* 2016;95(1):368–376.
37. Llorente JL, López F, Suárez C, Hermsen MA. Sinonasal carcinoma: clinical, pathological, genetic and therapeutic advances. *Nat Rev Clin Oncol.* 2014;11(8):460–472.
38. Scangas GA, Eloy JA, Lin DT. The role of chemotherapy in the management of sinonasal and ventral skull base malignancies. *Otolaryngol Clin North Am.* 2017;50(2):433–441.
39. Suarez C, Llorente JL, Fernandez De Leon R, et al. Prognostic factors in sinonasal tumors involving the anterior skull base. *Head Neck.* 2004;26(2):136–144.
40. Reiersen DA, Pahilan ME, Devaiah AK. Meta-analysis of treatment outcomes for sinonasal undifferentiated carcinoma. *Otolaryngol—Head Neck Surg Off J Am Acad Otolaryngol-Head Neck Surg.* 2012;147(1):7–14.
41. Bossi P, Saba NF, Vermorken JB, et al. The role of systemic therapy in the management of sinonasal cancer: a critical review. *Cancer Treat Rev.* 2015;41(10):836–843.
42. Hanna EY, Cardenas AD, DeMonte F, et al. Induction chemotherapy for advanced squamous cell carcinoma of the paranasal sinuses. *Arch Otolaryngol Head Neck Surg.* 2011;137(1):78–81.
43. Ock C-Y, Keam B, Kim TM, et al. Induction chemotherapy in head and neck squamous cell carcinoma of the paranasal sinus and nasal cavity: a role in organ preservation. *Korean J Intern Med.* 2016;31(3):570–578.
44. LoRusso P, Tapazoglou E, Kish JA, et al. Chemotherapy for paranasal sinus carcinoma. A 10-year experience at Wayne State University. *Cancer.* 1988;62(1):1–5.
45. Hoffmann TK. Systemic therapy strategies for head-neck carcinomas: current status. *GMS Curr Top Otorhinolaryngol Head Neck Surg.* 2012;11:Doc03.

46. Ow TJ, Bell D, Kupferman ME, et al. Esthesioneuroblastoma. *Neurosurg Clin North Am.* 2013;24(1):51–65.
47. Su SY, Bell D, Ferrarotto R, et al. Outcomes for olfactory neuroblastoma treated with induction chemotherapy. *Head Neck.* 2017;39(8):1671–1679.
48. Modesto A, Blanchard P, Tao YG, Rives M, Janot F, Serrano E, et al. Multimodal treatment and long-term outcome of patients with esthesioneuroblastoma. *Oral Oncol.* 2013;49(8):830–834.
49. Gay LM, Kim S, Fedorchak K, et al. Comprehensive genomic profiling of esthesioneuroblastoma reveals additional treatment options. *Oncologist.* 2017;22(7):834–842.
50. Likhacheva A, Rosenthal DI, Hanna E, et al. Sinonasal neuroendocrine carcinoma: impact of differentiation status on response and outcome. *Head Neck Oncol.* 2011;3:32.
51. Lian B, Si L, Cui C, et al. Phase II randomized trial comparing high-dose IFN-α2b with temozolomide plus cisplatin as systemic adjuvant therapy for resected mucosal melanoma. *Clin Cancer Res.* 2013;19(16):4488–4498.

20

Evaluation and Treatment of Metastatic Lymphadenopathy From an Unknown Primary

Shirin Attarian
Richard Blake Ross
Shlomo A. Koyfman
Missak Haigentz, Jr.

Head and neck cancer with unknown primary (HNCUP) is defined as the presence of metastatic tumor in a neck lymph node with no identifiable primary site. HNCUP historically has accounted for about 10% of new cases of head and neck cancers (1); however, with new diagnostic technologies, including positron emission tomography (PET) with fluorodeoxyglucose (FDG-PET) with or without CT, the incidence of HNCUP is now reported at 1% to 3%. Many patients with head and neck cancer initially present with a neck mass, with the primary site of origin readily identified with the appropriate evaluation, and therefore, HNCUP is a diagnosis of exclusion.

It should be noted that neck lymphadenopathy is a common patient presentation in primary care offices, and most cases are benign (Table 20.1). Malignancy must be differentiated from benign neoplasms or infectious disorders by cytological or pathological diagnosis (Table 20.2). This chapter will discuss the etiology, evaluation, and current management recommendations of HNCUP, focusing on squamous cell carcinomas with unknown primary (SCCUP). As human papillomavirus (HPV)–associated SCCUP is a newly recognized clinical entity, separate discussion is provided on its epidemiology, diagnostic considerations, and treatment.

CLINICAL EVALUATION

HNCUP is a diagnosis of exclusion, and complete head and neck evaluation must be performed in an effort to identify a primary tumor. When a mass is discovered in the head and neck that is a concern for malignancy, the diagnostic evaluation should include a comprehensive history and physical examination including fiberoptic endoscopy, fine-needle aspiration (FNA) of the mass, high-quality diagnostic imaging, and panendoscopy. Advanced age, smoking history, and large, hard, and immobile nodes are more causes for concerns for malignancy. Figure 20.1 demonstrates the recommended diagnostic evaluation algorithm for HNCUP. It is important to note that in any person middle aged or older, a pathologically enlarged cervical lymph node, especially with central necrosis or cystic appearance, should be considered cancer until proved otherwise.

TABLE 20.1

Differential Diagnosis of Cervical Lymphadenopathy

Benign	Malignant
Acute/chronic local infections	Head and neck squamous cell carcinoma (SCC)
HIV	Salivary gland cancers
Infectious mononucleosis	Lymphomas (Hodgkin and non-Hodgkin)
Benign neoplasms (e.g., schwannoma, paraganglioma, lipoma)	Thyroid cancer
	Skin cancer (SCC or melanoma)
	Sarcoma
	Cancers of remote primary site (e.g., lung, gastrointestinal tract)

TABLE 20.2

Incidence of Different Pathologies of a Cervical Mass With Unknown Primary

Type	Incidence (%)
Nonspecific lymphadenopathy	33
Tuberculous lymphadenitis	24
Metastatic lymphadenopathy	19
Lymphoma	16
Specific lymphadenitis (nontuberculous)	8

Source: Adapted From Ref. (2). Moor JW, Murray P, Inwood J. Diagnostic biopsy of lymph nodes of the neck, axilla, and groin: rhyme, reason, or chance? *Ann R Coll Surg Engl.* 2008;90(3): 221–225.

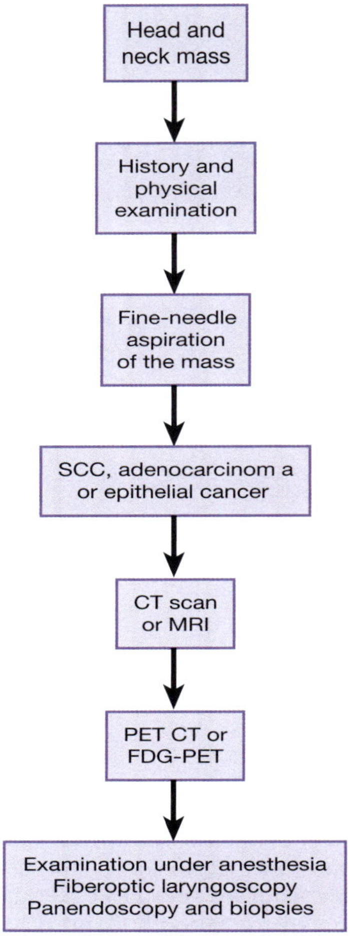

FIGURE 20.1 Diagnostic approach to the patient with a head and neck mass.

FDG, fluorodeoxyglucose; SCC, squamous cell carcinoma.

HISTORY AND PHYSICAL EXAMINATION

A detailed medical history should be taken, including history of any previous malignancies, notably of skin cancers. Physical examination should include a thorough examination of the scalp and non-hair-bearing skin for evidence of cutaneous malignancy, a frequent cause of metastatic cervical lymphadenopathy.

The location of cervical lymph node metastases can offer clues for finding the location of the primary tumor and may guide the initial evaluation. Nearly 40% of SCCUP present with a single enlarged lymph node that is most commonly located in level II, suggesting an occult oropharyngeal primary tumor location. Lymphadenopathy in level III, without involvement of level II, suggests a primary site in the supraglottic larynx or hypopharynx. Tumors of the lip and oral cavity usually metastasize to lymph nodes in levels I to III, whereas metastases from oropharyngeal, hypopharyngeal, and laryngeal sites and the thyroid tend to appear lower in the jugular chain (levels II–IV) or, centrally, in level VI. Cervical lymph node metastases localized to level V are commonly of nasopharyngeal or cutaneous origin. Enlarged parotid nodes should direct the search for a primary tumor of cutaneous or salivary origin. Bilateral cervical lymph node metastases should focus attention on the nasopharynx, base of tongue, hypopharynx, and midline structures.

Approximately 50% of masses limited to level IV and the supraclavicular fossa are from a primary tumor arising below the clavicle. The most common malignancies below the clavicles that metastasize to neck lymph nodes are cancers of the breast, lung, kidney, cervix, and testis. The lymph nodes in the left supraclavicular region have afferent drainage that includes the thorax, abdomen, and pelvis, and as a consequence left-sided metastases from primary cancers from these sites are common. The left supraclavicular node, as described by the 19th century pathologists Virchow and Troisier, is known as Virchow's node and is characteristically involved in gastric carcinoma. Involvement of right-sided neck nodes from remote primary tumors may be associated with mediastinal involvement (3).

Other clinical symptoms at presentation should direct the evaluation of the primary tumor site. For example, hoarseness may suggest involvement of the vocal cords, and rapid enlargement of a neck mass may suggest lymphoma.

DIAGNOSTIC SAMPLING (BIOPSY)

FNA of the lymph node is the preferred initial approach to diagnosis of carcinomas, though core-needle or fresh excisional lymph node biopsies for pathological architecture remain standard for suspected lymphoma diagnoses. In addition to cytological diagnoses, FNA samples can be evaluated by immunohistochemical methods (on cell blocks, when sufficient cells are available) and when indicated, by flow cytometry (for suspected lymphoma), calcitonin measurements (for medullary thyroid cancers), or molecular testing for suspected thyroid cancers. Nondiagnostic FNA results should be repeated under radiologic guidance (e.g., ultrasound or CT guided). Importantly, as FNA can frequently have insufficient material needed to perform molecular testing for viral causes, we frequently repeat a core-needle biopsy.

Open biopsy is discouraged because of the possibility of disruption of fascial planes that act as a natural barrier to tumor spread and because of possible interference with a planned neck dissection in the future, if deemed appropriate for definitive therapy. It is also discouraged because of increased morbidity. When necessary, open biopsy should be performed by a surgeon prepared for a neck dissection as part of the same procedure, if indicated (4).

Because of the heterogeneity of possible malignancies in the differential diagnosis, including tumors of major and minor salivary glands as well as other remote, infraclavicular sites, nonsquamous cytopathology (e.g., adenocarcinoma) without a clear primary site on imaging studies should prompt consideration for additional tumor sampling and consultation with expert pathologists.

Once the FNA shows SCC, adenocarcinoma, or other epithelial cancer and no primary site has been identified, additional imaging studies, if not already performed, are required. If this does not reveal a primary tumor, FDG-PET or integrated PET/CT should be done, and if still not conclusive, examination under anesthesia should be performed to evaluate the sinuses, nasal cavity, nasopharynx, pharyngeal walls, base of tongue, larynx, and hypopharynx. Biopsies of the likely mucosal primary sites should be performed, including a tonsillectomy. Many primary cancers are identified after tonsillectomy; however, the therapeutic benefit of this surgery is uncertain (see following text) (5–7).

ROLE OF MOLECULAR TESTING

Most SCCUP cases are positive for HPV (8,9); only about 10% are HPV negative by p16 immunohistochemical analysis (IHC) or high-risk HPV DNA by in situ hybridization (ISH). As up to 80% of oropharyngeal SCC and 20% to 25% of sino-nasal tract SCC are related to transcriptionally active HPV, a finding of HPV-positive disease may aid in localizing possible primary mucosal tumors and in guiding cancer therapy (10).

However, there are a number of limitations to widespread HPV-testing, and specifically p16 testing, in SCCUP cases, justifying caution. Among mucosal SCC cases, positive p16 IHC has been a validated surrogate HPV marker in oropharyngeal primaries; outside this anatomic site, the specificity of p16 overexpression is low or has not been established, and the prognostic value of p16-positive disease has not been proved. Nevertheless, it is critically important in SCCUP with level II (particularly cystic) nodes, as this is almost certainly an indication of an occult oropharyngeal primary. As such, if the FNA reveals SCC but has insufficient cellularity with which viral testing can be accomplished, we frequently pursue a core-needle biopsy as a means of attaining more tissue for p16/EBV (Epstein–Barr virus) testing. Prior studies have shown a negligibly low rate of tumor seeding with core-needle biopsy (11).

Although p16 is generally an accepted surrogate marker for HPV-positive disease of a presumed occult oropharyngeal primary, there are other diseases that can stain positively for p16 and even the more specific HPV DNA testing. There appears to be an increasing incidence of p16/HPV-associated nasopharyngeal cancer, which has led some to advocate covering the nasopharynx as a potential primary site in p16-positive SCCUP (12). Similarly, cutaneous SCC of the head and neck can metastasize to cervical nodes and can demonstrate p16 and even HPV positivity (13).

OTHER TESTS

A growing number of commercially available tumor-based gene expression profiling tests are available to aid detection for the origin of cancers of unknown origin (e.g., CancerTYPE ID, RosettaGX Cancer Origin, and Tissue of Origin). Although these tests do include head and neck cancer as a site of origin, the usefulness of these evaluations is limited in the setting of SCC metastases to cervical lymph nodes, and the tests cannot as yet differentiate primaries from specific mucosal sites and subsites within the head and neck.

RADIOGRAPHIC IMAGING

CT and MRI with contrast are usually the first line of imaging for patients with HNCUP, although iodinated contrast agent should be avoided if differentiated thyroid cancer remains a diagnostic consideration (given the therapeutic role of postoperative radioactive iodine). If CT and MRI do not identify a primary tumor, FDG-PET or integrated PET/CT (either skull base to midthigh, or whole body imaging) is the next step.

Both PET and PET/CT scans improve the diagnosis in the search for the primary tumor in cases of HNCUP. Prior studies have indicated that PET/CT may increase the chance of detection of a primary site from 25% to 55% (14), and current widespread use of PET imaging has likely resulted in a decreased frequency of HNCUP diagnoses in recent series. Integrated PET/CT is superior to PET in the detection of the primary site of clinically occult tumors (15). Some practitioners prefer to use PET/CT as the initial imaging step; however, it is important to note that structural and anatomic information can be lost if the CT component is of low resolution or performed without contrast. As such, we recommend obtaining diagnostic quality contrast-enhanced CT or MRI in addition to functional imaging. An additional advantage of PET imaging is the ability to diagnose occult or distant tumors and metastatic disease.

In particular, it is recommended to perform PET/CT prior to panendoscopy or mucosal biopsies. If a biopsy or deep examination or manipulation of the tissues is performed prior to PET/CT, the scan will show FDG uptake in those areas because of inflammation from the procedures, and the specificity of the imaging is decreased. In addition, PET/CT before panendoscopy might increase the diagnostic yield in the HNCUP population, leading to more targeted, and therefore less morbid, treatment (14).

All HNCUP patients should undergo examination under anesthesia, including panendoscopy with tonsillectomy and blind biopsies of mucosal sites (15).

ROLE OF TONSILLECTOMY

Historically, it has been noticed that many SCCUP patients have occult tonsillar primaries, resulting in a recommendation for tonsillectomy in the evaluation of these patients. Given our current understanding of oncogenic HPV infection and its involvement in oropharyngeal carcinogenesis, with common presentations of small primary tumors and bulky, often cystic lymphadenopathy, it should not be a surprise that many SCCUP cases are in fact HPV-related oropharyngeal cancers. If a primary tumor is not found by the above initial approaches, ipsilateral or bilateral tonsillectomy and sampling of the base of tongue can be considered as the next steps in diagnosis. In a study by Waltonen et al. (7) the overall yield of finding an occult primary carcinoma in the tonsil was 3.2% for deep tonsil biopsies vs. 29.6% for tonsillectomies. However, random tonsillar biopsies and unilateral versus bilateral tonsillectomies remain controversial (16).

Some experts recommend bilateral tonsillectomy over unilateral tonsillectomy. The dominant hypothesis behind this suggestion is that bilateral tonsillectomy has a low rate of complications, and there is a chance of missing a contralateral tonsillar primary if a bilateral removal is not done. Furthermore, there is a theoretical advantage that subsequent examinations for cancer surveillance may be facilitated by a greater symmetry on physical examination after bilateral tonsillectomy.

Similar to palatine tonsillectomy, recent studies have suggested that lingual tonsillectomy during workup for an unknown primary can improve the ability to identify a primary (17). Historically, lingual tonsillectomy was performed through open surgery; however, in recent years transoral robotic surgery (TORS) has been used. TORS can significantly improve the ability to identify and resect the occult primary site and thereby decrease the intensity of and morbidities associated with adjuvant chemoradiotherapy in a subset of patients (18). However, whether more precise identification and resection using TORS will result in improved outcomes remains unknown and further studies are needed in this area.

TREATMENT APPROACHES

As appropriate cancer treatment depends on the primary tumor site, AJCC/UICC (American Joint Committee on Cancer/ Union for International Cancer Control) stage grouping, and histopathological type as well as molecular test features, treatment of HNCUP should only be initiated after the evaluations described earlier are carried out. In principle, treatment should always be directed to the site of origin of the suspected primary tumor. Our discussion in the following text focuses on treatment approaches for SCCUP, with specific discussion and considerations for HPV-associated disease.

The AJCC 8th edition has modified the staging system for oropharynx cancer and made minor changes for HPV/p16 negative disease and major changes for patients with HPV/p16 positive disease. However, it is crucial to recognize that the new stage groupings are associated with prognosis and NOT treatment recommendations. These outcomes are based on treatment algorithms that were tailored to the AJCC 7 system and as such, treatment recommendations in this chapter will reflect AJCC 7 staging.

TREATMENT OF HPV-NEGATIVE SCCUP

Surgery and radiotherapy are the main treatment options for early and locoregionally advanced head and neck SCC. Most patients are treated with multimodality therapy. Multimodality therapy for limited disease may include initial resection followed by adjuvant radiation with or without concurrent chemotherapy or initial sequential or concurrent chemoradiotherapy with or without planned neck dissection.

NECK DISSECTION

The initial surgical treatment for SCC is neck dissection (4). The decision regarding the type of neck dissection should be individualized and based on the extent of nodal disease. Selective neck dissection is preferred, as all five levels of the neck are rarely at risk. Therefore, classical radical neck dissection is rarely indicated (19).

Surgery alone for SCCUP management may be appropriate for a limited number of patients. Management of SCCUP with surgery alone requires identification of patients at low risk for mucosal emergence and regional recurrence. Mucosal emergence has been reported to be as high as 25% in historical series (20). Therefore surgery monotherapy for SCCUP is typically reserved only for patients who may be elderly or compromised in whom minimal treatment is preferred. In these select cases, surgery alone may be appropriate in patients with a single involved lymph node without evidence of extranodal extension (Table 20.3). However, adjuvant radiotherapy to the neck and covering the potential mucosal primary sites has become standard practice in most institutions.

RADIOTHERAPY

Unilateral radiotherapy is not as commonly used as bilateral treatment in both definitive and adjuvant settings. Although mucosal emergence and contralateral neck recurrence seem to be rare after unilateral radiotherapy, it is a departure from standard practice (4).

Although the majority of single-institution retrospective studies comparing the involved field and elective neck irradiation did not show any advantage for more extensive radiotherapy, there are reports of improved regional control after nodal resection and bilateral neck irradiation over ipsilateral neck radiotherapy. The European Organisation for Research and Treatment of Cancerconducted a phase III trial (EORTC 22205) comparing comprehensive bilateral neck and mucosal radiation to 50 Gy, followed by a 10-Gy boost to the ipsilateral neck with ipsilateral neck radiation to 60 Gy alone. The trial was closed after 2 years because of poor accrual, and no results have been reported. Given the lack of data, firm conclusions cannot be drawn.

TABLE 20.3

Recommended Treatment for Occult Primary Head and Neck Cancers Based on Extent of Nodal Involvement

Involved Lymph Nodes	Recommended Treatment
Single lymph node, 3 cm or smaller	Single modality treatment, surgery or RT
Single lymph node, greater than 3 cm but less than 6 cm	1. Favorable risk factor profile*: single-modality therapy, surgery or RT
	2. Unfavorable risk factors† but no ENE: surgery plus RT or definitive RT
	3. ENE: primary chemoradiotherapy; if complete metabolic response is not achieved based on PET/CT at week 12, proceed to surgery
Multiple ipsilateral lymph nodes, none larger than 6 cm	Neck dissection followed by adjuvant RT or primary chemoradiotherapy followed by PET/CT after 12 weeks
Bilateral lymph nodes, none larger than 6 cm	Primary chemoradiotherapy followed by PET/CT after 12 weeks
Any lymph node greater than 6 cm	1. ENE present: primary chemoradiotherapy followed by PET/CT after 12 weeks
	2. No ENE present: surgery followed by RT

*Favorable risk factors: p16 positive, smoking history <10 pack-years, and no evidence of ENE.
†Lack of favorable risk factors.
ENE, extranodal extension; RT, radiation therapy.

In clinical practice, candidates for bilateral neck radiotherapy are patients with suspected primary tumors located close to the midline or those with extensive nodal disease putting the contralateral neck at increased risk for occult nodal metastases or with bilateral nodes. The advantage of bilateral radiotherapy must be weighed against the morbidity induced and the limitations of salvage surgery and reirradiation in case of recurrence or second primary (19). In the intensity-modulated radiation therapy (IMRT) era, bilateral neck irradiation carries a much lower risk of significant morbidity than conventional techniques, and therefore remains standard treatment for SCCUP.

CHEMORADIOTHERAPY

Systemic chemotherapy is generally employed in two settings, to intensify locoregional treatment for local control or for palliation of regionally advanced disease with or without systemic metastasis. Although chemotherapy as a single treatment modality may be reasonable for palliative therapy of patients with clear evidence of distant metastases at diagnosis, most patients with SCCUP, similar to other patients with locoregionally advanced head and neck SCC of known primary sites, can be treated with curative intent approaches to include chemoradiotherapy. However, current evidence for chemoradiotherapy in SCCUP patients is limited to retrospective series, as there are no large randomized prospective clinical trials evaluating the efficacy of chemotherapy in SCCUP. Additionally, most of these studies are small and did not differentiate between HPV-positive and HPV-negative disease, further limiting interpretation of results.

Shehadeh et al. (21) conducted a retrospective review of patients treated from 1995 to 2002 for SCCUP. Thirty-seven patients were treated with neck dissection, bilateral neck irradiation, and three cycles of concurrent high-dose cisplatin (at 100 mg/m^2 intravenously, every 3 weeks). With a median follow-up of 42 months among the survivors, very few patients had regional recurrence (5%) or distant failure (11%), and 89% of patients were alive. They concluded that the addition of concurrent cisplatin chemotherapy to adjuvant radiotherapy given after neck dissection results in high rates of regional disease control and may prolong survival.

Rödel et al. (22) reviewed the charts of 58 patients treated from 1986 to 2006. Thirteen of 22 patients (59%) with advanced nodal disease (N2b–N3, AJCC/UICC 7th Edition) treated initially by surgery and adjuvant radiotherapy developed distant metastases on follow-up, whereas this was the case in only 4 of 11 patients (36%) with advanced nodal disease treated initially by surgery and concurrent chemoradiotherapy. Neck dissection followed by chemoradiotherapy was associated with the best 3-year and 5-year locoregional control rates.

In contrast, Ligey and colleagues (23) retrospectively analyzed 95 patients with SCCUP who had undergone different combinations of neck dissection, radiotherapy, and chemotherapy. With a median follow-up of 3.3 years, the investigators observed no difference in locoregional control (p = .639) and no difference in survival (p = .493) when chemotherapy was added to the treatment plan. Chen et al. (24) reported a retrospective review of 60 patients with histologically proven SCCUP. Forty-five patients (75%) underwent surgery as the initial treatment. All patients received continuous-course external-beam radiation therapy delivered daily using conventional fractionation. Concurrent cisplatin-based chemotherapy was administered to 32 patients (53%). No advantage to overall survival, locoregional control, and progression-free survival was found in any subset of patients. A significant increase in grade 3 acute (59% vs. 25%) and late (47% vs. 14%) toxicity was associated with concurrent cisplatin (p value <.001, for both).

In the absence of high level of evidence data, current treatment guidelines (National Comprehensive Cancer Network [NCCN]) support the use of chemoradiotherapy for high-risk disease, either as primary therapy or in the postoperative setting, similar to that justified for locoregional disease of known primary site.

TREATMENT PRINCIPLES

1. If any concern for ECE exists, primary chemoradiotherapy should be administered, followed by a PET/CT at 12 weeks, and if positive, neck dissection should be undertaken.
2. Follow-up PET or CT scan should be performed after about 12 weeks of chemoradiotherapy, and if complete metabolic response has not been achieved, neck dissection should be considered.

Table 20.3 provides a summary of recommended treatment by extent of lymph node involvement.

CASE 20.1: HPV-NEGATIVE SCCUP

A 53-year-old man with history of hypertension, hyperlipidemia, more than 30 pack-years of smoking, and distant history of cocaine and inhaled heroin use, but no intravenous drug abuse presented with an enlarging right-sided neck mass over 1 month. Fiberoptic laryngoscopy did not reveal any abnormalities. He underwent FNA of the mass, pathological examination confirmed SCC, and p16 immunohistochemistry on the cell block was negative. FDG-PET and diagnostic CT imaging showed a 5.3 cm × 3.9 cm × 4.6 cm hypermetabolic right-sided neck mass inseparable from the sternocleidomastoid muscle (Figure 20.2), but no evidence of other hypermetabolic lymphadenopathy or other distant metastatic disease.

He underwent a right-sided tonsillectomy and multiple random biopsies of the oropharynx and nasopharynx, which were negative for carcinoma, and his tumor was staged as N2a disease by AJCC 7th Edition (though now N3b (ECS+) by 8th Edition staging, now in effect). He was treated with concurrent cisplatin-based chemoradiotherapy (receiving 70 Gy to right neck mass, 60 Gy to ipsilateral and retropharyngeal nodes at risk levels I to V, and 54 Gy to contralateral neck nodes) and subsequently underwent a posttherapy neck dissection with reconstruction at 8 weeks, for salvage of gross residual disease.

(continued)

CASE 20.1: HPV-NEGATIVE SCCUP (*continued*)

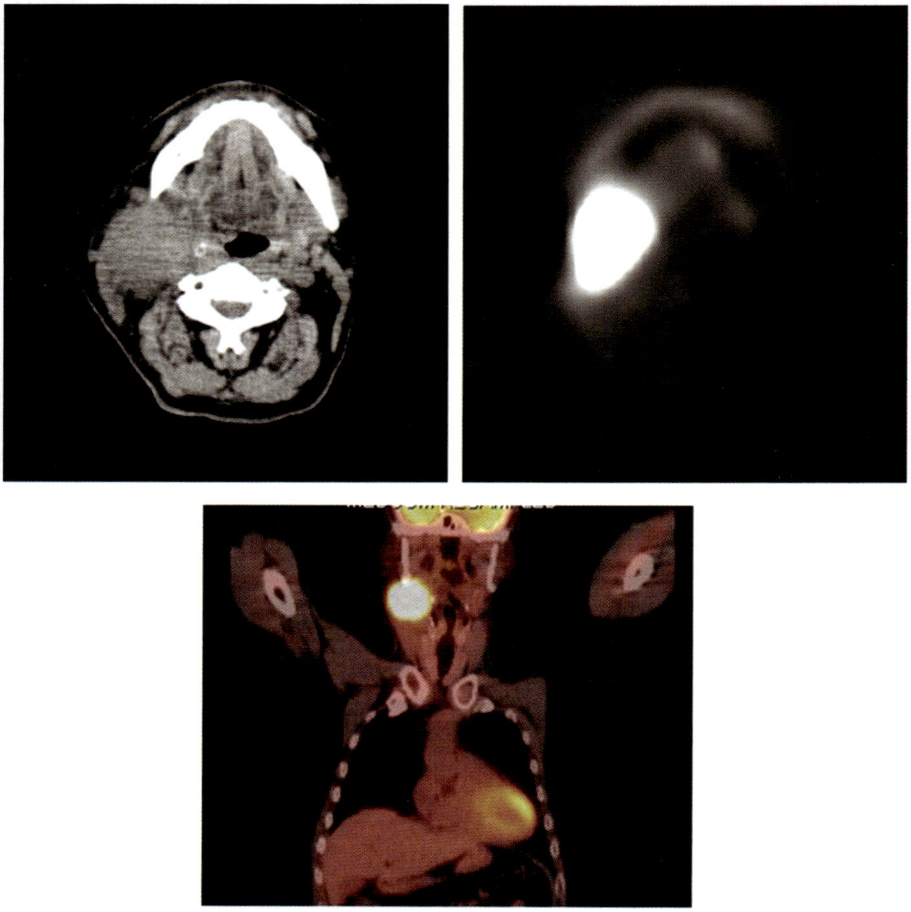

FIGURE 20.2 Diagnostic CT and FDG-PET imaging showing a 5.3 cm × 3.9 cm × 4.6 cm hypermetabolic right-sided neck mass inseparable from the sternocleidomastoid muscle.

SPECIFIC CONSIDERATIONS IN P16/HPV-POSITIVE DISEASE

EPIDEMIOLOGY AND OUTCOMES

Recently, there has been a paradigm shift in the epidemiology for head and neck cancer because of an increase in the incidence of HPV-associated SCC. A retrospective single-institutional study published in 2016 found that in recent years there has been an increasing incidence of SCCUP along with an increased proportion of patients with HPV-associated disease at a rate of 90% (8). Part of this phenomenon may be because of an increasing number of patients with HPV-positive oropharyngeal cancer who initially present as an unknown primary cancer, but have their primary tumor discovered at the time of tonsillectomy and/or tongue base biopsy/resection. However, even among those patients in whom a primary site is never identified despite an extensive workup, they are most likely to demonstrate HPV-positive disease in their lymph nodes and have a demographic profile similar to HPV-positive oropharyneal cancer (9).

HPV-positive SCCUP tends to have a better prognosis and increased disease-free survival than HPV-negative SCCUP, regardless of the extent of disease in the neck or mode of treatment (25). One retrospective study reports patients with HPV-positive SCCUP who were treated with a transoral approach plus or minus adjuvant radiotherapy had a 5-year disease-specific survival rate of 98% and overall survival rate of 97% when the primary was detected (n = 58) and a 100% 5-year overall survival rate when the primary was not detected (n = 7) (26). The strongest significant beneficial prognostic factor for patients with HPV-positive SCCUP is absence of ECE (9).

The 8th Edition AJCC/UICC staging system for head and neck cancers, now in effect, classifies p16 positive occult primary tumors as T0 oropharyngeal cancers. The reader is encouraged to refer to Chapter 13 for additional discussion on epidemiology, staging and treatment of HPV-associated oropharyngeal cancers.

IMAGING WORKUP CONSIDERATIONS

The advancement of contrast-enhanced CT imaging has increased the identification of the site of primary tumors not discovered on physical examination. A CT of the neck with contrast that demonstrates level II cystic nodes is highly consistent with HPV-positive disease. Although FDG-PET and PET/CT is standard in this setting, it has specific limitations in this context as well. As there is a strong physiologic background uptake of FDG in the oropharynx, especially in the palatine and lingual tonsillar region, it can obscure the discovery of a small primary in this location (27).

SURGICAL WORKUP CONSIDERATIONS

Diagnostic tonsillectomy should be performed over directed biopsy as a first step after a primary tumor for HPV-positive SCCUP, as the detection rate is tenfold higher (7). It is common for unilateral tonsillectomy when there is ipsilateral neck disease, and bilateral resection when there is bilateral neck disease. We recommend bilateral tonsillectomy regardless of extent of disease in the neck because of the possibility of bilateral disease either due to synchronous primaries or local spread (28–30). Furthermore, future interpretation of PET scans is facilitated owing to the loss of physiologic uptake of the tonsils. Studies with the aim of determining how often tonsillectomy leads to the discovery of the primary in initial SCCUP report rates of 29.6% and 39%; however, these cohorts are not exclusively p16 positive (7,31).

TRANSORAL LINGUAL TONSILLECTOMY

If the tonsils are negative for the primary tumor, it is overwhelmingly likely that the primary is in the base of tongue. Blind biopsying of the oropharynx is common procedure; however, the yield is limited. Some groups are performing lingual tonsillectomy (hemi or full) using TORS, a technique that can uncover primary tumors in the oropharynx via margin-negative resection with relatively low morbidity (32). Mehta et al. report that using the TORS technique uncovered 90% of primaries (mean diameter of 0.9 cm) in the base of the tongue after a negative diagnostic tonsillectomy (33). TORS could reduce the radiation dose to surrounding sites and may even justify elimination of radiotherapy in some cases. It is unknown if volume reductions due to TORS has significantly decreased toxicity rates. A recent study from Washington University employing TORS for 65 p16+ SCCUP patients was published with a primary detection rate of 89% (26). Forty-seven of those patients had subsequent adjuvant radiation with 36 sparing the primary site as the disease was resected with a negative margin. Five-year disease-specific survival rates were 98% in the detected group in and 100% in the undetected group. A review of transoral techniques reported an overall detection rate of 80% using transoral techniques, with a 72% rate of detection after lingual tonsillectomy when all other techniques failed to locate the primary. Hemorrhage (5%) was the most common adverse effect, with no deaths in 139 patients (17).

TREATMENT CONSIDERATIONS

In patients in whom the primary is eventually discovered, and it is no longer considered a cancer of unknown primary, follow normal algorithms for the known primary with a few notable exceptions.

1. In a patient managed with neck dissection who meets criteria for adjuvant radiation and the primary is discovered in the tonsil or base of tongue and resected with negative margins, the need for primary site radiotherapy is questionable. Similarly, even if the primary is only biopsied, the volume of treatment, which normally would have included the entire tongue base, may be

reduced. As discussed earlier, reduction of volumes after negative resection has not significantly affected survival rates (26).
2. Discovery of a primary lateralized tonsil cancer or a small base of tongue cancer far off the midline may raise the possibility of treating only the ipsilateral neck with radiotherapy if the extent of neck disease is limited. While this is controversial in the unknown primary setting, it may be more commonly pursued in a case of a known lateralized primary tumor.
3. If the primary is uncovered at the time of palatine ± lingual tonsillectomies and concurrent neck dissection, a patient with multiple known involved lymph nodes could be treated with adjuvant radiotherapy alone without the use of chemotherapy in the absence of ECE.
4. For patients with obvious clinical extranodal extension at presentation, the benefit of upfront neck dissection is limited as it leads to trimodality therapy with an associated increase in cost and morbidity as compared to primary chemoradiotherapy.

In patients with HPV-associated SCCUP in whom the primary tumor is never discovered despite extensive workup as detailed earlier, several important principles guide treatment.

1. Typically, after removal of both palatine tonsils, only the tongue base is targeted in most cases. Controversy exists regarding whether the nasopharynx should also be targeted as a potential mucosal primary site as p16-positive nasopharyngeal cancer is becoming a more commonly recognized entity (12). Some counter that even when the treatment of the nasopharynx is omitted, the nasopharynx receives incidental dose of around 50 Gy due to the coverage of the lateral pharyngeal nodes in the elective nodal volume, which may be sufficient in HPV-positive disease.
2. Because HPV-positive SCCUP behaves very similar to HPV-positive oropharyngeal cancer, levels II to IV and ipsilateral lateral pharyngeal nodes should be targeted in all patients, while level IB and V nodes can often be spared in the absence of multilevel nodal disease due to low risk of involvement (34). There may also be a benefit in avoiding coverage of the contralateral pharyngeal nodes in cases with clinically uninvolved contralateral neck nodes, although this may be a concern in an unknown primary setting knowing the nasopharynx is a potential primary site (35).
3. Consideration can be given to ipsilateral neck radiation only in patients with limited nodal involvement. While this is not currently the commonly accepted practice, several retrospective series have reported contralateral failures of <10% when the contralateral neck was spared in this context (4,36,37).
4. The dose to the putative mucosal sites being targeted with radiation varies across institutions. Some argue 50 to 54 Gy to be sufficient for microscopic disease, while others continue to use the historical standard of 60 Gy (4).
5. Patients with limited nodal involvement (AJCC 7th Edition N1-N2b disease) and a modest smoking history and patients with known T1-T3 primary tumors are currently being enrolled in the NRG HN-002 phase II randomized de-intensification study investigating reduced-dose chemoradiation versus reduced-dose accelerated radiation alone. One could argue that patients with p16-positive SCCUP who otherwise fit these criteria can be considered for treatment de-intensification as well in future studies, although this is not currently an acceptable standard option.

CONCLUSIONS

In the era of sensitive and specific PET/CT imaging, HNCUP diagnoses are relatively rare but remain challenging for patients and the treatment team. Although this cancer can often be highly curable (particularly for HPV-associated SCCUP), smoking cessation, supportive care, and survivorship are important areas of patient care (4,38). Efforts to identify the suspected primary tumor site are critical to direct appropriate cancer therapy and avoid toxicity associated with overtreatment.

To that end, advances in molecular testing for identification of primary tumor site and for risk stratification are eagerly anticipated. HPV testing of suspected SCC in current routine clinical use may indeed suggest occult oropharyngeal primaries and favorable prognoses, but may be limited by known frequent p16 staining of skin and some nasopharyngeal primaries. EBV is indicative of nasopharyngeal primary cancers. Although commercially available genetic tests

CASE 20.2: HPV-POSITIVE SCCUP

A 49-year-old Caucasian man with a 5 pack-year smoking history presented with a 3-week history of right cervical lymphadenopathy. He was treated with antibiotics by his primary care physician (PCP) without improvement. CT neck was obtained, which demonstrated a multilobulated cystic level II/III right-sided enlarged lymph node measuring 4.7 × 2.7 × 1.4 cm and another 1 × 1 cm right-sided level III lymph node (Figure 20.3A). No obvious primary was appreciated. FNA of the neck revealed atypical cells suspicious for carcinoma. PET/CT confirmed these areas of uptake without an obvious primary site or distant metastases. The patient was taken for an examination under anesthesia. Tonsillectomy and blind biopsies of the lingual tonsils were negative. A right-sided selective neck dissection (levels IB–IV) was completed. Pathological report revealed p16-positive SCC in a level II and in a level III lymph node, and 2 of 39 lymph nodes were involved without ECE. His nodal disease was classified as N2b per 7th Edition AJCC staging, though tumor would be pT0N1M0 (stage group I) according to the current 8th Edition staging for p16 positive oropharyngeal cancer. He received adjuvant radiotherapy to 60 Gy in 30 fractions to his right neck (levels IB–V) and base of tongue and 56 Gy in 30 fractions to the left levels II to IV electively (Figure 20.3B). More than 3 years after therapy, he is disease free with only grade 1 xerostomia.

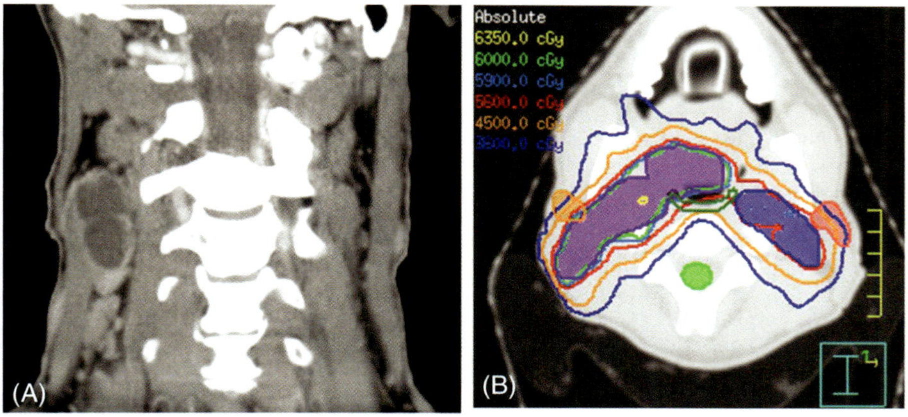

FIGURE 20.3 (A) CT neck demonstrating a multilobulated cystic level II/III right-sided lymph node measuring 4.7 × 2.7× 1.4 cm and a 1 × 1 cm right-sided level III lymph node. (B) Postoperative radiotherapy plan -60 Gy to the right neck (levels IB–V) and base of tongue and 56 Gy to the left levels II to IV

may offer assistance with identification of the primary tumor of origin in unknown primary cancers, limited data on such technologies is available, and current tests preclude differentiation of SCC from various systemic sites (i.e., head and neck vs. lung vs. cervical primaries); differentiation of nodal metastases from separate head and neck mucosal sites will require much additional research.

Specific molecular and microenvironment characteristics of tumors may also contribute to future treatment approaches. Next-generation sequencing technologies have already resulted in new biological understanding and newly approved therapies for a growing number of advanced malignancies and may influence future curative treatment paradigms. Although patients with SCC are yet to reap clear benefit from genetic approaches, the era of immunotherapy (with recently approved agents) is expected to revolutionize head and neck cancer care. The unique biology of HNCUP, namely, occult primaries with enhanced metastatic potential resulting in clinical evidence of cervical node involvement, is certainly of great scientific and clinical interest.

Most current clinical recommendations for management of HNCUP are based on expert consensus. This lack of high-level evidence-based treatment recommendations for HNCUP results from a paucity of clinical trials and a lack of ability to complete accrual to trials focused on this patient population. Furthermore, most phase III trials in the head and neck cancer literature exclude patients with unknown primaries. Given the rarity of this diagnosis and underrepresentation in studies, generating appropriate consensus on highly relevant clinical and scientific questions will be critical for future trial attempts for patients with HNCUP.

REFERENCES

1. Syrjänen S. Human papillomaviruses in head and neck carcinomas. *N Engl J Med*. 2007;356(19):1993–1995. doi:10.1056/NEJMe078004
2. Moor JW, Murray P, Inwood J. Diagnostic biopsy of lymph nodes of the neck, axilla and groin: rhyme, reason or chance? *Ann R Coll Surg Engl*. 2008;90(3):221–225.
3. Lopez F, Rodrigo JP, Silver CE, et al. Cervical lymph node metastases from remote primary tumor sites. *Head Neck*. 2016;38(Suppl 1):E2374–E2385.
4. Galloway TJ, Ridge JA. Management of squamous cancer metastatic to cervical nodes with an unknown primary site. *J Clin Oncol*. 2015;33(29):3328–3337.
5. Mendenhall WM, Mancuso AA, Amdur RJ, et al. Squamous cell carcinoma metastatic to the neck from an unknown head and neck primary site. *Am J Otolaryngol*. 2001;22(4):261–267.
6. Lapeyre M, Malissard L, Peiffert D, et al. Cervical lymph node metastasis from an unknown primary: is a tonsillectomy necessary? *Int J Radiat Oncol Biol Phys*. 1997;39(2):291–296.
7. Waltonen JD, Ozer E, Schuller DE, Agrawal A. Tonsillectomy vs. deep tonsil biopsies in detecting occult tonsil tumors. *Laryngoscope*. 2009;119(1):102–106.
8. Motz K, Qualliotine JR, Rettig E, et al. Changes in unknown primary squamous cell carcinoma of the head and neck at initial presentation in the era of human papillomavirus. *JAMA Otolaryngol Head Neck Surg*. 2016;142(3):223–228.
9. Keller LM, Galloway TJ, Holdbrook T, et al. p16 status, pathologic and clinical characteristics, biomolecular signature, and long-term outcomes in head and neck squamous cell carcinomas of unknown primary. *Head Neck*. 2014;36(12):1677–1684.
10. Bishop JA, Lewis JS Jr, Rocco JW, Faquin WC. HPV-related squamous cell carcinoma of the head and neck: an update on testing in routine pathology practice. *Semin Diagn Pathol*. 2015;32(5):344–351.
11. Shah KS,Ethunandan M. Tumour seeding after fine-needle aspiration and core biopsy of the head and neck–a systematic review. *Br J Oral Maxillofac Surg*. 2016;54(3):260–265.
12. Stenmark MH, McHugh JB, Schipper M, et al. Nonendemic HPV-positive nasopharyngeal carcinoma: association with poor prognosis. *Int J Radiat Oncol Biol Phys*. 2014;88(3):580–588.
13. McDowell LJ, Young RJ, Johnston ML, et al. p16-positive lymph node metastases from cutaneous head and neck squamous cell carcinoma: no association with high-risk human papillomavirus or prognosis and implications for the workup of the unknown primary. *Cancer*. 2016;122(8):1201–1208.
14. Rudmik L, Lau HY, Matthews TW, et al. Clinical utility of PET/CT in the evaluation of head and neck squamous cell carcinoma with an unknown primary: a prospective clinical trial. *Head Neck*. 2011;33(7):935–940.
15. Keller F, Psychogios G, Linke R, et al. Carcinoma of unknown primary in the head and neck: comparison between positron emission tomography (PET) and PET/CT. *Head Neck*. 2011;33(11):1569–1575.
16. Strojan P, Ferlito A, Medina JE, et al. Contemporary management of lymph node metastases from an unknown primary to the neck: I. A review of diagnostic approaches. *Head Neck*. 2013;35(1):123–132.
17. Fu TS, Foreman A, Goldstein, DP, et al. The role of transoral robotic surgery, transoral laser microsurgery, and lingual tonsillectomy in the identification of head and neck squamous cell carcinoma of unknown primary origin: a systematic review. *J Otolaryngol Head Neck Surg*. 2016;45(1):28.
18. Kang SY, Dziegielewski PT, Old MO, Ozer E. Transoral robotic surgery for carcinoma of unknown primary in the head and neck. *J Surg Oncol*. 2015;112(7):697–701.
19. Strojan P, Ferlito A, Langendijk JA, et al. Contemporary management of lymph node metastases from an unknown primary to the neck: II. a review of therapeutic options. *Head Neck*. 2013;35(2):286–293.
20. Nieder C, Gregoire V, Ang KK. Cervical lymph node metastases from occult squamous cell carcinoma: cut down a tree to get an apple? *Int J Radiat Oncol Biol Phys*. 2001;50(3):727–733.
21. Shehadeh NJ, Ensley JF, Kucuk O, et al. Benefit of postoperative chemoradiotherapy for patients with unknown primary squamous cell carcinoma of the head and neck. *Head Neck*. 2006;28(12):1090–1098.
22. Rodel RM, Matthias C, Blomeyer BD, et al. Impact of distant metastasis in patients with cervical lymph node metastases from cancer of an unknown primary site. *Ann Otol Rhinol Laryngol*. 2009;118(9):662–669.
23. Ligey A, Gentil J, Créhange G, et al. Impact of target volumes and radiation technique on loco-regional control and survival for patients with unilateral cervical lymph node metastases from an unknown primary. *Radiother Oncol*. 2009;93(3):483–487.

24. Chen AM, Farwell DG, Lau DH, et al. Radiation therapy in the management of head-and-neck cancer of unknown primary origin: how does the addition of concurrent chemotherapy affect the therapeutic ratio? *Int J Radiat Oncol Biol Phys*. 2011;81(2):346–352.
25. Dixon PR, Au M, Hosni A, et al. Impact of p16 expression, nodal status, and smoking on oncologic outcomes of patients with head and neck unknown primary squamous cell carcinoma. *Head Neck*. 2016;38(9):1347–1353.
26. Graboyes EM, Sinha P, Thorstad WL, et al. Management of human papillomavirus-related unknown primaries of the head and neck with a transoral surgical approach. *Head Neck*. 2015;37(11):1603–1611.
27. Rusthoven KE, Koshy M, Paulino AC. The role of fluorodeoxyglucose positron emission tomography in cervical lymph node metastases from an unknown primary tumor. *Cancer*. 2004;101(11):2641–2649.
28. Koch WM, Bhatti N, Williams MF, Eisele DW. Oncologic rationale for bilateral tonsillectomy in head and neck squamous cell carcinoma of unknown primary source. *Otolaryngol Head Neck Surg*. 2001;124(3):331–333.
29. Mackenzie K, Watson M, Jankowska P, et al. Investigation and management of the unknown primary with metastatic neck disease: United Kingdom National Multidisciplinary Guidelines. *J Laryngol Otol*. 2016;130(S2):S170–S175.
30. Rasband-Lindquist A, Shnayder Y, O'Neil M. Synchronous bilateral tonsillar squamous cell carcinoma related to human papillomavirus: two case reports and a brief review of the literature. *Ear Nose Throat J*. 2016;95(4–5):E30–E34.
31. Tanzler ED, Amdur RJ, Morris CG, et al. Challenging the need for random directed biopsies of the nasopharynx, pyriform sinus, and contralateral tonsil in the workup of unknown primary squamous cell carcinoma of the head and neck. *Head Neck*. 2016;38(4):578–581.
32. Chia SH, Gross ND, Richmon JD. Surgeon experience and complications with Transoral Robotic Surgery (TORS). *Otolaryngol Head Neck Surg*. 2013;149(6):885–892.
33. Mehta V, Johnson P, Tassler A, et al. A new paradigm for the diagnosis and management of unknown primary tumors of the head and neck: a role for transoral robotic surgery. *Laryngoscope*. 2013;123(1):146–151.
34. Sanguineti G, Califano J, Stafford E, et al. Defining the risk of involvement for each neck nodal level in patients with early T-stage node-positive oropharyngeal carcinoma. *Int J Radiat Oncol Biol Phys*. 2009;74(5):1356–1364.
35. Spencer CR, Gay HA, Haughey BH. Eliminating radiotherapy to the contralateral retropharyngeal and high level II lymph nodes in head and neck squamous cell carcinoma is safe and improves quality of life. *Cancer*. 2014;120(24):3994–4002.
36. Fakhrian K, Thamm R, Knapp S, et al. Radio(chemo) therapy in the management of squamous cell carcinoma of cervical lymph nodes from an unknown primary site. A retrospective analysis. *Strahlenther Onkol*. 2012;188(1):56–61.
37. Cuaron J, Rao S, Wolden S, et al. Patterns of failure in patients with head and neck carcinoma of unknown primary treated with radiation therapy. *Head Neck*. 2016;38(Suppl 1):E426–E431.
38. Rischin D, Ferris RL, Le QT. Overview of advances in head and neck cancer. *J Clin Oncol*. 2015;33(29):3225–3226.

21

Salivary Gland Malignancies

Cristina P. Rodriguez
Jessica L. Geiger
Jon Mallen-St. Clair
Patrick K. Ha
Sue S. Yom
Adam S. Garden
David J. Adelstein

EPIDEMIOLOGY AND HISTOLOGY

Salivary gland malignancies are a diverse group of neoplasms that arise from the secretory acinus and myoepithelial components of the paired major (parotid, sublingual, and submandibular) salivary glands and minor salivary glands located throughout the upper aerodigestive mucosa. Salivary gland cancers comprise approximately 6% of malignancies arising from the head and neck, and occur at an estimated rate of 3,000 cases annually in the United States (1). The median age at diagnosis of malignant salivary gland tumors is 60 years of age, with no apparent gender predisposition. Approximately 80% of salivary gland tumors arise from the parotid gland, and approximately 20% of them are malignant. In contrast, the proportion of malignant to benign tumors is significantly higher in the submandibular, sublingual, and minor salivary glands. The inherent infrequency and heterogeneity of this disease entity have posed challenges in the generation of prospective data and interpreting published literature. Similarly, causative risk factors have been difficult to establish, although a possible association between radiation exposure and the development of both benign and malignant salivary gland tumors has been suggested by observational studies (2,3).

The World Health Organization (WHO) classification includes 24 salivary gland cancer subtypes (Table 21.1) (4). Based on large series, the most frequently occurring subtypes are adenoid cystic carcinomas, mucoepidermoid carcinomas, and adenocarcinomas (5). Although squamous cell carcinomas (SCCs) of the parotid gland are included in this classification, the absence of squamous mucosa in salivary glands suggests that these most likely represent intraparotid nodal metastasis from cutaneous SCC. Specific salivary gland cancer subtypes are characterized by frequent immunohistochemical overexpression of specific molecular markers such as c-kit (adenoid cystic carcinomas), epidermal growth factor receptor (EGFR), Her-2 (salivary duct carcinoma), and androgen and estrogen receptors. These molecular markers represent potential therapeutic targets, and the clinical experience with targeted agents is discussed in the section on Targeted Therapy in Salivary Gland Malignancies of this chapter.

Salivary gland cancers are characterized by a broad spectrum of biologic behavior. Certain

TABLE 21.1

2005 World Health Organization (WHO) Malignant Salivary Gland Tumors

Acinic cell carcinoma
Mucoepidermoid carcinoma
Adenoid cystic carcinoma
Polymorphous low-grade adenocarcinoma
Epithelial-myoepithelial carcinoma
Clear cell carcinoma, not otherwise specified
Basal cell adenocarcinoma
Sebaceous carcinoma
Sebaceous lymphadenocarcinoma
Cystadenocarcinoma
Low-grade cribriform cystadenocarcinoma
Mucinous adenocarcinoma
Oncocytic carcinoma
Salivary duct carcinoma
Salivary duct carcinoma, not otherwise specified
Adenocarcinoma, not otherwise specified
Myoepithelial carcinoma
Carcinoma ex pleomorphic adenoma
Carcinosarcoma
Metastasizing pleomorphic adenoma
Squamous cell carcinoma
Large cell carcinoma
Lymphoepithelial carcinoma
Sialoblastoma

subsets demonstrate indolent growth, yet are progressive, as exemplified by adenoid cystic carcinomas; while others, such as salivary duct carcinoma, may be fulminating. The identification of distant metastases years after curative intent resection is a frequently described phenomenon in patients with adenoid cystic carcinomas. Consequently, there is relative insensitivity of this subset to traditional cytotoxic agents. A predictive histologic grading system exists for adenoid cystic carcinomas in which high-grade tumors characterized by a 30% or greater solid growth pattern (vs. cribriform) are associated with more aggressive disease biology and inferior survival outcomes (6). A similar grading system is used among adenocarcinomas and mucoepidermoid carcinomas, wherein higher histologic grade and differentiation can predict for more aggressive disease biology and adverse outcomes (7).

Advances in molecular profiling have led to insights into the mutational landscape of these tumors, as well as the identification of distinct subtypes not included in the current WHO classification. As an example, mammary analogue secretory carcinoma, a recently recognized salivary gland malignancy, is characterized by an *ETV6-NTRK3* fusion oncogene (8). Among adenoid cystic carcinomas, a balanced translocation between *MYB* and *NFIB* is frequently observed and is associated with higher rates of disease recurrence (9). In mucoepidermoid carcinomas, the t(11;19)(q21;p13) translocation resulting in a *MECT1-MAML2* fusion gene has been observed among lower grade tumors with more favorable prognosis (10).

DIAGNOSIS AND STAGING

The clinical presentation of a salivary gland malignancy is typically characterized by symptoms related to tumor invasion of surrounding structures; these findings can include a slowly or rapidly growing mass, pain, paresthesias or hyperesthesias, or facial weakness. Similarly, physical examination findings of motor weakness in the facial nerve distribution, cervical lymphadenopathy, and trismus should raise the clinical suspicion for malignancy and lead to tissue sampling. Histologic confirmation of a suspected salivary gland neoplasm is often obtained either intraoperatively or preoperatively with an in-office fine-needle aspiration, a well-established diagnostic procedure for major salivary gland tumors (11,12). It must be emphasized that histopathologic interpretation can be challenging in view of the morphologic diversity and rarity of these tumors as well as overlapping histologic staining with other epithelial malignancies. Therefore, independent review of ambiguous cases by a high-volume center with head and neck pathologic expertise may be necessary in certain cases.

Contrast-enhanced CT and MRI are the most frequently used modalities for staging the extent of the primary tumor and identifying clinically involved lymph nodes (13). Radiographic characteristics of a malignant salivary gland process include contrast enhancement, necrosis, bony invasion, and perineural spread. Salivary gland cancers arising from the paired parotid, sublingual, and submandibular glands are staged according to the American Joint Committee on Cancer (AJCC) version 8 staging system for major salivary glands (14). Those that arise from minor salivary glands are staged according to the AJCC staging system for the primary site of origin. Apart from prognostic information, staging provides valuable information on the extent of the primary tumor and involvement of cervical lymph nodes, which influences the resectability of these tumors.

PRINCIPLES OF SURGICAL MANAGEMENT

MANAGEMENT OF THE PRIMARY SITE AND NECK

Treatment recommendations regarding the surgical management of salivary gland tumors are almost entirely based on retrospective reviews. Most clinical guidelines have been established for parotid tumors, reflecting the higher prevalence of disease in this subsite. The cornerstone of treatment of these tumors is the complete removal of the mass with a cuff of normal tissue to obtain a negative margin, where possible, while maintaining the integrity of the facial nerve if not directly involved. This may involve peeling tumor off the facial nerve that is not invaded with the goal of a gross total resection. The extent of resection is determined by multiple tumor-specific factors including the biology of the tumor; the size, location, and relationship to the facial nerve; and invasion into local structures.

Surgical management of benign parotid neoplasms typically involves excision of the tumor including a cuff of normal tissue after identification and preservation of the facial nerve. When the tumor is located in the superficial lobe, this is accomplished with a superficial parotidectomy (15). If the tumor is located deep to the facial nerve, a total parotidectomy is performed with preservation of the facial nerve (16). All attempts to preserve the facial nerve should be attempted in the treatment of benign tumors.

Traditional surgical management of malignant parotid tumors depends on histologic differentiation, location, and size of the primary lesion. Similar to the management of benign masses, the surgical management of parotid malignancy also involves complete tumor resection with removal of a cuff of normal parotid tissue. Low-grade tumors confined to the superficial lobe of the parotid can be treated with a superficial parotidectomy. High-grade tumors are typically managed with a total parotidectomy with facial nerve preservation. However, select high-grade tumors located in the peripheral parotid can be treated with a superficial parotidectomy (5,17,18). T4 tumors that are invading adjacent structures may require resection of involved muscle, skin, or bone (mandible, zygoma, temporal bone). Reconstruction of these defects typically requires free tissue transfer. These patients are treated with postoperative radiation (19–21).

Facial nerve preservation is advocated when the nerve is functional prior to surgery. When necessary, because of proximity of the tumor to the facial nerve, dissection of a facial nerve branch off the tumor without a true cuff of normal tissue is typically performed. There have been reports that selective facial nerve sacrifice may improve local control and survival, with trends toward decreased quality of life (22), so one must balance these competing interests. In the event of a nonfunctional facial nerve preoperatively, or a nerve that is grossly invaded by tumor, resection of the facial nerve is recommended until it is cleared on frozen section. With malignant parotid tumors, facial nerve function is compromised in approximately 20% of patients on presentation (23). In cases of facial nerve sacrifice, immediate reconstruction using a cable graft of a cervical sensory nerve or the sural nerve is advocated (24,25).

The surgical management of submandibular salivary tumors is similar to those of the parotid gland. Approximately 50% of tumors within the submandibular gland are malignant. Benign lesions are removed with preservation of the nerves of importance in this region including the marginal mandibular branch of the facial nerve, the lingual nerve, and the hypoglossal nerve. Malignant tumors are removed en bloc with the affected glands, and, again, efforts are made to preserve the nerves in this region unless they are encased or directly involved with tumor (26).

The vast majority of sublingual gland tumors are malignant. The surgical management of these tumors typically involves resection of the involved gland, the floor of mouth, and the submandibular gland (27). In the event that invasion of the adjacent mandible or the lingual nerve is seen, the resection should include these structures.

Tumors of the minor salivary glands are mostly malignant and rare. The majority of these glands are located within the oral cavity, with a preponderance on the hard palate. Tumors that arise in these glands are typically managed surgically with a resection to include adequate margins.

Clinical or radiographic evidence of cervical lymph node involvement is managed by a neck dissection typically followed by postoperative radiotherapy (28). The neck dissection should include levels II and III at a minimum and I, IV, and V, if necessary. The majority of patients with parotid malignancy (~80%) do not present with nodal metastasis, and the role of elective neck dissection (ELND) in the N0 neck in parotid malignancy has been debated, especially when postoperative radiation therapy (PORT) is planned (29–31). A large meta-analysis was recently performed that established the presence of pathologic nodes in 23% of ELND (32), though this likely is related to the size and histology of the primary tumor. Treatment of the neck is therefore indicated with either selective neck dissection or radiation, resulting in a low rate of neck recurrence (5%) in these patients.

RESECTION OF METASTATIC SITES

The incidence of distant metastasis in salivary gland cancer upon presentation is relatively low. When distant metastasis does occur, it portends a poor prognosis with a median survival of 4 to 7 months (33). Risk factors for the ultimate development of distant metastasis are a histologic diagnosis of adenoid cystic carcinoma, salivary duct carcinoma, or high-grade mucoepidermoid carcinoma. Tumors that originate in the submandibular gland are also associated with an increased risk of distant metastasis. Salivary duct carcinoma may spread early both to lymph nodes and distant sites. In contrast, adenoid cystic carcinoma of the salivary gland is characterized by slow growth, locoregional recurrence and late distant metastasis, and a natural history that may span decades (34). Approximately 50% of patients develop distant metastatic disease, and the lung is the most frequent site (35–37). Lung metastasis is associated with relatively long survival when compared to other sites of distant metastasis (36). Given the indolent natural history and limited benefit of palliative chemotherapy to metastatic subsites (38), resection of adenoid cystic carcinoma pulmonary metastasis has been recently reviewed in retrospective studies (39,40). Though the overall effect on survival is unclear, in patients in which an R0 resection is feasible, there is an association with improved disease-free interval (39). Given the lack of effective systemic treatment for metastatic adenoid cystic carcinomas, the retrospective data supports lung metastasectomy using strict criteria including complete resectability of the metastatic lesion, adequate performance status, control of primary tumor, and absence of additional metastatic disease. In addition to pulmonary metastasectomy, the role of hepatic metastasectomy has been reported (41). Though our data regarding the role of metastasectomy in salivary gland cancer is limited to small case series, early evidence suggest it may be beneficial in well-defined clinical contexts.

PRINCIPLES OF RADIATION THERAPY (RT)

Definitive RT is not effective for most salivary cancers; thus, there are three principal roles of radiation in the management of salivary gland tumors: (a) adjuvant (postoperative) treatment to increase the probability of long-term locoregional control, for which it is very effective, (b) definitive treatment, in the uncommon scenario of unresectable disease, and (c) palliative treatment, typically for symptom control of disease at uncontrolled primary or metastatic sites. As the usual initial treatment of salivary gland tumors is surgery, in particular for neoplasms that present without distant metastatic disease, postoperative treatment is the most common scenario in which RT is deployed for these diseases.

RADIATION IN THE POSTOPERATIVE SETTING

Following surgery, the operative and pathologic findings are reviewed to determine if adjuvant radiation is necessary. Although the use of radiation for benign disease is a controversial issue in general, even patients with benign tumors may benefit from improved locoregional control with adjuvant radiation (42). For benign pleomorphic adenomas (BPAs), radiation is indicated in cases of recurrent tumors, particularly after "spillage" with multifocal or multicentric disease in patients not eligible for additional surgical salvage. Adjuvant radiation is rarely recommended for a resected BPA if it is a first occurrence, even in the setting of positive margins. The gains of radiation for benign disease should be balanced against the practicality of future repeat surgery, potential future risk to the facial nerve, and the age and expected disease course of the patient. There is a very small risk that over a very long disease course, BPA may metastasize or transform to a more aggressive carcinoma, but this is rare (1%).

For salivary gland carcinomas, the indications for recommending adjuvant radiation are quite broad, especially for locoregionally advanced disease, as there are significant long-term disease control benefits that accrue from the combination of surgery and RT.

The indications for postoperative radiation for salivary gland malignancies include:

1. T3/T4 disease
2. Positive or close resection margins
3. Extraglandular extension, particularly if this includes invasion of adjacent structures
4. High-grade histologic type
5. Perineural invasion, especially if it is clinically or radiographically present
6. Nodal involvement, especially if there is extranodal extension

While not an absolute indication, radiation is almost always recommended for adenoid cystic carcinomas arising in the major salivary glands. The locally infiltrative nature and neurotropism, including skip lesions, of this entity makes it likely that residual microscopic disease is present following resection even in the absence of traditional indications for PORT.

The design of the treatment volume to be targeted postoperatively with radiation will depend on the specific clinical, surgical, and pathologic aspects of the case. The tumor and operative bed will always be included as the highest priority. However, the selection of subclinical sites to be targeted will vary depending on the specific scenario. For high-grade tumors or tumors that have spread to cervical lymphatics, the ipsilateral neck will be treated (29,43,44). In the setting of a major salivary gland tumor, contralateral neck nodal metastases are rare; so with rare exceptions, only the side of the neck in which the tumor appeared will be treated.

As some salivary gland tumors have a propensity for perineural invasion, in particular adenoid cystic carcinoma, the specific nerves at risk from a tumor will be included in a radiation treatment plan whether or not perineural invasion is detected. The extent of nerve coverage to the skull base (and beyond, in some cases) is determined by the extent of perineural invasion, whether it is focal or extensive or clinically manifest, and whether large-caliber nerves or properly named nerves are involved. Thus, in parotid cancers without perineural invasion, the nerve is tracked at least to the stylomastoid foramen, whereas, for parotid cancers with extensive or clinically evident perineural involvement, the path of the facial nerve through the stylomastoid foramen to the geniculate ganglion is traced and will be given at least a subclinical dose. Preoperative MRI evaluation of the facial nerve is important; if portions in the temporal bone are abnormal, a temporal bone surgical procedure is indicated. Less frequently the auriculotemporal nerve can be involved, necessitating coverage of the cranial nerve (CN) V pathway. The lingual nerve, a branch of CN V3 (the mandibular nerve), and CN XII (the hypoglossal nerve) both course adjacent to the submandibular gland, and their respective pathways should be encompassed in the radiated area if perineural disease is found in a malignancy of the submandibular gland. Decisions about which nerves should be included when perineural spread is found in a minor salivary gland cancer depend on the specific anatomic location of the tumor.

Radiation techniques vary and are dependent both on the tools available to the oncologist and the site of disease. The ultimate goal of radiation is to treat the tissues suspected of harboring microscopic disease, while avoiding normal tissues that are not at risk. Techniques to accomplish a greater conformality of RT have evolved and continue to evolve. These techniques often involve a mix of photon radiation beams delivered at varying rotational angles, to distribute lower doses of radiation to surrounding nontargeted tissues, while delivering a desired high dose of accumulated radiation to the central targets. The evolution of these approaches began with a single en face x-ray or electron beam, progressing to mixed x-ray and electron beams to the current state of the art intensity-modulated radiation therapy (IMRT) for deeper tumors not eligible for mixed beam .

Electron therapy is sometimes used to treat salivary gland cancers. Depending on the energy (penetrating depth) of the electrons used, the radiation delivered with electrons has a fairly well defined range, with little radiation delivered beyond the range, resulting in a highly conformal dose distribution. High-energy electron beam skin dose is high, and the subsequent radiation dermatitis may be severe, so most often a “mixed beam” technique is used with 80% electrons and 20% x-rays. Thus, for parotid and submandibular cancers that are close to the surface, electron beam can be very appealing. When there is a free flap requiring radiation treatment to depths greater than can be reached by electrons, when nerve tracks require coverage, or if the skull base needs to be targeted, electrons may not be appropriate, so IMRT or proton techniques are used.

Radiation doses recommended for postoperative therapy have been principally based on empiric and retrospective data. The tumor bed is typically prescribed a dose of 60 Gy, the operative bed 56 to 57 Gy, and subclinical sites that have not been violated 50 to 54 Gy. In postoperative cases in which margins are positive, the area of concern is frequently boosted by an additional 6 Gy to a total dose of 66 Gy. Fractionation is usually conventional, that is, at 1.8 to 2.0 Gy per fraction (the latter given to the highest dose volume), with one fraction given daily for 5 days per week for 6 weeks; additional variations ensue if a boost is added. For an integrated IMRT plan, this means target volumes of 60, 57, and 54 Gy in 30 fractions that receive daily doses of 2, 1.9, and 1.8 Gy, respectively.

Treatment recommendations regarding the role of adjuvant radiation in the management of salivary gland tumors, similar to those governing the role of surgery, are almost entirely based on retrospective case series (45–49). Many of these single-institution retrospective series have demonstrated very high rates of local and regional control in patients treated with surgery and adjuvant radiation. Some are globally descriptive, while others are more specific for a narrower group of patients based either on the gland type (parotid, submandibular, or minor) or histologic characteristics. These studies are of two basic types; either they demonstrate very high control rates for relatively large patient cohorts treated with surgery and radiation, or they are comparative, demonstrating that a group of patients treated with radiation had improved disease control compared to a group treated with surgery only.

The use of combined chemoradiation is recommended for squamous cell cancers of the head and neck demonstrating "high-risk" features identified on pathologic examination (such as positive margins or extranodal extension), supported by the results of studies by Radiation Therapy Oncology Group (RTOG 9501) and European Organisation for Research and Treatment of Cancer (EORTC 22951). However, the utility of adding concurrent chemotherapy to adjuvant radiation in the postoperative setting for aggressive primary salivary gland malignancies is unknown. The literature is sparse and conflicted on this topic (50–52). A phase 2 cooperative group trial is ongoing and has recently been expanded into a phase 3 study, but as the results are not anticipated to be available for years, the role of concurrent therapy remains unclear at this time.

RADIATION FOR UNRESECTABLE OR MEDICALLY INOPERABLE DISEASE

It is uncommon to encounter a patient with salivary gland cancer who has technical or medical reasons for inoperability, and inoperability is most common with skull base adenoid cystic carcinomas that are not technically resectable with acceptable morbidity. In the absence of the ability to operate, radiation is often chosen by default. Small series have demonstrated some limited success in long-term disease control for patients treated with radiation (53,54), although the results are clearly inferior to those obtained in patients who are able to undergo initial surgical resection.

The principles of definitive-intent radiation, with regard to technique, target volumes, and dose, are fairly similar to those described for the postoperative setting. The tumor bed or gross target volume (GTV) is identified from clinical and radiologic findings. An additional margin is added to encompass potential clinical extension beyond what is appreciated on imaging (to form the clinical target volume, or CTV), and a further margin is based on the inaccuracies inherent in radiation delivery such as slight day-to-day patient positioning changes (to form the planning target volume, or PTV). When the gross tumor remains in situ, a full definitive dose, 70 Gy, is used.

Although concurrent chemoradiation is a standard of care in locally advanced SCC of the head and neck, with improved locoregional control and overall survival advantages over RT alone, the utility of concurrent chemoradiation in unresectable salivary gland cancer has not been studied prospectively. One small retrospective experience suggests this approach is feasible, with improved results as compared to historical RT-alone results, but the follow-up time is short (55). Given that RT alone has poor control for gross salivary cancer, a combined chemoradiation approach is often considered for those who can tolerate it and who have no other meaningful option.

There has been longstanding interest in particle therapy for the treatment of salivary gland cancers, especially for situations in which gross disease remains. In the 1970s and 1980s, neutron therapy was studied most extensively. The interest in neutrons was based on their property of a high linear energy transfer (LET) as compared to photon therapy. From a biologic perspective, it has been demonstrated that the mechanism of cellular damage is different from high LET particles as compared to lower LET energy delivered with photons and electrons. Based on preclinical models, it was thought that neutrons would overcome some of the radioresistance, because of either cell cycle dependence or hypoxia seen with photon radiation. Because of the higher LET of neutrons as compared to x-rays and electrons, neutrons lead to greater tumor cell kill for the same given dose. In general, the hopes of improved outcomes for all cancers thought to be radioresistant to standard therapy were not clearly confirmed with neutrons. However, for salivary gland cancers, particularly adenoid cystic carcinomas (56), neutrons did seem advantageous, and a small randomized trial (57) did show an advantage for neutron therapy. The main advantage is greater local control, but the toxicity was high, and there was no improvement in overall survival. Major critiques of this trial include its small size and the imbalance of populations among the arms. Furthermore, the major concern about neutron therapy is that it can be highly damaging to neural tissue, and one of the principal causes of inoperability is often intracranial involvement, via either direct extension or perineural spread.

Protons are another particle available in the RT menu, and they may have a role in the treatment of salivary gland cancers. At the present time, however, protons do not seem to have the markedly different biologic properties of other heavier particles, so a biologic advantage for protons in the treatment of salivary gland cancers remains speculative. The principal potential advantage of protons is physical in its ability to deliver the desired radiation to the target with a greater degree of conformality, thereby limiting the dose to adjacent normal tissues. For unresectable skull base cancers delivering 70 Gy by IMRT with x-rays might give excessive dose to adjacent dose-limiting critical normal structures. With IMRT, tumor underdosing may be accepted in order to minimize risk for a devastating complication. However, tighter dose distributions with protons may allow more safe delivery of high-dose RT while not overdosing those critical normal structures. Several small series reports, principally focused on adenoid cystic carcinomas, have been encouraging (58,59).

An additional particle of interest for the treatment of unresectable salivary cancers is carbon ion. In theory, carbon ions combine biologic (LET) advantages of neutrons (improved tumor kill) and the physical advantages (dose distribution) of protons (improved dose conformality). Similar to the proton literature, small retrospective series investigating carbon ion therapy, often delivered as a boost treatment following an initial photon-based IMRT course, appear promising, but carbon ion facilities are limited (60,61).

RADIATION FOR METASTATIC DISEASE

RT is also used for palliation of distant metastatic disease. The principles of radiation for metastatic salivary gland cancer are similar to those applied for more common malignancies. Short courses of radiation are recommended for pain caused by bony metastases or to reverse or prevent obstructive or neurologic symptoms from metastases to the lung, brain, or spinal cord.

These courses of radiation are typically 1 to 2 weeks long and are frequently effective in relieving pain and temporarily reducing compressive or obstructive threats from an advancing tumor mass, but in these situations RT is not expected to achieve long-term disease control in the absence of effective systemic therapy. The potential benefits of radiation-induced palliation should be balanced against the expected lifespan of the patient and the availability and efficacy of other potentially effective modalities, such as palliative surgical intervention and systemic therapy.

PRINCIPLES OF SYSTEMIC THERAPY

Presently, the role of systemic therapy in the treatment of salivary gland cancers in both the curative intent and palliative settings is largely undefined, although the preponderance of prospective literature with systemic agents is in the unresectable, recurrent, or metastatic setting. In general, systemic therapy trials in salivary gland cancers are difficult to interpret because of the small numbers and heterogeneous patient populations. The following section will review available data and ongoing trials investigating the utility of systemic therapy in this uncommon patient population.

SYSTEMIC THERAPY IN THE CURATIVE INTENT SETTING

Postoperative RT is considered the standard of care following surgical resection for locally advanced disease, described in the prior section of this chapter. High-grade features of disease, such as advanced T and N stages, positive surgical margins at resection, facial nerve paralysis, and perineural invasion have been associated with poor oncologic outcomes, suggesting a role for therapeutic intensification (62). Postoperative concurrent chemoradiation, an established therapeutic standard in resected head and neck SCC with positive surgical margins or extranodal extension (63,64), is an appealing approach in this high-risk salivary gland cancer subset. Single-institution report of various platinum-based chemoradiotherapy regimens demonstrated superior rates of locoregional control (61% vs. 44%) and overall survival (83% vs. 44%) when retrospectively compared to a stage-matched group of patients treated with postoperative radiation alone (65). These observations conflict with retrospective data obtained from the National Cancer Database (52) and a single-institution series (51) that observed no advantage to the administration of concurrent chemotherapy to postoperative radiation.

A large, prospective study in a cooperative group setting is an attractive mechanism for investigation, and a phase II/phase III NRG/RTOG study comparing postoperative RT alone to concurrent chemoradiotherapy with weekly cisplatin is ongoing (NCT01220583). This study, which includes only the most commonly occurring and highest risk resected salivary gland subtypes in an effort to limit the wide range of biologic heterogeneity, was originally opened to assess the feasibility of conducting such a trial in a disease as rare as salivary gland cancer. However, accrual exceeded expectations, and the trial reopened in an expanded phase III design to compare overall survival rates of patients receiving cisplatin and RT to those receiving RT alone in the adjuvant setting. A Chinese clinical trial is actively recruiting participants to evaluate two different concurrent chemoradiotherapy regimens in the adjuvant setting: cisplatin and RT versus cisplatin plus docetaxel and RT (NCT02776163).

SYSTEMIC THERAPY IN THE RECURRENT/METASTATIC SETTING

Among patients with incurable disease, systemic therapy is generally employed to attempt to reduce tumor burden and subsequently palliate or prevent impending tumor-related symptoms. Several conventional chemotherapeutic agents have been prospectively evaluated in this disease, including platinum agents, taxanes, vinorelbine, epirubicin, and gemcitabine (38,66–68). Gilbert et al. completed a phase II study of single agent paclitaxel in 45 patients with adenoid cystic carcinomas, adenocarcinomas, and mucoepidermoid carcinomas of the salivary gland. Although no objective responses were noted in the 14 patients with adenoid cystic carcinomas, 8 partial responses were observed in patients with non–adenoid cystic histologic features (68). A more contemporary study of eribulin mesylate, a novel microtubule inhibitor used in 29 patients with salivary gland malignancies (69), was recently reported,. One complete response was noted in an adenoid cystic cancer patient, 2 partial responses in an adenoid cystic and carcinoma ex pleomorphic adenoma, and 23 of the 29 patients had stable disease as best response.

Multiple combinations of chemotherapy agents have also been studied. A randomized phase II trial comparing single agent vinorelbine with the combination of vinorelbine and cisplatin demonstrated a higher response rate (45% vs. 19%) and more patients alive at 12 months with the combination chemotherapy, leading investigators to conclude that the combination was superior to the single agent (66). Another phase II study evaluated gemcitabine and platinum, though responses were observed in only 24% of the 32 patients treated (70).

These cytotoxic chemotherapy studies have in common small numbers, histologic heterogeneity, very low rates of objective responses, and the frequent observation of stable disease. The question of whether clinical benefit can be ascribed to drug activity or simply to the natural history of indolent tumors is currently unanswered. Likewise, the superiority of systemic therapy to best supportive care in the recurrent metastatic setting has not been explored in randomized studies.

In our practice, we typically reserve the use of single agent or combination chemotherapy in patients with aggressive or rapidly progressing salivary gland malignancies with imminent or heavy symptom burden and with adequate performance status. Because of the absence of a standard systemic therapy regimen, enrollment in a clinical trial, if available, is preferred in these clinical scenarios.

TARGETED THERAPY IN SALIVARY GLAND MALIGNANCIES

Salivary gland cancers can overexpress various immunohistochemical biomarkers that represent potential therapeutic targets. However, the clinical experience with these novel targeted agents in salivary gland cancers has been disappointing overall.

Overexpression of c-kit has been frequently observed in adenoid cystic carcinomas, and subsequently three phase II trials with the oral c-kit tyrosine kinase inhibitor imatinib have been completed and reported. One study observed 2 objective responses among 17 patients enrolled (71). Of the two other phase II studies, one by Pfeffer et al. (72) enrolled 10 patients, and Hotte et al. (73) treated 16 patients. In both studies no objective responses were noted. Wong et al. recently concluded a phase II study using the agent dasatinib, an oral multikinase inhibitor of c-kit, in 54 patients with c-kit overexpressing salivary gland cancers (74). Only one objective response was observed, with 50% of patients having stable disease as their best response. These agents' lack of activity is likely explained by the fact that c-KIT activating mutations, rarely present in adenoid cystic carcinoma, are biomarkers that predict response rather than overexpression (75).

Adenoid cystic carcinomas and mucoepidermoid carcinomas can demonstrate immunohistochemical overexpression of the epidermal growth factor receptor (EGFR) (76). Clinical trials testing the activity of EGFR directed therapy, namely, the oral tyrosine kinase inhibitor gefitinib and monoclonal antibody cetuximab, have yielded modest results (77,78). Though no objective responses were seen in these studies, 80% of patients treated with cetuximab achieved stable disease.

Several multikinase inhibitors with antiangiogenic properties due to vascular endothelial growth factor (VEGF) inhibition have also been studied in this disease. Sunitinib, active against VEGF, c-KIT, platelet-derived growth factor receptor (PDGFR), ret proto-oncogene (RET), and FMS-like tyrosine kinase 3 (FLT3), was studied in a phase 2 trial of 14 adenoid cystic carcinoma patients (79). Although no objective responses were seen, 85% of patients had stable disease with 62% of patients demonstrating prolonged tumor stabilization over 6 months. Similar experiences have been reported with sorafenib. Thomson et al. reported a phase II study of 23 adenoid cystic carcinoma patients, and observed an 11% response rate (80). Locati et al. treated 37 patients with salivary gland cancers and noted objective responses in 6 (16%) patients (81). Dovitinib, which inhibits the fibroblast growth factor receptor (FGFR), VEGF, and PDGFR was tested in a phase II trial of 35 adenoid cystic carcinomas, and only 2 partial responses were noted (82). A Korean study that enrolled 32 adenoid cystic carcinoma patients observed only 1 partial response (83). The experience with axitinib, a small molecule that inhibits VEGF, c-KIT, and PDGFR, was recently reported in a phase II study of 33 adenoid cystic carcinoma patients, 3 (9%) partial responses were observed (84).

Androgen receptor, estrogen receptor, and progesterone receptor overexpression has been observed in adenocarcinomas, salivary duct carcinomas (SDC), and carcinoma ex pleomorphic adenomas (85). Case reports of responses to the hormonal agents tamoxifen, anastrozole, goserelin, bicalutamide, and abiraterone in salivary gland malignancies have been published (86–89). Abiraterone, a CYP17 inhibitor, and enzalutamide, an androgen receptor inhibitor, are drugs approved for the treatment of prostate cancer and are currently being studied in phase II trials in patients with relapsed or metastatic salivary gland cancers (NCT02867852 and NCT02749903). Another study in active accrual is evaluating combinations cytotoxic chemotherapy with androgen deprivation therapy in patients with androgen receptor expressing salivary gland cancer in a randomized fashion (NCT01969578).

Her-2 can be overexpressed in salivary gland carcinomas, with the highest expression in salivary duct carcinomas (90). Prospective investigation of Her2 targeted therapy used as a single agent have had limited success. Haddad et al. reported results of a phase II study of trastuzumab in salivary gland cancers with 2+ or 3+ Her2 overexpression by immunohistochemistry (91). Among 14 patients enrolled on the study, only 1 patient with mucoepidermoid carcinoma achieved a partial response. Lapatinib, an oral EGFR and Her2 tyrosine kinase inhibitor, showed no objective responses among 40 patients treated on a phase II clinical trial (92).

In contrast, reports on the activity of Her2 directed therapy in combination with cytotoxic chemotherapy seem more encouraging. One case series included five patients with salivary duct carcinoma and HER2 expression who were treated with a combination of paclitaxel, carboplatin, and trastuzumab, a HER2-directed monoclonal antibody in the palliative setting (93). One patient achieved complete response, and two other patients had partial responses. The authors also reported two of the patients had received prior trastuzumab as a single agent and achieved prolonged disease control. Data from a single-arm phase II study of trastuzumab and docetaxel recently demonstrated a response rate of 76% in 31 patients with median progression-free survival of 9.8 months (94).

The development of immune checkpoint inhibitors and their demonstrated activity in both hematologic and epithelial malignancies has naturally generated interest in defining activity among rare tumors such as salivary gland cancers. Preliminary data with pembrolizumab, an anti-PD-1 monoclonal antibody (PD-1 = programmed cell death protein 1), was recently reported in a 26-patient salivary gland cancer cohort with >1% PDL-1 expression (PDL-1 = PD-1 ligand), and 3 partial responses were noted (95). Several studies are now exploring the use of PD-1 directed monoclonal antibodies either as a single agent or in combination (NCT02628067, NCT02538510, NCT02834013, NCT02636036).

CASE 21.1

A 64-year-old woman, with a remote past history of resected breast ductal carcinoma in situ, presented with right-sided facial weakness, which did not improve with an empiric course of corticosteroids. An MRI of the brain, done to rule out a stroke, revealed an infiltrating mass in the right parotid gland, with associated right-sided level II cervical adenopathy (Figure 21.1). A fine-needle aspiration of the parotid mass revealed "highly atypical cells with enlarged nuclei, coarse chromatin, nuclear membrane irregularities and mitotic figures consistent with a carcinoma." A chest radiograph was done to complete staging, revealing no abnormalities. The patient was deemed a candidate for surgical resection.

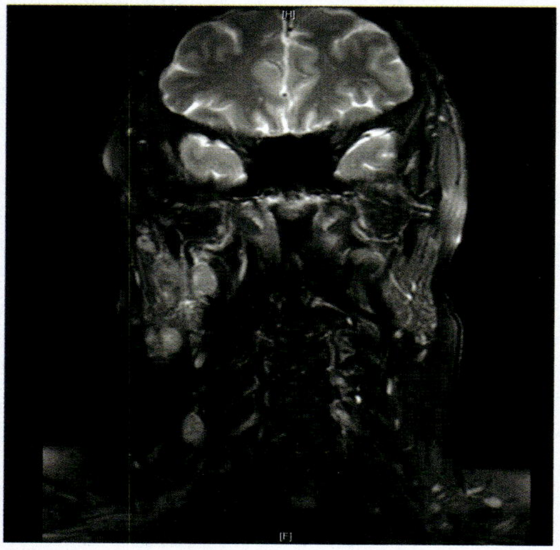

FIGURE 21.1 MRI at presentation revealing R sided cervical adenopathy.

The patient underwent a total parotidectomy and selective right-sided neck dissection. Final pathologic report from the resected specimen revealed a right parotid mass with a maximum dimension of 4.9 cm. Adenocarcinoma was present at the margin of resection, there was evidence of perineural involvement, and 8 intraparotid lymph nodes contained carcinoma. Fifteen of 20 resected lymph nodes from right levels II and III were positive for carcinoma with the largest being 3 cm in its greatest dimension with evidence of extracapsular extension. The patient recovered well from surgical resection and was referred to radiation oncology for postoperative RT.

The patient underwent radiation simulation, and CT imaging was obtained for restaging. Suspicious liver lesions were identified (Figure 21.2). A CT-guided biopsy confirmed the presence of metastatic adenocarcinoma, histologically identical to the resected primary tumor. The patient was subsequently treated in a clinical trial and received the investigational agent eribulin, to which she had a transient partial response. She developed intractable nausea and vomiting and was found to have extensive brain metastases, and was treated with palliative RT. She was subsequently enrolled in hospice care and died 9 months after her initial diagnosis.

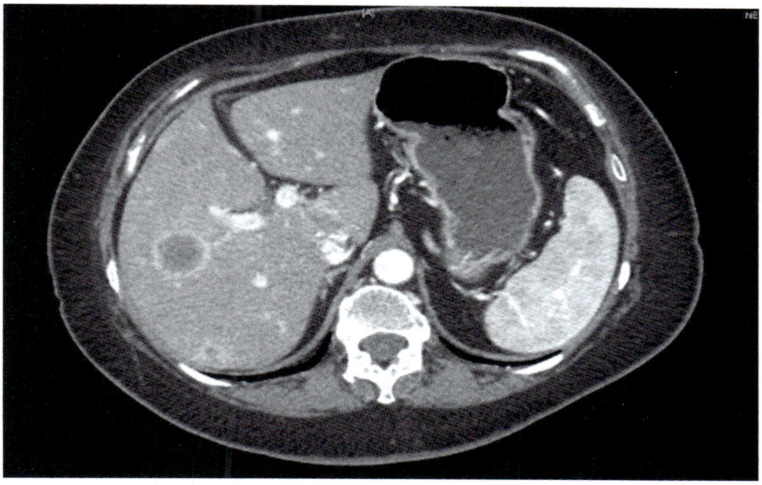

FIGURE 21.2 CT imaging revealing hepatic lesions suspicious for metastases.

CONCLUSIONS

It is clear that salivary gland cancers represent a disease entity in need of improved outcomes. Observations from previously completed clinical trials have underscored multiple challenges unique to this disease entity.

An attempt to control for heterogeneity of disease biology is a prerequisite for obtaining clinically meaningful results. Consequently, contemporary clinical trials are either narrowing eligible histologic features to those that demonstrate a fairly uniform aggressive disease biology or requiring objective clinical or radiographic progression in the months preceding trial enrollment.

Disease infrequency is a limiting factor in arriving at realistic trial sample sizes and completing accrual for these studies. In this regard, the cooperative group or cancer consortia may be ideal scenarios for studying these uncommon tumors. Eastern Cooperative Oncology Group (ECOG), RTOG/NRG, and EORTC have demonstrated prior success in the design, activation, and successful accrual in these trials.

Although objective responses to systemic therapy are rare, multiple cases of patients with remarkable responses to systemic or targeted therapy have been described. A greater understanding of the molecular profile of these outliers can potentially lead to identification of biomarkers for response and underscores the value of correlative tissue or serum collection as a component of prospective trials.

Finally, among uncommon tumors, site-agnostic molecular marker driven trial designs are gaining traction, spurred primarily by commercially available, reasonably priced, next-generation sequencing platforms that have fairly rapid turnaround times. There are now reports from single institutions suggesting success in identification of potential therapeutic targets when molecular profiling is employed for patients with salivary gland tumors (96,97). Two large ongoing federally funded clinical trials, MATCH (NCT02465060) and TAPUR (NCT02693535), are screening patient tumors using next-generation sequencing. Patients with an identified actionable mutation are assigned to a study arm with a corresponding targeted therapy. Apart from the clinical efficacy of these targeted treatments in rare cancers such as salivary gland malignancies, the successful completion of these trials will lead to valuable insights into the feasibility and cost effectiveness of the sequencing-based study designs.

REFERENCES

1. Carvalho AL, Nishimoto IN, Califano JA, Kowalski LP. Trends in incidence and prognosis for head and neck cancer in the united states: a site-specific analysis of the SEER database. *Int J Cancer*. 2005;114(5):806–816. doi:10.1002/ijc.20740
2. Boukheris H, Ron E, Dores GM, et al. Risk of radiation-related salivary gland carcinomas among survivors of hodgkin lymphoma: a population-based analysis. *Cancer*. 2008;113(11):3153–3159. doi:10.1002/cncr.23918
3. Boukheris H, Stovall M, Gilbert ES, et al. Risk of salivary gland cancer after childhood cancer: A report from the childhood cancer survivor study. *Int J Radiat Oncol Biol Phys*. 2013;85(3):776–783. doi:10.1016/j.ijrobp.2012.06.006
4. Barnes L, Eveson JW, Riechart P, Sidransky D. *World Health Organization Classification of Tumors. Pathology and Genetics of Head and Neck Tumours*. Lyon: IARC Press; 2005.
5. Spiro RH. Salivary neoplasms: overview of a 35-year experience with 2,807 patients. *Head Neck Surg*. 1986;8(3):177–184. doi:10.1002/hed.2890080309
6. Szanto PA, Luna MA, Tortoledo ME, White RA. Histologic grading of adenoid cystic carcinoma of the salivary glands. *Cancer*. 1984;54(6):1062–1069. doi:10.1002/1097-0142(19840915)54:6<1062::AID-CNCR2820540622>3.0.CO;2-E
7. Ghosh-Laskar S, Murthy V, Wadasadawala T, et al. Mucoepidermoid carcinoma of the parotid gland: factors affecting outcome. *Head Neck*. 2011;33(4):497–503. doi:10.1002/hed.21477
8. Connor A, Perez-Ordonez B, Shago M, et al. Mammary analog secretory carcinoma of salivary gland origin with the ETV6 gene rearrangement by FISH: expanded morphologic and immunohistochemical spectrum of a recently described entity. *Am J Surg Pathol*. 2012;36(1):27–34. doi:10.1097/PAS.0b013e318231542a
9. West RB, Kong C, Clarke N, et al. MYB expression and translocation in adenoid cystic carcinomas and other salivary gland tumors with clinicopathologic correlation. *Am J Surg Pathol*. 2011;35(1):92–99. doi:10.1097/PAS.0b013e3182002777
10. Okabe M, Miyabe S, Nagatsuka H, et al. *MECT1-MAML2* fusion transcript defines a favorable subset of mucoepidermoid carcinoma. *Clin Cancer Res*. 2006;12(13):3902–3907. doi:10.1158/1078-0432.CCR-05-2376
11. Zurrida S, Alasio L, Tradati N, et al. Fine-needle aspiration of parotid masses. *Cancer*. 1993;72(8):2306–2311. doi:10.1002/1097-0142(19931015)72:8<2306::AID-CNCR2820720804>3.0.CO;2-E
12. Wong DS, Li GK. The role of fine-needle aspiration cytology in the management of parotid tumors: a critical clinical appraisal. *Head Neck*. 2000;22(5):469–473. doi:10.1002/1097-0347(200008)22:53.0.CO;2-7
13. Thoeny HC. Imaging of salivary gland tumours. *Cancer Imaging*. 2007;7:52–62. doi:10.1102/1470-7330.2007.0008
14. Edge SB, Byrd DR, Compton CC, et al (eds). *AJCC Cancer Staging Manual*. 7th ed. New York, NY: Springer; 2010.
15. O'Brien CJ. Current management of benign parotid tumors–the role of limited superficial parotidectomy. *Head Neck*. 2003;25(11):946–952. doi:10.1002/hed.10312
16. Roh JL, Park CI. Function-preserving parotid surgery for benign tumors involving the deep parotid lobe. *J Surg Oncol*. 2008;98(1):42–45. doi:10.1002/jso.21082
17. Sullivan MJ, Breslin K, McClatchey KD, et al. Malignant parotid gland tumors: a retrospective study. *Otolaryngol Head Neck Surg*. 1987;97(6):529–533. doi:10.1177/019459988709700603
18. Scianna JM, Petruzzelli GJ. Contemporary management of tumors of the salivary glands. *Curr Oncol Rep*. 2007;9(2):134–138. doi:10.1007/s11912-007-0011-6
19. Bell RB, Dierks EJ, Homer L, Potter BE. Management and outcome of patients with malignant salivary gland tumors. *J Oral Maxillofac Surg*. 2005;63(7):917–928. doi:10.1016/j.joms.2005.03.006
20. Magnano M, Gervasio CF, Cravero L, et al. Treatment of malignant neoplasms of the parotid gland. *Otolaryngol Head Neck Surg*. 1999;121(5):627–632. doi:10.1016/S0194-5998(99)70070-7
21. Spiro RH. Changing trends in the management of salivary tumors. *Semin Surg Oncol*. 1995;11(3):240–245. doi:10.1002/ssu.2980110309
22. Iseli TA, Karnell LH, Preston TW, et al. Facial nerve sacrifice and radiotherapy in parotid adenoid cystic carcinoma. *Laryngoscope*. 2008;118(10):1781–1786. doi:10.1097/MLG.0b013e31817fae29
23. Terhaard C, Lubsen H, Tan B, et al. Facial nerve function in carcinoma of the parotid gland. *Eur J Cancer*. 2006;42(16):2744–2750. doi:10.1016/j.ejca.2006.06.010
24. Humphrey CD, Kriet JD. Nerve repair and cable grafting for facial paralysis. *Facial Plast Surg*. 2008;24(2):170–176. doi:10.1055/s-2008-1075832
25. Kimata Y, Sakuraba M, Hishinuma S, et al. Free vascularized nerve grafting for immediate facial nerve reconstruction. *Laryngoscope*. 2005;115(2):331–336. doi:10.1097/01.mlg.0000154753.32174.24
26. Kaszuba SM, Zafereo ME, Rosenthal DI, et al. Effect of initial treatment on disease outcome for patients with submandibular gland carcinoma. *Arch Otolaryngol Head Neck Surg*. 2007;133(6):546–550. doi:10.1001/archotol.133.6.546
27. Rinaldo A, Shaha AR, Pellitteri PK, et al. Management of malignant sublingual salivary gland tumors. *Oral Oncol*. 2004;40(1):2–5. doi:10.1016/S1368-8375(03)00104-0
28. Harish K. Management of primary malignant epithelial parotid tumors. *Surg Oncol*. 2004;13(1):7–16. doi:10.1016/j.suronc.2003.10.002
29. Armstrong JG, Harrison LB, Thaler HT, et al. The indications for elective treatment of the neck in cancer of the major salivary glands. *Cancer*. 1992;69(3):615–619. doi:10.1002/1097-0142(19920201)69:3<615::AID-CNCR2820690303>3.0.CO;2-9

30. Kelley DJ, Spiro RH. Management of the neck in parotid carcinoma. *Am J Surg*. 1996;172(6):695–697. doi:10.1016/S0002-9610(96)00307-8
31. Jackson GL. Management of the neck in parotid cancer. *Am J Surg*. 1998;175(5):435. doi:10.1016/S0002-9610(98)80043-3
32. Valstar MH, van den Brekel MW, Smeele LE. Interpretation of treatment outcome in the clinically node-negative neck in primary parotid carcinoma: a systematic review of the literature. *Head Neck*. 2010;32(10):1402–1411. doi:10.1002/hed.21316
33. Schwentner I, Obrist P, Thumfart W, Sprinzl G. Distant metastasis of parotid gland tumors. *Acta Otolaryngol*. 2006;126(4):340–345. doi:10.1080/00016480500401035
34. Bradley PJ. Adenoid cystic carcinoma of the head and neck: a review. *Curr Opin Otolaryngol Head Neck Surg*. 2004;12(2):127–132. doi:10.1097/00020840-200404000-00013
35. Kim KH, Sung MW, Chung PS, et al. Adenoid cystic carcinoma of the head and neck. *Arch Otolaryngol Head Neck Surg*. 1994;120(7):721–726. doi:10.1001/archotol.1994.01880310027006
36. Sung MW, Kim KH, Kim JW, et al. Clinicopathologic predictors and impact of distant metastasis from adenoid cystic carcinoma of the head and neck. *Arch Otolaryngol Head Neck Surg*. 2003;129(11):1193–1197. doi:10.1001/archotol.129.11.1193
37. van der Wal JE, Becking AG, Snow GB, van der Waal I. Distant metastases of adenoid cystic carcinoma of the salivary glands and the value of diagnostic examinations during follow-up. *Head Neck*. 2002;24(8):779–783. doi:10.1002/hed.10126
38. Laurie SA, Licitra L. Systemic therapy in the palliative management of advanced salivary gland cancers. *J Clin Oncol*. 2006;24(17):2673–2678. doi:10.1200/JCO.2005.05.3025
39. Locati LD, Guzzo M, Bossi P, et al. Lung metastasectomy in adenoid cystic carcinoma (ACC) of salivary gland. *Oral Oncol*. 2005;41(9):890–894. doi:10.1016/j.oraloncology.2005.04.014
40. Bobbio A, Copelli C, Ampollini L, et al. Lung metastasis resection of adenoid cystic carcinoma of salivary glands. *Eur J Cardiothorac Surg*. 2008;33(5):790–793. doi:10.1016/j.ejcts.2007.12.057
41. Park I, Lim SN, Yoon DH, et al. Metastasectomy for hepatic metastases from adenoid cystic carcinoma of the trachea. *Gut Liver*. 2009;3(2):127–129. doi:10.5009/gnl.2009.3.2.127
42. Barton J, Slevin NJ, Gleave EN. Radiotherapy for pleomorphic adenoma of the parotid gland. *Int J Radiat Oncol Biol Phys*. 1992;22(5):925–928. doi:10.1016/0360-3016(92)90789-K
43. Chen AM, Granchi PJ, Garcia J, et al. Local-regional recurrence after surgery without postoperative irradiation for carcinomas of the major salivary glands: implications for adjuvant therapy. *Int J Radiat Oncol Biol Phys*. 2007;67(4):982–987. doi:10.1016/j.ijrobp.2006.10.043
44. Lau VH, Aouad R, Farwell DG, et al. Patterns of nodal involvement for clinically N0 salivary gland carcinoma: refining the role of elective neck irradiation. *Head Neck*. 2014;36(10):1435–1439. doi:10.1002/hed.23467
45. Armstrong JG, Harrison LB, Spiro RH, et al. Malignant tumors of major salivary gland origin. A matched-pair analysis of the role of combined surgery and postoperative radiotherapy. *Arch Otolaryngol Head Neck Surg*. 1990;116(3):290–293. doi:10.1001/archotol.1990.01870030054008
46. Garden AS, El-Naggar AK, Morrison WH, et al. Postoperative radiotherapy for malignant tumors of the parotid gland. *Int J Radiat Oncol Biol Phys*. 1997;37(1):79–85. doi:10.1016/S0360-3016(96)00464-6
47. Garden AS, Weber RS, Ang KK, et al. Postoperative radiation therapy for malignant tumors of minor salivary glands. outcome and patterns of failure. *Cancer*. 1994;73(10):2563–2569. doi:10.1002/1097-0142(19940515)73:10<2563::AID-CNCR2820731018>3.0.CO;2-X
48. Storey MR, Garden AS, Morrison WH, et al. Postoperative radiotherapy for malignant tumors of the submandibular gland. *Int J Radiat Oncol Biol Phys*. 2001;51(4):952–958. doi:10.1016/S0360-3016(01)01724-2
49. Terhaard CH. Postoperative and primary radiotherapy for salivary gland carcinomas: indications, techniques, and results. *Int J Radiat Oncol Biol Phys*. 2007;69(2 Suppl):S52-S55. doi:10.1016/j.ijrobp.2007.04.079
50. Schoenfeld JD, Sher DJ, Norris CM Jr, et al. Salivary gland tumors treated with adjuvant intensity-modulated radiotherapy with or without concurrent chemotherapy. *Int J Radiat Oncol Biol Phys*. 2012;82(1):308–314. doi:10.1016/j.ijrobp.2010.09.042
51. Mifsud MJ, Tanvetyanon T, Mccaffrey JC, et al. Adjuvant radiotherapy versus concurrent chemoradiotherapy for the management of high-risk salivary gland carcinomas. *Head Neck*. 2016;38(11):1628–1633. doi:10.1002/hed.24484
52. Amini A, Waxweiler TV, Brower JV, et al. Association of adjuvant chemoradiotherapy vs radiotherapy alone with survival in patients with resected major salivary gland carcinoma: data from the national cancer data base. *JAMA Otolaryngol Head Neck Surg*. 2016;142(11):1100–1110. doi:10.1001/jamaoto.2016.2168
53. Chen AM, Bucci MK, Quivey JM, et al. Long-term outcome of patients treated by radiation therapy alone for salivary gland carcinomas. *Int J Radiat Oncol Biol Phys*. 2006;66(4):1044–1050. doi:10.1016/j.ijrobp.2006.06.050
54. Holtzman A, Morris CG, Amdur RJ, et al. Outcomes after primary or adjuvant radiotherapy for salivary gland carcinoma. *Acta Oncol*. 2017;56(3):484–489. doi:10.1080/0284186X.2016.1253863
55. Samant S, van den Brekel MW, Kies MS, et al. Concurrent chemoradiation for adenoid cystic carcinoma of the head and neck. *Head Neck*. 2012;34(9):1263–1268. doi:10.1002/hed.21905

56. Douglas JG, Laramore GE, Austin-Seymour M, et al. Neutron radiotherapy for adenoid cystic carcinoma of minor salivary glands. *Int J Radiat Oncol Biol Phys.* 1996;36(1):87–93. doi:10.1016/S0360-3016(96)00213-1
57. Griffin TW, Pajak TF, Laramore GE, et al. Neutron vs photon irradiation of inoperable salivary gland tumors: results of an RTOG-MRC cooperative randomized study. *Int J Radiat Oncol Biol Phys.* 1988;15(5):1085–1090. doi:10.1016/0360-3016(88)90188-5
58. Pommier P, Liebsch NJ, Deschler DG, et al. Proton beam radiation therapy for skull base adenoid cystic carcinoma. *Arch Otolaryngol Head Neck Surg.* 2006;132(11):1242–1249. doi:10.1001/archotol.132.11.1242
59. Bhattasali O, Holliday E, Kies MS, et al. Definitive proton radiation therapy and concurrent cisplatin for unresectable head and neck adenoid cystic carcinoma: a series of 9 cases and a critical review of the literature. *Head Neck.* 2016;38 Suppl 1:E1472–E1480. doi:10.1002/hed.24262
60. Jensen AD, Poulakis M, Nikoghosyan AV, et al. High-LET radiotherapy for adenoid cystic carcinoma of the head and neck: 15 years' experience with raster-scanned carbon ion therapy. *Radiother Oncol.* 2016;118(2):272–280. doi:10.1016/j.radonc.2015.05.010
61. Schulz-Ertner D, Nikoghosyan A, Jäkel O, et al. Feasibility and toxicity of combined photon and carbon ion radiotherapy for locally advanced adenoid cystic carcinomas. *Int J Radiat Oncol Biol Phys.* 2003;56(2):391–398. doi:10.1016/S0360-3016(02)04511-X
62. Terhaard CH, Lubsen H, Van der Tweel I, et al. Salivary gland carcinoma: independent prognostic factors for locoregional control, distant metastases, and overall survival: results of the Dutch head and neck oncology cooperative group. *Head Neck.* 2004;26(8):681–692; discussion 692–693. doi:10.1002/hed.10400
63. Bernier J, Domenge C, Ozsahin M, et al. Postoperative irradiation with or without concomitant chemotherapy for locally advanced head and neck cancer. *N Engl J Med.* 2004;350(19):1945–1952. doi:10.1056/NEJMoa032641
64. Cooper JS, Pajak TF, Forastiere AA, et al. Postoperative concurrent radiotherapy and chemotherapy for high-risk squamous-cell carcinoma of the head and neck. *N Engl J Med.* 2004;350(19):1937–1944. doi:10.1056/NEJMoa032646
65. Tanvetyanon T, Qin D, Padhya T, et al. Outcomes of postoperative concurrent chemoradiotherapy for locally advanced major salivary gland carcinoma. *Arch Otolaryngol Head Neck Surg.* 2009;135(7):687–692. doi:10.1001/archoto.2009.70
66. Airoldi M, Pedani F, Succo G, et al. Phase II randomized trial comparing vinorelbine versus vinorelbine plus cisplatin in patients with recurrent salivary gland malignancies. *Cancer.* 2001;91(3):541–547. doi:10.1002/1097-0142(20010201)91:3<541::AID-CNCR1032>3.0.CO;2-Y
67. Vermorken JB, Verweij J, de Mulder PH, et al. Epirubicin in patients with advanced or recurrent adenoid cystic carcinoma of the head and neck: a phase II study of the EORTC head and neck cancer cooperative group. *Ann Oncol.* 1993;4(9):785–788. doi:10.1093/oxfordjournals.annonc.a058665
68. Gilbert J, Li Y, Pinto HA, et al. Phase II trial of taxol in salivary gland malignancies (E1394): a trial of the eastern cooperative oncology group. *Head Neck.* 2006;28(3):197–204. doi:10.1002/hed.20327
69. Eaton KD, Goulart BG, Santana-Davila R, et al. Phase II trial of eribulin for recurrent or metastatic salivary gland cancers. *J Clin Oncol.* 2016;34(15 suppl):6095. doi:10.1200/JCO.2016.34.15_suppl.6095
70. Laurie SA, Siu LL, Winquist E, et al. A phase 2 study of platinum and gemcitabine in patients with advanced salivary gland cancer: a trial of the NCIC clinical trials group. *Cancer.* 2010;116(2):362–368. doi:10.1002/cncr.24745
71. Guigay JM, Bidault F, Temam S, et al. Antitumor activity of imatinib in progressive, highly expressing KIT adenoid cystic carcinoma of the salivary glands: a phase II study. *J Clin Oncol.* 2007;25(18 suppl):6086. doi:10.1200/jco.2007.25.18_suppl.6086
72. Pfeffer MR, Talmi Y, Catane R, et al. A phase II study of imatinib for advanced adenoid cystic carcinoma of head and neck salivary glands. *Oral Oncol.* 2007;43(1):33–36. doi:10.1016/j.oraloncology.2005.12.026
73. Hotte SJ, Winquist EW, Lamont E, et al. Imatinib mesylate in patients with adenoid cystic cancers of the salivary glands expressing c-kit: a Princess Margaret Hospital phase II consortium study. *J Clin Oncol.* 2005;23(3):585–590. doi:10.1200/JCO.2005.06.125
74. Wong SJ, Karrison T, Hayes DN, et al. Phase II trial of dasatinib for recurrent or metastatic c-KIT expressing adenoid cystic carcinoma and for nonadenoid cystic malignant salivary tumors. *Ann Oncol.* 2016;27(2):318–323. doi:10.1093/annonc/mdv537
75. Wetterskog D, Wilkerson PM, Rodrigues DN, et al. Mutation profiling of adenoid cystic carcinomas from multiple anatomical sites identifies mutations in the RAS pathway, but no KIT mutations. *Histopathology.* 2013;62(4):543–550. doi:10.1111/his.12050
76. Clauditz TS, Gontarewicz A, Lebok P, et al. Epidermal growth factor receptor (EGFR) in salivary gland carcinomas: potentials as therapeutic target. *Oral Oncol.* 2012;48(10):991–996. doi:10.1016/j.oraloncology.2012.05.005
77. Locati LD, Bossi P, Perrone F, et al. Cetuximab in recurrent and/or metastatic salivary gland carcinomas: a phase II study. *Oral Oncol.* 2009;45(7):574–578. doi:10.1016/j.oraloncology.2008.07.010
78. Jakob JA, Kies MS, Glisson BS, et al. Phase II study of gefitinib in patients with advanced salivary gland cancers. *Head Neck.* 2015;37(5):644–649. doi:10.1002/hed.23647
79. Chau NG, Hotte SJ, Chen EX, et al. A phase II study of sunitinib in recurrent and/or metastatic adenoid cystic carcinoma (ACC) of the salivary glands: current progress and challenges in evaluating molecularly targeted agents in ACC. *Ann Oncol.* 2012;23(6):1562–1570. doi:10.1093/annonc/mdr522
80. Thomson DJ, Silva P, Denton K, et al. Phase II trial of sorafenib in advanced salivary adenoid cystic carcinoma of the head and neck. *Head Neck.* 2015;37(2):182–187. doi:10.1002/hed.23577

81. Locati LD, Perrone F, Cortelazzi B, et al. A phase II study of sorafenib in recurrent and/or metastatic salivary gland carcinomas: translational analyses and clinical impact. *Eur J Cancer*. 2016;69:158–165. doi:10.1016/j.ejca.2016.09.022
82. Dillon PM, Petroni GR, Moskaluk C, et al. A phase II study of dovitinib in patients with recurrent or metastatic adenoid cystic carcinoma (ACC). *ASCO Meeting Abstracts*. 2015;33(15 suppl):e17092. doi:10.1200/jco.2015.33.15_suppl.e17092
83. Keam B, Kim SB, Shin SH, et al. Phase 2 study of dovitinib in patients with metastatic or unresectable adenoid cystic carcinoma. *Cancer*. 2015;121(15):2612–2617. doi:10.1002/cncr.29401
84. Ho AL, Sherman EJ, Fury MG, et al. Phase II study of axitinib in patients with progressive, recurrent/metastatic adenoid cystic carcinoma. *ASCO Meeting Abstracts*. 2014;32(15 suppl):6093. doi:10.1200/JCO.2007.11.8612
85. Nasser SM, Faquin WC, Dayal Y. Expression of androgen, estrogen, and progesterone receptors in salivary gland tumors. frequent expression of androgen receptor in a subset of malignant salivary gland tumors. *Am J Clin Pathol*. 2003;119(6):801–806. doi:10.1309/RVTP-1G0Q-727W-JUQD
86. Jaspers HC, Verbist BM, Schoffelen R, et al. Androgen receptor-positive salivary duct carcinoma: a disease entity with promising new treatment options. *J Clin Oncol*. 2011;29(16):e473-e476. doi:10.1200/JCO.2010.32.8351
87. Campos-Gomez S, Flores-Arredondo JH, Dorantes-Heredia R, et al. Case report: anti-hormonal therapy in the treatment of ductal carcinoma of the parotid gland. *BMC Cancer*. 2014;14:701. doi:10.1186/1471-2407-14-701
88. Elkin AD, Jacobs CD. Tamoxifen for salivary gland adenoid cystic carcinoma: report of two cases. *J Cancer Res Clin Oncol*. 2008;134(10):1151–1153. doi:10.1007/s00432-008-0377-3
89. Urban D, Rischin D, Angel C, et al. Abiraterone in metastatic salivary duct carcinoma. *J Natl Compr Canc Netw*. 2015;13(3):288–290. doi:10.6004/jnccn.2015.0040
90. Ettl T, Stiegler C, Zeitler K, et al. EGFR, HER2, survivin, and loss of pSTAT3 characterize high-grade malignancy in salivary gland cancer with impact on prognosis. *Hum Pathol*. 2012;43(6):921–931. doi:10.1016/j.humpath.2011.08.006
91. Haddad R, Colevas AD, Krane JF, et al. Herceptin in patients with advanced or metastatic salivary gland carcinomas. A phase II study. *Oral Oncol*. 2003;39(7):724–727. doi:10.1016/S1368-8375(03)00097-6
92. Agulnik M, Cohen EW, Cohen RB, et al. Phase II study of lapatinib in recurrent or metastatic epidermal growth factor receptor and/or erbB2 expressing adenoid cystic carcinoma and non adenoid cystic carcinoma malignant tumors of the salivary glands. *J Clin Oncol*. 2007;25(25):3978–3984. doi:10.1200/JCO.2007.11.8612
93. Limaye SA, Posner MR, Krane JF, et al. Trastuzumab for the treatment of salivary duct carcinoma. *Oncologist*. 2013;18(3):294–300. doi:10.1634/theoncologist.2012-0369
94. Takahashi H, Chihiro Fushimi TM, Matsuki T, et al. Trastuzumab and docetaxel for HER-2 positive unresectable salivary gland carcinoma: updated result of a phase II trial. 2016: American Head and Neck Society 9th International Conference on Head and Neck Cancer. Seattle, WA.
95. Cohen RB, Delord JP, Doi T, et al. Preliminary results for the advanced salivary gland carcinoma cohort of the phase 1b KEYNOTE-028 study of pembrolizumab. *J Clin Oncol*. 2016;34(15 suppl):6017. doi:10.1200/JCO.2016.34.15_suppl.6017
96. Ross JS, Wang K, Rand JV, et al. Comprehensive genomic profiling of relapsed and metastatic adenoid cystic carcinomas by next-generation sequencing reveals potential new routes to targeted therapies. *Am J Surg Pathol*. 2014;38(2):235–238. doi:10.1097/PAS.0000000000000102
97. Majewska H, Müller J, Lakis S, et al. Genomic profiling of salivary gland tumors identifies novel and targetable alterations. *Cancer Res*. 2016;76(14 suppl):3190. doi:0.1158/1538-7445.AM2016-3190

SECTION IV

Recurrent or Metastatic Disease

22

Locally Recurrent HNSCC: Salvage Surgery, Reirradiation

Antoine Eskander
Sharon A. Spencer
Corey J. Langer
Takashi Maruo
Ryuichi Hayashi
Sadamoto Zenda
James W. Rocco

Locoregionally recurrent head and neck cancers, which are defined as biopsy confirmed disease at the primary tumor site or in the regional nodal basin after a period of time during which the cancer was not detected, occurs in 30% to 40% of patients in the postcurative treatment setting (1), with approximately 20% to 30% occurring at the primary site and 10% to 15% in the regional nodal basin (2). Recurrent metastatic disease and second primary cancers occur in 20% to 30% of patients (1). The risk of second primary disease and locoregionally recurrent disease is nearly three- to fourfold greater in those patients who continue to use tobacco products and alcohol (3–5) and is generally more common in head and neck cancer than in other solid malignancies.

The ongoing risk of recurrent disease is a significant source of anxiety among patients treated for head and neck cancer, even among long-term survivors (6). Head and neck oncologists also experience similar concerns because treating patients with locoregionally recurrent disease is a challenge regardless of treatment modality, and outcomes are universally poor with a few exceptions (7). This chapter focuses on the role of salvage surgery and reirradiation for patients with locally and regionally recurrent squamous cell carcinoma (SCC) of the head and neck.

SCOPE OF PROBLEM

Locoregional failure occurs in 17% to 38% (8,9) with greater than 90% of recurrences occurring within the first 2 years after primary treatment (2). The scope of the problem is demonstrated in Table 22.1, where we have outlined the poor survival associated with head and neck cancer, particularly in those with advanced disease stage.

Close surveillance in the posttreatment period, usually every 3 months in the first year, every 4 months in the second year, every 6 months in the third year, and annually thereafter, is critical in picking up recurrences early. Evaluation should involve a thorough physical examination including inspection and palpation of the primary site and the regional basin

TABLE 22.1

Head and Neck Cancer Survival by Stage and Subsite

Subsite	Early Stage	Advanced Stage
Nasopharynx	96% (5-yr OS) (10)	62% (5-yr OS) (10)
Oral cavity	87% (5-yr DFS) (11)	67% (5-yr DFS) (11)
Oropharynx	93% (3-yr DSS) (12,13)	66% (5-yr DFS) (12,13)
Larynx	60%–67% (5-yr DFS) (14,15)	38% (5-yr DFS) (14,15)
Hypopharynx	57.5%–63.1% (5-yr DSS) (16)	22.0%–41.8% (5-yr DSS) (16)

1. DSS and DFS are different outcomes but often strongly correlated usually with a less than 5%–10% difference at 5 years in head and neck oncology.
2. DFS is used as a surrogate for locoregional control rates because these are not consistently reported across studies. Furthermore, in head and neck cancer, >90% of recurrences are locoregional.
3. This is a representative sampling of studies but is not meant to be a pooled analysis or systematic review.

DFS, disease-free survival; DSS, disease-specific survival; OS, overall survival.

in addition to visualization of mucosal surfaces with flexible fiberoptic nasolaryngoscopy (17). Patients should be counseled on risk factors including continued tobacco product and alcohol use.

Patients should be warned of the risk of recurrence, including signs and symptoms suggestive of recurrence, including but not limited to pain, otalgia, dysphagia, dysphonia, trismus, weight loss, and new lymphadenopathy. Patients should have access to and seek medical attention should they present with these signs or symptoms for early assessment and intervention.

EVALUATION AND PROGNOSIS

Once a patient has suspicion for recurrent disease, early biopsy is important to distinguish the diagnosis from scar, fibrosis, or inflammation. Sometimes, a diagnostic laryngoscopy under general anesthesia is required to confirm the diagnosis. Even if the patient is amenable to biopsy in an ambulatory setting, diagnostic laryngoscopy with esophagoscopy is our preferred practice because this allows for further assessment of the extent of disease and resectability, in addition to providing a thorough assessment for second primaries. If the disease is adjacent to or at the site of the previous cancer, this is considered locally recurrent, whereas if a different subsite is involved, this is considered a second primary cancer. The site of recurrence has significant prognostic implications.

Following a thorough history and physical examination, diagnostic imaging in the head and neck, in the form of CT or MRI, can provide additional valuable information regarding extent of the disease and resectability. The patient should also be fully restaged, which should include a CT scan of the chest to rule out synchronous pulmonary metastases. The use of positron emission tomography (PET) with CT (PET-CT) is routinely used by many centers to determine if there are any additional sites that require evaluation including the regional nodal basin; it is also an excellent tool to rule out distant metastases because the entire body is included in the scan. In the setting of isolated residual adenopathy in the neck, PET-CT is a particularly sensitive test and can be useful in the setting of isolated regional persistent/recurrent disease because if the neck disease is not metabolically active, it does not necessarily require a salvage neck dissection (18).

In their prospective study of 44 patients with head and neck cancer who received definitive chemoradiotherapy (CRT), Wang et al. reported that the sensitivity and specificity of the first post-CRT PET scan to detect residual primary tumors, performed at 12 to 17 weeks after the completion of CRT, were 100% and 91%, respectively (19). Several authors have reported that PET has superior accuracy to conventional imaging in assessing head and neck squamous cell carcinoma (HNSCC) patients after CRT. The sensitivity and specificity of PET in identifying persistent disease were 88% to 100% and 75% to 100%, respectively, compared with the 70% to 92% and 50% to 57% for CT and MRI, respectively (20–22). In contrast, other studies reported that PET had a high false-positive rate and suggested that PET should be added in the post-CRT evaluation of residual or recurrent cervical metastasis (23,24). With regard to the false-positive problem of PET, one meta-analysis reported that the correct diagnosis rate was high over 10 weeks after CRT (25), whereas other studies reported that a negative result 12 weeks after radiotherapy completion was more reliable than a negative result obtained at an earlier time point (26–28). On this basis, the use of PET to detect residual or recurrent head and neck cancer at 10 to 12 weeks after radiotherapy appears reasonable as an excellent rule-out (sensitive) test but with poor specificity, and therefore, positive results need careful further investigation to confirm locoregional recurrence. In general, reliance on a single modality is problematic, and recurrence or residual tumor after primary treatment should be carefully assessed using several modalities.

A number of factors determine the likelihood of successful salvage treatment. The disease-free interval, defined as the period between treatment of the initial tumor and the diagnosis of the recurrence, appears to be an important predictor of successful salvage (29–31). The longer this period, the better the outcome, particularly for those with more than 12 months elapsed after the completion of treatment (32). Other predictors include the local and regional extent of the initial tumor, the location of the recurrent tumor, and the initial treatment modality (or combination) used (29). Tumor stage is another strong predictor of successful salvage with T1/T2 tumors performing significantly better than T3/T4 tumors (33). Tumor subsite is a critical predictor of salvage success. A large series from Switzerland demonstrated that patients with recurrent laryngeal cancers have the best salvage rates (49%), while those with hypopharyngeal cancers had the lowest successful salvage rates (17%) (34). Patients with oral cavity and oropharyngeal cancers have intermediate salvage rates (33–35%) (34).

Quoted salvage rates are dependent on the quality of the workup; optimal evaluation should include an experienced head and neck oncologist, multidisciplinary consultation including tumor board discussion, thorough imaging reviewed by head and neck radiologists, and intraoperative assessment (35). Several studies have demonstrated a volume-outcome association in the surgical and nonsurgical management of head and neck cancers (36), and this effect is likely accentuated in the management of recurrent disease.

MANAGEMENT: GENERAL

Surgical salvage, when feasible, yields better survival outcomes for patients with recurrent HNSCC compared to radiotherapy or concurrent CRT and has long been the standard of care (30,35). However, when presenting the patient with treatment options it is important to weigh the survival benefit with the likely side effects of treatment as salvage treatment can pose significant implications on quality of life. Other possible treatment options with curative intent, particularly for those who are not surgical candidates, include radiotherapy (or reirradiation) and concurrent CRT. Palliative treatment can include radiotherapy or chemotherapy usually as single modality, with the goal of improving symptom control and increasing survival but generally without a chance for cure. The National Comprehensive Cancer Network (NCCN) guidelines have recommended enrolling patients in clinical trials in the setting of disease recurrence, particularly for those in whom a curative treatment approach has a very low likelihood of success and for those patients who do not wish to proceed with aggressive treatment (17). Human papillomavirus (HPV) status does not currently impact the management of primary or recurrent head and neck cancer according to the NCCN guidelines, despite having significant prognostic implications (17). The impact of HPV status on the success of salvage treatment has yet to be studied, but with the rising incidence of oropharyngeal HNSCC, this can be a topic for clinical trials moving forward.

We have organized the remainder of the chapter by treatment modality while discussing particular tumor subsites in each section, given the heterogeneity inherent in treating recurrent HNSCC. Nasopharyngeal recurrence is discussed separately with all treatment modalities discussed at one time, given its unique treatment approach in the salvage setting.

MANAGEMENT: SALVAGE SURGERY

Although salvage surgery, when recurrent disease is resectable, provides the best chance of cure, it is associated with significant morbidity and mortality (2). The morbidity and mortality rates in a systematic review with a pooled analysis are 39% and 5%, respectively. These rates are much higher than those observed for most head and neck procedures in the nonsalvage setting.

Not all patients are surgical candidates owing to either tumor or host factors. Tumor factors that preclude surgery include prevertebral fascia invasion, skull base invasion, and greater than 270-degree circumferential encasement of the internal carotid artery. Patient factors are discussed in depth in the reirradiation portion of this chapter.

LARYNGEAL CANCER RECURRENCE

Of all HNSCC subsites, laryngeal cancer recurrence has the best success with salvage surgery because patients present with early voice, airway, or swallowing dysfunction. Furthermore, the larynx possesses unique anatomic barriers to the spread of disease, unlike other head and neck mucosal sites. Lastly, particularly for the glottic subsite, there is limited lymphatic spread in early disease. In a thorough systematic review and meta-analysis on salvage surgery, early-stage recurrent disease had a pooled analysis 5-year survival rate of 85%, while the more advanced disease had a 5-year survival rate of 48% (2). A large single-institution study from MD Anderson Hospital demonstrated that the 5-year disease control and overall survival were 65% and 57%, respectively, for all comers (37). The most interesting finding from this study, however, is that patients with a short disease-free interval (<2 years) were more likely to develop a second recurrence after salvage laryngectomy and die from their disease. This, again, demonstrates the pronounced impact of the disease-free interval after definitive radiotherapy on disease control in the salvage setting. Patients with a >5 year disease-free interval had a higher disease control rate (92%) than those with a short (<2 year) disease-free interval.

The standard of care in recurrent laryngeal SCC remains total laryngectomy. This is particularly true for recurrent advanced (T3/T4) disease. However, early disease (T1/T2) may be amenable to conservation surgery in the form of transoral laser surgery and open partial laryngectomies (vertical or horizontal) with better results than total laryngectomy in appropriately selected patients (38). Reported survival in this latter group is excellent (93% 5-year disease-specific survival) (39). This is particularly true when transoral laser surgery is used after primary radiotherapy, although patients may require multiple laser resections to clear the disease (38,40,41). In advanced tumors (T3/T4), this sort of treatment is not recommended because of the significant risk of chondronecrosis, and because it yields a much lower chance of curing the disease (41).

Conservative open laryngeal surgery is contraindicated in patients with interarytenoid invasion, arytenoid fixation, extralaryngeal spread, subglottic extension, and pre-epiglottic space invasion (38). These patients require comprehensive and lengthy (months) rehabilitative programs to achieve adequate functional outcomes, decannulation, and oral intake without risk of developing aspiration pneumonia. Therefore, patients need to be motivated to undergo this sort of rehabilitation prior to proceeding with partial open laryngeal procedures. It is also important for patients in this group to demonstrate good pulmonary reserve. Based on these indications and contraindications, the number of patients qualifying for this type of salvage surgery is rather limited. Furthermore, the ablative technique requires advanced training and is not performed by all head and neck surgical oncologists.

For these reasons, total laryngectomy continues to be the gold standard and the most commonly performed laryngeal salvage procedure in the recurrent setting. It is indicated for advanced (T3/T4) recurrent disease in patients with poor pulmonary reserve and in those with a nonfunctioning larynx who are tracheostomy and gastrostomy tube dependent. Many patients with nonfunctioning larynx have severe chondronecrosis of the larynx, and in that setting, it is difficult to distinguish this complication from recurrent or persistent disease. In patients who have a nonfunctioning larynx with chondronecrosis, recurrent or persistent disease is often detected in the final laryngectomy specimen (42).

Reconstruction in the salvage laryngectomy setting is not always required if there is sufficient pharyngeal mucosa for a tensionless primary closure. Pharyngocutaneous fistula is the most common major wound complication in patients undergoing salvage laryngectomy and can be life threatening if not managed aggressively because the carotid arteries can be exposed in the wound. There is strong evidence to suggest that incorporating healthy nonirradiated mucosa into the pharyngeal closure in the form of a pectoralis major flap significantly decreases fistula rates (from 45% to 10%) (43). A study comparing a retrospective single center cohort to the Radiation Therapy Oncology Group (RTOG) 91-11 cohort demonstrated that free flap reconstruction for salvage laryngectomy did not decrease fistula rates, but that fistulas were smaller, did not result in exposed major vessels, and could be effectively managed with outpatient wound care (43). A more recent multi-institutional collaborative study demonstrated that regional/free flaps decreased the rate of fistula rates in the salvage setting compared to primary closure (34%) (44). Regional pectoralis major onlay graft without incorporation of the skin paddle into the pharynx had lower fistula rates (15%) when compared to free flaps incorporated into the pharyngeal closure as an inlay graft (25%). However, incorporating the flap into the pharyngeal closure results in lower stricture rates and gastrostomy tube dependence rates (45). Pharyngocutaneous fistula is associated with significantly increased hospital length of stay and delay in speech and swallowing functioning (44,45).

ORAL CAVITY CANCER RECURRENCE

Recurrence in the oral cavity happens equally locally, locoregionally, and regionally with only rare isolated metastatic disease (46–48); the locoregional recurrence rate, depending on the series, is 25% to 48% (30). Salvage treatment, typically with surgery, results in moderate (43%) 5-year survival results (2,48), although this rate is lower for local recurrences (39%) and combined locoregional recurrence (27%) (48).

Salvage surgery often requires a substantially larger resection of the previous surgical bed. The approach is often more extensive and should be tailored to the extent of the disease. A mandibulotomy can be useful for tumors in the posterior oral cavity, particularly if there is an extension to the oropharynx, although this is rarely required. More extensive surgery may involve a mandibulectomy if the tumor is abutting or invading the mandibular cortex. More extensive surgery in the oral cavity may also mean a total glossectomy, which is associated with poor functional outcomes despite advanced reconstructive techniques (49). On rare occasions, patients may require a total glossectomy with a total laryngectomy due to a significant supraglottic extension of the tumor. This is arguably one of the most functionally devastating operations performed for head and neck cancer as patients are often left unable to speak or swallow (49,50). Patients with recurrent disease, particularly if they have been previously irradiated, more often require reconstructive approaches to improve wound healing, although no studies have demonstrated improved wound healing with free tissue transfer in this group. Most patients with recurrent oral cavity HNSCC require a tracheotomy; however, in many practices, this is not always required and a well-secured nasal trumpet for 2 to 3 days postoperatively is often enough to bypass swelling in the oral cavity in the early postoperative period, even in patients receiving bulky free flap reconstructions, particularly if it is a lateralized defect (i.e., buccal mucosa or retromolar trigone).

OROPHARYNX RECURRENCE

Because of the epidemic rise in HPV-associated oropharyngeal cancer, despite excellent outcomes with radiotherapy with or without chemotherapy, there has also been an absolute rise in the number of treatment failures at this head and neck subsite (51). The rise in HPV-associated oropharyngeal cancer has led to improvements in survival; and HPV-positive patients have a lower rate of locoregional recurrence (14%) compared to HPV-negative patients (36.5%) (52,53). However, recurrent disease is associated with equally poor survival outcomes for HPV-positive and -negative patients (54–56). Sweeny et al. demonstrated that recurrence occurs more often in smokers, regardless of HPV status (56). Furthermore, despite aggressive treatment, 33% of patients developed a new recurrence after salvage surgery with a higher incidence among HPV-negative patients. Overall survival was lower among those with recurrent cervical metastases, advanced tumor stage, and dependence on gastrostomy tube postoperatively with an overall 5-year survival rate of only 23% (56). A systematic review and meta-analysis evaluating the efficacy, outcomes, and complication rates of different treatment modalities for recurrent and residual oropharyngeal carcinoma demonstrated that the pooled overall 5-year survival rate in this group was 23% (95% confidence interval [CI] 20% to 27%), although this rate was higher and improved with the treatment decade (57).

The same review demonstrated that salvage treatment with surgery was superior to radiation therapy (5-year pooled overall survival 26% vs. 16%, respectively; $p < .001$) (57). Despite this, recurrence-free survival remains quite poor in this group even with surgical salvage: 19% at 5 years (55). Predictors of survival include nodal disease at the time of recurrence, close or positive margins, and lymphovascular invasion. Currently, the NCCN guidelines do not recommend making treatment decisions based on HPV status for patients with oropharyngeal HNSCC, although a variety of clinical trials are assessing the possibility of de-escalating treatment in the HPV positive group (17). Little is known about the impact of de-escalating treatment in the recurrent setting, but acknowledging that patients with HPV-positive and -negative tumors have similar survival, albeit from small retrospective series with relatively small sample sizes, it is unlikely that HPV status would influence treatment approach in the recurrent setting.

Small tumors and limited disease can be managed with transoral resection; however, patients often present with treatment-related factors, including trismus and soft tissue fibrosis, which limit the success of this approach. These limitations affect the success of new techniques such as transoral robotic surgery (TORS); however, to date, the two studies assessing the use of TORS in this patient population have yielded excellent results (58,59). White et al. performed a multi-institution stage-matched pair analysis and demonstrated lower tracheotomy and gastrostomy tube use, shorter overall hospital stay, decreased operative time, less blood loss, and lower rates of positive margins among patients treated with TORS (n = 64) compared to matched pairs treated with open surgery (n = 64) (59). After controlling for disease stage, 2-year recurrence-free survival was significantly higher in the TORS group compared to the open surgery group (74% and 43%, respectively) (59). A more recent randomized study demonstrated low operative blood loss, low gastrostomy tube rates, low positive margin rate (6.7%), and comparable survival (median survival of 19 months) (58). These early results suggest that TORS may be useful in a subset of patients with recurrent oropharyngeal cancer, namely, those with limited T1/T2 disease, accessible tumor location, and favorable anatomy for good exposure (good neck extension, edentulous, no trismus, and appropriately arched palate). Further study is required; patients treated with this approach should be informed of the experimental nature of the use of this tool for the management of their disease. A clinical trial comparing TORS to open salvage surgery is unlikely to accrue sufficient patients; and additional retrospective series will ultimately provide the best available evidence to address this question.

For patients not amenable to TORS and with more advanced disease, the standard of care continues to be an open salvage procedure. This often requires a tracheotomy, mandibulotomy, or mandibulectomy and a free flap for reconstruction of the soft tissue with or without bony reconstruction. In this group there is a high tracheostomy and gastrostomy tube dependence, 15% and 65%, respectively (55). The complication rate in this group is high and a longer than usual length of hospital stay can be expected in those patients who have these complications (55). Furthermore, some of these patients, similar to those with advanced recurrent oral cancers, can require a total or near total glossectomy (sometimes with a total laryngectomy) to achieve negative margins; as previously mentioned this is associated with high morbidity and poor quality of life scores.

HYPOPHARYNX RECURRENCE

Of all of the head and neck cancer sites discussed, hypopharyngeal cancer has the worst survival and is associated with the poorest quality of life. There is often a high residual disease burden after curative treatment (20%), and 50% of first recurrences have regional or distant metastatic components (60). By 3 years, after primary curative treatment, 53% of patients have a local, locoregional, or regional recurrence. Although there is no difference in survival between primary surgery followed by adjuvant radiotherapy and primary radiotherapy (with or without chemotherapy) in patients with hypopharyngeal cancer (61), laryngeal preservation is higher in patients treated with nonsurgical approaches, which has led to an increased use of concurrent CRT as a primary approach in this patient population (62). However, the addition of chemotherapy to radiotherapy in this patient population has not improved survival compared to radiotherapy alone, although this remains controversial (62).

Many patients with hypopharyngeal cancer experience disease recurrence, and unfortunately this group has the lowest salvage rate (<20%) among recurrent HNSCC subsites

(34,63). Salvage surgery is the best treatment approach in the recurrent disease setting as demonstrated by Yasumatsu et al., who showed that salvage surgery followed by chemotherapy and/or radiotherapy resulted in a 79% 3-year disease-free survival rate, whereas there were no survivors among those treated with salvage chemotherapy and/or radiotherapy (64). However, surgical salvage is only possible in fewer than 1 in 4 patients (63). Successful surgical salvage is strongly correlated with T stage (T1 33%, T2 20%, T3 17%, T4 0%) (63). Initial stage IV disease and concurrent regional relapse predict worse outcomes in the salvage setting (65).

Local resection is rarely possible in recurrent hypopharyngeal cancer because of the aggressive nature of the disease, tumor invasion into adjacent vital structures, and the propensity for the disease to spread submucosally. Total laryngopharyngectomy is the salvage operation of choice requiring a circumferential reconstruction. Using this approach some groups have been able to achieve a 31% 5-year overall survival (66). However, this approach is associated with severe postoperative complications including a high rate of pharyngocutaneous fistula (50%) despite free flap reconstruction (63). Hypocalcemia occurs in 44% of patients and 15% have long-term pharyngeal stricture (66). The reconstruction of the defect in these patients is one of the most challenging, particularly in those patients with resected cervical esophageal submucosal disease. Both positive margins and free flap failure in the salvage setting are associated with poorer overall and disease-free survival (67).

NASOPHARYNGEAL CANCER (NPC) RECURRENCE

Radiotherapy with or without concurrent chemotherapy is very effective in the management of NPC, but nonetheless 8.3% of patients have local residual or recurrent tumor (68) and 1.6% have isolated regional failure (69). Close follow-up and early detection of recurrence or residual disease are critical to achieving good oncologic outcomes in this population.

Isolated neck recurrence in NPC is better treated with radical neck dissection (5-year local control of 66% and overall survival of 38%) (70) compared to reirradiation (5-year local control 51% and overall survival 19.7%); the latter is also associated with higher local complication rates (71). Radical neck dissection should include a thorough dissection of all nodal levels in the neck, particularly the posterior neck, because of a high rate of occult nodes in clinical node negative levels of the neck (72). Rarely, some patients with small localized neck recurrences may not require level I nodal dissection (73).

Residual or recurrent disease in the nasopharynx is typically managed with reirradiation but the radiation dose generally has to be higher than the original dose that failed to prevent local recurrence or capture residual tumor. Reirradiation is often combined with chemotherapeutic agents such as radiosensitizers in patients who can tolerate combined modality therapy. There are significant complications from this approach including but not limited to temporal lobe necrosis, multiple cranial neuropathies, and deafness, particularly with conventional radiotherapy techniques (74,75). Brachytherapy is an option in tumors that do not involve the eustachian tube cartilage and in small tumors that can be accessed for brachytherapy grain implantation. It is associated with better results than other radiotherapy techniques (intensity-modulated radiotherapy [IMRT] or stereotactic body radiotherapy [SBRT]) demonstrating 5-year local control rates of 87% for residual and 63% for recurrent NPC in the salvage setting (76).

Salvage surgery is reserved for cases in which reirradiation is not an option because of either tumor location or extent. Salvage surgery can be performed using one of two approaches: endoscopic or open (maxillary swing). Regardless of surgical approach, successful surgical salvage is heavily dependent on tumor removal with negative margins (77). Endoscopic approaches are only applicable to small tumors that can be easily accessed endoscopically with good margins, typically tumors of the posterior nasopharygeal wall.

The surgical standard of care for patients who do not qualify for reirradiation is a maxillary swing procedure, the only procedure that provides adequate exposure to the lateral nasopharynx. This procedure involves a Weber–Ferguson facial incision and three osteotomies: anterior maxillary wall (from the nasal bones to the lower zygomatic arch), on the hard palate just lateral to the lingual surface of the maxillary gingiva, and lastly between the maxillary tuberosity and the pterygoid plates posteriorly. With this approach the entire maxilla is opened and displaced laterally and an excellent open view of the nasopharynx is achieved. Encouraging results are achieved with this approach; 5-year local control, and overall survival has been as high as 74% and 56%, respectively, although surgical selection bias is likely (78).

Even when patients develop a second localized recurrence after initial salvage reirradiation with or without chemotherapy, surgical salvage appears to be a viable option in selected individuals with reasonable functional and survival outcomes (79).

NECK DISSECTION—SALVAGE SURGERY FOR REGIONALLY RECURRENT OR PERSISTENT DISEASE

Necks that have been previously treated with radiotherapy or surgery with no evidence of disease at the time of local recurrence do not necessarily need to be managed with neck dissection at the time of salvage surgery. An excellent study evaluated elective neck dissection in the clinically N0 setting in patients with isolated cervical recurrence and found a negligible rate of occult nodal metastases in this population (80). Furthermore, performing neck dissections in this patient population was associated with a high complication rate (40%). The neck should be treated if there is clinical evidence of disease or if the neck has never been treated in the past. Even when the neck has been previously treated, the neck is nearly always surgically explored for free flap donor vessels given that many patients require free flap reconstruction in the recurrent disease setting.

ISOLATED NECK RECCURENCE

With increased uptake of organ preservation approaches, there is a rise in the need to manage the neck in the posttreatment setting for residual and recurrent disease. PET-CT in the posttreatment setting, usually 1 to 3 months after completion of radiotherapy, has been used by some but with poor specificity. It is, however, a useful adjunct when trying to avoid neck dissection in this population as it is rarely negative when viable tumor remains in the neck (negative predictive value of 97%) (81). When there is a complete response to treatment and the initial disease was not bulky (N1), there is no need to dissect the neck. However, with high volume disease (N2 or greater), the decision is controversial. Neck dissection in this setting is often planned at the outset of treatment because the likelihood of a complete response is low and the results with salvage surgery are poor. In our practice, these patients are observed; if there is evidence of residual disease or if the neck has PET avid activity, the neck is dissected.

Salvage neck dissection for isolated neck recurrence is associated with poor outcomes; however, patients with recurrent N1 disease and those treated with primary surgery tend to have better salvage outcomes (32). A delay between completion of treatment and emergence of recurrence (>6 months) is also associated with improved outcomes (82). The management of the neck is preferably surgical because it is associated with better 3-year overall survival (36%) compared to nonsurgical salvage with chemoradiotherapy (12%) (32). One study showed that without surgical salvage the median survival is only 6 months (83). Whether the neck has been previously treated also influences survival. Once series documented a 5-year disease-free survival rate of 32% for unilateral nodal recurrence in a previously untreated neck, but only 18% for those with a previously treated neck (83). The most important predictor of poor outcomes in this group is evidence of extracapsular spread in the salvage neck dissection specimen; in this setting adjuvant radiotherapy or chemoradiotherapy is beneficial (82,84).

MANAGEMENT: REIRRADIATION

In the locoregionally recurrent disease setting, there are three distinct roles for reirradiation. Reirradiation can be used as an adjuvant treatment after salvage surgery; it can be used as the primary modality of treatment for patients who are not candidates for surgery but are candidates for curative treatment; and finally, it can be used in the palliative setting for symptom control. In this section we discuss the indications, contraindications, and outcomes with each of these approaches.

A substantial portion of previously irradiated patients with locoregional head and neck cancer recurrence present with unresectable recurrence. Surgery is precluded in cases in which there is prevertebral fascia invasion, skull base invasion, and greater than 270-degree circumferential encasement of the internal carotid artery. In the setting of primary management of head and neck cancer, carotid artery sacrifice is performed with reasonable results. Carotid sacrifice in the setting of salvage surgery is associated with significant complications and poor outcomes and therefore is rarely recommended (85). Palliative treatment is often the most appropriate recommendation. Many patient factors preclude the use of salvage surgery. Patients with a high perioperative mortality risk, from myocardial infarction or stroke, are not good surgical salvage candidates. Patients on irreversible anticoagulants (with the exception of aspirin), which cannot be stopped because of recent revascularization procedures, are also not good surgical candidates, but can undergo definite reirradiation. Some patients in the salvage setting elect to undergo reirradiation over salvage surgery for personal reasons, but because of the aforementioned evidence of poorer disease-free and overall survival, this approach is less favored.

Careful patient selection is required to minimize treatment-related morbidity and mortality. Common selection criteria include patients who have been out from primary radiotherapy for more than 6 months, have an ECOG of 0 to 2, and can receive additional therapy without exceeding a cumulative dose to the spinal cord of 50 to 60 Gy (86). Patients whose disease recurs within 6 months of radiation are typically not candidates for reirradiation as their tumor is likely radioresistant and further irradiation would provide little benefit. This is particularly true for patients who have who received concurrent chemotherapy with their radiotherapy. Radiosensitizing chemotherapy is typically considered to overcome radioresistance. Other strategies that have shown success in this setting include altered fractionation schedules and brachytherapy (87,88). Patients whose disease recurs at >1 year appear to have a longer progression-free interval but treatment-related mortality and morbidity can be seen in 10% and 33% (severe), respectively (35).

Every attempt is made to minimize the planning target volumes (PTVs) because 96% of failures recur within the irradiated volume and 4% occur outside the high-dose volumes (89). The neck is not usually electively treated because of the high morbidity and low risk of regional disease when the neck has been previously treated.

Guidelines or consensus on the dose and scheme that should be used in the reirradiation setting are lacking. Favorable results have been reported with doses of 60 Gy (87,90). The largest and most recent series on this topic analyzed 166 patients who were treated with a median dose of 66 Gy; this group has advocated for this dose in the reirradiation setting (91). However, the results are universally poor with 2-year overall survival and disease-free survival rates of 25% and 20%, respectively. Most concerning was that one fifth (20%) of patients died of treatment-related toxicity. Prior CRT has been shown to be a negative predictor of overall survival, whereas surgery prior to reirradiation, full dose reirradiation, and a longer radiotherapy interval portend better overall survival outcomes.

REIRRADIATION AFTER SURGICAL SALVAGE

Reirradiation after surgical salvage is a feasible, safe, and important adjunct treatment. A single randomized trial has investigated this question looking at patients who have had macroscopic complete resection of their recurrent head and neck cancer and then been randomized to CRT (60 Gy; 5-fluorouracil and hydroxyurea) or watchful waiting (92). This resulted in improved disease-free survival (hazard ratio [HR] 1.68 95% CI 1.13 to 2.50) but not overall survival with an increase in both acute and late toxicity in the CRT arm. For this reason, there is a huge variability in radiation oncologists' practice. Most advocate for some postsurgical salvage reirradiation when there are high-risk features such as positive margins, extracapsular spread, perineural invasion, or lymphovascular invasion (93). With this approach, 3-year locoregional control and overall survival rates have been reported as high as 74% and 44%, respectively. Others have advocated that postsurgical salvage reirradiation be reserved only for those with positive margins or extracapsular extension (35), while others feel that all surgical salvage patients are high risk and warrant some form of reirradiation (94). This question has not been fully addressed and randomized trials are warranted to assess the impact of reirradiation dose as well as the impact of adding chemotherapy to reirradiation in the postsurgical salvage setting. We suspect that although chemotherapy is an important radiosensitizer to overcome radioresistance in the reirradiation setting, the lack of difference in overall survival between groups is due to the additional toxicity associated with chemotherapy. Although this has not been specifically assessed in the recurrent HNSCC setting, it has been shown to be true particularly in patients over the age of 70 (95).

REIRRADIATION WITHOUT SALVAGE SURGERY

Although reirradiation without salvage surgery is less ideal than salvage surgery, it is sometimes the only treatment available for some patients owing to patient or tumor factors. Although many studies have suggested that this approach with or without concurrent chemotherapy can produce long-term survival (96–98), there has never been a trial comparing reirradiation with or without chemotherapy to chemotherapy alone. A trial to study this question is unlikely to accrue enough patients to answer the question.

Proton beam therapy (PBT) also holds promise in reducing treatment-related morbidity in reirradiation. Proton beams are characterized by their rapid fall-off at the distal end of the Bragg peak and sharp lateral penumbra, depending on energy, depth, and delivery (99). These physical characteristics give proton beam therapy better dose distribution than x-ray irradiation, and PBT is now deemed a feasible and effective treatment modality that provides curative high-dose irradiation to the tumor volume without increasing normal tissue toxicity.

Nevertheless, only a few retrospective studies of reirradiation in clinical practice have yet appeared (100). A prospective trial to compare PBT with IMRT or other radiation techniques in previously irradiated patients with local recurrence is urgently required.

IMRT is associated with superior locoregional progression-free survival compared to external beam radiotherapy (52% vs. 20%; $p < .01$) (101). Stereotactic body radiotherapy (SBRT) has also been investigated with acceptable results because it can reduce PTV margin using image-guided high-precision repositioning (102). SBRT allows for hypofractionation with the delivery of large doses in fewer fractions and is best administered where there is low-volume well-visualized disease (103–105). Despite a lower mean dose (35 Gy), one study demonstrated that the 1-year and 2-year local control rates were 51% and 31%, respectively. More importantly, there were no grade 4 or 5 treatment-related toxicities (103). Reirradiation with a dose up to 50 Gy in five fractions is feasible with a higher dose being associated with improved locoregional control rates and higher tumor volume benefiting from a larger total dose (106). A recent systematic review demonstrated that the 1-year overall survival rates with SBRT are similar to those for chemotherapy alone and concurrent conventionally fractioned CRT (107).

Reirradiation is associated with significant morbidity with at least one third of patients experiencing grade 3 to 4 toxicity. With reirradiation there is the risk of osteoradionecrosis, fistulas, skin/wound breakdown, stroke and major vessel rupture, and necrosis (108). Risks of severe complications are lower when patients have had a longer disease-free interval before reirradiation and when the PTV is low (<100 cm^3) (109). Another study reported equally poor outcomes with a 46% 1-year overall survival and 75% of patients experiencing grade 3 to 4 toxicity (96).

PALLIATIVE REIRRADIATION

There are limited data comparing palliative reirradiation and palliative chemotherapy; however, historically, palliative reirradiation was reserved for symptom control. Now with the advent of SBRT, palliative radiotherapy produces comparable survival and toxicity results to palliative chemotherapy (107). SBRT has a natural advantage compared to conventionally fractioned radiotherapy in that treatment can be provided in three to five high-dose fractions and can take less than 2 weeks. This results in a lower overall dose and, therefore, decreased acute toxicity. Higher dose per fraction schedules are associated with significant late effects but this may not be relevant in the palliative population.

MANAGEMENT: ADDITION OF CHEMOTHERAPY TO REIRRADIATION

A brief discussion is warranted in this chapter about the use of chemotherapy with reirradiation, although the next chapter (Chapter 23) is dedicated to this topic and will address it in far more detail.

Many trials have studied concurrent CRT in the salvage setting and different chemotherapeutic combinations have been devised for this indication. To date, no studies have compared these regimens head to head. In this setting, it is also important to distinguish those studies evaluating chemoradiation in the adjuvant setting after surgical salvage from those employing definitive chemotherapy and reirradiation as primary treatment in those patients whose recurrences prove unresectable. We suggest that well-vetted institutional protocols with an established safety record be used until such studies are completed. Ideally, as part of these protocols, the agent used should be one to which the patient is treatment-naive. There is evidence supporting the addition of chemotherapy to reirradiation in patients who have extracapsular extension, with one study demonstrating a significant improvement in 5-year disease-specific survival (47%)

compared to salvage surgery alone (15%) or salvage surgery with adjuvant radiotherapy alone (36%) (84). Positive margins are also a key indication for postsurgical salvage chemotherapy with reirradiation; however, no study has specifically examined its impact in this population.

One of the best-studied regimens consists of 5-fluorouracil and hydroxyurea in combination with reirradiation; this offers a potential advantage in that it omits cisplatin, which is often administered in the primary treatment setting. However, this combination of medications has not yielded especially promising results and continues to be associated with poor outcomes (90,91). A variety of other combinations have been studied such as cisplatin alone or with 5-fluorouracil and hydroxyurea (110), cisplatin and paclitaxel (111), carboplatin/paclitaxel (112), and docetaxel/cisplatin (113).

One study, spearheaded by the RTOG, evaluated split-course reirradiation (1.5 Gy twice daily × 5 every other week to a total dose of 60 Gy) in combination with daily low-dose radiosensitizing cisplatin and paclitaxel as primary therapy for unresectable locoregional recurrence, with growth factor support given during the nontreatment weeks (111). The median prior radiation dose was 65.4 Gy. Of 105 patients enrolled, 74% completed chemotherapy. However, grade 4 or worse acute toxicity occurred in 28%, with 8 treatment-related deaths; 5 in the acute setting and 3 as outpatients (including two carotid hemorrhages). Median survival time was 12.1 months, with 1- and 2-year overall survival rates of 50.2% and 25.9%, respectively. An attempt to compare this regimen to chemotherapy alone in the setting of unresectable locoregional recurrence was aborted because of poor accrual.

Table 22.2 lists some of the new clinical trials investigating the role of targeted therapy and immunotherapy in the salvage setting, sometimes in combination with the previously described chemotherapeutic agents with or without concurrent radiotherapy. There is substantial interest in immunotherapy, and early results suggest that this approach may be useful in patients with recurrent HNSCC. In a phase 3 trial for patients with recurrent HNSCC whose disease progressed within 6 months after platinum-based chemotherapy, patients were randomized to receive single agent nivolumab (an anti-PD-1 [programmed cell death protein 1] monoclonal antibody) versus single agent systematic therapy (methotrexate, docetaxel, or cetuximab) (114). Overall survival, the primary end point, was significantly better in the nivolumab arm than with standard therapy, 36% and 17%, respectively (p = .01). These results are promising and have led to the approval of nivolumab in recurrent/metastatic HNSCC after platinum "failure." In this context, either alone or in combination with a variety of targeted therapies currently undergoing investigation, we suspect that the recurrent head and neck cancer patient of the future will almost certainly be much more treatable as time goes on. Nonetheless, surgery still offers the best chance of cure and reirradiation with chemotherapy should be reserved for the adjuvant setting or for those with unresectable tumor.

CONCLUSIONS

Management of locoregionally recurrent HNSCC is challenging, and outcomes are generally poor with the exception of recurrent laryngeal carcinoma and NPC. Typically, the best management approach is surgical salvage followed by radiation or reirradiation using IMRT/SBRT. Chemotherapy can be added for patients with positive margins or extracapsular spread. Palliative radiotherapy and chemotherapy, separately or together, are also options for incurable disease.

TABLE 22.2

Active Clinical Trials Studying Targeted Therapies (Recurrent HNSCC)*

Target	Clinical Trial Name
EGFR-R	Phase I/II Dose Escalation Trial of Induction and Concomitant Erlotinib and Celecoxib With Radiation Therapy for Treatment of Poor Prognosis Head and Neck Cancer, Including Re-irradiation (NCT00970502)

(continued)

TABLE 22.2 (*continued*)

Active Clinical Trials Studying Targeted Therapies (Recurrent HNSCC)*

PD-1	A Phase 3 Clinical Trial of Pembrolizumab (MK-3475) in First Line Treatment of Recurrent/ Metastatic HNSCC (NCT02358031)
EGFR-R	Phase II Study of the Combination of Panitumumab With Paclitaxel as First-line Treatment of Subjects With Metastatic or Recurrent Head and Neck Cancer (NCT01264328)
PD-1	A Phase II Trial of Reirradiation Combined With Open Label MK-3475 (Pembrolizumab) in Patients With Locoregional Inoperable Recurrence or Second Primary HNSCC (NCT02358031)
PI3K	A Phase II, Multicenter Trial Aiming to Evaluate the Clinical Interest of a Monotherapy With BKM120, a PI3K Inhibitor in Patient With Metastatic Head and Neck Cancer Recurrent or Progressive Under Platin and Cetuximab-based Chemotherapy (NCT01737450)
PD-1	A Single Arm Phase I/II Study of MK-3475 Combined With Vorinostat for Recurrent Unresectable and/or Metastatic Squamous Cell Head and Neck Cancer and Recurrent Unresectable and/or Metastatic Salivary Gland Malignacies (NCT02538510)
PD-1 and CTLA-4	A Phase III Randomized, Open-label, Multi-center, Global Study of MEDI4736 Alone or in Combination With Tremelimumab Versus Standard of Care in the Treatment of First-line Recurrent or Metastatic Squamous Cell Head and Neck Cancer Patients (NCT02551159)
PD-1, CTLA-4 and EGFR-R	An Open Label, Randomized, Two Arm Phase III Study of Nivolumab in Combination With Ipilimumab Versus Extreme Study Regimen (Cetuximab + Cisplatin/Carboplatin + Fluorouracil) as First Line Therapy in Recurrent or HNSCC (NCT02741570)
PD-1	Immunomodulation of Pembrolizumab Plus Docetaxel for the Treatment of Recurrent or Metastatic (R/M) HNSCC After Platinum Failure (NCT02718820)
PD-1 and CTLA-4	A Double-Blind, Randomized, Two Arm Phase 2 Study of Nivolumab in Combination With Ipilimumab Versus Nivolumab in Combination With Ipilimumab Placebo in Recurrent or Metastatic HNSCC (NCT02823574)

*This list is not inclusive but includes a range of the newest trials (115).

HNSCC, head and neck squamous cell carcinoma.

CASE 22.1: RECURRENT HYPOPHARYNGEAL HNSCC

At the age of 43, a 100 pack-year male smoker presented with a T2N2bM0 (stage IVA) SCC of the right piriform sinus. He underwent primary concurrent CRT with cisplatin and 50 Gy to the hypopharynx and bilateral neck sites with an additional 20 Gy boost to the primary site and the involved ipsilateral nodes.

He unfortunately developed a right cervical regional recurrence 9 months after completion of concurrent CRT. He underwent salvage modified radical neck dissection, which successfully cleared gross residual disease, but required sacrifice of the internal jugular vein. Pathologic examination revealed a single 1.3 cm positive node with extracapsular extension. Therefore, he received additional adjuvant treatment with 66 Gy and cetuximab.

Unfortunately, this resulted in chondronecrosis of his larynx and a large pharyngocutaneous fistula Figure 22.1. On physical examination, the greater cornu of the hyoid bone, the lateral border of the thyroid cartilage, and the thyroarytenoid joint were exposed. The cutaneous defect was approximately 7 cm craniocaudally and 4 cm laterally.

The patient opted to undergo a total laryngopharyngectomy because he had a nonfunctional larynx. The pathologic examination did not reveal any residual tumor. At the end of the ablation he had a total laryngopharyngectomy defect as well as a large 10 × 10 cm skin defect. He underwent a butterfly tubed reconstruction for pharyngeal reconstruction and to cover the cutaneous defect.

(*continued*)

CASE 22.1: RECURRENT HYPOPHARYNGEAL HNSCC (*continued*)

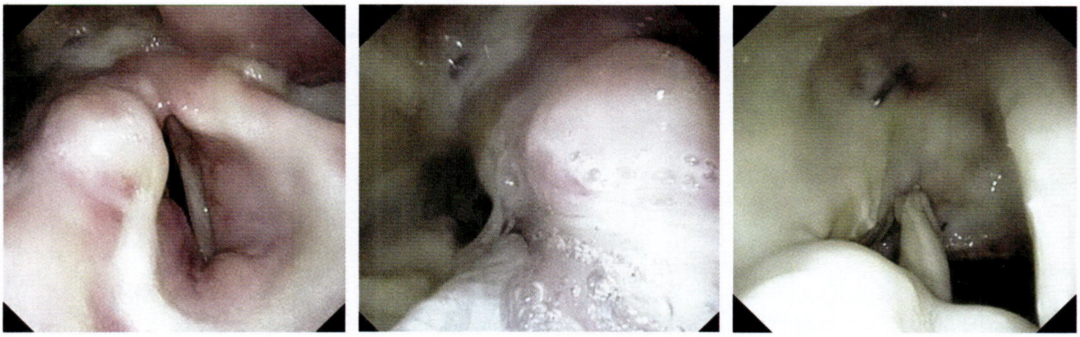

(A) (B) (C)

FIGURE 22.1 (A) Left piriform sinus ulceration and mucositis after reirradiation with chronic aspiration. (B) Deep right hypopharyngeal ulceration communication with skin (pharyngocutaneous fistula). (C) Further down in pharyngocutaneous fistula tract from endolaryngeal view demonstrating the exposed thyroarytenoid joint and cutaneous edges.

CASE 22.2: RECURRENT TONGUE BASE HNSCC DESPITE TRIPLE MODALITY TREATMENT

At the age of 67, an 80 pack-year male smoker presented with a T1N1M0 (stage III) HPV-positive SCC of the left tongue base and lateral pharyngeal wall. This was treated with a transoral robotic resection and a left selective neck dissection (levels II–IV). His final pathologic examination demonstrated a moderately differentiated 1.8 × 1.8 × 1.4 endophytic moderately differentiated SCC with close superior and deep margins despite a re-resection of the deep margin. There was evidence of angiolymphatic invasion but not perineural invasion. The neck specimen demonstrated 1 out of 43 involved nodes (2.8 cm) with 2 mm of extracapsular extension (ECE).

Because of the margin status and the ECE, the patient underwent adjuvant concurrent CRT with 66 Gy in 33 fractions with concurrent weekly carboplatin.

Fourteen months after the completion of treatment, he presented with the left floor of the mouth and tongue fullness and associated tenderness. A transcervical suprahyoid base of tongue fine-needle aspiration biopsy was performed after reviewing his CT scan (see Figure 22.2A–C). This confirmed recurrent SCC centered on the left tongue base but crossing midline measuring 3.16 × 3.61 × 2.40 cm with no concurrent neck disease (cT2N0M0).

A surgical salvage was attempted. This included a tracheotomy, lingual release approach resection of the entire floor of mouth, total glossectomy, and partial pharyngectomy. The left neck had been previously treated with both surgery and radiotherapy and was only minimally explored surgically as part of the resection, completing a level IA/IB neck dissection. The right neck was addressed surgically with a selective neck dissection (levels I–IV). He was reconstructed with a rectus abdominus perforator based fasciocutaneous free flap.

His final pathologic examination demonstrated a 3.8 × 2.8 × 1.8 cm endophytic moderately differentiated HPV-positive SCC with lymphovascular and perineural invasion. Both positive lymph nodes were in level I and were continguous with the tumor mass (pT2N2b). The remainder of the neck dissection did not reveal any lymphatic spread (2 out of 48 positive lymph nodes).

(*continued*)

CASE 22.2: RECURRENT TONGUE BASE HNSCC DESPITE TRIPLE MODALITY TREATMENT (*continued*)

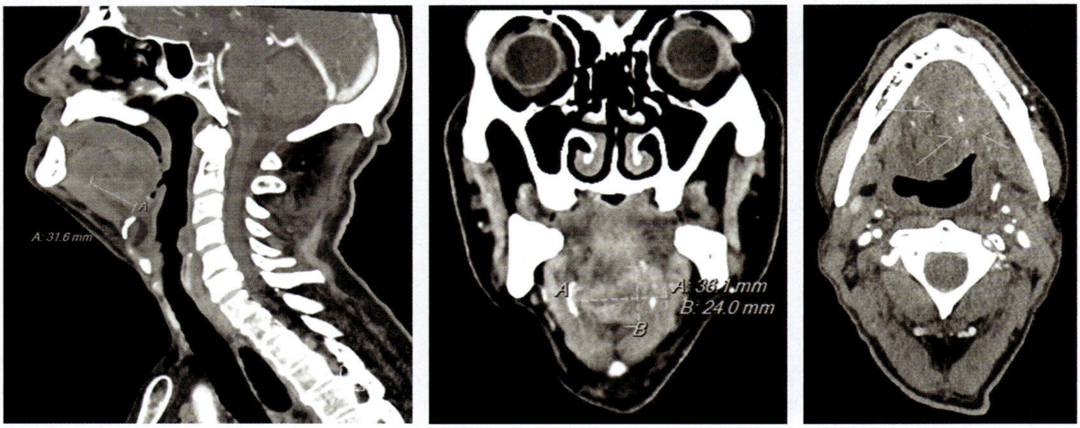

(A) (B) (C)

FIGURE 22.2 CT scan with contrast for recurrent base of tongue tumor: (A) sagittal; (B) coronal; (C) axial.

Intraoperatively the superior pre-epiglottic space margin was highly suspicious for SCC. After a re-resection of this region an intraoperative frozen section negative margin was achieved. Final pathologic examination demonstrated the re-resection specimen was negative.

After extensive discussion at the multidisciplinary tumor board, it was decided that reirradiation would benefit this patient given the advanced stage of recurrence and the perineural invasion demonstrated on final pathologic examination. Furthermore, the free flap reconstruction provided healthy vascularized tissue to the previously irradiated oropharyngeal and oral tissues.

CASE 22.3: RECURRENT LARYNGEAL CANCER

A 68-year-old woman presented with recurrent laryngeal cancer. Her initial treatment was primary radiotherapy, standard external beam treatment, 20 years prior with 70 Gy over 35 fractions. She then developed a second primary esophageal cancer 10 years after treatment of her laryngeal cancer with radiotherapy. She received a thoracolaparoscopic esophagectomy and three field lymphadenectomy, through a posterior mediastinal approach with gastric tube reconstruction.

During outpatient follow-up, the patient reported hoarseness at 8 years after esophageal surgery. Endoscopic findings showed left recurrent nerve palsy and tumor at the left vocal cord. Biopsy was done immediately, and the tumor in the laryngeal ventricle was diagnosed as SCC (T3N0MO). Endoscopic and CT findings are shown in Figure 22.3A and B.

We diagnosed this case as recurrent laryngeal cancer, not iatrogenic secondary laryngeal carcinoma, because the tumor occurred in nearly the same area previously treated for laryngeal cancer. Salvage total laryngectomy with pectoralis major musculocutaneous flap pharyngeal reconstruction and left neck dissection were planned. Findings of the surgery are shown in Figure 22.3C–F.

The postoperative course encountered no complications such as leakage, wound infection, or necrosis of the flap, and the patient was discharged 27 days after surgery.

(*continued*)

CASE 22.3: RECURRENT LARYNGEAL CANCER (*continued*)

Some key points to consider during salvage total laryngectomy are:

1. Avoid producing any unnecessary dead space and adding unnecessary surgical scar.
2. Reduce the range of skin flap elevation as much as possible.
3. Set the skin flap layer to deeper than usual, and make the flap thicker to maintain blood circulation in the skin flap.
4. When dead space is suspected preoperatively, consider the addition of reconstructive surgery to fill the dead space with tissue having good circulation.

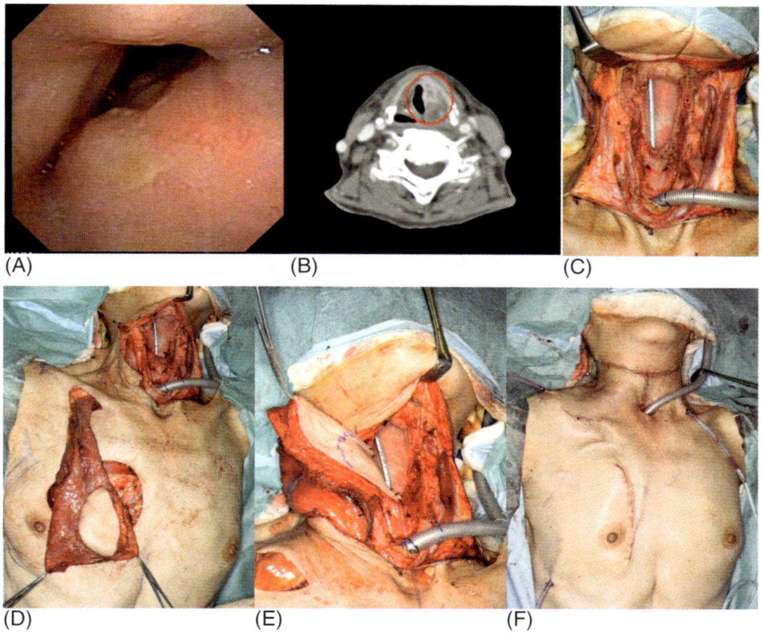

FIGURE 22.3 (A) The main tumor is in the left laryngeal ventricle, and had a poor margin and rough surface. (B) The main tumor extends from the laryngeal ventricle to the paraglottic space. (C) After resection. Surgery avoided the production of unnecessary dead space. (D) Elevation of the PMMC flap. (E) Suturing of the PMMC flap to the pharyngeal defect. (F) Closing the surgery incision.

REFERENCES

1. Marur S, Forastiere AA. Head and neck cancer: changing epidemiology, diagnosis, and treatment. *Mayo Clin Proc*. 2008;83(4):489–501. doi:10.4065/83.4.489
2. Goodwin WJ Jr. Salvage surgery for patients with recurrent squamous cell carcinoma of the upper aerodigestive tract: when do the ends justify the means? *Laryngoscope*. 2000;110(3 Pt 2 Suppl 93):1–18.
3. Day GL, Blot WJ, Shore RE, et al. Second cancers following oral and pharyngeal cancers: role of tobacco and alcohol. *J Natl Cancer Inst*. 1994;86(2):131–137.
4. Do KA, Johnson MM, Doherty DA, et al. Second primary tumors in patients with upper aerodigestive tract cancers: joint effects of smoking and alcohol (United States). *Cancer Causes Control*. 2003;14(2):131–138.
5. Leon X, del Prado Venegas M, Orus C, et al. Influence of the persistence of tobacco and alcohol use in the appearance of second neoplasm in patients with a head and neck cancer. A case-control study. *Cancer Causes Control*. 2009;20(5):645–652.
6. Campbell BH, Marbella A, Layde PM. Quality of life and recurrence concern in survivors of head and neck cancer. *Laryngoscope*. 2000;110(6):895–906.
7. Bloebaum M, Poort L, Bockmann R, Kessler P. Survival after curative surgical treatment for primary oral squamous cell carcinoma. *J Craniomaxillofac Surg*. 2014;42(8):1572–1576.

8. Brockstein B, Haraf DJ, Rademaker AW, et al. Patterns of failure, prognostic factors and survival in locoregionally advanced head and neck cancer treated with concomitant chemoradiotherapy: a 9-year, 337-patient, multi-institutional experience. *Ann Oncol.* 2004;15(8):1179–1186.
9. Posner MR, Hershock DM, Blajman CR, et al. Cisplatin and fluorouracil alone or with docetaxel in head and neck cancer. *N Engl J Med.* 2007;357(17):1705–1715.
10. Su SF, Han F, Zhao C, et al. Treatment outcomes for different subgroups of nasopharyngeal carcinoma patients treated with intensity-modulated radiation therapy. *Chin J Cancer.* 2011;30(8):565–573.
11. Noble AR, Greskovich JF, Han J, et al. Risk factors associated with disease recurrence in patients with stage III/IV squamous cell carcinoma of the oral cavity treated with surgery and postoperative radiotherapy. *Anticancer Res.* 2016;36(2):785–792.
12. O'Sullivan B, Huang SH, Perez-Ordonez B, et al. Outcomes of HPV-related oropharyngeal cancer patients treated by radiotherapy alone using altered fractionation. *Radiother Oncol.* 2012;103(1):49–56.
13. Denis F, Garaud P, Bardet E, et al. Final results of the 94-01 French Head and Neck Oncology and Radiotherapy Group randomized trial comparing radiotherapy alone with concomitant radiochemotherapy in advanced-stage oropharynx carcinoma. *J Clin Oncol.* 2004;22(1):69–76.
14. De Santis RJ, Poon I, Lee J, et al. Comparison of survival between radiation therapy and trans-oral laser microsurgery for early glottic cancer patients; a retrospective cohort study. *J Otolaryngol Head Neck Surg.* 2016;45(1):42.
15. Forastiere AA, Zhang Q, Weber RS, et al. Long-term results of RTOG 91-11: a comparison of three nonsurgical treatment strategies to preserve the larynx in patients with locally advanced larynx cancer. *J Clin Oncol.* 2013;31(7):845–852.
16. Hoffman HT, Karnell LH, Shah JP, et al. Hypopharyngeal cancer patient care evaluation. *Laryngoscope.* 1997;107(8):1005–1017.
17. National Comprehensive Cancer Network. NCCN Clinical Practice Guidelines in Oncology: Head and Neck Cancers. United States: NCCN; 2016 June 5, 2016. Report No. V1.2016.
18. Yoo J, Henderson S, Walker-Dilks C. Evidence-based guideline recommendations on the use of positron emission tomography imaging in head and neck cancer. *Clin Oncol (R Coll Radiol).* 2013;25(4):e33–e66.
19. Wang YF, Liu RS, Chu PY, et al. Positron emission tomography in surveillance of head and neck squamous cell carcinoma after definitive chemoradiotherapy. *Head Neck.* 2009;31(4):442–451.
20. Anzai Y, Carroll WR, Quint DJ, et al. Recurrence of head and neck cancer after surgery or irradiation: prospective comparison of 2-deoxy-2-[F-18]fluoro-D-glucose PET and MR imaging diagnoses. *Radiology.* 1996;200(1):135–141.
21. Fischbein NJ, AAssar OS, Caputo GR, et al. Clinical utility of positron emission tomography with 18F-fluorodeoxyglucose in detecting residual/recurrent squamous cell carcinoma of the head and neck. *AJNR Am J Neuroradiol.* 1998;19(7):1189–1196.
22. Farber LA, Benard F, Machtay M, et al. Detection of recurrent head and neck squamous cell carcinomas after radiation therapy with 2-18F-fluoro-2-deoxy-D-glucose positron emission tomography. *Laryngoscope.* 1999;109(6):970–975.
23. Yao M, Smith RB, Hoffman HT, et al. Clinical significance of postradiotherapy [18F]-fluorodeoxyglucose positron emission tomography imaging in management of head-and-neck cancer-a long-term outcome report. *Int J Radiat Oncol Biol Phys.* 2009;74(1):9–14.
24. Tan A, Adelstein DJ, Rybicki LA, et al. Ability of positron emission tomography to detect residual neck node disease in patients with head and neck squamous cell carcinoma after definitive chemoradiotherapy. *Arch Otolaryngol Head Neck Surg.* 2007;133(5):435–440.
25. Isles MG, McConkey C, Mehanna HM. A systematic review and meta-analysis of the role of positron emission tomography in the follow up of head and neck squamous cell carcinoma following radiotherapy or chemoradiotherapy. *Clin Otolaryngol.* 2008;33(3):210–222.
26. Kapoor V, Fukui MB, McCook BM. Role of 18FFDG PET/CT in the treatment of head and neck cancers: posttherapy evaluation and pitfalls. *AJR Am J Roentgenol.* 2005;184(2):589–597.
27. Greven KM, Williams DW 3rd, McGuirt WFS, et al. Serial positron emission tomography scans following radiation therapy of patients with head and neck cancer. *Head Neck.* 2001;23(11):942–946.
28. Yao M, Graham MM, Smith RB, et al. Value of FDG PET in assessment of treatment response and surveillance in head-and-neck cancer patients after intensity modulated radiation treatment: a preliminary report. *Int J Radiat Oncol Biol Phys.* 2004;60(5):1410–1418.
29. Ganan L, Lopez M, Garcia J, et al. Management of recurrent head and neck cancer: variables related to salvage surgery. *Eur Arch Otorhinolaryngol.* 2016;273(12):4417–4424.
30. Schwartz GJ, Mehta RH, Wenig BL, et al. Salvage treatment for recurrent squamous cell carcinoma of the oral cavity. *Head Neck.* 2000;22(1):34–41.
31. Stell PM. Time to recurrence of squamous cell carcinoma of the head and neck. *Head Neck.* 1991;13(4):277–281.
32. Lim JY, Lim YC, Kim SH, et al. Factors predictive of successful outcome following salvage treatment of isolated neck recurrences. *Otolaryngol Head Neck Surg.* 2010;142(6):832–837.
33. Kim AJ, Suh JD, Sercarz JA, et al. Salvage surgery with free flap reconstruction: factors affecting outcome after treatment of recurrent head and neck squamous carcinoma. *Laryngoscope.* 2007;117(6):1019–1023.
34. Matoscevic K, Graf N, Pezier TF, Huber GF. Success of salvage treatment: a critical appraisal of salvage rates for different subsites of HNSCC. *Otolaryngol Head Neck Surg.* 2014;151(3):454–461.
35. Zafereo M. Surgical salvage of recurrent cancer of the head and neck. *Curr Oncol Rep.* 2014;16(5):386.

36. Eskander A, Merdad M, Irish JC, et al. Volume-outcome associations in head and neck cancer treatment: a systematic review and meta-analysis. *Head Neck*. 2014;36(12):1820–1834.
37. Sandulache VC, Vandelaar LJ, Skinner HD, et al. Salvage total laryngectomy after external-beam radiotherapy: a 20-year experience. *Head Neck*. 2016;38(Suppl 1):E1962–E1968.
38. Holsinger FC, Funk E, Roberts DB, Diaz EM Jr. Conservation laryngeal surgery versus total laryngectomy for radiation failure in laryngeal cancer. *Head Neck*. 2006;28(9):779–784.
39. Ganly I, Patel SG, Matsuo J, et al. Results of surgical salvage after failure of definitive radiation therapy for early-stage squamous cell carcinoma of the glottic larynx. *Arch Otolaryngol Head Neck Surg*. 2006;132(1):59–66.
40. de Gier HH, Knegt PP, de Boer MF, et al. CO2-laser treatment of recurrent glottic carcinoma. *Head Neck*. 2001;23(3):177–180.
41. Steiner W, Vogt P, Ambrosch P, Kron M. Transoral carbon dioxide laser microsurgery for recurrent glottic carcinoma after radiotherapy. *Head Neck*. 2004;26(6):477–484.
42. Rowley H, Walsh M, McShane D, et al. Chondroradionecrosis of the larynx: still a diagnostic dilemma. *J Laryngol Otol*. 1995;109(3):218–220.
43. Fung K, Teknos TN, Vandenberg CD, et al. Prevention of wound complications following salvage laryngectomy using free vascularized tissue. *Head Neck*. 2007;29(5):425–430.
44. Patel UA, Moore BA, Wax M, et al. Impact of pharyngeal closure technique on fistula after salvage laryngectomy. *JAMA Otolaryngol Head Neck Surg*. 2013;139(11):1156–1162.
45. Withrow KP, Rosenthal EL, Gourin CG, et al. Free tissue transfer to manage salvage laryngectomy defects after organ preservation failure. *Laryngoscope*. 2007;117(5):781–784.
46. Ho AS, Kraus DH, Ganly I, et al. Decision making in the management of recurrent head and neck cancer. *Head Neck*. 2014;36(1):144–151.
47. Koo BS, Lim YC, Lee JS, Choi EC. Recurrence and salvage treatment of squamous cell carcinoma of the oral cavity. *Oral Oncol*. 2006;42(8):789–794.
48. Yuen AP, Wei WI, Lam LK, et al. Results of surgical salvage of locoregional recurrence of carcinoma of the tongue after radiotherapy failure. *Ann Otol Rhinol Laryngol*. 1997;106(9):779–782.
49. Lin DT, Yarlagadda BB, Sethi RK, et al. Long-term functional outcomes of total glossectomy with or without total laryngectomy. *JAMA Otolaryngol Head Neck Surg*. 2015;141(9):797–803.
50. Rigby MH, Hayden RE. Total glossectomy without laryngectomy—a review of functional outcomes and reconstructive principles. *Curr Opin Otolaryngol Head Neck Surg*. 2014;22(5):414–418.
51. Gross ND, Hanna EY. The role of surgery in the management of recurrent oropharyngeal cancer. *Recent Results Cancer Res*. 2017;206:197–205.
52. Ang KK, Harris J, Wheeler R, et al. Human papillomavirus and survival of patients with oropharyngeal cancer. *N Engl J Med*. 2010;363(1):24–35.
53. Roosli C, Studer G, Stoeckli SJ. Salvage treatment for recurrent oropharyngeal squamous cell carcinoma. *Head Neck*. 2010;32(8):989–996.
54. Guo T, Rettig E, Fakhry C. Understanding the impact of survival and human papillomavirus tumor status on timing of recurrence in oropharyngeal squamous cell carcinoma. *Oral Oncol*. 2016;52:97–103.
55. Patel SN, Cohen MA, Givi B, et al. Salvage surgery for locally recurrent oropharyngeal cancer. *Head Neck*. 2016;38(Suppl 1):E658–E664.
56. Sweeny L, Rosenthal EL, Clemons L, et al. Outcomes after surgical salvage for recurrent oropharyngeal squamous cell carcinoma. *Oral Oncol*. 2016;60:118–124.
57. Jayaram SC, Muzaffar SJ, Ahmed I, et al. Efficacy, outcomes, and complication rates of different surgical and nonsurgical treatment modalities for recurrent/residual oropharyngeal carcinoma: a systematic review and meta-analysis. *Head Neck*. 2016;38(12):1855–1861.
58. Dabas S, Dewan A, Ranjan R, et al. Salvage transoral robotic surgery for recurrent or residual head and neck squamous cell carcinoma: a single institution experience. *Asian Pac J Cancer Prev*. 2015;16(17):7627–7632.
59. White H, Ford S, Bush B, et al. Salvage surgery for recurrent cancers of the oropharynx: comparing TORS with standard open surgical approaches. *JAMA Otolaryngol Head Neck Surg*. 2013;139(8):773–778.
60. Hall SF, Groome PA, Irish J, O'Sullivan B. The natural history of patients with squamous cell carcinoma of the hypopharynx. *Laryngoscope*. 2008;118(8):1362–1371.
61. Hall SF, Groome PA, Irish J, O'Sullivan B. Radiotherapy or surgery for head and neck squamous cell cancer: establishing the baseline for hypopharyngeal carcinoma? *Cancer*. 2009;115(24):5711–5722.
62. Hall SF, Griffiths R. Did the addition of concomitant chemotherapy to radiotherapy improve outcomes in hypopharyngeal cancer? A population-based study. *Curr Oncol*. 2016;23(4):266–272.
63. Taki S, Homma A, Oridate N, et al. Salvage surgery for local recurrence after chemoradiotherapy or radiotherapy in hypopharyngeal cancer patients. *Eur Arch Otorhinolaryngol*. 2010;267(11):1765–1769.
64. Yasumatsu R, Nakashima T, Toh S, et al. Salvage of recurrent hypopharyngeal carcinoma after primary curative treatment. *Acta Otolaryngol*. 2013;133(10):1110–1116.
65. Omura G, Saito Y, Ando M, et al. Salvage surgery for local residual or recurrent pharyngeal cancer after radiotherapy or chemoradiotherapy. *Laryngoscope*. 2014;124(9):2075–2080.
66. Clark JR, de Almeida J, Gilbert R, et al. Primary and salvage (hypo)pharyngectomy: analysis and outcome. *Head Neck*. 2006;28(8):671–677.
67. Fakhry N, Chamorey E, Michel J, et al. Salvage circular laryngopharyngectomy and radial forearm free flap for recurrent hypopharyngeal cancer. *Laryngoscope*. 2013;123(4):910–915.

68. Ng WT, Lee MC, Hung WM, et al. Clinical outcomes and patterns of failure after intensity-modulated radiotherapy for nasopharyngeal carcinoma. *Int J Radiat Oncol Biol Phys*. 2011;79(2):420–428.
69. Lee AW, Sze WM, Au JS, et al. Treatment results for nasopharyngeal carcinoma in the modern era: the Hong Kong experience. *Int J Radiat Oncol Biol Phys*. 2005;61(4):1107–1116.
70. Sham JS, Choy D. Nasopharyngeal carcinoma: treatment of neck node recurrence by radiotherapy. *Australas Radiol*. 1991;35(4):370–373.
71. Wei WI, Lam KH, Ho CM, et al. Efficacy of radical neck dissection for the control of cervical metastasis after radiotherapy for nasopharyngeal carcinoma. *Am J Surg*. 1990;160(4):439–442.
72. Wei WI, Ho CM, Wong MP, et al. Pathological basis of surgery in the management of postradiotherapy cervical metastasis in nasopharyngeal carcinoma. *Arch Otolaryngol Head Neck Surg*. 1992;118(9):923,9; discussion 930.
73. Khafif A, Ferlito A, Takes RP, Thomas Robbins K. Is it necessary to perform radical neck dissection as a salvage procedure for persistent or recurrent neck disease after chemoradiotherapy in patients with nasopharyngeal cancer? *Eur Arch Otorhinolaryngol*. 2010;267(7):997–999.
74. Lam KS, Ho JH, Lee AW, et al. Symptomatic hypothalamic-pituitary dysfunction in nasopharyngeal carcinoma patients following radiation therapy: a retrospective study. *Int J Radiat Oncol Biol Phys*. 1987;13(9):1343–1350.
75. Lee AW, Ng SH, Ho JH, et al. Clinical diagnosis of late temporal lobe necrosis following radiation therapy for nasopharyngeal carcinoma. *Cancer*. 1988;61(8):1535–1542.
76. Choy D, Sham JS, Wei WI, et al. Transpalatal insertion of radioactive gold grain for the treatment of persistent and recurrent nasopharyngeal carcinoma. *Int J Radiat Oncol Biol Phys*. 1993;25(3):505–512.
77. Vlantis AC, Tsang RK, Yu BK, et al. Nasopharyngectomy and surgical margin status: a survival analysis. *Arch Otolaryngol Head Neck Surg*. 2007;133(12):1296–1301.
78. Wei WI, Chan JY, Ng RW, Ho WK. Surgical salvage of persistent or recurrent nasopharyngeal carcinoma with maxillary swing approach—critical appraisal after 2 decades. *Head Neck*. 2011;33(7):969–975.
79. Wei WI, Kwong DL. Recurrent nasopharyngeal carcinoma: surgical salvage vs. additional chemoradiation. *Curr Opin Otolaryngol Head Neck Surg*. 2011;19(2):82–86.
80. Temam S, Koka V, Mamelle G, et al. Treatment of the N0 neck during salvage surgery after radiotherapy of head and neck squamous cell carcinoma. *Head Neck*. 2005;27(8):653–658.
81. Sjovall J, Chua B, Pryor D, et al. Long-term results of positron emission tomography-directed management of the neck in node-positive head and neck cancer after organ preservation therapy. *Oral Oncol*. 2015;51(3):260–266.
82. Chung EJ, Lee SH, Baek SH, et al. Clinical outcome and prognostic factors after salvage surgery for isolated regional squamous cell carcinoma recurrences. *Head Neck*. 2015;37(11):1612–1617.
83. Wong LY, Wei WI, Lam LK, Yuen AP. Salvage of recurrent head and neck squamous cell carcinoma after primary curative surgery. Head Neck. 2003;25(11):953–959.
84. Leon X, Rigo A, Farre N, et al. Prognostic significance of extracapsular spread in isolated neck recurrences in head and neck squamous cell carcinoma patients. *Eur Arch Otorhinolaryngol*. 2017:274(1):527–533.
85. Ozer E, Agrawal A, Ozer HG, Schuller DE. The impact of surgery in the management of the head and neck carcinoma involving the carotid artery. *Laryngoscope*. 2008;118(10):1771–1774.
86. Nieder C, Grosu AL, Andratschke NH, Molls M. Proposal of human spinal cord reirradiation dose based on collection of data from 40 patients. *Int J Radiat Oncol Biol Phys*. 2005;61(3):851–855.
87. Langendijk JA, Bourhis J. Reirradiation in squamous cell head and neck cancer: recent developments and future directions. *Curr Opin Oncol*. 2007;19(3):202–209.
88. Seiwert TY, Salama JK, Vokes EE. The concurrent chemoradiation paradigm–general principles. *Nat Clin Pract Oncol*. 2007;4(2):86–100.
89. Popovtzer A, Gluck I, Chepeha DB, et al. The pattern of failure after reirradiation of recurrent squamous cell head and neck cancer: implications for defining the targets. *Int J Radiat Oncol Biol Phys*. 2009;74(5):1342–1347.
90. Spencer SA, Wheeler RH, Peters GE, et al. Concomitant chemotherapy and reirradiation as management for recurrent cancer of the head and neck. *Am J Clin Oncol*. 1999;22(1):1–5.
91. Choe KS, Haraf DJ, Solanki A, et al. Prior chemoradiotherapy adversely impacts outcomes of recurrent and second primary head and neck cancer treated with concurrent chemotherapy and reirradiation. *Cancer*. 2011;117(20):4671–4678.
92. Janot F, de Raucourt D, Benhamou E, et al. Randomized trial of postoperative reirradiation combined with chemotherapy after salvage surgery compared with salvage surgery alone in head and neck carcinoma. *J Clin Oncol*. 2008;26(34):5518–5523.
93. Kasperts N, Slotman BJ, Leemans CR, et al. Results of postoperative reirradiation for recurrent or second primary head and neck carcinoma. *Cancer*. 2006;106(7):1536–1547.
94. De Crevoisier R, Domenge C, Wibault P, et al. Full dose reirradiation combined with chemotherapy after salvage surgery in head and neck carcinoma. *Cancer*. 2001;91(11):2071–2076.
95. Pignon JP, Bourhis J, Domenge C, Designe L. Chemotherapy added to locoregional treatment for head and neck squamous-cell carcinoma: three meta-analyses of updated individual data. MACH-NC Collaborative Group. Meta-Analysis of Chemotherapy on Head and Neck Cancer. *Lancet*. 2000;355(9208):949–955.

96. Goldstein DP, Karnell LH, Yao M, et al. Outcomes following reirradiation of patients with head and neck cancer. *Head Neck*. 2008;30(6):765–770.
97. Dawson LA, Myers LL, Bradford CR, et al. Conformal re-irradiation of recurrent and new primary head-and-neck cancer. *Int J Radiat Oncol Biol Phys*. 2001;50(2):377–385.
98. Vargo JA, Heron DE, Ferris RL, et al. Examining tumor control and toxicity after stereotactic body radiotherapy in locally recurrent previously irradiated head and neck cancers: implications of treatment duration and tumor volume. *Head Neck*. 2014;36(9):1349–1355.
99. Urie MM, Sisterson JM, Koehler AM, et al. Proton beam penumbra: effects of separation between patient and beam modifying devices. *Med Phys*. 1986;13(5):734–741.
100. Romesser PB, Cahlon O, Scher ED, et al. Proton beam reirradiation for recurrent head and neck cancer: multi-institutional report on feasibility and early outcomes. *Int J Radiat Oncol Biol Phys*. 2016;95(1):386–395.
101. Lee N, Chan K, Bekelman JE, et al. Salvage re-irradiation for recurrent head and neck cancer. *Int J Radiat Oncol Biol Phys*. 2007;68(3):731–740.
102. Baliga S, Kabarriti R, Ohri N, et al. Stereotactic body radiotherapy for recurrent head and neck cancer: a critical review. *Head Neck*. 2017;39(3):595–601.
103. Rwigema JC, Heron DE, Ferris RL, et al. Fractionated stereotactic body radiation therapy in the treatment of previously-irradiated recurrent head and neck carcinoma: updated report of the University of Pittsburgh experience. *Am J Clin Oncol*. 2010;33(3):286–293.
104. Heron DE, Ferris RL, Karamouzis M, et al. Stereotactic body radiotherapy for recurrent squamous cell carcinoma of the head and neck: results of a phase I dose-escalation trial. *Int J Radiat Oncol Biol Phys*. 2009;75(5):1493–1500.
105. Karam I, Poon I, Lee J, et al. Stereotactic body radiotherapy for head and neck cancer: an addition to the armamentarium against head and neck cancer. *Future Oncol*. 2015;11(21):2937–2947.
106. Rwigema JC, Heron DE, Ferris RL, et al. The impact of tumor volume and radiotherapy dose on outcome in previously irradiated recurrent squamous cell carcinoma of the head and neck treated with stereotactic body radiation therapy. *Am J Clin Oncol*. 2011;34(4):372–379.
107. Strom T, Wishka C, Caudell JJ. Stereotactic body radiotherapy for recurrent unresectable head and neck cancers. *Cancer Control*. 2016;23(1):6–11.
108. Machtay M, Rosenthal DI, Chalian AA, et al. Pilot study of postoperative reirradiation, chemotherapy, and amifostine after surgical salvage for recurrent head-and-neck cancer. *Int J Radiat Oncol Biol Phys*. 2004;59(1):72–77.
109. Lee JY, Suresh K, Nguyen R, et al. Predictors of severe long-term toxicity after re-irradiation for head and neck cancer. *Oral Oncol*. 2016;60:32–40.
110. Salama JK, Vokes EE, Chmura SJ, et al. Long-term outcome of concurrent chemotherapy and reirradiation for recurrent and second primary head-and-neck squamous cell carcinoma. *Int J Radiat Oncol Biol Phys*. 2006;64(2):382–391.
111. Langer CJ, Harris J, Horwitz EM, et al. Phase II study of low-dose paclitaxel and cisplatin in combination with split-course concomitant twice-daily reirradiation in recurrent squamous cell carcinoma of the head and neck: results of Radiation Therapy Oncology Group Protocol 9911. *J Clin Oncol*. 2007;25(30):4800–4805.
112. Marwaha A, Choong NW, Firat S. Clinical efficacy and tolerability of continuous course reirradiation with concurrent weekly carboplatin-paclitaxel for locally recurrent, nonmetastatic squamous cell carcinoma of the head and neck. *J Clin Oncol*. 2010;28:7s (Abstract #5518).
113. Hehr T, Classen J, Belka C, et al. Reirradiation alternating with docetaxel and cisplatin in inoperable recurrence of head-and-neck cancer: a prospective phase I/II trial. *Int J Radiat Oncol Biol Phys*. 2005;61(5):1423–1431.
114. Ferris RL, Blumenschein G Jr, Fayette J, et al. Nivolumab for recurrent squamous-cell carcinoma of the head and neck. *N Engl J Med*. 2016;375(19):1856–1867.
115. Clinical Trials on Recurrent Head and Neck Cancer [Internet]. Bethesda, Maryland, USA: U.S. National Institutes of Health; 2016 [updated November 1, 2016; cited November 6, 2016]. https://clinicaltrials.gov/ct2/results?term=recurrent+head+and+neck+-cancer&recr=Open.

23

Recurrent or Metastatic HNSCC: Systemic Therapy

Tomohiro Enokida
Susumu Okano
Makoto Tahara

Despite aggressive surgery with or without adjuvant therapy, or multidisciplinary approaches, approximately half the patients with head and neck squamous cell carcinoma (HNSCC) develop recurrent disease (10% to 20% of early stage HNSCC and 50% of locally advanced [LA] HNSCC) (1–4). Patients with recurrent or metastatic (R/M) HNSCC have a poor prognosis, with median overall survival (OS) of approximately 4 months with best supportive care (BSC) (5). Only a small fraction of patients with R/M HNSCC can be treated with curative intent, and the vast majority of this population receives palliative systemic therapy. The choice of a systemic regimen is based on whether the patient has received prior treatment as part of a combined modality approach postoperatively or for functional organ preservation as part of the initial management or whether the patient had previously received systemic therapy for metastatic or locoregional recurrent disease. Combination therapy with cetuximab (Cmab) plus platinum (cisplatin, CDDP; or carboplatin, CBDCA) plus 5-fluorouracil (5-FU) followed by maintenance Cmab has shown the best results so far in terms of overall response rate (ORR), progression-free survival (PFS), and OS in the first-line treatment of R/M HNSCC (6,7). There are some variations of this regimen (which is referred to as ERBITUX in first-line Treatment of REcurrent or MEtastatic head and neck cancer—EXTREME regimen), such as substitution of 5-FU for taxanes (e.g., docetaxel, DTX; or paclitaxel, PTX) (8,9). In clinical practice, other combinations, such as a taxane or CDDP plus Cmab, are also sometimes used as first-line treatment for R/M HNSCC (10). Among other treatment options, monotherapy and a combination regimen using either or both conventional cytotoxic chemotherapy and molecular targeted drugs are available. Patients who are ineligible for the EXTREME regimen or other Cmab-based first-line treatments and those who progress on these regimens have limited therapeutic options; these include monotherapy with methotrexate (MTX), DTX, PTX, or Cmab (11,12). Patients who progress relatively early in their disease course after the last administered dose of a platinum agent (within 6 months as a general guide) have been referred to as "platinum-refractory." It is commonly understood that they should be treated with non-platinum-containing regimen after that date. Immune checkpoint inhibitors (ICIs) are a relatively new option for those patients with progressive disease (PD) after an initial chemotherapy regimen which will be reviewed here. Although these widen treatment options, the order in which these agents are used requires careful consideration if a maximally effective and tolerable multiline continuum of care is to be achieved. In addition, this chapter will also review several special settings. Human papillomavirus (HPV) has a prognostic role and may affect sensitivity to a certain treatment. Elderly patients can also obtain similar benefit from antitumor treatment albeit with increased toxicity. With R/M nasopharyngeal cancer (NPC), the first randomized phase III trial showed the superiority of gemcitabine (GEM) and CDDP to infusional 5-FU and CDDP, which has long been regarded as the standard of care (Figure 23.1). This review highlights the evidence-based data to propose and support a current best management practices for the systemic therapy of patients with R/M HNSCC to maximize survival without worsening quality of life or jeopardizing toxicities. The details of other therapeutic modalities, such as radiation therapy and surgery, are described in other chapters.

ACTIVE AGENTS IN HNSCC

CYTOTOXIC AGENTS

The most common chemotherapy drugs used for advanced HNSCC include platinum agents (e.g., CDDP and CBDCA), taxanes (e.g., PTX and DTX), and antimetabolites (e.g., MTX and 5-FU).

Platinum Agents (Cisplatin, Carboplatin)

CDDP is still one of the most commonly used standard agents for R/M disease, and offers a single-agent ORR of approximately 30% (13–15). Most single-agent studies have used doses of 80 to 120 mg/m^2, given as an intravenous bolus at 3- to 4-week intervals. One small randomized trial that compared CDDP at 120 mg/m^2 versus 60 mg/m^2 as a bolus found no evidence of CDDP dose dependency (16). A randomized 2 × 2 factorial design trial of CDDP and bleomycin in 116 patients with R/M HNSCC showed that CDDP prolonged median survival significantly by 10 weeks as compared with BSC (17). Carboaplatin (CBDCA) is a second-generation platinum analog. As a single agent, CBDCA has shown ORRs of 20% to 26% (18–21). CBDCA may be preferable for some patients on account

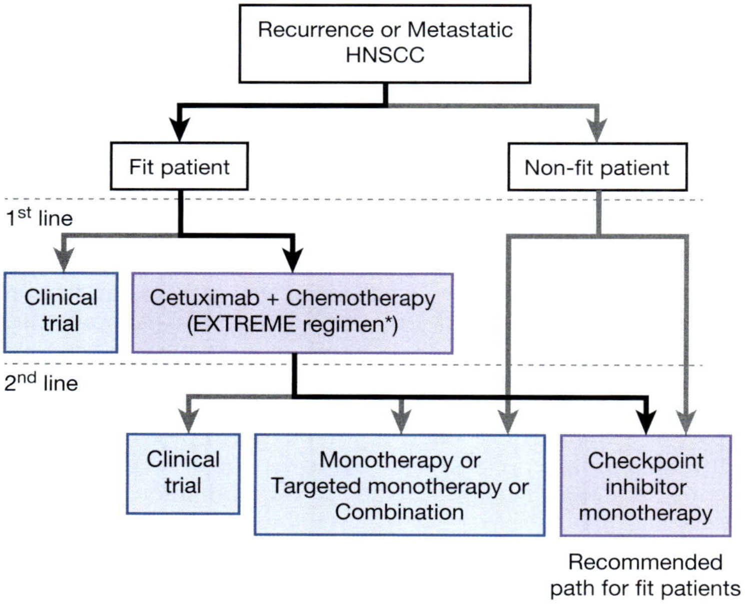

FIGURE 23.1 Continuum of care for R/M HNSCC. There are now multiple lines of treatment that constitute a continuum of care. HNSCC, head and neck squamous cell carcinoma; CT, chemotherapy; EXTREME, cetuximab plus cisplatin/carboplatin plus 5-fluorouracil followed by maintenance cetuximab. *EXTREME regimen is supported by phase III trial evidence. Other first-line options include TPEx (cisplatin, docetaxel, and cetuximab), PCE (paclitaxel, carboplatin, and cetuximab), cetuximab + cisplatin, cetuximab + paclitaxel, and other platinum-based treatment.

EXTREME, erbitux in first line treatment of recurrent or metastatic head and neck cancer; R/M HNSCC, recurrent of metastatic head and neck squamous cell carcinoma.

Source: Modified from Argiris A, Harrington KJ, Tahara M, et al. Evidence-based treatment options in recurrent and/or metastatic squamous cell carcinoma of the head and neck. *Front Oncol*. 2017;7:72.

of its lower neurotoxicity, nephrotoxicity, and nausea and vomiting than CDDP, albeit it does result in more myelosuppression (20,22–24). However, conclusive direct comparisons of CDDP and CBDCA as single agents in this patient population are lacking. A Southwest Oncology Group (SWOG) trial showed similar survival (7 months vs. 5 months) for CDDP plus 5-FU versus CBDCA plus fluorouracil in the metastatic recurrent setting, with a nonstatistically significant improvement in ORR (32% vs. 21%) (25). Although CBDCA is often considered to be less effective than CDDP in head and neck cancer, direct evidence for this in R/M HNSCC is scant. On the other hand, it has been demonstrated that CDDP plus fluorouracil is more effective than CBDCA plus fluorouracil as neoadjuvant treatment in LA (stage IV-M0) head and neck cancer (22).

Taxanes (Paclitaxel, Docetaxel)

PTX is currently biosynthesized by diterpene plants and exerts its cytotoxic effects by promoting microtubule assembly and eventually disrupting mitosis and cell death. Single-agent activity for R/M HNSCC in phase II trials demonstrated an encouraging ORR range of 20% to 40%. Previous studies of high-dose triweekly PTX (200 to 250 mg/m^2) in patients with advanced or R/M HNSCC demonstrated an ORR of 35% to 40%, which was associated with severe neuropathy and myelosuppression (26,27). In a phase II trial of weekly PTX in 74 patients with R/M HNSCC (28), an ORR of 29.0% was observed. Median duration of response, median time to progression, and median survival time were 7.4 months, 3.4 months, and 14.3 months, respectively. Although no randomized study has been published (6), these findings suggest that weekly PTX offers promising efficacy with acceptable tolerance in R/M HNSCC. DTX is a semisynthetic taxane analog that also possesses significant activity in HNSCC. Several single-agent phase II studies in chemotherapy-naive patients with R/M HNSCC yielded ORRs of 21% to 42% (29–31). Guardiola et al. reported the results of a randomized phase II study that compared DTX with MTX in patients with recurrent HNSCC (32). Response rate was significantly higher in the DTX arm, with an ORR of 27% versus 15% in the MTX arm. In contrast, no significant differences between the arms were seen in either OS or time to progression. A lower dose of DTX (60 mg/m^2, every 3 to 4 weeks) was evaluated in 63 patients. Previously treated patients showed a 17.9% (10/56) response rate, whereas treatment-naive patients showed a 57.1% (4/7) response rate (33). No direct comparison of PTX with DTX as monotherapy in the treatment of HNSCC has been reported.

Antimetabolites (Methotrexate, 5-Fluorouracil)

Antimetabolites are substances that compete with, replace, or inhibit a specific metabolite of tumor cells. Weekly administration of 40 to 60 mg/m^2 produces the best response rates; higher dosages and more frequent administration do not improve the rate or duration of response (34). In previous reports, ORRs and median OS to MTX monotherapy as first-line treatment was 10% to 15% and 3.9 to 5.6 months, respectively. Currently, the agent is considered the standard of care in second-line setting of R/M HNSCC (35–37). 5-FU administered as an infusion in conjunction with CDDP achieved superior tumor response rates to bolus delivery in head and neck cancer (38). ORR and median OS to 5-FU monotherapy as first-line treatment was 15% and 6.1 months, respectively (15). Currently, the agent is used with CDDP and cetuximab (Cmab) as a standard of care in the first-line setting. Capecitabine and S-1, oral 5-FU anticancer agents, have shown certain effects in the treatment of previously treated R/M HNSCC. The respective ORR and PFS were 24.2% and 4.8 months for capecitabine (39), 27% and 4.2 months for S-1 (40), respectively.

ANTI-EGFR TARGETED AGENTS (CETUXIMAB, PANITUMUMAB)

HNSCC tumors are greatly affected by dysregulation of the epidermal growth factor receptor (EGFR) pathway and high EGFR expression is associated with poor outcome (41). Cmab, an immunoglobulin G subclass 1 (IgG1) monoclonal antibody (mAb), targets the EGFR by preventing its ligand-mediated activation and dimerization. This in turn inhibits the proliferation of tumor cells and leads to their apoptosis (42–44). Furthermore, the IgG1 isotype brings about Cmab-induced antibody-dependent cell-mediated cytotoxicity (ADCC), in which immune cells target and kill cells coated in IgG1 or other antibody isotypes (42,45,46). In addition to its apoptosis-inducing, EGFR-blocking activity, Cmab directs the ADCC mechanism at tumor cells, using primarily natural killer cells to maximize antitumor effects (43,47–49). The contribution of ADCC to Cmab's antitumor activity has not been widely evaluated in clinical trials, but recent studies have revealed a correlation between the efficacy of Cmab and high ADCC, suggesting that ADCC contributes to the antitumor activity of Cmab (50,51). Further, several studies have shown an immunomodulatory effect of EGFR monoclonal antibodies by some such tumor antigen-specific T cell activation as a result of T cell activation by interaction with antigen-presenting cells (52,53).

Single-agent Cmab in a platinum-refractory setting showed a major ORR of 13% in a phase II study (12). Cmab has been shown to enhance the antitumor activity of CDDP without any effect on its pharmacokinetic profile (54,55). The Eastern Cooperative Oncology Group (ECOG) conducted a randomized placebo-controlled trial using CDDP with or without Cmab in first-line R/M HNSCC (56). The addition of Cmab to CDDP resulted in significantly higher response rates in the CDDP plus Cmab arm than in the CDDP-alone arm (26% vs. 10%; p = .029). However, no significant difference was seen in the primary end point of PFS (4.1 months vs. 3.4 months; p = .27) or secondary end point of OS (9.2 months vs. 8 months; p = .18). In this trial, patients who fail on platinum therapy within 3 months were excluded. A subsequent phase III trial by Vermorken et al. (EXTREME trial) showed that Cmab confers survival benefits in combination with platinum-based chemotherapy in the first-line treatment of R/M HNSCC (7). This trial is described in detail later in this chapter. Meanwhile, a phase II study in patients with HNSCC demonstrated that the combination of Cmab and CDDP could not show apparent clinical benefit in patients with documented disease recurrence and tumor progression within 3 months of platinum (3). The results obtained by reintroducing platinum in combination with Cmab did not appear to differ from the results obtained by treatment with Cmab alone after platinum failure (57).

IMMUNE CHECKPOINT INHIBITORS: ICIs (NIVOLUMAB, PEMBROLIZUMAB)

ICIs represent a new class of therapeutic agents in cancer. Tumor cells act to prevent their detection and elimination by the immune system of the host by disrupting a particular immunosuppressive pathway, termed the inhibitory checkpoint (48,58). ICIs are expected to be particularly promising in tumors that highly express endogenous PD-L1 (programmed death ligand 1), including HNSCC. Pembrolizumab and nivolumab are monoclonal antibodies (pembrolizumab, humanized; nivolumab, human) targeting PD-1 that have been recently approved by the Food and Drug Administration (FDA) as monotherapy for platinum-refractory HNSCC. The available data on the efficacy of ICIs in HNSCC concern anti-PD-1 therapy and were derived from trials with platinum-refractory and second- or later-line R/M HNSCC patient populations predominantly with an Eastern Cooperative Oncology Group (ECOG) Performance Status (PS) of 0 or 1, as of this writing. Studies to evaluate anti-PD-1 therapy in other settings, such as the first-line setting, and to test novel agents targeting the other immunoinhibitory (e.g., LAG3) or -stimulatory (e.g., OX-40) molecules are also ongoing (59). Research to explore predictive factors is an indispensable way of identifying patients who will benefit from treatment, because patients who receive a clinical benefit from ICIs tend to have a longer response than is generally expected from conventional standard chemotherapy (60–62). Furthermore, it is also necessary to examine when to stop treatment in responders.

CURRENT TREATMENT ACCORDING TO CLINICAL SETTING

PRINCIPLES OF MANAGEMENT

The appropriate treatment for R/M HNSCC should be determined by the patient's status (e.g., performance status, organ function, medical comorbid conditions). Other determinants for consideration include the presence or absence of symptoms, pace of disease progression, goals of care, and benefits of therapy. The only multidrug regimen to demonstrate a survival advantage is platinum/5-FU/Cmab, which should be used as the standard of care for otherwise healthy patients with platinum-sensitive disease requiring an objective response. From the viewpoint of platinum sensitivity, prior therapy is also important factor. Patients who progress within 6 months after the last administered dose of a platinum agent (CDDP or CBDCA) in either the LA or R/M setting are not suitable for platinum re-treatment. These patients have been referred to as "platinum-refractory" (or EXTREME-ineligible). Because treatment options for patients with platinum-refractory disease and for those in second-line R/M HNSCC are similar, these two patient subgroups will be discussed here together and termed "second line" (63–65). BSC alone is often appropriate for patients with poor performance status and comorbid conditions. Despite decades of active research into multiple novel agents, survival remains poor, and clinical trial participation (including elderly patients) should accordingly be routinely offered and encouraged.

FIRST-LINE TREATMENT OPTIONS IN R/M HNSCC

Cetuximab Plus Platinum (Cisplatin or Carboplatin) Plus 5-Fluorouracil (5-FU) Followed by Maintenance Cetuximab (the EXTREME Regimen)

For decades prior to the introduction of the EXTREME regimen (platinum, 5-FU, Cmab, followed by maintenance Cmab until PD or toxicity), no experimental treatments yielded any significant increase in survival in patients with R/M HNSCC. The EXTREME trial was a randomized phase III trial of platinum-based chemotherapy with or without Cmab as first-line therapy for R/M HNSCC, published in 2008 (7). Four hundred and forty-two eligible patients were randomly assigned at a 1:1 ratio to receive CDDP (100 mg/m^2 on day 1) or CBDCA (AUC [area under the curve] 5 on day 1) plus fluorouracil (1,000 mg/m^2/day for 4 days) every 3 weeks for a maximum of six cycles, either alone (chemotherapy-alone group) or in combination with Cmab (400 mg/m^2 initially, then 250 mg/m^2 per week) for a maximum of six cycles. Patients with stable disease (SD) who received chemotherapy plus Cmab continued to receive Cmab until disease progression or unacceptable toxic effects. The main exclusion criteria were surgery or irradiation within the previous 4 weeks, or previous systemic therapy unless part of a multimodal treatment for LA disease that had been completed > 6 months before study entry. The primary end point of the EXTREME trial was OS. The trial included otherwise healthy patients with R/M HNSCC, with 88% at ECOG PS 0-1 (Karnofsky score ≥80) and 12% at ECOG PS 2 (Karnofsky score <80), who were not candidates for local therapy. The addition of Cmab to platinum-based chemotherapy significantly prolonged median OS, from 7.4 months to 10.1 months (hazard ratio [HR] = 0.80 p = .04), and also prolonged median PFS from 3.3 months to 5.6 months (p <.001) and increased the ORR from 20% to 36% (odds ratio [OR] = 2.33 [95% CI, 1.50–3.60]; p <.001). There was a similar improvement in PFS attributable to Cmab in patients treated with CDDP plus fluorouracil and those given CBDCA plus fluorouracil, and there was no apparent difference in results between patients treated with the two platinum regimens. Of note, this study regimen was the first to show an improvement in PFS and OS in patients with R/M HNSCC. The most common grade 3 or 4 adverse events in the chemotherapy-alone and Cmab groups were anemia (19% and 13%, respectively), neutropenia (23% and 22%), and thrombocytopenia (11% in both groups). Adding Cmab to chemotherapy significantly increased sepsis (p = .02) and skin reaction (p < .001), although for the most part, there was no significant difference in the overall incidence of grade 3 or 4 adverse events between the groups.

Finally, the QoL Questionnaire-Core 30 (QLQ-C30) showed a significant improvement in global health status/QoL score in the Cmab group (p = .0415) but no treatment differences in the social functioning scale (66). For QLQ-Head and Neck 35 (QLQ-H&N35), mean score in the chemotherapy and Cmab group was not significantly worse than the mean chemotherapy group score for all symptom scales and post-baseline visits. At cycle 3, some symptom scores (pain, swallowing, speech problems, and social eating) significantly were favored in the chemotherapy and Cmab group. Given the cumulative toxicity of CDDP, substitution of CBDCA is often necessary and acceptable. The role of Cmab in first-line R/M HNSCC in patients who have previously received Cmab for LA HNSCC has not been fully evaluated, although responsiveness to re-treatment in these patients has been reported (67).

Because there is no randomized clinical trial (RCT) of chemotherapy with or without Cmab maintenance, the role of Cmab maintenance remains controversial. In a retrospective study of 31 patients with R/M HNSCC, Cmab plus chemotherapy followed by maintenance with biweekly Cmab led to a SD rate of 52%, partial response (PR) rate of 39%, and complete response (CR) rate of 9% (68). Furthermore, there is evidence that maintenance therapy until PD with biweekly Cmab as a single agent following the EXTREME regimen is also well tolerated with good compliance (relative dose intensity = 82%) (68,69). It is important to note that the addition of panitumumab (Pmab), a fully human anti-EGFR IgG2 monoclonal antibody with weak ADCC activity, to CDDP and 5-FU showed a statistically significant improvement in PFS (5.8 months vs. 4.6 months; HR = 0.780; p = .0036) and ORR (36% vs. 25%; OR = 1.69; p = .0065), but not in the primary end point of OS (11.1 months vs. 9.0 months; HR = 0.873; p = .1403) in a phase III trial (SPECTRUM study) (70). Given that Pmab is a very potent EGFR inhibitor, the differential outcomes between EXTREME study and SPECTRUM study might be explained by the different nature of ADCC stimulation.

Alternative Regimen in the First-Line Setting

Cmab plus platinum (CDDP or CBDCA) plus taxane followed by maintenance Cmab could be the optional regimen in this setting. The combination of CDDP, DTX, and Cmab (TPE regimen), for which biweekly Cmab was continued until PD after four cycles of TPE, has been evaluated in the first-line setting of R/M HNSCC (GORTEC 2008–03 study) (8). ORR and OS were 44.4% and 14 months, respectively. Six cycles of CBDCA, PTX, and Cmab combination (PCE) followed by Cmab maintenance until PD or toxicity was also examined. ORR was 40% and median OS was 14.7 months. Further, a phase II trial of weekly Cmab and PTX (80 mg/m^2) in 46 patients with R/M HNSCC who were platinum-refractory or -ineligible has demonstrated promising data (59). ORR was 54%, with a CR rate of 22%, and disease control rate (DCR) of 80%. Median PFS was 4.2 months, and median OS was 8.1 months, comparable with historical controls (71). Currently, substitution of taxane for 5-FU should be done with caution, because this combination has not been actively compared against the current standard, the EXTREME regimen. However, the TPE regimen is currently being compared with the EXTREME regimen in the first-line setting (NCT02268695). Randomized phase II trial of platinum and DTX with or without erlotinib (EGFR-TKIs) showed addition of erlotinib to first-line platinum and DTX significantly improved PFS and OS (72). This regimen may warrant further evaluation in phase III trial.

Status of ICI Clinical Trials for First-Line Treatment

ICIs such as nivolumab, pembrolizumab, and durvalumab are currently being investigated in the first-line R/M HNSCC setting for fit patients, and the EXTREME regimen has been chosen as a comparator arm in several recently opened phase III trials. Nivolumab in combination with the anti–CTLA-4 antibody ipilimumab is being compared with the EXTREME regimen in the CheckMate 651 trial (73) (NCT02741570). In contrast, pembrolizumab is being investigated as a monotherapy as well as in combination with chemotherapy for first-line R/M HNSCC (KEYNOTE-048 study). Finally, durvalumab is under examination as a monotherapy and in combination with the anti–CTLA-4 antibody tremelimumab (the KESTREL study). As of this writing, however, no results from these trials are yet available, and the use of ICIs in first-line R/M setting is therefore not recommended outside clinical trial settings (60,74–77).

SECOND-LINE AND PLATINUM-REFRACTORY OPTIONS IN R/M HNSCC

Generally, patients who experience disease progression within 6 months of the last dose of platinum in either LA or R/M settings are not optimal candidates for platinum re-treatment. These patients have been referred to as "platinum-refractory" (or EXTREME-ineligible). Some studies of first-line chemotherapy have excluded patients having received prior chemotherapy for LA disease within 3 or 4 months (56,78). Re-treatment with platinum in the setting of platinum-refractory disease increases toxicity without improving efficacy outcomes (57,79). These patients are most commonly treated with single-agent chemotherapy or BSC. Patients who receive BSC for the sole purpose of symptom management also attain a median OS of around 5 months (80). Against this background, pembrolizumab and nivolumab were newly approved by the FDA in 2016 for use in patients with R/M HNSCC who progress on or after platinum-based chemotherapy.

ICI Therapy for Second-Line Treatment

KEYNOTE-012, a nonrandomized phase 1b trial of pembrolizumab monotherapy, enrolled 192 patients. The first 60 patients were selected for PD-L1–positive tumors and treated with 10 mg/kg pembrolizumab intravenously every 2 weeks (Cohort B). Among Cohort B patients,

70% had received two or more lines of therapy. For this cohort, median PFS and OS were 2 and 13 months, respectively. The remaining 132 patients were enrolled irrespective of tumor PD-L1 expression and treated with pembrolizumab at a fixed dose of 200 mg intravenously every 3 weeks (Cohort B2) (61,74,81). In Cohort B2, 18% had not received prior therapy in the R/M setting, while 57% had received two or more lines of therapy. These patients achieved a median PFS of 2 months and median OS of 8 months. The observed ORR was 18% in both cohorts. Subgroup analyses in KEYNOTE-012 demonstrated higher OS and ORR in patients with ≥1% PD-L1–expressing tumors who had received one or more doses of pembrolizumab (61,82). When immune cells were included in the PD-L1 expression analysis, ORR rose to 22% in patients with PD-L1–expressing tumors but dropped to 4% in those with <1% PD-L1 expression. On post hoc analysis, furthermore, patients with less pretreatment (no more than two previous treatment lines) showed a higher ORR than those with heavy pretreatment (32% vs. 16%, respectively). In addition, patients with a lower amount of disease showed improved response (36% vs. 14%, respectively) compared to patients with higher doses. Small-volume disease was defined in one study as being a disease with less than the median of the sum of the size of the lesions, where the median was 96 mm (10–664 mm). CheckMate 141 was a phase III trial that enrolled 361 patients with R/M HNSCC, of any tumor PD-L1 expression status, who had disease progression within 6 months after platinum-based chemotherapy (37). This trial compared nivolumab 3 mg/kg every 2 weeks to the investigator's selected standard therapy, namely MTX, DTX, or Cmab. Nivolumab monotherapy provided better OS than standard therapy, with a median OS of 7.5 months versus 5.1 months for standard therapy and an HR for death of 0.70 (p = .01). Median PFS in the two arms was similar, however, at 2 months for nivolumab and 2.3 months for standard therapy, and an HR of disease progression or death of 0.89 (p = .32). Further, ORR was 13.3% for nivolumab versus 5.8% for standard therapy. Of note, the rate of PFS at 6 months was 19.7% with nivolumab versus 9.9% for standard therapy, contrasting with the rate of OS at 1 year of 36% for nivolumab and 16.6% for standard therapy. This study was terminated ahead of schedule due to the superiority of the nivolumab arm compared to the control arm (83). Positive tumor PD-L1 expression appeared to have resulted in a greater numerical survival benefit in those patients who received nivolumab versus the investigator's choice therapy, with an HR of 0.55 (95% CI, 0.36–0.83) in patients with tumors expressing ≥1% PD-L1 versus 0.89 (95% CI, 0.54–1.45) in those patients whose tumors expressed <1% PD-L1 (37,75). Although PD-L1–positive tumors showed somewhat higher tumor responses when compared with PD-L1–negative tumors, the trial could not show apparent interactions between tumor PD-L1 expression status and treatment (84). Safety findings from studies of ICI with available data have indicated that pembrolizumab and nivolumab have a favorable and tolerable toxicity profile compared with standard therapies in second-line and platinum-refractory R/M HNSCC. Treatment-related events occurred in 58.9% (grade 3–4 in 13.1%) and 62% (grade 3–4 in 9%) of patients in CheckMate 141 and KEYNOTE-012, respectively (37,81). These frequencies are closely similar to the safety data reported from 576 advanced melanoma patients who received nivolumab (85). With regard to patient-reported outcomes from CheckMate 141, quality of life measures such as social functioning and pain revealed stabilization or slight improvement, whereas monochemotherapy with the investigator's choice resulted in a clinically meaningful exacerbation in many of these measures (37). ORRs to ICIs remain around the 20% mark in second-line patients with R/M HNSCC unselected for tumor PD-L1 expression status. As described earlier, the data continue to suggest that there is potential correlation of PD-L1 expression with better efficacy of ICIs. Nevertheless, the correlation is not very strong or definitive, and no other reliable biomarker for effectively selecting optimally responsive patient subgroups has yet been identified (48,62). A potential biomarker of response to ICIs is the interferon-γ (IFN-γ) six-gene signature (*CXCL9*, *CXCL10*, *IDO1*, *IFNG*, *HLA-DRA*, and *STAT1*). This signature was identified in the KEYNOTE-001 study, in which 18 melanoma patients were treated with pembrolizumab, and validated in the KEYNOTE-012 study, in which 43 HNSCC patients and 33 gastric cancer patients were treated with pembrolizumab (86,87). In the KEYNOTE-012 study, a higher IFN-γ six-gene score was significantly associated with response to pembrolizumab monotherapy and correlated with longer PFS and OS. This gene signature may reflect the so-called "T cell inflamed type" or "non–T cell inflamed type," which is related to the therapeutic effect of anti-PD-1 therapy (87,88). In contrast, the six-gene score showed no correlation with HPV status in any way. Other trials of ICI monotherapy are also investigating second-line R/M HNSCC. Ongoing trials with pembrolizumab include KEYNOTE-040 and MASTERKEY232 (combination pembrolizumab and talimogene laherparepvec in second-line and platinum-refractory R/M HNSCC). Upcoming nivolumab trials in HNSCC include CheckMate 714 (mixed population of patients with platinum-refractory and first-line R/M HNSCC). Finally, ongoing trials with durvalumab include the phase 2 HAWK study (monotherapy in second-line, PD-L1–positive R/M HNSCC following a single platinum-based treatment) and the phase 3 EAGLE study (monotherapy or combination with tremelimumab in second-line R/M HNSCC following a single platinum-based treatment) (60,75,76,89,90).

Chemotherapy

Available and frequently used cytotoxic agents for second-line therapy in R/M HNSCC include MTX, DTX, and PTX. Combination therapy generally does not show better results than monotherapy in second-line treatment for patients with R/M HNSCC. A phase II trial of irinotecan (CPT-11) and DTX, which recruited patients with good PS in second-line treatment returned poor results, with an ORR of 3% and median survival of 5 months (65). In addition, other randomized phase II trials conducted to date have suggested no difference in survival between these monotherapies (32,37). Thus, cytotoxic agents are usually used as a single agent in second treatment, such as MTX monotherapy, with ORR of 6% and median OS of 6 months (35,36). Before ICIs appeared in daily practice, a retrospective report in a cohort of 117 patients described the outcome after Cmab and platinum-containing pretreatment (91). Among the 117 patients treated for R/M HNSCC with first-line platinum and Cmab-based systemic therapy, 63 patients (54%) did not reach second-line treatment and 5 were not assessable for response, and only 49 patients were included in analysis. The regimen used in second-line therapy was mainly MTX (55%), the majority of which was monotherapy. ORR was 8%, with 33% showing SD. Median PDS and OS were 81 days and 184 days, respectively. Although the Checkmate 141 trial was not designed to compare the three regimens used in the comparator arm, DTX appeared slightly numerically superior to MTX with regard to OS, and possibly Cmab also, albeit that the Cmab group included only 15 patients.

Anti-EGFR Therapy

As monotherapy for platinum-refractory R/M HNSCC populations, Cmab monotherapy has been tested in two phase II clinical trials. ORRs were 10% and 13% and disease control rates while on Cmab monotherapy were as high as 50%, while median OS was between 5 and 6 months (12,13). Cmab monotherapy is currently approved in the United States but has not yet been compared with BSC. Adding platinum to Cmab in this setting has not been considered to improve efficacy. Cmab plus CDDP or CBDCA in platinum-refractory patients within 50 days of the last platinum dose of the previous regimen in the R/M setting achieved ORRs of 10% with a median OS of around 6 months (79). Herbst et al. also reported an ORR to Cmab plus CDDP of 6% and a median OS of 4.3 months in patients with platinum-refractory disease if PD occurred within 90 days of the last platinum dose prior to entering the study (3). Meanwhile, Cmab plus taxane is another treatment option in the second-line setting. The combination of Cmab and PTX has shown ORRs of 38% to 55% and median OS of 7.6 to 10 months (92–94). Cmab plus DTX given to patients with R/M HNSCC after failure of platinum-based therapy resulted in 11% of patients achieving PRs and 40% achieving disease control, and median OS was 6.7 months (95). Moreover, retrospective analysis of a biweekly Cmab and DTX regimen in patients not suitable for platinum doublet treatment showed equivalent results (96), with an ORR, DCR, PFS, and OS of 12.9%, 41.9%, 4.0 months, and 8.3 months, respectively. In contrast, other anti-EGFR therapies have failed to show promising efficacy. Second-line Pmab monotherapy yielded an ORR of 4% and a median OS of 5.1 months (97). Zalutumumab, an anti-EGFR antibody, also failed to prolong OS compared with BSC alone (many patients received MTX in the control arm) in a patient population with platinum-refractory R/M HNSCC, as described above (80). EGFR tyrosine kinase inhibitors such as afatinib and gefitinib have also yielded modest efficacy. LUX-Head & Neck 1 was a randomized phase III trial comparing afatinib versus MTX in fit patients with R/M HNSCC who had progressed on or after first-line platinum-based therapy. When compared with the efficacy of MTX monotherapy described earlier, afatinib was associated with an improved PFS compared with MTX (median PFS: 2.6 vs. 1.7 months; $p = .03$). However, afatinib yielded a median OS of 6.8 months (vs. no improvement), with an ORR of 10% (35). Accordingly, afatinib offers no survival advantage over MTX in these patients and should not be considered an evidence-based approach in second-line therapy. Cohen et al. evaluated the association of ERBB-related biomarkers and p16 on the antitumor activity of afatinib and MTX to identify the subsets of patients who would most benefit from afatinib therapy (98). They showed that afatinib had a higher response rate in EGFR-directed therapy–naive patients with p16-negative tumors (27.5% vs. 4.8%) and patients with p16-negative and EGFR-amplified tumors (15.5% vs. 0%). In contrast to this, there were no responders among patients with p16-positive disease. Another phase II trial showed comparable efficacy with some toxicity profile differences between Cmab and afatinib (99). Similar results were obtained from a randomized phase III trial with gefitinib. Patients who had progressed on or were not fit for standard first-line therapy received DTX plus a placebo or DTX plus gefitinib. ORRs for the DTX plus placebo versus DTX plus gefitinib arms were 6.2% and 12.5%, respectively, with a nonsignificant improvement in median OS of 1.3 months (from 6.0 to 7.3 months) (100).

PI3K/AKT/mTOR Inhibition

Phosphatidylinositol 3-kinase (PI3K), Akt (a serine/threonine kinase also known as PKB), and mammalian target of rapamycin (mTOR) are three major junctions in the pathway. Because the PI3K/Akt/mTOR pathway is a downstream signaling cascade of EGFR, activation of this pathway contributes to treatment resistance and disease progression in HNSCC (101). Indeed, approximately 20% of HNSCCs harbor mutations in the *PIK3CA* gene, making this the most commonly mutated gene in the pathway (102). Buparlisib (BKM120), a pan-PI3K inhibitor, plus PTX treatment was compared to a placebo plus PTX regimen in platinum-pretreated patients with one or two previous lines of therapy in the R/M HNSCC setting (the BERIL-1 trial). A statistically significant difference in the primary end point of PFS (median PFS 4.6 months vs. 3.4 months; $p = .011$) and secondary end point of ORR (39% vs. 14%; $p = .00031$) were observed. Temsirolimus, an mTORC1 inhibitor, was evaluated as a single agent in a phase II trial, which enrolled patients who were platinum and Cmab-refractory with a primary end point of PFS rate at 12 weeks of therapy (103). Although no objective responses were noted, a PFS rate of 40% at 12 weeks and a high safety profile were reported. Everolimus, an oral selective tyrosine kinase inhibitor of the mTOR protein, was also evaluated as a single agent in a single-arm phase II study enrolling patients who failed at least one prior therapy. There have been no major successes in response rate with 0% and prognosis; median PFS and OS were 1.5 and 4.5 months, respectively (104). On the other hand, the combination of temsirolimus plus erlotinib was poorly tolerated in patients with platinum-refractory R/M HNSCC, suggesting the need for caution in using mTOR and EGFR targeting therapy (105).

SPECIAL POPULATIONS

HUMAN PAPILLOMAVIRUS

Retrospective data show the value of HPV as an independent favorable prognostic factor in R/M HNSCC. The 181 patients with stage III to IV oropharyngeal cancer recruited in Radiation Therapy Oncology Group (RTOG) trials 0129 or RTOG 0522 with a known tumor p16 status (p16-positive, $n = 105$; p16-negative, $n = 76$) as well as disease progression after receiving platinum-based chemoradiotherapy (CRT) were candidates for retrospective analysis of the association of tumor p16 status with OS after disease progression (106). The patients with p16-positive oropharyngeal cancer had significantly improved survival rates compared with the p16-negative patients (2-year OS, 54.6% vs. 27.6%; median, 2.6 vs. 0.8 years; $p < .001$). Further, p16-positive tumor status reduced risk of death after disease progression (HR, 0.48; 95% CI [0.31–0.74]) after adjustment for tumor stage and smoking status. Similarly, the 64 patients with R/M HNSCC enrolled onto ECOG protocol 1395 (E1395) or E3301 who had known tumor HPV status (HPV-positive, $n = 11$; HPV-negative, $n = 53$) were eligible for retrospective analysis of the association between HPV status, and ORR and OS. The patients with HPV-positive HNSCC had significantly improved ORR and OS compared with HPV-negative patients (ORR, 55% v 19%; $p = .022$, median OS, 11.9 vs. 6.7 months; $p < .001$). In multivariate analysis, the

HR for OS was 2.69 for HPV-negative versus HPV-positive status (95% CI [1.01–7.20]; $p = .048$), favoring HPV-positive patients (107). The impact of tumor HPV status on outcome in patients with R/M HNSCC receiving the EXTREME regimen was retrospectively examined. Four hundred and sixteen tumor samples were available for p16 and HPV analysis, of which 10% were p16-positive and 5% were HPV-positive. Adding Cmab to chemotherapy improved survival, irrespective of tumor p16 or HPV status (108). Moreover, the prognostic value of HPV status seems to remain consistent in patients under treatment with ICIs. In CheckMate 141, patients with p16-positive tumors experienced a numerically larger magnitude of benefit from nivolumab treatment than patients with p16-negative tumors in terms of OS (p16-positive [HR=0.56] and p16-negative [HR=0.73] (75). Subgroup analyses of response rates to pembrolizumab by HPV status revealed an ORR in patients with HPV-positive disease of 22% versus 16% in patients with HPV-negative disease in the KEYNOTE-055 study, and 32% versus 14%, respectively, in the KEYNOTE-012 study (60,81). Importantly, however, these effects of tumor PD-L1 expression and HPV status lack the strength required to influence ICI therapy, and it is important to remember that patients with R/M HNSCC currently should be treated similarly, irrespective of HPV status. Nevertheless, these studies illustrate the importance of HPV stratification in future clinical trials. The current lack of data will strongly influence the analysis of future randomized trials.

MANAGEMENT OF UNFIT PATIENTS

A patient with an ECOG PS of 0 or 1 will generally receive the EXTREME regimen as first-line treatment, because this regimen is the only multidrug regimen to show a survival advantage and should be used as the standard of care for such fit patients. On the other hand, a patient with an ECOG PS of 2 would generally be treated with a single-agent therapy in the first-line setting. The regimens include targeted therapeutics, such as Cmab or cytotoxic chemotherapy agents, including MTX, DTX, PTX, CBDCA, 5-FU, and capecitabine (109–111). Some clinical studies have enrolled patients with an ECOG PS of 2: one was a phase 3 trial that compared gefitinib with MTX, while a second compared DTX with or without gefitinib (the IMEX trial) and a third compared DTX with or without gefitinib. All three studies failed to show survival benefits with these newer therapies over standard monotherapy with MTX or a taxane (36,100). Currently, Cmab and MTX monotherapy is being compared as first-line treatment in the unfit elderly (≥70 years of age) with R/M HNSCC in a randomized phase III trial (ELAN-UNFIT, NCT01884623). Given the preferable toxicity profile of ICIs, the use of ICIs as monotherapy for the treatment of unfit patients is appraisable. However, it should be recognized that ICIs as monotherapy have low activity and that the majority of patients progress at first reevaluation. Accordingly, symptomatic patients with a PS of 2 due to disease may experience rapid deterioration.

ELDERLY POPULATION

In general, most clinical trials use an age level of 70 years to define the elderly (112). However, chronological age does not always reflect individual organ function, and life expectancy is not always absolutely predicted by the risk of treatment-related adverse events. Thus, for fragile patients with poor performance status or comorbid conditions, a single-drug regimen or BSC would be offered irrespective of their actual age, as described previously. In the United States, 54% of malignant head and neck cancer cases occur in patients older than 65 years of age, and this proportion is expected to rise to 66% by 2030 (113). Considering this, treatment of this population urgently warrants more careful consideration. There have been many attempts to explore how chronological age affects benefit and safety profiles of treatment in both first- and second-line settings. As one example, a combined analysis of two phase III trials (ECOG 1393 and 1395) was conducted to evaluate outcomes in elderly patients (70 years or older) with head and neck cancer undergoing palliative platinum-doublet chemotherapy (112). Results showed no statistically significant differences in ORR (28% vs. 33%), median time to progression (5.25 months vs. 4.8 months), median OS (5.3 months vs. 8 months), or 1-year survival (26% vs. 33%) between elderly and younger patients, respectively. However, a significantly higher incidence of severe adverse events, including nephrotoxicity, diarrhea, and thrombocytopenia was observed in the elderly population. In the EXTREME trial, patients aged 65 years and over accounted for 17% of the total number of patients enrolled. Subgroup analysis of this cohort showed that the survival advantage given by adding Cmab to platinum/5-FU chemotherapy was not statistically significant (median OS 9.1 and 7.8 months; HR = 1.07, 95% CI, 0.65–1.77), in contrast to the young population (7). With regard to second-line treatment for R/M HNSCC, the population aged 65 years or older enrolled in the LUX-Head and Neck 1 trial accounted for 27% of the total number of patients. The PFS benefit with afatinib versus MTX was equivalent in patients aged 65 years or older (2.8 months vs. 2.3 months; HR = 0.68, 95%CI, 0.45–1.03, *p* = .061) and younger patients (2.6 months vs. 1.6 months; HR = 0.79; 95% CI, 0.62–1.01, *p* = .052), with no excessive toxicity in the elderly (114). On the other hand, a phase III trial that compared docetaxel with or without gefitinib, showed survival benefits of combination therapy in patients younger than 65 years (100). With regard to immunotherapy, particularly immunity checkpoints, these drugs may induce a durable response even in patients with refractory disease and are believed to have a relatively low incidence of serious adverse events. Promising results were presented from early clinical trials exploring nivolumab in the CHECKMATE-141 trial; in this trial, nivolumab improved median OS in platinum-refractory R/M-HNSCC compared with single-agent chemotherapy or Cmab and was the first drug ever to improve OS in these patients. Of the 361 enrolled patients, 113 (31%) were 65 years or older. Unfortunately, the survival benefit of nivolumab observed in patients aged 65–74 years did not reach statistical significance (HR = 0.93, 95% CI, 0.56–1.54), and the benefit was thus limited to their younger counterparts (76). Reports of patients treated with nivolumab show no apparent difference in the incidence of immune-related toxicities between younger and older patients (115). Meanwhile, a meta-analysis used data for 5,265 patients from nine randomized controlled trials (RCTs) of ICI to compare the efficacy of ICIs between younger and older patients. When patients were dichotomized into younger and older groups with an age cut-off of 65–70 years, ICIs improved OS in both younger (HR = 0.75, 95% CI, 0.68–0.82) and older (HR = 0.73, 95% CI, 0.62–0.87) groups. Moreover, an improvement in PFS was observed in both younger (HR = 0.58, 95% CI, 0.40–0.84) and older (HR = 0.77, 95% CI, 0.58–1.01) patients. The benefit in OS with ICIs was significant in both younger and older patients with a cut-off age of 65–70 years (116). In addition, given the need to better predict chemotherapeutic toxicity in this population, a predictive model was developed to identify risk factors for chemotherapy-induced toxicity in 500 elderly patients aged 65 years or older with median age of 74 years. This scoring system allowed patients to be classified as high (83%), intermediate (52%), or low risk (30%) for grade 3 to 5 chemotherapy toxicity ($p < .001$) (117). Most recently, this classification was externally validated in 250 independent patients similarly aged 65 years or older, with median age of 73 years. Risk of toxicity increased with increasing risk score (36.7% low, 62.4% medium, 70.2% high risk; $p < .001$). The AUC of the receiver-operating characteristic curve (ROC) was 0.65 (95% CI, 0.58–0.71), which was not statistically different from that of the development cohort (HR = 0.72, 95% CI, 0.68–0.77, *p* = .09). The author concluded that the predictive model should be considered when discussing the risks and benefits of chemotherapy with older adults (118). In summary, these results suggest that the benefits of systemic therapy are present even in the elderly. Nevertheless, given concerns about toxicity, further efforts to improve safety are required.

NASOPHARYNGEAL CANCER

Radiation therapy (RT) or CRT has become the primary treatment of early or locoregionally advanced NPC (119,120). However, about one third of these patients have treatment failure due to distant metastasis (121). NPC is a highly chemosensitive tumor, and the high response rate of 80% has been reported for several regimens based on CDDP. Thus, systemic chemotherapy is often used in patients with R/M disease. Fluorouracil and CDDP are generally regarded as standard first-line chemotherapy regimens for these patients but have not been compared directly with the best supportive regimen. Zhang et al. reported the first randomized controlled trial in the R/M setting (122). This study compared two widely used CDDP-containing doublet chemotherapy regimens and covered a major gap in the management of patients with R/M NPC. With the primary end point of PFS, the results established the superiority of gemcitabine over 5-FU by infusion as companion to the CDDP backbone. Regarding adverse events, the CDDP/gemcitabine (GEM) group experienced greater hematological toxicity than the group treated with CDDP/5-FU (neutropenia, 23% vs. 13%, $p = .0251$; thrombocytopenia, 13% vs. 2%; $p = .0007$). In contrast, patients in the CDDP/5-FU group experienced a greater incidence of grade 3 and above mucositis (15% vs. 0%; $p < .0001$). Nevertheless, the incidence of serious adverse events attributed to treatment was similarly low between the two groups, at 4% versus 6%. For other nonhematologic toxicities, results in the two groups were otherwise identical. Furthermore, CDDP/GEM's ability to be administered in the outpatient setting makes it advantageous in terms of logistics and patient convenience. In a retrospective trial, no difference in PFS or OS was observed between doublet and triplet platinum-containing regimens (123). Considering that a prospective phase II trial of PTX, CBDCA, and GEM also showed substantial toxic effects but no substantial improvement in efficacy, triplet regimens should not be given in this setting (124). DTX, capecitabine, and GEM monotherapy are suitable second-line therapies in platinum-resistant disease, with reported ORRs of 30%–40% (125–127). Doublet combinations (GEM plus vinorelbine, CDDP plus pemetrexed) have been investigated in this setting, but ORR and time to disease progression with these regimens are no better than those obtained with monotherapy (125,127). Among molecular-targeted therapies, inhibition of EGFR or vascular endothelial growth factor (VEGF) has shown clinical efficacy in patients with platinum-refractory disease. In a multicenter phase II clinical trial of 60 heavily pretreated NPC patients who progressed after pre-platinum-based chemotherapy, the ORR and DCR to Cmab in combination with CBDCA was 12% and 48% respectively (128). Agents targeting VEGF, such as sorafenib, pazopanib, famitinib, sunitinib, and axitinib, have demonstrated promising clinical activities in NPC, with clinical benefit in 37% to 74% of cases (129–133). However, one issue for VEGF inhibition concerns the increase in risk of bleeding: 13 patients (64%) treated with sunitinib who had previously received curative RT to the nasopharynx/neck experienced hemorrhagic events. Previous RT to the thorax was significantly associated with hemoptysis. In addition, two patients with local tumor infiltration into the carotid sheath developed lethal epistaxis/hematemesis during the first cycle of sunitinib, likely due to internal carotid bleeding after tumor shrinkage. It is therefore suggested that patients with disease recurrence or invasion to the major vasculature within a previously irradiated area should be excluded from trials of VEGF inhibitors (132,134).

Epstein–Barr virus (EBV) is present in virtually almost all patients with poorly differentiated (WHO type II) and undifferentiated non-NPC (WHO type III). Viral antigens expressed by tumor cells are therefore attractive targets for immunotherapy via recognition of expressed viral antigens (EBNA1, latent membrane protein 1 [LMP1], and LMP2). Adoptive transfer of cytotoxic T cells (CTLs) specific for EBV antigens has been tested in several clinical studies: Results demonstrate that administration of EBV-specific CTLs to patients with advanced NPC is feasible and induces a virus antigen-specific immune response and is associated with objective response and disease control (135,136). Autologous dendritic cell (DC) vaccination is also being studied. DCs are antigen-presenting cells that play a critical role in the activation of naive $CD4^+$ and $CD8^+$ T cells. Following ex vivo generation and maturation, the cells are pulsed with tumor antigens and then administered. A vaccine of DCs pulsed with peptides derived from LMP2 has been evaluated in 16 NPC patients with local recurrence or distant metastasis. Nine patients showed the elicitation or boosting of peptide-specific T-cell responses, and two showed partial tumor reduction (137). PD-L1 expression was detected in 95% of NPC patients (132/139) and high expression of PD-L1 or PD-1 and PD-L1 was associated with disease-free survival (138). Antibodies that inhibit the interaction of PD-1 with its ligand are now undergoing clinical trial. Among these, KEYNOTE-028 (NCT 02054806) is being conducted as a randomized phase 1b study of pembrolizumab in patients with PD-L1–positive advanced solid tumors. Among 27 heavily pretreated patients in the NPC cohort, 7 patients experienced PR and 14 had SD. Best ORR was 25.9% (95% CI, 11.1–46.3). Responses were reasonably durable, with a median of 10.8 months (139). Based upon these results, KEYNOTE-122 (NCT02611960), a study of pembrolizumab versus standard of care treatment (capecitabine, GEM, or DTX) for the treatment of R/M NPC, is now being initiated. In addition, a phase II trial of nivolumab in R/M NPC is also ongoing (NCT02339558).

PROGNOSTIC/PREDICTIVE FACTORS

Great efforts have been taken to identify prognostic and predictive factors in patients with R/M HNSCC. Indeed, several biomarkers such as HPV infection have been proposed, as described earlier. Argiris and Forastiere revealed that high or moderate tumor differentiation and a primary tumor in the oral cavity or the hypopharynx were determined as unfavorable prognostic factors for OS of the patients treated with cisplatin doublets (140). Patient's status and previous treatment have also been attracting attention. Subgroup analysis of the EXTREME study indicated patients with young age or better PS (Karnofsky score ≥80) might benefit from adding Cmab to chemotherapy (7). In the SPECTRUM trial, weight loss of more than 5% during the last 6 months and prior platinum chemotherapy were identified as independent negative prognostic factors (70). These factors seem worthwhile to take into consideration when selecting an optimal treatment for individual patient and performing trials.

CONCLUSIONS

The EXTREME regimen has been in use for more than 10 years as standard treatment for R/M HNSCC in the first-line setting. In addition, ICI monotherapy has shown promising therapeutic effects in the second and later line and in the platinum-refractory setting. Looking forward, promising clinical effects are expected for molecular targeted drugs other than Cmab. Meanwhile, ongoing evaluation of treatment for elderly patients and unfit patients is required. With R/M NPC, the first randomized controlled trial showed the superiority of gemcitabine over infusional 5-FU as companion to the CDDP backbone and provided long-sought data about the optimal chemotherapy regimen in first-line treatment of the disease. We emphasize that our treatment goal is to maximize patient survival while retaining maximum quality of life. Accordingly, our future activities should seek optimal combinations and sequencing of those drugs that are already available, and those introduced in the future. Participation of patients in clinical trials should be strongly encouraged when possible (including elderly patients and unfit cases). Finally, the identification of clinically useful predictive biomarkers is also urgently needed.

REFERENCES

1. Zhang XF, Yang HS, Lee J, et al. MicroRNA-related genetic variations as predictors for risk of second primary tumor and/or recurrence in patients with early-stage head and neck cancer. *Carcinogenesis.* 2010;31:2118–2123. doi:10.1093/carcin/bgq177
2. Argiris A, Karamouzis MV, Raben D, Ferris RL. Head and neck cancer. *Lancet.* 2008;371:1695–1709. doi:10.1016/S0140-6736(08)60728-X
3. Herbst RS, Arquette M, Shin DM, et al. Phase II multicenter study of the epidermal growth factor receptor antibody cetuximab and cisplatin for recurrent and refractory squamous cell carcinoma of the head and neck. *J Clin Oncol.* 2005;23:5578–5587. doi:10.1200/JCO.2005.07.120
4. Cho BC, Keum KC, Shin SJ, et al. Weekly docetaxel in patients with platinum-refractory metastatic or recurrent squamous cell carcinoma of the head and neck. *Cancer Chemother Pharmacol.* 2009;65:27–32. doi:10.1007/s00280-009-0999-4
5. Kowalski LP, Carvalho AL. Natural history of untreated head and neck cancer. *Eur J Cancer.* 2000;36:1032–1037. doi:10.1016/S0959-8049(00)00054-X
6. Vermorken JB, Specenier P. Optimal treatment for recurrent/metastatic head and neck cancer. Ann Oncol. 2010;21(Suppl 7):vii252–vii261. doi:10.1093/annonc/mdq453
7. Vermorken JB, Mesia R, Rivera F, et al. Platinum-based chemotherapy plus cetuximab in head and neck cancer. *N Engl J Med.* 2008;359:1116–1127. doi:10.1056/NEJMoa0802656
8. Guigay J, Fayette J, Dillies AF, et al. Cetuximab, docetaxel, and cisplatin as first-line treatment in patients with recurrent or metastatic head and neck squamous cell carcinoma: a multicenter, phase II GORTEC study. *Ann Oncol.* 2015;26:1941–1947. doi:10.1093/annonc/mdv268
9. Tahara M Kiyota N, Yokota T, et al. Phase II trial of combination treatment with paclitaxel, carboplatin and cetuximab (PCE) as first-line treatment in patients with recurrent and/or metastatic squamous cell carcinoma of the head and neck (CSPOR-HN02). *Ann Oncol.* 2018. [Epub ahead of print] doi:10.1093/annonc/mdy040.
10. Argiris A, Harrington KJ, Tahara M, et al. Evidence-based treatment options in recurrent and/or metastatic squamous cell carcinoma of the head and neck. *Front Oncol.* 2017;7:72. doi:10.3389/fonc.2017.00072
11. Price KA, Cohen EE. Current treatment options for metastatic head and neck cancer. *Curr Treat Options Oncol.* 2012;13:35–46. doi:10.1007/s00405-012-1998-3
12. Vermorken JB, Trigo J, Hitt R, et al. Open-label, uncontrolled, multicenter phase II study to evaluate the efficacy and toxicity of cetuximab as a single agent in patients with recurrent and/or metastatic squamous cell carcinoma of the head and neck who failed to respond to platinum-based therapy. *J Clin Oncol.* 2007;25:2171–2177. doi:10.1200/JCO.2006.06.7447

13. Wheeler RH. Chemotherapy of patients with recurrent head and neck cancers. In: Jacobs C, ed. *Carcinomas of the Head and Neck: Evaluation, Management*. Boston, MA: Kluwer Academic; 1990:171–193.
14. Hong WK, Schaefer S, Issell B, et al. A prospective randomized trial of methotrexate versus cisplatin in the treatment of recurrent squamous cell carcinoma of the head and neck. *Cancer*. 1983;52:206–210. doi:10.1002/1097-0142(19830715)52:2<206::AID-CNCR2820520204>3.0.CO;2-J
15. Jacobs C, Lyman G, Velez-Garcia E, et al. A phase III randomized study comparing cisplatin and fluorouracil as single agents and in combination for advanced squamous cell carcinoma of the head and neck. *J Clin Oncol*. 1992;10:257–263. doi:10.1200/JCO.1992.10.2.257
16. Veronesi A, Zagonel V, Tirelli U, et al. High-dose versus low-dose cisplatin in advanced head and neck squamous carcinoma: a randomized study. *J Clin Oncol*. 1985;3:1105–1108. doi:10.1200/JCO.1985.3.8.1105
17. Morton RP, Rugman F, Dorman EB, et al. Cisplatinum and bleomycin for advanced or recurrent squamous cell carcinoma of the head and neck: a randomised factorial phase III controlled trial. *Cancer Chemother Pharmacol*. 1985;15:283–289. doi:10.1007/BF00263902
18. Eisenberger M, Hornedo J, Silva H, et al. Carboplatin (NSC-241-240): an active platinum analog for the treatment of squamous-cell carcinoma of the head and neck. *J Clin Oncol*. 1986;4:1506–1509. doi:10.1200/JCO.1986.4.10.1506
19. de Andres Basauri L, Lopez Pousa A, Alba E, Sampedro F. Carboplatin, an active drug in advanced head and neck cancer. *Cancer Treat Rep*. 1986;70:1173–1176.
20. Al-Sarraf M, Metch B, Kish J, et al. Platinum analogs in recurrent and advanced head and neck cancer: a Southwest Oncology Group and Wayne State University Study. *Cancer Treat Rep*. 1987;71:723–726.
21. Inuyama Y, Togawa K, Morita M, et al. Phase II study of carboplatin in head and neck cancer. *Gan To Kagaku Ryoho*. 1988;15:2131–2138.
22. De Andres L, Brunet J, Lopez-Pousa A, et al. Randomized trial of neoadjuvant cisplatin and fluorouracil versus carboplatin and fluorouracil in patients with stage IV-M0 head and neck cancer. *J Clin Oncol*. 1995;13:1493–1500. doi:10.1200/JCO.1995.13.6.1493
23. Welkoborsky HJ, Bleier R, Wissen-Siegert I. Antineoplastic effectiveness and unwanted side effects of polychemotherapy of extensive oro- and hypopharyngeal cancers–results of a prospective therapy study with 5-FU/cisplatin versus 5-FU/carboplatin. *Laryngorhinootologie*. 1992;71:261–266. doi:10.1055/s-2007-997292
24. Ebeling O, Eckel HE, Volling P, et al. Cisplatin/5-FU versus carboplatin/5-FU. 5 year follow-up. *HNO*. 1994;42:629–635.
25. Forastiere AA, Metch B, Schuller DE, et al. Randomized comparison of cisplatin plus fluorouracil and carboplatin plus fluorouracil versus methotrexate in advanced squamous-cell carcinoma of the head and neck: a Southwest Oncology Group study. *J Clin Oncol*. 1992;10:1245–1251. doi:10.1200/JCO.1992.10.8.1245
26. Smith RE, Thornton DE, Allen J. A phase II trial of paclitaxel in squamous cell carcinoma of the head and neck with correlative laboratory studies. *Semin Oncol*. 1995;22:41–46.
27. Forastiere AA, Shank D, Neuberg D, et al. Final report of a phase II evaluation of paclitaxel in patients with advanced squamous cell carcinoma of the head and neck: an Eastern Cooperative Oncology Group trial (PA390). *Cancer*. 1998;82:2270–2274. doi:10.1002/(SICI)1097-0142(19980601)82:11<2270::AID-CNCR24>3.0.CO;2-Q
28. Tahara M, Minami H, Hasegawa Y, et al. Weekly paclitaxel in patients with recurrent or metastatic head and neck cancer. *Cancer Chemother Pharmacol*. 2011;68:769–776. doi:10.1007/s00280-010-1550-3
29. Catimel G, Verweij J, Mattijssen V, et al. Docetaxel (Taxotere): an active drug for the treatment of patients with advanced squamous cell carcinoma of the head and neck. EORTC Early Clinical Trials Group. *Ann Oncol*. 1994;5:533–537. doi:10.1093/oxfordjournals.annonc.a058908
30. Dreyfuss AI, Clark JR, Norris CM, et al. Docetaxel: an active drug for squamous cell carcinoma of the head and neck. *J Clin Oncol*. 1996;14:1672–1678. doi:10.1200/JCO.1996.14.5.1672
31. Couteau C, Chouaki N, Leyvraz S, et al. A phase II study of docetaxel in patients with metastatic squamous cell carcinoma of the head and neck. *Br J Cancer*. 1999;81:457–462. doi:10.1038/sj.bjc.6690715
32. Guardiola E, Peyrade F, Chaigneau L, et al. Results of a randomised phase II study comparing docetaxel with methotrexate in patients with recurrent head and neck cancer. *Eur J Cancer*. 2004;40:2071–2076. doi:10.1016/j.ejca.2004.05.019
33. Inuyama Y, Kataura A, Togawa K, et al. Late phase II clinical study of RP56976 (docetaxel) in patients with advanced/recurrent head and neck cancer. *Gan To Kagaku Ryoho*. 1999;26:107–116.
34. Muggia FM, Rozencweig M, Louie AE. Role of chemotherapy in head and neck cancer: systemic use of single agents and combinations in advanced disease. *Head Neck Surg*. 1980;2:196–205. doi:10.1002/hed.2890020305
35. Machiels JP, Haddad RI, Fayette J, et al. Afatinib versus methotrexate as second-line treatment in patients with recurrent or metastatic squamous-cell carcinoma of the head and neck progressing on or after platinum-based therapy (LUX-Head & Neck 1): an open-label, randomised phase 3 trial. *Lancet Oncol*. 2015;16:583–594. doi:10.1016/S1470-2045(15)70124-5
36. Kushwaha VS, Gupta S, Husain N, et al. Gefitinib, Methotrexate and Methotrexate plus 5-Fluorouracil as palliative treatment in recurrent head and neck squamous cell carcinoma. *Cancer Biol Ther*. 2015;16:346–351. doi:10.4161/15384047.2014.961881
37. Ferris RL, Blumenschein G Jr, Fayette J, et al. Nivolumab for recurrent squamous-cell carcinoma of the head and neck. *N Engl J Med*. 2016;375:1856–1867. doi:10.1056/NEJMoa1602252

38. Lokich JJ. Optimal schedule for 5-fluorouracil chemotherapy. Intermittent bolus or continuous infusion? *Am J Clin Oncol.* 1985;8:445–448.
39. Martinez-Trufero J, Isla D, Adansa JC, et al. Phase II study of capecitabine as palliative treatment for patients with recurrent and metastatic squamous head and neck cancer after previous platinum-based treatment. *Br J Cancer.* 2010;102:1687–1691. doi:10.1038/sj.bjc.6605697
40. Park S, Lee S,Park J, et al. Phase II study of oral S-1 in pretreated patients with recurrent or metastatic head and neck cancer. *J Clinl Oncol.* 2008;26:17007. doi:10.1200/jco.2008.26.15_suppl.17007
41. Agulnik M. New approaches to EGFR inhibition for locally advanced or metastatic squamous cell carcinoma of the head and neck (SCCHN). *Med Oncol.* 2012;29:2481–2491. doi:10.1007/s12032-012-0159-2
42. Trivedi S, Srivastava RM, Concha-Benavente F, et al. Anti-EGFR targeted monoclonal antibody isotype influences antitumor cellular immunity in head and neck cancer patients. *Clin Cancer Res.* 2016;22:5229–5237. doi:10.1158/1078-0432.CCR-15-2971
43. Veluchamy JP, Spanholtz J, Tordoir M, et al. Combination of NK cells and cetuximab to enhance anti-tumor responses in RAS mutant metastatic colorectal cancer. *PLOS ONE.* 2016;11:e0157830. doi:10.1371/journal.pone.0157830
44. Li S, Schmitz KR, Jeffrey PD, et al. Structural basis for inhibition of the epidermal growth factor receptor by cetuximab. *Cancer Cell.* 2005;7:301–311. doi:10.1016/j.ccr.2005.03.003
45. Teillaud J-L. *Antibody-Dependent Cellular Cytotoxicity (ADCC)*.2012. In: eLS. John Wiley & Sons Ltd, Chichester. http://www.els.net. doi:10.1002/9780470015902.a0000498.pub2
46. Ferris RL, Jaffee EM, Ferrone S. Tumor antigen-targeted, monoclonal antibody-based immunotherapy: clinical response, cellular immunity, and immunoescape. *J Clin Oncol.* 2010;28:4390–4399. doi:10.1200/JCO.2009.27.6360
47. Kurai J, Chikumi H, Hashimoto K, et al. Antibody-dependent cellular cytotoxicity mediated by cetuximab against lung cancer cell lines. *Clin Cancer Res.* 2007;13:1552–1561. doi:10.1158/1078-0432.CCR-06-1726
48. Schoppy DW, Sunwoo JB. Immunotherapy for head and neck squamous cell carcinoma. *Hematol Oncol Clin North Am.* 2015;29:1033–1043. doi:10.1016/j.hoc.2015.07.009
49. Taylor RJ, Saloura V, Jain A, et al. Ex vivo antibody-dependent cellular cytotoxicity inducibility predicts efficacy of cetuximab. *Cancer Immunol Res.* 2015;3:567–574. doi:10.1158/2326-6066.CIR-14-0188
50. Lo Nigro C, Ricci V, Vivenza D, et al. Evaluation of antibody-dependent cell-mediated cytotoxicity activity and cetuximab response in KRAS wild-type metastatic colorectal cancer patients. *World J Gastrointest Oncol.* 2016;8:222–230. doi:10.4251/wjgo.v8.i2.222
51. Lattanzio L, Denaro N, Vivenza D, et al. Elevated basal antibody-dependent cell-mediated cytotoxicity (ADCC) and high epidermal growth factor receptor (EGFR) expression predict favourable outcome in patients with locally advanced head and neck cancer treated with cetuximab and radiotherapy. *Cancer Immunol Immunother.* 2017;66:573–579. doi:10.1007/s00262-017-1960-8
52. Srivastava RM, Lee SC, Andrade Filho PA, et al. Cetuximab-activated natural killer and dendritic cells collaborate to trigger tumor antigen-specific T-cell immunity in head and neck cancer patients. *Clin Cancer Res.* 2013;19:1858–1872. doi:10.1158/1078-0432.CCR-12-2426
53. Ferris RL. Immunology and immunotherapy of head and neck cancer. *J Clin Oncol.* 2015;33:3293–3304. doi:10.1200/JCO.2015.61.1509
54. Fan Z, Baselga J, Masui H, Mendelsohn J. Antitumor effect of anti-epidermal growth factor receptor monoclonal antibodies plus cis-diamminedichloroplatinum on well established A431 cell xenografts. *Cancer Res.* 1993;53:4637–4642.
55. Baselga J, Pfister D, Cooper MR, et al. Phase I studies of anti-epidermal growth factor receptor chimeric antibody C225 alone and in combination with cisplatin. *J Clin Oncol.* 2000;18:904–914. doi:10.1200/JCO.2000.18.4.904
56. Burtness B, Goldwasser MA, Flood W, et al. Phase III randomized trial of cisplatin plus placebo compared with cisplatin plus cetuximab in metastatic/recurrent head and neck cancer: an Eastern Cooperative Oncology Group study. *J Clin Oncol.* 2005;23:8646–8654. doi:10.1200/JCO.2005.02.4646
57. Vermorken JB, Herbst RS, Leon X, et al. Overview of the efficacy of cetuximab in recurrent and/or metastatic squamous cell carcinoma of the head and neck in patients who previously failed platinum-based therapies. *Cancer.* 2008;112:2710–2719. doi:10.1002/cncr.23442
58. Baksh K, Weber J. Immune checkpoint protein inhibition for cancer: preclinical justification for CTLA-4 and PD-1 blockade and new combinations. *Semin Oncol.* 2015;42:363–377. doi:10.1053/j.seminoncol.2015.02.015
59. Assal A, Kaner J, Pendurti G, Zang X. Emerging targets in cancer immunotherapy: beyond CTLA-4 and PD-1. *Immunotherapy.* 2015;7:1169–1186. doi:10.2217/imt.15.78
60. Bauml J, Seiwert TY, Pfister DG, et al. Preliminary results from KEYNOTE-055: Pembrolizumab after platinum and cetuximab failure in head and neck squamous cell carcinoma (HNSCC). *ASCO.* 2016;34, (suppl):6011. doi:10.1200/JCO.2016.34.15_suppl.6011
61. Seiwert TY, Burtness B, Mehra R, et al. Safety and clinical activity of pembrolizumab for treatment of recurrent or metastatic squamous cell carcinoma of the head and neck (KEYNOTE-012): an open-label, multicentre, phase 1b trial. *Lancet Oncol.* 2016;17:956–965. doi:10.1016/S1470-2045(16)30066-3
62. Delyon J, Maio M, Lebbe C. The ipilimumab lesson in melanoma: achieving long-term survival. *Semin Oncol.* 2015;42:387–401. doi:10.1053/j.seminoncol.2015.02.005

63. Patil VM, Noronha V, Joshi A, et al. Metronomic chemotherapy in platinum-insensitive failures and/or early failures postmultimodality management in oral cancers. *Indian J Med Paediatr Oncol*. 2015;36:161–165. doi:10.4103/0971-5851.166725
64. Saloura V, Cohen EE, Licitra L, et al. An open-label single-arm, phase II trial of zalutumumab, a human monoclonal anti-EGFR antibody, in patients with platinum-refractory squamous cell carcinoma of the head and neck. *Cancer Chemother Pharmacol*. 2014;73:1227–1239. doi:10.1007/s00280-014-2459-z
65. Argiris A, Buchanan A, Brockstein B, et al. Docetaxel and irinotecan in recurrent or metastatic head and neck cancer: a phase 2 trial of the Eastern Cooperative Oncology Group. *Cancer*. 2009;115:4504–4513. doi:10.1002/cncr.24528
66. Mesia R, Rivera F, Kawecki A, et al. Quality of life of patients receiving platinum-based chemotherapy plus cetuximab first line for recurrent and/or metastatic squamous cell carcinoma of the head and neck. *Ann Oncol*. 2010;21:1967–1973. doi:10.1093/annonc/mdq077
67. Knutzen G, Subbiah S. Cetuximab rechallenge and monotherapy in patients with squamous cell carcinoma of the head and neck. *Case Rep Oncol*. 2015;8:503–508. doi:10.1159/000441019
68. Bossi P, Kornek G, Lanzetta G, et al. Safety and feasibility of every-other-week maintenance cetuximab after first-line chemotherapy in patients with recurrent or metastatic head and neck squamous cell cancer. *Head Neck*. 2013;35:1471–1474. doi:10.1002/hed.23170
69. Guigay J, Peyrade F, Petre-Lazar B, et al. Cetuximab relative dose intensity (RDI) in recurrent/metastatic (R/M) squamous cell carcinoma of the head and neck (SCCHN): first observational prospective study in unselected patients (DIRECT trial). *Ann Oncol*. 2014;25(Suppl 4):iv344. doi:10.1093/annonc/mdu340.11
70. Vermorken JB, Stohlmacher-Williams J, Davidenko I, et al. Cisplatin and fluorouracil with or without panitumumab in patients with recurrent or metastatic squamous-cell carcinoma of the head and neck (SPECTRUM): an open-label phase 3 randomised trial. *Lancet Oncol*. 2013;14:697–710. doi:10.1016/S1470-2045(13)70181-5
71. Hitt R, Irigoyen A, Cortes-Funes H, et al. Phase II study of the combination of cetuximab and weekly paclitaxel in the first-line treatment of patients with recurrent and/or metastatic squamous cell carcinoma of head and neck. *Ann Oncol*. 2012;23:1016–1022. doi:10.1093/annonc/mdr367
72. William WN, Feng L, Kies MS, et al. Randomized, double-blind, placebo-controlled, phase II trial of first-line platinum/docetaxel with or without erlotinib (E) in patients (pts) with recurrent and/or metastatic (R/M) head and neck squamous cell carcinomas (HNSCCs). *J Clin Oncol*. 2017;35:6017. doi:10.1200/JCO.2017.35.15_suppl.6017
73. Argiris A, Gillison M,Ferris RL, et al. A randomized, open-label, phase 3 study of nivolumab in combination with ipilimumab vs extreme regimen (cetuximab + cisplatin/carboplatin + fluorouracil) as first-line therapy in patients with recurrent or metastatic squamous cell carcinoma of the head and neck-CheckMate 651. *Ann Oncol*. 2016;27:1016TiP. doi:10.1093/annonc/mdw376.68
74. Mehra R ST, Mahipal A, et al. Efficacy and safety of pembrolizumab in recurrent/metastatic head and neck squamous cell carcinoma (R/M HNSCC): Pooled analyses after long-term follow-up in KEYNOTE-012. *J Clin Oncol*. 2016;34(suppl):6012. doi:10.1200/JCO.2016.34.15_suppl.6012
75. Ferris RL, Blumenschein GR, Fayette J, et al. Further evaluations of nivolumab (nivo) versus investigator's choice (IC) chemotherapy for recurrent or metastatic (R/M) squamous cell carcinoma of the head and neck (SCCHN): CheckMate 141. *J Clin Oncol*. 2016;34(suppl):6009. https://meetinglibrary.asco.org/record/129273/abstract
76. Gillison ML, Blumenschein GR, Fayette J, et al. Nivolumab (nivo) vs investigator's choice (IC) for recurrent or metastatic (R/M) head and neck squamous cell carcinoma (HNSCC): CheckMate-141. *Cancer Res*. 2016;76(suppl). Available from http://cancerres.aacrjournals.org/content/76/14 Supplement/CT099
77. Seiwert TY, Weiss J, Baxi SS, et al. A phase 3, randomized, open-label study of first-line durvalumab (MEDI4736) ± tremelimumab versus standard of care (SoC; EXTREME regimen) in recurrent/metastatic (R/M) SCCHN: KESTREL. *J Clin Oncol*. 2016;34(suppl). doi:10.1200/JCO.2016.34.15_suppl.TPS6101
78. Argiris A, Li S, Savvides P, et al. Phase III randomized trial of chemotherapy with or without bevacizumab (B) in patients (pts) with recurrent or metastatic squamous cell carcinoma of the head and neck (R/M SCCHN): Survival analysis of E1305, an ECOG-ACRIN Cancer Research Group trial. *J Clin Oncol*. 2017;35:6000. doi:10.1200/JCO.2017.35.15_suppl.6000
79. Baselga J, Trigo JM, Bourhis J, et al. Phase II multicenter study of the antiepidermal growth factor receptor monoclonal antibody cetuximab in combination with platinum-based chemotherapy in patients with platinum-refractory metastatic and/or recurrent squamous cell carcinoma of the head and neck. *J Clin Oncol*. 2005;23:5568–5577. doi:10.1200/JCO.2005.07.119
80. Machiels JP, Subramanian S, Ruzsa A, et al. Zalutumumab plus best supportive care versus best supportive care alone in patients with recurrent or metastatic squamous-cell carcinoma of the head and neck after failure of platinum-based chemotherapy: an open-label, randomised phase 3 trial. *Lancet Oncol*. 2011;12:333–343. doi:10.1016/S1470-2045(11)70034-1
81. Chow LQ, Haddad R, Gupta S, et al. Antitumor activity of pembrolizumab in biomarker-unselected patients with recurrent and/or metastatic head and neck squamous cell carcinoma: results from the phase Ib KEYNOTE-012 expansion cohort. *J Clin Oncol*. 2016;34:3838–3845. doi:10.1200/JCO.2016.68.1478

82. Chow LQM Mehra R, Haddad RI, et al. Biomarkers and response to pembrolizumab (pembro) in recurrent/metastatic head and neck squamous cell carcinoma (R/M HNSCC). *J Clin Oncol*. 2016;34(suppl):6010. doi:10.1200/ JCO.2016.34.15_suppl.6010
83. CheckMate-141, a Pivotal Phase 3 Opdivo (nivolumab) Head and Neck Cancer Trial, Stopped Early. 2016. Available from https://news.bms.com/press-release/checkmate-141-pivotal-phase-3-opdivo-nivolumab-head-and-neck-cancer-trial-stopped-early
84. Carbognin L, Pilotto S, Milella M, et al. Differential activity of nivolumab, pembrolizumab and MPDL3280A according to the tumor expression of programmed death-ligand-1 (PD-L1): sensitivity analysis of trials in melanoma, lung and genitourinary cancers. *PLOS ONE*. 2015;10:e0130142. doi:10.1371/journal.pone.0130142
85. Weber JS, Hodi FS, Wolchok JD, et al. Safety profile of nivolumab monotherapy: a pooled analysis of patients with advanced melanoma. *J Clin Oncol*. 2017;35:785–792. doi:10.1200/JCO.2015.66.1389
86. Mark Ayers JL, Nebozhyn M, Murphy E, et al. Relationship between immune gene signatures and clinical response to PD-1 blockade with pembrolizumab (MK-3475) in patients with advanced solid tumors. *J Immunother Cancer*. 2015;3(Suppl 2):P80. doi:10.1186/2051-1426-3-S2-P80
87. Tanguy Y, Seiwert BB, Weiss J, et al. Inflamed-phenotype gene expression signatures to predict benefit from the anti-PD-1 antibody pembrolizumab in PD-L1+ head and neck cancer patients. *J Clin Oncol*. 2015;33(suppl):6017. doi:10.1200/jco.2015.33.15_suppl.6017
88. Gajewski TF, Louahed J, Brichard VG. Gene signature in melanoma associated with clinical activity: a potential clue to unlock cancer immunotherapy. *Cancer J*. 2010;16:399–403. doi:10.1097/PPO.0b013e3181eacbd8
89. Zandberg DP, Jarkowski A, Emeribe UA, et al. A phase 2, multicenter, single-arm, global study of MEDI4736 monotherapy in patients with recurrent or metastatic (R/M) squamous cell carcinoma of the head and neck (SCCHN): HAWK (NCT02207530). *J Clin Oncol*. 2015;33. doi:10.1200/jco.2015.33.15_suppl.tps6086
90. Ferris RL, Even C, Haddad R, et al. Phase III, randomized, open-label study of durvalumab (MEDI4736) monotherapy, or durvalumab + tremelimumab, versus standard of care (SoC), in recurrent or metastatic (R/M) squamous cell carcinoma of the head and neck (SCCHN): EAGLE. *J Immunother Cancer*. 2015;3(Suppl 2):P150. doi:10.1186/2051-1426-3-S2-P150
91. Siano M, Resteghini C, Cau MC, et al. Outcome of systemic treatments after first line platinum and cetuximab treatment in patients with recurrent/metastatic (RM) head and neck squamous cell cancer (HNSCC): a retrospective analysis. *Eur J Cancer*. 2015;51:S578. doi:10.1016/S0959-8049(16)31603-3
92. Jimenez B, Trigo JM, Pajares BI, et al. Efficacy and safety of weekly paclitaxel combined with cetuximab in the treatment of pretreated recurrent/metastatic head and neck cancer patients. *Oral Oncol*. 2013;49:182–185. doi:10.1016/j.oraloncology.2012.09.003
93. Sosa AE, Grau JJ, Feliz L, et al. Outcome of patients treated with palliative weekly paclitaxel plus cetuximab in recurrent head and neck cancer after failure of platinum-based therapy. *Eur Arch Otorhinolaryngol*. 2014;271:373–378. doi:10.1007/s00405-013-2537-6
94. Peron J, Ceruse P, Lavergne E, et al. Paclitaxel and cetuximab combination efficiency after the failure of a platinum-based chemotherapy in recurrent/metastatic head and neck squamous cell carcinoma. *Anticancer Drugs*. 2012;23:996–1001. doi:10.1007/s00405-013-2537-6
95. Knoedler M, Gauler TC, Gruenwald V, et al. Phase II study of cetuximab in combination with docetaxel in patients with recurrent and/or metastatic squamous cell carcinoma of the head and neck after platinum-containing therapy: a multicenter study of the Arbeitsgemeinschaft Internistische Onkologie. *Oncology*. 2013;84:284–289. doi:10.1159/000345453
96. Posch D, Fuchs H, Kornek G, et al. Docetaxel plus cetuximab biweekly is an active regimen for the first-line treatment of patients with recurrent/metastatic head and neck cancer. *Sci Rep*. 2016;6:32946. doi:10.1038/srep32946
97. Rischin D, Spigel DR, Adkins D, et al. PRISM: phase 2 trial with panitumumab monotherapy as second-line treatment in patients with recurrent or metastatic squamous cell carcinoma of the head and neck. *Head Neck*. 2016;38(Suppl 1):E1756–E1761. doi:10.1002/hed.24311
98. Cohen EEW, Licitra LF, Fayette J, et al. Biomarker analysis in recurrent and/or metastatic head and neck squamous cell carcinoma (R/M HNSCC) patients (pts) treated with second-line afatinib versus methotrexate (MTX): LUX-Head & Neck 1 (LUX-H&N1). *J Clin Oncol*. 2015;33(suppl):6023. doi:10.1200/jco.2015.33.15_suppl.6023
99. Seiwert TY, Fayette J, Cupissol D, et al. A randomized, phase II study of afatinib versus cetuximab in metastatic or recurrent squamous cell carcinoma of the head and neck. *Ann Oncol*. 2014;25:1813–1820. doi:10.1093/annonc/mdu216
100. Argiris A, Ghebremichael M, Gilbert J, et al. Phase III randomized, placebo-controlled trial of docetaxel with or without gefitinib in recurrent or metastatic head and neck cancer: an eastern cooperative oncology group trial. *J Clin Oncol*. 2013;31:1405–1414. doi:10.1200/JCO.2012.45.4272
101. Simpson DR, Mell LK, Cohen EE. Targeting the PI3K/AKT/mTOR pathway in squamous cell carcinoma of the head and neck. *Oral Oncol*. 2015;51:291–298. doi:10.1016/j.oraloncology.2014.11.012
102. Lui VW, Hedberg ML, Li H, et al. Frequent mutation of the PI3K pathway in head and neck cancer defines predictive biomarkers. *Cancer Discov*. 2013;3:761–769.
103. Grunwald V, Keilholz U, Boehm A, et al. TEMHEAD: a single-arm multicentre phase II study of temsirolimus in platin- and cetuximab refractory recurrent and/or metastatic squamous cell carcinoma of the head and neck (SCCHN) of the German SCCHN Group (AIO). *Ann Oncol*. 2015;26:561–567. doi:10.1158/2159-8290.CD-13-0103

104. Geiger JL, Bauman JE, Gibson MK, et al. Phase II trial of everolimus in patients with previously treated recurrent or metastatic head and neck squamous cell carcinoma. *Head Neck*. 2016;38:1759–1764. doi:10.1002/hed.24501
105. Bauman JE, Arias-Pulido H, Lee SJ, et al. Phase II study of temsirolimus and erlotinib in patients (pts) with recurrent/metastatic (R/M), platinum-refractory head and neck squamous cell carcinoma (HNSCC). *J Clin Oncol*. 2013;49:461–467. doi:10.1016/j.oraloncology.2012.12.016
106. Fakhry C, Zhang Q, Nguyen-Tan PF, et al. Human papillomavirus and overall survival after progression of oropharyngeal squamous cell carcinoma. *J Clin Oncol*. 2014;32:3365–3373. doi:10.1200/JCO.2014.55.1937
107. Argiris A, Li S, Ghebremichael M, et al. Prognostic significance of human papillomavirus in recurrent or metastatic head and neck cancer: an analysis of Eastern Cooperative Oncology Group trials. *Ann Oncol*. 2014;25:1410–1416. doi:10.1093/annonc/mdu167
108. Vermorken JB, Psyrri A, Mesia R, et al. Impact of tumor HPV status on outcome in patients with recurrent and/or metastatic squamous cell carcinoma of the head and neck receiving chemotherapy with or without cetuximab: retrospective analysis of the phase III EXTREME trial. *Ann Oncol*. 2014;25:801–807. doi:10.1093/annonc/mdt574
109. National Comprehensive Cancer Network. Head and neck cancers. NCCN clinical practice guidelines in oncology. 2016; Version 2.
110. Peyrade F, Cupissol D, Geoffrois L, et al. Systemic treatment and medical management of metastatic squamous cell carcinoma of the head and neck: review of the literature and proposal for management changes. *Oral Oncol*. 2013;49:482–491. doi:10.1016/j.oraloncology.2013.01.005
111. Gregoire V, Lefebvre JL, Licitra L, et al. Squamous cell carcinoma of the head and neck: EHNS-ESMO-ESTRO clinical practice guidelines for diagnosis, treatment and follow-up. *Ann Oncol*. 2010;21(Suppl 5):v184–v186. doi:10.1093/annonc/mdq185
112. Argiris A, Li Y, Murphy BA, et al. Outcome of elderly patients with recurrent or metastatic head and neck cancer treated with cisplatin-based chemotherapy. *J Clin Oncol*. 2004;22:262–268. doi:10.1200/JCO.2004.08.039
113. Smith BD, Smith GL, Hurria A, et al. Future of cancer incidence in the United States: burdens upon an aging, changing nation. *J Clin Oncol*. 2009;27:2758–2765. doi:10.1200/JCO.2008.20.8983
114. Clement PM, Gauler T, Machiels JP, et al. Afatinib versus methotrexate in older patients with second-line recurrent and/or metastatic head and neck squamous cell carcinoma: subgroup analysis of the LUX-Head & Neck 1 trial. *Ann Oncol*. 2016;27:1585–1593. doi:10.1093/annonc/mdw151
115. Harpreet Singh GK, Maher VE, Beaver JA, et al. FDA subset analysis of the safety of nivolumab in elderly patients with advanced cancers. *J Clin Oncol*. 2016;34(suppl):10010. doi:10.1200/JCO.2016.34.15_suppl.10010
116. Nishijima TF, Muss HB, Shachar SS, Moschos SJ. Comparison of efficacy of immune checkpoint inhibitors (ICIs) between younger and older patients: a systematic review and meta-analysis. *Cancer Treat Rev*. 2016;45:30–37. doi:10.1016/j.ctrv.2016.02.006
117. Hurria A, Togawa K, Mohile SG, et al. Predicting chemotherapy toxicity in older adults with cancer: a prospective multicenter study. *J Clin Oncol*. 2011;29:3457–3465. doi:10.1200/JCO.2011.34.7625
118. Hurria A, Mohile S, Gajra A, et al. Validation of a prediction tool for chemotherapy toxicity in older adults with cancer. *J Clin Oncol*. 2016;34:2366–2371. doi:10.1200/JCO.2015.65.4327
119. Guan Y, Liu S, Wang HY, et al. Long-term outcomes of a phase II randomized controlled trial comparing intensity-modulated radiotherapy with or without weekly cisplatin for the treatment of locally recurrent nasopharyngeal carcinoma. *Chin J Cancer*. 2016;35:20. doi:10.1186/s40880-016-0081-7
120. Lee N, Harris J, Garden AS, et al. Intensity-modulated radiation therapy with or without chemotherapy for nasopharyngeal carcinoma: radiation therapy oncology group phase II trial 0225. *J Clin Oncol*. 2009;27:3684–3690. doi:10.1200/JCO.2008.19.9109
121. Yang L, Hong S, Wang Y, et al. Development and external validation of nomograms for predicting survival in nasopharyngeal carcinoma patients after definitive radiotherapy. *Sci Rep*. 2015;5:15638. doi:10.1038/srep15638
122. Zhang L, Huang Y, Hong S, et al. Gemcitabine plus cisplatin versus fluorouracil plus cisplatin in recurrent or metastatic nasopharyngeal carcinoma: a multicentre, randomised, open-label, phase 3 trial. *Lancet*. 2016;388:1883–1892. doi:10.1016/S0140-6736(16)31388-5
123. Jin Y, Shi YX, Cai XY, et al. Comparison of five cisplatin-based regimens frequently used as the first-line protocols in metastatic nasopharyngeal carcinoma. *J Cancer Res Clin Oncol*. 2012;138:1717–1725. doi:10.1007/s00432-012-1219-x
124. Leong SS, Wee J, Tay MH, et al. Paclitaxel, carboplatin, and gemcitabine in metastatic nasopharyngeal carcinoma: a Phase II trial using a triplet combination. *Cancer*. 2005;103:569–575. doi:10.1002/cncr.20804
125. Foo KF, Tan EH, Leong SS, et al. Gemcitabine in metastatic nasopharyngeal carcinoma of the undifferentiated type. *Ann Oncol*. 2002;13:150–156. doi:10.1093/annonc/mdf002
126. Chua DT, Sham JS, Au GK. A phase II study of capecitabine in patients with recurrent and metastatic nasopharyngeal carcinoma pretreated with platinum-based chemotherapy. *Oral Oncol*. 2003;39:361–366. doi:10.1016/S1368-8375(02)00120-3
127. Ngeow J, Lim WT, Leong SS, et al. Docetaxel is effective in heavily pretreated patients with disseminated nasopharyngeal carcinoma. *Ann Oncol*. 2011;22:718–722. doi:10.1093/annonc/mdq425

128. Chan AT, Hsu MM, Goh BC, et al. Multicenter, phase II study of cetuximab in combination with carboplatin in patients with recurrent or metastatic nasopharyngeal carcinoma. *J Clin Oncol.* 2005;23:3568–3576. doi:10.1200/JCO.2005.02.147
129. Elser C, Siu LL, Winquist E, et al. Phase II trial of sorafenib in patients with recurrent or metastatic squamous cell carcinoma of the head and neck or nasopharyngeal carcinoma. *J Clin Oncol.* 2007;25:3766–3773. doi:10.1200/JCO.2006.10.2871
130. Lim WT, Ng QS, Ivy P, et al. A Phase II study of pazopanib in Asian patients with recurrent/metastatic nasopharyngeal carcinoma. *Clin Cancer Res.* 2011;17:5481–5489. doi:10.1158/1078-0432.CCR-10-3409
131. Huang Y, Zhang L, Pan J-J, et al. A phase II, multicenter, open-label, single-arm trial of famitinib in patients with advanced recurrent and/or metastatic nasopharyngeal carcinoma (NPC) after two previous treatment regimens. *J Clin Oncol.* 2013;31:6026. doi:10.1200/jco.2013.31.15_suppl.6026
132. Hui EP, Ma BB, King AD, et al. Hemorrhagic complications in a phase II study of sunitinib in patients of nasopharyngeal carcinoma who has previously received high-dose radiation. *Ann Oncol.* 2011;22:1280–1287. doi:10.1093/annonc/mdq629
133. Hui EP, Ma B, Mo F, et al. A phase II study of axitinib in patients with recurrent or metastatic nasopharyngeal carcinoma (NPC). *J Clin Oncol.* 2015;33(suppl):6031. doi:10.1200/jco.2015.33.15_suppl.6031
134. Soria JC, Deutsch E. Hemorrhage caused by antiangiogenic therapy within previously irradiated areas: expected consequence of tumor shrinkage or a warning for antiangiogenic agents combined to radiotherapy? *Ann Oncol.* 2011;22:1247–1249. doi:10.1093/annonc/mdq775
135. Straathof KC, Bollard CM, Popat U, et al. Treatment of nasopharyngeal carcinoma with Epstein-Barr virus–specific T lymphocytes. *Blood.* 2005;105:1898–1904. doi:10.1182/blood-2004-07-2975
136. Comoli P, Pedrazzoli P, Maccario R, et al. Cell therapy of stage IV nasopharyngeal carcinoma with autologous Epstein-Barr virus-targeted cytotoxic T lymphocytes. *J Clin Oncol.* 2005;23:8942–8949. doi:10.1200/JCO.2005.02.6195
137. Lin CL, Lo WF, Lee TH, et al. Immunization with Epstein-Barr Virus (EBV) peptide-pulsed dendritic cells induces functional CD8+ T-cell immunity and may lead to tumor regression in patients with EBV-positive nasopharyngeal carcinoma. *Cancer Res.* 2002;62:6952–6958. Available from http://cancerres.aacrjournals.org/content/62/23/6952.full-text.pdf
138. Zhang J, Fang W, Qin T, et al. Co-expression of PD-1 and PD-L1 predicts poor outcome in nasopharyngeal carcinoma. *Med Oncol.* 2015;32:86. doi:10.1007/s12032-015-0501-6
139. Hsu C, Lee S, Ejadi S, et al. Antitumor activity and safety of pembrolizumab in patients with PD-L1-positive nasopharyngeal carcinoma: Interim results from a phase 1b study. *Ann Oncol.* 2015;26:93–102. Available from http://oncologypro.esmo.org/Meeting-Resources/ESMO-Asia-2015-Congress/Antitumor-activity-and-safety-of-pembrolizumab-in-patients-with-PD-L1-positive-nasopharyngeal-carcinoma-Interim-results-from-a-phase-1b-study
140. Argiris A, Li Y, Forastiere A. Prognostic factors and long-term survivorship in patients with recurrent or metastatic carcinoma of the head and neck. *Cancer.* 2004;101:2222–2229. doi:10.1002/cncr.20640

SECTION V

Supportive Care and Special Patient Groups

24

Oral Complications

Rajesh V. Lalla
Douglas E. Peterson

The treatment of head and neck cancer (HNC) can result in a number of secondary effects in the oral cavity. Radiation therapy (RT), in particular, causes significant oral toxicity. Chemotherapy used concurrently can aggravate toxicities, while chemotherapy used sequentially can independently cause oral complications. Surgery is also linked to some oral complications, including pain and dysphagia (discussed in Chapter 25). More recently, use of immunotherapy for HNC treatment has led to unique oral complications often but not exclusively involving the oral mucosa. This chapter presents some of the common oral complications seen in HNC patients receiving RT and chemotherapy.

ORAL MUCOSITIS

Oral mucositis refers to inflamed and ulcerative lesions of the oral mucosa as a side effect of systemic chemotherapy or RT to the head and neck (HN) region (1). Most patients receiving therapeutic RT for HNC develop some degree of oral mucositis (2). The severity is largely dependent on the fields of RT and total RT dose. Chemotherapy concurrent with HN RT further aggravates the severity of oral mucositis (3). Oral mucositis may also be seen as a consequence of induction chemotherapy prior to RT, when used. The mechanisms involved in the pathobiology of oral mucositis include direct damage from radiation or chemotherapy to basal epithelial cells, generation of damaging reactive oxygen species, activation of transcription factors such as nuclear factor-κB (NFκB) and of inflammatory pathways such as the cyclooxygenase (COX) pathway, and the upregulation of proinflammatory cytokines such as tumor necrosis factor-α (TNF-α) and interleukin 1β (IL-1β) (4).

Oral mucositis initially presents as erythema of the oral mucosa, which can progress to erosion and ulceration (1). The ulcerations are often covered by a pseudomembrane (Figure 24.1). Nonkeratinized oral tissues including the buccal mucosa and lateral tongue are commonly affected. In patients receiving the standard 6- to 7-week course of RT for HNC, onset of oral mucositis occurs by the second or third week of RT, and severity worsens with increasing dose of radiation. The lesions typically persist for several weeks after the end of RT, depending on their size.

The primary morbidity of oral mucositis is the intense pain typically associated with ulcerative lesions. Owing to the pain, patients with severe oral mucositis may be unable to maintain oral hygiene and to continue eating by mouth. Therefore, they are often fed through a gastrostomy tube. HNC patients with oral mucositis are significantly more likely to have weight loss of 5% or more (3). Impaired nutrition impacts healing and resistance to infection and leads to a general failure to thrive. The pain and nutritional compromise adversely impact quality of life (QOL) (5). Ulcerative oral mucositis gets colonized by oral microflora and is sometimes complicated by local infection such as herpes simplex virus (HSV) infection and candidiasis. Oral mucositis also results in increased costs associated with pain management, gastrostomy

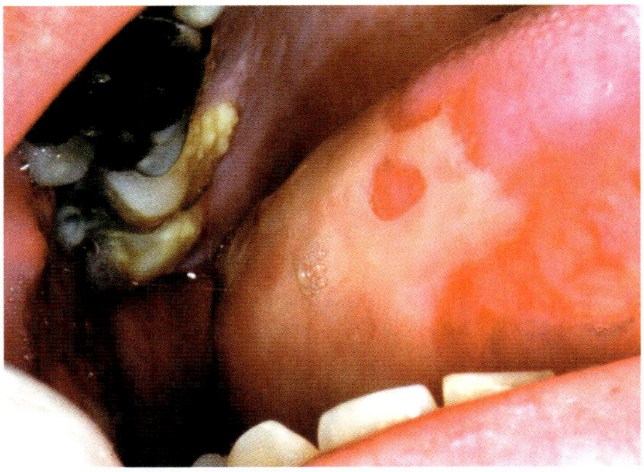

FIGURE 24.1 A large oral mucositis lesion on the right lateral tongue of a patient receiving radiation therapy for head and neck cancer. Note the yellowish pseudomembrane covering much of the ulceration and the surrounding erythema.

tubes with liquid diet supplements, secondary infections, and hospitalizations (3). Perhaps most significantly, severe mucositis can necessitate undesirable interruptions in cancer therapy. In one study, 11% of patients receiving RT for HNC had unplanned breaks in RT because of severe mucositis (6). Such modifications in cancer therapy can negatively impact cancer prognosis (7).

Symptom management of oral mucositis is largely focused on pain control. Many centers use a mouth rinse containing a topical anesthetic such as lidocaine, often in combination with other agents such as diphenhydramine and an antacid coating agent (often referred to as "magic" or "miracle" mouthwash). In a recent multicenter, randomized trial of patients undergoing definitive HN RT, both a mouthwash containing lidocaine/diphenhydramine/antacid and a doxepin mouthwash significantly reduced short-term oral pain as compared to placebo. The mouthwash containing lidocaine/diphenhydramine/antacid reduced mouth pain between 5 to 30 minutes after use. The doxepin mouthwash reduced mouth pain between 30 and 60 minutes after use but was associated with drowsiness and fatigue (8). A number of commercial topical coating agents are also marketed for oral mucositis, but there is inadequate evidence to support their use. Sucralfate is a well-studied generic topical coating agent, and evidence demonstrates that it is not effective for prevention or treatment of oral mucositis secondary to chemotherapy or RT (9). Regardless of use of topical agents, most patients with ulcerative oral mucositis need systemic opioids to achieve adequate pain control.

Evidence-based clinical practice guidelines for the prevention and management of oral and gastrointestinal mucositis have been developed by the Multinational Association of Supportive Care in Cancer/International Society of Oral Oncology (MASCC/ISOO) (10). These guidelines include recommendations (based on higher level evidence), suggestions (based on lower level evidence), or a determination of "no guideline possible," in cases of inadequate or conflicting evidence (11,12). For patients undergoing RT for HNC, the MASCC/ISOO guidelines include a recommendation in favor of benzydamine mouthwash to prevent oral mucositis in HNC patients receiving moderate-dose RT (up to 50 Gy) without concomitant chemotherapy; a suggestion that oral care protocols be used to prevent oral mucositis in all age groups and across all cancer treatment modalities; a suggestion that low-level laser therapy be used to prevent oral mucositis in HNC patients undergoing RT without concomitant chemotherapy; a suggestion that that 0.2% morphine mouthwash may be effective to treat pain due to oral mucositis in patients receiving chemoradiation for HNC; a suggestion that 0.5% doxepin mouthwash may be effective to treat pain due to oral mucositis; and a suggestion that systemic zinc supplements administered orally may be of benefit to prevent oral mucositis in oral cancer patients receiving RT or chemoradiation. The full guidelines statements are presented in Table 24.1.

HYPOSALIVATION AND XEROSTOMIA

Hyposalivation refers to objectively measured reduction in salivary flow, while xerostomia refers to a subjective complaint of a dry mouth. The inclusion of the major salivary glands in the fields of RT causes cellular senescence and resulting hypofunction (13). The severity and persistence of salivary hypofunction depend on the volume of salivary gland tissue in the radiation fields, unilateral versus bilateral treatment, and RT dose (14). A reduction in salivary flow may be seen as early as the first week of RT, with about 80% of HN RT patients reporting some degree of subjective xerostomia during RT (14). The stimulated salivary flow rate typically

TABLE 24.1

MASCC/ISOO EVIDENCE-BASED CLINICAL PRACTICE GUIDELINES FOR ORAL MUCOSITIS SECONDARY TO CANCER THERAPY

RECOMMENDATIONS *IN FAVOR* OF AN INTERVENTION (i.e., strong evidence supports effectiveness in the treatment setting listed)

1. The panel *recommends* that 30 minutes of oral cryotherapy be used to prevent oral mucositis in patients receiving bolus 5-fluorouracil chemotherapy (Level of Evidence II).
2. The panel *recommends* that recombinant human keratinocyte growth factor-1 (KGF-1/palifermin) be used to *prevent* oral mucositis (at a dose of 60 µg/kg per day for 3 days prior to conditioning treatment and for 3 days post-transplant) in patients receiving high-dose chemotherapy and total body irradiation, followed by autologous stem cell transplantation, for a hematological malignancy (Level of Evidence II).
3. The panel *recommends* that low-level laser therapy (wavelength at 650 nm, power of 40 mW, and each square centimeter treated with the required time to a tissue energy dose of 2 J/cm2), be used to *prevent* oral mucositis in patients receiving hematopoietic stem cell transplantation conditioned with high-dose chemotherapy, with or without total body irradiation (Level of Evidence II).
4. The panel *recommends* that patient-controlled analgesia with morphine be used to *treat* pain due to oral mucositis in patients undergoing hematopoietic stem cell transplantation (Level of Evidence II).
5. The panel *recommends* that benzydamine mouthwash be used to *prevent* oral mucositis in patients with head and neck cancer receiving moderate dose radiation therapy (up to 50 Gy), without concomitant chemotherapy (Level of Evidence I).

SUGGESTIONS *IN FAVOR* OF AN INTERVENTION (i.e., weaker evidence supports effectiveness in the treatment setting listed)

1. The panel *suggests* that oral care protocols be used to *prevent* oral mucositis in all age groups and across all cancer treatment modalities (Level of Evidence III).
2. The panel *suggests* that oral cryotherapy be used to *prevent* oral mucositis in patients receiving high-dose melphalan, with or without total body irradiation, as conditioning for hematopoietic stem cell transplantation (Level of Evidence III).
3. The panel *suggests* that low-level laser therapy (wavelength around 632.8 nm) be used to *prevent* oral mucositis in patients undergoing radiotherapy, without concomitant chemotherapy, for head and neck cancer (Level of Evidence III).
4. The panel *suggests* that transdermal fentanyl may be effective to *treat* pain due to oral mucositis in patients receiving conventional or high-dose chemotherapy, with or without total body irradiation (Level of Evidence III).
5. The panel *suggests* that 0.2% morphine mouthwash may be effective to *treat* pain due to oral mucositis in patients receiving chemoradiation for head and neck cancer (Level of Evidence III).
6. The panel *suggests* that 0.5% doxepin mouthwash may be effective to *treat* pain due to oral mucositis (Level of Evidence IV).
7. The panel *suggests* that systemic zinc supplements administered orally may be of benefit to *prevent* oral mucositis in oral cancer patients receiving radiation therapy or chemoradiation (Level of Evidence III).

RECOMMENDATIONS *AGAINST* AN INTERVENTION (i.e., strong evidence indicates lack of effectiveness in the treatment setting listed)

1. The panel *recommends* that PTA (polymyxin, tobramycin, amphotericin B) and BCoG (bacitracin, clotrimazole, gentamicin) antimicrobial lozenges and PTA paste *not* be used to *prevent* oral mucositis in patients receiving radiation therapy for head and cancer (Level of Evidence II).

(continued)

TABLE 24.1 (*continued*)

MASCC/ISOO EVIDENCE-BASED CLINICAL PRACTICE GUIDELINES FOR ORAL MUCOSITIS SECONDARY TO CANCER THERAPY

2. The panel *recommends* that iseganan antimicrobial mouthwash *not* be used to *prevent* oral mucositis in patients receiving high-dose chemotherapy, with or without total body irradiation, for hematopoietic stem cell transplantation (Level of Evidence II), or in patients receiving radiation therapy or concomitant chemoradiation for head and neck cancer (Level of Evidence II).
3. The panel *recommends* that sucralfate mouthwash *not* be used to *prevent* oral mucositis in patients receiving chemotherapy for cancer (Level of Evidence I), or in patients receiving radiation therapy (Level of Evidence I) or concomitant chemoradiation (Level of Evidence II) for head and neck cancer.
4. The panel *recommends* that sucralfate mouthwash *not* be used to *treat* oral mucositis in patients receiving chemotherapy for cancer (Level of Evidence I), or in patients receiving radiation therapy (Level of Evidence II) for head and neck cancer.
5. The panel *recommends* that intravenous glutamine *not* be used to *prevent* oral mucositis in patients receiving high-dose chemotherapy, with or without total body irradiation, for hematopoietic stem cell transplantation (Level of Evidence II).

SUGGESTIONS *AGAINST* AN INTERVENTION (i.e., weaker evidence indicates lack of effectiveness in the treatment setting listed)

1. The panel *suggests* that chlorhexidine mouthwash *not* be used to *prevent* oral mucositis in patients receiving radiation therapy for head and neck cancer (Level of Evidence III).
2. The panel *suggests* that granulocyte macrophage–colony stimulating factor (GM-CSF) mouthwash *not* be used to *prevent* oral mucositis in patients receiving high-dose chemotherapy, for autologous or allogeneic stem cell transplantation (Level of Evidence II).
3. The panel *suggests* that misoprostol mouthwash *not* be used to *prevent* oral mucositis in patients receiving radiation therapy for head and neck cancer (Level of Evidence III).
4. The panel *suggests* that systemic pentoxifylline, administered orally, *not* be used to *prevent* oral mucositis in patients undergoing bone marrow transplantation (Level of Evidence III).
5. The panel *suggests* that systemic pilocarpine, administered orally, *not* be used to *prevent* oral mucositis in patients receiving radiation therapy for head and neck cancer (Level of Evidence III), or in patients receiving high-dose chemotherapy, with or without total body irradiation, for hematopoietic stem cell transplantation (Level of Evidence II).

Source: The MASCC/ISOO Evidence-Based Clinical Practice Guidelines For Oral Mucositis Secondary To Cancer Therapy is used with the permission from the Multinational Association for Supportive Care in Cancer.

shows a further drop between 1 to 3 months after RT, with the potential for some degree of longer-term recovery. The use of intensity-modulated radiation therapy (IMRT) allows for better salivary gland protection. However, recent data from patients receiving IMRT or newer modalities demonstrate a 60% decline in stimulated salivary flow from before RT to 6 months after RT, with a partial recovery by 18 months, resulting in a net 40% decline (15). Patients commonly complain of a dry mouth and difficulty in eating and speaking. RT to the parotid glands also results in reductions in the serous content of saliva, resulting in a thicker more viscous saliva, which is more difficult to swallow.

Preventive measures include radiation sparing of the salivary glands when possible. It has been reported that keeping RT doses to the parotid glands below 26 to 30 Gy leads to reduced severity of salivary hypofunction and significant recovery of salivary flow over time (14). A recent study has reported that stem and progenitor cells of rat parotid salivary gland are predominantly located in the major ducts. Interestingly, the radiation dose to this region in humans was predictive of salivary gland function at 1 year after RT (16). Further development of this work may identify a new strategy for salivary gland protection. The use of intravenous amifostine during the RT period is Food and Drug Administration

(FDA) approved to reduce incidence of moderate-to-severe xerostomia in patients undergoing postoperative RT for HNC, where the radiation port includes a substantial portion of the parotid glands (17). The mechanism is believed to be via scavenging of damaging free oxygen radicals.

Treatment of hyposalivation includes symptomatic management via frequent sipping of water or use of artificial saliva or other oral lubricants such as Biotene Oral Balance gel. Some stimulation of salivary flow may be achieved via use of sugar-free chewing gum or lemon candy. Pilocarpine tablets have been approved by the FDA for the treatment of dry mouth for salivary hypofunction caused by HN RT (18). Pilocarpine acts as a cholinergic agonist and is effective in stimulating salivary flow if functional salivary gland tissue remains. Cevimeline is another cholinergic agonist that is also available.

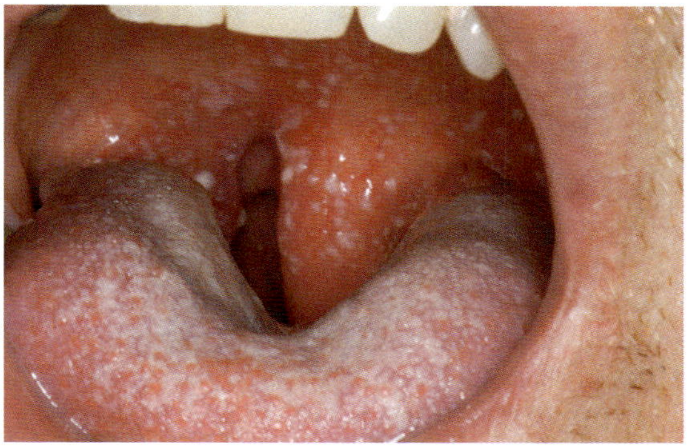

FIGURE 24.2 Pseudomembranous candidiasis in a patient receiving radiation therapy for head and neck cancer. Note the white pseudomembranous lesions on the dorsal tongue, soft palate, uvula, and tonsillar pillar.

ORAL CANDIDIASIS

Oral candidiasis is a clinical fungal infection, most commonly caused by *Candida albicans*. Thirty-five percent or more of healthy individuals may carry *Candida albicans* as a component of the normal oral flora, without any clinical disease (19). This percentage is further increased in immunocompromised populations such as patients with cancer (20,21). A systematic review reported that the weighted prevalence of oral fungal colonization during and after HN RT is 70% to 75% (20). The main factor that predisposes this population to developing clinical oral candidiasis is hyposalivation, since saliva normally washes away the fungal organisms. Immunosuppression (due to drugs or disease) imbalances in the oral flora (e.g., secondary to antibiotics) and local tissue damage (mucositis) further increase the risk (22). The weighted prevalence of clinical oral candidiasis in HN RT patients has been reported as 7.5% before RT, 37.4% during treatment, and 32.6% after RT (20).

Oral candidiasis exists in several different clinical forms, as described in the following list (23). Most forms of oral candidiasis are typically asymptomatic, and patients may be unaware of its presence.

1. Pseudomembranous candidiasis (thrush)
   This is the most widely recognized form of oral candidiasis (24). It appears as white or yellow pseudomembranes on the oral mucosal surface (Figure 24.2). These pseudomembranes are adherent but can be removed with some pressure. The underlying mucosa is usually erythematous and inflamed. It often occurs on the tongue, buccal mucosa, soft palate, and pharyngeal areas.
2. Erythematous candidiasis

- Erythematous candidiasis appears as red atrophic areas of the oral mucosa, without any white pseudomembranes. It often occurs on the hard palate and the dorsum of the tongue, where it can result in an atrophic smooth-appearing tongue. Common predisposing factors include the use of broad-spectrum antibiotics and steroid inhalers. Patients may complain of a burning sensation.
- Denture stomatitis is a form of erythematous candidiasis that occurs under a removable denture. It usually affects the palatal surface under a maxillary denture. The boundaries of the lesion correspond to the tissue within the denture margins. Denture stomatitis occurs in patients who do not remove their dentures at night and in patients who do not clean their dentures regularly (25).
- Median rhomboid glossitis is a form of erythematous candidiasis that presents as a characteristic oval to rhomboid erythematous patch along the midline of the dorsum of the tongue (26). Predisposing factors include smoking and use of steroid inhalers. On occasion, a similar erythematous lesion may be seen on the palate, in the area contacted by the affected part of the tongue.

3. Angular cheilitis
   Angular cheilitis refers to a mixed fungal and bacterial infection of the corners of the mouth. It appears as a red, fissured, and sometimes crusted area of the mucosa. It may also affect the adjacent skin at the corners of the mouth. Predisposing factors include denture wearing, loss of teeth, and vitamin deficiencies (27). Angular cheilitis may be seen in association with intraoral candidiasis, especially denture stomatitis, but can also occur alone. Patients may complain of discomfort when opening the mouth wide.
4. Chronic hyperplastic candidiasis
   This is an uncommon form of oral candidiasis, characterized by the presence of a white hyperkeratotic plaque that cannot be wiped off. It has been reported on the buccal mucosa and lateral tongue. There is controversy about the malignant potential of such lesions (28).

Prevention of oral candidiasis includes measures to address hyposalivation as described above and maintenance of good oral hygiene, including denture hygiene when applicable. Treatment of oral candidiasis includes the use of topical antifungals such as clotrimazole troches, nystatin rinse, and miconazole buccal tablet (Oravig) (22,29). Systemic fluconazole is also used, particularly in immunocompromised patients.

TASTE CHANGES

Taste dysfunction is a common complaint in HNC patients. In some cases, systemic chemotherapy can be associated with transient taste changes, including a metallic taste during/shortly after chemotherapy administration. More commonly, patients undergoing HN RT report altered taste (dysgeusia) or decreased taste (hypogeusia). The inclusion of the dorsal tongue in the radiation field increases risk for taste alterations owing to the concentration of taste receptors on this surface. RT can lead to taste changes via direct damage to taste cells, damage to nerves supplying taste buds, and reducing flow of saliva (which plays an important role in carrying tastants in food to their receptors). A recent study of 73 oropharyngeal cancer patients receiving IMRT with concurrent chemotherapy found that severe dysgeusia was reported by 50% at 1 month after RT, 40% at 3 months, 22% at 6 months, and 23% at 12 months. The radiation dose to the oral cavity and tongue was associated with severe dysgeusia, with a mean oral cavity D_{50} dose over 53 Gy found to be predictive of severe dysgeusia at 3 months after RT (30).

Prevention of taste changes may include reduction of dose to the oral cavity and tongue when feasible. As the above data demonstrate, taste sensation does slowly recover for most affected patients in the months following RT. Measures to address hyposalivation can be helpful. Treatment with zinc sulfate has been tried but with inconsistent results. A phase III double-blind, placebo-controlled study found no benefit of zinc sulfate for taste changes in HN RT patients (31).

OSTEORADIONECROSIS

Osteoradionecrosis (ORN) of the jaw refers to mandibular or maxillary bone exposed through the overlying mucosa or skin for at least 3 months, as a result of the effects of high-dose RT (32). Bone exposure associated with tumor recurrence is excluded from this definition. ORN of the jaw is a different entity from osteonecrosis of the jaw secondary to bisphosphonates and other medications (called medication-related osteonecrosis of the jaw—MRONJ). ORN is thought to be due to the effects of radiation on bone and blood vessels. Marx and Johnson proposed that radiation results in the formation of tissue that is hypoxic, hypocellular, and hypovascular (33). A more recent theory proposes that ORN is a result of radiation-induced fibrosis and atrophy, resulting in fragile and poorly vascularized tissues (34). Under certain conditions, these states can result in tissue breakdown and chronic nonhealing exposed bone (Figure 24.3). It can slowly progress leading to pain, infection, and pathological fracture.

The risk of ORN is lifelong and dose-dependent. Most cases occur in the mandible at sites that have either directly received greater than 5,000 cGy radiation or are anterior and unilateral to more posterior mandibular sites that have received this level of radiation. The majority of cases, but not all, occur following trauma from dental extractions or ill-fitting dentures (32). Poor oral hygiene and periodontal disease are also considered to be risk factors for ORN, especially in cases without a specific inciting event. A wide range of ORN prevalence has been reported in the literature,

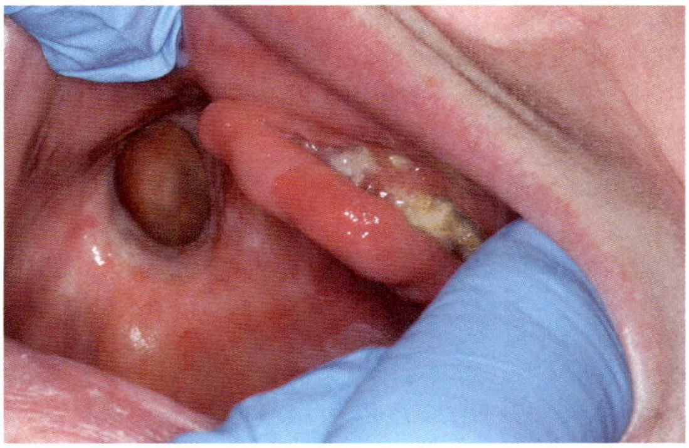

FIGURE 24.3 Osteoradionecrosis in a patient receiving radiation therapy for head and neck cancer. Note the exposed bone in the left maxilla and the surgical defect in the palate.

ranging from 0% to 22% (32). A systematic review reported a weighted ORN prevalence of 7.4% after older RT modalities (35). It has been suggested that the incidence of ORN may be lower with IMRT than with older RT modalities (36,37). A recently published retrospective review from Memorial Sloan Kettering Cancer Center reported that 4.3% of HN IMRT patients developed ORN during a median follow-up time of 52 months (38). A prospective Radiation Therapy Oncology Group (RTOG-022) study reported an ORN incidence of 6% in oropharyngeal cancer patients receiving 66 Gy at a fraction size of 2.2 Gy over 6 weeks, without chemotherapy (39).

To prevent ORN, it is now standard of care for patients who are to receive high-dose RT to the jaws to be referred for a pre-RT dental evaluation. Teeth with a poor prognosis are extracted before the start of RT, to avoid post-RT extractions and associated risk of ORN (32). However, the extraction of teeth just before the start of RT can also lead to ORN, especially if sufficient time is not allowed for healing prior to start of RT. Data published by Marx and Johnson showed that incidence of ORN was lessened if teeth were removed at least 14 days before start of RT (33). Therefore, providers attempt to leave a 14-day healing period between pre-RT dental extractions and start of RT. Dental extractions are avoided after RT in high-dose areas. If necessary, some centers use prophylactic hyperbaric oxygen (HBO) therapy to reduce ORN risk. However, the evidence for its efficacy is conflicting (40,41), and access to the technology as well its associated cost can be significant barriers to its use. Other preventive measures include minimizing trauma and achieving primary closure of the surgical site.

Management of ORN depends on its extent and severity. In early cases, conservative management consisting of local irrigation, topical and systemic antibiotics, avoiding trauma, and maintenance of good oral hygiene can promote healing and resolution (42). If there is sequestrating bone, gentle debridement and removal of sequestrum is performed. Recent data have suggested that pentoxyfylline and tocopherol can help resolve early-stage ORN via their antifibrotic activity (43). In cases that progress further, surgical resection of the affected bone may be necessary. HBO therapy is commonly used in such cases, again with conflicting evidence for efficacy (40,41).

REDUCED MOUTH OPENING/ TRISMUS

Reduced mouth opening refers to the inability to open the mouth wide. Trismus refers to severely restricted mouth opening (maximal mouth opening of 35 mm or less). Reduced mouth opening has been reported in 0% to 100% of HNC patients, depending on tumor site, extension, and treatment modalities (44). Possible causes of trismus include tumor involvement or extension, surgery, and RT, affecting the muscles of mastication and temporomandibular joint (45). Radiation-induced fibrosis of the muscles of mastication can lead to a progressive reduction in the range of mandibular motion. Dose of RT over 50 Gy to the masticatory structures increases the risk, with greater risk reported for parotid and nasopharyngeal cancers (46). An overall reduction of 18% to 32% in mouth opening has been reported after HN RT (47). Over time, reduced mouth opening may improve, worsen, or stay the same. Patients may report pain on mouth opening and difficulty with food intake, speech, and oral hygiene.

Exercise therapy involving range-of-motion exercises is the main component of prevention and management of trismus. This should be started soon after surgery and during HN RT. The use of simple aids such as tongue depressors can be useful. Commercial devices such as the Therabite Jaw Motion Rehabilitation System and the Dynasplint Trismus System are also available. If conservative treatment fails, a coronoidectomy may be considered (44).

DENTAL CARIES

Dental caries refers to breakdown of tooth structure as a consequence of acid production by bacteria that colonize the tooth surface. It presents as discoloration and cavitation of the tooth structure. Dental caries is asymptomatic in its initial stages but can lead to sensitivity and pain once the carious lesion deepens. Patients who have undergone HN RT have been found to be at significantly increased risk for dental caries, sometimes referred to as "radiation caries" in this population (48). This increased risk is mainly due to the effects of RT on the salivary glands. Saliva plays an important role in washing away food particles that provide a food source for the acid-producing bacteria. The loss of this natural cleansing in patients with hyposalivation promotes caries activity. Furthermore, patients with hyposalivation have been found to have a shift to a more cariogenic mouth flora (49). Saliva also contains some natural antibacterial substances and mineralizing components, which normally act to increase caries resistance (50).

The prevention of dental caries in HN RT patients includes measures to address salivary hypofunction as described previously. In addition, the use of prescription strength topical fluoride strengthens the tooth structure and makes it more resistant to caries (51). This can be used as a brush-on toothpaste (such as Prevident 5000 plus) or as a gel used in plastic trays fabricated by a dentist. Other measures to reduce caries risk include limiting the consumption of sugars, avoiding frequent snacking, maintaining good oral hygiene, and brushing/flossing after meals. The treatment of dental caries includes removal of the carious tissue and replacement with a restorative material. In advanced cases, root canal treatment, placement of a crown, or extraction of the tooth may be necessary.

PERIODONTAL DISEASE

Periodontal disease refers to inflammation and destruction of the soft and hard tissues that surround the teeth. It is caused by the effects of a chronic bacterial infection. The initial stage is called gingivitis, which presents as inflamed and erythematous gums, which may be swollen. The more advanced stage is called periodontitis, which includes destruction of the attachment fibers and bone holding the tooth in place. Thus, advanced periodontal disease may result in mobility and loss of teeth. The literature on periodontal disease in patients who have received HN RT is relatively sparse. Three small studies have reported worsening of periodontal disease following older RT modalities (52–54). Initial data from an ongoing multicenter study in patients receiving IMRT or newer modalities indicate that the number of sites with periodontal disease is significantly increased by 2 years after RT (15). The reasons for this increased risk after HN RT may include changes in cellularity, vascularity, and decreased healing/remodeling potential of the soft tissue and bone, as well as effects of hyposalivation including changes in the oral flora (54). The difficulty in maintaining oral hygiene because of the effects of oral mucositis and surgery may also contribute.

Prevention of periodontal disease includes oral hygiene maintenance (regular brushing and flossing) as well as professional dental cleanings at 6-month or more frequent intervals. Treatment of periodontal disease includes deeper dental cleanings (including root surface debridement), periodontal surgery, and the use of antibacterial agents including chlorhexidine mouthwash (such as Peridex or Periogard). In severe cases, extraction of teeth may be necessary.

IMMUNOTHERAPY FOR HNC CANCER

Immunotherapy for treatment of malignant disease, including HNC, represents a strategic new direction in oncology (55). This technology modifies the patient's immune system by a variety of mechanisms, including immune enhancement, suppression, or induction, depending upon the type of agent (56). In addition to primary treatment with immunotherapy, the potential value for neoadjuvant immunotherapy is equally exciting, and holds promise for several clinical benefits including but not limited to tumor downsizing, early management of risk of metastatic dissemination, conversion to resection disease, and early selection of patients likely to respond to subsequent treatment (57).

Despite the considerable opportunity associated with these agents, their use has resulted in a range of toxicities, including those involving the oral cavity (58). Fortunately, these toxicities are often less severe than is typically observed in patients receiving high-dose cancer therapy.

Given the often-unique characteristics of these sequelae, the term "immune-related adverse events" (irAEs) has arisen within the literature (56). irAES involving the oral cavity appear to occur in approximately 10% of patients receiving a single checkpoint inhibitor.

Two principal oral irAEs associated with single-agent checkpoint inhibitors as reported in the recent literature include (56,58):

- Lichenoid mucosal lesions. These lesions are the most common oral adverse sequela of these agents, and typically include an inflammatory component characterized by erythema or tissue sloughing.
- Xerostomia as reported by approximately 5% of patients. However, there is need for further study of the potential impact of these agents relative to producing objective salivary hypofunction, as well as subsequent development of oral mucosal infection, dysgeusia, and mucosal trauma.

Given the only recent emergence of these oral toxicities in clinical practice, management of these conditions of necessity draw upon treatment protocols utilized in other cancer patient cohorts with similar types of toxicities. For example:

- The patient with clinically symptomatic lichenoid lesions can be managed with nonmedicated coating agents and high potent topical or orally administered steroids, depending upon severity of the condition.
- The patient with dry mouth/potential salivary hypofunction can be managed as described previously in this chapter ("Hyposalivation and Xerostomia"; "Oral Candidiasis").

It is important to note that these toxicities, while directly associated with immunotherapy in HNC patients, may be masked in clinical expression by the more severe and direct effects of HN radiation and chemotherapy on oral tissues.

REFERENCES

1. Lalla RV, Saunders DP, Peterson DE. Chemotherapy or radiation-induced oral mucositis. *Dent Clin North Am*. 2014;58(2):341–349. doi:10.1016/j.cden.2013.12.005
2. Vera-Llonch M, Oster G, Hagiwara M, Sonis S. Oral mucositis in patients undergoing radiation treatment for head and neck carcinoma. *Cancer*. 2006;106(2):329–336.
3. Elting LS, Cooksley CD, Chambers MS, Garden AS. Risk, outcomes, and costs of radiation-induced oral mucositis among patients with head-and-neck malignancies. *Int J Radiat Oncol Biol Phys*. 2007;68(4):1110–1120.
4. Al-Dasooqi N, Sonis ST, Bowen JM, et al. Emerging evidence on the pathobiology of mucositis. *Support Care Cancer*. 2013;21(7):2075–2083.
5. Duncan GG, Epstein JB, Tu D, et al. Quality of life, mucositis, and xerostomia from radiotherapy for head and neck cancers: a report from the NCIC CTG HN2 randomized trial of an antimicrobial lozenge to prevent mucositis. *Head Neck*. 2005;27(5):421–428.
6. Trotti A, Bellm LA, Epstein JB, et al. Mucositis incidence, severity and associated outcomes in patients with head and neck cancer receiving radiotherapy with or without chemotherapy: a systematic literature review. *Radiother Oncol*. 2003;66(3):253–262.
7. Rosenthal DI. Consequences of mucositis-induced treatment breaks and dose reductions on head and neck cancer treatment outcomes. *J Support Oncol*. 2007:5(9 Suppl 4):23–31.
8. Miller RC, Le-Rademacher J, Sio TTW, et al. A phase III, randomized double-blind study of doxepin rinse versus magic mouthwash versus placebo in the treatment of acute oral mucositis pain in patients receiving head and neck radiotherapy with or without chemotherapy (Alliance A221304). *Int J Radiat Oncol Biol Phys*. 2016:96(2 (Supplement):938.
9. Saunders DP, Epstein JB, Elad S, et al. Systematic review of antimicrobials, mucosal coating agents, anesthetics, and analgesics for the management of oral mucositis in cancer patients. *Support Care Cancer*. 2013:21(11):3191–3207.
10. Lalla RV, Bowen J, Barasch A, et al. MASCC/ISOO clinical practice guidelines for the management of mucositis secondary to cancer therapy. *Cancer*. 2014:120(10):1453–1461.
11. Bowen JM, Elad S, Hutchins RD, et al. Methodology for the MASCC/ISOO mucositis clinical practice guidelines update. *Support Care Cancer*. 2013:21(1):303–308.
12. Elad S, Bowen J, Zadik Y, et al. Development of the MASCC/ISOO clinical practice guidelines for mucositis: considerations underlying the process. *Support Care Cancer*. 2013:21(1):309–312.
13. Marmary Y, Adar R, Gaska S, et al. Radiation-induced loss of salivary gland function is driven by cellular senescence and prevented by IL6 modulation. *Cancer Res*. 2016:76(5):1170–1180.
14. Jensen SB, Pedersen AM, Vissink A, et al. A systematic review of salivary gland hypofunction and xerostomia induced by cancer therapies: prevalence, severity and impact on quality of life. *Support Care Cancer*. 2010:18(8):1039–1060.
15. Lalla RV, Sollecito T, Treister N, et al. Oral complications after radiation therapy for head and neck cancer. *J Dent Res*. 2017:96(Spec Issue A: 2632355).
16. van Luijk P, Pringle S, Deasy JO, et al. Sparing the region of the salivary gland containing stem cells preserves saliva production after radiotherapy for head and neck cancer. *Sci Transl Med*. 2015:7(305):305ra147.

17. Brizel DM, Wasserman TH, Henke M, et al. Phase III randomized trial of amifostine as a radioprotector in head and neck cancer. *J Clin Oncol*. 2000:18(19):3339–3345.
18. Rieke JW, Hafermann MD, Johnson JT, et al. Oral pilocarpine for radiation-induced xerostomia: integrated efficacy and safety results from two prospective randomized clinical trials. *Int J Radiat Oncol Biol Phys*. 1995:31(3):661–669.
19. Darwazeh AM, Hammad MM, Al-Jamaei AA. The relationship between oral hygiene and oral colonization with Candida species in healthy adult subjects. *Int J Dent Hyg*. 2010:8(2):128–133.
20. Lalla RV, Latortue MC, Hong CH, et al. A systematic review of oral fungal infections in patients receiving cancer therapy. *Support Care Cancer*. 2010:18(8):985–992.
21. Dongari-Bagtzoglou A, Dwivedi P, Ioannidou E, et al. Oral candida infection and colonization in solid organ transplant recipients. *Oral Microbiol Immunol*. 2009:24(3):249–254.
22. Bensadoun RJ, Patton LL, Lalla RV, Epstein JB. Oropharyngeal candidiasis in head and neck cancer patients treated with radiation: update 2011. *Support Care Cancer*. 2011:19(6):737–744.
23. Lalla RV, Patton LL, Dongari-Bagtzoglou A. Oral candidiasis: pathogenesis, clinical presentation, diagnosis and treatment strategies. *J Calif Dent Assoc*. 2013;41(4):263–268.
24. Fotos PG, Hellstein JW. Candida and candidosis. Epidemiology, diagnosis and therapeutic management. *Dent Clin North Am*. 1992;36(4):857–878.
25. Glass RT, Bullard JW, Hadley CS, et al. Partial spectrum of microorganisms found in dentures and possible disease implications. *J Am Osteopath Assoc*. 2001:101(2):92–94.
26. Goregen M, Miloglu O, Buyukkurt MC, et al. Median rhomboid glossitis: a clinical and microbiological study. *Eur J Dent*. 2011;5(4):367–372.
27. Rose JA. Folic-acid deficiency as a cause of angular cheilosis. *Lancet*. 1971:2(7722):453–454.
28. Sitheeque MA, Samaranayake LP. Chronic hyperplastic candidosis/candidiasis (candidal leukoplakia). *Crit Rev Oral Biol Med*. 2003:14(4):253–267.
29. Lalla RV, Bensadoun RJ. Miconazole mucoadhesive tablet for oropharyngeal candidiasis. *Expert Rev Anti Infect Ther*. 2011;9(1):13–17.
30. Sapir E, Tao Y, Feng F, et al. Predictors of dysgeusia in patients with oropharyngeal cancer treated with chemotherapy and intensity modulated radiation therapy. *Int J Radiat Oncol Biol Phys*. 2016;96(2):354–361.
31. Halyard MY, Jatoi A, Sloan JA, et al. Does zinc sulfate prevent therapy-induced taste alterations in head and neck cancer patients? Results of phase III double-blind, placebo-controlled trial from the North Central Cancer Treatment Group (N01C4). *Int J Radiat Oncol Biol Phys*. 2007;67(5):1318–1322.
32. Buglione M, Cavagnini R, Di Rosario F, et al. Oral toxicity management in head and neck cancer patients treated with chemotherapy and radiation: dental pathologies and osteoradionecrosis (Part 1) literature review and consensus statement. *Crit Rev Oncol Hematol*. 2016;97:131–142.
33. Marx RE, Johnson RP. Studies in the radiobiology of osteoradionecrosis and their clinical significance. *Oral Surg Oral Med Oral Pathol*. 1987;64(4):379–390.
34. Delanian S, Lefaix JL. The radiation-induced fibroatrophic process: therapeutic perspective via the antioxidant pathway. *Radiother Oncol*. 2004;73(2):119–131.
35. Peterson DE, Doerr W, Hovan A, et al. Osteoradionecrosis in cancer patients: the evidence base for treatment-dependent frequency, current management strategies, and future studies. *Support Care Cancer* 2010;18(8):1089–1098.
36. Ben-David MA, Diamante M, Radawski JD, et al. Lack of osteoradionecrosis of the mandible after intensity-modulated radiotherapy for head and neck cancer: likely contributions of both dental care and improved dose distributions. *Int J Radiat Oncol Biol Phys*. 2007:68(2):396–402.
37. Studer G, Graetz KW, Glanzmann C. In response to Dr. Merav A. Ben-David et al. ("Lack of osteoradionecrosis of the mandible after IMRT," Int J Radiat Oncol Biol Phys 2007:In Press). *Int J Radiat Oncol Biol Phys*. 2007;68(5):1583–1584.
38. Owosho AA, Tsai CJ, Lee RS, et al. The prevalence and risk factors associated with osteoradionecrosis of the jaw in oral and oropharyngeal cancer patients treated with intensity-modulated radiation therapy (IMRT): the memorial sloan kettering cancer center experience. *Oral Oncol*. 2017:64:44–51.
39. Eisbruch A, Harris J, Garden AS, et al. Multi-institutional trial of accelerated hypofractionated intensity-modulated radiation therapy for early-stage oropharyngeal cancer (RTOG 00-22). *Int J Radiat Oncol Biol Phys*. 2010:76(5):1333–1338.
40. Sultan A, Hanna GJ, Margalit DN, et al. The use of hyperbaric oxygen for the prevention and management of osteoradionecrosis of the jaw: a Dana-Farber/Brigham and Women's Cancer center multidisciplinary guideline. *Oncologist*. 2017:22(3):343–350.
41. Bennett MH, Feldmeier J, Hampson N, et al. Hyperbaric oxygen therapy for late radiation tissue injury. *Cochrane Database Syst Rev*. 2012(5):CD005005.
42. Rice N, Polyzois I, Ekanayake K, et al. The management of osteoradionecrosis of the jaws—a review. *Surgeon*. 2015;13(2):101–109.
43. Patel V, Gadiwalla Y, Sassoon I, et al. Use of pentoxifylline and tocopherol in the management of osteoradionecrosis. *Br J Oral Maxillofac Surg*. 2016:54(3):342–345.
44. Rapidis AD, Dijkstra PU, Roodenburg JL, et al. Trismus in patients with head and neck cancer: etiopathogenesis, diagnosis and management. *Clin Otolaryngol*. 2015;40(6):516–526.
45. Satheeshkumar PS, Mohan MP, Jacob J. Restricted mouth opening and trismus in oral oncology. *Oral Surg Oral Med Oral Pathol Oral Radiol*. 2014;117(6):709–715.
46. Johnson J, van As-Brooks CJ, Fagerberg-Mohlin B, Finizia C. Trismus in head and neck cancer patients in Sweden: incidence and risk factors. *Med Sci Monit*. 2010;16(6):CR278-82.

47. Goldstein M, Maxymiw WG, Cummings BJ, Wood RE. The effects of antitumor irradiation on mandibular opening and mobility: a prospective study of 58 patients. *Oral Surg Oral Med Oral Pathol Oral Radiol Endod*. 1999;88(3):365–373.
48. Gupta N, Pal M, Rawat S, et al. Radiation-induced dental caries, prevention and treatment—a systematic review. *Natl J Maxillofac Surg*. 2015;6(2):160–166.
49. Brown LR, Dreizen S, Handler S, Johnston DA. Effect of radiation-induced xerostomia on human oral microflora. *J Dent Res*. 1975;54(4):740–750.
50. Hicks J, Garcia-Godoy F, Flaitz C. Biological factors in dental caries: role of saliva and dental plaque in the dynamic process of demineralization and remineralization (part 1). *J Clin Pediatr Dent*. 2003;28(1):47–52.
51. Carey CM. Focus on fluorides: update on the use of fluoride for the prevention of dental caries. *J Evid Based Dent Pract*. 2014;14:95–102.
52. Ammajan RR, Joseph R, Rajeev R, et al. Assessment of periodontal changes in patients undergoing radiotherapy for head and neck malignancy: a hospital-based study. *J Cancer Res Ther*. 2013;9(4):630–637.
53. Marques MA, Dib LL. Periodontal changes in patients undergoing radiotherapy. *J Periodontol*. 2004:75(9):1178–1187.
54. Epstein JB, Lunn R, Le N, Stevenson-Moore P. Periodontal attachment loss in patients after head and neck radiation therapy. *Oral Surg Oral Med Oral Pathol Oral Radiol Endod*. 1998;86(6):673–677.
55. Chan KK, Glenny AM, Weldon JC, et al. Interventions for the treatment of oral and oropharyngeal cancers: targeted therapy and immunotherapy. *Cochrane Database Syst Rev*. 2015(12):CD010341. doi:10.1002/14651858.CD010341.pub2
56. Rapoport BL, van Eeden R, Sibaud V, et al. Supportive care for patients undergoing immunotherapy. *Support Care Cancer*. 2017;25(10):3017–3030.
57. Hanna GJ, Adkins DR, Zolkind P, Uppaluri R. Rationale for neoadjuvant immunotherapy in head and neck squamous cell carcinoma. *Oral Oncol*. 2017;73:65–69.
58. Vigarios E, Epstein JB, Sibaud V. Oral mucosal changes induced by anticancer targeted therapies and immune checkpoint inhibitors. *Support Care Cancer*. 2017;25(5):1713–1739.

25

Dysphagia in Patients With Head and Neck Cancer

Katherine A. Hutcheson

Jan S. Lewin

Dysphagia is a priority issue in head and neck cancer (HNC) (1). Swallowing function is a leading driver of quality of life in survivorship (2,3), and has the potential to adversely affect the health of patients (4,5). Malnutrition and aspiration pneumonia are both recognized as potentially life-threatening sequelae of dysphagia in this population. This chapter will review normal and disordered swallowing, risk and morbidities associated with dysphagia in HNC, methods to evaluate swallowing function, and management of dysphagia.

NORMAL SWALLOWING

OVERVIEW OF SWALLOWING

Swallowing is a complex sensorimotor function typically described in four phases as detailed in Table 25.1: (a) oral preparatory, (b) oral, (c) pharyngeal, and (d) esophageal (6). HNC and its treatment can adversely impact all phases of swallowing, but in general, the oropharyngeal phases are most commonly affected.

During the oropharyngeal phases of swallowing, five cranial nerves (V, VII, IX, X, XII) and more than two dozen paired muscles function under control of the medullary central pattern generator (CPG) simultaneously close the airway and nasal port, open the esophagus, and propel a bolus from the mouth through the pharynx for a successful swallow. Cranial nerves V (trigeminal), IX (glossopharyngeal), and the superior laryngeal nerve (SLN) branch of X (vagus) provide sensory feedback to the CPG for swallowing. In turn, complex motor output integrates facial (VII), masticatory (V), lingual (XII), submental (V), palatal (X), laryngeal (X), and pharyngeal (IX, X) musculature for oropharyngeal swallowing. This complex system serves to redirect the respiratory tract temporarily into an alimentary tract for safe and efficient clearance of a bolus through the pharynx (7). In deglutology, swallowing *safety* refers to keeping a bolus out of the airway (i.e., avoidance of high grade laryngeal penetration or aspiration), whereas swallowing *efficiency* refers to how fully and quickly one clears a bolus through the mouth and pharynx. Normal pharyngeal clearance occurs within 31 to 138 milliseconds with 24 to 128 milliseconds of overlapping apnea while the airway is closed (8).

DYSPHAGIA IN HNC: RISK AND ASSOCIATED MORBIDITIES

DYSPHAGIA IN HNC

Dysphagia in HNC is a heterogeneous, multifactorial issue. The risk, severity, and pathophysiology of dysphagia vary widely depending on the clinical scenario and patient characteristics. Among the most important patient factors impacting swallowing are age and comorbid medical conditions. Critical tumor and

TABLE 25.1

Phases of Swallowing

Phase	Function
Oral preparatory	Intake, containment, preparation, and formation of the bolus in the oral cavity
Oral	Anterior to posterior clearance of bolus through mouth to pharynx
Pharyngeal	Clearance of bolus through pharynx into esophagus (includes airway closure and bolus propulsion)
Esophageal	Clearance of bolus through esophagus to stomach

Source: From Logemann JA. Introduction: definitions and basic principles of evaluation and treatment of swallowing disorders. In: Logemann JA. *Evaluation and Treatment of Swallowing Disorders*. 2nd ed. Austin, TX: Pro-Ed; 1998:13–52.

treatment factors include tumor location and size (marked by T classification) and the modality and intensity of treatment (e.g., dose/volume of radiation fields, surgical technique/field, and chemotherapy agent/schedule).

Age

Presbyphagia refers to age-related deterioration in swallowing function. Presbyphagia is thought to reflect loss of the *functional reserve* as sarcopenia and frailty increase with age (9,10). Because swallowing is a submaximal task (i.e., swallowing requires less than maximum capacity of the muscle), presbyphagia represents changes in swallowing that occur as the physiologic reserve (i.e., the difference between maximum capacity and swallowing force) gets smaller. Healthy aging populations have longer latency to swallow onset (11), greater respiratory/swallowing incoordination (11,12), and longer swallowing apnea (11,12) than younger counterparts.

In HNC populations, age at diagnosis is an independent prognosticator of chronic dysphagia and aspiration pneumonia (13–16). This is not only relevant to elderly patients diagnosed with HNC. For instance, the threshold at which risk of chronic fluoroscopy-detected aspiration, stricture, or chronic gastrostomy increases after oropharyngeal chemoradiation is only age >62 at diagnosis (14). Preliminary internal data from the authors' institution also suggest that dysphagia probabilities as a function of swallowing organ-at-risk (OAR) dose rise steadily with each decade of age at diagnosis. This can be interpreted to indicate that the ability to functionally compensate for the impact of 50 Gy to, for instance, the pharyngeal constrictor OAR diminishes as one ages. In the HNC population, this may mean that diminished functional reserve in aging patients makes it harder to overcome or compensate for local treatment effects on the swallowing mechanism. Personalized dysphagia management in the HNC population very likely needs to account for age at diagnosis.

Pretreatment Dysphagia

Tumors arising in the head and neck can adversely impact swallowing function, even prior to cancer treatment. Tumor size and location drive the nature and severity of baseline dysphagia. Many patients with small primary tumors (T1-T2) do not report dysphagia symptoms at baseline. Among symptomatic patients with small primary tumors (T1-T2), clinical experience suggests mild tumor-associated dysphagia symptoms may be present but the swallow is typically functional to safely continue oral intake. In contrast, larger T3 or T4 tumors arising in critical swallowing regions such as the supraglottic larynx, hypopharynx, or deep muscles of the tongue may cause unsafe, high-grade dysphagia necessitating pretreatment feeding tube support.

Baseline functional status predicts functional recovery after treatment. In general, high-grade baseline dysphagia is a poor prognosticator for functional organ preservation. For instance, the authors have previously published 100% chronic gastrostomy dependence among the subset of patients who begin definitive chemoradiation for advanced stage laryngeal cancers with fluoroscopy detected chronic aspiration requiring liquid restrictions (i.e., feeding tube or thick liquids) prior to treatment (17). Likewise, baseline vocal fold fixation that occurs in a subset of patients with advanced stage laryngeal/hypopharyngeal tumors is associated with almost sevenfold increased risk of chronic gastrostomy (6% with mobile larynx vs. 35% with fixed larynx) (18).

Posttreatment Dysphagia

Swallowing outcomes after HNC vary widely. Early-stage disease treated with single-modality therapy is associated with lower risk of severe, chronic dysphagia (19). More common in this subset of HNC patients is acute dysphagia after single-modality laryngeal preservation surgeries (e.g., supraglottic laryngectomy) or single-modality wide-field radiation therapy. Severe and chronic dysphagia is more commonly expected after multimodality treatment (19). Multimodality therapy provides optimal control of locoregionally advanced HNCs but with the trade-off for greater risk of functionally limiting chronic dysphagia.

Attempting to estimate the frequency of posttreatment dysphagia broadly in the HNC population is fraught with uncertainty. Dysphagia rates are reported using many clinical end points such as feeding tube dependence, fluoroscopy-detected aspiration, aspiration pneumonia, and stricture, each with complementary but distinct frequencies of occurrence. For this reason, this chapter summarizes each of these commonly reported end points separately.

Aspiration

Aspiration in HNC survivors may result from surgical resection or sensorimotor disruption of laryngopharyngeal functions that prevent the airway from fully closing during a swallow or cause incomplete bolus clearance prompting aspiration of postswallow bolus residue. With exception of partial laryngeal surgeries or vocal fold paralyses with which aspiration *during* the swallow is common due to laryngeal insufficiency (20), in most HNC subgroups, aspiration most often occurs *after* the swallow from residual bolus in the laryngeal vestibule or pharynx.

Ineffective or absent cough is common, reported in at least half of aspirators in various HNC populations (17,21,22). Given that a high proportion of aspiration events are silent, there is general agreement that aspiration is underreported in clinical studies that only test symptomatic patients. Still, there is great variability in the incidence of posttreatment aspiration reported, even in series that systematically examine all patients regardless of symptoms, with fluoroscopy-detected aspiration reported in 7% to 62% of patients treated with multimodality nonsurgical therapies (13,23–25) and 25% to 34% of those treated with primary surgery for advanced HNC (26).

Feeding Tube Dependence

Feeding tube dependence is the most frequently reported swallowing-related end point in published literature in HNC populations. This likely reflects, at least in part, the simplicity of the measure and the fact that it is readily available in the medical record. Feeding tube utilization metrics include *placement* (i.e., "ever tube") and *dependency* (prolonged use in cancer survivorship, e.g., "1-year gastrostomy rates"). Feeding tube utilization remains common in populations treated with multimodality therapy for advanced stages of HNC, but is usually temporary. It is critical to recognize that feeding tube metrics are nonspecific, particularly in acute posttreatment setting, and not sensitive to oropharyngeal dysphagia in long-term follow-up. That is, in the acute treatment period, feeding tubes are placed for various reasons beyond physical dysphagia, such as in periods when postsurgical pain or mucositis precludes adequate oral alimentation despite adequate oropharyngeal swallow function. This is also the case in periods when swallow function is intact but not allowed until the surgical wound has sufficiently healed. In contrast, after acute recovery, in long-term follow-up, patients with severe dysphagia often elect to eat despite their challenges. In other words, placement of a feeding tube in the acute treatment period does not equate to oropharyngeal dysphagia, and absence of a feeding tube in the long-term follow-up does not equate to functional swallowing (27).

Aspiration Pneumonia

Pneumonia is a potentially life-threatening consequence of aspiration. Prevalence of pneumonia within 3 years of diagnosis historically reported using administrative Surveillance, Epidemiology and End Results (SEER)–Medicare data from 1992 to 1999 was approximately 8% to 10% among patients treated with a single modality (surgery or radiation therapy alone) and approximately 15% in patients treated with multimodality strategies (surgery plus radiation or chemoradiation) (19). More recent estimates in subsets of HNC survivors include 23.8% 5-year cumulative incidence of aspiration pneumonia after chemoradiation for all sites of HNC based on SEER-Medicare data (2000–2009) (4), and 20% actuarial risk at 3 years based on clinical trial results from the University of Michigan's swallowing-optimized intensity-modulated radiation therapy (IMRT) method for oropharyngeal cancers (5). Aspiration pneumonia is also a leading contributor to noncancer-related deaths in HNC survivorship. In a single-institution report, it was the source of 8% of all deaths after definitive radiation therapy and 19% of noncancer-related deaths (28). SEER-Medicare analysis also

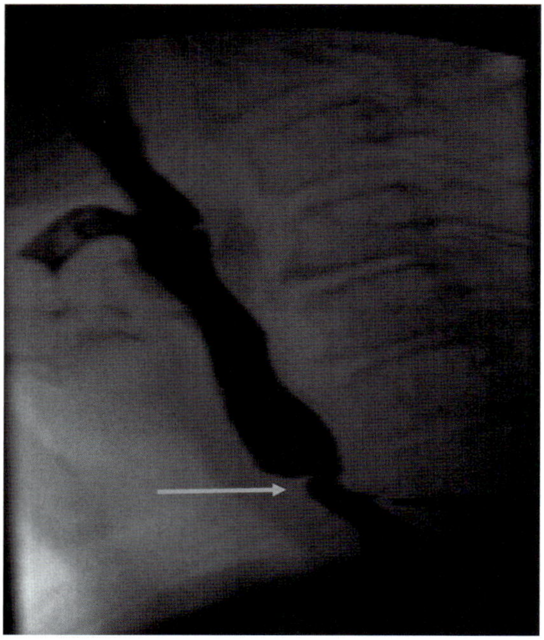

FIGURE 25.1 Example post-radiation stricture on modified barium swallow (MBS) study

reported striking mortality estimates including 42% increased risk of death associated with aspiration pneumonia in HNC survivorship (4).

Stricture

Pharyngoesophageal stricture (Figure 25.1) is a rare, but potentially crippling source of dysphagia after HNC. Stricture results when scarring proliferates in the distal pharynx or esophageal inlet after benign mucosal injury (e.g., in response to acute mucositis) (29). Strictures in HNC survivors are typically reported in populations treated with radiation therapy in excess of 50 Gy to the esophageal inlet or after total laryngectomy (30,31). Systematic review of published work from 1989 to 2008 reported overall risk of stricture after radiation therapy at 7% with higher risk subsets including patients treated with concurrent chemotherapy or older methods of IMRT not shielding the esophageal inlet (32). After total laryngectomy, risk of stricture was estimated using single-institution data at 19% with higher risk among patients requiring circumferential pharyngeal reconstruction (31). Although stricture represents an anatomic source of dysphagia that is amenable to dilation or surgical intervention, it is critical to recognize that stricture almost always coexists with physiologic dysphagia. As such, outcomes of dilation or surgery are likely optimized when coupled with behavioral swallowing therapies, directed in North America by speech language pathologists.

EVALUATION OF DYSPHAGIA

PROTOCOL FOR MULTIDIMENSIONAL EVALUATION OF DYSPHAGIA

Multidimensional assessment is the best practice to comprehensively assess swallowing function. At a minimum, ***physical/physiologic function***, ***functional performance*** status of the patient (i.e., what an individual routinely eats), and ***patient's perceived function*** should be examined. Components of multidimensional dysphagia evaluation are illustrated in Figure 25.2.

FUNCTIONAL STATUS MEASURES

Functional status of the patient pertains to his or her level of oral intake as well as the feeding tube and tracheostomy status of the patient. Quantitative measures of functional status are detailed in Table 25.2. The Performance Status Scale—Head and Neck (PSS-HN) is widely used to standardize the rating of the functional status of the patient (33). This brief semistructured interview rates three domains: (a) 10-point

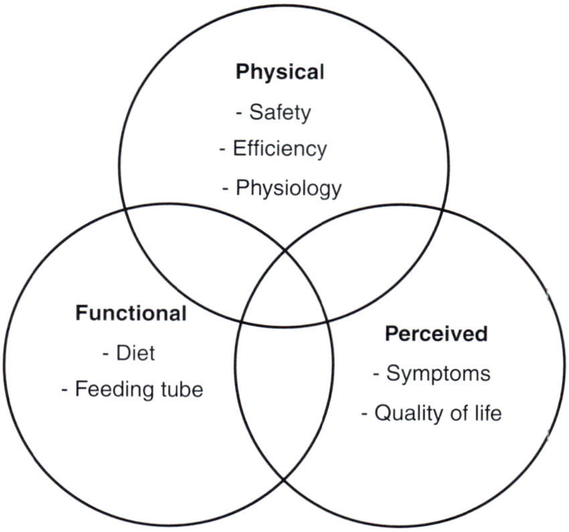

FIGURE 25.2 Components of multidimensional swallowing evaluation.

TABLE 25.2

Measures of Swallowing-Related Functional Status

Measure	Description
FOIS (34)	Functional Oral Intake Scale: 7-point ordinal grade of oral intake (nothing by mouth [NPO] to full oral). Accounts for partial tube dependence.
PSS-HN (33)	Performance Status Scale—Head and Neck Cancer: normalcy of diet is a 10-point ordinal grade (NPO to full oral). Does not account for partial tube dependence. Eating in public is 5-point ordinal grade measuring where and with whom one eats.
CTCAE (35)	Common Terminology Criteria for Adverse Events: dysphagia item is a 5-point grade combining oral intake status (tube fed to full oral) with dysphagia symptoms reported to a clinician.

Note: All functional status measures are clinician-rated based on patient/proxy interview.

normalcy of diet, (b) 5-point public eating, and (c) 5-point understandability of speech. The PSS-HN can be incorporated into the patient's interview during routine assessment to quantify dysphagia-related functional status. PSS-HN does not account for partial feeding tube dependence, so adjunctive questions should be considered to systematically ascertain feeding tube status and manner of use. Another option for quantifying oral intake status is the 7-point Functional Oral Intake Scale (FOIS) (34). Contrary to the PSS-HN, lower level FOIS categories account for partial feeding tube dependence. FOIS likely better discriminates more severe degrees of dysphagia, whereas PSS-HN may better discriminate selective restrictions among higher functioning groups of patients with dysphagia. Because dysphagia grading using the National Cancer Institute's Common Toxicity Criteria for Adverse Events (CTCAE) relies largely on oral diet alteration or feeding tube dependence for classification (35), CTCAE dysphagia grades are likely best considered a functional status measure.

PATIENT-REPORTED OUTCOME MEASURES

Measuring individuals' perception of their swallowing function and quality of life (QOL) is a critical aspect of patient-centered care. In recent decades, several dysphagia-specific patient-reported outcomes (PROs) were developed, validated, and translated for this purpose. Three dysphagia-specific PRO measures that focus on swallowing are detailed in Table 25.3 (36–38), and swallowing is included as a domain of most multisymptom PRO inventories designed for HNC (39,40). The MD Anderson Dysphagia Inventory (MDADI) is the most commonly reported swallowing-focused PRO in published HNC literature, quantifying physical, emotional, and functional domains of swallowing-related QOL. Eat-10 and Sydney Swallowing Questionnaire (SSQ) are not HNC specific, but dysphagia-specific PROs focusing primarily on dysphagia symptoms. Recent work highlights the complementary information provided by QOL (i.e.,

TABLE 25.3

Selected Swallowing-Related Patient-Reported Outcome Measures

Measure*	Description
MDADI (37)	20-item PRO questionnaire of swallowing-related QOL (three domains: physical, functional, emotional)
SSQ (38)	17-item PRO questionnaire of swallowing symptoms
EAT-10 (36)	10-item PRO questionnaire of swallowing symptoms
MDASI-HN (39)	28-item PRO multisymptom questionnaire including two swallowing-related items (problems swallowing/chewing; choking on foods/liquids)
VHNSS (40)	28-item PRO multisymptom questionnaire including seven swallowing-related items

*See text discussion for further description of each measure.
PRO, patient-reported outcome; QOL, quality of life.

MDADI) and symptom (i.e., SSQ) PROs for dysphagia, particularly among higher functioning subgroups with mild to moderate dysphagia symptoms who do not universally report QOL impact of dysphagia (41). In addition to a noninvasive, patient-centered option to track outcomes, PRO questionnaires offer a standardized way to help clinicians identify the primary concerns of patients. Incorporating these questionnaire instruments into routine clinical practice is extremely valuable when establishing patient-centered therapy goals.

CLINICAL AND INSTRUMENTAL SWALLOWING EVALUATIONS

The severity and pathophysiology of swallowing dysfunction must be established using instrumental examinations or imaging studies. Swallowing is an exquisitely complex task involving internal structures best visualized using instrumentation. Videofluoroscopy (i.e., radiographic assessment of swallowing also known as the *modified barium swallow (MBS)* study; Figures 25.3 and 25.4) and endoscopy (known as *fiberoptic endoscopic evaluation of swallowing, FEES;* Figures 25.5 and 25.6) are the cornerstone for instrumental assessment of the oropharyngeal swallow. A clinical or bedside swallow evaluation by the speech pathologist often precedes instrumental assessment. Validated metrics should be applied to quantify results of clinical and instrumental swallowing examinations.

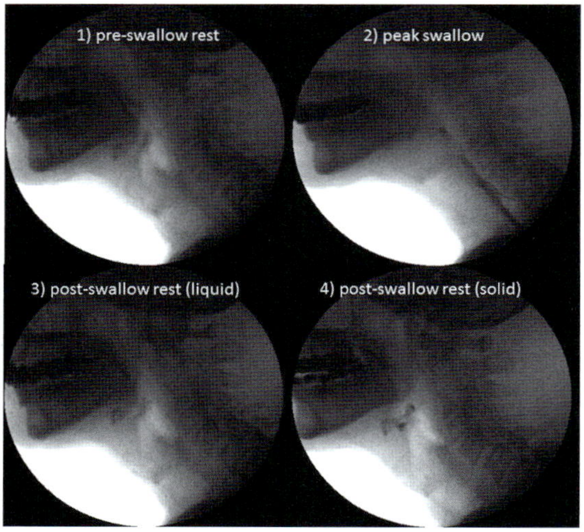

FIGURE 25.3 Example modified barium swallow (MBS) study from patient with a functional swallow.

Note near complete pharyngeal constriction and complete laryngeal vestibule closure at peak swallow (frame 2). Note clear airway and negligible residue post-swallow (frames 3 and 4).

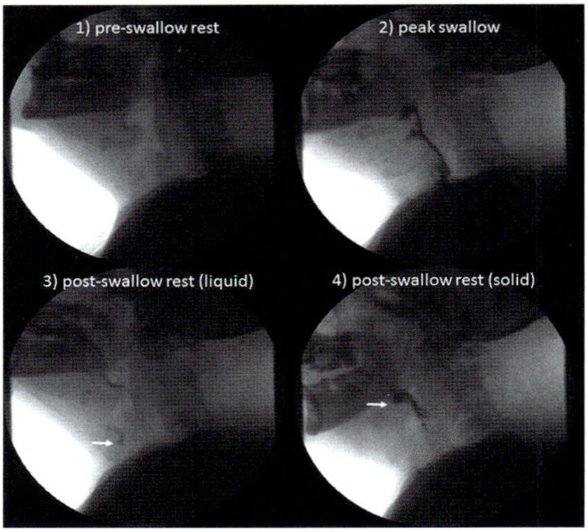

FIGURE 25.4 Example modified barium swallow (MBS) study from patient with severe dysphagia.

Note incomplete pharyngeal constriction and laryngeal vestibule closure peak swallow (frame 2). Laryngeal vestibule residue aspirated post-swallow (frame 3) and solid food residue in valleculae and pharynx (frame 4).

Clinical Swallow Evaluation

Logemann (42) first developed methods and minimal standards to conduct a clinical or bedside swallow evaluation. The clinical examination includes assessment of the oral structures, swallowing-related cranial nerve function, and administration of bolus trials during which the swallow is externally palpated and signs of dysphagia and aspiration may be detected. In clinical practice, the bedside or clinical observation of a “natural” eating environment (i.e., without instrumentation) is invaluable. Yet, as a measure of dysphagia, the clinical examination is often challenged because, in many settings, it fails to provide quantitative or objective benchmarks. For this reason, a number of noninvasive tools have been developed and validated as quantitative metrics that can be obtained in the clinic or at the bedside (without instrumentation). For instance, standardized methods to clinically test a patient during bolus trials include the 3-ounce water screen (43), the Toronto bedside swallowing screening test (44), and the water swallow test (WST) (45). These methods all seek to quantify or screen an individual’s capacity

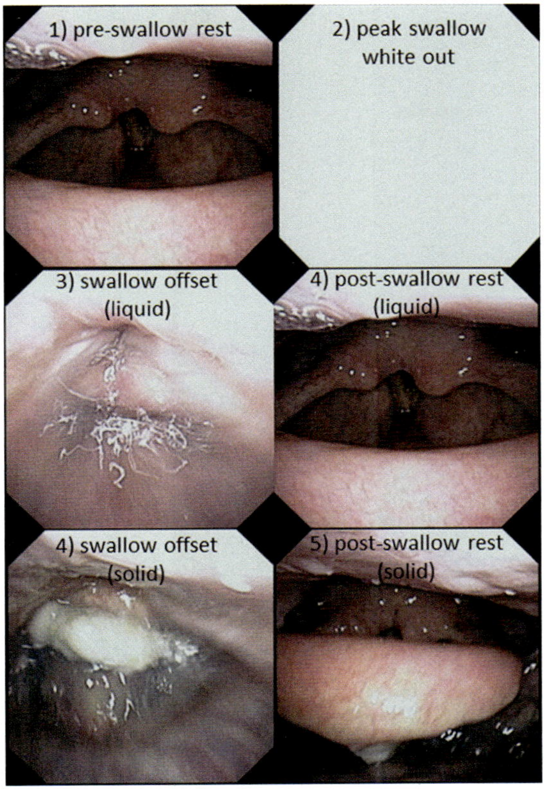

FIGURE 25.5 Example fiberoptic endoscopic evaluation of swallowing (FEES) from patient with a functional swallow.

Frames 1-4 represent a liquid bolus swallow without penetration or aspiration. Note typical white out at peak swallow as the pharynx is maximally constricted around the endoscope. Frames 4-5 demonstrate mild vallecular residue on the cracker bolus visualized both at swallow offset and post-swallow rest.

to swallow a large-volume bolus challenge. Normative ranges of performance on some of these measures allow clinicians a benchmark to contribute to their clinical decision making. The Mann Assessment of Swallow Ability (MASA) (46) is an index measure comprised of a checklist of observations obtained during the clinical swallow evaluation. MASA weights features of the oral mechanism examination, neurocognitive abilities, functional status, and bolus trials to derive a summary score and is validated in cancer populations (MASA-C) (47). Finally, there is promise that affordable, noninvasive adjunctive measures of nonbolus tasks, such as cough strength testing (48–50), electrical impedance myography (51), spontaneous swallowing frequency (52), or tongue strength measures (53,54), may serve as quantitative parameters or functional surrogates that can be tracked longitudinally to improve the yield of clinical swallowing examinations.

Modified Barium Swallow

Videofluoroscopy is widely considered the most popular method of instrumental swallowing assessment among speech pathologists. During videofluoroscopy, the patient is administered contrast enhanced bolus trials of various consistencies while a dynamic x-ray records bolus passage from the mouth through the cervical esophagus.

Tremendous progress has been made to standardize the method since adoption of the MBS study into speech-language pathology (SLP) practice more than three decades ago (55–60). Diagnostic observations from MBS are only reproducible and reliably quantified when clinicians adhere to a standard acquisition protocol. Critical elements of MBS standardization include, among many, the concentration of contrast agent(s), the bolus protocol, frame rate (temporal resolution), and instructions provided to the patient during the examination. A uniform bolus protocol must be efficient to minimize radiation exposure (per ALARA [as low as reasonably achievable] principle) (61) yet comprise a sufficient range of consistencies that represent a range of food types. As a foundational step in developing the Modified Barium Swallow Impairment Profile (MBSImP), Martin-Harris and colleagues (55) developed and assessed a consensus-derived, standard bolus protocol. The recommended bolus protocol from MBSImP includes measured-volumes and natural "cup sip" presentations of thin liquid barium (Varibar, Bracco Diagnostics Inc., Monroe Township, NJ), pudding thick barium, and a dry solid bolus.

Dozens of videofluoroscopic measures quantify MBS results including bolus-based measures (such as the penetration-aspiration scale, PAS (62) and the Dynamic Imaging Grade of Swallowing Toxicity, DIGEST) (63), physiologic ratings (such as MBSImP) (55), temporal scales (such as Oropharyngeal Swallow Efficiency, OPSE) (64), and kinematics or morphometrics (including numerous hyoid kinematic parameters (65–67), the Computational Assessment of Swallowing Mechanics, CASM, and the Pharyngeal Constriction Ratio, PCR).

The field has yet to adopt a core set of measures to report from MBS in HNC trials. The authors propose that the selection of MBS measures

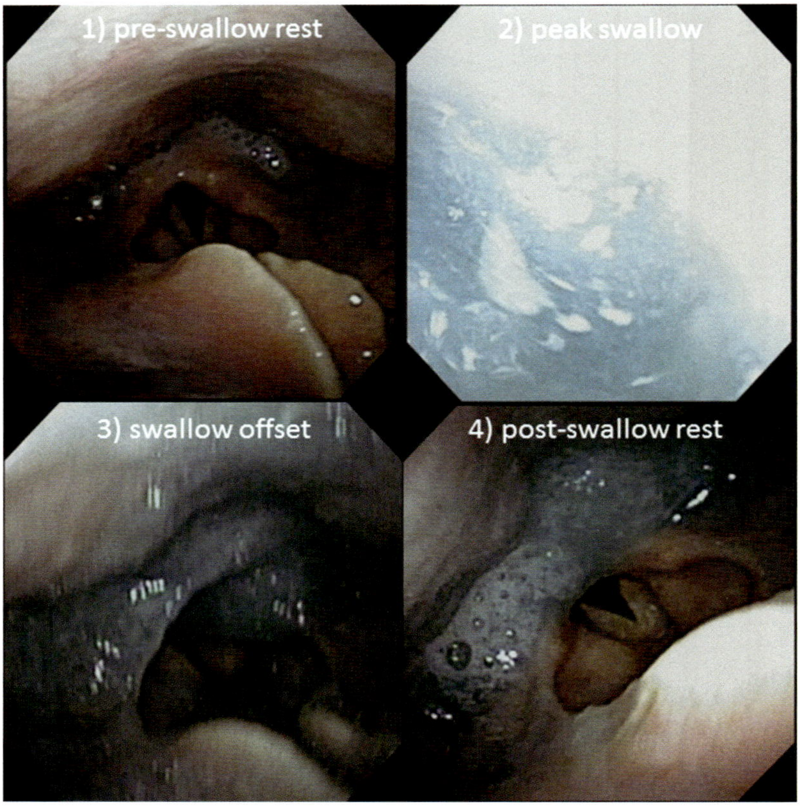

FIGURE 25.6 Example fiberoptic endoscopic evaluation of swallowing (FEES) from patient with severe dysphagia.

Note saliva pooling in piriform sinuses and supraglottic fibrosis pre-swallow (frame 1), absence of typical white out at peak swallow indicating incomplete pharyngeal constriction (frame 2), and severe post-swallow residue (frames 3-4).

depends on the intended goal. For studies seeking to quantify the severity of dysphagia, DIGEST provides a functional bolus-derived MBS classification of pharyngeal dysphagia on a 5-point ordinal scale analogous to the familiar CTCAE toxicity grading (0 = none; 1 = mild; 2 = moderate; 3 = severe; 4 = profound/life-threatening). DIGEST classifies severity of dysphagia based on both safety and efficiency of bolus clearance through the pharynx. In contrast, the PAS, commonly used to rank severity of dysphagia in this population considers safety but not efficiency. For studies that seek to quantify and characterize the pathophysiology of dysphagia using results of the MBS, the authors propose use of morphometric or kinematic measures that include the anterior (i.e., submental suprahyoid muscles) and proximal sling (i.e., longitudinal pharyngeal muscles that shorten pharynx and lift the larynx) of hyolaryngeal excursion (e.g., CASM, Figure 25.7), pharyngeal constriction (e.g., PCR that combines velopharyngeal seal, pharyngeal constriction, and tongue base retraction into a single surrogate of pharyngeal propulsion), and esophageal inlet opening. Kinematic and morphometric measures historically required labor-intensive, frame-by-frame analysis by a trained rater, but semiautomated processes are rapidly evolving to simplify this method (65,67,68).

Fiberoptic Endoscopic Evaluation of Swallowing

FEES was first described as an endoscopic alternative for instrumental oropharyngeal swallow evaluation by Langmore and colleagues over 25 years ago (69). Advantages relative to videofluoroscopy include the ability to visualize (without radiation exposure) the tumor, surgical defects, reconstruction, and postradiation

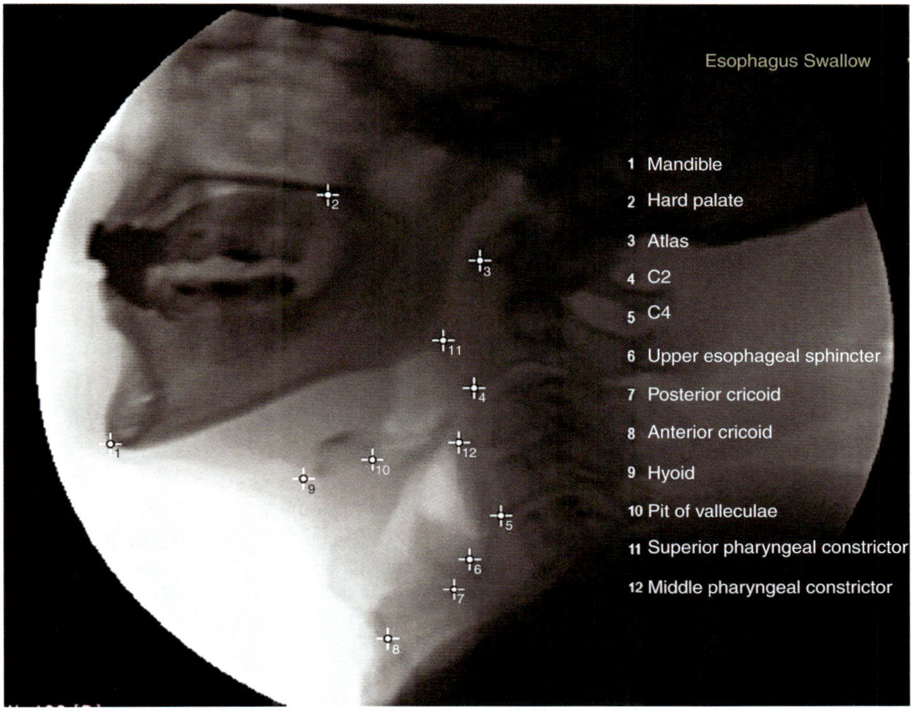

FIGURE 25.7 Example modified barium swallow (MBS) study frame annotated for computational analysis of swallowing mechanics (CASM).

soft tissue morphology of the palate, pharynx, and larynx at rest, during swallows, and during nonswallow tasks such as phonation, Valsalva, and coughing. Secretions and sensation can also be assessed. With portable equipment that does not require x-ray, FEES is also useful for serial studies and even daily therapeutic biofeedback programs (69–76). A disadvantage of FEES is the inability to directly observe oral or esophageal functions and peak swallow "white-out" that obstructs visualization of the laryngopharynx while the pharynx constricts around the endoscope during the swallow. Comparative studies find FEES and MBS comparable in terms of detecting airway penetration and pharyngeal residue (77–80) although far fewer quantitative FEES methods are available to use this method in research.

High-Resolution Manometry

Complex pressure dynamics underlie bolus movement through the pharynx during swallowing. Manometry uses endoscopic catheters to directly measure pressure propagation during swallows. High-resolution manometry (HRM) uses up to 43 closely spaced (≤1 cm), solid-state, circumferential pressure sensors that record contact pressures with high temporal resolution (50 Hz). HRM outputs spatiotemporal plots demonstrating patterns of pressure propagation over time (81) (Figure 25.8). Impedance sensors can simultaneously record surrogates of bolus presence and residue, as well as upper esophageal sphincter (UES) distention during swallowing (82–91). HRM is broadly adopted as a gastrointestinal (GI) motility study, and the popular Chicago Classification System assigns motility diagnoses using an algorithm of pressure features from HRM (92). Pharyngeal HRM is gaining ground with various laboratories describing methods to quantify regional pharyngeal pressures and UES outlet obstruction (86,93–98). It is possible to simultaneously acquire HRM with MBS, FEES, or even electromyography (EMG) recording (99), but these pairings are typically reserved for research procedures. In the clinic, HRM serves primarily as an adjunct study to characterize pathophysiology of dysphagia in complex cases and as a tool for biofeedback during swallowing therapy (95).

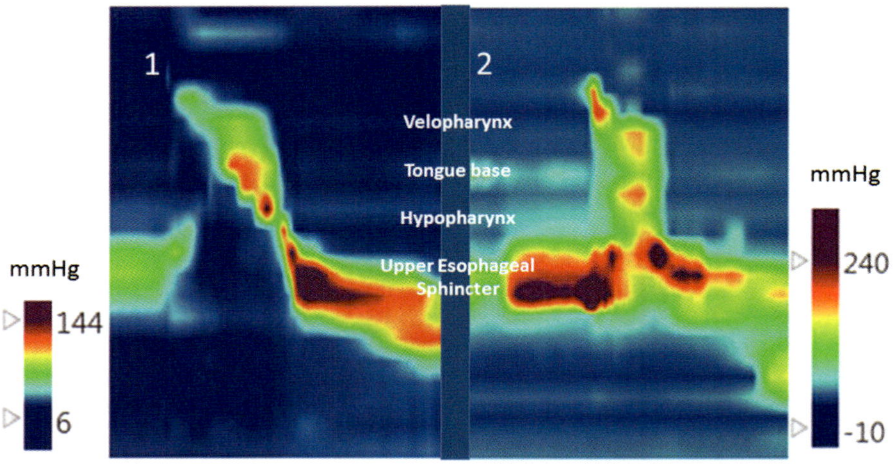

FIGURE 25.8 Spatiotemporal plots from pharyngeal high resolution manometry (HRM).

Examples of normal pharyngeal pressure propagation during 10 mL swallow in 33 year old female (frame 1), and abnormal pharyngeal pressure pattern during 10 mL swallow in a 66 year male status post hemiglossectomy, neck dissection and postoperative radiation therapy (frame 2). Note static high UES pressure indicating poor to no UES relaxation as well as weak and incoordinated pharyngeal contractions.

Courtesy of Dr. Tim McCulloch at the University of Wisconsin.

MANAGEMENT OF DYSPHAGIA

MULTIDISCIPLINARY TEAM

Multidisciplinary care has long been considered best practice in HNC. Cancer therapy is directed jointly by a head and neck surgeon, radiation oncologist, and medical oncologist. The same multidisciplinary approach is required for dysphagia management in HNC. Dysphagia rehabilitation is a team sport. Dysphagia does not exist in isolation but instead coexists with various problems such as:

Communication impairments (dysphonia, dysarthria or resonance disturbance)

Head and neck lymphedema (interstitial soft tissue swelling)

Trismus (restricted mouth opening)

Neck and shoulder dysfunction (weakness, stiffness, or impaired range of motion)

Salivary dysfunction (xerostomia or thick mucus)

Ototoxicity (hearing loss)

These diverse functional problems require assessment and management by multiple specialists including, among others:

Speech-language pathologists

Otolaryngologists/head and neck surgeons

Physical therapists

Dental oncologists and maxillofacial prosthodontists

Dietitians

Gastroenterologists

Audiologists

The following sections focus on proactive and reactive management of ***swallowing function***, but it is imperative to screen for and address all affected functional domains to achieve the best QOL outcomes. Common symptoms such as pain and fatigue may limit survivors' capacity or motivation to perform or enjoy routine daily activities. While beyond the scope of this chapter, proactive symptom management and supportive care, particularly pain management, form a critical component of multidisciplinary care necessary to achieve optimal swallowing outcomes. For example, prophylactic neuropathic pain management during chemoradiation for oropharyngeal cancer patients has been shown to significantly correlate with better posttreatment functioning (100).

PRINCIPLES OF SWALLOWING REHABILITATION

Two principal components of effective swallowing rehabilitation in HNC patients are (a) mobilize early and often (i.e., "use it or lose it") and (b) mass practice of functional activity (i.e., high-intensity or frequent swallowing practice).

Fields of rehabilitation, sports medicine, and exercise science define the principles of effective exercise therapy and neuromuscular retraining. Intensity and specificity are critical features. Therapy must be specific to the target, following the clinical adage that "swallowing is the best therapy for swallowing," but must also force the neuromuscular system beyond its usual level of activity. Swallowing is a submaximal task. That is, the force generated during swallowing is well below the maximum capacity of the system. Thus, therapy must push the functional activity beyond typical intensity. Therapy can be intensified by (a) more frequent or longer repetitions and (b) resistive loading (101).

Skill training is an emerging area in dysphagia rehabilitation. Skill training can be conceived as a more structured extension of compensatory techniques that speech pathologists have historically prescribed. In skill training, principles of motor learning are used to habituate behaviors that facilitate safe and efficient bolus clearance. Central to this therapy is the acknowledgment that not all patients with dysphagia have oropharyngeal weakness and not all weakness can be fixed. Instead, or in addition to weakness, coordination, timing, and motor planning for swallow can be impaired. Structured, skill-based training programs aimed at improving timing and coordination of the swallowing sequence using principles of motor learning often incorporate biofeedback (102,103). For example, Martin-Harris and colleagues recently reported promising results of a phase II single-arm clinical trial that integrated a novel biofeedback paradigm to train chronic aspirators after radiation therapy to swallow at the optimal point in the respiratory cycle (103).

PROACTIVE DYSPHAGIA THERAPY: USE IT OR LOSE IT

Disuse of swallowing muscles, temporary or chronic, occurs during treatment for HNC. Pharyngeal immobilization can occur when postsurgical restrictions mandate that patients remain NPO (taking nothing orally) while the surgical wound heals or during radiation therapy when patients stop eating for prolonged periods because of acute toxicities such as mucositis and odynophagia. Regardless of the source, immobilization prompts disuse atrophy that encourages adverse neuromuscular remodeling and likely exacerbates dysfunction related to soft tissue edema and fibrosis (104,105). Skeletal muscles in other regions begin to show evidence of disuse atrophy just hours after immobilization. Myoarchitecture changes rapidly with a decrease in muscle mass, infiltration of adipose tissue, and unfavorable redistribution of fiber types. Over time, disuse atrophy manifests as a reduced muscle strength, increased fatigability, and aberrant motor control. The extent of injury is dependent on the degree of disuse. For these reasons, early and more frequent mobilization of swallowing muscles should equate to more normal muscle composition and function after treatment—"use it or lose it" (104,105).

The "use it or lose it" premise is supported by work in which, relative to sham exercise or no exercise conditions, patients randomized to proactive swallowing exercise during chemoradiation had significantly less deterioration in genioglossus, hyoglossus, and mylohyoid muscle mass and composition per T2-weighted MRI (106). For these reasons, proactive swallowing therapy is increasingly favored over the outdated practice of placing a feeding tube and waiting to start swallow therapy until a patient feels better. Models for proactive swallowing therapy in populations treated with radiation or surgery are detailed in the sections that follow.

Model for Proactive Swallowing Therapy in Patients Treated With Radiation Therapy

Preventive swallowing therapy is considered best practice for patients treated with wide-field radiation therapy (i.e., to bilateral neck) for HNC (107,108). Acute radiation therapy toxicities including mucositis, salivary dysfunction, and dysgeusia make it difficult or at least unpleasant to eat. For this reason, at least half of patients require temporary feeding tube placement during treatment (109,110), and even those who avoid a tube usually stop eating solid foods. When patients stop eating normal foods, it is suggested that loss of the normal load of swallowing prompts varying degrees of disuse atrophy. Thus, proactive swallowing therapy follows the "use it or lose it" philosophy to mitigate muscular wasting and remodeling that occurs after even brief intervals of nonuse. Proactive swallowing therapy encourages persistent use of the swallowing musculature by (a) avoiding NPO intervals during treatment and (b) adhering to swallowing exercise. Benefits of swallowing activity (*eat* and *exercise*) are reported in numerous randomized trials and observational studies. Early implementation of manual therapies, recently reported in a small case series, may offer a new extension of proactive therapy models for dysphagia in the future (106,111,112).

Several randomized trials report benefit of ***preventive swallowing exercise*** during chemoradiation (106,113–115). A sham-controlled trial found a 36% absolute risk reduction for loss of functional swallow ability in patients randomized to active swallow exercise during chemoradiation (106). Other favorable outcomes reported in association with preventive exercise include superior swallowing-related QOL (116,117); better tongue base and epiglottic inversion (118); larger postchemoradiation muscle mass and T2 signal intensity on MRI of the genioglossus, mylohyoid, and hyoglossus muscles (106); shorter duration of gastrostomy (111); and greater return to normal oral diet levels (111). Methodologic inconsistencies preclude meta-analyses and a recent Cochrane review found inconclusive evidence from mostly small, single-site data (119).

Observational studies suggest the benefit of continuing oral intake during radiation therapy and avoiding even brief NPO intervals. For instance, NPO intervals of just 2 weeks significantly and independently predict lower swallowing-related QOL scores in long-term survivorship after chemoradiation (median: 4.7 years) (120). Multidisciplinary symptom management likely helps patients safely maintain oral intake. In case-control analysis, prophylactic neuropathic pain management was associated with lower pain scores, decreased PEG utilization, and decreased aspiration after chemoradiation (100). Authors of this study posited less pain allowed patients to keep eating and adhere to exercises, and ultimately conferred a physiologic advantage in preserved swallowing function on MBS.

Patients often ask if they can just *eat* or *exercise*. That is, patients and providers alike wonder if there is added benefit of doing exercises if they are still eating during radiation therapy. Multivariate models suggest that *eat* and *exercise* independently and significantly predict for better short- and long-term swallowing-related outcomes (111).

A practical, evidence-based approach to implement preventive swallowing therapy includes at a minimum:

1. Pretreatment referral to a speech pathologist for baseline evaluation (preferably including instrumental examination) and training on swallow exercise
2. On-treatment swallowing therapy with a speech pathologist to monitor swallowing and adjust swallow exercise program as needed as toxicities increase
3. Posttreatment speech pathology evaluation (preferably using instrumental examination)

The radiation swallowing pathway developed by MD Anderson is depicted in Figure 25.9.

POSTSURGICAL REHABILITATION

Swallowing outcomes after head and neck surgery vary widely. Critical factors that affect postsurgical swallowing outcomes include (a) location/size of resection, (b) surgical approach, (c) closure technique, and (d) management of the neck.

Location: It is natural that the size and location of the primary tumor will dictate the nature and degree of swallowing problems after surgery. Functional loss after surgery can be predicted by asking: (a) What is the functional role of the structure to be resected? How much will be resected (per T stage)? Does the surgical bed extend to swallowing-relevant adjacent structures?

Approach: Open surgical procedures via a transmandibular or transoral approach are more likely to damage swallowing-relevant structures adjacent to the primary tumor. Among these, suprahyoid elevators in the floor of mouth region are commonly disrupted in conventional open resections with downstream effects on airway closure and esophageal opening. Functional advantages of transoral resections have been demonstrated in many comparative observational studies. A common theme is that swallowing recovery is earlier after transoral surgery compared to open surgery (121).

Closure: Closure techniques that do not tether or restrict mobility of remnant structures empirically facilitate the best functional outcome. When reconstruction is required to cover vessels or fill a large defect, the ideal balance is

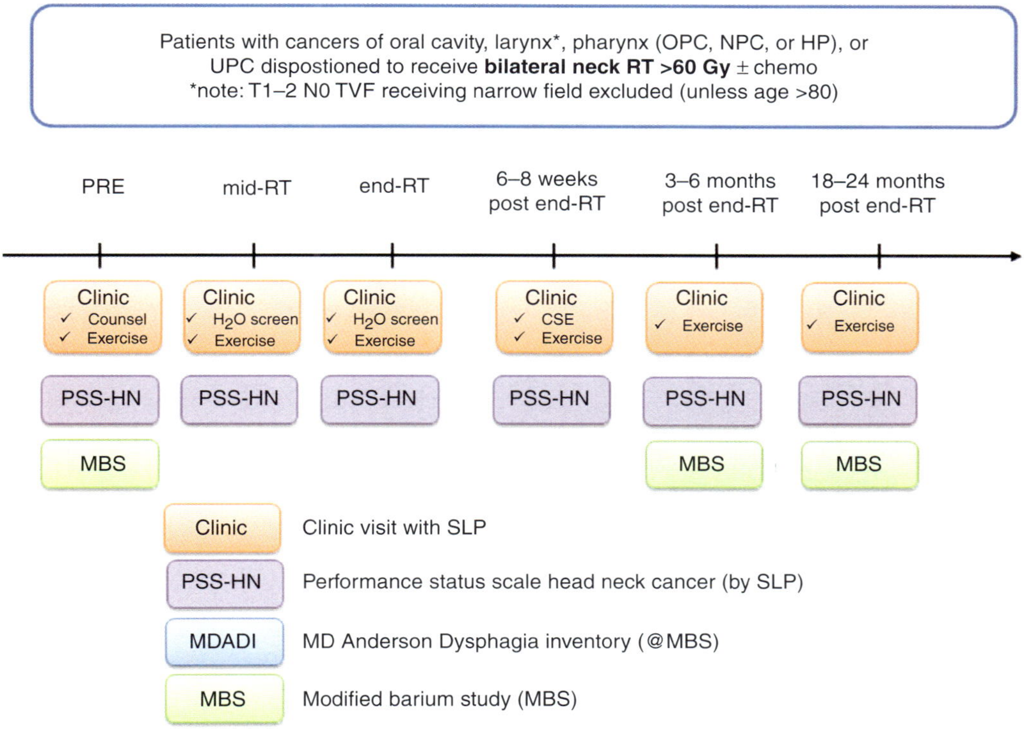

FIGURE 25.9 MD Anderson Cancer Center model for speech pathology radiation swallowing pathway.

OPC, oropharyngeal cancer; NPC, nasopharyngeal cancer; HP, hypopharyngeal cancer; UPC, unknown primary cancer; Gy, Gray; TVF, true vocal fold; RT, radiation therapy; CSE, clinical swallow evaluation; SLP, speech-language pathologist

to reconstitute the missing bulk while retaining as much mobility as possible in the remaining structures.

Neck management: Neck dissection is thought to add morbidity, particularly in the areas of neck fibrosis, lymphedema, and neck and shoulder range of motion with downstream QOL implications (122). The impact of neck dissection on swallowing outcomes is less consistent in published literature. After chemoradiation, for instance, limited neck dissections did not significantly increase likelihood of severe, clinically detected dysphagia using markers of chronic gastrostomy, aspiration, or stricture (122).

Model for Proactive Postsurgical Dysphagia Management in HNC

Proactive, postsurgical dysphagia management also follows the "use it or lose it" adage. In this scenario, swallowing rehabilitation follows the logical steps depicted in Figure 25.10.

INTENSIVE THERAPY METHODS FOR PERSISTENT OR REFRACTORY DYSPHAGIA

Despite best efforts to prevent dysphagia, still probably at least 30% of patients develop moderate to severe persisting or late dysphagia after multimodality HNC treatment. Intensive swallowing therapy is typically indicated in this setting. A distinguishing component of intensive, clinician-directed dysphagia therapy is a progressive paradigm of therapy tasks. Progressive methods iteratively increase the complexity, intensity, or load of a therapy task as skill or strength improves. Resistive loading of swallowing musculature is obviously not as simple as adding another weight to the barbell in the gym. Popular methods used to increase the resistive load of swallowing of the oral and pharyngeal muscles include (a) ***device-driven*** methods and (b) ***bolus-driven*** paradigms. Regardless of the model of intensive therapy selected, the authors generally wait to begin intensive "loading" until acute mucosal injury

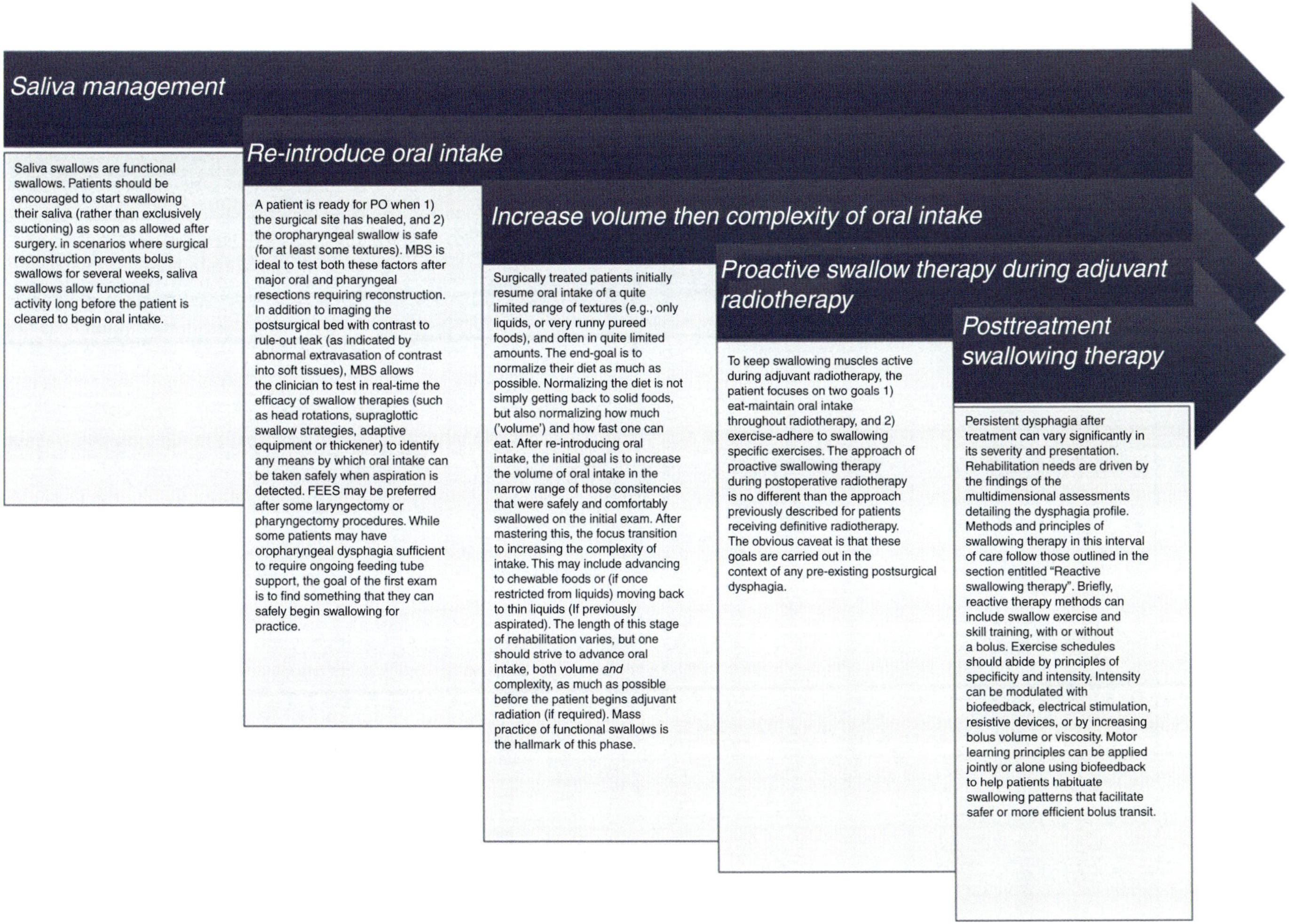

FIGURE 25.10 Model for proactive postsurgical dysphagia management in HNC.

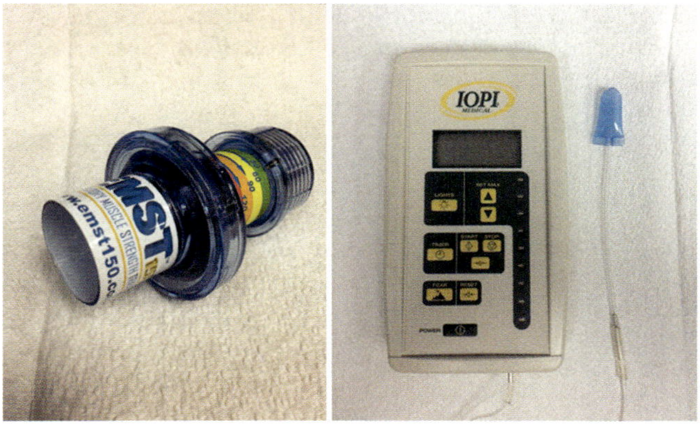

FIGURE 25.11 Example resistive exercise devices used adjunctively in dysphagia management.
Expiratory muscle strength training respiratory resistive device used for airway protection exercise (left) and Iowa Oral Pressure Instrument used for lingual strengthening (right).

is sufficiently healed to allow pain-free swallows and the patient is disease-free.

Device-Driven Therapies

With device-driven therapy, biofeedback, resistance, or neuromuscular electrical stimulation is applied to augment the intensity of swallowing exercise. Biofeedback devices like tongue-resistance bulbs or surface EMG take a reading of muscle activity during a functional task. Patients watch their performance in real time and try to meet a specified level of intensity during the exercise task. Goals are set based on a percentage of their peak force and increased as strength improves. Exercise principles guide the pace of loading using biofeedback devices. Biofeedback-driven exercise typically starts at roughly 60% intensity (i.e., 60% of the patient's maximum ability) and peaks at 80% intensity (101). Efficacy of device-driven biofeedback therapies is suggested in a number of case series in patients with dysphagia related to HNCs and other pathologies (123,124).

Resistive exercise devices offer another option to augment the intensity of swallowing-related exercises (Figure 25.11). Resistive devices are typically used during nonswallow tasks. Two primary examples include lingual resistance devices during a tongue press (e.g., the Iowa Oral Pressure Instrument, IOPI, or Swallow Strong isometric Progressive Resistance Oral, i-PRO), and expiratory resistance during a blowing task (e.g., Expiratory Muscle Strength Training, EMST). IOPI and iPRO are associated with improved lingual strength, penetration/aspiration scores, and manometric pharyngeal pressures during swallowing in case series (124–126). EMST is associated with stronger subglottic pressure generation that may assist cough to expel aspiration, and swallowing-related muscle activation during resistive exercise including velopharyngeal closure, hyolaryngeal excursion, and pharyngeal shortening (99,127,137).

Neuromuscular electrical stimulation (NMES) is another popular device that can be paired with swallowing therapy in an effort to enhance neuromuscular recruitment. NMES transmits low-voltage current through bipolar surface electrodes on the skin, triggering a nerve to activate sensory responses and muscular contraction. NMES is a long-established practice in rehabilitation medicine for upper and lower extremity motor function of large skeletal muscles (128,129). Conflicting data have been reported with regard to the potential benefit of electrical stimulation in swallowing rehabilitation. Mechanistic studies from the intramural Laryngeal Study Section of the National Institutes of Health (NIH) suggest that variable response to NMES for dysphagia may relate to the greater activation of swallowing antagonist musculature that are superficial to deep swallowing muscle targets and therefore are stimulated to a greater degree during NMES (130). A recently published multisite, randomized, sham-controlled clinical trial found no added therapeutic benefit of current models of NMES over traditional swallowing exercise in HNC patients with chronic, moderate-severe dysphagia after chemoradiation (131). Thus, at present, the role of current NMES systems in dysphagia rehabilitation for HNC is not supported by the most rigorous available published work.

Bolus-Driven Therapies

A bolus-driven model of progressive resistance dysphagia therapy was developed and published out of the University of Florida and named the McNeil Dysphagia Therapy Program (MDTP) in honor of the first patient to successfully complete the program. In MDTP, clinicians systematically navigate patients up and down a food hierarchy to increase the workload of swallowing exercise using increasing volume or viscosity of the bolus to progressively load the swallow task (132). A patient first masters, then must maintain the ideal swallowing form while increasing the volume and viscosity of what he is eating in daily, clinician-directed 1-hour therapy sessions for 3 weeks. Promising results of bolus-driven MDTP are reported in small case series (133). Bolus-driven methods were found superior to device-driven therapy (using surface electromyography [sEMG]) in a matched case-control comparison (132). Regardless of the method or techniques applied, mass practice of functional tasks under conditions that require progressive work over time is the hallmark of successful swallowing rehabilitation programs in patients who develop persistent, refractory, or late moderate to severe dysphagia after HNC treatment.

Boot Camp Swallowing Therapy

Device-driven and bolus-driven therapies may be delivered in a "boot camp" type of schedule in which patients participate in a short, intense series of daily therapy sessions over a 2- to 3-week period. In case-control comparison, bolus-driven boot camp models (i.e., MDTP) outperformed device-driven therapy. Patients treated with bolus-driven therapy were significantly more likely to have reduced aspiration, less gastrostomy dependence, and better diet levels after therapy compared to those who participated in device-driven therapy with sEMG biofeedback (132). On the basis of these results and relevance of functionally driven therapy, the authors prefer bolus-driven "boot camp" therapy whenever possible. Other medical/surgical (e.g., dilation, myotomy, botulinum toxin injections), prosthetic (e.g., dentures, palatal lift), and device-driven methods (e.g., IOPI, iPRO, EMST) are ideally incorporated prior to beginning the bolus-driven segment of boot camp in effort to optimize the system for best functional gains with bolus.

SPECIAL CONSIDERATIONS FOR LATE DYSPHAGIA

Early dysphagia is now characterized reasonably well with prospective data. The same is not true for late effects of therapy. Prospective late effects data are rare and are certainly not robust among patients treated with highly conformal radiation therapy, minimally invasive surgery, or emerging biologic agents. Most late-effects data derive from single-institution cross-sectional samples or small case series. Commonly referenced on this topic is the report of Machtay and colleagues based on pooled analysis of three Radiation Therapy Oncology Group (RTOG) chemoradiation trials reporting 43% incidence of grade 3 to 4 (severe) late laryngopharyngeal toxicity attributable to treatment (134). Late dysphagia was also common in a prospective late effects clinic of 5-year survivors of accelerated radiation therapy with concurrent cisplatin; 23% had silent aspiration and 85% had restricted diets (22). Notably, both of these studies report findings of two-dimensional (2D) and three-dimensional (3D) conformal methods that have largely been replaced by more conformal methods such as IMRT, volumetric modulated arc therapy (VMAT), and proton therapy. These data also do not distinguish chronic/persistent dysphagia from late-onset dysphagia, which is notable because there appears to be clinically significant distinctions in these scenarios.

Late-onset radiation-associated dysphagia (late-RAD) is a particularly challenging form of dysphagia in long-term survivors. Late-RAD has a different time course than classic RAD. With late-RAD, patients enjoy functional oropharyngeal swallowing for many years after acute toxicities resolve before presenting back with clinically significant delayed dysphagia. The authors' initial case series characterizing late-RAD reported median latency of 9 years (135). Late-RAD is presumably rare with an estimated prevalence of <10% in the first 10 years of survivorship, but it is associated with late-onset cranial neuropathies and severe dysphagia that is refractory to conventional nonsurgical therapies (136). Silent aspiration and global lingual and laryngopharyngeal paresis are the norm in patients with late-RAD. Bleak outcomes of late-RAD (66% prevalence of pneumonia in late-RAD series) and limited functional gains observed to date with conventional therapy motivate investigations into novel therapies.

CONCLUSIONS

Swallowing function substantially impacts health and quality of life in HNC survivorship. Multidimensional swallowing evaluation methods should combine instrumental assessments of physical dysphagia, standardized oral intake measures of functional status, and PRO instruments to quantify perceived symptoms and QOL. Optimization of swallowing outcomes mandates close attention to age, comorbidity, baseline functionality, disease, and treatment burden. Proactive models of swallowing therapy are best practice in both surgically and nonsurgically treated patients. Intensive, structured therapy programs are expected to provide best outcomes for those patients who, despite preventive services, develop persistent (chronic or late) moderate to severe dysphagia after treatment.

REFERENCES

1. Wilson JA, Carding PN, Patterson JM. Dysphagia after nonsurgical head and neck cancer treatment: patients' perspectives. *Otolaryngol Head Neck Surg*. 2011;145(5):767–771. doi:10.1177/0194599811414506
2. Goepfert RP, Fuller CD, Gunn GB, et al. Symptom burden as a driver of decisional regret in long-term oropharyngeal cancer survivors. *Head Neck*. 2017;39(11):2151–2158.
3. Hunter KU, Schipper M, Feng FY, et al. Toxicities affecting quality of life after chemo-IMRT of oropharyngeal cancer: prospective study of patient-reported, observer-rated, and objective outcomes. *Int J Radiat Oncol Biol Phys*. 2013;85(4):935–940.
4. Xu B, Boero IJ, Hwang L, et al. Aspiration pneumonia after concurrent chemoradiotherapy for head and neck cancer. *Cancer*. 2015;121(8):1303–1311.
5. Hunter KU, Lee OE, Lyden TH, et al. Aspiration pneumonia after chemo-intensity-modulated radiation therapy of oropharyngeal carcinoma and its clinical and dysphagia-related predictors. *Head Neck*. 2014;36(1):120–125.
6. Logemann JA. Introduction: definitions and basic principleswallowing disorders. In: Logemann JA. *Evaluation and Treatment of Swallowing Disorders*. 2nd ed. Austin, TX: Pro-Ed; 1998:13–52.
7. Kendall K. Anatomy and physiology of deglutition. In: Leonard R, Kendall K, eds. *Dysphagia Assessment and Treatment Planning: A Team Approach*. 2nd ed. Abingdon, Oxfordshire, UK: Plural Publishing; 2008.
8. Molfenter SM, Steele CM. Temporal variability in the deglutition literature. *Dysphagia*. 2012;27(2):162–177.
9. Wakabayashi H. Presbyphagia and sarcopenic dysphagia: association between aging, sarcopenia, and deglutition disorders. *J Frailty Aging*. 2014;3(2):97–103.
10. Ney DM, Weiss JM, Kind AJ, et al. Senescent swallowing: impact, strategies, and interventions. *Nutr Clin Prac*. 2009;24(3):395–413.
11. Wang CM, Chen JY, Chuang CC, et al. Aging-related changes in swallowing, and in the coordination of swallowing and respiration determined by novel non-invasive measurement techniques. *Geriatr Gerontol Int*. 2015;15(6):736–744.
12. Leslie P, Drinnan MJ, Ford GA, et al. Swallow respiratory patterns and aging: presbyphagia or dysphagia? *J Gernontol A Biol Sci Med Sci*. 2005;60(3):391–395.
13. Soderstrom K, Nilsson P, Laurell G, et al. Dysphagia—results from multivariable predictive modelling on aspiration from a subset of the ARTSCAN trial. *Radiother Oncol*. 2017;122(2):192–199.
14. MD Anderson Head Neck Cancer Symptom Working Group. Beyond mean pharyngeal constrictor dose for beam path toxicity in non-target swallowing muscles: Dose-volume correlates of chronic radiation-associated dysphagia (RAD) after oropharyngeal intensity modulated radiotherapy. *Radiother Oncol*. 2016;118(2):304–314.
15. Chiesa Estomba CM, Betances Reinoso FA, Lorenzo Lorenzo AI, et al. Functional outcomes of supraglottic squamous cell carcinoma treated by transoral laser microsurgery compared with horizontal supraglottic laryngectomy in patients younger and older than 65 years. *Acta Otorhinolaryngol Ital*. 2016;36(6):450–458.
16. Caudell JJ, Schaner PE, Meredith RF, et al. Factors associated with long-term dysphagia after definitive radiotherapy for locally advanced head-and-neck cancer. *Int J Radiat Oncol Biol Phys*. 2009;73(2):410–415.
17. Hutcheson KA, Barringer DA, Rosenthal DI, et al. Swallowing outcomes after radiotherapy for laryngeal carcinoma. *Arch Otolaryngol Head Neck Surg*. 2008;134(2):178–183.
18. Solares CA, Wood B, Rodriguez CP, et al. Does vocal cord fixation preclude nonsurgical management of laryngeal cancer? *Laryngoscope*. 2009;119(6):1130–1134.
19. Francis DO, Weymuller EA Jr, Parvathaneni U, et al. Dysphagia, stricture, and pneumonia in head and neck cancer patients: does treatment modality matter? *Ann Otol Rhinol Laryngol*. 2010;119(6):391–397.
20. Lewin JS. Functional analysis of swallowing outcomes after supracricoid partial laryngectomy. *Head Neck*. 2008;30(5):559–566.
21. Nguyen NP, Moltz CC, Frank C, et al. Effectiveness of the cough reflex in patients with aspiration following radiation for head and neck cancer. *Lung*. 2007;185(5):243–248.

22. Rutten H, Pop LA, Janssens GO, et al. Long-term outcome and morbidity after treatment with accelerated radiotherapy and weekly cisplatin for locally advanced head-and-neck cancer: results of a multidisciplinary late morbidity clinic. *Int J Radiat Oncol Biol Phys.* 2011;81:923–929.
23. Hutcheson KA, Lewin JS, Holsinger FC, et al. Long-term functional and survival outcomes after induction chemotherapy and risk-based definitive therapy for locally advanced squamous cell carcinoma of the head and neck. *Head Neck.* 2014;36(4):474–480.
24. Eisbruch A, Lyden T, Bradford CR, et al. Objective assessment of swallowing dysfunction and aspiration after radiation concurrent with chemotherapy for head-and-neck cancer. *Int J Radiat Oncol Biol Phys.* 2002;53(1):23–28.
25. Agarwal J, Palwe V, Dutta D, et al. Objective assessment of swallowing function after definitive concurrent (chemo)radiotherapy in patients with head and neck cancer. *Dysphagia.* 2011;26(4):399–406.
26. Borggreven PA, Verdonck-de Leeuw I, Rinkel RN, et al. Swallowing after major surgery of the oral cavity or oropharynx: a prospective and longitudinal assessment of patients treated by microvascular soft tissue reconstruction. *Head Neck.* 2007;29(7):638–647.
27. Goepfert RP, Lewin JS, Barrow MP, et al. Grading dysphagia as a toxicity of head and neck cancer: Differences in severity classification based on MBS DIGEST and clinical CTCAE grade. *Dysphagia.* 2017;Aug 23 [Epub ahead of print].
28. Szczesniak MM, Maclean J, Zhang T, et al. Persistent dysphagia after head and neck radiotherapy: a common and under-reported complication with significant effect on non-cancer-related mortality. *Clin Oncol (R Coll Radiol).* 2014;26(11):697–703.
29. Prisman E, Miles BA, Genden EM. Prevention and management of treatment-induced pharyngo-oesophageal stricture. *Lancet Oncol.* 2013;14(9):e380–e386.
30. Caglar HB. Dose to larynx predicts for swallowing complications after intensity-modulated radiotherapy. *Int J Radiat Oncol Biol Phys.* 2008;72(4):1110–1118.
31. Sweeny L, Golden JB, White HN, et al. Incidence and outcomes of stricture formation postlaryngectomy. *Otolaryngol Head Neck Surg.* 2012;146(3):395–402.
32. Wang JJ, Goldsmith TA, Holman AS, et al. Pharyngoesophageal stricture after treatment for head and neck cancer. *Head Neck.* 2012;34(7):967–973.
33. List MA, Ritter-Sterr C, Lansky SB. A performance status scale for head and neck cancer patients. *Cancer.* 1990;66(3):564–569.
34. Crary MA, Mann GD, Groher ME. Initial psychometric assessment of a functional oral intake scale for dysphagia in stroke patients. *Arch Phys Med Rehabil.* 2005;86(8):1516–1520.
35. Common Terminology Criteria for Adverse Events (CTCAE). v4.03 ed. Bethesda, MD: National Institutes of Health, National Cancer Institute, Department of Health and Human Services; 2010.
36. Belafsky PC, Mouadeb DA, Rees CJ, et al. Validity and reliability of the Eating Assessment Tool (EAT-10). *Ann Otol Rhinol Laryngol.* 2008;117(12):919–924.
37. Chen AY, Frankowski R, Bishop-Leone J, et al. The development and validation of a dysphagia-specific quality-of-life questionnaire for patients with head and neck cancer: the M. D. Anderson dysphagia inventory. *Arch Otolaryngol Head Neck Surg.* 2001;127(7):870–876.
38. Dwivedi RC, St Rose S, Chisholm EJ, et al. Evaluation of swallowing by Sydney Swallow Questionnaire (SSQ) in oral and oropharyngeal cancer patients treated with primary surgery. *Dysphagia.* 2012;27(4):491–497.
39. Rosenthal DI, Mendoza TR, Chambers MS, et al. Measuring head and neck cancer symptom burden: the development and validation of the M. D. Anderson symptom inventory, head and neck module. *Head Neck.* 2007;29(10):923–931.
40. Murphy BA, Dietrich MS, Wells N, et al. Reliability and validity of the Vanderbilt Head and Neck Symptom Survey: a tool to assess symptom burden in patients treated with chemoradiation. *Head Neck.* 2010;32(1):26–37.
41. Quon H, Hui X, Cheng Z, et al. Complementary role of Sydney Swallow Questionnaire (SSQ) and MD Anderson Dysphagia Inventory (MDADI) in developing a comprehensive multidimensional patient-reported outcome (PRO) evaluation of head and neck cancer (HNC) treatment-related outcomes. *Int J Radiat Oncol Biol Phys.* 2016;96(2 supplement):E537–E538.
42. Logemann JA. Instrumental techniques for the study of swallowing. In: Logemann JA. *Evaluation and Treatment of Swallowing Disorders.* 2nd ed. Austin, TX: Pro-Ed; 1998:53–70.
43. Suiter DM, Leder SB. Clinical utility of the 3-ounce water swallow test. *Dysphagia.* 2008;23(3):244–250.
44. Martino R, Silver F, Teasell R, et al. The Toronto Bedside Swallowing Screening Test (TOR-BSST): development and validation of a dysphagia screening tool for patients with stroke. *Stroke.* 2009;40(2):555–561.
45. Patterson JM, McColl E, Carding PN, et al. Swallowing performance in patients with head and neck cancer: a simple clinical test. *Oral Oncol.* 2009;45(10):904–907.
46. Mann G. *MASA: The Mann Assessment of Swallowing Ability.* Clifton Park, NY: Singular; 2002.
47. Carnaby GD, Crary MA. Development and validation of a cancer-specific swallowing assessment tool: MASA-C. *Support Care Cancer.* 2014;22(3):595–602.
48. Wheeler Hegland K, Troche MS, Brandimore AE, et al. Comparison of voluntary and reflex cough effectiveness in Parkinson's disease. *Parkinsonism Relat Disord.* 2014;20(11):1226–1230.
49. Kallesen M, Psirides A, Huckabee ML. Comparison of cough reflex testing with videoendoscopy in recently extubated intensive care unit patients. *J Crit Care.* 2016;33:90–94.
50. Miles A, Moore S, McFarlane M, et al. Comparison of cough reflex test against instrumental assessment of aspiration. *Physiol Behav.* 2013;118:25–31.
51. Shellikeri S, Yunusova Y, Green JR, et al. Electrical impedance myography in the evaluation of the tongue musculature in amyotrophic lateral sclerosis. *Muscle Nerve.* 2015;52(4):584–591.

52. Crary MA, Sura L, Carnaby G. Validation and demonstration of an isolated acoustic recording technique to estimate spontaneous swallow frequency. *Dysphagia*. 2013;28(1):86–94.
53. Yoshida M, Kikutani T, Tsuga K, et al. Decreased tongue pressure reflects symptom of dysphagia. *Dysphagia*. 2006;21(1):61–65.
54. Butler SG, Stuart A, Leng XY, et al. The relationship of aspiration status with tongue and handgrip strength in healthy older adults. *J Gerontol Ser A Biol Sci Med Sci*. 2011;66(4):452–458.
55. Martin-Harris B, Brodsky MB, Michel Y, et al. MBS measurement tool for swallow impairment-MBSImp: establishing a standard. *Dysphagia*. 2008;23(4):392–405.
56. Bonilha HS, Humphries K, Blair J, et al. Radiation exposure time during MBSS: influence of swallowing impairment severity, medical diagnosis, clinician experience, and standardized protocol use. *Dysphagia*. 2013;28(1):77–85.
57. Stoeckli SJ, Huisman TA, Seifert B, et al. Interrater reliability of videofluoroscopic swallow evaluation. *Dysphagia*. 2003;18(1):53–57.
58. Stokely SL, Molfenter SM, Steele CM. Effects of barium concentration on oropharyngeal swallow timing measures. *Dysphagia*. 2014;29(1):78–82.
59. Logemann J. *Manual for the Videofluoroscopic Study of Swallowing*. London: Taylor & Francis; 1986.
60. Lefton-Greif M, Carson K, Pinto J, et al. A novel tool for standardization of videofluoroscopic swallowing assessment in bottle-fed children. Presented at the 24th Annual Dysphagia Research Society Meeting; 2016; Tucson, AZ.
61. The International Commission on Radiological Protection. Implications of commission recommendations that doses be kept as low as readily achievable. ICRP publication 22; 1973.
62. Rosenbek JC, Robbins JA, Roecker EB, et al. A penetration-aspiration scale. *Dysphagia*. 1996;11(2):93–98.
63. Hutcheson K, Barringer D, Knott J, et al. Dynamic Imaging Grade of Swallowing Toxicity (DIGEST): scale development and validation. Presented at the 24th Annual Dysphagia Research Society Meeting; 2016; Tucson, AZ.
64. Rademaker AW, Pauloski BR, Logemann JA, et al. Oropharyngeal swallow efficiency as a representative measure of swallowing function. *J Speech Hear Res*. 1994;37(2):314–325.
65. Kellen PM, Becker DL, Reinhardt JM, et al. Computer-assisted assessment of hyoid bone motion from videofluoroscopic swallow studies. *Dysphagia*. 2010;25(4):298–306.
66. Molfenter SM, Steele CM. Use of an anatomical scalar to control for sex-based size differences in measures of hyoid excursion during swallowing. *J Speech Hear Res*. 2014;57(3):768–778.
67. Thompson TZ, Obeidin F, Davidoff AA, et al. Coordinate mapping of hyolaryngeal mechanics in swallowing. *J Vis Exp*. 2014;87:51476.
68. Leonard R, Belafsky PC, Rees CJ. Relationship between fluoroscopic and manometric measures of pharyngeal constriction: the pharyngeal constriction ratio. *Ann Otol Rhinol Laryngol*. 2006;115(12):897–901.
69. Langmore SE, Schatz K, Olson N. Endoscopic and videofluoroscopic evaluations of swallowing and aspiration. *Ann Otol Rhinol Laryngol*. 1991;100(8):678–681.
70. Kidder TM, Langmore SE, Martin BJ. Indications and techniques of endoscopy in evaluation of cervical dysphagia: comparison with radiographic techniques. *Dysphagia*. 1994;9(4):256–261.
71. Leder SB. Serial fiberoptic endoscopic swallowing evaluations in the management of patients with dysphagia. *Arch Phys Med Rehabil*. 1998;79(10):1264–1269.
72. Leder SB, Sasaki CT, Burrell MI. Fiberoptic endoscopic evaluation of dysphagia to identify silent aspiration. *Dysphagia*. 1998;13(1):19–21.
73. Manor Y, Mootanah R, Freud D, et al. Video-assisted swallowing therapy for patients with Parkinson's disease. *Parkinsonism Relat Disord*. 2013;19(2):207–211.
74. Bastian RW. The videoendoscopic swallowing study: an alternative and partner to the videofluoroscopic swallowing study. *Dysphagia*. 1993;8(4):359–367.
75. Hoppers P, Holm SE. The role of fiberoptic endoscopy in dysphagia rehabilitation. *J Head Trauma Rehabil*. 1999;14(5):475–485.
76. Denk DM, Kaider A. Videoendoscopic biofeedback: a simple method to improve the efficacy of swallowing rehabilitation of patients after head and neck surgery. *ORL J Otorhinolarngol Relat Spec*. 1997;59(2):100–105.
77. Kelly AM, Drinnan MJ, Leslie P. Assessing penetration and aspiration: how do videofluoroscopy and fiberoptic endoscopic evaluation of swallowing compare? *Laryngoscope*. 2007;117(10):1723–1727.
78. da Silva AP, Lubianca Neto JF, et al. Comparison between videofluoroscopy and endoscopic evaluation of swallowing for the diagnosis of dysphagia in children. *Otolaryngol Head Neck Surg*. 2010;143(2):204–209.
79. Wu CH, Hsiao TY, Chen JC, et al. Evaluation of swallowing safety with fiberoptic endoscope: comparison with videofluoroscopic technique. *Laryngoscope*. 1997;107(3):396–401.
80. Kelly AM, Leslie P, Beale T, et al. Fibreoptic endoscopic evaluation of swallowing and videofluoroscopy: does examination type influence perception of pharyngeal residue severity? *Clin Otolaryngol*. 2006;31(5):425–432.
81. Fox MR, Bredenoord AJ. Oesophageal high-resolution manometry: moving from research into clinical practice. *Gut*. 2008;57(3):405–423.
82. Lee TH, Lee JS, Hong SJ, et al. Impedance analysis using high-resolution impedance manometry facilitates assessment of pharyngeal residue in patients with oropharyngeal dysphagia. *J Neurogastroenterol Motil*. 2014;20(3):362–370.
83. Lee TH, Lee JS, Park JW, et al. High-resolution impedance manometry facilitates assessment of pharyngeal residue and oropharyngeal dysphagic mechanisms. *Dis Esophagus*. 2014;27(3):220–229.

84. Omari T, Kritas S, Cock C. New insights into pharyngo-esophageal bolus transport revealed by pressure-impedance measurement. *Neurogastroenterol Motil.* 2012;24(11):e549–e556.
85. Omari TI, Dejaeger E, Tack J, et al. An impedance-manometry based method for non-radiological detection of pharyngeal postswallow residue. *Neurogastroenterol Motil.* 2012;24(7):e277–e284.
86. Omari TI, Dejaeger E, Van Beckevoort D, et al. A novel method for the nonradiological assessment of ineffective swallowing. *Am J Gastroenterol.* 2011;106(10):1796–1802.
87. Omari TI, Ferris L, Dejaeger E, et al. Upper esophageal sphincter impedance as a marker of sphincter opening diameter. *Am J Physiol Gastrointest Liver Physiol.* 2012;302(9):G909–G913.
88. Omari TI, Jones CA, Hammer MJ, et al. Predicting the activation states of the muscles governing upper esophageal sphincter relaxation and opening. *Am J Physiol Gastrointest Liver Physiol.* 2016;310(6):G359–G366.
89. Omari TI, Rommel N, Szczesniak MM, et al. Assessment of intraluminal impedance for the detection of pharyngeal bolus flow during swallowing in healthy adults. *Am J Physiol Gastrointest Liver Physiol.* 2006;290(1):G183–G188.
90. Szczesniak MM, Rommel N, Dinning PG, et al. Intraluminal impedance detects failure of pharyngeal bolus clearance during swallowing: a validation study in adults with dysphagia. *Neurogastroenterol Motil.* 2009;21(3):244–252.
91. Szczesniak MM, Rommel N, Dinning PG, et al. Optimal criteria for detecting bolus passage across the pharyngo-oesophageal segment during the normal swallow using intraluminal impedance recording. *Neurogastroenteral Motil.* 2008;20(5):440–447.
92. Fox MR, Pandolfino JE, Sweis R, et al. Inter-observer agreement for diagnostic classification of esophageal motility disorders defined in high-resolution manometry. *Dis Esophagus.* 2015;28(8):711–719.
93. Hoffman MR, Jones CA, Geng Z, et al. Classification of high-resolution manometry data according to videofluoroscopic parameters using pattern recognition. *Otolaryngol Head Neck Surg.* 2013;149(1):126–133.
94. Jones CA, Hoffman MR, Geng Z, et al. Reliability of an automated high-resolution manometry analysis program across expert users, novice users, and speech-language pathologists. *J Speech Lang Hear Res.* 2014;57(3):831–836.
95. Knigge MA, Thibeault S, McCulloch TM. Implementation of high-resolution manometry in the clinical practice of speech language pathology. *Dysphagia.* 2014;29(1):2–16.
96. Mielens JD, Hoffman MR, Ciucci MR, et al. Automated analysis of pharyngeal pressure data obtained with high-resolution manometry. *Dysphagia.* 2011;26(1):3–12.
97. Mielens JD, Hoffman MR, Ciucci MR, et al. Application of classification models to pharyngeal high-resolution manometry. *J Speech Lang Hear Res.* 2012;55(3):892–902.
98. Omari TI, Papathanasopoulos A, Dejaeger E, et al. Reproducibility and agreement of pharyngeal automated impedance manometry with videofluoroscopy. *Clin Gastroenterol Hepatol.* 2011;9(10):862–867.
99. Hutcheson KA, Hammer MJ, Rosen SP, et al. Expiratory muscle strength training evaluated with simultaneous high resolution manometry and electromyography. *Laryngoscope.* 2017;127(4):797–804.
100. Starmer HM, Yang W, Raval R, et al. Effect of gabapentin on swallowing during and after chemoradiation for oropharyngeal squamous cell cancer. *Dysphagia.* 2014;29(3):396–402.
101. Burkhead LM, Sapienza CM, Rosenbek JC. Strength-training exercise in dysphagia rehabilitation: principles, procedures, and directions for future research. *Dysphagia.* 2007;22(3):251–265.
102. Athukorala RP, Jones RD, Sella O, et al. Skill training for swallowing rehabilitation in patients with Parkinson's disease. *Arch Phys Med Rehabil.* 2014;95(7):1374–1382.
103. Martin-Harris B, McFarland D, Hill EG, et al. Respiratory-swallow training in patients with head and neck cancer. *Arch Phys Med Rehabil.* 2015;96(5):885–893.
104. Kasper CE, Talbot LA, Gaines JM. Skeletal muscle damage and recovery. *AACN Clin Issues.* 2002;13(2):237–247.
105. Clark BC. In vivo alterations in skeletal muscle form and function after disuse atrophy. *Med Sci Sports Exerc.* 2009;41(10):1869–1875.
106. Carnaby-Mann G, Crary MA, Schmalfuss I, et al. "Pharyngocise": randomized controlled trial of preventative exercises to maintain muscle structure and swallowing function during head-and-neck chemoradiotherapy. *Int J Radiat Oncol Biol Phys.* 2012;83(1):210–219.
107. Starmer H, Gourin C, Lua LL, et al. Pretreatment swallowing assessment in head and neck cancer patients. *Laryngoscope.* 2011;121(6):1208–1211.
108. Starmer HM, Gourin CG. Is speech language pathologist evaluation necessary in the nonoperative treatment of head and neck cancer? *Laryngoscope.* 2013;123(7):1571–1572.
109. Setton J, Lee NY, Riaz N, et al. A multi-institution pooled analysis of gastrostomy tube dependence in patients with oropharyngeal cancer treated with definitive intensity-modulated radiotherapy. *Cancer.* 2015;121(2):294–301.
110. Bhayani MK, Hutcheson KA, Barringer DA, et al. Gastrostomy tube placement in patients with oropharyngeal carcinoma treated with radiotherapy or chemoradiotherapy: factors affecting placement and dependence. *Head Neck.* 2013;35(11):1634–1640.
111. Hutcheson KA, Bhayani MK, Beadle BM, et al. Eat and exercise during radiotherapy or chemoradiotherapy for pharyngeal cancers: use it or lose it. *JAMA Otolaryngol Head Neck Surg.* 2013;139(11):1127–1134.
112. Krisciunas GP, Golan H, Marinko LN, et al. A novel manual therapy program during radiation therapy for head and neck cancer—our clinical experience with 5 patients. *Clin Otolaryngol.* 2015;41(4):425–431.

113. Kotz T, Federman AD, Kao J, et al. Prophylactic swallowing exercises in patients with head and neck cancer undergoing chemoradiation: a randomized trial. *Arch Otolaryngol Head Neck Surg.* 2012;138(4):376–382.
114. Retel VP, van der Molen L, Hilgers FJ, et al. A cost-effectiveness analysis of a preventive exercise program for patients with advanced head and neck cancer treated with concomitant chemo-radiotherapy. *BMC Cancer.* 2011;11:475.
115. van der Molen L, van Rossum MA, Burkhead LM, et al. A randomized preventive rehabilitation trial in advanced head and neck cancer patients treated with chemoradiotherapy: feasibility, compliance, and short-term effects. *Dysphagia.* 2011;26(2):155–170.
116. Shinn EH, Basen-Engquist K, Baum G, et al. Adherence to preventive exercises and self-reported swallowing outcomes in post-radiation head and neck cancer patients. *Head Neck.* 2013;35(12):1707–1712.
117. Kulbersh BD, Rosenthal EL, McGrew BM, et al. Pretreatment, preoperative swallowing exercises may improve dysphagia quality of life. *Laryngoscope.* 2006;116(6):883–886.
118. Carroll WR, Locher JL, Canon CL, et al. Pretreatment swallowing exercises improve swallow function after chemoradiation. *Laryngoscope.* 2008;118(1):39–43.
119. Perry A, Lee SH, Cotton S, et al. Therapeutic exercises for affecting post-treatment swallowing in people treated for advanced-stage head and neck cancers. *Cochrane Database Syst Rev.* 2016;8:CD011112.
120. Gillespie MB, Brodsky MB, Day TA, et al. Swallowing-related quality of life after head and neck cancer treatment. *Laryngoscope.* 2004;114(8):1362–1367.
121. Hutcheson KA, Holsinger FC, Kupferman ME, et al. Functional outcomes after TORS for oropharyngeal cancer: a systematic review. *Eur Arch Otorhinolaryngol.* 2015;272(2):463–471.
122. Hutcheson KA. Does adjuvant neck dissection increase risk of chronic dysphagia after oropharyngeal IMRT? Presented at the 5th World Congress of the International Federation of Head and Neck Oncologic Societies (IFHNOS) and the Head and Neck Society (AHNS) Annual Meeting; 7/30/2014; New York, NY.
123. Crary MA, Carnaby Mann GD, et al. Functional benefits of dysphagia therapy using adjunctive sEMG biofeedback. *Dysphagia.* 2004;19(3):160–164.
124. Juan J, Hind J, Jones C, McCulloch T, et al. Case study: application of isometric progressive resistance oropharyngeal therapy using the Madison Oral Strengthening Therapeutic device. *Top Stroke Rehabil.* 2013;20(5):450–470.
125. Robbins J, Gangnon RE, Theis SM, et al. The effects of lingual exercise on swallowing in older adults. *J Am Geriatr Soc.* 2005;53(9):1483–1489.
126. Robbins J, Kays SA, Gangnon RE, et al. The effects of lingual exercise in stroke patients with dysphagia. *Arch Phys Med Rehabil.* 2007;88(2):150–158.
127. Wheeler-Hegland KM, Rosenbek JC, Sapienza CM. Submental sEMG and hyoid movement during Mendelsohn maneuver, effortful swallow, and expiratory muscle strength training. *J Speech Lang Hear Res.* 2008;51(5):1072–1087.
128. Cauraugh J, Light K, Kim S, et al. Chronic motor dysfunction after stroke: recovering wrist and finger extension by electromyography-triggered neuromuscular stimulation. *Stroke.* 2000;31(6):1360–1364.
129. Kimberley TJ, Lewis SM, Auerbach EJ, et al. Electrical stimulation driving functional improvements and cortical changes in subjects with stroke. *Exp Brain Res.* 2004;154(4):450–460.
130. Humbert IA, Poletto CJ, Saxon KG, et al. The effect of surface electrical stimulation on hyolaryngeal movement in normal individuals at rest and during swallowing. *J Appl Physiol.* 2006;101(6):1657–1663.
131. Langmore SE, McCulloch TM, Krisciunas GP, et al. Efficacy of electrical stimulation and exercise for dysphagia in patients with head and neck cancer: a randomized clinical trial. *Head Neck.* 2016;38(Suppl 1):E1221–E1231.
132. Carnaby-Mann GD, Crary MA. McNeill dysphagia therapy program: a case-control study. *Arch Phys Med Rehabil.* 2010;91(5):743–749.
133. Crary MA, Carnaby GD, LaGorio LA, et al. Functional and physiological outcomes from an exercise-based dysphagia therapy: a pilot investigation of the McNeill Dysphagia Therapy Program. *Arch Phys Med Rehabil.* 2012;93(7):1173–1178.
134. Machtay M, Moughan J, Trotti A, et al. Factors associated with severe late toxicity after concurrent chemoradiation for locally advanced head and neck cancer: an RTOG analysis. *J Clin Oncol.* 2008;26(21):3582–3589.
135. Hutcheson KA, Lewin JS, Barringer DA, et al. Late dysphagia after radiotherapy-based treatment of head and neck cancer. *Cancer.* 2012;118(23):5793–5799.
136. Hutcheson KA, Yuk M, Hubbard R, et al. Delayed lower cranial neuropathy after oropharyngeal intensity-modulated radiotherapy: a cohort analysis and literature review. *Head Neck.* 2017;39(8):1516–1523.
137. Hutcheson KA, Barrow MP, Plowman EK, et al. Expiratory muscle strength training for radiation-associated aspiration after head and neck cancer: a case-series. *Laryngoscope.* 2017. PMID: 28833185.

26

Quality of Life Assessment and Patient-Reported Outcomes in Head and Neck Cancer

Minh Tam Truong

Lisa Ann Kachnic

The treatment of head and neck cancer (HNC) involves a complex multidisciplinary approach wherein survival, function, and quality of life (QOL) should be balanced to determine the optimal management for each individual patient. The World Health Organization (WHO) in 1948 originally declared health to be "a state of complete physical, mental and social well-being, and not merely the absence of disease and infirmity" (1). WHO defines QOL as "individuals' perception of their position in life in the context of culture and value systems in which they live, and in relation to their goals, expectations, standards, and concerns" (2). As such, it is important to recognize that the treatment of HNC may impact many vital patient functions including voice/speech, hearing/balance, taste/eating/swallowing, and cosmesis, all of which may have a significant impact on a patient's QOL and survivorship.

Health-related quality of life (HRQOL) is a complex multidimensional concept which describes the patient's perception of the effects of disease and treatment, and its impact on the individual's physical functioning, psychological and social well-being, his or her personal beliefs, level of independence, and his or her relationship to the environment. Evaluating QOL involves measuring multiple domains, which include cognitive, social, emotional, and psychological well-being, as well as physical and role functioning. For the purpose of this chapter, QOL will refer to HRQOL.

QOL is ideally measured using patient-reported outcome (PRO) instruments, which use the patient's self-report of the effects of disease and treatment on his or her health and well-being, without the interference of another person's opinion. Many PRO instruments have been developed over the past few decades, which have been designed to measure changes in a patient's report of health through signs, symptoms, function, or complex multidimensional concepts. This is in contrast to toxicity, which refers to signs or symptoms related to treatment and is a subset of morbidity, which may be related to treatment or disease effect (3). Toxicity and adverse event reporting have traditionally been used as a clinician-graded measure, although there is now increasing interest to develop and use patient-reported toxicity scales.

Early-stage HNC is often treated by a single modality treatment such as surgery or radiation therapy alone, while locally advanced HNC requires combined modality therapy using either primary surgery followed by adjuvant radiation with/without chemotherapy based on pathological risk factors, or by primary chemoradiotherapy (CRT). The optimal sequencing of therapy requires a team-based approach incorporating evidence-based medicine and taking into account patient factors, decision preferences of the patient and family, and consideration of acute and long-term functional outcome and QOL (4,5).

Treatment for HNC is associated with significant acute and late toxicity potentially impacting many critical functions in the head and neck region. Surgery may be associated with acute and long-term sequelae relating to voice/speech, eating/swallowing, cosmesis, and neck/shoulder function. Radiation therapy is associated with a constellation of acute and late toxicities, including xerostomia, mucositis, dysphagia, hearing and taste impairment, and neck fibrosis, all of which may be enhanced by concurrent chemotherapy or biologic therapy administration. The effect of such treatment on QOL from the patient's perspective using PROs has emerged as an important end point in clinical investigations over the past two decades, and PROs have been extensively used on many randomized controlled clinical trials. Yet, clinical trials have primarily focused on survival as the primary end point, while QOL has usually been studied as a secondary end point, along with clinician-graded toxicity. Although physician-reported toxicity may detect and grade adverse clinical events, it fails to provide the patient's perspective on how a treatment affects the patient. Hence, PROs have become of increasing interest as we focus more on a personalized approach to medicine. Furthermore, as there are multiple treatment options with contrasting toxicity profiles, PRO data may be invaluable in guiding optimal individualized treatment decisions.

Therefore, the focus of this chapter is to examine the importance of QOL and PROs in HNC. We describe the commonly used instruments, discuss how PROs are incorporated into HNC trial design, present relevant data from recent studies, and emphasize how PROs guide clinical practice and inform HNC patient survivorship.

WHY MEASURE QUALITY OF LIFE AND PATIENT-REPORTED OUTCOMES IN HNC?

Clinical trials for locally advanced HNC over the past two decades have focused on treatment intensification by various combinations of surgery, radiation, chemotherapy, and biologic therapies. Meta-analyses have demonstrated survival gains using primary CRT over radiation alone (6). However, further treatment intensification efforts have failed to improve survival, yet have shown substantial increases in toxicity (7–9). These clinical trials included primary survival end points combined with important secondary functional outcomes and QOL.

PROs and QOL data may inform patients and providers to select the optimal treatment when there are multiple different management options available. PROs may also provide an improved insight and understanding of the patient's expectation and experience of cancer treatment and, as such, may be used as a primary end point in clinical trials to select the best treatment when survival outcomes are expected to be equivalent. Yet, despite the important information that PROs provide, there are many challenges in routinely incorporating these instruments into clinical practice and trials. Significant barriers include cost, infrastructure requirements, increasing time required to administer the test, patient burden, compliance, and handling of missing data. There are also inherent potential biases in how the patient answers the questionnaires, including responders bias, adaptation bias, and patient's change of internal frame of reference (10,11).

Increasingly, in the era of electronic health records (EHRs), PROs are also being incorporated into routine clinical practice as part of the EHR for initial screening, monitoring of treatment, evaluating patient-focused care, facilitating communication between multidisciplinary teams, and evaluating the quality of care (12). It is recognized that the patient's perspective using PROs is important in evaluating disease and treatment outcome, and provides an important perspective in conjunction with objective measures and clinician-graded evaluation. In the management of HNC, symptoms from the cancer and its treatments may cause significant patient distress. For example, CRT may cause acute nausea, alterations in taste and smell, mucositis leading to significant oral pain, odynophagia, and malnutrition. In the long term, consequential late sequelae, such as xerostomia and dysphagia, may have functional consequences for dental health, normalcy of diet and nutrition, and ability to socialize and eat in public (13,14).

It is important to recognize that symptoms from cancer therapy are often found in clusters, and measuring a symptom in isolation may not provide the full picture of the burden of treatment or disease on the patient. Studies have shown that CRT for patients with HNC have been found to be associated with two stable symptom clusters: head and neck–specific symptoms (radiodermatitis, dysphagia, radiomucositis, dry mouth, pain, taste disturbance, and fatigue), and a second cluster including gastrointestinal side effects (nausea, vomiting, and dehydration) (15). These symptoms can cause both acute and long-term deterioration of QOL in HNC survivors. How these symptom clusters impact the patient may be referred to as "symptom burden." Symptom burden measures the symptom severity and the patient's perception of the impact of the symptoms reported (16). Patient-reported symptom burden is a subset of QOL that may be incorporated into clinical trials to evaluate new treatments without measuring other QOL domains, and has been shown to provide additive, and sometimes discrepant, information from the toxicity that has been reported by the physician.

The United States, National Cancer Institute's Common Terminology Criteria for Adverse Events (NCI-CTCAE) reporting system is routinely used by physicians and on clinical trials to measure toxicity or adverse medical events. There are other toxicity scoring systems such as the National Cancer Institute of Canada–Common Toxicity Criteria (NCIC-CTC), Radiation Therapy Oncology Group (RTOG) Grading System, the Late Effects Normal Tissue/Subjective, Objective, Management, and Analytic (LENT–SOMA) (17), and the Danish Head and Neck Cancer Study Group (DAHANCA) toxicity scoring system. These scoring systems are effective in objective assessments of toxicity, but have varying sensitivity for subjective patient end points. The DAHANCA observer-based toxicity scoring system was noted to have low sensitivity to subjective end points (18). A patient-reported version of the LENT–SOMA was compared to the validated QOL instrument—the European Organisation for Research and Treatment of Cancer Core Questionnaire (EORTC QLQ-C30 version 3) and their 35-item head-and-neck module (H&N35) evaluating pain, swallowing, dental pain, dry mouth, opening mouth, and analgesic requirements; good concordance was noted between the PRO-LENT–SOMA and EORTC QLQ-H&N35, except for analgesic end points (19). The PRO-LENT–SOMA was noted, however, to be reliable in detecting patient-reported late effects of radiation therapy. In a retrospective pooled analysis of 2,279 cancer patients from 14 EORTC randomized controlled trials, six cancer symptoms (pain, fatigue, vomiting, nausea, diarrhea, and constipation) were analyzed to evaluate the extent of agreement between the clinician and patient symptom scoring (20). In this study, patient-reported fatigue differed from clinician-reported scores. For the six cancer symptoms evaluated at baseline, the clinician and patient scores both contributed independently and positively to the predictive accuracy of outcomes. For the prediction of overall survival, both patient and clinician scores had greater predictive accuracy than models that considered clinician scores alone for fatigue, vomiting, nausea, and constipation, hence highlighting the importance of measuring PROs, in addition to clinician scoring, in predicting outcomes.

Given this discrepancy between physician and patient reporting of toxicity, patient-reported toxicity scoring systems are being developed. The PRO version of the CTCAE (PRO-CTCAE) has been validated and tested for reliability and responsiveness in 975 patients with cancer undergoing chemotherapy and/or radiation therapy (21). In the HNC population, a study evaluating CRT compared the NCI-CTCAE to the PRO-CTCAE, and found a high concordance between patient-reported and practitioner-reported symptom severity at baseline, when symptoms were absent, but as toxicity increased during therapy, it was noted that clinician-reported toxicity was significantly lower than patient-reported toxicity. Symptoms such as fatigue and anxiety were not well documented by clinician-graded objective measures (22). As the patient-reported scoring system is quite new and is being evaluated in ongoing prospective HNC trials, our validated instruments for measuring QOL and PROs in HNC continue to be of paramount importance.

DEVELOPMENT AND SCORING METHODS OF QOL INSTRUMENTS

Measuring QOL requires the development and validation of questionnaires used for assessing QOL in the population of interest. Statistical and psychometric techniques are used to confirm that the test is valid and performs in a manner that is expected. The research question and hypothesis must be clearly defined, and then the appropriate QOL tool which will best answer the research question both qualitatively and quantitatively in the target population should be selected. The objective of using a QOL instrument is to alert the clinician to symptoms or side effects from the patient's perspective, and its effect on QOL (23). Finally, a QOL instrument is dependent on the language spoken by the patients and the cultural context of their environment. Many QOL instruments have been translated and then validated in different patient populations to determine if the instrument is linguistically and culturally relevant to the population studied.

When an instrument is developed, it is tested for reliability, validity, responsiveness, interpretability, and patient burden. Reliability refers to the degree in which an instrument is reproducible, stable, and is free from measurement error. Internal consistency reliability is the degree to which the items in a multi-item instrument are interrelated. Test-retest reliability is the ability for the instrument to be reproducible and provide consistency of scores over time in a stable population. Validity is the degree to which an instrument measures the concept it is aiming to measure. Content validity is the extent to which the instrument contains the most relevant and important aspects of a dimension of interest. Construct validity is the extent to which an instrument measures the concept that it is designed to measure in relation to other measures. Criterion validity refers to the degree to which scores of an instrument relate to a "gold standard." Responsiveness is the ability of an instrument to detect a clinically significant important change (a change that is meaningful to the patient). Sensitivity is the ability of an instrument to detect between group differences. Responsiveness and sensitivity may be assessed by effect size statistics, using ratios of mean changes of differences in standard deviations. Interpretability refers to how understandable the QOL scores are (23).

To help interpret the scores, the QOL instruments aim to detect a minimum important difference (MID), which is defined as the smallest difference in score that a patient perceives as important, that may lead to a change in the patient's management (24). There are different statistical methods to measure the MID, including patient rating of change, anchor-based (where groups are anchored to performance status or another QOL instrument), or distribution-based (using 33% to 50% of the standard deviation, or one standard error of measurement, or effect size). The MID may vary by the population studied. The clinically meaningful MID of a QOL instrument is often estimated as being at least 5% to 10% of the instrument range. Ringash et al. demonstrated, using the Functional Assessment of Cancer Therapy-Head and Neck Cancer instrument (FACT-H&N), a minimum 4.3% (range, 4%–6%) increase in score for a positive MID, and a 8.6% (range, 6%–14%) decrease in score for a negative MID, in patients with laryngeal cancer (25,26). Similarly, Cella et al. found that clinical meaningful group score changes in global QOL are often small for QOL improvements from baseline, whereas worsening global QOL is often associated with much larger negative score changes (27). Patient factors that may influence these changes in score include adaptation to disease, responder shift, and responder bias. Hutcheson et al. evaluated the MD Anderson Dysphagia Inventory (MDADI) questionnaire (scored out of 100) for swallowing-related QOL in 1,136 patients with HNC. Using anchor-based methods, a 10-point difference between groups in composite MDADI scores was identified as clinically meaningful (28). As such, when comparing different treatments, if survival or disease control end points are thought to be equivalent, then appropriately powered QOL or PRO designed end points, using the MID between treatment groups, may be used to determine which treatment is superior.

One of the caveats of QOL research is how to handle missing data. There are many causes of missing data, including incomplete or incorrect data collection, missing forms, patient fatigue due to burden of the number of questions or number of instruments, patients being too sick to complete forms, and QOL being considered as an optional component of a clinical study. In addition, QOL data are time sensitive, and collection of QOL outside the study window also contributes to missing data. Unlike survival data, QOL data cannot be obtained retrospectively. Missing data negatively impact the statistical analysis of QOL assessments, and potentially introduce bias into the study sample. Statistical methods to handle missing data also make certain assumptions; missing data may be assumed to be missing completely at random or not missing at random. Several statistical methods may be used to impute such missing data (23).

COMMON QOL INSTRUMENTS USED IN HNC

Common validated QOL and PRO instruments used in HNC (although not an exhaustive list) include the EORTC QLQ-C30 version 3.0 and its 35-item Head-and-Neck module (EORTC QLQ-H&N35) (29); the Functional Assessment of Cancer Therapy General Questionnaire (FACT-G) and its 12-item Head and Neck specific scale (FACT-H&N) (30,31); the University of Washington 15-item QOL Questionnaire (UW-QOL) (32); the MD Anderson Symptom Inventory (MDASI) and its nine-item Head and Neck Cancer module (MDASI-HN) (33,34); the new 22-item National Comprehensive Cancer Network–Functional Assessment of Cancer Therapy–Head and Neck Cancer Symptom Index (NFHNSI-22) (35); the 22-item Head and Neck Radiotherapy Questionnaire (HNRQ) (36); and the five-item EuroQol (EQ-5D) (37), a health utility instrument. The various instruments are reviewed in Table 26.1.

The EORTC QLQ-C30/H&N35 consists of a 30-item self-reporting questionnaire developed to assess overall QOL of patients with cancer, and a 35-item HNC-specific module (38). Version 3 is the most recent version. The QLQ-30 is grouped into five functional subscales (role, physical, cognitive, emotional, and social functioning), three multi-item symptom

TABLE 26.1

Frequently Used PRO Instruments for HNC

Instrument	General QOL Items	HNC Specific Items	Indication	Time to Complete (Minutes)
EORTC QLQ-C30/H&N35 (29)	30	35	QOL from surgery, radiation, and chemotherapy	15–20
FACT-H&N (30,31)	27 FACT-G	12	QOL from surgery, radiation, and chemotherapy	5–10
UW-QOL (32)	3	12	QOL and symptom burden from surgery and radiation	5–10
MDASI-HN (33,34)	19	9	Symptom burden from surgery, radiation, and chemotherapy	5–10
NFHNSI-22 (35)	3	19	Symptom burden and QOL from surgery, radiation, and chemotherapy; tailored for advanced disease	5–10
HNRQ (36)	3	22	Acute symptom burden and QOL from radiotherapy in patients with locally advanced HNC	5–10
EQ-5D™ (37)	5 + VAS	0	Health utilities; quality adjusted survival	1–5

EORTC QLQ-C30/H&N35, the European Organisation for Research and Treatment of Cancer Core Questionnaire (EORTC QLQ-C30 version 3.0) and the 35-item head-and-neck module (H&N35); EQ-5D™, the 5-item heath utilities instrument of the EuroQol Group; FACT-G, the Functional Assessment of Cancer Therapy–General instrument; FACT-H&N, the Functional Assessment of Cancer Therapy–Head and Neck Cancer instrument; HNC, Head and Neck Cancer; HNRQ, Head and Neck Radiotherapy Questionnaire; MDASI-HN, the MD Anderson Symptom Inventory Head and Neck Cancer module; NFHNSI-22, the National Comprehensive Cancer Network–Functional Assessment of Cancer Therapy–Head and Neck Cancer Symptom Index; QOL, Quality of Life; UW-QOL, the University of Washington Questionnaire; VAS, Visual Analogue Scale.

scales (fatigue, pain, and nausea and vomiting), individual questions concerning common symptoms in cancer patients, and two questions assessing overall QOL. This copyrighted instrument has been translated and validated into over 100 languages and is used in more than 3,000 studies worldwide. The H&N35 module is specific for multimodality HNC therapy and contains an additional 35 questions. Both of the scales and single-item measures range in score from 0 to 100; a high scale score represents a higher response/functioning level (better QOL). The time for administration is about 7 to 10 minutes for each instrument. The EORTC recently developed a 43-item H&N module, which is an update of the QLQ-H&N35. This instrument is currently undergoing psychometric testing in large international groups of patients (39). Permission to use the EORTC scales may be obtained at http://groups.eortc.be/qol/eortc-qlq-c30.

The self-administered FACT-H&N consists of the 27-item FACT-G that assesses patient function in four domains: physical, social/family, emotional, and functional well-being, and 12 additional HNC specific symptom items. Each item is rated on a 0 to 4 Likert type scale, and then combined to produce subscale scores for each domain, as well as a global QOL score. Higher scores represent better QOL, and the maximum score of 144 reflects the best possible QOL. A clinically significant change in score is represented by an increase of approximately 6 units or a decrease of 12 units. This copyrighted instrument has been translated and validated into more than 50 languages. Version 4 is the most current version. This instrument takes about 5 to 10 minutes to complete. Permission to use the FACT questionnaires may be obtained at http://www.facit.org/FACITOrg/Questionnaires.

Investigators from the University of Washington, Seattle, developed the self-administered University of Washington Questionnaire (UW-QOL) to specifically address problems incurred by patients with HNC following surgery (32). Version 4 is the most current version of the UW-QOL and consists of 12 single item domains (pain, appearance, activity, recreation, swallowing, chewing, speech, shoulder, taste, saliva, mood, and anxiety), having between three and six response options. There are also three general QOL questions. The questionnaire focuses on current patient health and QOL within the past 7 days. Each of the domain-specific items is scored from 0 (worst QOL) to 100 (best QOL). A clinical significant change in score is approximately six to seven points. The UW-QOL takes less than 5 minutes to complete. The instrument, although originally developed at the University of Washington, has subsequently been extensively researched by Professor Simon Rogers at Aintree Head and Neck Cancer Centre. More information on this questionnaire may be obtained at http://www.headandneckcancer.co.uk/For+professionals/Quality+of+Life+(QOL)/Quality+of+Life+Questionnaires.aspx.

The MD Anderson Symptom Inventory (MDASI) is a self-administered multisymptom PRO measure for clinical and research use. The MDASI's 13 core items (pain, fatigue, nausea, disturbed sleep, distress, shortness of breath, lack of appetite, drowsiness, dry mouth, sadness, vomiting, difficulty remembering, and numbness or tingling) include symptoms found to have the highest frequency and severity in patients with various cancers and treatment types. There are also six interference items (general activity, mood, walking ability, normal work, relations with other people, and enjoyment of life). This inventory uses a 0 to 10 numerical rating scale (NRS) to assess the severity of symptoms and interference. The MDASI assesses the severity of symptoms at their worst in the last 24 hours, with 0 being "not present" and 10 being "as bad as you can imagine." The MDASI Head and Neck Module (MDASI-HN) was developed for patients with HNC. Nine items consistent with symptoms specific to the HNC population were identified, including mucus in the mouth and throat, difficulty swallowing/chewing, choking/coughing, difficulty with voice/speech, skin pain/burning/rash, constipation, problems with tasting food, mouth/throat sores, and problems with teeth or gums. The MSASI and MDASI-HN copyrights are held by the University of Texas MD Anderson Cancer Center and administered by MDASI's developer, Charles S. Cleeland, PhD. Each instrument takes 5 to 10 minutes to complete. Permission to use the MDASI questionnaires may be obtained at https://www.mdanderson.org/research/departments-labs-institutes/departments-divisions/symptom-research/symptom-assessment-tools/md-anderson-symptom-inventory-head-and-neck-cancer-module.html.

The National Comprehensive Cancer Network–Functional Assessment of Cancer Therapy–Head and Neck Cancer Symptom Index-22 (NFHNSI-22) is the newest addition to the PRO literature (35). This 22-item questionnaire is the first symptom index developed through both qualitative and quantitative methodologies to assess advanced HNC symptoms. The items are categorized into disease-related symptoms, treatment side effects, and general function and well-being. It measures symptom burden and the relative importance from a patient perspective, but also takes into account the rankings of importance and causality of symptoms from the oncologist's perspective. The NFHNSI-22 takes 5 to 10 minutes to complete. Permission to use the NFHNSI-22 questionnaires may be obtained at http://www.facit.org/FACITOrg/Questionnaires.

The Head and Neck Radiotherapy Questionnaire (HNRQ) is a 22-item instrument that was designed to measure patient-reported acute radiation–related morbidity and QOL (36). This instrument encompasses six domains (oral cavity–mouth, throat, skin, digestive function, energy, and psychosocial), and a global score using a 7-point Likert scale from 0 to 6 (a higher score representing worse symptoms and worse QOL). The questionnaire takes approximately 5 to 10 minutes to complete. The maximal score is 132. The instrument is in the public domain and was developed at McMaster's University by Dr. George Browman.

The EQ-5D is a trademark of the EuroQol Group and was originally designed to complement other instruments, but is now increasingly used as a "standalone" measure to assess a patient's current health status. The EQ-5D is a two-part patient self-administrated questionnaire that takes approximately 1 to 5 minutes to complete. The first part consists of five items covering five dimensions: mobility, self-care, usual activities, pain/discomfort, and anxiety/depression. The EQ-5D-3L version grades each dimension on three levels: 1—no problems, 2—moderate problems, and 3—extreme problems. The EQ-5D-5L version grades each dimension on five levels: 1—no problems, 2—slight problems, 3—moderate problems, 4—severe problems, and 5—unable to/extreme problems for all dimensions. Health states are defined by the combination of the leveled responses to the five dimensions. The second part is a visual analogue scale (VAS) valuing current health state, measured on a 20-cm 10-point interval scale. Worst health state is scored as 0 at the bottom of the scale, and best health state is scored as 100 at the top. Both the five-item index score and the VAS score are transformed into a utility score between 0 "worst health state" and 1 "best health state." The index score or the VAS score may be used in a quality-adjusted survival analysis depending on the health state(s) of interest. The EQ-5D is available in over 125 languages, and can be accessed at http://www.euroqol.org.

OTHER SYMPTOM- OR SITE-SPECIFIC QOL INSTRUMENTS USED IN HNC

A National Cancer Institute Symptom Management and QOL Clinical Trials Planning Meeting performed a review of QOL domains in HNC clinical trials through a PubMed search (40). Investigators identified 29 symptoms and 9 domains from which 10 HNC-specific core symptoms and 2 HRQOL domains were identified including swallowing, oral pain, skin changes, dry mouth, dental health, opening mouth/trismus, taste, excess/thick mucus/saliva, shoulder disability/motion, voice/hoarseness, social domain, and functional domain. These items were deemed important for evaluation on future clinical HNC trials (40).

To evaluate these important HNC core symptoms, there are a variety of symptom-specific PRO instruments available, including the MDADI (41); the Swallow Quality of Life Questionnaire (SWAL-QOL) (42); the Sydney Swallow Questionnaire (SSQ) (43); the Deglutition Handicap Index (DHI) (44); the Dysphagia Handicap Index (DHI') (45,46); Eating Assessment Tool (EAT-10) (47); the Voice Handicap Index (VHI, VHI-10) (48); the Voice-Related Quality of Life instrument (VR-QOL) (49,50); the University of Michigan Xerostomia-Related Quality of Life Scale (XeQOLS) (51); the Dermatology Life Quality Index (DLQI) (52); the Functional Assessment of Cancer Therapy–Epidermal Growth Factor Receptor Inhibitor 18 (FACT-EGFR-18) (53) to specifically address dermatologic symptoms from EGFR inhibitors; the Oral Health Impact Profile (OHIP) (54); the Chemosensory Complaints Score (CCS) to measure taste and smell alterations (55); the Hearing Handicap Inventory for Adults (HHIA) (56); the Neck Dissection Impairment Index (NDII) (57); the Shoulder Pain and Disability Index (SPADI) (58); the Shoulder Disability Questionnaire (SDQ) (59); Constant's Shoulder Score (CS) (60); and the Disabilities of the Arm, Shoulder, and Hand Questionnaire (DASH, QuickDASH)

(61) to measure patient reported QOL related to injury from neck dissection.

Disease-specific modules also are available for patients with different sites of HNC such as nasopharyngeal cancer (NPC). Patients with NPC have a unique disease presentation and treatment-related sequelae due to frequent skull base and cranial nerve involvement (62). At present, NPC-specific instruments include the FACIT nasopharyngeal-specific QOL subscale (FACT-NP) (63), and the 30-item QOL-NPC, version 2 (64). The FACT-NP uses the core set of questions from FACT-G with 16 additional NPC-specific items including eating, swallowing, mouth dryness, appetite, taste, voice quality, communication, appearance, pain, neck movement, tinnitus, hearing, vision, smell, and nasal blockage. This instrument was validated in the endemic population and is available in traditional and simplified Chinese. Currently, the FACT-NP is being used on NRG Oncology HN001, A Randomized Phase II and Phase III Study of Individualized Treatment for Nasopharyngeal Carcinoma Based on Biomarker Epstein Barr Virus (EBV) Deoxyribonucleic Acid (DNA) (65). Table 26.2 describes the frequently used symptom- and disease-specific PRO instruments for HNC.

QOL AS A PROGNOSTIC FACTOR IN HNC

Baseline QOL data, in addition to a multitude of clinical factors, have been found to be an independent variable predicting outcomes for a variety of cancer types including HNC. In a meta-analysis of individual QOL data for 11 different cancer types across 30 EORTC randomized controlled trials conducted between 1986 and 2004, the QOL parameters of physical functioning, pain, and appetite loss, in addition to the sociodemographic and clinical

TABLE 26.2

Frequently Used Symptom- and Disease-Specific PRO Instruments for HNC

Instrument	Symptom/ Disease	Number of Items	Indication	Time to Complete (Minutes)
MDADI (41)	Swallowing	20	Swallowing-related QOL and symptom burden from surgery, radiation, and chemotherapy	10
SWAL-QOL (66)	Swallowing	44	Swallowing-related QOL and symptom burden from surgery, radiation, and chemotherapy	15
SSQ (43)	Swallowing	17	Swallowing-related QOL and symptom burden from surgery, radiation, and chemotherapy	5–10
DHI (45,46)	Swallowing	25	Swallowing-related QOL and symptom burden from surgery, radiation, and chemotherapy	10–15
DHI' (44)	Swallowing	30	Swallowing-related QOL from surgery, radiation, and chemotherapy	10–15
EAT-10 (47)	Swallowing	10	Swallowing-related QOL from surgery, radiation, and chemotherapy	5
VHI, VHI-10 (48)	Voice	VHI = 30 VHI-10 = 10	Voice-related QOL from surgery or radiation	VHI: 15 VHI-10: 5

(continued)

TABLE 26.2 (*continued*)

Frequently Used Symptom- and Disease-Specific PRO Instruments for HNC

Instrument	Symptom/ Disease	Number of Items	Indication	Time to Complete (Minutes)
VR-QOL (49,50)	Voice	10	Voice-related QOL from surgery or radiation	5
XeQOLS (51)	Dry mouth	15	Salivary gland dysfunction and xerostomia-related QOL	5–10
DLQI (52)	Skin changes	12	Skin-related QOL and symptom burden from radiation and chemotherapy/biologic therapy	5–10
FACT-EGFR-18 (53)	Skin, eye, hair changes	18	QOL and symptom burden from EGFR inhibitor/biologic therapy	5–10
OHIP (54)	Oral health	49	Oral health–related QOL	20
CCS (55)	Taste/smell	15	Taste and smell symptom burden from radiation and chemotherapy	5–10
HHIA (56)	Hearing	25	Hearing-related QOL from surgery, chemotherapy, and radiation	10–15
NDII (57)	Shoulder	10	Shoulder symptoms and QOL from neck dissection	5–10
SPADI (58)	Shoulder	13	Shoulder symptoms and QOL from neck dissection	10
SDQ (59)	Shoulder	16	Shoulder symptoms and QOL from neck dissection	10–12
CS (60)	Shoulder	8	Shoulder pain, activity, and range of motion (clinician graded) after neck dissection	10
DASH, *Quick*DASH (61)	Upper extremity	DASH: 30 *Quick*DASH: 11	Upper extremity activities from neck dissection and radiation	DASH: 15 *Quick*DASH: <5
FACT-NP (63)	NPC	16	QOL and symptom burden from chemoradiation for NPC	10
QOL-NPC, version 2 (64)	NPC	26	QOL and symptom burden from chemoradiation for NPC in Chinese patients	10–15

CCS, Chemosensory Complaints Score; CS, Constant's Shoulder Score; DASH, Disabilities of the Arm, Shoulder, and Hand Questionnaire; DHI, Deglution Handicap Index; DHI', Dysphagia Handicap Index; DLQI, Dermatology Life Quality Index; EAT-10, Eating Assessment Tool; FACT-EGFR-18, Functional Assessment of Cancer Therapy–Epidermal Growth Factor Receptor 18; FACT-NP, Functional Assessment of Cancer Therapy–Nasopharyngeal; HHIA, Hearing Handicap Inventory for Adults; MDADI, MD Anderson Dysphagia Inventory; NDII, Neck Dissection Impairment Index; NPC, nasopharyngeal cancer; OHIP, Oral Health Impact Profile; QOL, quality of life; *Quick*DASH, the shortened DASH instrument; SDQ, Shoulder Disability Questionnaire; SPADI, Shoulder Pain and Disability Index; SSQ, Sydney Swallow Questionnaire; SWAL-QOL, Swallow Quality of Life Questionnaire; VHI, Voice Handicap Index; VHI-10, Voice Handicap Index-10 items; VR-QOL, Voice-Related Quality of Life Questionnaire; XeQOLS, University of Michigan Xerostomia-Related Quality of Life Scale.

factors of age, sex, and distant metastases, were all predictive for overall survival, whereas WHO performance status was not (67). Consideration of the three QOL parameters, as well as sociodemographic and clinical data, increased the predictive accuracy of prognosis of overall survival by 6%, relative to sociodemographic and clinical characteristics alone, in this large dataset of 10,108 patients. In a systematic review of 19 studies of QOL in HNC, van Nieuwenhuizen et al. found a strong association between pretreatment physical function, change in global QOL, and survival, from pretreatment to 6 months posttreatment (68). There was, however, no association between other QOL domains, including role, emotional, cognitive, social, and mental health well-being, with survival. In a retrospective QOL pooled analysis from the RTOG of the randomized RTOG 90-03 trial (evaluating four definitive radiation fractionation schedules in patients with locally advanced HNC) and the RTOG 91-11 trial (a comparison of three nonsurgical treatment strategies to preserve the larynx in patients with locally advanced larynx cancer), FACT-HN QOL data were available for 1093 patients (69). The baseline FACT-HN score was independently predictive of locoregional control ($p = .0038$), but not overall survival, with the functional well-being domain being most predictive on multivariate analysis ($p = .0004$) (69). Using the same dataset, emotional well-being was not found to be an independent predictor for survival (70).

In a prospective QOL substudy of chemoradiation trials RTOG 0129 (a randomized phase III trial of concurrent chemoradiation with cisplatin, randomizing to standard fractionation versus accelerated concomitant boost radiation for patients with stage III to IV HNC) and RTOG 0522 (a randomized phase III trial of concurrent accelerated radiation and cisplatin versus concurrent accelerated radiation, cisplatin, and cetuximab for patients with stage III and IV HNC), investigators demonstrated the prognostic significance of baseline QOL and functional data on overall survival (71,72). In RTOG 0129, for every one-point increase in baseline score on both the HNRQ and the Spitzer Quality of Life Index (SQLI), where a higher score indicates better QOL, there was a significantly associated lower hazard of death ($p < .001$ and $p = .004$, respectively) (71). Similarly, RTOG 0522 demonstrated that for every 10-point increase in baseline FACT-HN score and EQ-5D index, there was also a significantly associated lower hazard of death ($p = .0009$ and $p = .0004$, respectively) (72). In addition, baseline QOL scores using the HNRQ and SQLI in RTOG 0129, and FACT-HN in RTOG 0522 substudies, were independently correlated with better overall survival, progression-free survival, and locoregional control (71,72).

Prospective QOL in locally advanced HNC has been recently reported for 320 patients treated on the Canadian Cancer Trials Group HN.6 trial, a randomized phase III study of standard fractionated radiation therapy with concurrent cisplatin versus accelerated fractionated radiation therapy with the epidermal growth factor receptor (EGFR) inhibitor panitumumab (73). QOL was collected at baseline, at completion of radiation, and then at 2, 4, 6, 12, 24, and 36 months following radiation using the FACT-H&N, the MDADI, and the SWAL-QOL. The secondary QOL hypothesis was a six-point improvement in FACT-H&N scores from baseline to 1 year in the panitumumab arm. Baseline QOL scores did not significantly differ by treatment arm. At 1 year, no QOL difference was seen between arms in FACT-H&N change from baseline. Therefore, neither progression-free survival (the primary end point of this trial) nor QOL was improved in locally advanced HNC with the addition of the anti–EGFR inhibitor panitumumab (73). Patient-reported swallowing outcomes are reported later in this chapter.

QOL has also been analyzed in randomized trials specific to different sites of HNC. In laryngeal cancer, a retrospective analysis of QOL was performed for patients treated on the landmark Veterans Affairs Laryngeal Cancer Study 268 (VA Larynx Study) that established larynx preservation with chemotherapy and radiation as a standard of care. Patients with stage III and IV laryngeal cancer were randomized to laryngectomy followed by radiation versus induction chemotherapy followed by radiation. Forty-six (71%) of the 65 surviving patients who could be retrospectively contacted completed QOL items using the University of Michigan Head and Neck Quality of Life (HNQOL) instrument, the Medical Outcomes Studies Short-Form 36 (SF-36) general health survey, the Beck Depression Inventory, as well as smoking and alcohol consumption surveys (74). Patients randomized to larynx preservation experienced significantly better QOL scores on the SF-36 mental health domain than the surgery and radiation group, and also had better HNQOL pain scores. Compared with patients who underwent laryngectomy, patients with intact larynges also experienced significantly less bodily pain, better scores on the SF-36 mental health instrument, better HNQOL emotion scores, and less depression on the Beck Inventory.

In oropharyngeal cancer (OPC), RTOG randomized trials have demonstrated the prognostic significance of baseline QOL in association with human papillomavirus (HPV) status (identified through in situ hybridization or p16 immunohistochemistry on tumor tissues) (71,72). QOL data from both the RTOG 0129 and RTOG 0522 trials (described above) demonstrated better baseline and 1-year QOL and performance status in patients with p16 positive OPC compared to p16 negative OPC. In RTOG 0522, patients with p16-positive OPC showed higher baseline, and 1-year FACT-HN total scores, physical function, and HNC additional items, as compared to patients with p16-negative disease. Patients with p16-positive OPC, however, were noted to have both a greater deterioration in QOL scores during treatment, as well as a faster recovery in QOL after treatment, as compared to p16-negative patients. Similar findings for patients with p16-positive OPC were demonstrated in the Trans-Tasman Radiation Oncology Group TROG-02.02 HeadSTART trial (a phase III evaluation of the hypoxic cytotoxin tirapazamine with cisplatin, and radiation versus cisplatin and radiation for advanced HNC), which reported acute decline in FACT-HN scores after CRT despite having higher baseline QOL (75). Table 26.3 summarizes the published multicenter randomized trials in HNC with inclusion of QOL and PROs as important secondary end points.

Several studies have shown that patients with HPV-positive OPC have a significantly improved overall and disease-free survival compared to patients with HPV-negative OPC (76–81). Currently, HPV-related OPC is treated similarly to stage-matched OPC. However, because tumor HPV status is strongly associated with therapeutic response and survival, as compared with p16-negative OPC, less intensive use of radiation therapy or chemotherapy (treatment "de-intensification") is under investigation for low or good risk OPC (defined as HPV-positive OPC, with ≤ 10 pack-year smoking history, or HPV-positive OPC with >10 pack-years smoking, but only N0-N2a disease) (76). Because the RTOG 0129, RTOG 0522, and TROG-02.02 HeadSTART studies demonstrated that patients with p16-positive OPC experience a greater decline in QOL and greater symptom burden during CRT, as compared to P16-negative OPC, evaluating patient-reported symptom burden and QOL will be critical to de-intensification research efforts. These trials and their QOL end points are presented in Table 26.4 later in this chapter.

In nasopharyngeal cancer, global QOL before and after treatment has also been found to be prognostic for survival outcome (83,84). In a Taiwanese study of 347 patients with NPC receiving conformal radiation therapy, pretreatment QOL scores using the EORTC QLQ-C30 and EORTC QLQ-H&N35 instruments showed that physical and role functioning, as well as three symptoms scales (fatigue, pain, and appetite loss), predicted for distant metastases on multivariate analysis after adjusting for age, sex, smoking, and cancer stage (83). Physical functioning was the most powerful predictor of overall and distant metastases-free survival. Of note, Karnofsky Performance Status (KPS) was not prognostic for survival on multivariate analysis. Similarly, 1-year post-treatment QOL was able to predict survival in 273 NPC patients from the same center (84). Multivariate analysis demonstrated that physical functioning, fatigue, and appetite loss were all predictive of disease-specific and overall survival ($p < .05$). These datasets suggest that QOL at baseline and after treatment may be a better prognostic marker than physician-graded performance status. As such, baseline QOL or PRO scores should be considered, in lieu of KPS or ECOG performance status, as a stratification factor on clinical trials.

IMPACT OF RADIATION THERAPY TECHNIQUE ON QOL

Intensity-modulated radiotherapy (IMRT) represented a major technological advance in treatment planning and radiation delivery over the past decade. IMRT is an advanced form of three-dimensional conformal radiotherapy (3DCRT) in which beam intensity may be modulated to create nonuniform dose distribution to maximize target coverage of the tumor and spare adjacent organs at risk. In HNC, IMRT was originally used to decrease the radiation dose to the parotid gland with the aim of reducing long-term xerostomia and improving xerostomia-related QOL. Initially, the utility of these technical improvements was

TABLE 26.3

Multicenter Randomized Trials With Inclusion of QOL and PRO as Secondary End Points

Study Name	Study Design	QOL Analysis	QOL Instrument(s)	QOL Findings
RTOG 90-03 (69,70)	Stage III-IV HNC Randomized to: 1. Standard RT fractionation 2. Split course accelerated RT 3. Hyperfractionated RT 4. Accelerated concomitant boost RT	Retrospective pooled analysis of RTOG 90-03 and 91-11	FACT-H&N	Emotional well- being not a predictor of survival; pretreatment QOL predicts locoregional control but not OS
RTOG 91-11 (69,70)	Stage T3-T4 small volume laryngeal cancer Randomized to: 1. Induction chemotherapy followed by RT alone 2. Concurrent CRT 3. RT alone	Retrospective pooled analysis of RTOG 90-03 and 91-11	FACT-H&N	Emotional well- being not a predictor of survival; pretreatment QOL predicts locoregional control but not OS
RTOG 0129 (71)	Stage III-IV HNC Randomized to: 1. Accelerated RT-cisplatin 2. Standard fractionation RT-cisplatin	Prospective substudy with additional QOL consent Longitudinal QOL	HNRQ; SQLI	No clinically meaningful difference in QOL between arms; p16-positive OPC associated with higher QOL than p16-negative OPC; pretreatment QOL is a prognostic marker for OS
RTOG 0522 (72)	Stage III-IV HNC Randomized to: 1. Accelerated RT-cisplatin 2. Accelerated RT-cisplatin + cetuximab	Prospective substudy with additional QOL consent of longitudinal QOL	FACT-H&N; EQ-5D	No clinically meaningful difference in QOL between arms; p16-positive OPC associated with higher QOL than p16-negative OPC; pretreatment QOL is a prognostic marker for OS
Trans-Tasman Radiation Oncology Group TROG-02.02 HeadSTART (75,82)	Stage III-IV HNC Randomized to: 1. RT-cisplatin 2. RT-cisplatin + tirapazamine	Prospective substudy of longitudinal QOL	FACT-H&N	No clinically meaningful difference in QOL between arms; p16-positive OPC associated with higher QOL than p16-negative OPC

(continued)

TABLE 26.3 (*continued*)

Multicenter Randomized Trials With Inclusion of QOL and PRO as Secondary Endpoints

Study Name	Study Design	QOL Analysis	QOL Instrument(s)	QOL Findings
VA Larynx Study (74)	Stage T3-T4 laryngeal cancer Randomized to: 1. Total laryngectomy followed by RT 2. Induction chemotherapy followed by RT alone	Retrospective cross-sectional QOL	University of Michigan HNQOL; SF-36; Beck Depression Inventory	Laryngeal preservation associated with better QOL, less pain, better mental health, better emotional QOL, and less depression
Canadian Cancer Trials Group study HN.6 (73)	Stage III-IV HNC Randomized to: 1. RT-cisplatin 2. Accelerated RT-panitumumab	Prospective longitudinal QOL	FACT-H&N MDADI SWAL-QOL	No QOL differences between arms

CT, chemotherapy; EQ-5D™, 5-item heath utilities instrument of the EuroQol Group; FACT-H&N, Functional Assessment of Cancer Therapy–Head and Neck Cancer instrument; HNC, head and neck cancer; HNQOL, University of Michigan Head and Neck Quality of Life instrument; HNRQ, Head and Neck Radiotherapy Questionnaire; MDADI, the MD Anderson Dysphagia Inventory; OPC, oropharyngeal cancer; OS, overall survival; QOL, quality of life; RT, radiation therapy; RTOG, Radiation Therapy Oncology Group; SF-36, Medical Outcomes Studies Short-Form 36 general health survey; SQLI, Spitzer Quality of Life Index; SWAL-QOL, Swallow Quality of Life Questionnaire; TROG, Trans-Tasman Radiation Oncology Group; VA, Veterans Affairs.

in question because of the significant increased costs of IMRT without improvements in survival. However, several key randomized trials addressed these concerns after demonstrating the superiority of IMRT over 3DCRT with respect to HNC physician-graded toxicity and patient-reported QOL, while maintaining equivalent disease control and survival (85–87). Table 26.5 summarizes these randomized trials assessing QOL using parotid-sparing IMRT.

The PARSPORT (CRUK/03/005) trial was a multicenter phase III randomized trial study performed in the United Kingdom assessing 3DCRT versus IMRT in patients with stage I-IVA HNC (85). The primary end point was the proportion of patients with grade 2 or worse xerostomia at 12 months assessed by the LENT–SOMA scale. Patient-reported QOL, an important secondary end point of this study, was also collected at baseline, 2 weeks, and then at 3, 6, 12, 18, and 24 months after radiation therapy using the EORTC QLQ-C30/H&N35 version 3 and the modified xerostomia questionnaire. At 12 and 24 months, a decrease in global QOL was noted in both arms, although a consistently higher QLQ30 Global and H&N35 dry mouth QOL score was reported in patients who received IMRT. However, it is important to note that these QOL differences between the two groups at 24 months were clinically but not statistically significant.

An unexpected finding from the PARSPORT (CRUK/03/005) trial was a statistically significant increase in acute fatigue (clinician graded) in patients who were treated with IMRT as compared to 3DCRT. The investigators attributed this finding to dosimetric central nervous system (CNS) factors. The posterior fossa, brainstem, cerebellum, pituitary gland, pineal gland, hypothalamus, hippocampus, and basal ganglia were retrospectively contoured. Both maximum and mean radiation doses were significantly higher for the posterior fossa, brainstem, and cerebellum in patients who reported grade 2 or higher acute fatigue, as compared to those who did not ($p \leq 0.01$) (88). In this study, it was suggested that both higher CNS radiation dose and volume were associated with higher levels of fatigue in patients with HNC. A subsequent study in patients with NPC confirmed this association between IMRT dosimetry to CNS structures and clinician-measured fatigue (89). Dosimetric variables to the CNS structures (brainstem, cerebellum, pituitary gland,

TABLE 26.4

Recently Closed or Ongoing HPV-Positive Oropharyngeal Cancer "De-intensification" Trials With QOL End Points

Study Name [Clinical Trials.gov Identifier]	Study Design	Eligibility	QOL Instruments	QOL End Point
RTOG 1016 (120) [NCT01302834] Closed to accrual	Phase III randomized trial of: 1. IMRT 70 Gy accelerated over 6 weeks with high-dose cisplatin 2. IMRT 70 Gy accelerated over 6 weeks with cetuximab	T1-2 N2a-N3 or T3-4 any N M0	EORTC- QLQ/H&N35; EQ-5D; PRO-CTCAE-H&N; Work Status Questionnaire; HHIA-S	Primary: Comparable 5-year OS Secondary: QOL, swallowing, patient-reported adverse events, work status, hearing, and cost effectiveness at baseline, end of treatment, and at 3, 6, and 12 months from the end of treatment
TROG 12.01 [NCT01855451] (121) Ongoing	Phase III randomized trial of: 1. IMRT 70 Gy standard fractionation with weekly cisplatin 2. IMRT 70 Gy standard fractionation with cetuximab	Stage III (excluding T1-2 N1) or stage IV (excluding T4, N3, and distant metastasis) if smoking history of < 10 pack-years. If >10 pack-years, nodal disease must be N0-N2a	MDASI-HN; MDADI; FACT-H&N; HHIA-S; Depression Anxiety HADs; EQ-5D-5; Return to Work Questionnaire	Primary: To compare the area under the curve of symptom severity between arms from baseline to week 20 (13 weeks after completion of radiotherapy) using MDASI-HN
De-ESCALaTE HPV Study UK (122) [NCT01874171] Closed to accrual	Phase III randomized trial of: 1. IMRT 70 Gy in 35 fractions with high-dose cisplatin 2. IMRT 70 Gy in 35 fractions with cetuximab	Stage III-IVa (T3N0-T4N0 and T1N -1-T4N3)	EORTC-QLQ C30 and H&N35; MDADI; EQ-5D	Primary: Overall acute and late grade 3-5 CTCAE v4 toxicity Secondary: QOL and swallowing up to 2 years from end of treatment, cost effectiveness, disease-free survival, recurrence, metastases
NRG HN002 (123) [NCT02254278] Closed to accrual	Phase II Randomized Trial of: 1. IMRT 60 Gy in 6 weeks and weekly cisplatin 2. IMRT 60 Gy in 5 weeks alone	T1-T2, N1-N2b or T3, N0-N2b M0	MDADI; UW-QOLv4; Return to Work Questionnaire	Primary: 2-year progression-free survival of >= 85% without unacceptable swallowing (MDADI >60) toxicity at 1 year Secondary: Change in total MDADI score at 6 months, 1, and 2 years

(continued)

TABLE 26.4 (*continued*)

Recently Closed or Ongoing HPV-Positive Oropharyngeal Cancer “De-intensification” Trials With QOL End Points

Study Name [Clinical Trials.gov Identifier]	Study Design	Eligibility	QOL Instruments	QOL End Point
ECOG 3311 (124) [NCT01898494] Ongoing	Phase IIb of TORS and risk adapted IMRT to: 1. TOS alone low risk 2. Low-dose IMRT 50 Gy over 5 weeks 3. Standard dose IMRT 60 Gy over 6 weeks and cisplatin 4. Standard dose IMRT 60 Gy over 6 weeks and cisplatin	T1-2, N1-2b	MDADI; FACT-HN; VHI-10; NDII	Primary: 2-year progression-free survival Secondary: 2 year MDADI scores, QOL, voice quality, neck function, CTCAE v4 adverse effects, overall survival
ORATOR [NCT01590355] (126) Ongoing	Phase II randomized to: 1. IMRT 70 Gy over 7 weeks with/without chemotherapy 2. TORS with ND	T1-2, N0-2, <4 cm node	MDADI	Primary: 1 year MDADI scores Secondary: Overall and progression-free survival, MSADI at 6-month intervals for 5 years, CTCAE v4 toxicity
EORTC ‘Best of’ (119,127) [NCT02984410] Ongoing	Phase III randomized to: 1. IMRT 66-70 Gy over 6 weeks 2. Transoral surgery (TORS, TLM, CTOS)	T1-T2, N0 M0	MDADI	Primary: Change in the MDADI score at 4.5, 6, 9, and 12 months after randomization
CRUK-PATHOS (125) [NCT02215265] Ongoing	Phase II/III TORS then risk adapted randomization to: 1. Observation 2. IMRT 60 Gy over 6 weeks 3. IMRT 50 Gy over 5 weeks 4. IMRT 60 Gy over 6 weeks with cisplatin	T1-T3 N0-N2b M0	MDADI; EORTC-QLQ C30 and H&N35	Primary phase II: MDADI score at 12 months Secondary: QOL, CTCAE v4 toxicity, overall and disease-free survival

CRUK-PATHOS, Cancer Research United Kingdom–Post-operative Adjuvant Treatment for HPV-positive Tumors; CTOS, conventional transoral surgery; De-ESCALaTE, Determination of Cetuximab Versus Cisplatin Early and Late Toxicity Events in HPV+ OPSCC; ECOG, Eastern Cooperative Oncology Group; EORTC-QLQ/H&N35, EORTC QLQ-C30/H&N35, the European Organization for Research and Treatment of Cancer Core Questionnaire (EORTC QLQ-C30 version 3.0) and the 35-item head-and-neck module (H&N35); EQ-5D-5L, 5-item heath utilities instrument of the EuroQol Group, 5L version; FACT-H&N, Functional Assessment of Cancer Therapy–Head and Neck; HHIA-S, Hearing Handicap Inventory for Adults-Screening tool; IMRT, intensity modulated radiation therapy; MDADI, MD Anderson Dysphagia Inventory; MDASI-HN, MD Anderson Dysphagia Inventory for Head and Neck; ND, neck dissection; ORATOR, Randomized Trial for Early-stage Squamous Cell Carcinoma of the Oropharynx: Radiotherapy vs Trans-oral Robotic Surgery; OS, overall survival; PORT, postoperative radiation therapy; QOL, quality of life; RTOG, Radiation Therapy Oncology Group; TLM, transoral microsurgery; TORS, transoral robotic surgery; TROG, Trans-Tasman Radiation Oncology Group.

TABLE 26.5

Randomized Parotid Sparing IMRT Studies With QOL End Points

Study Name	Study Design	QOL Analysis	QOL Instrument(s) Used	QOL Findings
PARSPORT (CRUK/03/005) (85)	Stage I-IVA HNC Randomized to: 1. 3D-CRT 2. IMRT	Prospective longitudinal QOL	EORTC QLQ-C30/H&N35; Xerostomia Questionnaire	Higher QLQ-C30 Global QOL and improved H&N35 dry mouth scores in IMRT group; however, at 24 months, group differences remained clinically but not statistically significant
Rathod et al. Tata Memorial Hospital (87)	Stage I-IVA HNC Randomized to: 1. 3D-CRT 2. IMRT	Prospective pre- and posttreatment QOL	EORTC QLQ-C30/H&N35	Emotional, role, and social functioning scores, as well as dry mouth, opening mouth, sticky saliva, pain, senses, and QOL domains all higher or improved with IMRT
Pow et al. University of Hong Kong (86)	T2, N0/N1, M0 NPC Randomized to: 1. 3D-CRT 2. IMRT	Prospective longitudinal QOL	EORTC QLQ-C30/H&N35	Global health scores improved in both arms; 12-month subscale scores for role function, bodily pain, and physical function all improved in the IMRT group

3D-CRT, three-dimensional conformal radiotherapy; EORTC QLQ-C30/H&N35, European Organisation for Research and Treatment of Cancer Core Questionnaire (EORTC QLQ-C30 version 3) and the 35-item head-and-neck module (H&N35); HNC, head and neck cancer; IMRT, intensity-modulated radiation therapy; NPC, nasopharyngeal cancer; QOL, quality of life; RT, radiation therapy; XQ, Xerostomia Questionnaire.

pineal gland, hypothalamus, hippocampus, and basal ganglia) were associated with increased grade 2 or higher fatigue, and these investigators hypothesized that the possible underlying mechanism of radiation-induced fatigue may be pituitary-related hormonal function or disruption of connections between these critical CNS structures (89). While these two studies used clinician-measured fatigue in their analyses, patient-reported fatigue has been demonstrated in up to 75% of patients receiving radiation for HNC (90). More recent datasets have shown that using PROs for measuring fatigue may have greater predictive accuracy than clinician scores alone (20).

Rathod et al. prospectively evaluated QOL outcomes in patients with HNC treated with IMRT versus 3DCRT in a randomized trial of 60 patients, of whom 58 patients completed the QOL questionnaires at baseline and at each subsequent 3-month visit up to 24 months (87). QOL was evaluated using the EORTC QLQ-C30 version 3 and the EORTC QLQ-H&N35. Both arms were well balanced in terms of patient characteristics and baseline QOL. Patients in the IMRT arm had superior QOL in emotional and role functioning (12 months, p = .008) and social contact (24 months, p = .03). For symptom-specific QOL, dry mouth (at 6, 12, and 18 months), as well as mouth opening (at 6 and 24 months), were both improved in the IMRT arm, as compared to patients treated with 3DCRT ($p < .05$). Other patient-reported symptoms were also improved in at least one time point after IMRT as compared to 3DCRT, including sticky saliva, pain, swallowing, senses, sexuality, feeling ill, and insomnia. In addition, none of the QOL domains were worse in the IMRT arm as compared to the 3DCRT group, and disease outcomes for locoregional control and survival were not significantly different between the two arms.

Pow et al. from the University of Hong Kong conducted a randomized study of IMRT versus 3DCRT in 51 patients with NPC (86). Stimulated whole and parotid saliva flow were measured together with QOL using the SF-36, the EORTC QLQ-C30 version 3, and the EORTC QLQ-H&N35 at baseline, and then at 2, 6, and 12 months after radiation therapy (86). The IMRT group demonstrated improved QOL related to speech (at 6 and 12 months) and swallowing (at 12 months), but worse problems with the senses at 2 months posttreatment. The IMRT group also experienced fewer issues with sticky saliva and coughing. Interestingly, while there was a marked decrease in salivary flow in the 3DCRT group, there was a trend for improvement in patient-reported dry mouth with IMRT, but this did not reach statistical significance. Differences between objective measures and QOL outcomes in these studies may be multifactorial, and may also be in part due to patient expectations and readjusting to a new baseline after therapy (91).

Pow et al. subsequently reported the measured parotid and whole salivary flow, as well as QOL using the SF-36, the EORTC QLQ-C30 version 3, the EORTC QLQ-H&N35, and the Oral Health Impact Profile Questionnaire completed at baseline and 2, 6, 12, 18, and 24 months after IMRT on 57 patients with early-stage NPC that received IMRT (92). Parotid saliva flow fully recovered at 1 year after IMRT, and recovery was maintained in longer follow-up. Whole salivary flow recovered to 40% of baseline at 1 year after IMRT. QOL decreased after IMRT, most notably at 2 months, with significant recovery at 6 months. At 12 and 24 months after IMRT, most QOL subscales returned to baseline. However, persistent oral symptoms using the Oral Health Impact Profile Questionnaire remained at 2 years indicating incomplete recovery (92).

Patients with HNC often have significant weight loss and tumor shrinkage during radiation resulting in set-up inaccuracies that may necessitate IMRT re-planning. To address this finding, IMRT re-planning was evaluated by Yang et al. in 129 patients with NPC (93). Forty-three patients who underwent IMRT without re-planning were compared to 86 patients who received IMRT re-planning performed prior to the 25th fraction of radiation. Patients' QOLs were evaluated using the EORTC QLQ-C30 version 3 and the EORTC QLQ-H&N35 prior to treatment, at the end of treatment, and then at 1, 3, 6, and 12 months after IMRT. Patients who underwent IMRT re-planning had a statistically significant improved 2-year locoregional control, as well as higher global QOL, role and social functioning, and less patient-reported dyspnea, constipation, diarrhea, and appetite problems. Patients who did not receive re-planning had worse PROs with speech, social contact, teeth, mouth opening, sticky saliva, and dry mouth. It is postulated that the effects of mucositis and pain medication requirements may have influenced patient-reported appetite, diarrhea, and constipation.

While IMRT for HNC has resulted in marked improvements in various QOL end points as demonstrated in multiple studies (85–87,93–95), as well as dosimetric improvements in normal tissue sparing reducing the severity of clinician-reported treatment toxicities, whether these improvements in QOL using IMRT are cost effective was evaluated in the PARSPORT (CRUK/03/005) trial (96). Using Markov modeling, IMRT with reduced xerostomia and dysphagia symptoms was not found to be cost-effective in the first 2 years following treatment as compared to 3DCRT. However, over 15 years, IMRT was deemed to be more cost-effective over the patient's lifetime assuming that the benefits of IMRT persisted over time (96).

Proton beam radiation is gaining increasing interest as the next technological delivery advancement in the management of HNC. Although similar survival is expected with proton beam radiation, the toxicity and QOL end points are both of primary interest. PRO data from prospective registries comparing IMRT to intensity modulated proton radiotherapy (IMPT) have shown that patients with OPC experienced less symptom burden at 3 months posttreatment, particularly for appetite and taste, when treated with IMPT as compared to IMRT, using the MDASI-HN instrument (97).

SWALLOWING-RELATED QOL IN HNC

Oropharyngeal dysphagia after HNC treatment is a major morbidity that may have devastating consequences on function and QOL in HNC survivors. Furthermore, the functional morbidity of dysphagia after multimodality treatment may contribute to noncancer deaths, such as complications from malnutrition and aspiration, which may offset any survival gains from treatment intensification (98,99). Multiple factors are thought to contribute to the severity of oropharyngeal dysphagia, including different types of surgery, radiation dosimetric factors (such as the mean dose and volume to the larynx and pharyngeal constrictors), and the addition of concurrent chemotherapy or biologic therapy. Perhaps the most commonly used validated PRO swallowing instrument is the MDADI, a 20-item self-administered patient-reported dysphagia-specific instrument consisting of global, emotional, functional, and physical subscales (Table 26.2). The MDADI has been validated in patients with HNC in single-institution series (41), and is currently being used on several prospective multicenter randomized clinical trials. Other validated swallowing QOL instruments currently used in ongoing trials include the SWAL-QOL (66), the SSQ (43), the DHI (44), the DHI' (45), and EAT-10 (47). Please refer to Table 26.2 for a more detailed description. A comparison of the psychometric properties of the MDADI and three dysphagia instruments—the DHI, DHI', and the SWAL-QOL—has been performed (46). The SWAL-QOL, a 44-item QOL tool for dysphagia covering 10 QOL concepts—food selection, burden, mental health, social function, fear, eating duration, eating desire, communication, sleep, and fatigue—was found to have the strongest rating in terms of content validity and interpretability (66).

The Canadian Cancer Trials Group study HN.6 (a prospective randomized trial comparing standard fractionation radiation with cisplatin [arm A] and altered fractionation with panitumumab [arm B]) used the MDADI and SWAL-QOL to measure swallowing-related QOL as a secondary end point (73). Even though no survival or QOL differences using the FACT-H&N were found between the arms, a similar decline in QOL in the last week of radiation (from baseline) was seen in both arms (A/B) in the MDADI Physical (−40.4, −33.9, $p = .045$), and SWAL-QOL Eating Duration (−61.2, −51.2, $p = .02$), Eating Desire (−53.3, −43.9, $p = .031$) and Mental Health domain (−42, −32.6, $p = .009$). The QOL response analyses with SWAL-QOL and MDADI were similar, with two thirds of patients experiencing worsening of swallowing at every time point from baseline to 2 months posttreatment. Improved, stable, and worsening QOL was reported at 12 months posttreatment in 19%, 13%, and 67% using the SWAL-QOL, and in 23%, 8%, and 69% using the MDADI in arm A, with corresponding rates of 17%, 17%, and 66% for SWAL-QOL, and 25%, 7%, and 68% for MDADI in arm B (73).

The SSQ is a 17-item patient-reported swallowing-specific instrument measuring patient-reported swallowing function rather than QOL in patients with HNC. The individual questions are scored on a 100-mm VAS. The total score is calculated from the sum of the individual scores, where a higher score indicates more severe swallowing impairment. This instrument was validated by Dwivedi et al. in a cohort of 31 patients with oral cancer and OPC after treatment (43). A higher score indicates worse swallowing function. In a study of patients with oral and OPC, mean composite SSQ scores (SD) for patients with base of tongue, oral tongue, and tonsillar cancer were 663.8 (382.8), 456.2 (407.6), and 283.0 (243.1), respectively ($p = .005$). More advanced disease stage and older age were associated with worse swallowing impairment, represented by higher SSQ scores. For patients with advanced, compared to early-stage HNC, the SSQs were 918.1 (319.5) versus 344.8 (292.1) ($p \leq .001$); for patients <60 years versus ≥60 years of age, scores were 549.3 (415.1) versus 314.0 (247.3) ($p = .02$); and for patients with reconstruction versus without reconstruction, scores were 676.5 (410.5) versus 331.9 (286.5) ($p = .002$) (100).

IMPACT OF IMRT ON SWALLOWING-RELATED QOL

Poor swallowing outcomes after HNC radiation therapy have been attributed to higher mean radiation dose to the swallowing muscles including the pharyngeal constrictors, glottis, supraglottic larynx, and esophagus (101). Swallowing outcomes have been assessed by patient-reported measures, clinician-graded toxicity, percutaneous endoscopic gastrostomy tube rates, and objective measures such as videofluoroscopy (102,103). In a prospective single-arm study of 73 patients with OPC from the University of Michigan, treated with pharyngeal constrictor, laryngeal, and parotid sparing IMRT, patient, clinician, and objective swallowing measures were compared. Patient-reported swallowing was measured using the Eating Domain of the HNQOL and the Swallowing Question from the UW-QOL. Dysphagia worsened acutely 1 to 3 months after radiation with observer- and patient-reported scores, and gradually recovered by 1 year (104). In a subsequent report with more than 6 years of median follow-up, excellent long-term patient-reported swallowing was demonstrated when pharyngeal constrictor and parotid sparing IMRT was performed (102). HRQOL was reported as stable or improved at 2 years, and new late toxicities beyond 2 years were uncommon. Eleven percent and 14% of patients reported "moderate" or "severe" long-term worsening in HNQOL pain and overall other domains, respectively, which were shown to be associated with higher mean radiation dose to the cervical esophagus, larynx, and pharyngeal constrictors (102).

Bhide et al. retrospectively evaluated superior, middle, and inferior pharyngeal constrictor, and suprahyoid muscle radiation dose in 50 patients with HNC treated with induction chemotherapy followed by CRT (105). One-year clinician-graded swallowing toxicity and swallowing PROs using the MDADI was available for 37 patients. There was a significant correlation between observer-rated RTOG graded dysphagia and all MDADI parameters. At 1-year posttreatment, the investigators were not able to detect a statistically significant correlation between pharyngeal constrictor radiation dose and objective measurements of dysphagia and patient-reported MDADI parameters. However, the study was limited by its small sample size and retrospective grading of clinician-observed dysphagia.

Levendag et al. examined the relationship between pharyngeal constrictor radiation dose, observer-reported dysphagia, and patient-reported swallowing, using the EORTC-QLQ/H&N35 and MDADI, in 81 patients with OPC treated with CRT using both IMRT and 3DCRT (106). A dose-effect relationship was found with an increase in the probability of clinician-graded dysphagia of 19% for every 10-Gy increase in mean radiation dose above 55 Gy to the superior and middle pharyngeal constrictors. At a mean follow-up of 18 months, RTOG grade 3 and 4 dysphagia (determined from chart review) was found in 23% of patients, and poor swallowing outcomes reflected by a total MDADI score of ≤50 was found in 26% of patients. A significant correlation was also noted between observer-rated grade 3 and 4 dysphagia and MDADI total scores, such that MDADI scores of ≤50 were considered equivalent to clinician-graded 3 or 4 dysphagia. In addition, the scores of several EORTC-QLQ/H&N35 items (question 35 = swallowing liquids, 36 = pureed, 37 = solids) and the general MDADI was found to be associated with the superior and middle constrictor radiation dose, and the scores of EORTC-QLQ/H&N35 (questions 37 = swallowing solids and 38 = aspiration) were associated with radiation dose to the inferior constrictor.

Because swallowing involves more than the pharyngeal constrictors, the MD Anderson Head and Neck Cancer Symptom Working Group have sought to identify additional swallowing muscle dose thresholds for late radiation-induced dysphagia in a cohort of 300 OPC patients (107). These muscle groups include the inferior, middle, and superior constrictors, medial and lateral pterygoids, anterior and posterior digastrics, intrinsic tongue muscles, mylo/geniohyoid complex, genioglossus, masseter, buccinator, palatoglossus, and cricopharyngeus. In this cohort, 11% experienced late radiation-induced dysphagia. A recursive partitioning analysis was used to identify dose-volume data associated with late dysphagia. Investigators identified the mylo/geniohyoid complex (volume receiving ≥69 Gy, V69), genioglossus (V35), anterior digastric (V60), middle constrictor (V49), and superior constrictor (V70) dose thresholds to be associated with late dysphagia.

These interesting datasets informed the ongoing DARS trial (CRUK/14/014) from the Institute of Cancer Research in London (108). This prospective phase III randomized multicenter study is evaluating dysphagia-optimized intensity-modulated radiotherapy (Do-IMRT) versus standard intensity-modulated radiotherapy (S-IMRT) in patients with HNC to determine if optimizing the treatment plan to specific dose constraints to the pharyngeal constrictors with Do-IMRT will lead to an improvement in long-term swallowing function without an associated detriment on disease-specific survival. The primary end point of this trial is a patient-centered outcome using the difference in the mean MDADI composite score, measured at 1 year after radiation. Secondary end points include prospective and longitudinal evaluation of clinician-graded and patient-reported swallowing and QOL outcomes, locoregional control, and overall survival (108).

Swallowing QOL using MDADI data has also recently been assessed retrospectively using pooled data from three prospective HNC clinical trials of "de-intensification" in p16-positive OPC cancers (ECOG 3311, NRG HN002, and CRUK PATHOS) (109). MDADI was collected at baseline and at least one posttreatment interval available in the trial databases. The overall mean baseline MDADI composite score was 90.1, dropping to 74.6 at 6 months posttreatment (p <.0001), and rising to 78.5 (p <.0001) and 83.1 (p = .002) at 12 and 24 months, respectively, relative to baseline. This represented a clinically meaningful decline in MDADI scores at 6 months that partially recovered by 24 months (6 vs. 24 months, p = .05). Poor MDADI scores (defined as composite score <60) were reported in only 4%, 11%, 15%, and 9% of patients at baseline and at 6, 12, and 24 months, respectively. This analysis is important as it is the first to define baseline and posttreatment MDADI scores in HPV-positive low-risk OPC patients, some of whom were treated with dose de-escalated IMRT, and has helped to inform PRO primary end point hypotheses for de-intensification studies in this population (Table 26.4).

IMPACT OF SURGERY AND SURGICAL TECHNIQUE ON SWALLOWING-RELATED QOL

Comparison of swallowing outcomes between CRT and surgery, with respect to swallowing-related QOL, are difficult given the lack of randomized studies. Attempts to compare primary CRT to primary surgery in randomized trials have either been underpowered or failed to accrue (110,111). In a systematic review of QOL in HNC patients treated with surgical resection with or without adjuvant radiation, Rathod et al. performed a MEDLINE and EMBASE search and found 302 reports, of which 26 studies met quality criteria (112). Criteria included inclusion of a priori hypothesis (present in only 8%) accounting for missing data statistics (present in 8%), reporting of QOL time interval (performed in 35%), and providing rationale of the instrument selection (done in 53% of studies). QOL including physical/social functioning and symptom domains deteriorated with either surgery or radiation, with gradual recovery to baseline in both modalities. It is important to note that more extensive surgical resection was associated with worse QOL.

As such, increasing interest in transoral surgical techniques including transoral robotic surgery (TORS), transoral microsurgery (TLM), or conventional transoral surgery (CTOS) has emerged over the past decade for OPC with excellent disease control and promising swallowing-related QOL outcomes in single-institution retrospective observational studies (113–119). Patients undergoing transoral surgery for early-stage OPC have an initial drop in swallowing-related QOL in the immediate postoperative period, particularly affecting the global and physical subscales, with recovery of scores observed at 6 months and returning to baseline by 1 year (113–119). As a result of these small series showing promising disease control and swallowing outcomes, a number of phase II/III studies are currently evaluating transoral surgical techniques in good-risk OPC patients with the intent of decreasing long-term swallowing morbidity and improving QOL (Table 26.4).

EVALUATION OF SWALLOWING PROs ON RECENTLY CLOSED AND ONGOING PROSPECTIVE TRIALS

Swallowing PROs are currently being evaluated on several prospective, randomized, multi-institutional studies of treatment de-intensification in low-risk OPC. The general study designs include comparing cisplatin to the EGFR inhibitor cetuximab concurrently with radiation (120–122); assessing reduced dose radiation with or without chemotherapy either in the definitive setting (123) or postoperative setting after transoral surgery using TORS, TLM, or CTOS (124,125); and evaluating optimal radiation therapy versus optimal minimally invasive surgical techniques. The overarching goal of these trials is to achieve high survival, as well as excellent patient-reported swallowing and QOL for the individualized management of low-risk OPC. Because survival outcomes are expected to be equivalent on these studies, swallowing QOL primary end points have been designed for several of these efforts (ORATOR, CRUK-PATHOS and EORTC "Best of" trials). Table 26.4 summarizes these de-intensification trials.

NECK DISSECTION, SHOULDER FUNCTION, AND QOL

For patients with HNC undergoing neck dissection, shoulder dysfunction due to trauma to the spinal accessory nerve or resection of the sternocleidomastoid muscle has been shown to significantly impair the patient's shoulder function (57). There are several patient-reported shoulder-specific instruments to measure the effect of neck dissection on QOL including the 10-item Neck Dissection Impairment Index (NDII) (57), the 16-item Shoulder Disability Questionnaire (SDQ) (59), the 13-item Shoulder Pain Disability Index (SPDI) (58), the 30-item Disabilities of the Arm, Shoulder and Hand Questionnaire (DASH), and the 11-item shortened version *Quick*DASH (61,128), which specifically measures the effect of shoulder dysfunction on QOL (129). The UW-QOL version 4 contains one question pertaining to shoulder function and is also an effective screening tool to measure patient-reported neck stiffness, pain, weakness, or change in work/hobbies related to shoulder problems (130). A double-blinded randomized study of the extent of supraomohyoid neck dissection comparing level IIa versus IIb dissections in 57 patients with stage T1 or T2 clinically node negative oral cavity cancer demonstrated both functional and QOL changes associated with the extent of dissection using electromyography, nerve conduction studies, the shoulder domain of the UW-QOL version 4, and the NDII, performed prior to surgery, 6 weeks after surgery, and then 6 months after surgery (131). The primary outcome was functional data from electromyography and nerve conduction studies of the trapezius muscle. Shoulder QOL was a secondary end point. A greater mean fall in trapezius muscle M-response was found in patients who had level IIb dissections indicating higher morbidity. The change in M-amplitude from baseline to 6 weeks, and from baseline to 6 months, was strongly associated with changes in shoulder-related QOL using the UW-QOL shoulder domain and the NDII.

In a cross-sectional survey of 181 patients with cT1-2 oral cavity cancer undergoing watchful waiting, sentinel lymph node biopsy, supraomohyoid neck dissection, or modified radical neck dissection, shoulder morbidity and health utilities were examined using the SDQ and the EQ-5D at any point after their treatment (132). Mean shoulder disability scores were progressively higher (or worse) after surgery (8.64, 10.57, 18.92, and 33.66), correlating with more extensive surgery (watchful waiting, sentinel lymph node biopsy, supraomohyoid neck dissection, and modified radical neck dissection, respectively). After adjusting for age, gender, and time since treatment, the corresponding EQ-5D mean health utilities were 0.804, 0.863, 0.834, and 0.794, respectively (a higher score indicating higher state of health). Patients with shoulder complaints had a lower mean health utility of 0.78, as compared to patients without shoulder complaints (0.90), and patients undergoing sentinel lymph node biopsy reported high health utility. These shoulder QOL data support less invasive neck surgery if oncologic outcomes can be maintained.

VOICE-RELATED QOL IN PATIENTS WITH LARYNGEAL CANCER

Patients with laryngeal and hypopharyngeal cancer have unique QOL concerns relating to voice, speech, and swallowing outcomes. In early-stage T1 glottic cancer, surgical (transoral microlaser excision) and radiation outcomes are thought to be equivalent in terms of local control, although no randomized data exist to validate this belief. As such, differences in QOL or PROs with each approach are of paramount importance. In a review of the literature on voice quality following definitive treatment for T1 glottic cancer, Greulich et al. identified 18 studies that used the Voice Handicap Index (VHI), a 30-item questionnaire, to evaluate voice outcomes after surgery or radiation (133). A meta-analysis was performed on eight of these studies, 362 patients in total, and demonstrated no significant differences in VHI scores between patients who received surgery versus those treated with radiation. Of the eight studies, two described improved voice quality following radiation, and none reported improved voice outcomes after resection (133).

In locally advanced laryngeal cancer, the VA Larynx Study (74,134) and RTOG 91-11 trial (99,135) both demonstrated that organ preservation using chemotherapy and radiation could be used instead of total laryngectomy in T3 and small volume T4 laryngeal cancer. In a prospective phase II study from the University of Michigan, 97 patients with locally advanced laryngeal cancer underwent induction chemotherapy for one cycle and then were assessed for response (136). Patients who were responders went onto CRT, while nonresponders were treated with immediate total laryngectomy. Comparisons of voice-related QOL were made between patients with an intact larynx, laryngectomy, and early versus late salvage laryngectomy. Further comparisons of the study population were also made with normative data (using published data from a population of facial cosmetic surgery patients without a known voice disorder). The 10-item Voice-Related QOL Measure (V-RQOL) was evaluated at least 8 months after treatment (49). Patients with an intact larynx had higher mean V-RQOL scores indicating better QOL, as compared to those receiving laryngectomy, although lower than normative data. Patients with intact larynx also experienced higher social-emotional (p = .007), and physical functioning (p = .03) scores compared to total laryngectomy (TL) patients. Patients with an intact larynx were also more likely to have high rates of oral intake alone without nutritional supplements. Patients with lower T3 stage, organ preservation, and longer duration since treatment all had significantly higher V-RQOL scores (136).

INTEGRATING WEB-BASED PLATFORMS AND ELECTRONIC TECHNOLOGY TO OBTAIN QOL ASSESSMENTS

Traditionally, QOL data have been collected in paper format. More recently, electronic and web-based platforms have been developed to facilitate the collection of PROs. Such technology allows patients to fill out questionnaires on computers or mobile devices, which has been demonstrated to improve compliance and reduce missing data on clinical trials (137). In practice, there is also increasing interest in using electronic PROs as part of routine cancer care, and in integrating PROs into existing electronic medical health records in order to obtain real-time patient-reported data, which may enhance clinical history and examination findings. Furthermore, real-time electronic PROs may improve communication between the patient and provider, allow providers to monitor longitudinal QOL, and potentially implement early intervention to mitigate any patient-reported side effects (90).

INTEGRATING QOL DATA INTO CLINICAL PRACTICE

A cross-sectional survey of oncologists from Canada, the United Kingdom, and the Australian clinical trials network was conducted to determine if QOL information from clinical trials was incorporated into clinical practice (138). With a 30% response rate representing 396 oncologists, 73% found trial QOL data to be valuable, but only 45% used the data to inform clinical practice and guide decision making, owing to the perceived barriers of lack of time, understanding, and generalizability of the results. Most respondents preferred the QOL data to be reported simultaneously in the same journal with the main trial results, and 39% of respondents felt confident in interpreting clinically meaningful change of QOL data. To improve integration of important QOL data into clinical decision making and routine practice, strategies are warranted to enhance dissemination, and to promote the interpretability and clinical relevance of the data combined with other outcomes.

PROs AND HNC SURVIVORSHIP

Improvements in multimodality therapy, as well as a rise in the incidence of low-risk HPV-related OPC, have enhanced the survivorship of patients with HNC. In addition to the treatment-related morbidity and changes in QOL already discussed in this chapter, sequelae from therapy, such as a tracheotomy, in HNC can lead to high levels of psychological distress, depression, and anxiety (139). Depression in patients with HNC has been noted to be as high as 19% in a SEER-Medicare cohort of 3,466 patients with HNC (140). In this series, patients with HNC were identified using ICD-O-3 (*International Classification of Diseases for Oncology*) codes, and depression was identified using ICD-9-CM (*International Classification of Diseases, Ninth Revision, Clinical Modification*) codes from Medicare claims. Patients who had a diagnosis of depression prior to cancer diagnosis had a 1.55 times greater hazard ratio (HR) of any death compared to patients who did not receive a diagnosis of depression. Patients who were diagnosed with depression after cancer diagnosis had 1.4 times greater HRof any death. For cancer-specific death, multivariate analysis showed that patients with a depression diagnosis, either before (HR 1.49; 95% CI, 1.27, 1.76) or after (HR 1.38; 95% CI, 1.16, 1.65) cancer diagnosis, were significantly associated with cancer death, compared to patients without depression.

Investigators from Princess Margaret Cancer Centre performed a retrospective cross-sectional survey of 158 patients with HNC at any point during their cancer survivorship course, using the 35-item patient-reported Cancer Survivors' Unmet Needs Measure (CaSUN) (141,142). They found 61% of patients reported at least one unmet need on the CaSUN. The mean number of unmet needs was 5.8 ± 8.9. The most common unmet needs were "I need to know that all my doctors talk to each other to coordinate my care" and "I need help to manage my concerns about the cancer coming back" in 32% and 26% of respondents, respectively. On multivariate analysis, factors associated with increased unmet needs in survivorship were younger age, earlier survivorship phase, and worse QOL. Similar findings were demonstrated in another retrospective multi-institutional cross-sectional survey of 597 patients with HNC in Australia. These investigators found that approximately 50% of patients reported having received little or no information regarding coping with stress and anxiety during survivorship, and 56% reported minimal information concerning psychosexual health or the availability of patient support groups (143).

Taken together, these data suggest that patients with HNC are often unprepared for the long-term lifestyle changes after therapy and perceive a lack of adequate information, support, and advice in the survivorship period (144). With increasing availability of Internet and electronic medical records, data obtained from QOL end points are informing the development of patient information packets to address these unmet needs and concerns of HNC survivors. There are also web-based QOL resources available to patients. Rogers et al. recently analyzed long-term UW-QOL data collected over a 19-year period from 2,624 patients with HNC in the United Kingdom (145). Data from this extensive cohort are divided into subgroups according to age, stage, disease, and treatment received. Through a novel interactive web-based platform (http://www.headandneckcancer.co.uk/For+patients/What+will+I+be+like.aspx), providers and patients can search the database on specific items including pain, appearance, activity, recreation, swallowing, chewing, speech, shoulder, taste, saliva, mood, and anxiety to determine patient-reported expectations of treatment using QOL data from patients who are matched for age, gender, site, stage of disease, and treatment received. However, with the plethora of web-based information available, it is often difficult to discern the scientific accuracy of HNC survivorship information (145). Best et al. used validated online health information instruments (146,147) and *Journal of the American Medical Association* (*JAMA*) benchmarking (148) to validate the accuracy of HNC website information (149). Only 40 of 160 websites ranked by Google were suitable for analysis, seven (17.5%) met *JAMA* benchmarks, and only 28 websites included reference to QOL factors and survivorship. The authors concluded that the quality of online health information for patients with HNC is highly variable, and that healthcare providers should continue to guide their patients in accessing useful and accurate online resources (149,150).

CONCLUSIONS

QOL and PROs in HNC have been extensively studied in single-institution and randomized multicenter clinical trials. Baseline and longitudinal QOL and patient-reported symptom burden in HNC provides prognostic information that may inform conventional survival end points, as well as survivorship from the patient's perspective. QOL and PROs may also be used to determine the superiority of different therapeutic approaches, when survival outcomes are expected to be equivalent, such as in the ongoing treatment "de-intensification" trials for HPV-related low-risk cancers. Further work is warranted to integrate QOL and PROs data into clinical decision making by healthcare providers and patients, as well as to incorporate PROs into routine clinical practice with the goal of potentially facilitating early therapeutic intervention. As information technology and electronic platforms evolve, a more seamless integration of QOL and PROs into standard practice and trial enrollment may improve the collection, analysis, and interpretation of QOL data in patients with HNC, and further promote patient-centered precision care.

REFERENCES

1. Constitution of the world health organization. http://www.Who.Int/governance/eb/who_constitution_en.Pdf.
2. Measuring quality of life. http://www.Who.Int/mental_health/media/68.Pdf.
3. Ringash J, Bernstein LJ, Cella D, et al. Outcomes toolbox for head and neck cancer research. *Head Neck*. 2015;37:425–439. doi:10.1002/hed.23561
4. Fleissig A, Jenkins V, Catt S, Fallowfield L. Multidisciplinary teams in cancer care: are they effective in the uk? *Lancet Oncol*. 2006;7:935–943. doi:10.1016/S1470-2045(06)70940-8

5. Shah BA, Qureshi MM, Jalisi S, et al. Analysis of decision making at a multidisciplinary head and neck tumor board incorporating evidence-based national cancer comprehensive network (NCCN) guidelines. *Pract Radiat Oncol.* 2016;6(4):248–254. doi:10.1016/j.prro.2015.11.006
6. Pignon JP, le Maitre A, Maillard E, Bourhis J. Meta-analysis of chemotherapy in head and neck cancer (mach-nc): an update on 93 randomised trials and 17,346 patients. *Radiother Oncol.* 2009;92:4–14. doi:10.1016/j.radonc.2009.04.014
7. Nguyen-Tan PF, Zhang Q, Ang KK, et al. Randomized phase iii trial to test accelerated versus standard fractionation in combination with concurrent cisplatin for head and neck carcinomas in the radiation therapy oncology group 0129 trial: long-term report of efficacy and toxicity. *J Clin Oncol.* 2014;32:3858–3866. doi:10.1200/jco.2014.55.3925
8. Ang KK, Zhang Q, Rosenthal DI, et al. Randomized phase iii trial of concurrent accelerated radiation plus cisplatin with or without cetuximab for stage iii to iv head and neck carcinoma: RTOG 0522. *J Clin Oncol.* 2014;32:2940–2950. doi:10.1200/jco.2013.53.5633
9. Haddad R, O'Neill A, Rabinowits G, et al. Induction chemotherapy followed by concurrent chemoradiotherapy (sequential chemoradiotherapy) versus concurrent chemoradiotherapy alone in locally advanced head and neck cancer (paradigm): a randomised phase 3 trial. *Lancet Oncol.* 2013;14:257–264. doi:10.1016/s1470-2045(13)70011-1
10. Rogers SN. Quality of life for head and neck cancer patients—has treatment planning altered? *Oral Oncol.* 2009;45:435–439. doi:10.1016/j.oraloncology.2008.11.006
11. Rogers SN. Improving quality-of-life questionnaires in head and neck cancer. *Expert Rev Qual LifeCancer Care.* 2016;1:61–71. doi:10.1080/23809000.2016.1142357
12. User's guide to implementing patient-reported outcomes assessment in clinical practice. http://www.Isoqol.Org/userfiles/file/usersguide.Pdf.
13. List MA, Siston A, Haraf D, et al. Quality of life and performance in advanced head and neck cancer patients on concomitant chemoradiotherapy: a prospective examination. *J Clin Oncol.* 1999;17:1020–1028. doi:10.1200/jco.1999.17.3.1020
14. List MA, Mumby P, Haraf D, et al. Performance and quality of life outcome in patients completing concomitant chemoradiotherapy protocols for head and neck cancer. *Qual Life Res.* 1997;6:274–284.
15. Xiao C, Hanlon A, Zhang Q, et al. Symptom clusters in patients with head and neck cancer receiving concurrent chemoradiotherapy. *Oral Oncol.* 2013;49:360–366. doi:10.1016/j.oraloncology.2012.10.004
16. Cleeland CS. Symptom burden: multiple symptoms and their impact as patient-reported outcomes. *J Natl Cancer Inst Monogr.* 2007;37:16–21. doi:10.1093/jncimonographs/lgm005
17. Denis F, Garaud P, Bardet E, et al. Late toxicity results of the GORTEC 94-01 randomized trial comparing radiotherapy with concomitant radiochemotherapy for advanced-stage oropharynx carcinoma: comparison of LENT/SOMA, RTOG/EORTC, and NCI-CTC scoring systems. *Int J Radiat Oncol Biol Phys.* 2003;55:93–98. doi:10.1016/s0360-3016(02)03819-1
18. Jensen K, Bonde Jensen A, Grau C. The relationship between observer-based toxicity scoring and patient assessed symptom severity after treatment for head and neck cancer. A correlative cross sectional study of the dahanca toxicity scoring system and the EORTC quality of life questionnaires. *Radiother Oncol.* 2006;78:298–305. doi:10.1016/j.radonc.2006.02.005
19. Ho KF, Farnell DJ, Routledge JA, et al. Comparison of patient-reported late treatment toxicity (LENT-SOMA) with quality of life (EORTC QLQ-C30 and QLQ-H&N35) assessment after head and neck radiotherapy. *Radiother Oncol.* 2010;97:270–275. doi:10.1016/j.radonc.2010.01.017
20. Quinten C, Maringwa J, Gotay CC, et al. Patient self-reports of symptoms and clinician ratings as predictors of overall cancer survival. *J Natl Cancer Inst.* 2011;103:1851–1858. doi:10.1093/jnci/djr485
21. Dueck AC, Mendoza TR, Mitchell SA, et al. Validity and reliability of the us national cancer institute's patient-reported outcomes version of the common terminology criteria for adverse events (pro-ctcae). *JAMA Oncol.* 2015;1:1051–1059. doi:10.1001/jamaoncol.2015.2639
22. Falchook AD, Green R, Knowles ME, et al. Comparison of patient- and practitioner-reported toxic effects associated with chemoradiotherapy for head and neck cancer. *JAMA Otolaryngol Head Neck Surg.* 2016;142:517–523. doi:10.1001/jamaoto.2016.0656
23. Walters SJ. *Quality of Life Outcomes in Clinical Trials and Health-Care Evaluation.* Chichester, UK: John Wiley & Sons, Ltd, Chichester, UK; 2009.
24. King MT. A point of minimal important difference (mid): a critique of terminology and methods. *Expert Rev Pharmacoecon Outcomes Res.* 2011;11:171–184. doi:10.1586/erp.11.9
25. Ringash J, O'Sullivan B, Bezjak A, Redelmeier DA. Interpreting clinically significant changes in patient-reported outcomes. *Cancer.* 2007;110:196–202. doi:10.1002/cncr.22799
26. Ringash J, Bezjak A, O'Sullivan B, Redelmeier DA. Interpreting differences in quality of life: the fact-h&n in laryngeal cancer patients. *Qual Life Res* 2004;13:725–733. doi:10.1023/b:qure.0000021703.47079.46
27. Cella D, Hahn EA, Dineen K. Meaningful change in cancer-specific quality of life scores: differences between improvement and worsening. *Qual Life Res* 2002;11:207–221.
28. Hutcheson KA, Barrow MP, Lisec A, et al. What is a clinically relevant difference in mdadi scores between groups of head and neck cancer patients? *Laryngoscope.* 2016;126:1108–1113. doi:10.1002/lary.25778
29. Aaronson NK, Ahmedzai S, Bergman B, et al. The European Organization for Research and Treatment of Cancer QLQ-C30: a quality-of-life instrument for use in international clinical trials in oncology. *J Natl Cancer Inst.* 1993;85:365–376. doi:10.1093/jnci/85.5.365
30. Cella DF, Tulsky DS, Gray G, et al. The functional assessment of cancer therapy scale: development and validation of the general measure. *J Clin Oncol.* 1993;11:570–579. doi:10.1200/jco.1993.11.3.570

31. D'Antonio LL, Zimmerman GJ, Cella DF, Long SA. Quality of life and functional status measures in patients with head and neck cancer. *Arch Otolaryngol Head Neck Surg*. 1996;122:482–487. doi:10.1001/archotol.1996.01890170018005
32. Hassan SJ, Weymuller EA Jr. Assessment of quality of life in head and neck cancer patients. *Head Neck*. 1993;15:485–496. doi:10.1002/hed.2880150603
33. Rosenthal DI, Mendoza TR, Chambers MS, et al. Measuring head and neck cancer symptom burden: the development and validation of the M. D. Anderson symptom inventory, head and neck module. *Head Neck*. 2007;29:923–931. doi:10.1002/hed.20602
34. Rosenthal DI, Mendoza TR, Chambers MS, et al. The M. D. Anderson symptom inventory-head and neck module, a patient-reported outcome instrument, accurately predicts the severity of radiation-induced mucositis. *Int J Radiat Oncol Biol Phys*. 2008;72:1355–1361. doi:10.1016/j.ijrobp.2008.02.072
35. Pearman TP, Beaumont JL, Paul D, et al. Evaluation of treatment- and disease-related symptoms in advanced head and neck cancer: validation of the national comprehensive cancer network-functional assessment of cancer therapy-head and neck cancer symptom index-22 (NFHNSI-22). *J Pain Symptom Manage*. 2013;46:113–120. doi:10.1016/j.jpainsymman.2012.06.004
36. Browman GP, Levine MN, Hodson DI, et al. The head and neck radiotherapy questionnaire: a morbidity/quality-of-life instrument for clinical trials of radiation therapy in locally advanced head and neck cancer. *J Clin Oncol*. 1993;11:863–872. doi:10.1200/jco.1993.11.5.863
37. About eq-5d. http://www.Euroqol.Org/about-eq-5d.Html.
38. Sherman AC, Simonton S, Adams DC, et al. Assessing quality of life in patients with head and neck cancer: cross-validation of the european organization for research and treatment of cancer (eortc) quality of life head and neck module (QLQ-H&N35). *Arch Otolaryngol Head Neck Surg*. 2000;126:459–467. doi:10.1001/archotol.126.4.459
39. Singer S, Araujo C, Arraras JI, et al. Measuring quality of life in patients with head and neck cancer: update of the EORTC QLQ-H&N module, phase III. *Head Neck*. 2015;37:1358–1367. doi:10.1002/hed.23762
40. Chera BS, Eisbruch A, Murphy BA, et al. Recommended patient-reported core set of symptoms to measure in head and neck cancer treatment trials. *J Natl Cancer Inst*. 2014;106(7). doi:10.1093/jnci/dju127.
41. Chen AY, Frankowski R, Bishop-Leone J, et al. The development and validation of a dysphagia-specific quality-of-life questionnaire for patients with head and neck cancer: the M. D. Anderson dysphagia inventory. *Arch Otolaryngol Head Neck Surg*. 2001;127:870–876. doi:ooa00162 [pii]
42. McHorney CA, Martin-Harris B, Robbins J, Rosenbek J. Clinical validity of the swal-qol and swal-care outcome tools with respect to bolus flow measures. *Dysphagia*. 2006;21:141–148. doi:10.1007/s00455-005-0026-9
43. Dwivedi RC, St Rose S, Roe JW, et al. Validation of the sydney swallow questionnaire (ssq) in a cohort of head and neck cancer patients. *Oral Oncol*. 2010;46:e10–e14. doi:10.1016/j.oraloncology.2010.02.004
44. Woisard V, Andrieux MP, Puech M. Validation of a self-assessment questionnaire for swallowing disorders (deglutition handicap index). *Rev Laryngol Otol Rhinol (Bord)*. 2006;127:315–325.
45. Silbergleit AK, Schultz L, Jacobson BH, et al. The dysphagia handicap index: development and validation. *Dysphagia*. 2012;27:46–52. doi:10.1007/s00455-011-9336-2
46. Timmerman AA, Speyer R, Heijnen BJ, Klijn-Zwijnenberg IR. Psychometric characteristics of health-related quality-of-life questionnaires in oropharyngeal dysphagia. *Dysphagia*. 2014;29:183–198. doi:10.1007/s00455-013-9511-8
47. Belafsky PC, Mouadeb DA, Rees CJ, et al. Validity and reliability of the eating assessment tool (EAT-10). *Ann Otol Rhinol Laryngol*. 2008;117:919–924. doi:10.1177/000348940811701210
48. Rosen CA, Lee AS, Osborne J, et al. Development and validation of the voice handicap index-10. *Laryngoscope*. 2004;114:1549–1556. doi:10.1097/00005537-200409000-00009
49. Hogikyan ND, Sethuraman G. Validation of an instrument to measure voice-related quality of life (V-RQOL). *J Voice*. 1999;13:557–569. doi:10.1016/s0892-1997(99)80010-1
50. Portone CR, Hapner ER, McGregor L, et al. Correlation of the voice handicap index (VHI) and the voice-related quality of life measure (V-RQOL). *J Voice*. 2007;21:723–727. doi:10.1016/j.jvoice.2006.06.001
51. Henson BS, Inglehart MR, Eisbruch A, Ship JA. Preserved salivary output and xerostomia-related quality of life in head and neck cancer patients receiving parotid-sparing radiotherapy. *Oral Oncol*. 2001;37:84–93. doi:10.1016/s1368-8375(00)00063-4
52. Finlay AY, Khan GK. Dermatology life quality index (DLQI)—a simple practical measure for routine clinical use. *Clin Exp Dermatol*. 1994;19:210–216. doi:10.1111/j.1365-2230.1994.tb01167.x
53. Wagner LI, Berg SR, Gandhi M, et al. The development of a functional assessment of cancer therapy (FACT) questionnaire to assess dermatologic symptoms associated with epidermal growth factor receptor inhibitors (FACT-EGFRI-18). *Support Care Cancer*. 2013;21:1033–1041. doi:10.1007/s00520-012-1623-4
54. Slade GD, Spencer AJ. Development and evaluation of the oral health impact profile. *Community Dent Health*. 1994;11:3–11.
55. Alvarez-Camacho M, Gonella S, Ghosh S, et al. The impact of taste and smell alterations on quality of life in head and neck cancer patients. *Qual Life Res*. 2016;25:1495–1504. doi:10.1007/s11136-015-1185-2
56. Newman CW, Weinstein BE, Jacobson GP, Hug GA. The hearing handicap inventory for adults: psychometric adequacy and audiometric correlates. *Ear Hear*. 1990;11:430–433. doi:10.1097/00003446-199012000-00004

57. Taylor RJ, Chepeha JC, Teknos TN, et al. Development and validation of the neck dissection impairment index: a quality of life measure. *Arch Otolaryngol Head Neck Surg.* 2002;128:44–49. doi:10.1001/archotol.128.1.44
58. Breckenridge JD, McAuley JH. Shoulder pain and disability index (SPADI). *J Physiother.* 2011;57:197. doi:10.1016/s1836-9553(11)70045-5
59. van der Heijden GJ, Leffers P, Bouter LM. Shoulder disability questionnaire design and responsiveness of a functional status measure. *J Clin Epidemiol.* 2000;53:29–38. doi:10.1016/s0895-4356(99)00078-5
60. Constant CR, Murley AH. A clinical method of functional assessment of the shoulder. *Clin Orthop Relat Res.* 1987;(214):160–164. doi:10.1097/00003086-198701000-00023
61. Hudak PL, Amadio PC, Bombardier C. Development of an upper extremity outcome measure: the DASH (disabilities of the arm, shoulder and hand) [corrected]. The upper extremity collaborative group (UECG). *Am J Ind Med.* 1996;29:602–608. doi:10.1002/(sici)1097-0274(199606)29:6<602::aid-ajim4>3.0.co;2-l
62. Fang FM, Chiu HC, Kuo WR, et al. Health-related quality of life for nasopharyngeal carcinoma patients with cancer-free survival after treatment. *Int J Radiat Oncol Biol Phys.* 2002;53:959–968. doi:10.1016/s0360-3016(02)02838-9
63. Tong MCF, Lo PSY, Wong KH, et al. Development and validation of the functional assessment of cancer therapy nasopharyngeal cancer subscale. *Head Neck-J Sci Spec.* 2009;31:738–747. doi:10.1002/hed.21023
64. Su Y, Mo CW, Cheng WQ, et al. Development and validation of quality of life scale of nasopharyngeal carcinoma patients: the QOL-NPC (version 2). *Health Qual Life Outcomes.* 2016;14:76. doi:10.1186/s12955-016-0480-0
65. NRG-HN001 protocol information. https://www.Rtog.Org/clinicaltrials/protocoltable/studydetails.Aspx?Study=1305.
66. McHorney CA, Robbins J, Lomax K, et al. The SWAL-QOL and SWAL-CARE outcomes tool for oropharyngeal dysphagia in adults: III. Documentation of reliability and validity. *Dysphagia.* 2002;17:97–114. doi:10.1007/s00455-001-0109-1
67. Quinten C, Coens C, Mauer M, et al. Baseline quality of life as a prognostic indicator of survival: A meta-analysis of individual patient data from eortc clinical trials. *Lancet Oncol.* 2009;10:865–871. doi:10.1016/s1470-2045(09)70200-1
68. van Nieuwenhuizen AJ, Buffart LM, Brug J, et al. The association between health related quality of life and survival in patients with head and neck cancer: a systematic review. *Oral Oncol.* 2015;51:1–11. doi:10.1016/j.oraloncology.2014.09.002
69. Siddiqui F, Pajak TF, Watkins-Bruner D, et al. Pretreatment quality of life predicts for locoregional control in head and neck cancer patients: a radiation therapy oncology group analysis. *Int J Radiat Oncol Biol Phys.* 2008;70:353–360. doi:10.1016/j.ijrobp.2007.06.024
70. Coyne JC, Pajak TF, Harris J, et al. Emotional well-being does not predict survival in head and neck cancer patients: a radiation therapy oncology group study. *Cancer.* 2007;110:2568–2575. doi:10.1002/cncr.23080
71. Xiao C, Zhang Q, Nguyen-Tan PF, et al. Quality of life and performance status from a substudy conducted within a prospective phase 3 randomized trial of concurrent standard radiation versus accelerated radiation plus cisplatin for locally advanced head and neck carcinoma: NRG oncology RTOG 0129. *Int J Radiat Oncol Biol Phys.* 2017;97:667–677. doi:10.1016/j.ijrobp.2016.07.020
72. Truong MT, Zhang Q, Rosenthal DI, et al. Quality of life and performance status from a substudy conducted within a prospective phase 3 randomized trial of concurrent accelerated radiation plus cisplatin with or without cetuximab for locally advanced head and neck carcinoma: NRG oncology radiation therapy oncology group 0522. *Int J Radiat Oncol Biol Phys.* 2017;97:687–699. doi:10.1016/j.ijrobp.2016.08.003
73. Ringash J, Waldron JN, Siu LL, et al. Quality of life and swallowing with standard chemoradiotherapy versus accelerated radiotherapy and panitumumab in locoregionally advanced carcinoma of the head and neck: a phase III randomised trial from the Canadian Cancer Trials Group (HN.6). *Eur J Cancer.* 2017;72:192–199. doi:10.1016/j.ejca.2016.11.008
74. Terrell JE, Fisher SG, Wolf GT. Long-term quality of life after treatment of laryngeal cancer. The Veterans Affairs Laryngeal Cancer Study Group. *Arch Otolaryngol Head Neck Surg.* 1998;124:964–971. doi:10.1001/archotol.124.9.964
75. Ringash J, Fisher R, Peters L, et al. Effect of p16 status on the quality-of-life experience during chemoradiation for locally advanced oropharyngeal cancer: a substudy of randomized trial trans-tasman radiation oncology group (TROG) 02.02 (headstart). *Int J Radiat Oncol Biol Phys.* 2017;97:678–686. doi:10.1016/j.ijrobp.2016.03.017
76. Ang KK, Harris J, Wheeler R, et al. Human papillomavirus and survival of patients with oropharyngeal cancer. *N Engl J Med.* 2010;363:24–35. doi:10.1056/nejmoa0912217
77. Fakhry C, Westra WH, Li S, et al. Improved survival of patients with human papillomavirus-positive head and neck squamous cell carcinoma in a prospective clinical trial. *J Natl Cancer Inst.* 2008;100:261–269. doi:10.1093/jnci/djn011
78. Gillison ML, Koch WM, Capone RB, et al. Evidence for a causal association between human papillomavirus and a subset of head and neck cancers. *J Natl Cancer Inst.* 2000;92:709–720.
79. Lassen P, Eriksen JG, Krogdahl A, et al. The influence of hpv-associated p16-expression on accelerated fractionated radiotherapy in head and neck cancer: evaluation of the randomised DAHANCA 6&7 trial. *Radiother Oncol.* 2011;100:49–55. doi:10.1016/j.radonc.2011.02.010

80. Posner MR, Lorch JH, Goloubeva O, et al. Survival and human papillomavirus in oropharynx cancer in tax 324: a subset analysis from an international Phase III trial. *Ann Oncol.* 2011;22:1071–1077. doi:10.1093/annonc/mdr006
81. Rischin D, Young RJ, Fisher R, et al. Prognostic significance of p16ink4a and human papillomavirus in patients with oropharyngeal cancer treated on trog 02.02 Phase III trial. *J Clin Oncol.* 2010;28:4142–4148. doi:10.1200/jco.2010.29.2904
82. Canis M, Weiss BG, Ihler F, et al. Quality of life in patients after resection of pt3 lateral tongue carcinoma: microvascular reconstruction versus primary closure. *Head Neck.* 2016;38:89–94. doi:10.1002/hed.23862
83. Fang FM, Tsai WL, Chien CY, et al. Pretreatment quality of life as a predictor of distant metastasis and survival for patients with nasopharyngeal carcinoma. *J Clin Oncol.* 2010;28:4384–4389. doi:10.1200/jco.2010.28.8324
84. Tsai WL, Chien CY, Huang HY, et al. Prognostic value of quality of life measured after treatment on subsequent survival in patients with nasopharyngeal carcinoma. *Qual Life Res.* 2013;22:715–723. doi:10.1007/s11136-012-0213-8
85. Nutting CM, Morden JP, Harrington KJ, et al. Parotid-sparing intensity modulated versus conventional radiotherapy in head and neck cancer (parsport): a phase 3 multicentre randomised controlled trial. *Lancet Oncol.* 2011;12:127–136. doi:10.1016/s1470-2045(10)70290-4
86. Pow EH, Kwong DL, McMillan AS, et al. Xerostomia and quality of life after intensity-modulated radiotherapy vs. Conventional radiotherapy for early-stage nasopharyngeal carcinoma: initial report on a randomized controlled clinical trial. *Int J Radiat Oncol Biol Phys.* 2006;66:981–991. doi:10.1016/j.ijrobp.2006.06.013
87. Rathod S, Gupta T, Ghosh-Laskar S, et al. Quality-of-life (qol) outcomes in patients with head and neck squamous cell carcinoma (hnscc) treated with intensity-modulated radiation therapy (imrt) compared to three-dimensional conformal radiotherapy (3d-crt): evidence from a prospective randomized study. *Oral Oncol.* 2013;49:634–642. doi:10.1016/j.oraloncology.2013.02.013
88. Gulliford SL, Miah AB, Brennan S, et al. Dosimetric explanations of fatigue in head and neck radiotherapy: an analysis from the parsport phase iii trial. *Radiother Oncol.* 2012;104:205–212. doi:10.1016/j.radonc.2012.07.005
89. Powell C, Schick U, Morden JP, et al. Fatigue during chemoradiotherapy for nasopharyngeal cancer and its relationship to radiation dose distribution in the brain. *Radiother Oncol.* 2014;110:416–421. doi:10.1016/j.radonc.2013.06.042
90. Niska JR, Halyard MY, Tan AD, et al. Electronic patient-reported outcomes and toxicities during radiotherapy for head-and-neck cancer. *Qual Life Res.* 2017;26(7):1721–1731. doi:10.1007/s11136-017-1528-2
91. Carr AJ, Gibson B, Robinson PG. Measuring quality of life: Is quality of life determined by expectations or experience? *BMJ.* 2001;322:1240–1243. doi:10.1136/bmj.322.7296.1240
92. Pow EH, Kwong DL, Sham JS, et al. Can intensity-modulated radiotherapy preserve oral health-related quality of life of nasopharyngeal carcinoma patients? *Int J Radiat Oncol Biol Phys.* 2012;83:e213–e221. doi:10.1016/j.ijrobp.2011.12.040
93. Yang H, Hu W, Wang W, et al. Replanning during intensity modulated radiation therapy improved quality of life in patients with nasopharyngeal carcinoma. *Int J Radiat Oncol Biol Phys.* 2013;85:e47–e54. doi:10.1016/j.ijrobp.2012.09.033
94. Fang FM, Chien CY, Tsai WL, et al. Quality of life and survival outcome for patients with nasopharyngeal carcinoma receiving three-dimensional conformal radiotherapy vs. intensity-modulated radiotherapy—a longitudinal study. *Int J Radiat Oncol Biol Phys.* 2008;72:356–364. doi:10.1016/j.ijrobp.2007.12.054
95. Liu K, Han Y, Ma B. The study of clinical long-term effect and prognostic factors in nasopharyngeal carcinoma after intensity modulated radiation therapy. *Lin Chung Er Bi Yan Hou Tou Jing Wai Ke Za Zhi.* 2013;27:1177–1183.
96. Kohler RE, Sheets NC, Wheeler SB, et al. Two-year and lifetime cost-effectiveness of intensity modulated radiation therapy versus 3-dimensional conformal radiation therapy for head-and-neck cancer. *Int J Radiat Oncol Biol Phys.* 2013;87:683–689. doi:10.1016/j.ijrobp.2013.08.011
97. Sio TT, Lin HK, Shi Q, et al. Intensity modulated proton therapy versus intensity modulated photon radiation therapy for oropharyngeal cancer: first comparative results of patient-reported outcomes. *Int J Radiat Oncol Biol Phys.* 2016;95:1107–1114. doi:10.1016/j.ijrobp.2016.02.044
98. Cooper JS, Zhang Q, Pajak TF, et al. Long-term follow-up of the RTOG 9501/intergroup phase iii trial: postoperative concurrent radiation therapy and chemotherapy in high-risk squamous cell carcinoma of the head and neck. *Int J Radiat Oncol Biol Phys.* 2012;84:1198–1205. doi:10.1016/j.ijrobp.2012.05.008
99. Forastiere AA, Zhang Q, Weber RS, et al. Long-term results of RTOG 91-11: a comparison of three nonsurgical treatment strategies to preserve the larynx in patients with locally advanced larynx cancer. *J Clin Oncol.* 2013;31:845–852. doi:10.1200/jco.2012.43.6097
100. Dwivedi RC, St Rose S, Chisholm EJ, et al. Evaluation of swallowing by Sydney Swallow Questionnaire (SSQ) in oral and oropharyngeal cancer patients treated with primary surgery. *Dysphagia.* 2012;27:491–497. doi:10.1007/s00455-012-9395-z
101. Feng FY, Kim HM, Lyden TH, et al. Intensity-modulated radiotherapy of head and neck cancer aiming to reduce dysphagia: early dose-effect relationships for the swallowing structures. *Int J Radiat Oncol Biol Phys.* 2007;68:1289–1298. doi:10.1016/j.ijrobp.2007.02.049

102. Vainshtein JM, Moon DH, Feng FY, et al. Long-term quality of life after swallowing and salivary-sparing chemo-intensity modulated radiation therapy in survivors of human papillomavirus-related oropharyngeal cancer. *Int J Radiat Oncol Biol Phys.* 2015;91:925–933. doi:10.1016/j.ijrobp.2014.12.045
103. Eisbruch A, Kim HM, Feng FY, et al. Chemo-imrt of oropharyngeal cancer aiming to reduce dysphagia: swallowing organs late complication probabilities and dosimetric correlates. *Int J Radiat Oncol Biol Phys* 2011;81:e93–e99. doi:10.1016/j.ijrobp.2010.12.067
104. Feng FY, Kim HM, Lyden TH, et al. Intensity-modulated chemoradiotherapy aiming to reduce dysphagia in patients with oropharyngeal cancer: clinical and functional results. *J Clin Oncol.* 2010;28:2732–2738. doi:10.1200/jco.2009.24.6199
105. Bhide SA, Gulliford S, Kazi R, et al. Correlation between dose to the pharyngeal constrictors and patient quality of life and late dysphagia following chemo-IMRT for head and neck cancer. *Radiother Oncol.* 2009;93:539–544. doi:10.1016/j.radonc.2009.09.017
106. Levendag PC, Teguh DN, Voet P, et al. Dysphagia disorders in patients with cancer of the oropharynx are significantly affected by the radiation therapy dose to the superior and middle constrictor muscle: a dose-effect relationship. *Radiother Oncol.* 2007;85:64–73. doi:10.1016/j.radonc.2007.07.009
107. MD Anderson head and neck cancer symptom working group. Beyond mean pharyngeal constrictor dose for beam path toxicity in non-target swallowing muscles: dose-volume correlates of chronic radiation-associated dysphagia (rad) after oropharyngeal intensity modulated radiotherapy. *Radiother Oncol.* 2016;118:304–314.
108. Petkar I, Rooney K, Roe JW, et al. Dars: a Phase III randomised multicentre study of dysphagia- optimised intensity-modulated radiotherapy (DO-IMRT) versus standard intensity- modulated radiotherapy (s-IMRT) in head and neck cancer. *BMC Cancer.* 2016;16:770. doi:10.1186/s12885-016-2813-0
109. Goepfert RP, Lewin JS, Barrow MP, et al. Long-term, prospective performance of the md anderson dysphagia inventory in "low-intermediate risk" oropharyngeal carcinoma after intensity modulated radiation therapy. *Int J Radiat Oncol Biol Phys.* 2017;97:700–708. doi:10.1016/j.ijrobp.2016.06.010
110. Iyer NG, Tan DS, Tan VK, et al. Randomized trial comparing surgery and adjuvant radiotherapy versus concurrent chemoradiotherapy in patients with advanced, nonmetastatic squamous cell carcinoma of the head and neck: 10-year update and subset analysis. *Cancer.* 2015;121:1599–1607. doi:10.1002/cncr.29251
111. Soo KC, Tan EH, Wee J, et al. Surgery and adjuvant radiotherapy vs concurrent chemoradiotherapy in stage III/IV nonmetastatic squamous cell head and neck cancer: a randomised comparison. *Br J Cancer.* 2005;93:279–286. doi:10.1038/sj.bjc.6602696
112. Rathod S, Livergant J, Klein J, et al. A systematic review of quality of life in head and neck cancer treated with surgery with or without adjuvant treatment. *Oral Oncol.* 2015;51:888–900. doi:10.1016/j.oraloncology.2015.07.002
113. Hurtuk AM, Marcinow A, Agrawal A, et al. Quality-of-life outcomes in transoral robotic surgery. *Otolaryngol Head Neck Surg.* 2012;146:68–73. doi:10.1177/0194599811421298
114. Dziegielewski PT, Teknos TN, Durmus K, et al. Transoral robotic surgery for oropharyngeal cancer: long-term quality of life and functional outcomes. *JAMA Otolaryngol Head Neck Surg.* 2013;139:1099–1108. doi:10.1001/jamaoto.2013.2747
115. Choby GW, Kim J, Ling DC, et al. Transoral robotic surgery alone for oropharyngeal cancer: quality-of-life outcomes. *JAMA Otolaryngol Head Neck Surg.* 2015;141:499–504. doi:10.1001/jamaoto.2015.0347
116. Ling DC, Chapman BV, Kim J, et al. Oncologic outcomes and patient-reported quality of life in patients with oropharyngeal squamous cell carcinoma treated with definitive transoral robotic surgery versus definitive chemoradiation. *Oral Oncol.* 2016;61:41–46. doi:10.1016/j.oraloncology.2016.08.004
117. Sinclair CF, McColloch NL, Carroll WR, et al. Patient-perceived and objective functional outcomes following transoral robotic surgery for early oropharyngeal carcinoma. *Arch Otolaryngol Head Neck Surg.* 2011;137:1112–1116. doi:10.1001/archoto.2011.172
118. Funk GF, Karnell LH, Christensen AJ, et al. Comprehensive head and neck oncology health status assessment. *Head Neck.* 2003;25:561–575. doi:10.1002/hed.10245
119. Leonhardt FD, Quon H, Abrahao M, et al. Transoral robotic surgery for oropharyngeal carcinoma and its impact on patient-reported quality of life and function. *Head Neck.* 2012;34:146–154. doi:10.1002/hed.21688
120. Phase III trial of radiotherapy plus cetuximab versus chemoradiotherapy in hpv-associated oropharynx cancer. https://www.Rtog.Org/clinicaltrials/protocoltable/studydetails.Aspx?Study=1016.
121. Weekly cetuximab/rt vs weekly cisplatin/rt in hpv-associated oropharyngeal squamous cell carcinoma (hpvoropharynx). http://www.Trog.Com.Au/trog-1201-hpv.
122. Determination of epidermal growth factor receptor inhibitor (cetuximab) versus standard chemotherapy (cisplatin) early and late toxicity events in human papillomavirus positive oropharyngeal squamous cell carcinoma. http://www2.Warwick.Ac.Uk/fac/med/research/hscience/ctu/trials/cancer/deescalate.
123. NRG-HN002: a randomized phase ii trial for patients with p16 positive, non-smoking associated, locoregionally advanced oropharyngeal cancer, NCT02254278. https://www.Nrgoncology.Org/clinical-trials/nrg-hn002.
124. ECOG-ACRIN Cancer Research Group. E3311 Phase II randomized trial of transoral surgical resection followed by low-dose or standard-dose IMRT in resectable p16+ locally advanced oropharynx cancer.

http://ecog-acrin.Org/clinical-trials/e3311-educational-materials.
125. Owadally W, Hurt C, Timmins H, et al. Pathos: a Phase II/III trial of risk-stratified, reduced intensity adjuvant treatment in patients undergoing transoral surgery for human papillomavirus (HPV) positive oropharyngeal cancer. *BMC Cancer.* 2015;15:602. doi:10.1186/s12885-015-1598-x
126. Palma A. A Phase II randomized trial for early-stage squamous cell carcinoma of the oropharynx: Radiotherapy vs trans-oral robotic surgery (orator). 2016. https://clinicaltrials.Gov/ct2/show/nct01590355.
127. European Organisation for Research and Treatment of Cancer. Study assessing the "best of" radiotherapy vs the "best of" surgery in patients with oropharyngeal carcinoma (best of). 2016. https://clinicaltrials.Gov/ct2/show/nct02984410.
128. Goldstein DP, Ringash J, Irish JC, et al. Assessment of the disabilities of the arm, shoulder, and hand (DASH) questionnaire for use in patients after neck dissection for head and neck cancer. *Head Neck.* 2014;37:234–242. doi:10.1002/hed.23593
129. Goldstein DP, Ringash J, Bissada E, et al. Evaluation of shoulder disability questionnaires used for the assessment of shoulder disability after neck dissection for head and neck cancer. *Head Neck.* 2013;36:1453–1458. doi:10.1002/hed.23490
130. Rogers SN, Scott B, Lowe D. An evaluation of the shoulder domain of the university of washington quality of life scale. *Br J Oral Maxillofac Surg.* 2007;45:5–10. doi:10.1016/j.bjoms.2006.09.007
131. Parikh S, Tedman BM, Scott B, et al. A double blind randomised trial of iib or not iib neck dissections on electromyography, clinical examination, and questionnaire-based outcomes: a feasibility study. *Br J Oral Maxillofac Surg.* 2012;50:394–403. doi:10.1016/j.bjoms.2011.09.007
132. Govers TM, Schreuder WH, Klop WM, et al. Quality of life after different procedures for regional control in oral cancer patients: cross-sectional survey. *Clin Otolaryngol.* 2016;41:228–233. doi:10.1111/coa.12502
133. Greulich MT, Parker NP, Lee P, et al. Voice outcomes following radiation versus laser microsurgery for t1 glottic carcinoma: systematic review and meta-analysis. *Otolaryngol Head Neck Surg.* 2015;152:811–819. doi:10.1177/0194599815577103
134. Wolf GT, Fisher SG, Hong WK, et al. Induction chemotherapy plus radiation compared with surgery plus radiation in patients with advanced laryngeal cancer. *N Engl J Med* 1991;324:1685–1690.
135. Forastiere AA, Goepfert H, Maor M, et al. Concurrent chemotherapy and radiotherapy for organ preservation in advanced laryngeal cancer. *N Engl J Med.* 2003;349:2091–2098. doi:10.1056/nejmoa031317
136. Fung K, Lyden TH, Lee J, et al. Voice and swallowing outcomes of an organ-preservation trial for advanced laryngeal cancer. *Int J Radiat Oncol Biol Phys.* 2005;63:1395–1399. doi:10.1016/j.ijrobp.2005.05.004
137. Movsas B, Hunt D, Watkins-Bruner D, et al. Can electronic web-based technology improve quality of life data collection? Analysis of radiation therapy oncology group 0828. *Pract Radiat Oncol.* 2014;4:187–191. doi:10.1016/j.prro.2013.07.014
138. Rouette J, Blazeby J, King M, et al. Integrating health-related quality of life findings from randomized clinical trials into practice: an international study of oncologists' perspectives. *Qual Life Res.* 2015;24:1317–1325. doi:10.1007/s11136-014-0871-9
139. Ninu MB, Miccinesi G, Bulli F, et al. Psychological distress and health-related quality of life among head and neck cancer patients during the first year after treatment. *Tumori.* 2016;102:96–102. doi:10.5301/tj.5000448
140. Rieke K, Schmid KK, Lydiatt W, et al. Depression and survival in head and neck cancer patients. *Oral Oncol.* 2017;65:76–82. doi:10.1016/j.oraloncology.2016.12.014
141. Giuliani M, McQuestion M, Jones J, et al. Prevalence and nature of survivorship needs in patients with head and neck cancer. *Head Neck* 2016;38:1097–1103. doi:10.1002/hed.24411
142. Hodgkinson K, Butow P, Hunt GE, et al. The development and evaluation of a measure to assess cancer survivors' unmet supportive care needs: The casun (cancer survivors' unmet needs measure). *Psychooncology.* 2007;16:796–804. doi:10.1002/pon.1137
143. Jabbour J, Milross C, Sundaresan P, et al. Education and support needs in patients with head and neck cancer: a multi-institutional survey. *Cancer.* 2017;123(11):1949–1957. doi:10.1002/cncr.30535
144. Newell R, Ziegler L, Stafford N, Lewin RJ. The information needs of head and neck cancer patients prior to surgery. *Ann R Coll Surg Engl.* 2004;86:407–410. doi:10.1308/147870804722
145. Rogers SN, Hogg ES, Cheung WK, et al. The use of health related quality of life data to produce information sheets for patients with head and neck cancer. *Ann R Coll Surg Engl.* 2015;97:359–363. doi:10.1308/003588415x14181254789448
146. Minervation validation instrument for health care web sites. http://www.minervation.com/wp-content/uploads/2011/04/Minervation-LIDA-instrument-v1-2.pdf.
147. Charnock D, Shepperd S. Learning to discern online: applying an appraisal tool to health websites in a workshop setting. *Health Educ Res.* 2004;19:440–446. doi:10.1093/her/cyg046
148. Silberg WM, Lundberg GD, Musacchio RA. Assessing, controlling, and assuring the quality of medical information on the internet: caveant lector et viewor–let the reader and viewer beware. *JAMA.* 1997;277:1244–1245.
149. Best J, Muzaffar J, Mitchell-Innes A. Quality of information available via the internet for patients with head and neck cancer: are we improving? *Eur Arch Otorhinolaryngol.* 2015;272:3499–3505. doi:10.1007/s00405-014-3349-z
150. Ni Riordain R, McCreary C. Head and neck cancer information on the internet: type, accuracy and content. *Oral Oncol.* 2009;45:675–677. doi:10.1016/j.oraloncology.2008.10.006

27

Management of Head and Neck Cancers in the Elderly

Jessica L. Geiger
Julie E. Bauman

Tobacco and alcohol use and persistent oral human papillomavirus (HPV) infection are well-established, important risk factors for the development of head and neck cancer (HNC). Previous irradiation to the head and neck region, occupational exposure, poor oral hygiene, and chronological age are other considerations that may contribute to HNC carcinogenesis. The molecular, cellular, and physiologic changes that impact the natural aging process influence the development of cancer, including the concepts of free radical formation and cellular senescence (1,2). Similarly, these age-related changes not only influence the behavior of cancer and its response to therapy, but the underlying frailty of the patient, therefore posing unique and often complicated challenges in caring for the elderly cancer patient.

Although there is no consensus on the definition of an elderly patient, the chronological age of 65 years or more is generally accepted (3). The percentage of elderly people in the Western Hemisphere is gradually increasing, and the number of adults aged 65 years or more is expected to more than double to over 88 million in 2050 according to the U.S. Census Bureau (4). As such, the number of people annually diagnosed with cancer is expected to increase significantly since most malignancies are age-dependent. This holds true for HNC: Among patients aged 65 and older, the incidence of cancers of the larynx, pharynx, and oral cavity are projected to increase from 27,000 in 2010 to 44,000 in 2030 (5). Even without the projected increase in number of HNC cases in the coming decades, approximately 25% of current HNC patients fall into the elderly category based on chronological age in a number of studies (6–8).

Approximately two thirds of all HNC patients present with locoregionally advanced disease (9), requiring aggressive curative-intent therapy that warrants multidisciplinary care and multimodal treatment consisting of a combination of surgical resection, radiation therapy, and systemic chemotherapy. Despite the high numbers of elderly patients presenting with HNC, there are no defined treatment paradigms for this patient population, and numerous studies show elderly patients with HNC are less likely to receive curative therapy compared with younger patients based on age alone (10–12). Furthermore, elderly patients are frequently underrepresented in clinical trials. This is despite a median age of 65 years for patients diagnosed with cancer of the larynx from 2009 to 2013 according to the Surveillance, Epidemiology and End Results (SEER) database (13). In the two large cooperative groups studies that established trimodality therapy for locally advanced HNC, the median age for patients enrolled was 57 years, and less than 5% of patients were over the age of 70 (14,15). Many trials include an upper age limit for enrollment of 70 years old, although one-fourth of patients with HNC are older than 70 (7).

The treatment of HNC has evolved over the past several years, from minimally invasive surgical techniques to intensity-modulated radiation therapy (IMRT) to molecular and immune-targeted systemic therapies. These improvements have benefited patients of all ages, and ongoing research seeks to improve outcomes in this disease while also minimizing treatment-related toxicities. The purpose of this chapter is to highlight important aspects unique to the care of elderly patients and to inform the reader of recent strategies in the management of HNC in this patient population.

ASSESSING THE ELDERLY PATIENT

Although chronological age is recognized as a risk factor for the development of many cancers, including HNC, the exact impact of age as a prognostic factor is unclear. Factors related to advanced age that may potentially lead to increased cancer incidence include cumulative environmental exposures, deficient DNA repair mechanisms, reduced immune surveillance, and increased mutation rate (16). Elderly patients with HNC are also more likely to have a second primary malignancy compared with younger patients (17,18). However, a SEER database analysis of patients with HNC revealed no statistically significant difference in overall or disease-specific survival in patients with respect to age when stratified by stage (19). Additional retrospective and prospective data also support similar survival outcomes in elderly patients compared with younger patients (20–22). This suggests other factors may be more relevant criteria to consider than simply chronological age when approaching treatment of HNC in elderly patients (23). Such factors include frailty, the presence and severity of medical comorbid conditions, nutrition, the presence of certain geriatric syndromes, socioeconomic issues, polypharmacy, and overall functional status. Together, these factors are included in the Comprehensive Geriatric Assessment (CGA), as seen in Table 27.1. The CGA is a multidimensional clinical tool used to assess physiologic reserve and identify limitations of an elderly person in order to develop a coordinated treatment plan in effort to maximize overall health (24,25). This instrument better describes a "functional" age—a significant parameter for treatment planning that should be considered when making decisions regarding treatment—rather than the chronological age of the patient.

TABLE 27.1

Components of the Comprehensive Geriatric Assessment (CGA)

Functional Capacity	Cognition
Mood	Polypharmacy
Social support	Financial concerns
Goals of care	Nutrition/weight change
Living situation	Dentition
Comorbid conditions	Geriatric syndromes

Source: Adapted from Stuck AE, Siu AL, Wieland GD, et al. Comprehensive geriatric assessment: a meta-analysis of controlled trials. *Lancet*. 1993;342(8878):1032–1036.

Frailty is a condition used to describe the severe decline in physiologic reserve that renders the patient unable to tolerate any further stress. The phenotype of frailty is based upon a clinical assessment of various health measurements such as weakness, endurance, and activity levels as measured by grip strength, walking time, and self-reported level of exhaustion, among other factors (26).

Medical comorbid conditions are defined as the presence of additional concurrent illnesses and disorders that are independent of the patient's underlying disease for which treatment is sought (27). The presence, type, and severity of comorbidity may impact the selection and administration of treatment and overall prognosis in elderly HNC patients, as suggested by several studies (28–30). Several instruments have been studied and validated to assess the effect of individual comorbid conditions on overall survival. One such instrument, the Charlson Comorbidity Index (Table 27.2), assigns an individual score to various conditions depending on the risk of dying associated with each one. The sum total is then calculated to predict the 1-year mortality for that patient (31). Another model, proposed by Hurria and colleagues, has been used to objectively assess the risk for chemotherapy toxicity in elderly cancer patients by balancing comorbid conditions and potential adverse effects related to treatment (32). These tools are utilized to help

TABLE 27.2

Charlson Comorbidity Index

Condition	Assigned Weights for Diseases
Myocardial infarction	1
Heart failure	1
Cerebrovascular disease	1
Dementia	1
Chronic pulmonary disease	1
Connective tissue disease	1
Ulcer disease	1
Mild liver disease	1
Diabetes	1
Hemiplegia	2
Moderate/severe renal disease	2
Diabetes with end-organ damage	2
Any tumor	2
Leukemia	2
Lymphoma	2
Moderate/severe liver disease	3
Metastatic solid tumor	6
AIDS	6
Weighted comorbidity classes	
Low	0 points
Medium	1–2 points
High	3–4 points
Very high	≥5 points

predict those elderly patients who are more likely to have poor outcomes during and after HNC treatment due to other competing medical diseases and conditions.

Geriatric syndromes refer to common health conditions in older adults that do not fit into distinct organ-based categories and frequently have multiple underlying causes. Depression, delirium, and dementia are included in this description, in addition to falls, osteoporosis, and failure to thrive. The prevalence of such syndromes appears to be higher in elderly cancer patients than age-matched patients who do not have an underlying malignancy, and the presence of a geriatric syndrome negatively impacts overall survival (33).

Other considerations in the assessment of an elderly HNC patient include evaluation of nutritional status and socioeconomic issues. Unintentional weight loss is a marker of frailty, and malnutrition may be a substantial issue for older patients who live alone or in an institution and are unable to independently prepare meals. It is important to be aware of the patient's living situation as many elderly patients are also caring for a sick spouse, or may be widowed and living alone with little social support. Medical insurance coverage and other financial considerations may also factor into the decision of treatment.

Polypharmacy refers to the use of at least five prescription medications and is another important factor to consider within the elderly patient population (34). It is estimated that 50% of Medicare beneficiaries receive at least five medications (35). One study revealed this figure to be even higher with 84% of older adults with cancer receiving at least 5 prescription medications and 43% receiving at least 10 medications (36). Although the term "polypharmacy" typically does not refer to the use of over-the-counter medications or herbal supplements, the use of these products should also be documented as they may interact with prescribed medications and lead to adverse events. While the use of such products within the elderly patient population has increased from 14% in 1998 to 63% in 2010 (37,38), most patients do not routinely volunteer this information when questioned about medication use (39).

There are a number of reasons elderly patients are discordantly impacted by polypharmacy. First, older patients have physiologic changes in the metabolism of medications, which can lead to toxicity and adverse events if metabolic clearance is delayed, or ineffective therapy in the case of the administration of pro-drugs. Older patients may also have an increased sensitivity to common side effects of certain medications, such as opioids (40), which are commonly used in the management of HNC. The risk for drug-drug interactions is increased with polypharmacy, and the use of multiple medications may lead to difficulties with compliance or adherence. The latter is compounded by the potential for increased prevalence of baseline visual or cognitive difficulties in elderly patients, a factor not always considered in younger patients.

Finally, the overall functional status and reserve of an elderly patient play prominent roles in approaching the management of HNC. Functional status is sometimes assessed in terms of performance measures, utilizing such tools as the Karnofsky performance status or Eastern Cooperative Oncology Group (ECOG) performance status scales, but may also involve assessment of organ function, frailty, and presence of comorbid conditions (23). The ability to perform activities of daily living and other measurements of physical strength, such as a steady ambulatory gait and a strong hand grip, are predictors of survival, as demonstrated and accepted across many cultures, with patients who display these characteristics generally living longer than age-matched individuals who have lost these abilities (41–43).

All of the abovementioned factors must be considered when approaching the management of an elderly patient with HNC, whether in the curative setting or when the intention of therapy is palliative in nature. Many of these issues may be evaluated in all HNC patients regardless of age; however recognizing some of these special circumstances in an elderly patient is paramount to balancing the goal of therapy with overall quality of life and toxicities of treatment.

MODALITIES OF THERAPY IN THE ELDERLY HNC PATIENT

The approach to any HNC patient is almost always multidisciplinary in nature, involving head and neck surgeons, radiation oncologists, and medical oncologists; however, further specialties are just as crucial to the success of HNC treatment, including prophylactic and rehabilitative treatment of swallowing and speaking disorders by speech and language pathologists, nutritional support by dietitians and nutritionists, recognition and remediation of difficult social support by social workers, and often interventions by pain management specialists. The first step in management is to define the goal of therapy: curative or palliative. Regardless of therapeutic intention, the management of HNC in elderly patients is often much more complex than treatment in younger patients because of the high toxicity associated with locoregional therapy, frequently requiring a combination of two or more treatment modalities. Therefore, the optimal management strategy should be carefully considered in each individual elderly HNC patient to balance the benefits of cancer-directed therapy with the potential adverse effects to avoid toxicities and significant post-treatment clinical decline.

SURGERY

Surgery has been the backbone of HNC treatment in both early-stage resectable disease as well as locally advanced tumors where improvements and innovations in microsurgical technique have allowed for reconstructive procedures affording better clinical and cosmetic outcomes. Despite multiple studies indicating that a surgical approach in elderly patients is feasible, well-tolerated, and associated with good functional outcomes, such procedures are less often utilized when compared with younger patients with similar disease burden (12,44–46). Retrospective studies matching older HNC patients undergoing major head and neck surgery with a younger cohort have shown no difference in survival end points (47–49). The perioperative systemic complications following surgical resection are mixed, however, with a higher rate of cardiovascular pulmonary complications often found in elderly patients compared with younger patients (50,51).

Advances in minimally invasive surgery for HNC are being readily adopted to address the need for reduction in postoperative complications while maintaining adequate tumor resection and reducing collateral damage to the surrounding tissues. This is especially important in elderly patients, and may afford the opportunity for such patients to undergo a surgical resection who otherwise would be considered medically unfit to withstand surgical intervention. Such advances include microsurgical resection with use of robotic surgery or endoscopic laser procedures. The use of robotics in surgery began in the 1980s in the field of neurosurgery (52), and the da Vinci robot (Intuitive Surgical Inc., Sunnyvale, CA) was approved by the Food and Drug Administration (FDA) in 1997 for use in laparoscopic general surgery. In 2006, transoral robotic surgery (TORS) was utilized to resect tongue base tumors from three patients in the context of a prospective clinical trial (53). Shortly thereafter, supraglottic partial laryngectomies and radical tonsillectomies were performed, with no reported complications, and the authors noted improvement in surgical exposure and greater magnification with use of robotic technique (54,55). Since then, it is estimated that over 3 million patients have benefited from the use of robotic surgery in HNC. The current use of TORS in HNC at various sites of the upper aerodigestive tract has been well established and is considered a safe procedure with good functional and quality of life outcome measures as reported by many institutions (56–60). Other benefits of TORS are the reduced operation time and preservation of oropharyngeal function in a majority of cases. While the use of TORS is being actively investigated in several ongoing clinical trials, including a large cooperative group trial in efforts to reduce toxicity for HPV-related oropharyngeal cancer that has a better prognosis (NCT 01898494), its application in the elderly population is also attractive given the benefits of shorter operative times and better functional outcomes.

The surgical management of clinically node-negative HNC remains controversial, with many studies reporting the rate of occult metastasis at 20% to 30%, making lymph node dissection unnecessary in a majority of patients (61–64). The surgical morbidity associated with neck dissections is especially risky in elderly patients, and strategies to improve the complications associated with the surgical procedure are warranted. The omission of an elective neck dissection altogether is a consideration in the attempt to shorten duration of surgical time and lessen surgical complications; however, this decision runs the risk of undertreating such patients. The risk of undertreatment was highlighted in a French study involving 260 patients over the age of 80 with oral cavity cancer in which neck dissections were omitted in 69% of cases. In this study, 40% of patients with early-stage disease who did not have a neck dissection had disease recurrence in the neck nodes compared with only 6% of those who had undergone the procedure, demonstrating the undertreatment of a substantial number of patients (65).

One way to possibly overcome the risk of inadequately treating an elderly HNC patient while potentially avoiding an unnecessary surgical procedure is by performing the less morbid procedure of sentinel lymph node biopsy. While pretreatment imaging with various modalities such as CT, MRI, and PET may accurately clinically stage a majority of patients, there are imaging limitations regarding micrometastatic disease within small lymph nodes. Therefore, the sentinel lymph node biopsy may improve staging of lymph node metastatic disease histologically with better accuracy (66). Several studies reported diagnostic reliability of sentinel lymph node biopsy in patients with HNC, and a meta-analysis of 26 studies validated sentinel lymph node biopsy as a diagnostic technique to accurately stage regional metastatic disease (67).

The benefits seen in practical use of these minimally invasive surgical procedures are difficult to extrapolate to elderly HNC patients given the paucity of older patients included in these studies and reports. All of the 12 studies involving TORS currently open include elderly patients, but it remains to be seen whether patients with advanced age are actually accrued. Strategies to enroll such patients on clinical trials are encouraged.

Reconstructive surgery with microvascular free flaps has been shown to be feasible and safe in elderly HNC patients in multiple studies (68–70). Microvascular reconstructive surgery success rates are similar among all HNC patients regardless of age. However, postoperative complications (medical and surgical) are more prevalent in elderly HNC patients and may be directly related to the presence and severity of other comorbid conditions rather than age alone (45,71,72). One retrospective review of 53 patients with an average age of 85 years who were surgically treated for a head and neck malignancy at a tertiary care center revealed no perioperative deaths or failure of free flap reconstruction (73). Cardiovascular disease was the most common comorbid condition (43%), and the most prevalent postsurgical complications were cardiovascular (15%), infection (19%), and delirium (11%). Over three quarters of patients did not report any major limitations to their activities of daily living, and the authors concluded that age alone should not be a primary factor considered in the surgical management of HNC patients.

In summary, surgery as part of the treatment plan for elderly patients with HNC should involve careful consideration and selection of patients based on factors other than chronological age. Characteristics of surgery, such as type and extent of procedure and duration of anesthesia time, need to be considered along with patient factors, including presence and severity of other medical comorbid conditions, functional status, required rehabilitation, quality of life, and the patient's personal philosophy toward his or her own disease and treatment. The potential need for further adjuvant therapy must also be taken into consideration. These factors reiterate the importance of the multidisciplinary approach warranted in elderly patients with HNC, not only for successful treatment, but also to optimize recovery and minimize treatment-related toxicities.

RADIATION THERAPY

Radiation therapy is a mainstay in the treatment of HNC, whether in locally advanced disease with curative intention or in the recurrent/metastatic setting where palliation is desired. Particularly in HNC, the use of radiation therapy allows for high rates of locoregional control of disease while preserving organ function that would otherwise be compromised with surgical intervention, such as speaking or swallowing. Radiation therapy is often used as a single modality in the treatment of early-stage glottic and oropharyngeal HNC, and radiation with concurrent chemotherapy is the accepted standard of care for nonoperative, locally advanced disease (16). The most widely accepted conventional fractionation of 1.8 to 2.0 Gy per fraction is delivered daily over the course of 6 to 7 weeks depending upon the definitive or adjuvant setting, treating to a total dose of 66 to 70 Gy for macroscopic disease and 50 to 60 Gy for prophylactic therapy. Radiation delivery and technique have evolved over the last several years in an attempt to minimize toxicities associated with this treatment while maintaining efficacy.

Radiation-related toxicity is mainly the result of the irradiation of normal tissue surrounding gross tumor, and the most commonly reported toxicities include xerostomia, mucositis, dysphagia, and odynophagia leading to weight loss and malnutrition, dysgeusia, and radiation dermatitis. These toxicities can result in unplanned breaks in radiation treatment, resulting in lower locoregional control and survival rates among HNC patients (74). Treatment-related toxicities are of specific concern in elderly HNC patients who may be frail and have comorbid conditions heightening their susceptibility to toxicity. Several retrospective studies supporting the use of radiation therapy in elderly HNC patients demonstrate effectiveness of therapy while maintaining treatment tolerability in this population (6,75–77). There is no correlation seen between age and cancer-specific outcome in these studies, whereas disease site and tumor stage were predictive. Furthermore, increased age was not associated with an increased risk of locoregional recurrence or decreased survival, and there was no interaction seen between age and need for treatment interruption or delay or severity of toxicities, though older patients were often treated with lower doses of radiation therapy (77). Modified dosing of radiation therapy was specifically evaluated in a cohort of very elderly patients with HNC, in which 23 patients aged 90 to 96 years were treated with individually planned radiation therapy dosing based on the stage of the disease and overall performance status of the patient; radiation therapy was not modified solely by chronological age (78). Definitive radiation therapy was completed in all patients with tolerable side effects, and the authors concluded that definitive radiation in conventional fractionation schedules should be considered in the very elderly patient population who displayed a good performance status.

Still, other studies suggest acute toxicity from conventional radiation therapy may limit delivery in elderly HNC patients. One retrospective study demonstrated equivalent survival rates between elderly and younger HNC patients 2 years after treatment with radiation therapy, though patients older than 75 years had rapidly decreased survival rates within the first 2 years following radiation therapy, suggesting increased acute toxicity may have been a factor (75). This finding was also supported by the largest reported HNC toxicity database, which included 1589 HNC patients enrolled in European Organisation for Research and Treatment of Cancer (EORTC) trials with 20% of patients aged 65 years or more and 2% greater than 75 years old (79). While there were no significant differences regarding survival, weight loss, or late toxicity occurrence between age groups, older patients had significantly more severe functional acute toxicity when compared with younger patients. The concern for acute treatment-related toxicities may factor into physicians' recommendations for radiation therapy in the adjuvant setting, with a French study demonstrating that less than half of elderly HNC patients eligible for adjuvant radiation therapy, according to guidelines, actually received such treatment (65).

Other radiation techniques have evolved in an effort to minimize toxicities to surrounding tissues, such as IMRT, delivering high doses of radiation to specific volumes and structures while reducing the dose and toxicity to adjacent nontarget tissues. Critical organs including the spinal cord, brachial plexus, and salivary glands can be spared with this technique, with improvements in late treatment-related toxicities. The PARSPORT trial, a phase 3 randomized study comparing parotid-sparing IMRT to conventional radiation in 90 patients with HNC, demonstrated significantly lower incidences of xerostomia at 12 and 24 months in the IMRT group in addition to improved recovery of saliva secretion and quality of life assessments (80).

Although no survival differences were seen between IMRT and conventional radiation therapy in the elderly patient population (81), other radiation techniques have shown a survival advantage in the overall HNC population, including elderly patients. Accelerated or hyperfractionated radiation therapy are two methods often utilized together to reduce overall treatment time by delivering more fractions of radiation therapy daily. Both methods are attractive alternatives to conventional radiation therapy in elderly patients, and meta-analyses have shown advantages in overall survival and tumor control. However, they also demonstrated increased rates of severe treatment-related toxicities and lower compliance with treatment, and the survival benefit was greater in younger patients (82,83). Utilizing these techniques in a split course, however, may mitigate the increase in toxicities related to radiation therapy while preserving the overall survival benefit seen with this delivery method. The split-course, accelerated, hypofractionated radiation therapy regimen consists of delivering 60 to 72 Gy in 20 to 24 fractions separated by a midcourse break of several weeks, allowing for toxicity recovery and disease reassessment. This regimen, studied at a single institution in 65 patients in whom a continuous course of conventional radiation therapy was deemed too toxic, was shown to be a safe, well-tolerated, and effective method of achieving durable locoregional disease control in patients with advanced age and significant comorbid conditions (84).

Still another advancement in radiation therapy is stereotactic body radiation therapy (SBRT), which aims to deliver very high doses of radiation therapy over one to five fractions while protecting the surrounding tissue environment. SBRT targets macroscopic tumor without prophylactic irradiation of the surrounding tissue and is therefore effective for smaller tumors and well tolerated owing to smaller treatment volumes. This technique has been widely applied to previously treated head and neck tumors, demonstrating promising local control in patients with recurrent disease when further conventional radiation therapy is limited (85–87). The smaller target volumes coupled with the short course of treatment is attractive for patients with advanced age, many comorbid conditions, or overall poor performance status. This is an exciting area of research with seven actively recruiting clinical trials (at time of publication) studying SBRT in HNC as either a single modality of therapy (NCT02474368, NCT02388932), following surgery (NCT02516969), or in combination with a variety of systemic agents (NCT02110992, NCT02057107, NCT02158234, NCT0268453).

In summary, advances in the type of radiation and delivery techniques have led to improved survival and toxicity profiles in patients with HNC. Use of radiation therapy, whether in the adjuvant, definitive, or palliative setting, has been shown to be effective and well tolerated in elderly patients. Further studies of SBRT and newer techniques including proton therapy may afford even better options in elderly patients with HNC.

SYSTEMIC THERAPY

Conventional cytotoxic chemotherapy is used in HNC patients in different settings, including as a concurrent radiosensitizing agent during adjuvant or definitive radiation therapy, as an induction regimen prior to definitive management with surgery or radiation, or as palliative therapy in the unresectable recurrent/metastatic setting. A variety of chemotherapeutic agents has shown activity in HNC, including platinum agents, taxanes, and antimetabolites, and these agents can be used as single-modality treatment or in combination with radiation or other therapies. Cetuximab, a monoclonal antibody that targets epidermal growth factor receptor (EGFR), was approved in 2006 for use in HNC and added to the repertoire of systemic therapies in this disease (88). EGFR is overexpressed in almost all head and neck squamous cell carcinomas (HNSCC) and is associated with a poor prognosis (89,90). Yet another modality of therapy, immune checkpoint inhibitors, has recently been approved in the unresectable/metastatic setting for HNSCC, further adding to treatment options in HNC.

The addition of concurrent systemic therapy to definitive radiation is the standard of care for the nonoperative management of locally advanced HNC, demonstrating a survival benefit (88,91,92). The optimal concurrent regimen has not been defined, though high-dose bolus cisplatin (100 mg/m^2 on days 1, 22, and 43) is considered the preferred treatment (92,93). This regimen requires an excellent performance status and minimal comorbid conditions and may not be the best approach in elderly HNC patients given the additional toxicities cisplatin chemotherapy confers, including myelosuppression, acute kidney injury, stomatitis, nausea and vomiting, and ototoxicity. Furthermore, late toxicities such as cervical fibrosis, osteoradionecrosis, and feeding tube dependence are more frequently reported in older patients (94,95). Alternative dosing schedules of cisplatin (30–40 mg/m^2 weekly; 6 mg/m^2 daily) have been substituted for bolus dosing because of improved tolerance (96–99). Though there is no direct comparison, weekly dosing is considered a reasonable option in patients who may not tolerate high-dose administration. Still other cytotoxic chemotherapies, such as carboplatin and paclitaxel, have radiosensitizing properties and have been proposed as further alternative options for concurrent chemoradiotherapy (100,101). However, it is unclear if these agents are as effective as cisplatin in this setting, though they tend to be better tolerated (102,103). Whether the addition of chemotherapy to definitive radiation therapy in elderly patients is beneficial is also unclear. A large meta-analysis of 87 trials showed the magnitude of benefit is less in older patients (16). Conversely, Ward and colleagues concluded the majority of elderly patients (defined as age >70 years) with locoregionally advanced HNC treated with definitive radiation therapy also receive systemic therapy, the use of which is associated with improved overall survival (104).

Cetuximab, an EGFR-targeting monoclonal antibody, is approved for concurrent treatment with radiation therapy for locally advanced HNC based on results from the Bonner randomized trial, which demonstrated improvement in locoregional control and reduced mortality compared to radiation therapy alone in patients with locally advanced disease (88). It remains unclear if concurrent cetuximab and radiation therapy is as effective as concurrent chemoradiotherapy with cisplatin, but cetuximab appears to have less toxicity than bolus cisplatin. This is supported by the compliance rate of 93% of patients receiving the prescribed cetuximab dose with concurrent definitive radiation therapy compared to 85% of patients who received all three planned doses of cisplatin in the Intergroup trial and only 70% in the Radiation Therapy Oncology Group (RTOG) 91-11 trial (91,92). Although all studies included patients of advanced age, the median age of patients included in these trials was in the sixth decade, further highlighting the difficulty in applying these results to elderly HNC patients. The more favorable toxicity profile and higher compliance rate of cetuximab has led to a shift in practice patterns, with cetuximab being the second most common radiosensitizing agent utilized after cisplatin (19% vs. 49%) (105).

The addition of concurrent cisplatin chemotherapy to postoperative radiation therapy has been shown to improve outcomes in selected patients with locally advanced HNC (14,15), and a meta-analysis of these trials identified the subgroups of patients who benefited from cisplatin chemotherapy were those with positive surgical margins and/or extranodal extension (106). As expected, it can be difficult to administer the full dose of chemotherapy prescribed during concurrent adjuvant therapy, with only 61% compliance reported (15). As in the definitive setting, cetuximab is an attractive radiosensitizing agent that may be better tolerated in the adjuvant setting, though it is unknown if the addition of cetuximab to postoperative radiation therapy will lead to improved outcomes compared to postoperative radiation therapy alone. This question is currently being addressed in a large cooperative group study enrolling patients with pathologic intermediate risk disease (NCT00956007). Regardless of chemotherapeutic agent, the added benefits of chemotherapy to definitive or adjuvant radiation is difficult to determine based on the fact that older patients are underrepresented in clinical studies.

Systemic therapy is the main form of treatment in recurrent/metastatic HNC that is no longer amenable to curative surgical or radiation therapy approaches. Platinum-based chemotherapy utilizing either cisplatin or carboplatin often combining with 5-fluorouracil has long been the standard frontline therapy in patients with inoperable recurrent/metastatic disease, and the addition of cetuximab to this chemotherapy doublet was shown to improve overall survival when given as first-line treatment in this setting (107). This regimen affords a 36% response rate and a 3-month improvement in median overall survival compared to platinum–fluorouracil therapy alone. While the addition of cetuximab to platinum-based chemotherapy demonstrated improved survival, both the experimental arm and the standard control chemotherapy arm both displayed significant treatment-related toxicities with 82% of patients in the cetuximab arm experiencing grade 3 or 4 toxicities compared with 76% in the control arm. Furthermore, the survival benefits of the addition of cetuximab to platinum–fluorouracil chemotherapy are inconclusive in the 17% of patients in the study aged 65 older. A combination of carboplatin with a taxane is also an acceptable frontline alternative with a more favorable toxicity profile (108). An analysis of two large phase 3 randomized trials conducted by ECOG comparing platinum-based chemotherapy regimens in patients 70 years or older versus younger patients revealed similar objective response rates and median time to progression among the two age groups (22). Despite the lack of difference in survival end points, the elderly patient group had a significantly higher incidence of severe toxicities, leading the authors to conclude more studies are necessary in the effort to ameliorate toxicities related to treatment, especially in elderly HNC patients.

The advent of immunotherapy with use of checkpoint inhibitors in HNC has brought promising results to the field of HNC with the approval of two programmed cell death 1 (PD-1) monoclonal antibodies in the recurrent/metastatic setting after failure of platinum chemotherapy (109,110). In these studies, treatment with pembrolizumab or nivolumab was well tolerated with reported grade 3 or higher toxicities of 17% and 13%, respectively, compared with 35% of patients treated with standard single-agent therapy in the nivolumab trial. Again, elderly patients were underrepresented in the studies (only 5% of patients were aged ≥75 years in the nivolumab study), but the results of these studies coupled with the more favorable side effect profile is promising for the treatment of elderly HNC patients.

FUTURE DIRECTIONS

Elderly patients with HNC have unique challenges related to the treatment of their cancer, and the aging U.S. population coupled with historically limited enrollment of elderly patients in clinical trials justifies the need for further studies to improve treatment in this disease. An active area of research in the treatment of locally advanced HNC is a de-escalation of therapy in attempt to balance favorable survival outcomes with minimizing treatment-related toxicities. Several larger cooperative group trials are seeking to accomplish this in a variety of ways, whether reducing radiation therapy dose or utilizing better-tolerated radiosensitizing agents. Although such studies are attractive trial designs for all patients with HNC, they are especially attractive to elderly patients, for whom treatment-related toxicity is a prioritizing concern.

Specifically, in HPV-related locally advanced oropharynx cancer, an RTOG trial is directly comparing concurrent chemoradiotherapy with radiation therapy plus cetuximab as definitive therapy (NCT01302834), and NRG Oncology is evaluating a modestly reduced dose of definitive radiation therapy with weekly cisplatin versus a modestly accelerated reduced dose of radiation therapy (NCT02254278). An ECOG study is evaluating patients undergoing TORS followed by low-dose or standard dose radiation therapy with or without chemotherapy, also in the HPV-positive oropharynx HNC patients (NCT01898494). While HPV-related oropharynx cancer is typically seen in younger patients, the incidence of oropharyngeal squamous cell carcinoma is increasing among elderly patients in the United States, likely driven by HPV-associated cancers, as the incidence of tobacco-associated HNCs are decreasing for elderly patients (111). Therefore, clinical studies investigating improved therapeutic strategies for elderly patients with HPV-related HNC are justified.

CONCLUSIONS

Treatment recommendations for the care of elderly HNC patients remains challenging for head and neck surgeons, radiation oncologists, and medical oncologists alike. Although elderly patients may not be specifically excluded from large cooperative group, practice-changing studies, elderly HNC patients have been largely underrepresented in such trials to date. Reasons for this are vast and include poor performance status, presence of multiple comorbid conditions, physician bias, frailty, and polypharmacy, among others. As such, further studies in elderly HNC patients are warranted to provide more specific treatment guidelines. There are many factors that favor older-specific clinical trials, as outlined by Sarris and colleagues: targeting results focused on elderly population, improved study accrual, study goals of studying toxicity and organ function, and increased likelihood of treating oncologists to enroll older patients on studies (112). There are also many factors that go against having trials focused on elderly HNC patients, including limiting the participation of older patients in trials with aggressive or newly studied agents, competing trials, inappropriately supporting the current age bias, and increasing expenses of conducting clinical trials.

HNC treatment is complex and involves a multidisciplinary approach with the expertise of many different medical specialties and support services. When approaching the elderly patient with HNC, there are even more complexities and special considerations that affect decision making. Evaluation for the presence and severity of medical comorbid conditions, assessment of the frailty index, and determination of functional status are crucial parts of the comprehensive geriatric assessment, which should be completed in every elderly HNC patient. Goals of therapy should be clearly identified, and age of the patient alone should not be the sole factor influencing clinical decision making, especially in the curative setting. Adapting treatment to minimize toxicities in elderly patients is essential, and advances in surgical and radiation therapy techniques have improved outcomes in elderly patients while preserving organ function and reducing morbidities related to treatment. Newer systemic agents with a more favorable side effect profile, including targeted therapies and immunotherapy, have also expanded the treatment repertoire for HNC patients. Still, there remains room for improvement in all aspects of treatment, and new therapeutic approaches for elderly patients are ongoing.

REFERENCES

1. Coppé JP, Kauser K, Campisi J, Beauséjour CM. Secretion of vascular endothelial growth factor by primary human fibroblasts at senescence. *J Biol Chem*. 2006;281(40):29568–29574. doi:10.1074/jbc.M603307200
2. Hekimi S,Lapointe J, Wen Y. Taking a "good" look at free radicals in the aging process. *Trends Cell Biol*. 2011;21(10):569–576.
3. World Health Organisation. *Definition of an Older or Elderly Person*; 2010.
4. Vincent GK, Velkoff VA. *The Next Four Decades, The Older Population in the United States: 2010–2050*. Current Population Reports. Washington, DC: US Census Bureau; 2010:25–1138.
5. Smith BD, Smith GL, Hurria A, et al. Future of cancer incidence in the United States: burdens upon an aging, changing nation. *J Clin Oncol*. 2009;27(17):2758–2765.
6. Huang SH, O'Sullivan B, Waldron J, et al. Patterns of care in elderly head-and-neck cancer radiation oncology patients: a single-center cohort study. *Int J Radiat Oncol Biol Phys*. 2011;79(1):46–51.
7. Kruse AL, Bredell M, Luebbers HT, Grätz KW. Head and neck cancer in the elderly: a retrospective study over 10 years (1999–2008). *Head Neck Oncol*. 2010;2:25.
8. Syrigos KN, Karachalios D, Karapanagiotou EM, et al. Head and neck cancer in the elderly: an overview on the treatment modalities. *Cancer Treat Rev*. 2009;35(3):237–245.
9. Argiris A, Eng C. Epidemiology, staging, and screening of head and neck cancer. *Cancer Treat Res*. 2003;114:15–60.
10. Bernardi D, Barzan L, Franchin G, et al. Treatment of head and neck cancer in elderly patients: state of the art and guidelines. *Crit Rev Oncol Hematol*. 2005;53(1):71–80.
11. Derks W, de Leeuw JR, Hordijk GJ, Winnubst JA. Reasons for non-standard treatment in elderly patients with advanced head and neck cancer. *Eur Arch Otorhinolaryngol*. 2005;262(1):21–26.
12. Sarini J, Fournier C, Lefebvre JL, et al. Head and neck squamous cell carcinoma in elderly patients: a long-term retrospective review of 273 cases. *Arch Otolaryngol Head Neck Surg*. 2001;127(9):1089–1092.
13. Howlader N, Noone AM, Krpacho M, et al. *SEER Cancer Statistics Review, 1975–2013*. Bethesda, MD: National Cancer Institute; 2016.
14. Bernier J, Domenge C, Ozsahin M, et al. Postoperative irradiation with or without concomitant chemotherapy for locally advanced head and neck cancer. *N Engl J Med*. 2004;350(19):1945–1952.
15. Cooper JS, Pajak TF, Forastiere AA, et al. Postoperative concurrent radiotherapy and chemotherapy for high-risk squamous-cell carcinoma of the head and neck. *N Engl J Med*. 2004;350(19):1937–1944.
16. Pignon JP, le Maître A, Maillard E, et al. Meta-analysis of chemotherapy in head and neck cancer (MACH-NC): an update on 93 randomised trials and 17,346 patients. *Radiother Oncol*. 2009;92(1):4–14.
17. Koch WM, Patel H, Brennan J, et al. Squamous cell carcinoma of the head and neck in the elderly. *Arch Otolaryngol Head Neck Surg*. 1995;121(3):262–265.
18. Verschuur HP, Irish JC, O'Sullivan B, et al. A matched control study of treatment outcome in young patients with squamous cell carcinoma of the head and neck. Laryngoscope. 1999;109(2 Pt 1):249–258.
19. Bhattacharyya N. A matched survival analysis for squamous cell carcinoma of the head and neck in the elderly. *Laryngoscope*. 2003;113(2):368–372.
20. Airoldi M, Cortesina G, Giordano C, et al. Postoperative adjuvant chemoradiotherapy in older patients with head and neck cancer. Arch Otolaryngol Head Neck Surg. 2004;130(2):161–166.
21. Lusinchi A, Bourhis J, Wibault P, et al. Radiation therapy for head and neck cancers in the elderly. *Int J Radiat Oncol Biol Phys*. 1990;18(4):819–823.

22. Argiris A, Li Y, Murphy BA, et al. Outcome of elderly patients with recurrent or metastatic head and neck cancer treated with cisplatin-based chemotherapy. *J Clin Oncol*. 2004;22(2):262–268.
23. Extermann M, Aapro M, Bernabei R, et al. Use of comprehensive geriatric assessment in older cancer patients: recommendations from the task force on CGA of the International Society of Geriatric Oncology (SIOG). *Crit Rev Oncol Hematol*. 2005;55(3):241–252.
24. Devons CA. Comprehensive geriatric assessment: making the most of the aging years. *Curr Opin Clin Nutr Metab Care*. 2002;5(1):19–24.
25. Stuck AE, Siu AL, Wieland GD, et al. Comprehensive geriatric assessment: a meta-analysis of controlled trials. *Lancet*. 1993;342(8878):1032–1036.
26. Fried LP, Tangen CM, Walston J, et al. Frailty in older adults: evidence for a phenotype. *J Gerontol A Biol Sci Med Sci*. 2001;56(3):M146–M156.
27. Extermann M, Aapro M. Assessment of the older cancer patient. *Hematol Oncol Clin North Am*. 2000;14(1):63–77, viii–ix.
28. Sanabria A, Carvalho AL, Vartanian JG, et al. Factors that influence treatment decision in older patients with resectable head and neck cancer. *Laryngoscope*. 2007;117(5):835–840.
29. Derks W, de Leeuw RJ, Hordijk GJ. Elderly patients with head and neck cancer: the influence of comorbidity on choice of therapy, complication rate, and survival. *Curr Opin Otolaryngol Head Neck Surg*. 2005;13(2):92–96.
30. Sanabria A, Carvalho AL, Vartanian JG, et al. Comorbidity is a prognostic factor in elderly patients with head and neck cancer. *Ann Surg Oncol*. 2007;14(4):1449–1457.
31. Charlson ME, Pompei P, Ales KL, MacKenzie CR. A new method of classifying prognostic comorbidity in longitudinal studies: development and validation. *J Chronic Dis*. 1987;40(5):373–383.
32. Hurria A, Togawa K, Mohile SG, et al. Predicting chemotherapy toxicity in older adults with cancer: a prospective multicenter study. *J Clin Oncol*. 2011;29(25):3457–3465.
33. Mohile SG, Fan L, Reeve E, et al. Association of cancer with geriatric syndromes in older Medicare beneficiaries. *J Clin Oncol*. 2011;29(11):1458–1464.
34. Ferner RE, Aronson JK. Communicating information about drug safety. *BMJ*. 2006;333(7559):143–145.
35. Tinetti ME, Bogardus ST Jr, Agostini JV. Potential pitfalls of disease-specific guidelines for patients with multiple conditions. *N Engl J Med*. 2004;351(27):2870–2874.
36. Nightingale G, Hajjar E, Swartz K, et al. Evaluation of a pharmacist-led medication assessment used to identify prevalence of and associations with polypharmacy and potentially inappropriate medication use among ambulatory senior adults with cancer. *J Clin Oncol*. 2015;33(13):1453–1459.
37. Qato DM, Wilder J, Schumm LP, et al. Changes in prescription and over-the-counter medication and dietary supplement use among older adults in the United States, 2005 vs 2011. *JAMA Intern Med*. 2016;176(4):473–482.
38. Kaufman DW, Kelly JP, Rosenberg L, et al. Recent patterns of medication use in the ambulatory adult population of the United States: the Slone survey. *JAMA*. 2002;287(3):337–344.
39. Eisenberg DM, Kessler RC, Foster C, et al. Unconventional medicine in the United States. Prevalence, costs, and patterns of use. *N Engl J Med*. 1993;328(4):246–252.
40. Gupta DK, Avram MJ. Rational opioid dosing in the elderly: dose and dosing interval when initiating opioid therapy. *Clin Pharmacol Ther*. 2012;91(2):339–343.
41. Syddall HE, Westbury LD, Dodds R, et al. Mortality in the Hertfordshire Ageing Study: association with level and loss of hand grip strength in later life. *Age Ageing*. 2016;46(3):407–412.
42. Nofuji Y, Shinkai S, Taniguchi Y, et al. Associations of walking speed, grip strength, and standing balance with total and cause-specific mortality in a general population of Japanese elders. *J Am Med Dir Assoc*. 2016;17(2):184.e1-7.
43. Leong DP, Teo KK, Rangarajan S, et al. Prognostic value of grip strength: findings from the Prospective Urban Rural Epidemiology (PURE) study. *Lancet*. 2015;386(9990):266–273.
44. Zabrodsky M, Calabrese L, Tosoni A, et al. Major surgery in elderly head and neck cancer patients: immediate and long-term surgical results and complication rates. *Surg Oncol*. 2004;13(4):249–255.
45. Grammatica A, Piazza C, Paderno A, et al. Free flaps in head and neck reconstruction after oncologic surgery: expected outcomes in the elderly. *Otolaryngol Head Neck Surg*. 2015;152(5):796–802.
46. Shuman AG, Patel SG, Shah JP, Korc-Grodzicki B. Optimizing perioperative management of geriatric patients with head and neck cancer. *Head Neck*. 2014;36(5):743–749.
47. McGuirt WF, Davis SP III. Demographic portrayal and outcome analysis of head and neck cancer surgery in the elderly. *Arch Otolaryngol Head Neck Surg*. 1995;121(2):150–154.
48. Clayman GL, Eicher SA, Sicard MW, et al. Surgical outcomes in head and neck cancer patients 80 years of age and older. *Head Neck*. 1998;20(3):216–223.
49. Kowalski LP, Alcantara PS, Magrin J, Parise Júnior O. A case-control study on complications and survival in elderly patients undergoing major head and neck surgery. *Am J Surg*. 1994;168(5):485–490.
50. Italiano A, Ortholan C, Dassonville O, et al. Head and neck squamous cell carcinoma in patients aged > or = 80 years: patterns of care and survival. *Cancer*. 2008;113(11):3160–3168.
51. Morgan RF, Hirata RM, Jaques DA, Hoopes JE. Head and neck surgery in the aged. *Am J Surg*. 1982;144(4):449–451.
52. Kwoh YS, Hou J, Jonckheere EA Hayati S. A robot with improved absolute positioning accuracy for CT guided stereotactic brain surgery. *IEEE Trans Biomed Eng*. 1988;35(2):153–160.
53. O'Malley BW Jr, Weinstein GS, Snyder W, Hockstein NG. Transoral robotic surgery (TORS) for base of tongue neoplasms. *Laryngoscope*. 2006;116(8):1465–1472.

54. Weinstein GS, O'Malley BW Jr, Snyder W, Hockstein NG. Transoral robotic surgery: supraglottic partial laryngectomy. *Ann Otol Rhinol Laryngol.* 2007;116(1):19–23.
55. Weinstein GS, O'Malley BW Jr, Snyder W, et al. Transoral robotic surgery: radical tonsillectomy. *Arch Otolaryngol Head Neck Surg.* 2007;133(12):1220–1226.
56. Hurtuk A, Agrawal A, Old M, et al. Outcomes of transoral robotic surgery: a preliminary clinical experience. *Otolaryngol Head Neck Surg.* 2011;145(2):248–253.
57. Hurtuk AM, Marcinow A, Agrawal A, et al. Quality-of-life outcomes in transoral robotic surgery. *Otolaryngol Head Neck Surg.* 2012;146(1):68–73.
58. Moore EJ, Henstrom DK, Olsen KD, et al. Transoral resection of tonsillar squamous cell carcinoma. *Laryngoscope.* 2009;119(3):508–515.
59. Moore EJ, Olsen KD, Kasperbauer JL. Transoral robotic surgery for oropharyngeal squamous cell carcinoma: a prospective study of feasibility and functional outcomes. *Laryngoscope.* 2009;119(11):2156–2164.
60. Ozer E, Waltonen J. Transoral robotic nasopharyngectomy: a novel approach for nasopharyngeal lesions. *Laryngoscope.* 2008;118(9):1613–1616.
61. Psychogios G, Mantsopoulos K, Bohr C, et al. Incidence of occult cervical metastasis in head and neck carcinomas: development over time. *J Surg Oncol.* 2013;107(4):384–387.
62. Rodrigo JP, Shah JP, Silver CE, et al. Management of the clinically negative neck in early-stage head and neck cancers after transoral resection. *Head Neck.* 2011;33(8):1210–1219.
63. Fasunla AJ, Greene BH, Timmesfeld N, et al. A meta-analysis of the randomized controlled trials on elective neck dissection versus therapeutic neck dissection in oral cavity cancers with clinically node-negative neck. *Oral Oncol.* 2011;47(5):320–324.
64. Goudakos JK, Markou K, Nikolaou A, et al. Management of the clinically negative neck (N0) of supraglottic laryngeal carcinoma: a systematic review. *Eur J Surg Oncol.* 2009;35(3):223–229.
65. Ortholan C, Lusinchi A, Italiano A, et al. Oral cavity squamous cell carcinoma in 260 patients aged 80 years or more. *Radiother Oncol.* 2009;93(3):516–523.
66. Melkane AE, Mamelle G, Wycisk G, et al. Sentinel node biopsy in early oral squamous cell carcinomas: a 10-year experience. *Laryngoscope.* 2012;122(8):1782–1788.
67. Thompson CF, St John MA, Lawson G, et al. Diagnostic value of sentinel lymph node biopsy in head and neck cancer: a meta-analysis. *Eur Arch Otorhinolaryngol.* 2013;270(7):2115–2122.
68. Tarsitano A, Pizzigallo A, Sgarzani R, et al. Head and neck cancer in elderly patients: is microsurgical free-tissue transfer a safe procedure? *Acta Otorhinolaryngol Ital.* 2012;32(6):371–375.
69. Derks W, De Leeuw JR, Hordijk GJ, Winnubst JA. Elderly patients with head and neck cancer: short-term effects of surgical treatment on quality of life. *Clin Otolaryngol Allied Sci.* 2003;28(5):399–405.
70. Malata CM, Cooter RD, Batchelor AG, et al. Microvascular free-tissue transfers in elderly patients: the leeds experience. *Plast Reconstr Surg.* 1996;98(7):1234–1241.
71. Shaari CM, Buchbinder D, Costantino PD, et al. Complications of microvascular head and neck surgery in the elderly. *Arch Otolaryngol Head Neck Surg.* 1998;124(4):407–411.
72. Pompei S, Tedesco M, Pozzi M, et al. Age as a risk factor in cervicofacial reconstruction. *J Exp Clin Cancer Res.* 1999;18(2):209–212.
73. Yang R, Lubek JE, Dyalram D, et al. Head and neck cancer surgery in an elderly patient population: a retrospective review. *Int J Oral Maxillofac Surg.* 2014;43(12):1413–1437.
74. Russo G, Haddad R, Posner M, Machtay M. Radiation treatment breaks and ulcerative mucositis in head and neck cancer. *Oncologist.* 2008;13(8):886–898.
75. Schofield CP, Sykes AJ, Slevin NJ, Rashid NZZ. Radiotherapy for head and neck cancer in elderly patients. *Radiother Oncol.* 2003;69(1):37–42.
76. Huguenin P, Sauer M, Glanzmann C, Lütolf UM. Radiotherapy for carcinomas of the head and neck in elderly patients. *Strahlenther Onkol.* 1996;172(9):485–488.
77. Schilcher B, Curschmann J. Clinical results of radiotherapy in 140 elderly patients treated at Basel University Hospital between 1980 and 1985. *Int J Radiat Oncol Biol Phys.* 1995;33(3):774.
78. Oguchi M, Ikeda H, Watanabe T, et al. Experiences of 23 patients > or = 90 years of age treated with radiation therapy. *Int J Radiat Oncol Biol Phys.* 1998;41(2):407–413.
79. Pignon T, Horiot JC, Van den Bogaert W, et al. No age limit for radical radiotherapy in head and neck tumours. *Eur J Cancer.* 1996;32A(12):2075–2081.
80. Nutting CM, Morden JP, Harrington KJ, et al. Parotid-sparing intensity modulated versus conventional radiotherapy in head and neck cancer (PARSPORT): a phase 3 multicentre randomised controlled trial. *Lancet Oncol.* 2011;12(2):127–136.
81. Yu JB, Soulos PR, Sharma R, et al. Patterns of care and outcomes associated with intensity-modulated radiation therapy versus conventional radiation therapy for older patients with head-and-neck cancer. *Int J Radiat Oncol Biol Phys.* 2012;83(1):e101-7.
82. Baujat B, Bourhis J, Blanchard P, et al. Hyperfractionated or accelerated radiotherapy for head and neck cancer. *Cochrane Database Syst Rev.* 2010(12):CD002026. doi:10.1002/14651858.CD002026
83. Bourhis J, Overgaard J, Audry H, et al. Hyperfractionated or accelerated radiotherapy in head and neck cancer: a meta-analysis. *Lancet.* 2006;368(9538):843–854.
84. Bledsoe TJ, Noble AR, Reddy CA, et al. Split-course accelerated hypofractionated radiotherapy (SCAHRT): a safe and effective option for head and neck cancer in the elderly or infirm. *Anticancer Res.* 2016;36(3):933–939.
85. Owen D, Iqbal F, Pollock BE, et al. Long-term follow-up of stereotactic radiosurgery for head and neck malignancies. *Head Neck.* 2015;37(11):1557–1562.

86. Siddiqui F, Patel M, Khan M, et al. Stereotactic body radiation therapy for primary, recurrent, and metastatic tumors in the head-and-neck region. *Int J Radiat Oncol Biol Phys*. 2009;74(4):1047–1053.
87. Siddiqui F, Raben D, Lu JJ, et al. Emerging applications of stereotactic body radiation therapy for head and neck cancer. Expert Rev Anticancer Ther. 2011;11(9):1429–1436.
88. Bonner JA, Harari PM, Giralt J, et al. Radiotherapy plus cetuximab for squamous-cell carcinoma of the head and neck. *N Engl J Med*. 2006;354(6):567–578.
89. Grandis JR, Tweardy DJ. Elevated levels of transforming growth factor alpha and epidermal growth factor receptor messenger RNA are early markers of carcinogenesis in head and neck cancer. *Cancer Res*. 1993;53(15):3579–3584.
90. Dassonville O, Formento JL, Francoual M, et al. Expression of epidermal growth factor receptor and survival in upper aerodigestive tract cancer. *J Clin Oncol*. 1993;11(10):1873–1878.
91. Forastiere AA, Goepfert H, Maor M, et al. Concurrent chemotherapy and radiotherapy for organ preservation in advanced laryngeal cancer. N Engl J Med. 2003;349(22):2091–2098.
92. Adelstein DJ, Li Y, Adams, GL, et al. An intergroup phase III comparison of standard radiation therapy and two schedules of concurrent chemoradiotherapy in patients with unresectable squamous cell head and neck cancer. *J Clin Oncol*. 2003;21(1):92–98.
93. Forastiere AA, Zhang Q, Weber RS, et al. Long-term results of Intergroup RTOG 91-11: A phase III trial to preserve the larynx-Induction cisplatin/5-FU and radiation therapy versus concurrent cisplatin and radiation therapy versus radiation therapy. *J Clin Oncol*. 2006;24(18_suppl):5517.
94. Machtay M, Moughan J, Trotti A, et al. Factors associated with severe late toxicity after concurrent chemoradiation for locally advanced head and neck cancer: an RTOG analysis. *J Clin Oncol*. 2008;26(21):3582–3589.
95. Caudell JJ, Schaner PE, Meredith RF, et al. Factors associated with long-term dysphagia after definitive radiotherapy for locally advanced head-and-neck cancer. *Int J Radiat Oncol Biol Phys*. 2009;73(2):410–415.
96. Newlin HE, Amdur RJ, Riggs CE, et al. Concomitant weekly cisplatin and altered fractionation radiotherapy in locally advanced head and neck cancer. *Cancer*. 2010;116(19):4533–4540.
97. Sharma A, Mohanti BK, Thakar A, et al. Concomitant chemoradiation versus radical radiotherapy in advanced squamous cell carcinoma of oropharynx and nasopharynx using weekly cisplatin: a phase II randomized trial. *Ann Oncol*. 2010;21(11):2272–2277.
98. Bachaud JM, Cohen-Jonathan E, Alzieu C, et al. Combined postoperative radiotherapy and weekly cisplatin infusion for locally advanced head and neck carcinoma: final report of a randomized trial. *Int J Radiat Oncol Biol Phys*. 1996;36(5):999–1004.
99. Jeremic B, Shibamoto Y, Stanisavljevic B, et al. Radiation therapy alone or with concurrent low-dose daily either cisplatin or carboplatin in locally advanced unresectable squamous cell carcinoma of the head and neck: a prospective randomized trial. *Radiother Oncol*. 1997;43(1):29–37.
100. Suntharalingam M, Haas ML, Conley BA, et al. The use of carboplatin and paclitaxel with daily radiotherapy in patients with locally advanced squamous cell carcinomas of the head and neck. *Int J Radiat Oncol Biol Phys*. 2000;47(1):49–56.
101. Haddad R, Sonis S, Posner M, et al. Randomized phase 2 study of concomitant chemoradiotherapy using weekly carboplatin/paclitaxel with or without daily subcutaneous amifostine in patients with locally advanced head and neck cancer. *Cancer*. 2009;115(19):4514–4523.
102. Lokich J, Anderson N. Carboplatin versus cisplatin in solid tumors: an analysis of the literature. *Ann Oncol*. 1998;9(1):13–21.
103. Go RS, Adjei AA. Review of the comparative pharmacology and clinical activity of cisplatin and carboplatin. *J Clin Oncol*. 1999;17(1):409–422.
104. Ward MC, Reddy CA, Adelstein DJ, Koyfman SA. Use of systemic therapy with definitive radiotherapy for elderly patients with head and neck cancer: a national cancer data base analysis. *Cancer*. 2016;122(22):3472–3483.
105. Ang KK, Chen A, Curran WJ Jr, et al. Head and neck carcinoma in the United States: first comprehensive report of the Longitudinal Oncology Registry of Head and Neck Carcinoma (LORHAN). *Cancer*. 2012;118(23):5783–5792.
106. Bernier J, Cooper JS, Pajak TF, et al. Defining risk levels in locally advanced head and neck cancers: a comparative analysis of concurrent postoperative radiation plus chemotherapy trials of the EORTC (#22931) and RTOG (# 9501). *Head Neck*. 2005;27(10):843–850.
107. Vermorken JB, Mesia R, Rivera F, et al. Platinum-based chemotherapy plus cetuximab in head and neck cancer. *N Engl J Med*. 2008;359(11):1116–1127.
108. Cohen EE, Lingen MW, Vokes EE. The expanding role of systemic therapy in head and neck cancer. *J Clin Oncol*. 2004;22(9):1743–1752.
109. Seiwert TY, Burtness B, Mehra R, et al. Safety and clinical activity of pembrolizumab for treatment of recurrent or metastatic squamous cell carcinoma of the head and neck (KEYNOTE-012): an open-label, multicentre, phase 1b trial. *Lancet Oncol*. 2016;17(7):956–965.
110. Ferris RL, Blumenschein G, Fayette J, et al. Nivolumab for recurrent squamous-cell carcinoma of the head and neck. *N Engl J Med*. 2016;375(19):1856–1867.
111. Zumsteg ZS, Cook-Wiens G, Yoshida E, et al. Incidence of oropharyngeal cancer among elderly patients in the United States. *JAMA Oncol*. 2016;2(12):1617–1623.
112. Sarris EG, Harrington KJ, Saif MW, Syrigos KN. Multimodal treatment strategies for elderly patients with head and neck cancer. *Cancer Treat Rev*. 2014;40(3):465–475.

Index